# ARCHIVES OF DISEASE IN CHILDHOOD





---

VOLUME XL, 1965



---

LONDON
**BRITISH MEDICAL ASSOCIATION**
TAVISTOCK SQUARE, W.C.1

## CONTENTS

No. 209. *FEBRUARY 1965*

PAGE

**An Inborn Defect of Intestinal Absorption of Certain Monosaccharides.** CHARLOTTE M. ANDERSON, K. R. KERRY, and R. R. W. TOWNLEY .. .. .. .. .. .. 1

**Studies in Osteopetrosis.** C. E. DENT, JEAN M. SMELLIE, and L. WATSON .. .. .. 7

**Urinary Excretion of Gonadotrophins with Particular Reference to Children.** W. FITSCHEN and BARBARA E. CLAYTON .. .. .. .. .. .. .. .. .. .. 16

**Lymphangiography and Chromosome Studies in Females with Lymphoedema and Possible Ovarian Dysgenesis.** P. F. BENSON, M. H. GOUGH, and P. E. POLANI .. .. .. .. .. 27

**The Renal Excretion of Hydrogen Ions in Infants and Children.** ALEXANDER PEONIDES, BARNETT LEVIN, and WINIFRED F. YOUNG .. .. .. .. .. .. .. .. .. 33

**A-β-lipoproteinaemia (Bassen-Kornzweig Syndrome). Report of a Case.** D. M. O. BECROFT, J. M. COSTELLO, and P. J. SCOTT .... .. .. .. .. .. .. .. 40

**A-β-lipoproteinaemia.** CONSTANCE C. FORSYTH, JUNE K. LLOYD, and AUDREY S. FOSBROOKE 47

**Megaloblastic Anaemia in Premature Infants.** O. P. GRAY and E. BLANCHE BUTLER .. 53

**Dyscephalia Mandibulo-oculo-facialis (Hallermann-Streiff Syndrome).** D. HOEFNAGEL and K. BENIRSCHKE .. .. .. .. .. .. .. .. .. .. .. 57

**The Respiratory Distress Syndrome of the Newborn: Immaturity Versus Prematurity.** PETER M. DUNN .. .. .. .. .. .. .. .. .. .. .. .. 62

**The Influence of Androgen Treatment on Ultimate Height in Males.** GEORGE L. FOSS .. 66

**Thyrotoxicosis in Children: A Follow-up Study.** T. MCKENDRICK AND G. H. NEWNS .. 71

**An Assessment of Gastric Acid Secretory Response with 'Maximal' Augmented Histamine Stimulation in Children with Peptic Ulcer.** O. P. GHAI, MEHARBAN SINGH, B. N. S. WALIA, and N. G. GADEKAR .. .. .. .. .. .. .. .. .. .. .. 77

**External Injury Causing Foetal Deformity.** E. HINDEN .. .. .. .. .. .. .. 80

**Partial Deletion of the Short Arms of a Chromosome of the 4-5 Group (Denver).** H. V. DYGGVE and MARGARETA MIKKELSEN .. .. .. .. .. .. .. .. .. .. 82

**Intrathoracic Kidney in a Premature Infant.** EMMANUEL SHAPIRA, EFRAIM FISHEL, and STANLEY LEVIN .. .. .. .. .. .. .. .. .. .. .. .. .. 86

**Fanconi's Anaemia with Hydrocephalus and Thyroid Abnormality.** RUTH LONDON, AHARON DRUKKER, and URI SANDBANK .. .. .. .. .. .. .. .. .. .. 89

**Obstetrical Paralysis Due to Ischaemia of the Spinal Cord.** J. HUME ADAMS and HECTOR M. CAMERON .. .. .. .. .. .. .. .. .. .. .. .. .. 93

**Conjugation Reactions in the Newborn Infant: The Metabolism of Para-aminobenzoic Acid.** MARKUS F. VEST and RENÉ SALZBERG .. .. .. .. .. .. .. .. .. 97

**Osteochondrodystrophia Deformans with Mucopolysaccharidosis.** S. VESTERMARK .. .. 106

**Editorial Notice** .. .. .. .. .. .. .. .. .. .. .. .. .. 111

**Book Reviews** .. .. .. .. .. .. .. .. .. .. .. .. .. 111

No. 210. *APRIL 1965*

**Review Article: the Undescended Testis.** J. H. JOHNSTON .. .. .. .. .. .. .. 113

**The Development of Heart Surgery in Children.** SIR RUSSELL BROCK .. .. .. .. 123

**The Surgery of Transposition of the Great Vessels.** A. G. BROM, H. V. D. SCHAAR, and J. NAUTA 128

**Pancreatitis in Childhood: Experience with 15 Cases.** W. HARDY HENDREN, JACOBUS M. GREEP, and ANTHONY S. PATTON .. .. .. .. .. .. .. .. .. .. .. 132

**The Role of Ventral Hernia in the Correction of Diaphragmatic Defects in the Newborn.** IRVING A. MEEKER, JR. and WILLIAM N. KINCANNON .. .. .. .. .. .. .. .. 146

PAGE

**Thalidomide Embryopathy and Limb Defects: Experiences in Habilitation of Children with Ectromelias.** WOLFGANG A. MAIER .. .. .. .. .. .. .. .. 154

**The Surgery of Infantile Obstructive Jaundice.** KEIJIRO SURUGA, ZENYA YAMAZAKI, SEIZO IWAI, KINJI NAGASHIMA, and WATARU MORI .. .. .. .. .. .. .. .. 158

**Intrahepatic Vascular and Bile-duct Systems as Related to Operative Treatment of Bile-duct Atresia.** WOLFGANG HASSE .. .. .. .. .. .. .. .. .. 162

**Hepatic Tumours in Childhood and Their Treatment by Major Hepatic Resection.** H. H. NIXON 169

**Polyps of the Colon Beyond the Reach of the Sigmoidoscope.** JEAN DUHAMEL and PIERRE BAUCHE 173

**Pseudo-Hirschsprung's Disease.** TH. EHRENPREIS .. .. .. .. .. .. .. .. 177

**Acquired Megacolon As a Complication of Recto-sigmoidectomy for Hirschsprung's Disease.** TH. EHRENPREIS .. .. .. .. .. .. .. .. .. .. .. 180

**Serum Lactic Dehydrogenase and Ribonuclease in the Diagnosis of Malignant Tumours in Children.** ALOJZY MACIEJEWSKI and HENRYK BOBIŃSKI .. .. .. .. .. .. .. 183

**Chylothorax in Infancy and Childhood: a Method of Treatment.** IAN KIRKLAND .. .. 186

**Late Results of the Operation for Coarctation in the Growing Child.** J. A. NOORDIJK, F. T. I. OEY, and H. M. P. VAN DEN BOOGAARD .. .. .. .. .. .. .. 192

**Oesophageal Stenosis Due to Reflux Oesophagitis.** JOSÉ BOIX-OCHOA and FRITZ REHBEIN 197

**Actinomycin D in Wilms' Tumour: Treatment of Lung Metastases.** RUSSELL HOWARD .. .. 200

**Functional Stenosis as a Cause of Pelvi-Ureteric Obstruction and Hydronephrosis.** L. BÄCKLUND, G. GROTTE, and A. REUTERSKIÖLD .. .. .. .. .. .. .. .. .. 203

**Lipoma of the Cauda Equina.** V. DUBOWITZ, J. LORBER, and R. B. ZACHARY .. .. .. 207

**Renal Vein Thrombosis in Infants.** ARIE D. VERHAGEN, JAMES P. HAMILTON, and MYRON GENEL 214

**Cervico-auricular Fistulae: a Review of Published Cases with a Report.** J. C. R. LINCOLN .. 218

**Internal Carotid Artery Occlusion in a Child.** S. A. MELLICK and P. D. PHELAN .. .. 224

**British Association of Paediatric Surgeons** .. .. .. .. .. .. .. .. 227

**Book Reviews** .. .. .. .. .. .. .. .. .. .. .. .. .. 231

No. 211. *JUNE 1965*

**The Use of Fibrinolytic Activators in Meningitis and Similar Conditions.** R. L. NEWMAN and G. T. STEWART .. .. .. .. .. .. .. .. .. .. .. .. 235

**A Study of the Immunoglobulins in Premature Infants.** J. C. HAWORTH, MAJORIE NORRIS, and LOUISE DILLING .. .. .. .. .. .. .. .. .. .. .. 243

**3β: 21-Dihydroxypregn-5-ene-20-one in Urine of Normal Newborn Infants and in Third Day Urine of Child with Deficiency of 3β-hydroxysteroid-dehydrogenase.** D. M. CATHRO, KATHLEEN BIRCHALL, F. L. MITCHELL, and CONSTANCE C. FORSYTH .. .. .. .. .. 251

**Aldosterone and 17-hydroxycorticosteroid Excretion Following Ramstedt's Operation.** WILLIAM HAMILTON .. .. .. .. .. .. .. .. .. .. .. .. 261

**The Placental Transfusion Syndrome in Monozygous Twins.** G. CORNEY and W. AHERNE .. 264

**Favism in England—Two More Cases.** J. M. HOLT and R. A. SLADDEN .. .. .. .. 271

**Gonadal Dysgenesis with Unusual Abnormalities.** K. HUGH-JONES, SHEILA J. WALLACE, JANET M. THORNBER, and N. B. ATKIN .. .. .. .. .. .. .. .. .. 274

**Neonatal Jaundice Associated with Familial G6PD Deficiency in Israel.** S. FREIER, K. MAYER, C. LEVENE, and A. ABRAHAMOV .. .. .. .. .. .. .. .. 280

**A Reliable Rapid Screening Test for Sulphatide Lipidosis.** BRIAN D. LAKE .. .. .. 284

**Neonatal Fits Associated with Hypomagnesaemia.** J. A. DAVIS, D. R. HARVEY, and J. S. YU 286

**The Osmotic Concentrating Ability in Healthy Infants and Children.** E. POLÁČEK, J. VOCEL, L. NEUGEBAUEROVÁ, M. ŠEBKOVÁ, E. VĚCHETOVÁ, with M. KŘIŠŤAN, and B. TROUSILOVÁ 291

PAGE

**Intellectual Impairment in Muscular Dystrophy.** VICTOR DUBOWITZ .. .. .. .. 296

**Cerebello-thalamo-spinal Degeneration in Infancy: An Unusual Variant of Werdnig-Hoffmann Disease.** R. M. NORMAN and J. M. KAY .. .. .. .. .. .. .. 302

**Methods of Routine Haemoglobinometry in Childhood: Evaluation of Copper Sulphate Densitometry.** HANAN COSTEFF .. .. .. .. .. .. .. .. .. .. 309

**Urinary White Cell Excretion in Childhood.** I. B. HOUSTON .. .. .. .. .. 313

**Histological Observations on Glycogen Reserves of the Foetus and Newborn Infant.** JEAN M. SCOTT .. .. .. .. .. .. .. .. .. .. .. .. .. 317

**Venous Pressure Measurement in Exchange Transfusion.** DENNIS COTTOM and MAUREEN YOUNG 323

**An Unusual Case of Subcutaneous Fat Necrosis in a Newly Born Infant.** W. S. CRAIG .. .. 326

**Choledochal Cyst: A Case Report and Discussion of Aetiology.** R. H. BURNELL and G. B. MARKEY 329

**Paediatric Pathology Club. Proceedings of the Tenth Annual Meeting** .. .. .. .. 332

**Book Reviews** .. .. .. .. .. .. .. .. .. .. .. .. .. 337

**Paediatric Research Society** .. .. .. .. .. .. .. .. .. .. .. 342

No. 212. *AUGUST 1965*

**Review Article: Iron Deficiency and Iron Overload.** R. SEPHTON SMITH .. .. .. .. .. 343

**A Deficiency State Arising in Infants on Synthetic Foods.** TREVOR P. MANN, K. MARGARET WILSON, and BARBARA E. CLAYTON .. .. .. .. .. .. .. .. 364

**Aetiology of Athetosis with Special Reference to Neonatal Asphyxia, Idiopathic Icterus, and ABO-Incompatibility.** P. PLUM .. .. .. .. .. .. .. .. .. .. 376

**Correction of Acidosis in the Resuscitation of the Collapsed Child.** M. E. DODSON and A. L STEAD .. .. .. .. .. .. .. .. .. .. .. .. .. 385

**Reversible Myocarditis Due to Chronic Lead Poisoning in Childhood.** RONALD FREEMAN .. 389

**Some Clinical Notes and Electroencephalographic Findings in Cerebral Palsy.** GRACE E. WOODS 394

**The Electrocardiogram in Respiratory Distress Syndrome: The Praecordial P wave as an Aid to Assessment.** G. J. SUTIN, RUTH HORNER, H. DE V. HEESE, and A. F. MALAN .. .. 402

**Fat Infiltration in the Tissues of the Newborn Infant.** W. AHERNE .. .. .. .. .. .. 406

**Biochemical, Pharmacological, and Histochemical Studies in Neuroblastoma.** P. P. ANTHONY, H. M. T. COLES, JOHN PRYSE-DAVIES, and LEONARD SINCLAIR .. .. .. .. .. .. 411

**The Excretion of 4-Hydroxy-3-Methoxy-Mandelic Acid by Children.** T. MCKENDRICK and R. W. H. EDWARDS .. .. .. .. .. .. .. .. .. .. 418

**Iatrogenic Lesions in Babies Following Umbilical Vein Catheterization.** JEAN M. SCOTT. .. 426

**Blood Chemistry of Normal Full-term Infants in the First 48 Hours of Life.** P. T. ACHARYA and W. W. PAYNE .. .. .. .. .. .. .. .. .. .. .. .. .. 430

**The Effect of Abnormal Birth on Blood Chemistry During the First 48 Hours of Life.** W. W. PAYNE and P. T. ACHARYA .. .. .. .. .. .. .. .. .. .. .. 436

**Normal/Trisomy 13-15 Mosaicism in Two Infants.** A. D. BAIN, J. INSLEY, D. M. DOUGLAS, I. K. GAULD, and H. A. SCOTT .. .. .. .. .. .. .. .. .. 442

**British Paediatric Association: Proceedings of the Thirty-sixth Annual Meeting** .. .. .. 446

**Book Reviews** .. .. .. .. .. .. .. .. .. .. .. .. .. 452

No. 213. *OCTOBER 1965*

**Cysts Arising in the Renal Corpuscle: A Microdissection Study.** THELMA J. BAXTER .. .. 455

**Cysts Arising in the Renal Tubules: A Microdissection Study.** THELMA J. BAXTER .. .. 464

**Intermittent Positive Pressure Respiration as a Treatment in Severe Respiratory Distress Syndrome.** M. DELIVORIA-PAPADOPOULOS, H. LEVISON, and P. R. SWYER .. .. .. .. .. 474

PAGE

**Blood Volume and Haematocrit Studies in Respiratory Distress Syndrome of the Newborn.** J. A. Inall, M. M. Bluhm, Margaret M. Kerr, T. A. Douglas, C. S. Hope, and J. H. Hutchison .. .. .. .. .. .. .. .. .. .. .. .. 480

**The Metabolic Error in Primary Hyperoxaluria.** T. D. R. Hockaday, J. E. Clayton, and L. H. Smith, Jr. .. .. .. .. .. .. .. .. .. .. .. .. 485

**Lactic Acidosis with Necrotizing Encephalopathy in two Sibs.** Helen E. Worsley, R. W. Brookfield, J. S. Elwood, R. L. Noble, and W. H. Taylor .. .. .. .. .. .. 492

**Infantile Neuroaxonal Dystrophy.** L. Crome and S. D. V. Weller .. .. .. .. 502

**The Insulin-Glucose Tolerance Test in Pituitary Growth Retardation.** Olav Trygstad .. 508

**Blood 5-Hydroxytryptamine Levels in the Newborn.** Meena Hazra, Sylvia Benson, and M. Sandler .. .. .. .. .. .. .. .. .. .. .. .. 513

**Biochemical Status of Healthy Premature Infants in the First 48 Hours of Life.** J. Yu, W. W. Payne, A. Ifekwunigwe, and J. Stevens .. .. .. .. .. .. .. 516

**The Jejunal Mucosa in Kwashiorkor.** David Burman .. .. .. .. .. .. .. 526

**Effect of Undernutrition in Early Life on Physical and Mental Development.** Vera Cabak and R. Najdanvic .. .. .. .. .. .. .. .. .. .. .. .. 532

**Infantile Hypercalcaemia and Cardiovascular Lesions: Evidence, Hypothesis, and Speculation.** Eric N. Coleman .. .. .. .. .. .. .. .. .. .. .. .. 535

**Accessory Lobe of Liver Presenting Through a Congenital Deficiency of Anterior Abdominal Wall.** George Johnstone .. .. .. .. .. .. .. .. .. .. .. .. 541

**Diverticulum of the Left Ventricle: Report of a Case.** El-Sayed El-Akkari, M. Kamal Badr El-Din, and A. Samir Kassem .. .. .. .. .. .. .. .. .. 545

**The Causes of Congenital Club Foot.** Eva D. Alderman .. .. .. .. .. .. .. 548

**Incubator-borne *Pseudomonas Pyocyanea* Infection in a Newborn Nursery.** Dinah Barrie .. 555

**Hand, Foot, and Mouth Diseases.** S. R. Meadow .. .. .. .. .. .. .. .. 560

**Dental Manifestations of Pseudohypoparathyroidism.** G. MacL. Ritchie .. .. .. 565

**Book Reviews** .. .. .. .. .. .. .. .. .. .. .. .. .. 573

No. 214. *DECEMBER 1965*

**Review Article: The Lungs at Birth.** L. B. Strang .. .. .. .. .. .. .. 575

**Excretion of Corticosteroids by Infants of Diabetic and Pre-diabetic Mothers.** D. Methven Cathro and Constance C. Forsyth .. .. .. .. .. .. .. .. .. 583

**Corticosteroids and Varicella: Six-year Experience in an Asthmatic Population.** Constantine J. Falliers and Elliot F. Ellis .. .. .. .. .. .. .. .. .. 593

**E (16-18) Trisomy Syndrome: Analysis of 13 Cases.** L. J. Butler, G. J. A. I. Snodgrass, N. E. France, L. Sinclair, and A. Russell .. .. .. .. .. .. .. 600

**Electroencephalographic Studies in Infants and Children with Hypothyroidism.** R. Harris, M. Della Rovere, and P. F. Prior .. .. .. .. .. .. .. .. 612

**Hyaline Membrane Disease: A Pathological Study of 55 Infants.** J. M. Lauweryns .. .. 618

**Acid-Base Changes Following Exchange Transfusion with Citrated Blood.** Mary Calladine, Douglas Gairdner, B. T. Naidoo, and D. H. Orrell .. .. .. .. .. .. 626

**Metabolic and Chromosomal Studies in Leprechaunism.** Anatole Dekaban .. .. .. 632

**Observations on Blood Pressure in Newborn Infants.** J. M. Gupta and J. W. Scopes .. .. 637

**Serial Acid-Base Determinations in Normal Premature and Full-term Infants During the First 72 Hours of Life.** A. F. Malan, A. Evans, and H. de V. Heese .. .. .. .. .. 645

**Effect of Penicillamine on Serum Iron.** J. M. Walshe and Valerie Patston .. .. .. 651

**Fatal Haemolytic Uraemic Syndrome and Idiopathic Hyperlipaemia in Monozygotic Twins.** S. Campbell and I. J. Carré .. .. .. .. .. .. .. .. .. 654

PAGE

**Nephrosis: A Clinical and Histological Study of 38 Children.** R. McLaren Todd and M. J. Bouton .. .. .. .. .. .. .. .. .. .. .. .. 659

**Effect of Blue Light on Hyperbilirubinaemia.** P. M. G. Broughton, E. J. R. Rossiter, C. B. M. Warren, G. Goulis, and P. S. Lord .. .. .. .. .. .. .. .. 666

**Head Circumference of Infants Related to Body Weight.** R. S. Illingworth and W. Lutz .. 672

**Mastocytosis: Report of a Case in a 15½-week-old Infant with Cutaneous and Generalized Skeletal Changes.** Arthur R. C. Cole .. .. .. .. .. .. .. .. .. 677

**Accuracy of the Sweat Test: Advantage of a Micromethod.** R. de Haller, J. de Haller, and P. Siegenthaler .. .. .. .. .. .. .. .. .. .. .. .. 684

**Laryngeal Stridor and Respiratory Obstruction Associated with Meningomyelocele.** J. S. Fitzsimmons .. .. .. .. .. .. .. .. .. .. .. .. 687

**Foetus in Foetu.** Edmund Y. C. Lee .. .. .. .. .. .. .. .. .. .. .. 689

**Syndrome of Incomplete Regional Achondroplasia (Ilium and Ribs) with Abdominal Muscle Dysplasia.** Emmanuel Shapira, Efraim Fischel, Shimon Moses, and Stanley Levin .. 694

**Book Reviews** .. .. .. .. .. .. .. .. .. .. .. .. 698

**Index 1965** .. .. .. .. .. .. .. .. .. .. .. .. 702

*Arch. Dis. Childh.*, 1965, **40**, 1.



# AN INBORN DEFECT OF INTESTINAL ABSORPTION OF CERTAIN MONOSACCHARIDES

BY

CHARLOTTE M. ANDERSON, K. R. KERRY,* and R. R. W. TOWNLEY

*From the Gastroenterological Research Unit, Royal Children's Hospital Research Foundation, Melbourne, Australia*

(RECEIVED FOR PUBLICATION AUGUST 17, 1964)

Since 1958 defective digestion of the disaccharide sugars has received increasing attention and hereditary congenital deficiencies of the enzymes, lactase, sucrase, and isomaltase, have been very convincingly demonstrated both clinically and by methods which estimate enzyme activity in small intestinal mucosa. The unhydrolysed and therefore predominantly unabsorbed disaccharide gives rise to diarrhoea, the stools being fluid, of an acid *p*H with a raised lactic acid and reducing sugar content. However, two groups of workers, Laplane, Polonovski, Etienne, Debray, Lods, and Pissarro (1962) and Lindquist and Meeuwisse (1962) have described infants in whom similar diarrhoea occurred when feedings were first instituted after birth, but in whom hydrolysis of the disaccharides appeared normal. These infants apparently could not absorb glucose or galactose, their diarrhoea ceasing only when feedings contained fructose as the source of sugar. The condition was also familial (Lindquist, Meeuwisse, and Melin, 1962).

This paper records a further family in which one infant was similarly affected and a sib was probably affected. The absorption of a number of disaccharides and monosaccharides was investigated and the results are discussed in relation to the mechanisms of sugar absorption.

### Case Report

Elizabeth, the second child of healthy young unrelated parents was born in November 1961, in a country town, following a pregnancy during which her mother was well except for mild glycosuria in the later months. The confinement was normal. Breast feeding was established, but on the third day of life the baby developed severe watery diarrhoea which continued despite the feeding being changed to a sweetened condensed milk formula.

The mother's first pregnancy had resulted in a male baby who developed similar diarrhoea at 3 days of age. This diarrhoea had persisted for the whole 3 months of the baby's life and despite numerous investigations and feeding changes no cause was found and the baby died in a state of inanition and chronic dehydration. A necropsy did not reveal any abnormal findings except the poor nutritional state. When the second infant developed identical symptoms the general practitioner, suspecting a metabolic cause, referred her to our centre.

On admission, the baby, now 7 days of age, was moderately dehydrated, and still passing very numerous fluid stools which were acid and accompanied by much flatus. She required intravenous resuscitation. Diarrhoea ceased when oral fluids were withheld, but recurred on giving a glucose and electrolyte mixture orally, though the significance of this was not grasped at the time. In view of the other sib's illness and the type of stools, lactase deficiency was suspected and as the infant was again becoming dehydrated the feeding was changed to a lactose-free formula 'Sobee' before further investigation was pursued. The diarrhoea abated a little but by no means ceased. However, hydration was maintained though the weight was stationary.

No pathogenic organisms were found in the stool. A 24-hour stool collection contained 4·8 g. fat and 850 mg. lactic acid. Per-oral suction biopsy of the duodenal mucosa was performed and disaccharidase enzyme activity tested by a previously published method (Anderson, Messer, Townley, and Freeman, 1963). To our surprise lactose was well hydrolysed by the intestinal mucosa as was sucrose and maltose. The histological appearance of the mucosa was also normal.

At this critical stage a colleague directed our attention to a letter in a recent issue of the *Lancet*, by Lindquist *et al.* (1962) in which was described an infant with a similar clinical history in whom they had also suspected lactase deficiency only to find this was not the diagnosis. The baby thrived only when it was given an artificially contrived feeding in which the source of sugar was fructose. We immediately placed our patient on this type of feeding and diarrhoea ceased within 24 hours. The baby began to gain weight at a relatively normal rate. Her progress has been followed for 18 months. She is starting to walk and talk, and is alert, cheerful, and seems of normal intellectual and physical development.

The fluid feedings have been a mixture containing sodium caseinate, fructose, butter fat, and water, mixed together in a vitamizer into a coarse emulsion. Until about 8 months of age the concentration of the various

* In receipt of a grant from the National Health and Medical Research Council of Australia.

constituents was as follows: sodium caseinate 3·5%, butter fat 4%, fructose 7·5%. Electrolytes were added to bring the sodium, potassium, and chloride content close to that of cows' milk. Calcium gluconate 1 g., in divided doses, was given each day to the child, and in the early months vitamins C, K, B12, and folic acid, were added to the normal amount of a multivitamin preparation.

Several attempts were made to change the feeding back to cows' milk. On each occasion diarrhoea occurred, and if three such feedings, at intervals of three hours, were given the weight loss could amount to 0·4 kg. The stools would become fluid and contain sugar and lactic acid in excess of normal.

At 6 months of age solid foods were introduced into the diet, these being at first confined to fruits (such as stewed apple, peach, or apricot), meat broth, and egg custard. Fructose was used as a sweetening agent and the artificial milk mixture to make the custard. Feeding these solids did not affect the stools, which at this stage consisted of one or two brown pasty bowel actions per day. After a few months a small amount of cereal was introduced and the mother learned by experience how much could be tolerated without causing the stools to become loose. At this stage the fructose content of the liquid feeding was decreased to 3·5%.

Now, at the age of 18 months, the child is taking meat, vegetables, fruit, eggs, a small amount of cereal, a little ice-cream, custard made from special milk mixture, all without effect on the stools. Honey is tolerated fairly well and is now being used as a sweetening agent in other foods instead of fructose. A small amount of cows' milk was introduced at 18 months of age and though the child did not like it she could take up to 4 ounces each day before the stools became very loose.

### Special Investigations

Once the patient was gaining weight following treatment with a glucose and galactose free diet, her tolerance to a number of sugars was tested. These included the monosaccharides, glucose, galactose, fructose, sorbose, mannose, xylose, and 3-0-methyl glucose, and the disaccharides lactose, sucrose, and maltose. Fructose and sorbose were obtained from Pfansteil Chemicals Inc., Waukegan, U.S.A., and 3-0-methyl glucose from L. Light and Son, England, and as a gift from Dr. R. K. Crane of Chicago. The remainder were from British Drug Houses. With the exception of L (+) sorbose all monosaccharides were in the D (+) form.

A 10% aqueous solution of the sugar (1·5 g./kg. body weight, except for 3-0-methyl glucose) was given by gavage after a preliminary fast of 4-5 hours. Blood samples were obtained at half-hourly intervals for 2 hours and levels of blood sugar were determined by the method of Nelson (1944) and Somogyi (1952).

While the patient was nursed on a metabolic bed, stools and urine were collected separately for at least 6 and sometimes 24 hours following each dose. Previous experience in other cases of sugar intolerance had shown that, after a single dose of the offending sugar, the passage of sugar in the stool was rapid and largely completed in 6 hours. Therefore inconvenience to the patient during the numerous tolerance tests was cut down by collecting for only 6 hours. Both stools and urine were deep frozen soon after any was passed and were kept so until estimations for sugar or lactic acid were carried out.

The faecal samples were thawed, their volume was measured, and then they were homogenized, the volume being made up to 1 litre with tap water. An aliquot was centrifuged and 50 ml. of the supernatant deproteinized with the zinc sulphate, barium hydroxide reagents of Somogyi (1945). If necessary the stools were decolorized with activated charcoal, but this step was avoided if chromatography showed that disaccharides were present. The solution was then centrifuged and the supernatant analysed for sugar and lactic acid content.

For total reducing substance the Nelson (1944) and Somogyi (1952) method was used; for glucose, the glucose oxidase method of Huggett and Nixon (1957) as modified by Dahlqvist (1961); for 3-0-methyl glucose, the anthrone method, and for lactic acid the method of Barker and Summerson (1941).

The type of reducing sugar found in the stools was determined by paper chromatography: 2 μl. of the solution was spotted on to Whatman No. 1 chromatography paper; descending chromatography was used and the solvent, ethyl acetate, pyridine, water (12 : 5 : 4), was allowed to drip from the end of a 30 cm. length of paper. An overnight run was sufficient to separate the sugars tested with the exception of sorbose, mannose, and fructose. Where it was necessary to resolve these sugars, phenol water (160 g. phenol plus 40 g. water) was used as the solvent. The spots were located by the silver nitrate reagent of Smith (1958).

The urine, after decolorization with activated charcoal, was also analysed by the above methods: 2 μl. of undiluted urine was used for urine chromatography.

The xylose absorption test was carried out by a method similar to that described by Clark (1962). The patient was fasted for 6 hours, then given a dose of xylose by gavage at the rate of 15 g./m.$^2$ of body surface area, as a 5% solution. Three doses of water each of 100 ml. were given at hourly intervals to encourage urine flow. Stools were collected for 6 hours and urine for 5 hours. Xylose was determined in all instances by the method of Roe and Rice (1948).

### Results

Table 1 illustrates the patient's response to cows' milk feedings. After three feedings of cows' milk with added lactose, instead of her special feedings, the stools became fluid, their volume increased, as did their reducing substance and lactic acid content, the former in excess of the latter. She lost 0·4 kg. body weight. Reducing substance equivalent to a considerable percentage of the administered sugar was found in the stool but it was shown by chromatography to be glucose and galactose, not lactose. The lactic acid content of the stool did not increase significantly until considerable amounts of sugar had already appeared in the stool indicating the diarrhoea to be 'osmotic' in origin.

Table 2 indicates the fate of the sugars which were given in individual test doses by recording the output of sugar and lactic acid in the stools, together with the maximum rise in blood reducing substances during two hours following the dose of sugar. Neither glucose nor galactose produced any rise in blood reducing substance and much of the sugar appeared in the subsequent stools, which were liquid. However, following a fructose dose no sugar appeared in the stool, the consistency of which was normal. The blood reducing substance rose slowly as is usual following fructose, normally a slowly absorbed monosaccharide.

The disaccharides lactose and maltose also showed little evidence of absorption. However, the sucrose dose was followed by some rise in blood reducing substance and less sugar in the faeces than followed the dose of lactose or maltose. After feeding a mixture of glucose and fructose very similar amounts of stool sugar were found. The feeding of sucrose was followed by a considerable rise in stool lactic acid—more than with any of the other sugars. A similar result was obtained on a second occasion.

Table 3 records the amount of sugar found in the stools and urine during 6 hours following a dose of the sugars mannose and sorbose. In each case the result obtained in a child of approximately the same age is recorded. Mannose, normally a poorly absorbed sugar, appeared in considerable quantity in the stool, with only a trace in the urine in both children. L-sorbose, a keto sugar, as is fructose, was moderately well absorbed by both patient and 'control', a small quantity of the dose appearing in the stools which did become more fluid, but some also appearing in the urine. The metabolism of absorbed sorbose in the body is not clearly known, but it seems that our patient was able to absorb this sugar in approximately the same way as another child who had no disturbance of sugar absorption.

TABLE 1

STOOL ANALYSIS DURING AND AFTER 3 FEEDINGS OF COWS' MILK GIVEN AT 3-HOURLY INTERVALS

| Hours After Initial Feed | Stool Volume (ml.) | Total 'Sugar' (g.) | Lactic Acid (mg.) | Fat (g.) |
|---|---|---|---|---|
| 1 | 35 | 0·012 | 8 | 0·5 |
| 5 | 240 | 3·9 | 143 | 1·6 |
| 10 | 245 | 4·2 | 494 | 1·7 |
| 24 | 130 | 0·5 | 154 | 2·6 |
| Total . . | 650 | 8·6 | 799 | 6·4 |

During the xylose tolerance test 10·5% of the dose of 5·1 g. was recovered from the urine. This result is at the lower end of the normal range quoted by Clark (1962). The mean absorption of 40 normal subjects tested by him was 24%.

In Table 4 the absorption of 3-0-methyl glucose by the patient is compared with that of three other children. The latter, two of whom suffered from fibrocystic disease of the pancreas, a disease in which sugar absorption is not usually disturbed, and one normal child, absorbed this sugar well, since it was almost quantitatively excreted in the urine. The

TABLE 2

'SUGAR' AND LACTIC ACID IN STOOLS COLLECTED FOR 6 HOURS AFTER DOSE OF INDIVIDUAL SUGARS, AND MAXIMUM RISE OF BLOOD 'SUGAR' DURING 2 HOURS

| Sugar Fed | | 'Sugar' in Stool | | Stool Lactic Acid (mg.) | Blood 'Sugar' Rise (mg./100 ml.) |
|---|---|---|---|---|---|
| Type | Amount (g.) | Type | Amount (g.) | | |
| Glucose | 7·0 | Glucose | 4·1 | 42 | 10 |
| Galactose | 7·0 | Galactose | 2·56 | 26 | 14 |
| Fructose | 7·0 | | 0·03 | 5 | 18 |
| Maltose | 7·3 | Glucose | 3·9 | 54 | 10 |
| Lactose | 7·0 | Glucose and galactose | 3·9 | 150 | 17 |
| Sucrose | 7·0 | Glucose (1·3 g.) | 1·5 | 320 | 31 |
| Fructose and glucose | 3·5 and 3·5 | Glucose (1·3 g.) | 1·4 | 11 | 11 |

TABLE 3

'SUGAR' IN STOOLS AND URINE COLLECTED FOR 6 HOURS AFTER DOSE OF MANNOSE AND SORBOSE, COMPARED IN EACH CASE WITH ANOTHER CHILD OF APPROXIMATELY THE SAME AGE

| | Sugar Fed | Amount (g.) | Stool Volume (ml.) | Stool 'Sugar' (g.) | Urine 'Sugar' (g.) |
|---|---|---|---|---|---|
| Patient | Mannose | 7·0 | 120 | 3·14 | No mannose |
| Control | Mannose | 9·3 | 385 | 3·5 | No mannose |
| Patient | Sorbose | 13·8 | 550 | 1·6 | 0·825 |
| Control | Sorbose | 7·9 | 560 | 2·44 | 0·316 |

TABLE 4

'SUGAR' IN URINE AND STOOLS COLLECTED FOR 24 HOURS AFTER FEEDING 3-0-METHYL GLUCOSE TO PATIENT AND THREE OTHER CHILDREN

| | Weight of Child (kg.) | Dose (g.) | Total 'Sugar' (g.) | | Glucose (g.) | |
|---|---|---|---|---|---|---|
| | | | Stool | Urine | Stool | Urine |
| Patient .. .. .. .. .. .. | 11·5 | 5 | 0·957 | 0·772 | 0·013 | 0·117 |
| Normal child .. .. .. .. .. | 9 | 5 | 0·025 | 5·36 | 0·009 | 0·012 |
| Fibrocystic disease of the pancreas .. | 7·5 | 5 | 0·437 | 3·5 | 0·010 | 0·011 |
| Fibrocystic disease of the pancreas .. | 11·5 | 17·5 | 0·595 | 16·2 | 0·067 | 0·692 |

stools were unaltered in consistency. However, the patient's absorption was grossly impaired, and during 24 hours a significant portion of the dose appeared in the stools which became liquid during the test period. A small quantity did appear in the urine together with a little glucose.

Random urine samples from the patient when she was taking cows' milk feedings always showed the presence of some glucose (90-145 mg./100 ml.). In normal babies of the same age and on similar feedings our experience has shown the level to be less than 30 mg./100 ml. As the patient's blood sugar was seldom above 100 mg./100 ml. intravenous glucose was given in an effort to raise the blood sugar to normal post-prandial levels. The glucose content of the urine increased when the blood sugar was between 100 and 160 mg./100 ml., indicating a probable lowering of renal threshold for glucose.

## Discussion

The clinical symptoms and results of investigations of this patient closely resemble those of the patients reported by Laplane *et al.* (1962) and Lindquist and Meeuwisse (1962), in that when the monosaccharides glucose and galactose and the disaccharides which contain these sugars (lactose, maltose, and sucrose) are fed, diarrhoea quickly develops. This leads to rapid loss of weight, dehydration, and electrolyte depletion, if the offending sugars are not removed from the diet. The stools become watery, acidic, and have a high sugar and lactic acid content. The diarrhoea may be severe enough to cause death in infancy. It seems likely that in the family we have studied another baby died of the condition. There were a number of deaths in infancy from chronic diarrhoea in the families of the patients described by Lindquist, Meeuwisse, and Melin (1963).

In contrast, the monosaccharide, fructose, is well absorbed by these patients, and when an artificial feeding containing this sugar together with a source of protein (casein) and fat (butter or corn oil) is fed they thrive and diarrhoea does not occur.

At the time when our patient presented for investigation only the brief report in a letter to the *Lancet* by Lindquist *et al.* (1962) from Northern Sweden was available to us, but subsequently we found the independent, but slightly earlier, description of two other such babies by Laplane *et al.* (1962) from France who had carried out their investigations along very similar lines and had come to virtually the same conclusions regarding the possible absorptive defect as did Lindquist and co-workers. To our knowledge the reports from these two groups of workers and ourselves are, as yet, the only recorded descriptions of this condition. It is interesting to note the similarity in methods of investigation and findings among three independent groups of workers at about the same time in three widely separated countries.

Regarding their absorption and transport across intestinal epithelial cells, monosaccharides are divided into two groups, i.e. those 'actively' absorbed against a concentration difference, and those 'passively' absorbed by a diffusion process (Wilson, 1962). It appears that the sugars belonging to the 'actively' absorbed group, such as glucose and galactose, are those affected in these patients, whereas fructose, of the 'passively' absorbed group, is dealt with normally.

In all patients described sucrose was better tolerated than other disaccharides, presumably because half the molecule is fructose. In support of this was the response obtained when we fed a mixture of glucose and fructose in equimolar amounts to our patient. Almost identical amounts of sugar appeared in the stools as with the equivalent dose of sucrose.

After feeding any of the disaccharides, stool chromatography showed only the constituent monosaccharides. Miller and Crane (1961) have demonstrated that the disaccharidase enzymes are located in the brush border of the intestinal epithelium and are not secreted into the lumen. In children with specific disaccharidase deficiencies, e.g. lactase or sucrase deficiencies, some of the particular disaccharide is found unsplit in the faeces (Auricchio, Dahlqvist, Mürset, and Prader, 1962; Auricchio, Rubino, Landolt, Semenza, and Prader, 1963). Therefore, in these monosaccharide intolerant patients, it seems that the disaccharides must be absorbed into or onto the brush border, hydrolysed, then the glucose and galactose passed back into the lumen. Crane (1962) believes that there are two regions in the brush border: the outer, where the disaccharidases are situated, and the inner, where the so-called active sodium-dependent transport of monosaccharides into the epithelial cell itself takes place. The handling of disaccharides by these patients supports this view.

The precise mechanism of active transport is as yet unknown but it is accepted to be sodium dependent, and related to the 'sodium pump'. It is also said to be 'carrier-mediated', but the carrier is unknown. Wilson (1962) summarizes the evidence so far available. There was no indication of any other disturbance of the 'sodium pump' mechanism in our patient. However, there was some evidence that glucose resorption in the kidney tubules was impaired and Lindquist and Meeuwisse (1962) have also suggested this but without very definite evidence. It has been suggested by workers studying Hartnup's disease, in which there is a disturbance of amino acid absorption in both the gut and the kidney tubule, that the normal mechanism of absorption may be the same in both situations. It is possible that the mechanism for glucose absorption is also the same in both situations.

Wilson (1962) when reviewing experimental work with animals regarding the specificity of the 'active' transport mechanism points out that the presence of a hydroxyl group on carbon atom 2 of the monosaccharide molecule is an essential feature. 3-0-methyl glucose, a synthetic sugar with this basic configuration, was shown by Csaky (1942) to have a similar rate of absorption to glucose but it is not metabolized, being rapidly passed out in the urine. This sugar was very poorly absorbed by our patient in comparison with other children, indicating again that the 'active' absorption mechanism is defective. The small amount that did appear in the urine may represent some passive diffusion of the sugar, which, as it is not metabolized, rapidly appears in the urine.

Mannose and xylose have been included among the sugars that are not actively absorbed. However, mannose is extremely poorly absorbed by humans and in our patient the response to a dose did not differ from that we obtained in normal children. Xylose was absorbed by our patient to about 50% of the mean normal absorption quoted by Clark (1962). However, recent work by Salomon, Allums, and Smith (1961) throws doubt on the acceptance of xylose as a purely passively absorbed sugar, indicating it may have some affinity for the glucose carrier.

The absorption of sorbose was tested because this is a 'keto' sugar which may have a furanose ring structure like fructose, while glucose and galactose are 'aldo' sugars with a pyranose ring structure. The latter is also said to be a characteristic of 'actively' absorbed sugars. We found the L form of sorbose (the D form was unavailable) to be slowly absorbed by normal children, and to be not completely metabolized as it appeared in the urine in significant quantity. Our patient absorbed L sorbose in a similar fashion to normal children.

Thus all data from the tests on absorption of sugars in our patient support the concept that the 'actively' absorbed sugars are not transported into or across the intestinal epithelial cell in a normal fashion, whereas the 'passively' absorbed sugars are. It seems that patients such as this might offer opportunities to study the 'active absorption' mechanism, to try to throw more light on the relation of the sodium pump and the identity of the 'mobile carrier system' postulated by Crane (1962).

Clinical management of these patients is largely confined to manipulation of the diet which has been described in some detail in this paper. As the child grows some carbohydrate containing the involved monosaccharides can be tolerated in the diet, but only trial and error will determine how much. As we believe that the diarrhoea caused by unabsorbed sugar is largely 'osmotic' in origin, the severity of the diarrhoea will depend on the concentration of unabsorbed sugar in the gut at any time. Diarrhoea or looseness of the stools can be kept to tolerable levels if the total intake of the offending carbohydrates is low and distributed throughout the daily meals. A personal communication from B. Lindquist and G. Meeuwisse (1964) revealed that one of their patients, a 36-year-old woman who had been discovered because she was a relative of a previously diagnosed patient, had been able to manipulate her own diet to avoid a carbohydrate or milk intake that caused troublesome diarrhoea. She was thin but healthy.

The condition appears to be familial and Lindquist *et al.* (1963) describe 4 proven cases in Northern Sweden, 3 of whom are related. In the families of these 3, which can be traced to a common ancestor, there were 6 deaths in infancy from chronic diarrhoea. They suggest that the pedigrees demonstrate an autosomal recessive type of inheritance of the disease. These patients therefore display yet another inborn error of metabolism, one in which the development of the 'active' transport mechanism of monosaccharides across epithelial cells is defective.

## Summary

A patient with symptoms closely resembling those

of disaccharide intolerance but in whom there was defective intestinal absorption of certain monosaccharides is described.

The monosaccharides affected were those described as absorbed 'actively' against a concentration difference, and included glucose, galactose, and 3-0-methyl glucose.

Disaccharides containing any of these monosaccharides also caused similar symptoms.

The passively absorbed sugar fructose was handled normally, and comprised the chief carbohydrate content of the child's diet.

Only two other reports of such patients are available, but the condition is familial and probably represents another inborn error of carbohydrate metabolism.

We are grateful to Mrs. Stebbing and to Miss Milroy for technical assistance; to the Infant Formula Room and Dietary Department for considerable help in constructing special diets; to the nursing staff who watched over the numerous metabolic collections; and to Dr. R. K. Crane who kindly gave us some 3-0-methyl glucose.

## References

Anderson, C. M., Messer, M., Townley, R. R. W., and Freeman, M. (1963). Intestinal sucrase and isomaltase deficiency in two siblings. *Pediatrics*, **31**, 1003.

Auricchio, S., Dahlqvist, A., Mürset, G., and Prader, A. (1962). Intestinal isomaltose deficiency in patients with hereditary sucrose and starch intolerance. *Lancet*, **1**, 1303.

——, Rubino, A., Landolt, M., Semenza, G., and Prader, A. (1963). Isolated intestinal lactase deficiency in the adult. *ibid.*, **2**, 324.

Barker, S. B., and Summerson, W. H. (1941). The colorimetric determination of lactic acid in biological material. *J. biol. Chem.*, **138**, 535.

Clark, P. A. (1962). The use of the d-xylose excretion test in children. *Gut*, **3**, 333.

Crane, R. K. (1962). Hypothesis for mechanism of intestinal active transport of sugars. *Fed. Proc.*, **21**, 891.

Csaky, T. (1942). Über die Rolle der Strucktur des Glucosemoleküls bei der Resorption aus dem Dünndarm. *Hoppe-Seylers Z. physiol. Chem.*, **277**, 47.

Dahlqvist, A. (1961). Determination of maltase and isomaltase activities with a glucose-oxidase reagent. *Biochem. J.*, **80**, 547.

Huggett, A. St. G., and Nixon, D. A. (1957). Use of glucose oxidase, peroxidase, and O-dianisidine in determination of blood and urinary glucose. *Lancet*, **2**, 368.

Laplane, R., Polonovski, C., Etienne, M., Debray, P., Lods, J. C., and Pissarro, B. (1962). L'intolérance aux sucres a transfert intestinal actif. (Ses rapports avec l'intolérance au lactose et le syndrome coeliaque.) *Arch. franç. Pédiat.*, **19**, 895.

Lindquist, B., and Meeuwisse, G. W. (1962). Chronic diarrhoea caused by monosaccharide malabsorption. *Acta paediat. (Uppsala)*, **51**, 674.

——, ——, and Melin, K. (1962). Glucose-galactose malabsorption. *Lancet*, **2**, 666.

——, ——, —— (1963). Osmotic diarrhoea in genetically transmitted glucose-galactose malabsorption. Proc. Swedish Paediatric Soc. *Acta paediat. (Uppsala)*, **52**, 217.

Miller, D., and Crane, R. K. (1961). The digestive function of the epithelium of the small intestine. II. Localization of disaccharide hydrolysis in the isolated brush border portion of intestinal epithelial cells. *Biochim. biophys. Acta (Amst.)*, **52**, 293.

Nelson, N. (1944). A photometric adaptation of Somogyi method for the determination of glucose. *J. biol. Chem.*, **153**, 375.

Roe, J. H., and Rice, E. W. (1948). A photometric method for the determination of free pentoses in animal tissues. *ibid.*, **173**, 507.

Salomon, L. L., Allums, J. A., and Smith, D. E. (1961). Possible carrier mechanism for the intestinal transport of d-xylose. *Biochem. biophys. Res. Commun.*, **4**, 123.

Somogyi, M. (1945). Determination of blood sugar. *J. biol. Chem.*, **160**, 69.

—— (1952). Notes on sugar determination. *ibid.*, **195**, 19.

Smith, I. (1958). *Chromatographic Techniques.* Heinemann, London.

Wilson, T. H. (1962). *Intestinal Absorption.* W. B. Saunders, Philadelphia.

*Arch. Dis. Childh.*, 1965, **40**, 7.

# STUDIES IN OSTEOPETROSIS

BY

C. E. DENT, JEAN M. SMELLIE, and L. WATSON

*From the Metabolic Ward and Paediatric Department, University College Hospital, London*

(RECEIVED FOR PUBLICATION JUNE 3, 1964)

Much attention has been paid to the rare, but spectacular bone disease known as osteopetrosis, Albers-Schönberg disease, or marble bones disease. It was first defined as a clinical entity in 1904 by Albers-Schönberg and the name osteopetrosis was introduced by Karshner in 1926. Many cases have since been reported and at intervals good review articles have appeared including those of McCune and Bradley (1934), Higinbotham and Alexander (1941), Pines and Lederer (1947), Seigman and Kilby (1950), Kneal and Sante (1951), and Hasenhuttl (1962). It is clear that the severe form presenting at birth is quite different clinically and genetically from the milder form which presents usually in adolescence or later (Turano, Fagan, and Corbo, 1954; Enell and Pehrson, 1958; Lièvre, Milhaud, and Camus, 1962). The severe congenital form is characterized by a remarkable homogeneity of greatly abnormal physical and radiological findings. All affected children show the same radiological findings in their bones and the same severe secondary haematological changes, consequent on the great reduction and in some cases almost complete obliteration of bone marrow. Most of the bone abnormalities can be immediately related to a quantitative, and perhaps also a qualitative, deficiency of osteoclasts as seen histologically (Kneal and Sante, 1951; Piatt, Erhard, and Araj, 1956; Engfeldt, Fajers, Lodin, and Pehrson, 1960). This is also shown by the persistence of too much calcified cartilage formed in the early chain of events of endochondral bone formation, and by a failure of remodelling of the bone during growth. As a result little or no bone marrow space is formed and the metaphyses show a characteristic club shape. Furthermore, the bone foramina, such as those through which the cranial nerves pass, fail to enlarge during growth, leading to a slow destruction of the nerves in question, yet another serious consequence of the osteoclastic deficiency.

Osteopetrosis of the severe form is inherited as if determined by an autosomal recessive gene (Enell and Pehrson, 1958). This fact, together with the clinical data, suggests very strongly that the disease is the result of an inborn error of metabolism. From this aspect, however, the literature makes depressing reading. No consistent biochemical abnormalities have yet been discovered that could have suggested a dysfunction of a single simple enzymic process. Plasma levels of calcium, phosphorus, and phosphatase are usually normal or inconsistently abnormal. No disorder closely linked to parathyroid or vitamin D dysfunction has been uncovered. Clearly, however, a hypofunctioning parathyroid gland could be invoked as a theoretical cause of the deficient osteoclastic activity. Likewise an oversensitivity to vitamin D may be present, for the radiographic appearances in osteopetrosis may resemble those in the severe form of 'idiopathic hypercalcaemia of infancy' (Fanconi, Girardet, Schlesinger, Butler, and Black, 1952), a disease in which such a mechanism may be involved.

A characteristic but puzzling feature of the untreated disease is that the bone radiographs of older survivors show signs of fluctuating activity of the osteosclerotic process. Commonly the club-shaped metaphyses show transverse alternating bands of greater and less density (Fairbank, 1948). Close examination shows that the less dense segments may show early signs of remodelling. According to our basic theory, such apparent fluctuations in true disease activity, in the face of a presumed constant genetic biochemical abnormality, indicate that the environment is also very much concerned in the disease pathogenesis (Dent, 1957), and suggest plausible forms of treatment. In this study we began from the premise that the modifying environmental factor was probably dietary and linked to calcium intake. Our tentative hypothesis was that the primary biochemical abnormality was an over-absorption of calcium from the diet resulting from an unidentified disordered mechanism. If this were so, profound changes in the development of the disease process should follow régimes aimed to produce

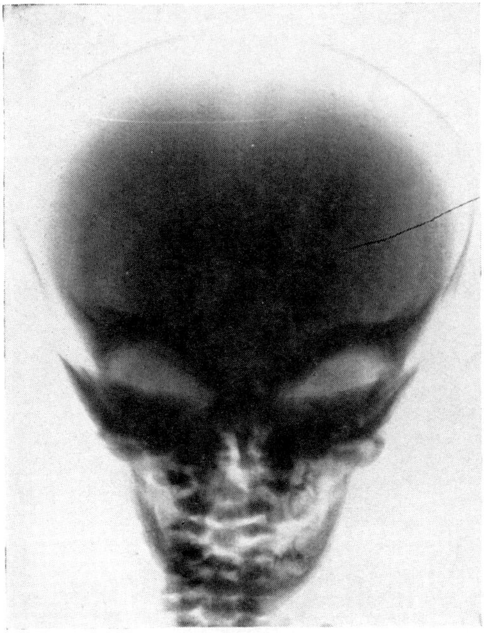

(a)

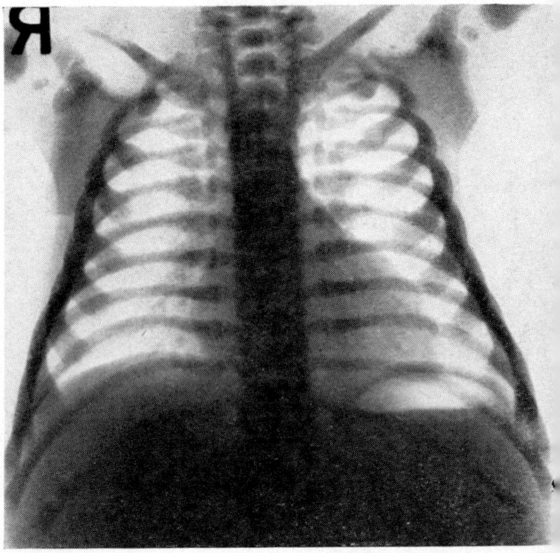

(b)

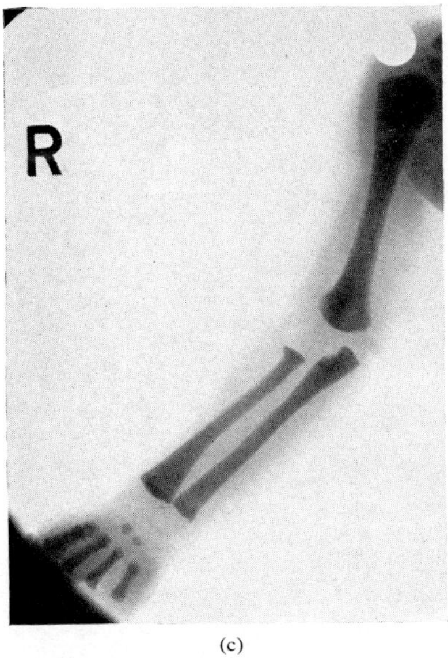


(c)

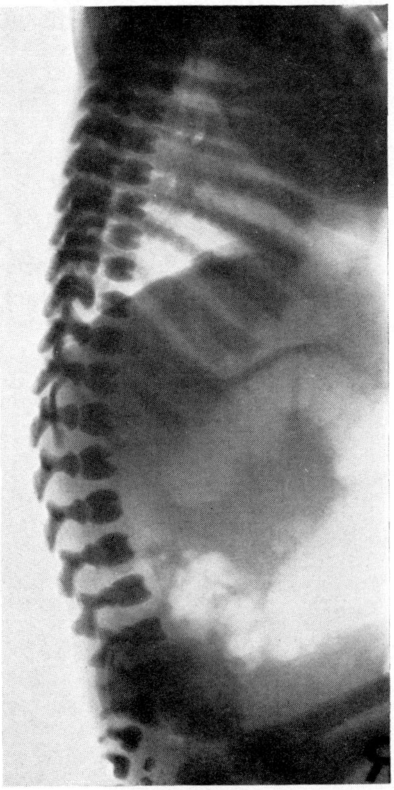

(d)

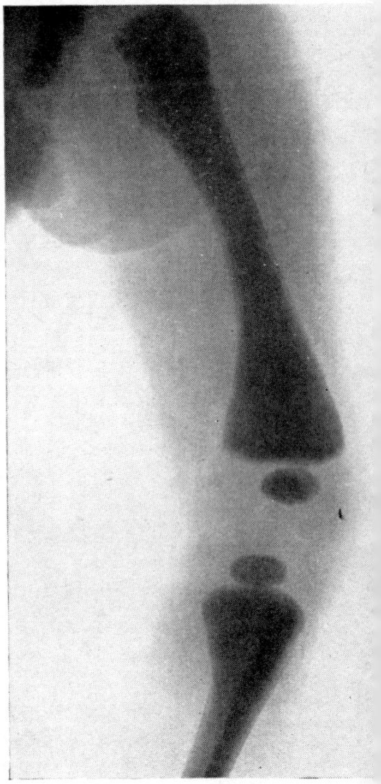

(e)

FIG. 1.—Bone radiographs when Kenneth was less than 1 year. (a) Skull at 4½ months; (b) chest at 4 months; (c) right arm at 4½ months; (d) lateral view of spine at 4½ months; (e) femur at 5 months.

calcium depletion. We are reporting here the effect in a child with osteopetrosis of treatment suggested by this basic hypothesis.

## Case Report

**History on Admission.** Kenneth M., the second child of normal parents, was born at term on September 1, 1957, with the assistance of forceps for a contracted pelvis. His birth weight was 7 lb. 6 oz. (3·4 kg.) and the only abnormality noted on initial examination was two erupted teeth which were extracted at 5 days.

He was noticeably pale from the age of 3 weeks and after confirmation of some degree of anaemia, treatment with oral iron and intramuscular vitamin $B_{12}$ was instituted with improvement. He also became snuffly, had frequent upper respiratory tract infections with cough, continuous rhinorrhoea, and consequent feeding difficulty. His mother noticed increasing prominence of his eyes and also of his scalp veins. He was fed on a standard evaporated milk schedule and solids were introduced from 2 months. Supplements of vitamins were added from 1 month in an approximate daily dosage of vitamin C, 25 mg. and vitamin D, 850 i.u.

At the age of 3 months, a radiological diagnosis of Albers-Schönberg disease was made at the U.S.A.F. Base Hospital, Ruislip, and he was transferred to the care of Dr. Bernard Schlesinger and one of us (C.E.D.) at University College Hospital on December 19, 1957.

The parents, aged 31 and 29 years, were unrelated, they and the patient's elder brother aged 2¼ years were normal. There was no family history of bone disease.

**Clinical Examination on Admission.** He was a pale baby (aged 3½ months) weighing 10 lb. 6 oz. (4·7 kg.) (3rd percentile), adequately nourished, with a relatively large head, short limbs, and a prominent abdomen. Length 24½ in. (61·5 cm.), upper segment 15½ in. (39 cm.), lower segment 9 in. (22·5 cm.), span 23 in. (57·5 cm.), head circumference 16½ in. (41·5 cm.).

He was snuffly, with a profuse mucopurulent nasal discharge. The bridge of the nose was depressed, accentuating the prominent eyes and there was frontal and parietal bossing. The anterior fontanelle was visibly full, pulsating, and measured about 5 cm. in diameter. The fontanelle tension was approximately 40 cm. water by tocodynamometer (Dr. C. N. Smyth). He was mouth-breathing with noisy respirations due to his pharyngeal secretions. The heart sounds were normal. The lower ribs were splayed by the distended abdomen in which the liver and spleen were palpable 4-5 cm. below the costal margin. There was no generalized lymphadenopathy. He appeared to hear, and he made sounds. The pupils reacted to light; the optic discs were grey without papilloedema, and the fundi were otherwise normal. He followed a slowly moving light with eye movements. The limb movements and his responses, the reflexes, and muscle tone appeared normal for his age.

**Preliminary Investigations.** Haemoglobin 57% (8·2 g./100 ml.). The blood smear showed numerous nucleated red cells, total white cell count 29,000/c.mm., the differential count showing neutrophils 52%, lymphocytes 35%, eosinophils 1%, immature cells 4%, and myelocytes 8%, platelets 89,000/c.mm. Routine examination of urine normal. Bone radiographs showed increased density with lack of cortico-medullary differentiation. The metaphyses were clubbed and showed longitudinal striations (Fig. 1a-e). Clear CSF of normal composition, under a pressure of 190 mm., was obtained by lumbar puncture. Plasma calcium varied from 8·5-9·5 mg./100 ml. with normal fractions (protein-bound calcium 2·7, complexed calcium 0·5, and ionized calcium 5·7 mg./100 ml.) (Dr. G. A. Rose). Plasma inorganic phosphorus 2·3-3·1 mg./100 ml., plasma alkaline phosphatase 25·8-31·5 K.A. units, blood urea 21 mg./100 ml. Serum proteins: total 8·1 g./100 ml., albumin 5·3 g./100 ml., globulin 2·8 g./100 ml. Serum was normal on electrophoresis. Urinary chromatography showed no abnormality of amino acid excretion. The urinary Sulkowitch reaction was low on repeated examinations and the 24-hour urinary calcium was 5 mg.

Many of the investigations and treatments carried out during a period of study lasting 5 years are summarized in Fig. 2. Fig. 3 shows his appearance at 2½ years. Fig. 4a and b shows the radiological appearances in the knees and wrists at the age of 5 years and a diagrammatic interpretation of the changes, correlated with dates, is shown in Fig. 5. Calcium balances are tabulated in the Table. For convenience, the further investigations, treatment, and progress will be considered in two parts, (A) the early studies performed before March 1960 and (B) the later ones after that date.

## (A) Investigations, Treatment, and Progress

**Ammonium Chloride.** Starting on January 16, 1958, a short trial of ammonium chloride in a daily dose of 0·5-1·0 g. was given in an attempt to increase urinary calcium excretion. The urinary *p*H fell from 6·7 to 5·5 without affecting the plasma bicarbonate of 21 mEq/l. The 24-hour calcium excretions were 15 mg. and 26 mg. on two occasions. The trial of ammonium chloride had to be abandoned on February 16, 1958, because of persistent anorexia and vomiting.

**Diet.** From January 16, 1958, at the age of 4½ months, a low calcium diet (approximately 200 mg. daily) was introduced in the form of Locasol (Trufood), and vitamin D additions were discontinued. After eight months on this intake his mother thought he was eating very little and attributed this to the Locasol which she exchanged for cows' milk, the daily calcium intake being increased to approximately 300 mg. After four months of this, Locasol was again substituted on our recommendation (Fig. 2).

**Transfusions.** Between the ages of 4 and 7 months, five transfusions of packed red cells were required (Fig. 2). The recurrent anaemia was undoubtedly being aggravated by withdrawal of blood for biochemical examination. After the age of 7 months the haemoglobin level was maintained between 80 and 100% (11·8-14·8 g./100 ml.), no further transfusions being required. The white cell

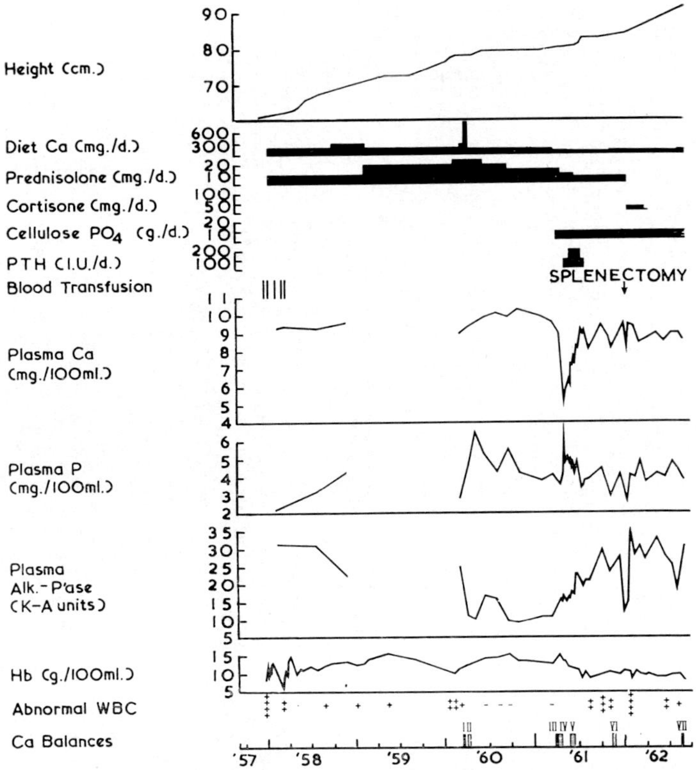


FIG. 2.—Clinical and biochemical data on Kenneth M. during the whole course of his study.

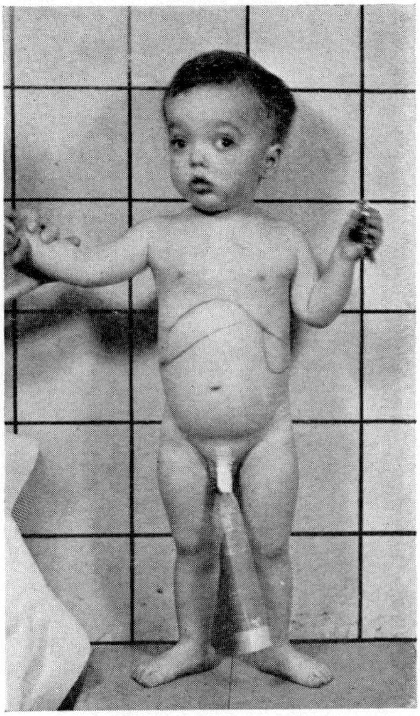

FIG. 3.—Kenneth M. at 2½ years. The outlines of the liver and spleen are marked.

count fell, circulating immature white cells virtually disappeared, and the platelet count returned to normal (Fig. 2).

**Corticosteroids.** On February 16, 1958, at the age of 5½ months prednisolone 10 mg. daily was started in the hope of prolonging the intervals between transfusions and

TABLE 1

CALCIUM BALANCES (IN SIX-DAY PERIODS) DURING VARIOUS THERAPY TRIALS

| Trial No. | Date | Daily Calcium Intake (mg.) | Daily Faecal Calcium (mg.) | Daily Urine Calcium (mg.) | Calcium Balance (mg./day) | Other Treatments |
|---|---|---|---|---|---|---|
| 1 | 11-16 March, 1960 | 282 | 75 | 113 | + 94 | Prednisolone 25 mg. daily |
| | 17-22 March, 1960 | 282 | 75 | 105 | + 102 | |
| 2 | 1-6 April, 1960 | 890 | 259 | 55 | + 576 | Prednisolone 25 mg. daily |
| | 7-12 April, 1960 | 890 | 238 | 45 | + 607 | |
| 3 | 22-27 March, 1961 | 97 | 10 | 15 | + 72 | Prednisolone 15 mg. daily |
| | 28 March-2 April, 1961 | 97 | 10 | 12 | + 75 | |
| 4 | 3-8 April, 1961 | 97 | 90 | 4 | + 3 | Prednisolone 15 mg. daily |
| | 9-14 April, 1961 | 97 | 99 | 3 | − 5 | Cellulose phosphate 10 g. daily |
| | 15-20 April, 1961 | 97 | 91 | 2 | + 4 | |
| 5 | 18-23 May, 1961 | 80 | 63 | 2 | + 15 | Prednisolone 10 mg. daily; Cellulose phosphate 10 g. daily; Parathormone 50 i.u., b.d. |
| | 24-29 May, 1961 | 80 | 54 | 2 | + 24 | Parathormone 100 i.u., b.d.; Cellulose phosphate 10 g. daily; Prednisolone 10 mg. daily |
| | 30 May-4 June, 1961 | 80 | 48 | 3 | + 29 | |
| | 5-10 June, 1961 | 80 | 47 | 2 | + 31 | |
| 6 | 11-16 Nov., 1961 | 84 | 86 | 3 | − 5 | Prednisolone 7·5 mg. daily |
| | 17-22 Nov., 1961 | 84 | 78 | 3 | + 3 | Cellulose phosphate 10 g. daily |
| 7 | 18-23 Aug., 1962 | 120 | 81 | 6 | + 33 | Cellulose phosphate 10 g. daily |
| | 24-29 Aug., 1962 | 120 | 90 | 11 | + 19 | |

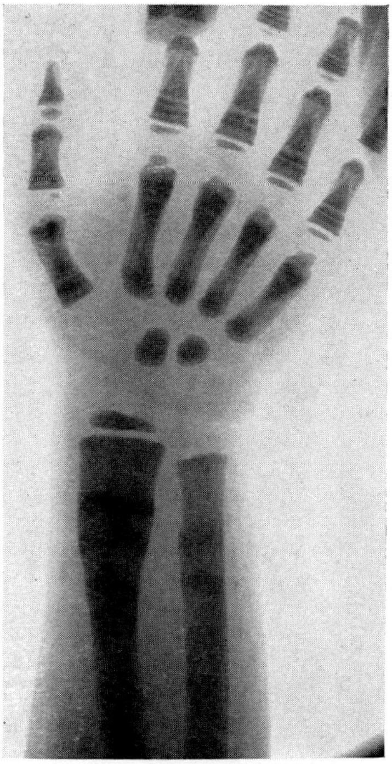

(a)

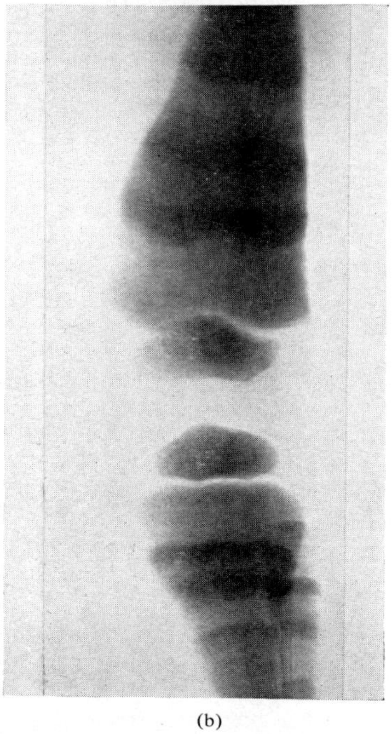

(b)

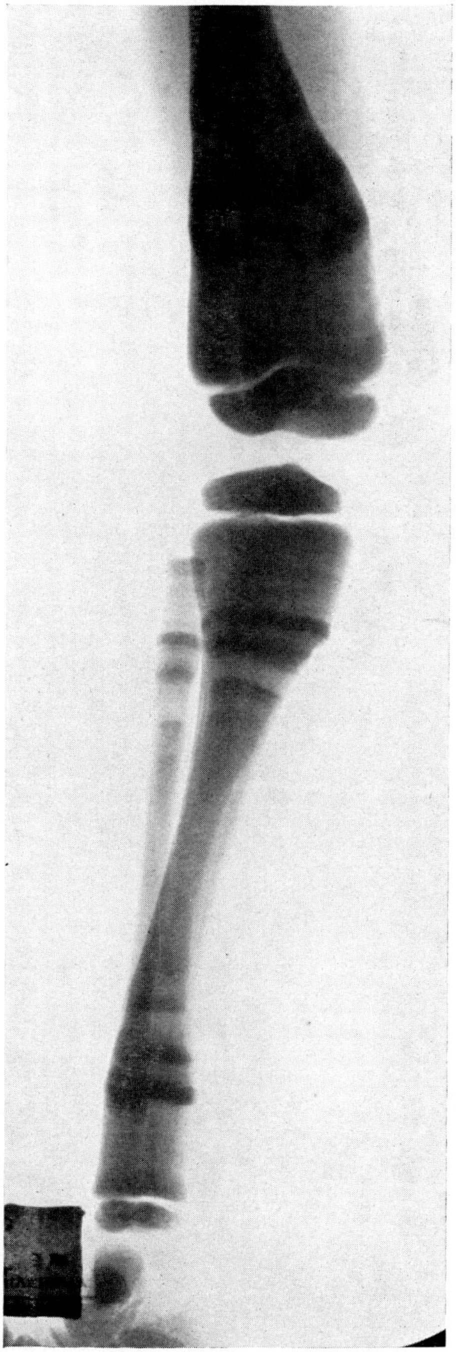

(c)

FIG. 4.—Bone radiographs when Kenneth was 5 years and over. (a) Right wrist at 5 years; (b) left knee at 5 years: the tracing shown on Fig. 5 is from a radiograph of one month later; (c) right leg at 5 years and 10 months.

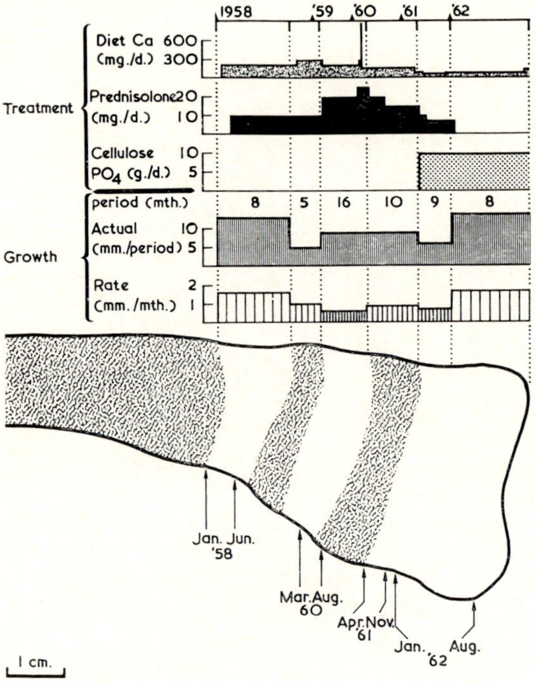


FIG. 5.—Tracing of left femur of Kenneth M. (Sept. 19, 1962). The datings shown have been derived from radiographs taken during his study. Changes in treatment and growth rate corresponding to this period of growth are shown above.

possibly reducing the mineralization of his bone. This dosage was continued for one year, increased to 20 mg. daily for a further year and then to 25 mg. daily for a further four months.

After four months of steroid therapy and low calcium diet the radiological appearances were encouraging (Fig. 5). The new bone formed was translucent with a suggestion of modelling both at the wrists and knees. During the next three months the new bone was slightly less translucent but the growth rate during this period was reasonably satisfactory (Fig. 5). In the next four-month period in which the calcium intake was increased from approximately 200 to 300 mg. daily the bone formed was very dense and growth rate appeared to slow down (Fig. 5).

After the dose of prednisolone was increased to 20 mg. daily there was a further deposition of less dense bone (Fig. 5). At the end of his second year of prednisolone therapy, at the age of 2 years and 5 months, his haemoglobin level had fallen to 64% (9·6 g./100 ml.) with reappearance of circulating immature cells and the prednisolone dosage was then increased to 25 mg. daily.

**Mile-stones.** Kenneth's general development was retarded though early and prolonged hospital admission and impaired vision may have contributed to this. He raised his head in the supine position at 6-7 months, sat at 1 year, stood and walked with support from 16 months and alone from 22 months. This was conducted on a wide base and with his legs externally rotated at the hips. He made noises from an early age and said 'Dad' from 1 year. He spoke three to four words with meaning from 18 months and proceeded to chatter continuously in a rather toneless voice.

The first dentition began to erupt at 10 months and continued irregularly. He continuously mouth-breathed because of the nasal discharge and poor airway and he dribbled saliva copiously. His eyes became less prominent but he developed a marked divergent strabismus by the age of 16 months. He could still appreciate light and darkness, apparently, reaching for toys and objects of support. At 19 months examination under anaesthesia confirmed bilateral optic atrophy. By 2 years 4 months he had a roving nystagmus and by 3 years there was no pupillary light reflex. Examination under anaesthesia then showed very atrophic discs but normal vasculature. He still succeeded in walking about in familiar surroundings remarkably well.

### (B) Investigations, Treatment, and Progress

On reviewing Kenneth's first 2½ years it was remarkable how much bone growth had varied both in rate and density (Fig. 5). It seemed that the first period of improvement in growth and bone density occurred when he was given a strict low calcium diet and a small dose of prednisolone and that radiological bone density increased and modelling failed to occur during the time when the mother allowed a little more calcium in the food. Increased prednisolone dosage produced improvement radiologically but an unsatisfactory rate of growth. It was clear that careful balance studies were now needed in addition to the other data to help assess these responses.

The investigations undertaken during this period included 6-day calcium and phosphorus balances at varying intervals and on different dietary calcium intakes with regular plasma calcium, phosphorus, and alkaline phosphatase estimations (Fig. 2) and fluoroscopy of the lower ends of radius and femur every few months (Fig. 5). Dietary intake of calcium and steroid dosage were adjusted in accordance with these data.

**Haematological Investigations and Treatment.** During 1960 and 1961 Kenneth's growth was most unsatisfactory (Figs. 2 and 5). It appeared that this was due in part to the prednisolone and the dosage was progressively lowered. After April 1961 there was a return of the anaemia and later of abnormal white cells in the peripheral blood (Fig. 2).

Radioisotope studies were then undertaken by Dr. T. A. J. Prankerd and Dr. A. J. Bowdler, who reported as follows.

'(1) *November 1961.* $^{51}Cr$ studies showed a marked reduction in the red cell life-span to approximately 4 days. The principal site of red cell destruction as indicated by surface counting was the spleen. $^{59}Fe$ studies showed rapid uptake and release by the spleen, maximal activity being found 24 hours after injection of the plasma-bound isotope. Surface counting over the lumbar spine and liver showed evidence of slight erythropoiesis; the spleen was, however, the most active site in this respect. The over-all erythropoietic rate appeared to be in excess of the normal requirement.

(2) *April 1962.* (3 months after splenectomy.) $^{51}Cr$ studies showed red cell survival at the lower limits of the normal range (T-half Cr 24 days). $^{59}Fe$ studies showed the liver to be the most active site of erythropoiesis. Anaemia at this time was due to impaired red cell production and not to haemolysis.

(3) *August 1962.* $^{59}Fe$ study showed the liver to be the most active site of erythropoiesis. No very active erythropoiesis was detectable in the lumbar spine or thigh.'

In view of the results of the isotope studies performed in November 1961 splenectomy was carried out on January 11, 1962 by Mr. G. L. Bunton. The spleen with splenunculus weighed 205 g. and histologically it showed active erythropoietic centres. Post-operatively cortisone was substituted for prednisolone and steroids were discontinued altogether in April 1962. The haemoglobin level settled between 9·2 and 9·9 g./100 ml. and circulating immature cells persisted.

There was a striking increase in growth rate and improvement in the radiological appearances when the steroids were stopped (Figs. 2 and 5).

**Diet and Calcium Balances** (Fig. 2 and Table). On a normal (890 mg. daily) calcium intake he was in strongly positive calcium balance (trial No. 2). On a low calcium intake (282 and 97 mg. daily) he remained in positive calcium balance (trials No. 1 and 3). It was only when cellulose phosphate (Balston Ltd.), 10 g. daily, was added to the very low calcium diet, 97 mg. daily, that approximate calcium balance was achieved (trial No. 4). Trial No. 6 showed that this effect was still maintained seven months later and trial No. 7 showed that with the greatly improved growth that followed splenectomy and withdrawal of steroid therapy he was still only in slightly positive balance with a slightly increased calcium intake (120 mg. daily).

In all these studies we had some difficulty in obtaining complete urine collections. This did not appreciably affect the calcium balance since urine calcium was always very low. Phosphorus balances reflected this uncertainty and are not, therefore, quoted here.

**Parathyroid Hormone.** Cellulose phosphate 10 g. daily was added to his other treatment in April 1961. So effective was this treatment in preventing gastro-intestinal absorption of calcium that one month after its start (in May 1961) Kenneth was admitted with severe hypocalcaemic tetany. The plasma calcium was 4·8 mg./100 ml., phosphorus 7·0 mg./100 ml. and alkaline phosphatase 10 K.A. units (Fig. 2).

The only change then introduced into his therapeutic régime was the addition of parathyroid hormone (Eli Lilly) by injection 50 units twice daily, increased after two weeks to 100 units twice daily. A small dose of vitamin D (about 900 i.u. daily) was also started.

There was rapid clinical improvement. The plasma calcium rose and returned to normal by mid-July when the parathyroid hormone was reduced and then stopped. There was no recurrence of tetany.

**Tetracycline.** Maintenance tetracycline was given throughout the five years to help control his recurrent upper respiratory tract infections.

**Radiology.** New bone formation was followed carefully in serial radiographs and the composite final picture is shown diagrammatically in Fig. 5. By correlating the dates on the corresponding graph it can be seen that the alternating bands of dense and translucent bone can be related to treatment. Dense bands correspond to periods of slightly increased calcium intake or of slow growth. The most recent bone growth is of normal density and shows some modelling. This took place during the 8-month period of vigorous dietary calcium depletion and withdrawal of prednisolone. No dense bands appeared during this period, but there was no apparent decrease in density of the bone already formed elsewhere and no evidence of medullary cavity formation. In some intermediate radiographs it was noted that the subperiosteal bone laid down in the shafts of long bones was also striated, in rough correspondence with the metaphysial changes.

**Growth and General Progress.** Rate of growth in height as measured clinically (Fig. 2), or radiologically (Fig. 5) was steadily decreasing from the age of 2 years. Almost no growth occurred while he was having 25 mg. prednisolone daily and very little in the following 19 months when he was having small doses. Following splenectomy and the withdrawal of steroid therapy he had a sudden and continuous growth spurt. He left our care in September 1962 to return home to the U.S.A. and then measured 36·5 in. (91·2 cm.). We are indebted for a later follow-up to Dr. Amos Christie (Vanderbilt University) who reported that in July 1963 his height was 39·5 in. (100 cm.), so that it is clear that the good progress shown during the last six months of our study has been maintained. A radiograph taken at this time is shown in Fig. 4c.

Kenneth's general condition remained satisfactory throughout. There was no deterioration in his haematological signs, and in spite of his divergent strabismus and bilateral optic atrophy he was able to walk around in familiar surroundings and was climbing and becoming more adventurous. He was able to hear, and joined in conversation with short sentences. Air studies of his ventricles were not undertaken though it was considered likely that he was hydrocephalic (head circumference 22·75 in. (57·7 cm.) at 5 years). At the age of 5 there was some mental and physical retardation, but special nursery schooling was already being considered for him at the time of his return home to the U.S.A.

## Discussion

For reasons mentioned in our introduction we have attempted to modify bone growth in this child by depleting him of bone mineral. We chose calcium depletion rather than phosphate, as calcium deficiency symptoms seemed more likely to be limited to the skeleton, and as calcium balances used to measure the efficiency of treatment are much easier to interpret than phosphorus balances. One of us (C.E.D.) had indeed attempted phosphate deprivation some years ago on another similar child. Aluminium hydroxide was given to bind the dietary phosphate, but the results were inconclusive probably because the phosphate absorption mechanism is so much more efficient than that for calcium (unpublished data).

Our early follow-up was difficult to interpret and largely unsuccessful because we did not realize that the child could utilize the calcium so efficiently even on low calcium diets. We were also giving fair doses of prednisolone, mainly to control the anaemia, but also hoping that perhaps this too would lessen gut absorption of calcium. When we discovered that the child was in positive balance on 100 mg. a day of calcium it was clear that even more severe calcium depletive measures needed to be taken. We, therefore, added the cellulose phosphate, then being currently used in this Department and by our colleagues at the Royal National Orthopaedic Hospital on adults with idiopathic hypercalcuria (Parfitt, Higgins, Nassim, Collins, and Hilb, 1964). This did make the calcium balance zero (Table), but this was still of no avail since bone growth at that time had practically ceased probably owing to the prednisolone. We were forced, therefore, to consider the haematological aspects more seriously. Our studies, giving similar results to those described by Sjölin (1959), suggested that splenectomy would be advisable since the spleen was destroying red cells faster than it was making them. Following splenectomy, we were able to withdraw the prednisolone slowly and bone growth became rapid soon after. The ensuing rapid deposition of less dense bone showing clear signs of remodelling can only be attributed to our therapy and it was furthermore encouraging to note how much better the child became clinically. Clearly a longer follow-up is necessary for fuller assessment of this therapy, but this is now out of our hands as the family has returned to their home in the U.S.A. We think, nevertheless, that the results of this study are sufficiently striking to recommend that it should be repeated on some further affected children and as soon as possible after diagnosis. Fortunately, this is usually in the first months of life owing to the conspicuous nature of the various disease manifestations. If prevention of some of the neurological complications could be achieved it would provide more striking evidence of effectiveness. A further study is also needed to try and distinguish the separate effects of the splenectomy and low calcium régime.

We wonder now how far this study may have contributed to our understanding of the disease pathogenesis. Clearly if a full clinical cure of the disease were to follow such a calcium-depleting régime begun soon after birth, this would strongly favour intestinal overabsorption of calcium as the only disorder. Such a cure would have to include the formation of normal bone marrow with normal peripheral blood, as well as the formation of normally structured bones and prevention of the blindness and other distressing neurological complications. Unfortunately, one known fact suggests already that this is an over-simplification, namely, the fact that the disease is already partly manifest at birth, indeed has been diagnosed radiologically *in utero* (Jenkinson, Pfisterer, Latteier, and Martin, 1943). This fact suggests either that the placenta shares the gut defect and in some way transfers too much calcium from the mother to the foetus, or, perhaps more likely, that the bones themselves (or rather the primary cartilage) have an increased ability to take up calcium from circulating body fluids thus manifesting a further basic biochemical defect. It is when the theoretical interpretation thus begins to be increasingly complicated, that our present concept of an inborn error of metabolism becomes helpful. This tells us that there must be a simple biochemical cause operating from the simple primary genetic defect, the multiplicity of clinical and other features being secondary to this. A moderately low calcium intake does not lead to a more than temporary negative calcium balance in most people since it is soon followed by compensating improvements in calcium absorption and decreased losses in the urine (Malm, 1958). Similarly under conditions of rapid bone growth, such as those during childhood, improved calcium absorption occurs. The underlying mechanism of these adaptations is ill understood but many have speculated on the possible blood-borne factor that would appear to be operating in these circumstances, normally correlating so very accurately the functions of gut, bones, and kidney. A gross overactivity of such a single factor could explain in our child the combination of excessive calcium deposition in metaphysial cartilage at the same time as the gut is overabsorbing dietary calcium, the two being as usual so accurately coordinated as to occur without change in plasma levels. The very low urine calcium in the presence of normal plasma levels could also be due to this action.

We are especially interested here to recall the temporary severe state of hypoparathyroidism which this child went through when first put on the full calcium-depleting régime. We have not yet put a normal child on this régime, but much experimental work suggests that a normal child would not manifest tetany owing to the very efficient parathyroid mechanism for maintaining plasma calcium levels. Adults certainly do not. We are not aware of tetany from a calcium-depleting régime being previously reported as a feature of marble bones disease. It suggests some previous mild parathyroid suppression, but the mechanism of this appears obscure since the child constantly showed substantially normal total, and on the one occasion tested, ionized plasma calcium levels. It has been postulated that the parathyroid glands produce at least two hormones, one regulating plasma calcium and phosphorus levels, the other directly controlling osteoclastic activity (Dent, 1962). If this is true it may be that our child when on a more normal calcium intake showed a parathyroid suppression, mainly concerning the osteoclast stimulating hormone. This theory fits well the known abnormalities in the bone histology and radiographs and suggests an explanation for the improvement we found in x-ray density and remodelling after some time on the severely calcium-poor régime (Fig. 5), during which parathyroid function was presumed to have become normal.

Clearly a long follow-up and trial of further cases is necessary for final appraisal of the possible benefits of this treatment, for it is theoretically inadequate in that it can claim to correct only one aspect of the disease process, namely, the overabsorption of calcium by the gut. It is vitally important to discover whether the other features of the disease may be modified should it be possible to apply the same treatment soon after birth.

## Summary

A child with the severe congenital form of osteopetrosis (Albers-Schönberg disease) has been studied from 3 months to 5 years of age.

The anaemia was controlled by adequate corticosteroid treatment but only at dosages that slowed or inhibited growth in stature.

Attempts were made to deplete the child of calcium by dietary means. Only partial control of bone density, as seen on radiographs, could at first be achieved. Calcium balances confirmed the suspected gross overpositivity. Excessive calcium absorption seems to be an important feature of the disease.

More severe calcium restriction did not produce negative balance. Addition of cellulose phosphate to the very low calcium diet made the balance zero, the child first going through a state of severe hypocalcaemic tetany as if parathyroid function had been previously suppressed. It may be that some of the disease manifestations can be explained on the basis of diminished action of parathyroid hormone on the bones.

Red cell studies showed that most of the active marrow was in the liver and spleen and most of the red cell destruction in the spleen. After splenectomy the red cell life-span markedly increased and it was possible to reduce and soon abandon corticosteroid therapy.

During the last months of the child's follow-up he continued on the strict calcium-depleting régime without corticosteroid therapy. He showed a large spurt in growth, became more lively and active, and laid down less dense bone which showed signs of remodelling.

The parents, both U.S. citizens on temporary stay in Britain, have asked us to record their gratitude to the National Health Service which bore the entire cost of this study in the ordinary course of its working. We thank the biochemists in the Metabolic Ward and Pathology Laboratories for performing the appropriate investigations.

### References

Albers-Schönberg, H. (1904). Röntgenbilder einer seltenen Knochenerkrankung. *Münch. med. Wschr.*, **51**, 365.

Dent, C. E. (1957). Foreword to Symposium on inborn errors of metabolism. *Amer. J. Med.*, **22**, 671.

—— (1962). Some problems of hyperparathyroidism. *Brit. med. J.*, **2**, 1419 and 1495.

Enell, H., and Pehrson, M. (1958). Studies on osteopetrosis. I. Clinical report of three cases with genetic considerations. *Acta paediat.* (*Uppsala*), **47**, 279.

Engfeldt, B., Fajers, C. M., Lodin, H., and Pehrson, M. (1960). Studies on osteopetrosis. III. Roentgenological and pathologic-anatomical investigations on some of the bone changes. *ibid.*, **49**, 391.

Fairbank, H. A. T. (1948). Osteopetrosis: osteopetrosis generalisata, marble bones, Albers-Schönberg's disease, osteosclerosis fragilitas generalisata. *J. Bone Jt Surg.*, **30-B**, 339.

Fanconi, G., Girardet, P., Schlesinger, B., Butler, N., and Black, J. (1952). Chronische Hypercalcämie, kombiniert mit Osteosklerose, Hyperazotämie, Minderwuchs und kongenitalen Missbildungen. *Helv. paediat. Acta*, **7**, 314.

Hasenhuttl, K. (1962). Osteopetrosis: review of the literature and comparative studies on a case with a twenty-four-year follow-up. *J. Bone Jt Surg.*, **44A**, 359.

Higinbotham, N. L., and Alexander, S. F. (1941). Osteopetrosis: four cases in one family. *Amer. J. Surg.*, **53**, 444.

Jenkinson, E. L., Pfisterer, W. H., Latteier, K. K., and Martin, M. (1943). A prenatal diagnosis of osteopetrosis. *Amer. J. Roentgenol.*, **49**, 455.

Karshner, R. G. (1926). Osteopetrosis. *ibid.*, **16**, 405.

Kneal, E., and Sante, L. R. (1951). Osteopetrosis (marble-bones): report of a case with special reference to early roentgenologic and pathological findings. *Amer. J. Dis. Child.*, **81**, 693.

Lièvre, J-A., Milhaud, G., and Camus, J-P. (1962). Ostéopétrose. Étude d'une famille comportant 12 sujets touchés en 4 générations: étude métabolique à l'aide du calcium radio-actif. *Rev. Rhum.*, **29**, 258.

McCune, D. J., and Bradley, C. (1934). Osteopetrosis (marble bones) in an infant: review of the literature and report of a case. *Amer. J. Dis. Child.*, **48**, 949.

Malm, O. J. (1958). Calcium requirement and adaptation in adult man. *Scand. J. clin. Lab. Invest.*, **10**, Suppl. 36.

Parfitt, A. M., Higgins, B. A., Nassim, J. R., Collins, J. A., and Hilb, A. (1964). Metabolic studies in patients with hypercalciuria. *Clin. Science*. In the press.

Piatt, A. D., Erhard, G. A., and Araj, J. S. (1956). Benign osteopetrosis: report of nine cases. *Amer. J. Roentgenol.*, **76**, 1119.

Pines, B., and Lederer, M. (1947). Osteopetrosis: Albers-Schönberg disease (marble bones). Report of a case and morphologic study. *Amer. J. Path.*, **23**, 755.

Seigman, E. L., and Kilby, W. L. (1950). Osteopetrosis: report of a case and review of recent literature. *Amer. J. Roentgenol.*, **63**, 865.

Sjölin, S. (1959), Studies on osteopetrosis. II. Investigations concerning the nature of the anaemia. *Acta paediat.* (*Uppsala*), **48**, 529.

Turano, A. F., Fagan, K. A., and Corbo, P. A. (1954). Variations in clinical manifestations of osteopetrosis: report of two cases. *J. Pediat.*, **44**, 688.

*Arch. Dis. Childh.*, 1965, **40**, 16.

# URINARY EXCRETION OF GONADOTROPHINS WITH PARTICULAR REFERENCE TO CHILDREN

BY

W. FITSCHEN* and BARBARA E. CLAYTON

*From the Department of Chemical Pathology, Hospital for Sick Children, Great Ormond Street, London*

(RECEIVED FOR PUBLICATION JUNE 24, 1964)

Until recently there has been fairly general agreement that gonadotrophins are not detectable in the urine during childhood. Table 1 summarizes the results of previous investigators in this field. Of the early workers, only Catchpole and Greulich (1943) have, in serial determinations, detected gonadotrophins in young girls. More recently, studies performed on pools of urine have indicated that gonadotrophins are excreted as early as 3 to 5 years in boys (Knappe, Dörner, and Stahl, 1961), and possibly in girls (Carletti and Kehyayan, 1962a, b), though the latter workers used combined pools for boys and girls. Full experimental details have not been published to substantiate the claim of Minkina (1961) that gonadotrophin excretion in girls aged 1-3 years is very much higher than in girls at or near the menarche.

In 1960, Landau, Schwartz, and Soffer suggested that children's urine contained an inhibitor for gonadotrophins. They observed inhibition of the response when extracts of children's urine were combined with extracts of known gonadotrophic potency. A later report (Soffer, Futterweit, and Salvaneschi, 1961) substantiated these observations, particularly with regard to children under 6 years of age. Soffer, Salvaneschi, and Futterweit (1962) claimed to have detected a factor in all age-groups that inhibited the action of human chorionic gonadotrophin (HCG), but failed to inhibit the uterine response to oestrone.

In view of the paucity both of positive results in young children and of results in terms of standard reference preparations, it seemed of value to investigate again the excretion of gonadotrophins in childhood. This was an essential preliminary to assessing gonadotrophin excretion in pathological conditions.

The increase in uterine weight of the immature mouse is regarded as the most sensitive end-point for the routine bio-assay of total urinary gonadotrophins (Rosemberg, 1961). Though methods commonly employed have involved multiple injections over a three-day period (Loraine and Brown, 1959), it was thought that the use of a single injection method such as that of Claringbold and Lamond (1957) might afford a more sensitive assay because a threshold dose would not be subdivided into sub-threshold doses. Since Lamond and Claringbold (1958) failed to demonstrate synergism between various gonadotrophins in an assay depending on the early response of the uterus after a single injection, it is likely that such an assay will more accurately reflect the total gonadotrophin present (follicle stimulating hormone (FSH) and luteinizing hormone (LH)). Brown and Billewicz (1962) showed that if enough time were allowed for growth and differentiation of the ovary (as in the usual three-day assay), the same uterine response was achieved by a wide variation in the total dose of gonadotrophin, using different proportions of FSH and LH. Thus extracts containing unknown proportions of FSH and LH could not be reliably assayed in an assay allowing extensive differentiation of the ovary, except at very low levels when the uterine response to FSH and LH was similar. Taking these facts into account, a more sensitive method for the assay of total urinary gonadotrophins has been developed.

In addition, luteinizing hormone (LH) has been estimated in children's urine using the ovarian ascorbic acid depletion assay, as modified by Schmidt-Elmendorff and Loraine (1962).

## Material and Methods

**Hormones Used in Assays.** These are listed below.

(1). Human menopausal gonadotrophin. International Reference Preparation (I.R.P.) (*Bull. Wld Hlth Org.*, 1960).

(2). Human chorionic gonadotrophin (HCG). The preparation used was gonadotrophin LH (Paines and Byrne, Ltd.).

(3). Human menopausal gonadotrophin (LAB-G). This preparation was extracted and purified from post-menopausal urine by the method of Loraine and Brown (1959). It was assayed in terms of I.R.P. using the modification of the mouse uterus method as described in this paper, and the following data were obtained.

* Present address: National Chemical Research Lab., P.O. Box 395, Pretoria, South Africa. Requests for reprints should be sent to Dr. B. Clayton.

TABLE 1

GONADOTROPHINS IN THE URINE OF CHILDREN

| Author | Response Used For Measurement | Urinary Gonadotrophins (units/24 hr.) | |
|---|---|---|---|
| | | Boys | Girls |
| Schörcher (1931) | Ovarian hyperaemia in immature mouse | Undetectable in boys and girls up to 20 yr. | |
| Saethre (1933) | Ovarian hyperaemia in immature mouse | | Undetectable in girls aged $11\frac{6}{12}$ to 14 yr. |
| Katzman and Doisy (1933, 1934) | Signs of oestrous in vagina and uterus | Undetectable in prepubertal boys and girls | |
| Catchpole, Greulich, and Sollenberger (1938) | Increase in mouse uterine weight | < 11 yr.: undetectable<br>12-16 yr.: 2-10 m.u. | |
| Nathanson, Towne, and Aub (1941) | Follicle growth in the immature mouse | < 13 yr.: undetectable | < 11 yr.: undetectable |
| Greulich, Dorfman, Catchpole, Solomon, and Culotta (1942) | Increase in mouse uterine weight | < 11 yr.: undetectable<br>13-14 yr.: 50% of cases gave a positive response<br>14 + yr.: 7-20 m.u. | |
| Catchpole and Greulich (1943) | Increase in mouse uterine weight | | Detectable in serial determinations on girls aged $4\frac{4}{12}$-14 yr. |
| Pedersen-Bjergaard and Tønnesen (1948a, b) | Changes in rat uterus | < 8 yr.: undetectable rising to 6 r.u. at 15 yr. | 3-12 yr.: 1 or < 1 r.u.<br>12-16 yr.: rising to 12 r.u. |
| Albert (1956) | Changes in immature rat ovary | Undetectable in prepubertal boys and girls | |
| Schwenk and Ohndorf (1957) | Changes in mouse uterus | < $12\frac{1}{2}$ yr.: undetectable | < 10 yr.: undetectable |
| Brown (1958) | Increase in mouse uterine weight | Pooled specimens<br>10-11 yr.: 2·9 mg. HMG 20A/l.<br>12-15 yr.: 3·5 mg. HMG 20A/l. | Pooled specimens<br>10-11 yr.: 8·2 mg. HMG 20A/l.<br>12-13 yr.: 7·3 mg. HMG 20A/l.<br>14-15 yr.: 14 mg. HMG 20A/l. |
| McArthur, Ingersoll, and Worcester (1958) | Repair of the ventral prostate in hypophysectomized rats | Interstitial cell stimulating hormone: positive in 2 boys aged 6 and 9 yr. | Interstitial cell stimulating hormone: positive in 1 girl aged 7 yr. |
| Johnsen (1959) | Changes in mouse uterus | Undetectable at 10 yr. | Undetectable at 9 yr. |
| Rosemberg (1960) | Changes in mouse uterus | Undetectable at 10 yr. | Undetectable at 10 yr. |
| Morató-Manaro, Cerviño, and Maggiolo (1960) | Mitosis count in the seminal vesicles of hypophysectomized rats | Interstitial cell stimulating hormone: undetectable in boys and girls of 7-9 yr. | |
| Kehyayan (1960) | Changes in immature mouse and rat uteri | < $10\frac{9}{12}$ yr.: undetectable | < $11\frac{6}{12}$ yr.: undetectable |
| Carletti, Kehyayan, and Perletti (1961) | Changes in immature mouse and rat uteri | Detectable in pooled urine from boys and girls of 6 to 8 yr. | |
| Carletti and Kehyayan (1962a, b) | Changes in rat uterus | Detectable in pooled urine from boys and girls of 3 to 6 yr. | |
| Knappe *et al.* (1961) | Changes in rat uterus | Pooled 3 to 5 yr.: detectable | |
| Minkina (1961) | Changes in mouse uterus | | Activity in girls 1 to 3 yr., much higher than in girls 12 to 13 yr. |

m.u. = mouse unit; r.u. = rat unit.

*Relative potency:* 1·00 mg. LAB-G = 0·77 mg. I.R.P.
*Errors:* Fiducial limits 0·60 to 0·93 mg. I.R.P. ($p = 0{\cdot}95$).
Index of precision, $\lambda = 0{\cdot}164$.

*Validity test:* t test for parallelism, $t = 0{\cdot}216$ (i.e. no significant deviation).

*Index of significance of slope b:* $g = 0{\cdot}083$ (i.e. significant).

(4). Luteinizing hormone (NIH-LH-S-1).*

**Extraction Method.** Extracts were prepared from complete 24-hour urine specimens (or multiples thereof) and from pooled random specimens of urine by the kaolin-acetone method of Albert (1956) as modified by Borth, Lunenfeld, and Menzi (1961), but using the adjustments of *p*H as described by Loraine and Brown (1959). Extracts were purified by salt-ethanol fractionation (stage 2, Albert, Kobi, Leiferman, and Derner, 1961).

For the assay of total urinary gonadotrophins and luteinizing hormone, the extracts were dissolved in 0·1 M borate buffer (*p*H 9) and 0·9% NaCl respectively, so that each mouse or rat received 0·25 or 0·2 ml., respectively.

0·1 *M borate buffer:* 100 ml. boric acid (6·18 g./l.) mixed with 42·6 ml. sodium hydroxide (4 g./l.).

**Animals.** Female mice, strain T/o, 19 to 22 days old and weighing 9 to 11 g., and female Sprague-Dawley rats aged 25 days and weighing 65 to 80 g. were obtained from Animal Suppliers (London) Ltd. They were maintained on a synthetic diet prepared from casein, lard, sucrose, salt mixture, and vitamins (H. Saunders, 1958, personal communication).

* Supplied by the Endocrinology Study Section, National Institutes of Health, Washington D.C., U.S.A., and prepared from sheep pituitary hormone.

**Statistical Evaluation of Results.** Slope (b), relative potency, fiducial limits of error, index of precision (λ), index of significance of regression, and validity of parallelism were calculated according to Gaddum (1953a, b) and Borth, Diczfalusy, and Heinrichs (1957).

**Genital and Secondary Sex Character Rating.** This was assessed according to Tanner (1955), but for various reasons it was not possible to do this in every child.

### Bio-assay of Total Urinary Gonadotrophins

Extracts were assayed by a modification of the mouse uterus test of Klinefelter, Albright, and Griswold (1943).

Each mouse received 0·1 i.u. HCG subcutaneously in 0·1 ml. 0·9% NaCl; 24 hours later the standard or extract was administered as a single injection, and the mice were killed by decapitation 40 to 44 hours later. The uteri were dissected out, placed in Bouin's fluid for 24 hours, cleaned, blotted dry, and weighed to the nearest 1 mg. on a torsion balance.

The design of the assays is described in the sections relating to the clinical investigations performed, dose-response curves for Standard being constructed using total dosages of LAB-G of 0·39 to 1·34 mg./mouse.

**Development of Method.**

(1). *Determination of the time of maximum response after a single injection of LAB-G:* in three separate investigations, a total of 68 mice were injected with 1·0 mg. LAB-G and killed in groups of four at intervals between 10 and 70 hours after injection.

The uterine responses obtained are shown in Fig. 1.

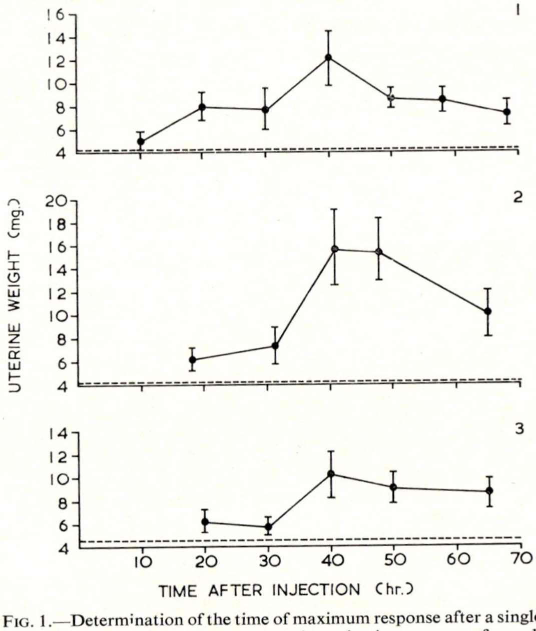


Fig. 1.—Determination of the time of maximum response after a single injection of LAB-G. Three separate investigations were performed. Each point = mean for 4 mice ± standard deviation. ---------- = control uterine weight.

Table 2

UTERINE WEIGHTS 40 TO 44 HOURS AFTER SINGLE INJECTION OF HCG

| Dose per Mouse (i.u.) | Mean Uterine Weight (mg. ± S.E.M.) |
|---|---|
| 0·10 | 3·8 ± 0·26 |
| 0·25 | 5·5 ± 1·07 |
| 0·50 | 6·0 ± 0·74 |
| 0·75 | 7·3 ± 0·71 |
| 1·0 | 9·7 ± 0·32 |
| Saline | 4·0 ± 0·32 |

The maximum response occurred at 40 hours, and in all subsequent experiments involving single injections the mice were killed 40 to 44 hours after injection of the material to be assayed.

(2). *Comparison of the size of the uterine response after single, as compared with multiple, injections:* 0·60 mg. LAB-G was injected into 2 groups of 8 mice. Group A received the total amount divided into 5 doses; 2 injections were given on both the first and second days, and one on the third day. The mice were killed 72 hours after the first injection. Group B received the total amount as a single injection, and the mice were killed 40 to 44 hours later. A control group of 5 mice, injected as in Group B, received saline only.

The mean uterine weights (± standard errors of the means) were as follows. Group A: 4·7 ± 0·4 mg.; Group B: 7·6 ± 0·3 mg.; and saline controls: 4·4 ± 0·4 mg.

The uterine weights in Group B were significantly greater than those of Group A ($p < 0 \cdot 005$).

(3). *Determination of a satisfactory priming dose of HCG:* mice, in groups of 5, were given single injections of HCG in doses of 0·10 to 1·0 i.u. per mouse; they were killed 40 to 44 hours later. The uterine weights are shown in Table 2. There was a significant increase ($p = 0 \cdot 05$) in uterine weight with 0·50 but not 0·25 i.u. per mouse, as compared with the saline-injected controls. The threshold dose therefore lay between 0·25 and 0·50 i.u. per mouse.

(4). *Effect of the length of time between the priming dose of HCG and injection of the test substance:* groups of 5

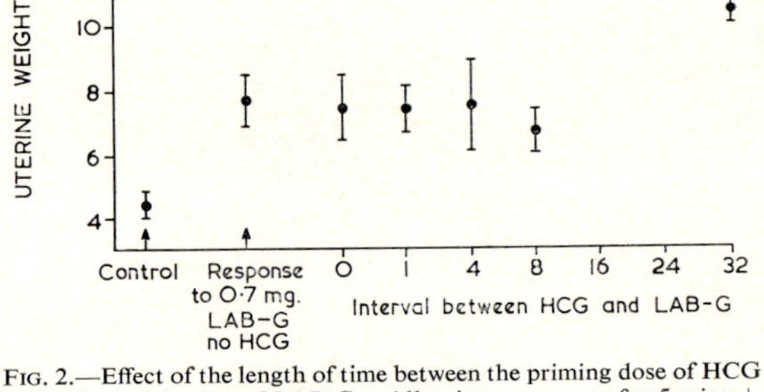


Fig. 2.—Effect of the length of time between the priming dose of HCG and a single injection of LAB-G. All points are means for 5 mice ± standard deviation.

TABLE 3

EFFECT OF SIZE OF PRIMING DOSE OF HCG

| Dose of HCG (i.u./mouse) | Dose of LAB-G (mg./mouse) | Uterine Weight ± S.E.M. | |
|---|---|---|---|
| 0·05 | 0·7 | 8·8 ± 1·3 | Not significantly different (p ≃ 0·15) |
| 0·10 | 0·7 | 11·4 ± 1·6 | |
| 0·10 | 1·0 | 14·5 ± 1·9 | Not significantly different (p ≃ 0·15) |
| 0·25 | 1·0 | 13·7 ± 1·5 | |

mice were primed with 0·10 i.u. HCG at intervals of 0 to 32 hours before a standard dose of 0·70 mg. LAB-G. The results are shown in Fig. 2. Maximum potentiation of response was achieved when the interval between HCG and LAB-G was 16 and 24 hours. In all subsequent assays, 24 hours was used as the priming interval.

(5). *Effect of the magnitude of the priming dose of HCG:* groups of 5 mice were primed with 0·05, 0·10, or 0·25 i.u. HCG, and 24 hours later 0·7 or 1·0 mg. LAB-G was injected. The results, given in Table 3, showed that variations in the size of the priming dose tested did not affect the uterine responses significantly. 0·10 i.u. HCG was selected as the priming dose in all subsequent experiments.

(6). *To study three different schedules of injection:* using 5 mice per group, LAB-G was injected in a total dosage of 0·2 to 1·0 mg. per mouse according to one of three schedules.

*Schedule A.* A single injection of LAB-G was given to mice pretreated 24 hours previously with 0·1 i.u. HCG. The mice were killed 40 to 44 hours after the last injection.

*Schedule B.* LAB-G was given in a single injection to untreated mice which were killed 40 to 44 hours later.

*Schedule C.* The total dose of LAB-G was divided into five, and administered to untreated mice. Two injections were given on both the first and second days, and one during the third day, and the mice were killed 72 hours after the first injection.

The results are given in Table 4, and recorded diagrammatically in Fig. 3, in which the logarithm of the total dose of LAB-G is plotted against the percentage increase in uterine weight, the control uterine weight being taken as 100%.

It was concluded that maximum sensitivity and the steepest dose-response line at low doses was achieved by using a single injection of LAB-G following pretreatment

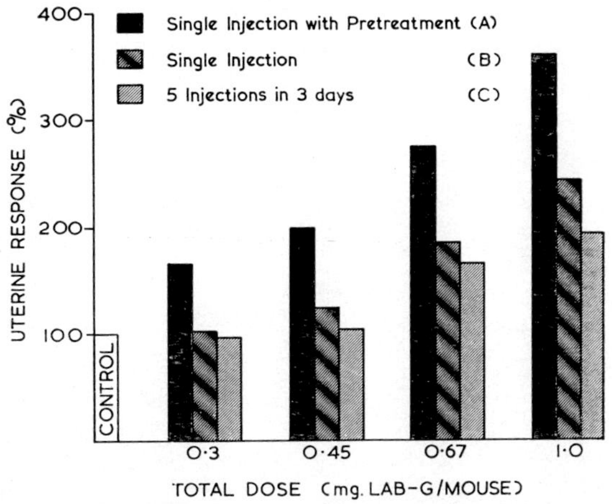


FIG. 3.—The effect of three different schedules of injection. The logarithm of the total dose of LAB-G is plotted against the percentage increase in uterine weight, the control uterine weight being taken as 100%.

with HCG. Schedule (a) has been used in all subsequent assays of total urinary gonadotrophin.

(7). *Ovarian histology with HCG, LAB-G, and HCG + LAB-G:* mice were injected and killed in groups of 4 according to the schedule illustrated in Fig. 4.

On sacrifice, the ovaries were fixed in 10% (v/v) formalin in saline, sectioned, and stained with haematoxylin and eosin. Ovaries from mice injected with 0·1 i.u. HCG only, showed slight follicular ripening at all time intervals compared with those from saline-injected controls. A similar but more marked effect was obtained with LAB-G at 24 hours. At 48 hours after LAB-G, extensive follicular stimulation and luteinization was seen. No difference in ovarian histology was noted between the groups injected with LAB-G and killed after the same time interval, with and without pretreatment with HCG.

(8). *Accuracy:* children's urine, in which no total gonadotrophin activity could be detected, was pooled. 20·0 mg. LAB-G dissolved in 2·0 ml. 0·1 M borate buffer was added to each of three 1 litre aliquots. These samples and a further 1 litre to which no LAB-G had been added, were extracted and purified. The purified extract from each sample was dissolved in 2·5 ml. 0·1 M borate buffer

TABLE 4

UTERINE RESPONSES USING THREE DIFFERENT SCHEDULES FOR INJECTION

| Total Dose LAB-G (mg./mouse) | Uterine Response (mg. ± S.E.M.) Schedule | | | Probability that Schedules Give Different Responses | |
|---|---|---|---|---|---|
| | A | B | C | A as compared with B | A as compared with C |
| 0 | 4·0 ± 0·4 | | | | |
| 0·3 | 6·6 ± 0·7 | 4·2 ± 0·2 | 3·8 ± 0·2 | ≃ 0·01 | ≃ 0·005 |
| 0·45 | 8·0 ± 0·5 | 5·0 ± 0·5 | 4·2 ± 0·8 | ≃ 0·002 | ≃ 0·005 |
| 0·67 | 11·0 ± 1·6 | 7·4 ± 0·5 | 6·6 ± 1·6 | ≃ 0·025 | ≃ 0·025-0·05 |
| 1·00 | 14·4 ± 2·0 | 9·8 ± 0·9 | 7·8 ± 1·2 | ≃ 0·025 | ≃ 0·01 |

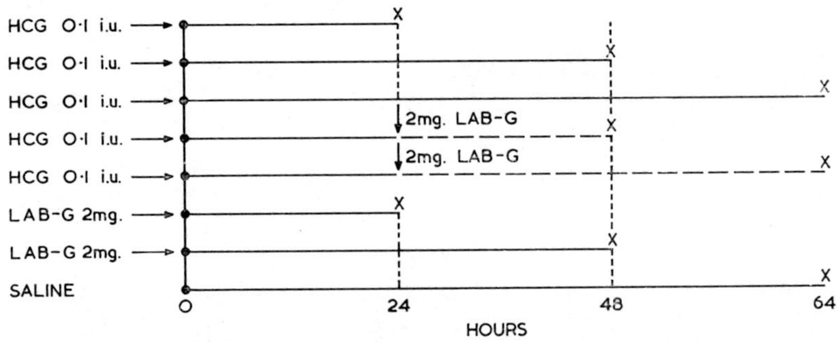


FIG. 4.—The schedule for injecting and killing the mice. × = killed; → = injection.

and assayed against LAB-G using 10 mice per group and a (2 + 1) assay design.

No gonadotrophic activity was detected in the urine containing no added LAB-G. Recoveries of added LAB-G are shown in Table 5.

Four samples of LAB-G, each of 10·0 mg., were purified by the salt-ethanol fractionation procedure, and assayed against LAB-G itself using 5 mice per group and a (2 + 1) assay design. Results are shown in Table 5.

TABLE 5

| Recovery (LAB-G in mg.) | 95% Fiducial Limits | Percentage Recovery |
|---|---|---|
| *Recovery of LAB-G after extraction and purification* (20·0 mg. LAB-G added to each litre of urine) | | |
| 10·5 | 5·5–17·7 | 52·5 |
| 11·5 | 6·2–17·4 | 57·5 |
| 13·4 | 6·4–21·8 | 67·0 |
| *Recovery of LAB-G after purification* (10·0 mg. samples of LAB-G were purified) | | |
| 7·1 | 2·9–12·5 | 71 |
| 8·1 | 3·3–14·9 | 81 |
| 8·5 | 4·2–14·3 | 85 |
| 10·5 | 4·5–18·1 | 105 |

In view of the number of steps involved and the errors inherent in the bio-assay, the recoveries were considered reasonably satisfactory.

(9). *Precision:* a pool of 4 litres of urine from normal men was divided into 4 aliquots which were extracted and purified. Each extract was assayed against LAB-G using a (2 + 1) assay design and 10 mice per group. The results, shown in Table 6, indicated satisfactory reproducibility.

The precision of the assay was satisfactory, Gaddum's $\lambda$ being $< 0{\cdot}2$ except on two occasions. Fiducial limits for assays are given in the relevant sections on clinical application of the method.

(10). *Toxicity of the purified extract:* no toxic effects were observed when purified extracts (equivalent to a 24-hour urine output) from children and adults were injected into individual mice. It was frequently possible to inject twice the equivalent of a 24-hour urine from a child into each mouse.

TABLE 6

REPRODUCIBILITY OF METHOD FOR ASSAYING TOTAL URINARY GONADOTROPHINS

| Urine Sample | Total Gonadotrophins in LAB-G (mg./l.) | Fiducial Limits of Assay (p = 0·95) | $\lambda$ |
|---|---|---|---|
| 1 | 3·56 | 1·47–6·25 | 0·139 |
| 2 | 3·35 | 1·36–6·08 | 0·151 |
| 3 | 3·92 | 1·89–6·57 | 0·135 |
| 4 | 4·04 | 1·71–7·19 | 0·151 |

Mean = 3·72 ± S.E.M. 0·15

(11). *Sensitivity:* over a period of two years, the mean control uterine weight of mice which received 0·1 i.u. HCG only, was consistently between 3·5 and 4·5 mg. Data with respect to three standard curves, selected at random from the results available, are shown in Table 7.

## Bio-assay of Luteinizing Hormone in Urine

Luteinizing hormone in urine was assayed by the method of ovarian ascorbic acid depletion, as modified by Schmidt-Elmendorff and Loraine (1962) using NIH-LH as a reference preparation. Symmetrical four-point assays with two dose levels of standard (S) and unknown (U) respectively were used, the log dose interval being $\log_{10}3$ (0·4771): 4 or 5 rats (8 or 10 ovaries) were used at each dose.

TABLE 7

DATA ON THREE STANDARD CURVES

| Dose/mouse (mg. LAB-G) | Mean Uterine Response for Group of 5 Mice ± Standard Deviation | | |
|---|---|---|---|
| | Curve 1 | Curve 2 | Curve 3 |
| 0·39 | 11·3 ± 2·1 | 10·6 ± 1·9 | 7·5 ± 2·9 |
| 0·59 | 17·1 ± 4·1 | 14·2 ± 3·8 | 10·5 ± 3·1 |
| 0·88 | 17·7 ± 6·2 | 17·9 ± 5·9 | 12·6 ± 2·9 |
| 1·34 | 27·1 ± 8·7 | 27·6 ± 7·0 | 20·6 ± 6·1 |
| Saline | 4·5 ± 1·0 | 5·7 ± 0·9 | 5·7 ± 1·2 |
| b | 28·24 | 30·75 | 24·34 |

TABLE 8

ASSAYS OF TOTAL URINARY GONADOTROPHIN EXCRETION

| Urine | Gonadotrophin Excretion per 24 hr. (mg. I.R.P.) | Fiducial Limits (p = 0·95) | λ | g | | p |
|---|---|---|---|---|---|---|
| Adult male | 6·1 | 4·5-8·1 | 0·12 | 0·0126 | 0·320 | 0·7-0·8 |
| Adult female | 6·7 | 4·5-9·9 | 0·13 | 0·4995 | 0·230 | 0·8 |
| Post-menarchal girls (pooled urine, 14-15 yr.) | 0·8 | 0·6-1·3 | 0·15 | 0·8190 | 0·138 | 0·8-0·9 |
| Pre-menarchal girls (pooled urine, 10-10½ yr.) | 0·3 | 0·2-0·5 | 0·20 | 0·1410 | 0·083 | 0·9-0·95 |
| Pre-adolescent boy, 8½ yr. | 0·5 | 0·3-0·9 | 0·23 | 0·1490 | 0·284 | 0·7-0·8 |

### Clinical Investigations and Results

**Four-point Assays for Total Gonadotrophins on Urine from Normal Subjects.** Assays using a (2 + 2) design and 5 mice per group were performed on extracts of urine from healthy subjects, both adults and children. All the assays were statistically valid and results are shown in Table 8.

**Excretion of Total Urinary Gonadotrophins in Normal Men and Women.** Pools of urine comprising 2 to 6 complete 24-hour collections from each subject were assayed for gonadotrophic activity using a 3 (standard) + 1 (unknown) design with 5 mice per group.

In 12 healthy men aged 18 to 40 years, total urinary gonadotrophins ranged from 3·8 to 18·1 mg. I.R.P./24 hr. with a mean of 7·7. Eight healthy women aged 18 to 35 years were studied, and 24-hour urine collections were made at random during the cycle and pooled for each subject, no attempt being made to follow changes during individual menstrual cycles. The mean excretion of total urinary gonadotrophins was 4·9 mg. I.R.P./24 hr. with a range of 2·7 to 7·05.

**Effect of Extracts from Urine of Children on Assay of Total Urinary Gonadotrophin.** In order to determine whether children's urine extracted by the method described contained an inhibitor to gonadotrophic activity, extracts of urine were added to a standard amount of 1·0 mg. LAB-G as shown in Table 9, and the mixture was assayed according to the usual procedure.

The uterine weights obtained are shown in Table 9. The extracts alone did not cause any increase in uterine weight. When combined with LAB-G they did not significantly alter the response to 1·0 mg. LAB-G. None of the mice showed evidence of toxicity in this experiment. There was no evidence to suggest that an inhibitor was present in extracts prepared from children's urine by the method already described.

**Total Urinary Gonadotrophin Excretion in Children Without Endocrinological Abnormalities.** The majority of assays were of 4 (standard) + 1 (unknown) design, using 5 mice at each dose level for the standard and 3 to 5 for the unknown, depending on the amount of extract available. The limit of sensitivity for each assay varied according to the amount of extract injected and the sensitivity of the mice. If the largest dose of extract injected failed to cause a positive response, the result was recorded as 'undetectable activity and less than *x* mg. I.R.P./24 hr.', the value of *x* varying with the sizes of the responses to the standard and the amount of extract injected. No toxic effects were observed when purified extracts equivalent to a 24-hour urine collection were injected into each mouse.

TABLE 9

EFFECT OF EXTRACTS FROM CHILDREN'S URINE ON TOTAL GONADOTROPHIC ACTIVITY

| Test | Material Assayed | | Number of Mice Tested | Mean Uterine Weight (mg. ± S.E.M.) | p |
|---|---|---|---|---|---|
| | LAB-G Added (mg.) | Urinary Extract | | | |
| 1 | 1·0 | Nil | 10 | 10·3 ± 0·90 | |
| 2 | 1·0 | From 24-hr. urine of 3-month-old boy | 5 | 9·6 ± 1·47 | For (1) and (2) ≃ 0·3 |
| 3 | 1·0 | From 400 ml. pooled urine from girls 7-9 yr. | 10 | 9·1 ± 1·18 | For (1) and (3) ≃ 0·25 |
| 4 | 1·0 | From 400 ml. pooled urine from boys 7-9 yr. | 10 | 10·6 ± 0·98 | For (1) and (4) ≃ 0·4 |
| 5 | Nil | From 400 ml. pooled urine from girls 7-9 yr. | 5 | 4·1 ± 0·34 | |
| 6 | Nil | From 400 ml. pooled urine from boys 7-9 yr. | 5 | 4·5 ± 0·41 | |
| 7 | Nil | Nil | 5 | 4·0 ± 0·35 | |

TABLE 10

EXCRETION OF TOTAL URINARY GONADOTROPHIN IN BOYS

| Patient | Chronological Age (yr.) | Genital and Secondary Sex Character Rating | | Total Urinary Gonadotrophin (mg. I.R.P./24 hr.) | Fiducial Limits (p = 0·95) |
|---|---|---|---|---|---|
| | | Genital | Pubic Hair | | |
| P.L. | 3/12 | 1 | 1 | < 0·3 | |
| R.A. | 6/12 | 1 | 1 | < 0·3 | |
| P.W. | 9/12 | 1 | 1 | 0·92 | 0·60-1 42 |
| R.W. | 1 11/12 | 1 | 1 | < 0·3 | |
| P.W. | 3 10/12 | 1 | 1 | 0·76 | 0·30-1·12 |
| G.S. | 4 6/12 | 1 | 1 | < 0·7 | |
| G.H. | 5 2/12 | — | — | < 0·5 | |
| D.S. | 5 2/12 | 1 | 1 | < 0·3 | |
| M.G. | 5 6/12 | — | — | 0·59 | 0·25-0·87 |
| L.B. | 5 9/12 | 1 | 1 | < 0·4 | |
| S.B. | 6 | 1 | 1 | < 0·3 | |
| M.P. | 7 | — | — | < 0·4 | |
| M.J. | 7 | 1 | 1 | < 0·3 | |
| M.Hu. | 7 | — | — | 3·14 | 2·04-5·50 |
| M.Hs. | 7 3/12 | 1 | 1 | < 0·04 | |
| M.R. | 7 3/12 | 1 | 1 | < 0·7 | |
| A.S. | 7 4/12 | 1 | 1 | < 0·5 | |
| R.S. | 7 9/12 | 1 | 1 | 0·76 | 0·49-1·18 |
| A.W. | 8 3/12 | 1 | 1 | 0·77 | 0·32-1·12 |
| G.S. | 8 5/12 | 1 | 1 | 0·80 | 0·58-1·25 |
| A.M. | 8 6/12 | — | — | 0·80 | 0·51-1·26 |
| L.L. | 8 6/12 | 1 | 1 | 0·94 | 0·71-1·16 |
| G.M. | 9 | — | — | < 0·3 | |
| R.D. | 9 6/12 | — | — | 0·32 | 0·13-0·45 |
| I.B. | 9 7/12 | — | — | < 0·5 | |
| P.F. | 9 9/12 | 3 | 1 | < 0·4 | |
| C.M. | 9 11/12 | 1 | 1 | < 0·3 | |
| A.H. | 10 | — | — | 0·43 | 0·19-0·87 |
| I.W. | 10 2/12 | 2 | 1 | 0·67 | 0·44-0·97 |
| A.G. | 11 | — | — | < 0·5 | |
| A.B. | 11 2/12 | 2 | 1 | < 0·4 | |
| D.F. | 11 9/12 | — | — | < 0·4 | |
| A.J. | 12 | — | — | 6·72 | 4·43-9·65 |
| R.D. | 12 2/12 | — | — | 0·31 | 0·09-0·49 |
| P.B. | 12 2/12 | — | — | 2·90 | 2·14-4·53 |
| A.M. | 12 7/12 | 5 | 4 | 1·86 | 1·32-2·65 |
| J.P. | 13 | — | — | < 0·4 | |
| R.O. | 13 | — | — | 4·23 | 2·32-7·52 |
| K.B. | 13 | — | — | < 0·5 | |
| J.B. | 13 1/12 | — | — | 1·36 | 0·66-2·28 |
| M.S. | 13 6/12 | 4 | 5 | 1·05 | 0·68-1·62 |
| S.B. | 13 9/12 | — | — | 0·59 | 0·28-0·88 |
| S.H. | 14 6/12 | — | — | 1·02 | 0·77-1·34 |
| J.S. | 14 7/12 | 4 | 4 | 0·58 | 0·34-0·80 |
| C.L. | 14 8/12 | — | — | 0·72 | 0·52-1·12 |
| P.D. | 15 | 5 | 4 | 3·30 | 2·42-4·72 |

— indicates 'not determined'.

Assays were performed on urine from 46 boys and 58 girls aged 3 months to 15 years 8 months. The results are given in Tables 10 and 11, and are shown diagrammatically in Fig. 5.

Measurable activity was obtained as early as 9 months in a boy and 1 year 10 months in a girl.

Serial determinations were made on 2- or 3-day pools of complete 24-hour urines, as follows.

(a). 5 premenarchal girls (M.M., L.O., A.P., A.H., and Y.Y.) all of whom had pre-adolescent secondary sex character rating.

(b). 1 post-menarchal girl (M.D.) with breast development rating, 3; and pubic hair rating, 4.

(c). 1 pre-adolescent boy (A.W.).

(d). 1 adolescent boy (J.S.) with genital development rating, 4; and pubic hair rating, 4.

In Y.Y. (7 yr. 10 mth. of age) no gonadotrophin activity was detected throughout a 30-day period of study. Results for M.M., L.O., A.H., M.D., A.W., A.P., and J.S. are shown in Fig. 6.

**Urinary Excretion of Luteinizing Hormone by Children without Endocrinological Abnormalities.** A series of assays was performed on pooled collections of urine from children of various age-groups. There were 6 to 8 children in each age-group, and the results are shown in Table 12. Toxic reactions were produced with urine from the higher age-groups, both boys and girls, even though the amount of extract injected was generally equivalent to less than 24-hour urine. In the lower age-groups the toxic effect (if any) was much less marked, even though the amount of extract injected into each rat exceeded the equivalent of 24-hour urine.

Assays were also performed on individual pools of 24-hour urines obtained from 12 children: 4 assays were invalid because of significant deviation from parallelism and 2 assays showed no depletion of ovarian ascorbic acid at the highest dose injected. Results of valid assays are shown in Table 12.

TABLE 11

EXCRETION OF TOTAL URINARY GONADOTROPHIN IN GIRLS

| Patient | Age (yr.) | Secondary Sex Character Rating | | Total Urinary Gonadotrophin (mg. I.R.P./24 hr.) | Fiducial Limits (p = 0·95) |
|---|---|---|---|---|---|
| | | Breast Development | Pubic Hair | | |
| M.M. | 1 10/12 | 1 | 1 | 0·51 | 0·14-0·80 |
| L.O. | 2 2/12 | 1 | 1 | 0·36 | 0·17-0·69 |
| L.H. | 3 2/12 | 1 | 1 | 1·07 | 0·60-1·87 |
| A.S. | 3 2/12 | 1 | 1 | < 0·3 | |
| S.E. | 3 4/12 | 1 | 1 | 0·47 | 0·21-0·81 |
| C.E. | 4 | — | — | < 0·4 | |
| C.O. | 5 1/12 | 1 | 1 | 0·34 | 0·13-0·50 |
| A.P. | 5 3/12 | 1 | 1 | 0·38 | 0·18-0·64 |
| A.A. | 5 8/12 | 1 | 1 | 0·51 | 0·28-0·89 |
| O.C. | 5 11/12 | 1 | 1 | 0·43 | 0·20-0·72 |
| S.O. | 6 3/12 | 1 | 1 | 0·42 | 0·28-0·67 |
| S.C. | 6 5/12 | 1 | 1 | < 0·5 | |
| K.W. | 6 7/12 | 1 | 1 | < 0·3 | |
| Y.Y. | 6 11/12 | 1 | 1 | < 0·3 | |
| B.C. | 7 1/12 | 1 | 1 | < 0·5 | |
| B.O. | 7 2/12 | 1 | 1 | 0·45 | 0·26-0·62 |
| L.N. | 7 2/12 | 1 | 1 | 0·45 | 0·23-0·77 |
| B.D. | 7 6/12 | 1 | 1 | 0·37 | 0·14-0·55 |
| S.R. | 7 11/12 | 1 | 1 | < 0·3 | |
| L.S. | 8 2/12 | 1 | 1 | < 0·3 | |
| I.C. | 8 4/12 | — | — | 0·59 | 0·62-0·85 |
| C.B. | 8 6/12 | 1 | 1 | < 0·4 | |
| M.W. | 8 10/12 | 1 | 1 | 0·42 | 0·26-0·80 |
| K.F. | 9 | — | — | < 0·4 | |
| J.M. | 9 3/12 | — | — | 0·44 | 0·23-0·78 |
| M.O. | 9 5/12 | 1 | 1 | < 0·5 | |
| A.H. | 9 5/12 | 1 | 1 | 0·51 | 0·28-0·91 |
| E.E. | 9 5/12 | 1 | 1 | 0·76 | 0·50-1·17 |
| P.B. | 9 5/12 | 2 | 1 | 0·38 | 0·18-0·57 |
| C.B. | 9 7/12 | 1 | 1 | 0·29 | 0·16-0·52 |
| T.S. | 9 10/12 | — | — | < 0·3 | |
| D.C. | 10 | — | — | < 0·3 | |
| Y.B. | 10 | — | — | 0·34 | 0·17-0·55 |
| J.B. | 10 1/12 | — | — | 0·59 | 0·43-0·73 |
| M.A. | 10 2/12 | 1 | 1 | 0·32 | 0·15-0·51 |
| C.E. | 10 3/12 | — | — | < 0·5 | |
| D.H. | 10 4/12 | 1 | 1 | 0·51 | 0·34-0·91 |
| J.G. | 10 6/12 | — | — | < 0·3 | |
| P.B. | 10 8/12 | — | — | 1·10 | 0·82-1·71 |
| P.O. | 10 8/12 | 1 | 1 | < 0·4 | |
| M.K. | 10 9/12 | 3 | 4 | 1·03 | 0·66-1·56 |
| S.B. | 11 2/12 | — | — | 0·50 | 0·15-0·93 |
| C.W. | 11 10/12 | — | — | 0·76 | 0·56-1·08 |
| L.W. | 12 | 2 | 2 | < 0·4 | |
| C.P. | 12 1/12 | 1 | 1 | 0·52 | 0·26-0·88 |
| C.R. | 12 2/12 | 2 | 3 | < 0·5 | |
| H.R. | 12 3/12 | — | — | 0·52 | 0·34-0·75 |
| P.W. | 12 3/12 | — | — | 0·75 | 0·41-1·34 |
| M.D. | 12 5/12 | 3 | 4 | 1·24 | 0·55-2·54 |
| S.I. | 12 9/12 | 4 | 3 | < 0·3 | |
| A.L. | 13 | — | — | 2·68 | 1·63-4·18 |
| P.R. | 13 4/12 | — | — | < 0·5 | |
| J.T. | 13 11/12 | — | — | < 0·5 | |
| E.G. | 14 | 4 | 3 | 0·80 | 0·53-1·16 |
| M.B. | 14 4/12 | 4 | 4 | 0·85 | 0·40-1·27 |
| C.W. | 14 11/12 | — | — | 0·38 | 0·18-0·57 |
| D.H. | 15 | — | — | 0·98 | 0·73-1·52 |
| B.S. | 15 8/12 | — | — | 0·51 | 0·29-1·89 |

— indicates 'not determined'.

## Discussion

The immature mouse uterus has been used as a reliable and sensitive end-point for the bio-assay of total urinary gonadotrophins. The extract has been administered as a single injection following pre-treatment of the mice with a sub-threshold dose of HCG.

From results published by other investigators (Borth *et al.*, 1961), it is clear that many strains of mice have a greater sensitivity to human menopausal gonadotrophin than the strain available for the present study, so that the method described could have even greater sensitivity.

The mechanism of potentiation with HCG remains obscure. The fact that simultaneous administration of HCG and LAB-G did not show any synergistic interaction raises the possibility that this phenomenon is only demonstrable when HCG is administered before an injection containing follicle-stimulating hormone. This aspect appears to have been over-looked in most studies on synergism because assays extending over several days have been used (Evans and Simpson, 1950).

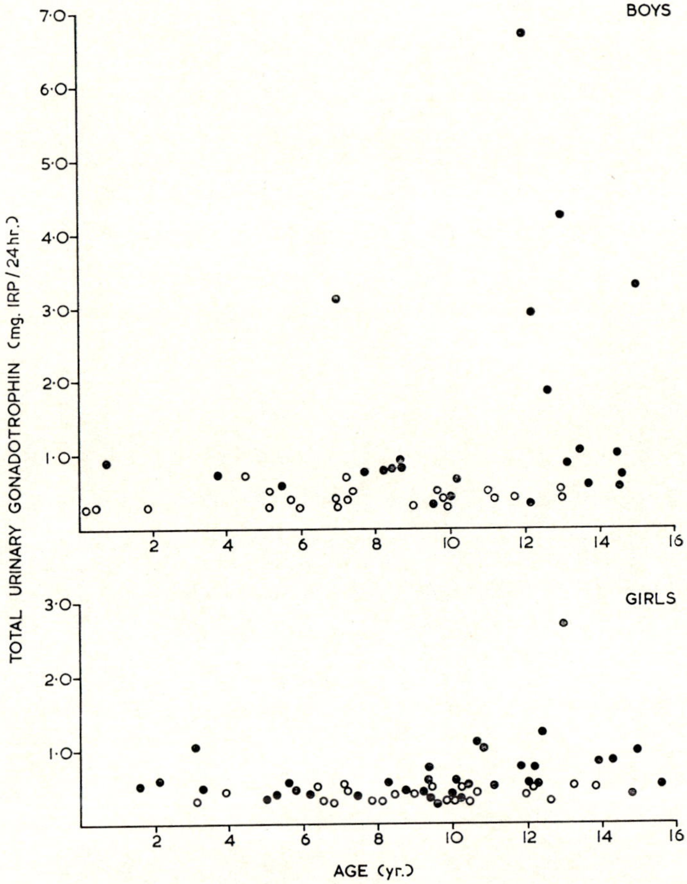


FIG. 5.—Total urinary gonadotrophin excretion in boys and girls.
● Total urinary gonadotrophin in mg. I.R.P./24 hours. ○ No gonadotrophin detected, and excretion is less than the value indicated.

The extraction and assay used in the present study gave reproducible results of reasonable accuracy. Recovery experiments showed results similar to those reported by Loraine and Brown (1959) and Heinrichs and Eulefeld (1960). This type of recovery can be criticized (Albert, 1956), because it is not certain that gonadotrophin added to raw urine or extracts will behave in the same way as it did initially in the original urine. The four-point assays with extracts of urine from pre-adolescent children and adults showed satisfactory similarity of response with the laboratory standard LAB-G which was obtained from post-menopausal urine. The levels found in men and women were similar to those reported by other investigators who used similar extraction procedures (Apostolakis, 1961; Brown, 1959a, b; Loraine and Bell, 1963).

Of 33 boys aged less than 12 years, measurable excretions of total urinary gonadotrophins were found in 13 of them, using pools of 24-hour urines from single subjects. The youngest boy with detectable amounts was only 9 months. In older boys aged 12 to 15 years, total urinary gonadotrophin was measurable in 12 of the 14 investigated. Serial determinations in a pre-adolescent boy (A.W.) indicated intermittent and/or considerable fluctuation in excretion, whereas a fairly constant excretion was found in an older adolescent boy (J.S.). Certainly below the age of 12 years, no clinical significance can be attached to a failure to demonstrate gonadotrophin in the urine, though a positive result may be of value.

Similar results were found in the girls though levels were generally lower than in the boys. Detectable excretion was found in 75% of the girls in the 0-6 year age-group. The more frequent undetectable levels (compared with boys) in the older age-groups may be due to the greater fluctua-

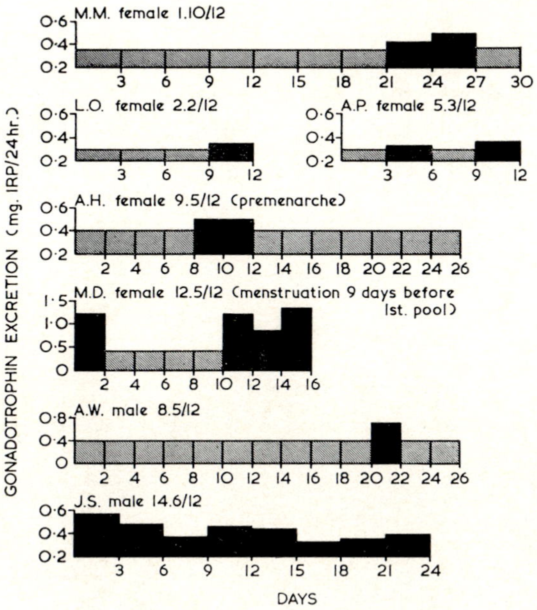


FIG. 6.—Serial determinations of the excretion of total urinary gonadotrophin in 7 children. Results are in mg. I.R.P./24 hours. The solid black area is total urinary gonadotrophin. The shaded area indicates no gonadotrophin, and excretion less than the value indicated.

tion in excretion as indicated by the serial determinations. Intermittent excretion was seen in M.M. aged 1 year and 10 months, and also in the post-menarchal subject studied (M.D., 12 years and 5 months). As with the boys, assays of total urinary gonadotrophin must be interpreted with these limitations in mind. In general, results for total

TABLE 12
ASSAY OF LUTEINIZING HORMONE IN CHILDREN'S URINE

| Patient | Age (yr.) | Excretion of Luteinizing Hormone (μg. NIH-LH/24 hr.) | Fiducial Limits (p = 0·95) | λ |
|---|---|---|---|---|
| *Boys:* | | | | |
| Pool | 0–6 | 0·89 | 0·35–1·47 | 0·28 |
| Pool | 6–8 | 0·26 | 0·04–0·53 | 0·34 |
| Pool | 10–12 | 1·14 | 0·29–2·16 | 0·33 |
| Pool | 12–15 | 6·59 | 2·38–11·70 | 0·34 |
| C.J. | 2 | 1·68 | 0·52–2·92 | 0·25 |
| A.B. | 11 | 2·30 | 1·04–3·98 | 0·24 |
| *Girls:* | | | | |
| Pool | 0–6 | Invalid assay: significant deviation from parallelism | | |
| Pool | 6–8 | 0·25 | 0·06–0·52 | 0·25 |
| Pool | 10–12 | 1·50 | 0·54–2·55 | 0·31 |
| Pool | 12–15 | 2·46 | 0·95–4·35 | 0·34 |
| M.M. | 2 | 1·06 | 0·27–1·97 | 0·29 |
| L.H. | 3 2/12 | <0·5 | — | — |
| S.B. | 11 | 1·98 | 1·11–3·56 | 0·21 |
| Y.B. | 12 | 2·09 | 1·14–3·10 | 0·25 |
| A.L. | 13 6/12 | <0·5 | — | — |

gonadotrophin excretion in children have not been related to a reference preparation. Brown (1958) studied children from 10 to 15 years and gave his results in mg. HMG 20/l. urine. He used pools composed of random samples of urine, so that his results cannot be interpreted in terms of individual 24-hour excretions. In contrast to the present results, he found more gonadotrophin in girls than in boys, his results for boys being similar to the ones reported in this study.

The ovarian ascorbic acid depletion assay of urinary extracts containing low levels of LH presented considerable difficulties. The large amount of extract that had to be injected produced toxic effects and resulted in death of some of the animals. The rather flat slope of the dose-response curve usually resulted in an unsatisfactory index of precision and wide fiducial limits. This is in accord with the results published by Schmidt-Elmendorff and Loraine (1962), though Bell, Mukerji, and Loraine (1964) have recently published a modification of the method overcoming all these difficulties.

In pooled urine from boys, measurable LH was found in all age-groups, the amount increasing with age. Similar results were seen in girls but the assay on the 0 to 6 year age-group was invalid. The results suggest that there may be a correlation between the onset of puberty and the excretion of LH, and this would be worth further investigation using the improved method of Bell *et al.* (1964).

No evidence suggesting a gonadotrophin inhibitor in children's urine has been found. The method of extraction and purification used in the present study is different from that of Soffer *et al.* (1961, 1962), and perhaps this explains the conflicting results.

The values, in terms of a reference preparation for gonadotrophin excretion in normal children, will enable the results found in pathological states, e.g. precocious puberty, to be better evaluated. Failure to demonstrate gonadotrophin in the urine of any particular child must be interpreted in the light of the findings in the normal child, and the other clinical and laboratory findings must be taken carefully into account.

**Summary**

The excretion of total urinary gonadotrophin was studied in endocrinologically normal boys and girls, and the results were expressed in terms of a standard reference preparation. Low amounts were frequently found in children's urine even before the age of puberty, the youngest boy being 9 months and girl 1 year and 10 months. The inability to detect gonadotrophin in any particular child must be interpreted with caution and in the light of the other clinical and laboratory findings. No inhibitor to urinary gonadotrophic activity could be demonstrated with the method of extraction and purification used in this study.

A method specific for luteinizing hormone was applied to pools of children's urine, and detectable amounts were present both before and after puberty. There was considerable variation in excretion among the few individuals studied separately.

We thank the Consultant Staff of The Hospital for Sick Children for permission to study their patients. The co-operation of the Nursing Staff in the collection of hundreds of 24-hour urines is greatly valued.

Dr. A. G. C. Renwick kindly helped in obtaining urine from patients at Tadworth Court. Mr. G. Crabb and Mr. D. Trafford gave invaluable technical assistance. One of us (W.H.E.F.) is indebted to The Joint Research Board of The Hospital for Sick Children and The Institute of Child Health for financial assistance during this study.

References

Albert, A. (1956). Human urinary gonadotrophin. *Recent Progr. Hormone Res.*, **12**, 227.

——, Kobi, J., Leiferman, J., and Derner, I. (1961). Purification of pituitary gonadotropin from urine of normal men. *J. clin. Endocr.*, **21**, 1.

Apostolakis, M. (1961). Experimentalle Grundlagen und klinische Bedeutung der Forschung auf dem Gebiet der menschlichen hypophysären Gonadotropine. *Klin. Wschr.*, **39**, 453.

Bell, E. T., Mukerji, S., and Loraine, J. A. (1964). A new bioassay method for luteinizing hormone depending on the depletion of rat ovarian cholesterol. *J. Endocr.*, **28**, 321.

Borth, R., Diczfalusy, E., and Heinrichs, H. D. (1957). Grundlagen der statistischen Auswertung biologischer Bestimmungen. *Arch Gynäk.*, **188**, 497.

——, Lunenfeld, B., and Menzi, A. (1961). Comparison of kaolin-acetone methods. In *Human Pituitary Gonadotropins*, ed. A. Albert, p. 13. Charles C. Thomas, Springfield, Illinois.

Brown, P. S. (1958). Human urinary gonadotrophins. I. In relation to puberty. *J. Endocr.*, **17**, 329.

—— (1959a). Human urinary gonadotrophins. II. In relation to the menstrual cycle, secondary amenorrhoea and the response to oestrogen. *ibid.*, **18**, 46.

—— (1959b). Urinary gonadotrophins in normal men. *Acta endocr. (Kbh.)*, **32**, 272.

——, and Billewicz, W. Z. (1962). The response of immature mice to mixtures of gonadotrophins. *J. Endocr.*, **24**, 65.

Carletti, B., and Kehyayan, E. (1962a). L'eliminazione urinaria delle gonadotropine nell 'età infantile. Studio di un gruppo di soggetti di 3-6 anni. *Minerva pediat.*, **14**, 21.

——, —— (1962b). Caratteristiche biologiche delle gonadotropine urinarie nell 'infanzia. Confronto fra gruppi di bambini di diversa età. *ibid.*, **14**, 786.

——, ——, and Perletti, L. (1961). Studio sulle caratteristiche biologiche e chimiche delle gonadotropine urinarie nell 'età infantile. *Folia endocr. (Roma)*, **14**, 388.

Catchpole, H. R., and Greulich, W. W. (1943). The excretion of gonadotrophic hormone by prepuberal and adolescent girls. *J. clin. Invest.*, **22**, 799.

——, ——, and Sollenberger, R. T. (1938). Urinary excretion of follicle stimulating hormone in young and adolescent boys. *Amer. J. Physiol.*, **123**, 32.

Claringbold, P. J., and Lamond, D. R. (1957). Optimum conditions for the biological assay of gonadotrophins. *J. Endocr.*, **16**, 86.

Evans, H. M., and Simpson, M. E. (1950). Physiology of the gonadotrophins. In *The Hormones, Physiology, Chemistry and Applications*, Vol. II, ed. G. Pincus and K. V. Thimann, p. 351. Academic Press, New York.

Gaddum, J. H. (1953a). Bioassays and mathematics. *Pharmacol. Rev.*, **5**, 87.

—— (1953b). Simplified mathematics for bioassays. *J. Pharm. Pharmacol.*, **5**, 345.

Greulich, W. W., Dorfman, R. I., Catchpole, H. R., Solomon, C. I., and Culotta, C. S. (1942). Somatic and endocrine studies of puberal and adolescent boys. *Monogr. Soc. Res. Child. Developm.*, 7, No. 3.

Heinrichs, H. D., and Eulefeld, F. (1960). Untersuchungen über die Extraktion von hypophysärem Gonadotropin aus Urin. *Acta endocr. (Kbh.)*, Suppl. 53.

Johnsen, S. G. (1959). A clinical routine-method for the quantitative determination of gonadotrophins in 24-hour urine samples. II: Normal values for men and women at all age groups from pre-puberty to senescence. *ibid.*, **31**, 209.

Katzman, P. A., and Doisy, E. A. (1933). A quantitative procedure for determining normal excretion of prolan. *Proc. Soc. exp. Biol. (N.Y.)*, **30**, 1188.

——, —— (1934). The quantitative determination of small amounts of gonadotropic material. *J. biol. Chem.*, **106**, 125.

Kehyayan, E. (1960). L'eliminazione urinaria delle gonadotropine dagli 8 ai 14 anni. *Minerva pediat.*, **12**, 1601.

Klinefelter, H. F., Jr., Albright, F., and Griswold, G. C. (1943). Experience with a quantitative test for normal or decreased amounts of follicle stimulating hormone in the urine in endocrinological diagnosis. *J. clin. Endocr.*, **3**, 529.

Knappe, G., Dörner, G., and Stahl, F. (1961). Nachweis hypophysärer Gonadotropine im Harn von Kindern. *Klin. Wschr.*, **39**, 971.

Lamond, D. R., and Claringbold, P. J. (1958). Joint action of gonadotrophic substances. *J. Endocr.*, **16**, 298.

Landau, B., Schwartz, H. S., and Soffer, L. J. (1960). Presence of a gonadotrophin-inhibiting factor in urine of young children. *Metabolism*, **9**, 85.

Loraine, J. A., and Bell, E. T. (1963). Hormone excretion during the normal menstrual cycle. *Lancet*, **1**, 1340.

——, and Brown, J. B. (1959). A method for the quantitative determination of gonadotrophins in the urine of non-pregnant human subjects. *J. Endocr.*, **18**, 77.

McArthur, J. W., Ingersoll, F. M., and Worcester, J. (1958). Urinary excretion of interstitial-cell stimulating hormone by normal males and females of various ages. *J. clin. Endocr.*, **18**, 460.

Minkina, A. I. (1961). Some findings on the biological activity and chemical composition of the gonadotrophic hormones in ontogenesis. Proc. 5th Int. Congr. Biochem., Moscow, **9**, 320.

Morató-Manaro, J., Cerviño, J. M., and Maggiolo, J. (1960). A method of determining interstitial-cell stimulating hormone in urine: some results in normal and pathological cases. In *Ciba Foundation Colloquia on Endocrinology*, Vol. 13, p. 238. Churchill, London.

Nathanson, I. T., Towne, L. E., and Aub, J. C. (1941). Normal excretion of sex hormones in childhood. *Endocrinology*, **28**, 851.

Pedersen-Bjergaard, K., and Tønnesen, M. (1948a). Oestrogenic, androgenic and gonadotrophic substances in the urine of normal women. Sex hormone analyses I. *Acta endocr. (Kbh.)*, **1**, 38.

——, —— (1948b). Sex hormone analyses II. The excretion of sexual hormones by normal males, impotent males, polyarthritics and prostatics. *Acta med. scand.*, Suppl. 213, 284.

Rosemberg, E. (1960). Urinary gonadotropin excretion measured by the mouse uterine response, employing estrone as the standard reference material. *J. clin. Endocr.*, **20**, 306.

—— (1961). End points of sensitivity. In *Human Pituitary Gonadotropins*, ed. A. Albert, p. 110. Charles C. Thomas, Springfield, Illinois.

Saethre, H. (1933). Über die Ausscheidung von Prolan im Harn in der Involutionsperiode bzw. im senium. *Klin. Wschr.*, **12**, 1727.

Schmidt-Elmendorff, H., and Loraine, J. A. (1962). Some observations on the ovarian ascorbic acid depletion method as a test for luteinizing hormone activity. *J. Endocr.*, **23**, 413.

Schörcher, F. (1931). Zur Physiologie und Pathologie der Prolanausscheidung im Harn bei Kindern und Jugendlichen. *Klin. Wschr.*, **10**, 2221.

Schwenk, A., and Ohndorf, H. (1957). Untersuchungen zur Endokrinologie der Pubertät. I. Mitteilung: Die Urinausscheidung der hypophysären Gonadotropine in der männlichen und weiblichen Pubertät. *Z. Kinderheilk*, **79**, 645.

Soffer, L. J., Futterweit, W., and Salvaneschi, J. (1961). A gonadotropin-inhibiting substance in the urine of normal young children. *J. clin. Endocr.*, **21**, 1267.

——, Salvaneschi, J., and Futterweit, W. (1962). A gonadotropin-inhibiting substance in the urine of normal subjects. *ibid.*, **22**, 532.

Tanner, J. M. (1955). *Growth at Adolescence*, p. 25 et seq. Blackwell, Oxford.

*Arch. Dis. Childh.*, 1965, **40**, 27.

# LYMPHANGIOGRAPHY AND CHROMOSOME STUDIES IN FEMALES WITH LYMPHOEDEMA AND POSSIBLE OVARIAN DYSGENESIS

BY

P. F. BENSON, M. H. GOUGH, and P. E. POLANI

*From the Paediatric Research Unit, Guy's Hospital Medical School, and the Professorial Surgical Unit, St. Thomas's Hospital Medical School, London*

(RECEIVED FOR PUBLICATION JULY 24, 1964)

In primary lymphoedema, lymphangiography has revealed abnormalities of the lymphatics. Kinmonth (1960), in a series of 192 patients, found hypoplasia of the lymphatic trunks in 65%, aplasia in 15%, varicose dilatation in 14%, and backflow of dye into the lymphatic dermal plexus in 6%. These findings suggested that primary lymphoedema was due to congenital error in the development of lymphatics.

Congenital peripheral oedema occurs in a proportion of patients with ovarian dysgenesis and allied disorders. A history of oedema was obtained in 45 out of 126 patients (35·7%) under the age of 16, but only in 4 of 120 (3·3%) over the age of 16 (Bishop, Lessof, and Polani, 1960); it was present in 9 of the 51 (17·6%) patients reported by Lindsten (1963).

The course of oedema in ovarian dysgenesis differs from that of other types of lymphoedema. Thus in primary lymphoedema, oedema is stationary or slowly progressive, while in ovarian dysgenesis it disappears in a few months or years in the majority of cases. Occasionally, however, it persists or recurs at puberty or after administration of oestrogens or anabolic steroids.

In this article we report the result of lymphangiography and chromosomal analysis in six patients with lymphoedema who were phenotypically female and who had clinical evidence of ovarian dysgenesis. Lymphangiography was carried out at St. Thomas's Hospital. Recent advances in the technique of lymphangiography have been published elsewhere (Gough, Guiney, and Kinmonth, 1963) and will not be repeated here. The chromosome analysis, after blood or skin culture, was carried out by one of us (P.E.P.) with the help of other members of the cytogenetics section of the Paediatric Research Unit, Guy's Hospital Medical School.

## Cases

**Case 1.** (P.R.U. 794). *Phenotypic female with congenital lymphoedema of hands and feet, webbing of neck. Sex chromosomes XO. Hypoplasia of lymphatic trunks of feet and of superficial lymphatics of legs. Anomalous lymph vessels at ankles.*

Congenital pitting oedema of hands and feet gradually subsided and disappeared by 3 years. She had been born after a normal pregnancy and delivery, weighing 2,800 g. Her parents and sister were healthy. The diagnosis of mild congenital hypertrophic pyloric stenosis was suspected clinically and supported by visualization of an elongated pylorus on barium meal studies. A brother had had congenital hypertrophic pyloric stenosis, confirmed at operation, and another brother had had the same condition diagnosed on clinical grounds. Her toe-nails were hypoplastic and she had webbing of the neck. At 9 months of age, she was 65·5 cm. tall (3rd percentile) and weighed 6·6 kg. (less than 3rd percentile).

*Chromosomes:* number 45; sex chromosomes complement XO; chromatin negative on nuclear sexing.

LYMPHANGIOGRAPHY. At 2 years and 10 months, incisions were made on the dorsum of each foot. A fine spongy network of lymphatics was seen in the subcutaneous tissue. Biopsy of this tissue confirmed the presence of multiple minute lymph vessels without valves. In the normal subject at this site there are three or four small discrete lymphatic vessels running in the subcutaneous tissue, immediately below the skin.

Further incisions were made in the skin over the dorsum of the ankles. On the left, several larger but abnormal lymphatics were seen that were too small to cannulate. On the right there were several vessels running superficial to the deep fascia before piercing it. In spite of the quantity of patent blue in the subcutaneous lymphatic plexus, these deep vessels were only slightly coloured, suggesting a poor circulation between the superficial and deep lymphatic systems. With the aid of a dissection microscope, a size 30 hypodermic needle was inserted in one of the vessels on the deep fascia, and 3·5 ml. of ultrafluid Lipiodol (Bengue) were injected.

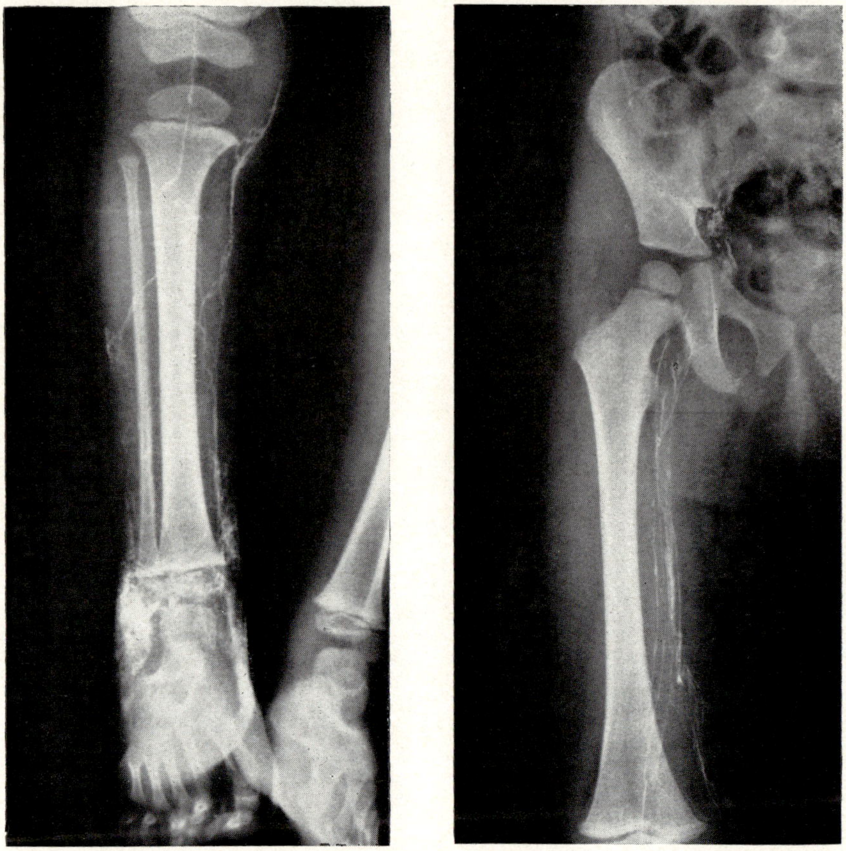

FIG. 1a and b.—X-ray lymphangiogram (Case 1) showing hypoplasia of superficial lymphatics with early filling of deep lymphatic vessels in leg and thigh. Aplasia of superficial inguinal glands. Compare normal lymphangiogram in Fig. 2.

Radiographs (Fig. 1a and b) showed contrast medium in the superficial plexus of the foot and lower leg, which, unlike those of the normal subject (Fig. 2), drained through the deep fascia to an apparently normal deep lymphatic system.

**Case 2.** (P.R.U. 144). *Phenotypic female with congenital lymphoedema of feet. Sex chromosomes XO. Hypoplasia of lymphatics of right leg, left leg not explored.*

Congenital pitting oedema of both feet, gradually subsided and disappeared by 4 years of age. She had been born after a normal pregnancy and delivery at full term, weighing 2,800 g. She was an only child of healthy parents. Hypoplasia of big toe-nail and aplasia of other toe-nails. Finger-nails were flat and on the left hand were spoon shaped. An intravenous pyelogram at 2 months of age showed bilateral bifid renal pelvis. The cardiovascular and other systems were normal. At 5 years 7 months, she was 103 cm. tall (5th percentile) and weighed 19·1 kg. (25th percentile).

*Chromosomes:* number 45; sex chromosomes complement XO; chromatin negative on nuclear sexing.

LYMPHANGIOGRAPHY. At 10 months of age, marked hypoplasia of the lymphatic tracts of the right leg was present, both on the dorsum of the foot and at the anterior aspect of the ankle. The left leg was not explored.

**Case 3.** (P.R.U. 393). *Phenotypic female with congenital lymphoedema of hand and feet. Sex chromosomes XO. Aplasia of lymphatics of the left leg and right foot. Hypoplasia of right leg.*

Congenital pitting oedema of right hand and both feet. Swelling of hand cleared by 9 months, but feet were still swollen at 3 years. She had been born at 44 weeks after normal pregnancy and delivery, weighing 3,200 g. The parents, brother, and sister were healthy. There was hypoplasia of the toe-nails. The cardiovascular and other systems were normal. When 33 months of age, she was 84 cm. tall (less than 3rd percentile) and weighed 12·7 kg. (25th percentile).

*Chromosomes:* number 45; sex chromosomes complement XO; chromatin negative on nuclear sexing.

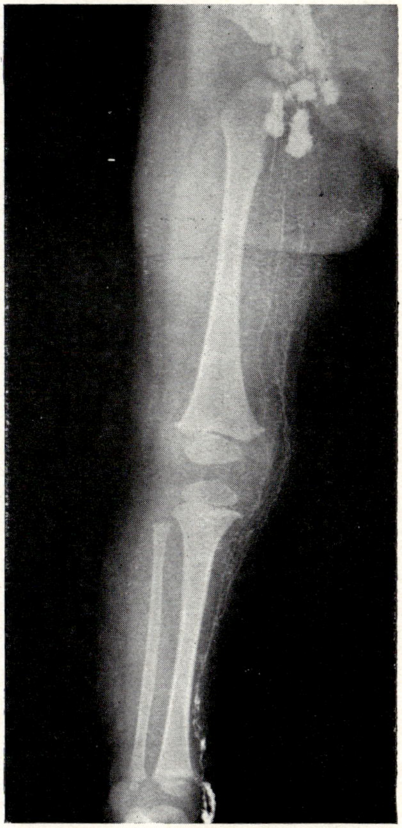

FIG. 2.—The appearance of normal superficial lymphatic trunks in child aged 5 months. Note filling of superficial lymphatic vessels and of superficial inguinal nodes.

LYMPHANGIOGRAPHY. At 2 years of age, no lymphatics were seen on the left side, either on the dorsum of the foot or at the ankle. No lymphatics were seen on the dorsum of the right foot, but a few hypoplastic vessels were present on the anterior aspect of the right ankle.

**Case 4.** (P.R.U. 1241). *Phenotypic female with congenital lymphoedema. Sex chromosomes XO. Aplasia of lymphatics of left foot. Extreme hypoplasia of lymphatics of right foot.*

Congenital lymphoedema of both feet and legs. The swelling on the left side was still present at 4 years of age, while on the right it had disappeared by 6 months. Her toe-nails were hypoplastic. She had been born at full term after a pregnancy complicated by pyelitis at 4 months. Her birth weight was 4·3 kg. Her parents and sister were healthy.

*Chromosomes:* number 45; sex chromosomes complement XO; chromatin negative on nuclear sexing.

LYMPHANGIOGRAPHY. At 3 years of age, dermal backflow occurred into vesicles below the left external malleolus. At exploration, no lymphatic tracts were seen on the dorsum of the left foot. On the dorsum of the right foot, a network of minute subcutaneous lymphatic tracts was seen. Some very small lymphatic tracts were seen at the ankle, which could not be cannulated.

**Case 5.** (P.R.U. 317). *Phenotypic female with bilateral congenital lymphoedema of hands and feet. Coarctation of aorta, webbing of neck. Sex chromosomes XO. Aplasia of lymphatics of feet and hypoplasia of superficial lymphatic vessels of legs. Anomalous lymphatic trunks of ankles.*

Congenital symmetrical lymphoedema of hands and feet, still present at 2½ years. Her parents and brother were healthy. She was born after a normal pregnancy and delivery weighing 2,800 g. She had probable coarctation of the aorta, moderate webbing of the neck, bilateral epicanthic folds, and hypoplastic nails. At 15 months of age, she was 81 cm. tall (90th percentile) and weighed 11·8 kg. (85th percentile).

*Chromosomes:* number 45; sex chromosomes complement XO; chromatin negative on nuclear sexing.

LYMPHANGIOGRAPHY. At 2 years and 8 months of age, dermal backflow occurred in both feet. No lymph vessels were seen through dorsal incisions in both feet. The subcutaneous tissue was spongy and vascular. At the ankles, the appearance was similar to that in Case 1, there being a few anomalous lymphatic vessels that were seen to pierce the deep fascia. These were too small for injection of radio-opaque material.

**Case 6.** (P.R.U. 1422). *Phenotypic female with congenital lymphoedema of both feet, double harelip, cleft palate, no secondary sexual characteristics, and primary amenorrhoea. Moderate webbing of the neck. Sex chromosomes XY. Hypoplasia of lymphatics of feet and ankles.*

Bilateral congenital lymphoedema of feet and legs which fluctuated in severity but persisted until last seen when she was 22. The father was healthy, but the mother, whose menarche had not occurred until the age of 20, had had a hysterectomy for oophoritis. The patient's sister had menarche at 17. There were no brothers. She had double harelip and complete cleft palate. She had never had any vaginal bleeding. At 20 years, an infantile uterus was felt rectally. There was no pubic or axillary hair and no development of breasts and nipples. There was moderate webbing of the neck, incurving of the fifth finger of the right hand, epicanthic folds and a soft basal cardiac systolic murmur, but no other abnormality of cardiovascular or other systems. At 21 years of age, she was 159 cm. tall and 24 kg. in weight. She was treated with ethinyl oestradiol 0·1 mg. daily three weeks out of four. Cyclical vaginal bleeding occurred and was accompanied by increase in weight and aggravation of oedema.

*Chromosomes:* number 46; sex chromosomes complement XY; chromatin negative on nuclear sexing.

LYMPHANGIOGRAPHY. Bilateral lower limb lymphangiography was performed under general anaesthetic at 20 years of age. Patent Blue was injected interdigitally

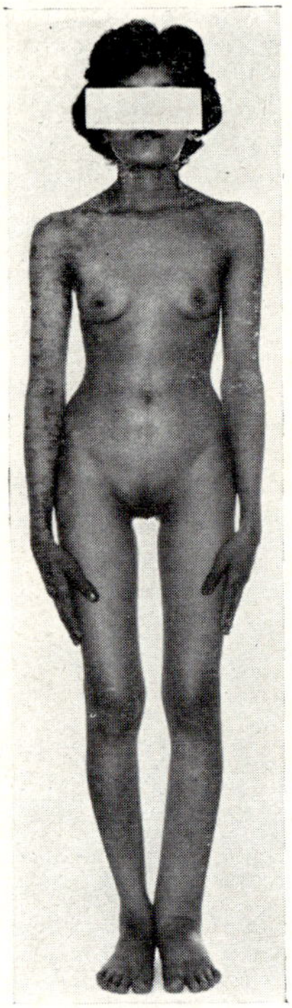

FIG. 3.—Case 7, aged 21. Normal development of breasts and nipples, scanty pubic hair, lymphoedema left leg.

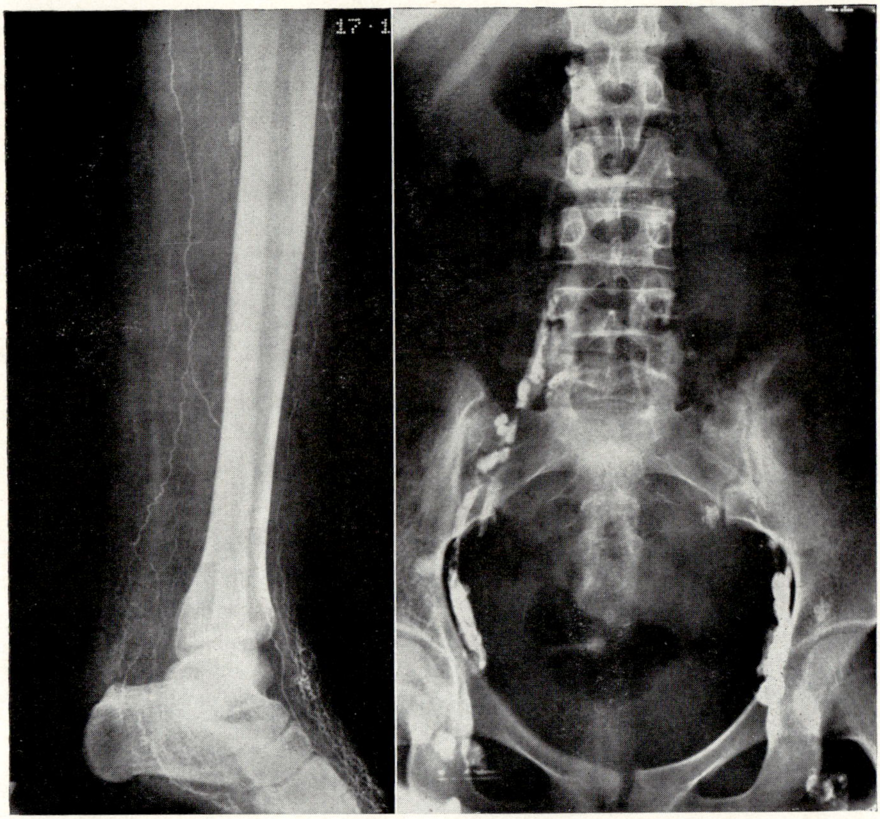

FIG. 4a and b.—X-ray lymphangiogram (Case 7) showing many small tortuous channels in left foot and calf, typical of distal obstruction. No filling of left common iliac or left para-aortic lymph nodes.

in each foot. There was an almost immediate appearance of dye in the dermal lymphatic plexus ('dermal backflow'), more pronounced on the right than the left. Exploration of the dorsum of both feet and ankles revealed extreme hypoplasia of the lymphatic trunks.

Radiographs after induction of pneumoperitoneum at 21 years of age confirmed the presence of a small uterus, but no ovaries were demonstrated.

**Case 7.** (P.R.U. 1139). *Phenotypic female. No axillary and scanty pubic hair. Absent uterus. Acute onset of lymphoedema of left leg. Hypoplasia of lymphatics of left foot and leg. Aplasia of left common iliac and para-aortic lymph nodes. Sex chromosomes XY.*

This girl from British Guiana was healthy until 7 years of age when she developed pain, redness, and swelling of her left leg below the knee. The onset was abrupt and cellulitis was diagnosed. Pain subsided over a few weeks and she was left with swelling. At 18 years of age, she had had vaginal bleeding on one occasion following intercourse. No further bleeding had occurred during the next three years. Her parents and one brother were healthy, but details of other relatives were unavailable. At 21 years of age, she was 155 cm. tall. Axillary hair was absent. There was scanty pubic hair, but otherwise the appearance of the external genitalia was that of a normal female. Breasts were developed, with normal development of nipples (Fig. 3). The uterus was not felt either during routine examination or under a general anaesthetic by Mr. K. J. R. Cuthbert, who found that the vagina ended blindly with a small area of thickening where one would expect the cervix to be. Reaching up from this, only a thin cord of tissue but no gonads could be felt.

No abnormality was present in her cardiovascular or other systems, her blood pressure being 140/80 mm. Hg.

*Chromosomes:* number 46; sex chromosomes complement XY; chromatin negative on nuclear sexing.

LYMPHANGIOGRAPHY. This was performed at 20 years of age. There was dermal backflow on the dorsum of the left foot, ankle, and calf. Dye was seen in the dermal plexus through an incision in the dorsum of the foot, but only two subcutaneous lymphatic tracts were seen, one normal in size and the other small. Ultrafluid Lipiodol was injected into the larger of the two tracts. Subsequent

TABLE 1

RELATION OF CLINICAL FEATURES TO FINDINGS ON LYMPHANGIOGRAPHY AND TO SEX CHROMOSOMES COMPLEMENT

| Case No. | Distribution of Oedema | Course of Oedema | Other Features | Sex Chromosomes | Lymphangiography |
|---|---|---|---|---|---|
| 1 | Hands and feet | Disappeared by 3 yr. | Congenital pyloric stenosis, webbing of neck | XO | Hypoplasia of superficial lymphatic vessels in both legs and feet; anomalous vessels |
| 2 | Feet | Disappeared by 4 yr. | Bifid pelvis both kidneys | XO | Hypoplasia right leg, left leg not explored |
| 3 | Right hand and feet | Still present in feet at 3 yr. | — | XO | Aplasia left leg and right foot, hypoplasia right leg |
| 4 | Feet | Right side disappeared at 6 mth.; left side present at 4 yr. | — | XO | Aplasia left foot; hypoplasia right foot and leg |
| 5 | Hands and feet | Present at 30 mth. | Coarctation, webbing of neck, epicanthic folds | XO | Aplasia both feet, hypoplasia both legs; anomalous vessels |
| 6 | Feet | Still present at 22 yr. | Double harelip, cleft palate, primary amenorrhoea, no secondary sexual characteristics | XY | Extreme hypoplasia both feet and ankles |
| 7 | Left leg | Still present at 21 yr. | Absent uterus, absent axillary hair, scanty pubic hair, breasts developed | XY | Hypoplasia left foot and leg; aplasia lymphatic left common iliac and left para-aortic lymph nodes |

radiographs (Fig. 4a), showed many small tortuous channels in the left foot and calf. The external iliac lymph nodes filled normally, but neither the left common iliac nor the left para-aortic glands had filled at either 2 or 24 hours (Fig. 4b). On the right side, lymphatic tracts appeared normal both visually and radiographically.

## Discussion

Results of our study are summarized in Table 1. All patients had hypoplasia or aplasia of the superficial lymphatic tracts of the lower limbs. In addition, two patients (Cases 1 and 5) had anomalous lymphatic channels in the ankles running on the outer aspect of the deep fascia before piercing it. After subcutaneous injection of Patent Blue in the interdigital spaces of the foot, these anomalous vessels were only a pale shade of blue in contrast to the deep colour observed in normal vessels. Subsequent radiographs of the lower limb showed filling of the deep lymph vessels (Fig. 1a and b), but not of the superficial trunks which are visualized in the normal subject (Fig. 2).

Obstructed lymphatic drainage due to congenital hypoplasia of the superficial lymphatic channels appears therefore to be a factor in the production of oedema in patients with gonadal dysgenesis. It is tempting to suggest that the presence of anomalous lymphatic channels connecting the hypoplastic superficial channels to the deep lymphatic system such as were demonstrated in two of our patients, may be a factor in the disappearance of oedema in the majority of patients with ovarian dysgenesis. Delayed or poor uptake of subcutaneous dye by the anomalous vessels, however, suggested that their compensating capacity was incomplete.

The cyclical increase of oedema while on periodic oestrogen therapy suggests that fluid retention may be another factor. Fluid retention is known to occur in women with normal ovarian function. During the menses, it may lead to oedema in normal women or to aggravation of oedema in women with primary lymphoedema.

An XO sex chromosomal complement was found in Cases 1-5, such as is found in the majority of patients with gonadal dysgenesis (Polani, 1961). Details of the cytological findings are in Table 2. In Case 6, the XY sex chromosomal complement was confirmed by blood cultures, and in Case 7 by both blood and skin cultures which failed to show any evidence of chromosome mosaicism. Testicular feminization syndrome was considered in the differential diagnosis of these two patients. In Case 6, the existence of associated congenital abnormalities, the presence of a uterus with occurrence of uterine bleeding during periodic oestrogen therapy and absence of family history militate against this diagnosis. However, in Case 7, the diagnosis of testicular feminization syndrome seems possible (see addendum). No uterus could be palpated at an examination under general anaesthesia, and there was definite breast development. The family history was incompletely known. We have been unable to find a previous report of lymphoedema occurring in testicular feminization syndrome.

The seven patients described in this paper were selected because they exhibited at least some of the

TABLE 2

RESULTS OF CHROMOSOMAL ANALYSIS

| Case No. | Sex Chromatin (oral smear) | No. of Tissue Investigations | | Chromosomes | | | | | |
|---|---|---|---|---|---|---|---|---|---|
| | | | | Count Distribution | | | | | Sex Chromosomes |
| | | Blood Culture | Skin Culture | Total Cell Count | < 45 | 45 | 46 | > 46 | |
| 1 | Negative | 4 | | 70 | 9 | 57 | 4 | — | XO |
| | | | 1 | 35 | 7 | 28 | — | — | XO |
| 2 | Negative | 2 | 0 | 68 | 3 | 65 | — | — | XO |
| 3 | Negative | 2 | 0 | 52 | 2 | 50 | — | — | XO |
| 4 | Negative | 1 | 0 | 51 | 1 | 50 | — | — | XO |
| 5 | Negative | 2 | 0 | 46 | 1 | 45 | — | — | XO |
| 6 | Negative | 2 | 0 | 62 | 2 | — | 60 | — | XY |
| 7 | Negative | 2 | | 56 | — | 1 | 55 | — | XY |
| | | | 1 | 38 | 2 | 2 | 34 | — | XY |

clinical features of ovarian dysgenesis and therefore no estimate can be made from them of the prevalence of sex chromosomal abnormalities in an unselected population of patients with lymphoedema.


## Summary

Seven phenotypic females with lymphoedema were investigated. Six were considered to have ovarian dysgenesis, the sex chromosomal complement being XO in five, and XY, without evidence of chromosome mosaicism, in one. No diagnosis was made in the seventh patient, whose sex chromosome complement was XY.

All seven patients had hypoplasia or aplasia of the superficial lymphatic vessels of the legs. In addition, two patients had anomalous lymphatic vessels connecting the hypoplastic superficial lymphatic vessels to the deep system. It is tentatively suggested that these channels may contribute towards the disappearance of oedema in patients with gonadal dysgenesis.


We are grateful to Dr. R. C. Mac Keith for referring Cases 2 and 3, and to Dr. D. Morris for Case 1; to Professor J. B. Kinmonth for allowing us to publish results of the lymphangiography; to Dr. F. Giannelli, Miss J. Northfield, and Dr. A. Taylor for their help in the chromosomal analysis, and to Miss M. McGuire for technical assistance with the cytological work.

REFERENCES


Bishop, P. M. F., Lessof, M. H., and Polani, P. E. (1960). Turner's syndrome and allied conditions. Memoirs of the Society for Endocrinology, 7, 162.

Gough, M. H., Guiney, E. J., and Kinmonth, J. B. (1963). Lymphangiography: New techniques and uses. *Brit. med. J.*, **1**, 1181.

Kinmonth, J. B. (1960). Some aspects of cardiovascular surgery. *J. roy. Coll. Surg. Edinb.*, 5, 287.

Lindsten, J. (1963). *The Nature and Origin of X Chromosome Aberrations in Turner's Syndrome*, p. 52. Almquist and Wiksell, Uppsala.

Polani, P. E. (1961). Turner's syndrome and allied conditions. *Brit. med. Bull.*, 17, 200.


## Addendum

In Case 7, the diagnosis of testicular feminization syndrome has recently been confirmed. At laparotomy (Professor J. B. Kinmonth), bilateral abdominal testes were found to be connected to the trigonal area of the bladder by two tubular structures interpreted as vasa deferentia. There was no uterus. The gonads were removed after their nature had been identified by histological examination of frozen sections.

*Arch. Dis. Childh.*, 1965, **40**, 33.

# THE RENAL EXCRETION OF HYDROGEN IONS IN INFANTS AND CHILDREN

BY

ALEXANDER PEONIDES, BARNETT LEVIN, and WINIFRED F. YOUNG
*From the Queen Elizabeth Hospital for Children, London*

(RECEIVED FOR PUBLICATION AUGUST 24, 1964)

The ability of the kidneys to excrete an acid urine is often assessed by correlating plasma carbon dioxide and urine *p*H. A low plasma $CO_2$ should be accompanied by a low urine *p*H, provided that respiratory function is normal. Buchanan and Komrower (1958) consider that the renal excretion of hydrogen ions is normal in children if urine *p*H falls below 5·0, after a single dose of 0·1 g./kg. of ammonium chloride has been given to produce metabolic acidosis. Under similar conditions, urine *p*H falls to below 5·2 in normal adults (Wrong and Davies, 1959). However, Elkinton, Huth, Webster, and McCance (1960) found that urine *p*H was not sufficient to differentiate latent cases of renal tubular acidosis in adults after prolonged administration of $NH_4Cl$. These authors suggested a quantitative assessment of the renal response to an ammonium chloride load by the 'hydrogen ion clearance index' calculated as the product of the total $H^+$ excreted in the urine (mEq/min./1·73 sq. m.) and the plasma $CO_2$ content (mEq/l.) in subjects after a continuous $NH_4Cl$ administration for 3-5 days. Abnormally low values of the index were considered to indicate renal acidosis. This index has not only proved a sensitive one in cases with latent renal tubular acidosis, but also useful in revealing the latent renal defect in otherwise normal relatives of patients with renal tubular acidosis, thus contributing to our knowledge of the genetics of the disease (Huth, Webster, and Elkinton, 1960).

In the present study the renal $H^+$ excretion on normal diet, as well as after the addition of $NH_4Cl$ for several days, has been investigated in order to determine values for the hydrogen ion clearance index in normal infants and children. Results from similar investigations in children with renal tubular acidosis and their relatives will be reported later.

### Subjects and Methods

Studies were carried out on 26 normal infants and children, mostly in-patients who had recovered from diseases not associated with renal or metabolic disturbances. No subjects with abnormal respiratory function, abnormal plasma electrolyte or blood urea levels, or abnormal urines were included. Where necessary urea and endogenous creatinine clearances were estimated, and found to be normal for their age.

Since little is known about younger infants after the neonatal period, it was thought desirable to divide the results now obtained into two groups, one including those children aged 1 year or less, and the other including children over 1 year old. The younger age-group consists of 12 infants, 6 girls and 6 boys, whose ages range from 2 to 11½ months, 3 of whom were only tested while on normal diets, 8 while on normal diets and also after $NH_4Cl$ had been added, and one only during $NH_4Cl$ administration. In each case, the infants were fed on a reconstituted dried cows' milk, with suitable semi-solid foods, except for one aged 2 months who was on the milk mixture only. The older group consists of 14 children, 5 girls and 9 boys, aged from 1 year 1 month to 16 years: 6 were tested both on normal diets and after $NH_4Cl$ had been added, and 8 only while $NH_4Cl$ was being given.

**Collection of Urine.** Urine was collected for a period of four to nine hours (average about six hours) during the day, each collection being accurately timed. Older children were asked to empty their bladder directly into chemically clean bottles or pots. The urine was collected from male infants by using Paul's tubing strapped around the penis, and from females by the use of a metabolic bed. The specimens were refrigerated and at the end of the test they were pooled and analysed immediately for *p*H, titratable acidity (TA), titratable acidity less bicarbonate ($TA - HCO_3^-$) and ammonia. In most cases the *p*H of the individual specimens of each collection was also determined. Fluid intake was increased whenever possible in order to augment the urine flow, and thus minimize the error from incomplete emptying of the bladder. Incomplete collections due to leakage around the tube, or specimens contaminated with faeces, were discarded.

A blood sample for plasma $CO_2$ content, and in some cases for blood *p*H, was taken about the middle of the period during which urine was collected and two or three hours after a meal.

TABLE 1

INFANTS AGED 2-11½ MONTHS: INDIVIDUAL RESULTS, MEANS, AND RANGE

| No. | Sex | Age (mth.) | Diet | Blood: Plasma $CO_2$ (mEq/l.) | Blood: Whole Blood *p*H | Urine*: *p*H Range | Urine*: *p*H Pooled Specimens | Urine* μEq/min./1·73 sq. m.: $NH_4^+$ | Urine* μEq/min./1·73 sq. m.: TA | Urine* μEq/min./1·73 sq. m.: TA − $HCO_3^-$ | Urine* μEq/min./1·73 sq. m.: Total $H^+$ | Urine*: % $NH_4^+$ in $NH_4^+$ + TA | $H^+$ Clearance Index |
|---|---|---|---|---|---|---|---|---|---|---|---|---|---|
| 1 | M | 2 | Normal | 19·0 | 7·36 | 5·7–6·3 | 5·8 | 18·7 | 35·3 | — | 54·0 | 34·6 | 1·02 |
| | | | Normal + $NH_4Cl$ | 18·3 | 7·35 | 5·0–5·2 | 5·0 | 26·3 | 40·8 | — | 67·1 | 39·2 | *1·23* |
| 2 | F | 3½ | Normal | 21·5 | | | 5·1 | 11·7 | 18·7 | — | 30·4 | 38·5 | 0·65 |
| 3 | M | 3½ | Normal | 21·0 | | 5·4–6·6 | 5·9 | 28·0 | 23·5 | — | 51·5 | 45·4 | 1·08 |
| | | 4 | Normal + $NH_4Cl$ | 18·5 | | 5·1–6·4 | 5·8 | 47·0 | 42·0 | — | 89·0 | 53·0 | *1·65* |
| 4 | F | 4 | Normal | 20·7 | | 6·4–7·3 | 6·7 | 7·3 | 3·6 | 1·1 | 8·4 | 67·0 | 0·16 |
| | | | Normal + $NH_4Cl$ | 15·5 | 7·36 | 5·3–6·4 | 5·8 | 62·0 | 20·6 | — | 82·6 | 75·0 | *1·28* |
| 5 | M | 4 | Normal | 19·5 | | 5·6–6·4 | 5·9 | 34·5 | 33·7 | — | 68·2 | 50·5 | 1·33 |
| | | 7 | Normal + $NH_4Cl$ | 20·0 | 7·45 | 4·7–5·3 | 4·9 | 100·0 | 72·0 | — | 172·0 | 58·1 | *3·44* |
| 6 | F | 4¼ | Normal | 19·0 | | 5·2–5·5 | 5·3 | 17·9 | 22·1 | — | 40·0 | 44·8 | 0·76 |
| 7 | M | 6 | Normal | 20·5 | 7·39 | 6·5–7·2 | 6·8 | 10·9 | 14·1 | 2·3 | 13·2 | 43·6 | 0·27 |
| | | | Normal + $NH_4Cl$ | 17·4 | 7·40 | 4·9–5·0 | 4·9 | 31·3 | 45·0 | — | 76·3 | 41·0 | *1·33* |
| 8 | M | 8 | Normal | 20·0 | 7·41 | 5·7–6·6 | 6·0 | 19·7 | 23·4 | — | 43·1 | 45·7 | 0·86 |
| 9 | F | 8 | Normal | 19·0 | 7·44 | 5·5–6·8 | 6·1 | 14·3 | 29·5 | — | 43·8 | 32·7 | 0·83 |
| | | | Normal + $NH_4Cl$ | 11·0 | 7·46 | 4·8–5·0 | 4·9 | 70·0 | 42·8 | — | 112·8 | 62·0 | *1·24* |
| 10 | F | 8⅔ | Normal | 19·3 | 7·39 | 5·4–5·9 | 5·6 | 31·5 | 41·7 | — | 73·2 | 43·0 | 1·41 |
| | | | Normal + $NH_4Cl$ | 11·0 | 7·30 | 4·6–5·0 | 4·8 | 59·4 | 49·6 | — | 109·0 | 54·4 | *1·20* |
| 11 | F | 9 | Normal | 19·5 | | | 5·3 | 30·3 | 35·2 | — | 65·5 | 46·3 | 1·28 |
| | | 9½ | Normal + $NH_4Cl$ | 18·0 | | 5·0–5·2 | 5·1 | 44·0 | 25·5 | — | 69·5 | 63·5 | *1·25* |
| 12 | M | 11½ | Normal + $NH_4Cl$ | 20·0 | | 5·2–5·3 | 5·2 | 50·0 | 44·5 | — | 94·5 | 53·0 | *1·89* |
| Mean .. | .. | .. | Normal | 19·9 | | | | 20·4 | 25·5 | — | 44·7 | 46·3 | 0·88 |
| Range .. | .. | .. | Normal | 19·0–21·5 | | | 5·1–6·8 | 7·3–34·5 | 3·6–41·7 | | 8·4–73·2 | 32·7–67·0 | 0·16–1·41 |
| Mean .. | .. | .. | Normal + $NH_4Cl$ | 16·6 | | | | 54·4 | 42·5 | — | 97·0 | 55·8 | 1·61 |
| Range .. | .. | .. | Normal + $NH_4Cl$ | 11·0–20·0 | | | 4·8–5·8 | 26·3–100·0 | 20·6–72·0 | | 67·1–172·0 | 39·2–75·0 | 1·20–3·44 |

TA = Titratable Acidity

* In all the Tables urinary excretions are expressed in μEq/min./1·73 sq. m. and not in mEq, as in text, because of the small amounts involved.

**Hydrogen Ion Loading.** The renal response to an added load of hydrogen ions was tested by giving $NH_4Cl$, usually for three days or in some cases for four or five days. Since the results in those few who had $NH_4Cl$ for the longer period did not differ significantly from the mean values of the majority who had been given it for three days, all the results have been analysed together. The dose of $NH_4Cl$ was from 6·0 to 9·0 g. (115-166 mEq)/day/1·73 sq. m., the actual dose being 1·0 to 7·5 g. day according to surface area. Each subject had the same amount daily, divided in three to four doses given with or after meals, to the younger children as a mixture in syrup, and to the older in uncoated capsules. No side-effects were observed apart from slight vomiting in three subjects on the second day of administration, but this was never severe enough to necessitate withdrawal of the $NH_4Cl$. A few of the older children were given the salt at home, but all came into hospital for the last day of the test. The urine was collected during the last day of $NH_4Cl$ administration as described above, blood being taken two to three hours after a meal, when the subject had already taken the first of the three or four daily doses of $NH_4Cl$.

The surface area was calculated from the height and weight using the Du Bois and Du Bois (1916) nomograms.

**Laboratory Methods.**

PLASMA $CO_2$ CONTENT. Approximately 1 ml. capillary blood, obtained by finger- or heel-prick, was collected dropwise in heparinized 2 × ⅜ in. test-tubes without paraffin oil. The plasma was then separated by centrifuging and kept for analysis within one to four hours. The $CO_2$ content was measured manometrically (Van Slyke and Neill, 1924).

BLOOD *p*H. This was determined on capillary blood collected in heparinized glass capillary tubes, both ends of which were sealed immediately after collection and examined within an hour after sampling. The *p*H was determined at 37° C. using a microcapillary glass electrode (Metrohm) and a *p*H meter with a Vibron electrometer (Electronic Instruments Ltd.).

URINE *p*H. This was determined at room temperature by external indicators using B.D.H. capillators.

AMMONIA. This was estimated by aeration and titration (Hawk, Oser, and Summerson, 1954).

*The titratable acidity* of the urine was determined by titration to *p*H 7·4 with N/20 NaOH. When the *p*H was greater than 6·2, titratable acidity minus bicarbonate (TA $-HCO_3^-$) was measured (Albright and Reifenstein, 1948).

CALCULATION.

*The Hydrogen Ion Clearance Index* = $H^+$ excretion (mEq/min./1·73 sq. m.) × plasma $CO_2$ content (mEq/l.). Where $H^+$ excretion = TA + $NH_4^+$ − $HCO_3^-$ each being expressed in mEq/min./1·73 sq. m.

## Results

The individual findings for the younger age-group are shown in Table 1 and for the older in Table 2.

A comparison of the results in the two groups shows that both on normal diet and after $NH_4Cl$ has been added, the plasma $CO_2$ was about 2 mEq/l. lower in the infants under 1 year. Urine *p*H was approximately the same in the two groups, as was the output of $NH_4^+$, though after $NH_4Cl$, this was a little higher in the older group. However, the urine of infants showed a higher titratable acidity than the children, both before and during $NH_4Cl$ administration and therefore a smaller proportion of $H^+$ was excreted as $NH_4^+$.

It is interesting to note that under normal dietary conditions the total $H^+$ excreted by the older age-group was about one-third less than the amount excreted by the infants. This may be explained by the fact that the diet of children contains less protein per kg. body weight than that of young infants who are being fed mainly on cows' milk, and the relatively large amount of phosphate in cows' milk also contributes to the excess of TA in the urine. After the acid load, the total $H^+$ in the urine of both groups was the same but the proportion of TA remained higher in infants, the children compensating by an increase in ammonia production.

There is no marked difference between the two age-groups in the mean values of the $H^+$ clearance index after $NH_4Cl$ administration, though by exclusion of one exceptionally high index in the infant group a

TABLE 2

CHILDREN AGED 1 YEAR AND 1 MONTH TO 16 YEARS: INDIVIDUAL RESULTS, MEANS, AND RANGE

| No. | Sex | Age (yr.) | Diet | Blood: Plasma $CO_2$ (mEq/l.) | Blood: Whole Blood *p*H | Urine: *p*H Range | Urine: *p*H Pooled Specimens | Urine µEq/min./1·73 sq. m.: $NH_4^+$ | Urine µEq/min./1·73 sq. m.: TA | Urine µEq/min./1·73 sq. m.: TA − $HCO_3^-$ | Urine µEq/min./1·73 sq. m.: Total $H^+$ | % $NH_4^+$ in $NH_4^+$ + TA | $H^+$ Clearance Index |
|---|---|---|---|---|---|---|---|---|---|---|---|---|---|
| 1 | F | 1 1/12 | Normal | 19·2 | 7·42 | | 5·7 | 23·4 | 24·2 | — | 47·6 | 49·3 | 0·92 |
| | | | Normal + $NH_4Cl$ | 14·0 | 7·37 | 4·8–5·8 | 5·3 | 111·0 | 53·8 | — | 164·8 | 67·5 | *2·30* |
| 2 | F | 1 4/12 | Normal + $NH_4Cl$ | 16·0 | 7·42 | 5·4–5·7 | 5·6 | 59·4 | 26·5 | — | 85·9 | 69·2 | *1·38* |
| 3 | F | 1 10/12 | Normal | 22·0 | 7·36 | 6·0–6·3 | 6·2 | 26·8 | 12·0 | — | 38·8 | 69·0 | 0·85 |
| | | | Normal + $NH_4Cl$ | 14·9 | 7·31 | 4·9–5·2 | 5·0 | 87·0 | 44·2 | — | 131·2 | 66·3 | *1·96* |
| 4 | M | 2 6/12 | Normal + $NH_4Cl$ | 21·0 | | 5·1–5·2 | 5·1 | 50·0 | 25·5 | — | 75·5 | 66·2 | *1·58* |
| 5 | M | 3 4/12 | Normal + $NH_4Cl$ | 16·8 | | 5·2–5·2 | 5·2 | 53·0 | 30·0 | — | 83·0 | 64·0 | *1·40* |
| 6 | M | 4 | Normal + $NH_4Cl$ | 18·5 | | | 4·8 | 65·0 | 33·3 | — | 98·3 | 66·0 | *1·82* |
| 7 | M | 4 | Normal + $NH_4Cl$ | 17·0 | | 4·9–5·1 | 5·0 | 71·8 | 26·0 | — | 97·8 | 73·4 | *1·66* |
| 8 | F | 4 8/12 | Normal + $NH_4Cl$ | 18·5 | | 5·0–5·7 | 5·3 | 70·0 | 30·0 | — | 100·0 | 70·0 | *1·85* |
| 9 | M | 5 | Normal + $NH_4Cl$ | 20·0 | | 5·1–5·2 | 5·1 | 45·7 | 27·0 | — | 72·7 | 63·0 | *1·45* |
| 10 | F | 5 3/12 | Normal | 25·8 | | | 7·2 | 18·2 | 2·0 | −7·9 | 10·3 | 90·0 | 0·26 |
| | | | Normal + $NH_4Cl$ | 21·3 | | | 4·7 | 48·2 | 13·9 | — | 62·1 | 77·6 | *1·32* |
| 11 | M | 5 9/12 | Normal | 24·8 | 7·40 | 5·2–5·4 | 5·3 | 11·2 | 18·9 | — | 30·1 | 37·2 | 0·74 |
| | | | Normal + $NH_4Cl$ | 21·4 | 7·37 | | 4·8 | 65·0 | 42·7 | — | 107·7 | 60·4 | *2·3* |
| 12 | M | 8 3/12 | Normal + $NH_4Cl$ | 17·5 | | 4·6–5·6 | 4·8 | 47·6 | 24·0 | — | 71·6 | 66·5 | *1·25* |
| 13 | M | 14 | Normal | 20·0 | 7·51 | 5·4–6·4 | 6·0 | 28·6 | 10·5 | — | 39·1 | 73·2 | 0·78 |
| | | | Normal + $NH_4Cl$ | 18·0 | 7·45 | 4·7–5·1 | 4·9 | 62·0 | 31·0 | — | 93·0 | 66·7 | *1·68* |
| 14 | M | 16 | Normal | 22·8 | 7·47 | 6·6–6·8 | 6·7 | 17·3 | 3·5 | −8·3 | 9·0 | 83·1 | 0·20 |
| | | | Normal + $NH_4Cl$ | 19·8 | 7·40 | 5·2–5·7 | 5·5 | 73·0 | 15·2 | — | 88·2 | 83·0 | *1·74* |
| Mean .. | .. | .. | Normal | 22·4 | | | | 20·9 | 11·9 | — | 29·2 | 64·0 | 0·63 |
| Range .. | .. | .. | Normal | 19·2–25·8 | | | 5·3–7·2 | 11·2–28·6 | 2·0–24·2 | — | 9·0–47·6 | 37·0–90·0 | 0·20–0·92 |
| Mean .. | .. | .. | Normal + $NH_4Cl$ | 18·2 | | | | 64·5 | 30·2 | — | 95·1 | 68·4 | 1·69 |
| Range .. | .. | .. | Normal + $NH_4Cl$ | 14·0–21·4 | | | 4·7–5·6 | 45·7–111·0 | 13·9–53·8 | — | 62·1–164·8 | 61·0–83·0 | 1·25–2·30 |

TA = Titratable acidity

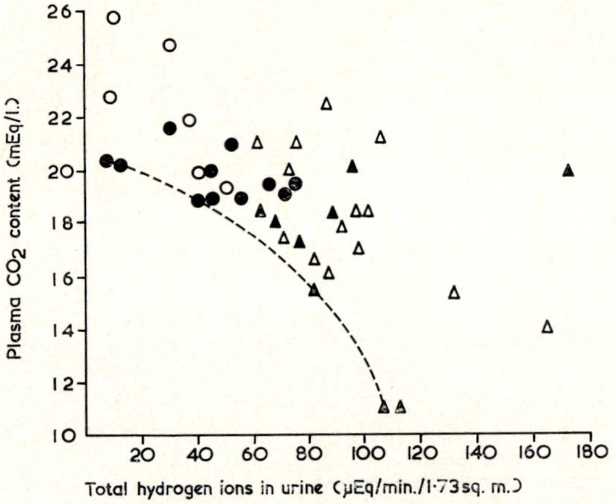


FIG. 1.—The relation of plasma $CO_2$ content to the rate of total hydrogen ion excretion in urine (infants and children). The interrupted line shows the limit of normal values.

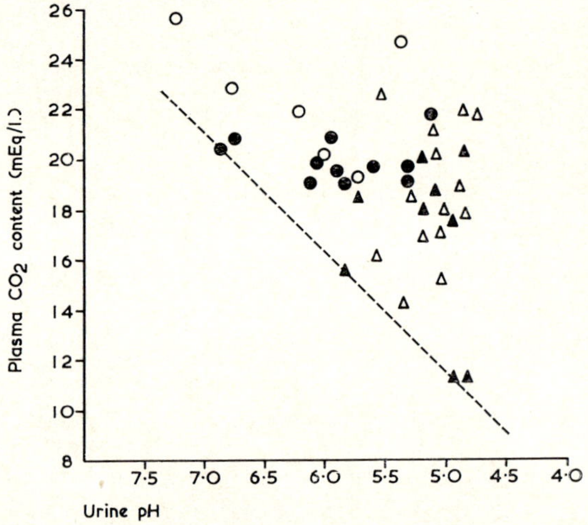


FIG. 2.—The relation of plasma $CO_2$ content to urine *p*H (infants and children). The interrupted line shows the limit of normal values. Symbols as in Fig. 1.

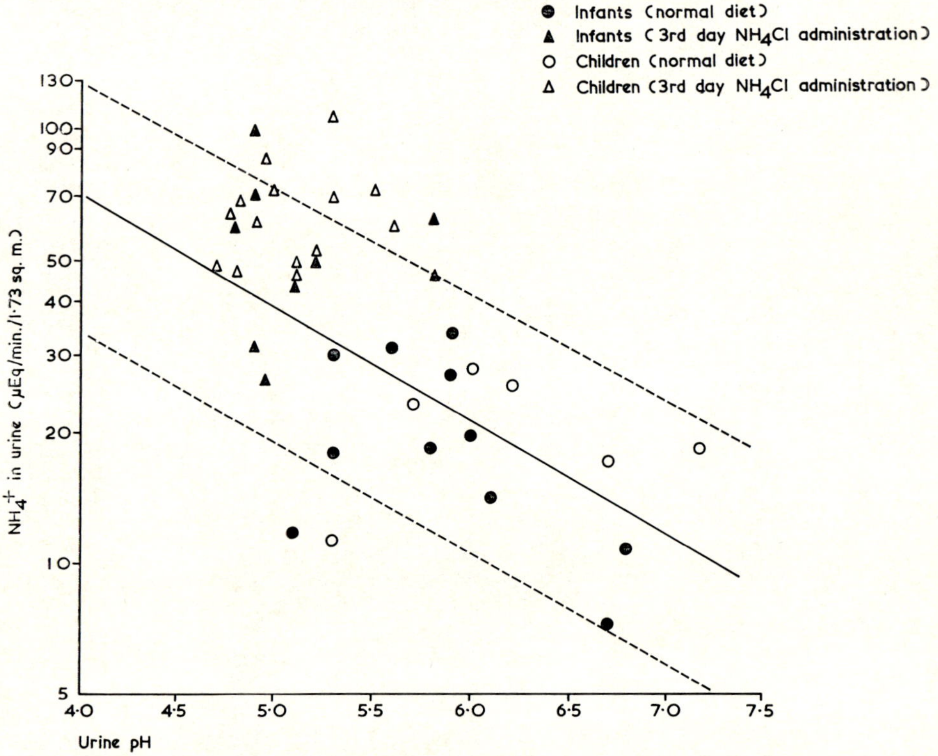


FIG. 3.—The relation of ammonium ion excretion to the *p*H of urine (infants and children). The bold line is the mean and the interrupted lines represent the 95% confidence limits for adults (Wrong, 1961). Symbols as in Fig. 1.

lower mean index would have been obtained. This is due to lower plasma $CO_2$ values rather than lower total $H^+$ excreted in the urine.

The index in subjects receiving a free diet varied widely. It can be very low or even negative if the diet is alkaline, when the subject is excreting more $HCO_3^-$ than $NH_4^+$ and TA together. In these cases the renal ability to excrete $H^+$ can be assessed by plotting the plasma $CO_2$ against total $H^+$ excreted in the urine. In Fig. 1 the results for both infants and children on normal diets and after $NH_4Cl$ administration have been plotted in this way. The interrupted line joining the lower points of the graph indicates the lower limit of the values for the infants: the lower normal limit for children is slightly higher than the one for infants. Infants or children whose values fall below this line may be considered abnormal as far as renal ability to excrete $H^+$ is concerned. Fig. 2 similarly shows the relation between plasma $CO_2$ and urine *p*H. Fig. 3 shows the $NH_4^+$ output in relation to urinary *p*H and includes also the normal limits and the mean for adults given by Wrong (1961). Under normal dietary conditions the values for all our control subjects except two—one infant and one child—fell within the normal limits for adults, while after stressing with $NH_4Cl$, several of them exceeded the upper limits of normal for adults.

The percentage of $H^+$ excreted as $NH_4^+$ is a useful index of ammonia production. Our lowest figure for this percentage is 32·7 in infants and 37 in children. McCance, Matheson, Gresham, and Elkinton (1960) consider that figures below 30% indicate impaired ammonia production. Two of the present subjects whose ratio of ammonia to urine *p*H was below the normal limits for adults (as shown in Fig. 3) also had a comparatively low percentage of $H^+$ excreted as $NH_4^+$, but this increased in one of them, who was tested after $NH_4Cl$, from 37·2 to 60·4%.

**Discussion**

Though the tests were arranged so that the results could be compared with those of Elkinton *et al.* (1960) for adults, there were difficulties in doing this, and the findings are not exactly comparable. Difficulties in obtaining accurate 24-hour specimens were avoided by using short periods of urine collections that did not require admission to hospital overnight. A further advantage in this procedure is that the urine could be analysed without delay, thus minimizing the risks of changes due to bacterial activity. Rates of daily $H^+$ excretion calculated from a short period of the day are probably not representative of the average rates for the whole 24 hours, measured by Elkinton *et al.* (1960), since urine passed at night tends to be more acid than that during the day. Furthermore, both the meals and the divided doses of $NH_4Cl$ administered during the collection period may have resulted in rapid and brief changes in the blood chemistry and the urine acidity, but blood for analysis was always taken at the same time after meals to offset this possibility.

The normal capillary plasma $CO_2$ content in this study ranged from 19-25·8 mEq/l., which is lower than the range given by Singer and Hastings (1948) for arterial plasma in adults. The dropwise collection of blood, and the omission of paraffin oil in the collecting tube may have contributed to these lower values. In this laboratory, blood is no longer collected under oil because of the practical difficulties, one of which is always ensuring adequate mixing of drops of capillary blood under oil. Gambino (1961) has drawn attention to the fact that mineral oil may result in big losses of $CO_2$ due to its high solubility in oil. The routine method in this laboratory is to equilibrate the specimen with alveolar air only if it is not analysed within three to four hours after its collection, but this hardly ever needed to be done in the present investigation.

For comparison, the findings from our infant group have been tabulated together with those from infants aged 2-10 months recorded in the literature (Table 3). Unfortunately as the technique and methods of investigation among the different authors have differed, the results may not be entirely comparable. Thus, Gordon, McNamara, and Benjamin (1948) and McCance *et al.* (1960) analysed 24-hour urine specimens, while Fomon, Harris, and Jensen (1959) used 12-hour night specimens of urine. The latter authors analysed venous blood and this gave higher values of $CO_2$ content in their series than in ours. The $H^+$ output of our infants is higher than in the breast-fed infants reported by Fomon *et al.* and in the artificially fed infants by McCance *et al.*, but it is much lower than that of the infants fed on cows' milk investigated by Gordon *et al.* (1948) and Fomon *et al.* (1959). Low $H^+$ excretion is to be expected in breast-fed infants compared with those who are artificially fed, but it is difficult to explain the large differences observed among infants fed artificially (Table 3), unless their diets were quite different, especially with regard to protein consumption.

The output of $H^+$ by our normal infants (66 mEq/24 hr./1·73 sq. m.) under normal dietary conditions is approximately the same as by two infants, aged 8 months and 1 year, studied by Widdowson and McCance (1958) (if their output is calculated per 1·73 sq. m. surface area, assuming each was of

TABLE 3

EXCRETION OF HYDROGEN IONS IN NORMAL INFANTS ON NORMAL DIET AND AFTER AMMONIUM CHLORIDE: PRESENT SERIES AND SOME PREVIOUSLY PUBLISHED FIGURES

| Author | Group (No.) | Age (mth.) | Diet | | Plasma $CO_2$ Content (mEq/l.) | Urine: µEq/min./1·73 sq. m. $NH_4^+$ | Urine: µEq/min./1·73 sq. m. TA | Urine: % of $NH_4^+$ in Total $H^+$ Excretion | $H^+$ Clearance Index |
|---|---|---|---|---|---|---|---|---|---|
| Gordon *et al.* (1948) | Infants | 2–4 | Cows' milk | Venous | 26·2 | 31·5 | 52·7 | 37·0 | 2·19 |
| | (3) | | Cows' milk + $NH_4Cl$ | Venous | 20·0 | 80·3 | 56·0 | 59·0 | 2·71 |
| Fomon *et al.* (1959) | Infants | 2–5½ | Cows' milk | Venous | 23·3 | 63·5 | 77·0 | 45·2 | 3·24 |
| | (4) | | Cows' milk + $NH_4Cl$ | Venous | 17·5 | 118·0 | 82·0 | 59·0 | 3·60 |
| Fomon *et al.* (1959) | Infants | 3½–4½ | Human milk | Venous | 25·6 | 15·8 | 6·2 | 70·8 | <0·56 |
| | (4) | | Human milk + $NH_4Cl$ | Venous | 15·5 | 48·9 | 13·6 | 79·8 | 0·97 |
| McCance *et al.* (1960) | Infants* | 10 | Normal diet | | | †17·7 | †14·4 | 55·0 | |
| | | | Human diet + $NH_4Cl$ | | | †37·2 | †21·0 | 64·0 | |
| Present Series | Infants (11) | 2–11½ | Artificially fed | Capillary | 19·9 | 20·4 | 25·5 | 46·3 | 0·88 |
| | (9) | | Artificially fed + $NH_4Cl$ | Capillary | 16·6 | 54·4 | 42·5 | 55·8 | 1·61 |

* The number of patients included is not stated. The series includes some infants studied by the authors, and others taken from published reports

† Calculated from authors' data.

TABLE 4

EFFECT OF $NH_4CL$ ADMINISTRATION ON RENAL EXCRETION OF HYDROGEN IONS: NORMAL INFANTS AND CHILDREN (PRESENT SERIES) AND PREVIOUSLY PUBLISHED VALUES IN ADULTS

| Author | Group (No.) | Age | | Mean Plasma $CO_2$ (mEq/l.) | Mean Total $H^+$ Excretion in Urine (µEq/min./1·73 sq. m.) | $H^+$ Clearance Index: Mean | $H^+$ Clearance Index: Range |
|---|---|---|---|---|---|---|---|
| Present series | Infants (9) | 2–11½ mth. | Capillary | 16·6 | 97·0 | 1·61 | 1·20–3·44 |
| Present series | Children (14) | 13 mth.–16 yr. | Capillary | 18·2 | 95·1 | 1·69 | 1·25–2·30 |
| Elkinton *et al.* (1960) | Adults (17) | | Venous (serum) | 20·7 | 100·0 | 2·07 | 1·40–3·40 |

normal body weight and height for age) and by adults reported by Elkinton *et al.* (1960). All are much higher than those for infants on the first, second, and eighth day of life (Widdowson and McCance, 1958).

The response to $NH_4Cl$ induced acidosis by both infants and children in our series (Table 4) is practically the same as that in adults (Elkinton *et al.*, 1960), though the clearance indices of adults are slightly higher owing to higher serum $CO_2$ levels. The present observations indicate that the kidneys of the children examined were able to cope as efficiently with the stress of $H^+$ added to normal feeding as those of adults. Hatemi and McCance (1961), investigating the response of newborn infants to a single dose of $NH_4Cl$, found that $H^+$ excretion was much less than in adults after a similar stress, the mean clearance indices in newborns being only 21% of their mean adult values. Our results now show that in the infant the specific renal function of acidifying the urine under stress has, presumably by a process of maturation, achieved adult level by about 3 months of age. Though the number of the younger infants examined in this series is not large enough to suggest the earliest age at which this maturation occurs in any individual, the results can be used as a basis for the assessment of acidosis of renal origin with increasing confidence over the age of 3 months.

## Summary

The renal ability to excrete hydrogen ions was assessed in 12 normal infants aged 2-11½ months and 14 children aged 1 year 1 month to 16 years on ordinary diets, and in most cases on the third day of continuous ammonium chloride administration. Titratable acidity and ammonium ion excretion in the urine and the carbon dioxide content in the plasma were determined within the same period, and from these values the hydrogen ion clearance index has been calculated for each child. The mean and range for the index in both age-groups, as well as the total hydrogen ions excreted/1·73 sq. m. surface area, were found to have reached adult levels.

It is considered that the values for these normal children are suitable to use as a standard that can be applied in assessing whether acidosis is, or is not, primarily of renal origin in children from the age of about 3 months.

REFERENCES

Albright, F., and Reifenstein, E. C., Jr. (1948). *The Parathyroid Glands and Metabolic Bone Disease.* Williams and Wilkins, Baltimore.

Buchanan, E. U., and Komrower, G. M. (1958). The prognosis of idiopathic renal acidosis in infancy with observations on urine acidification and ammonia production in children. *Arch. Dis. Childh.*, **33**, 532.

Du Bois, D., and Du Bois, E. F. (1916). Clinical calorimetry. X. A formula to estimate the approximate surface area if height and weight be known. *Arch. intern. Med.*, **17**, 863.

Elkinton, J. R., Huth, E. J., Webster, G. D., Jr., and McCance, R. A. (1960). The renal excretion of hydrogen ion in renal tubular acidosis. I. Quantitative assessment of the response to ammonium chloride as an acid load. *Amer. J. Med.*, **29**, 554.

Fomon, S. J., Harris, D. M., and Jensen, R. L. (1959). Acidification of the urine by infants fed human milk and whole cows' milk. *Pediatrics*, **23**, 113.

Gambino, S. R. (1961). Mineral oil and carbon dioxide. *Amer. J. clin. Path.*, **35**, 268.

Gordon, H. H., McNamara, H., and Benjamin, H. R. (1948). The response of young infants to ingestion of ammonium chloride. *Pediatrics*, **2**, 290.

Hatemi, N., and McCance, R. A. (1961). Renal aspects of acid-base control in the newly born. III. Response to acidifying drugs. *Acta paediat. (Uppsala)*, **50**, 603.

Hawk, P. B., Oser B. L., and Summerson, W. H. (1954). *Practical Physiological Chemistry*, 13th ed., p. 889. Churchill, London.

Huth, E. J., Webster, G. D., Jr., and Elkinton, J. R. (1960). The renal excretion of hydrogen ion in renal tubular acidosis. III. An attempt to detect latent cases in a family; comments on nosology, genetics and etiology of the primary disease. *Amer. J. Med.*, **29**, 586.

McCance, R. A., Matheson, W. J., Gresham, G. A., and Elkinton, J. R. (1960). The cerebro-ocular-renal dystrophies: a new variant. *Arch. Dis. Childh.*, **35**, 240.

Singer, R. B., and Hastings, A. B. (1948). An improved clinical method for the estimation of disturbances of the acid-base balance of human blood. *Medicine (Baltimore)*, **27**, 223.

Van Slyke, D. D., and Neill, J. M. (1924). The determination of gases in blood and other solutions by vacuum extraction and manometric measurement. *J. biol. Chem.*, **61**, 523.

Widdowson, E. M., and McCance, R. A. (1958). The development of acid-base control. In *Ciba Foundation. Colloquia on Ageing*, Vol. 4, p. 209. Churchill, London.

Wrong, O. (1961). Personal communication quoted by Berlyne, G. M. in Distal tubular function in chronic hydronephrosis. *Quart. J. Med.*, **30**, 339.

——, and Davies, H. E. F. (1959). The excretion of acid in renal disease. *Quart. J. Med.*, **28**, 259.

*Arch. Dis. Childh.*, 1965, **40**, 40.

# A-β-LIPOPROTEINAEMIA (BASSEN-KORNZWEIG SYNDROME)

## REPORT OF A CASE

BY

D. M. O. BECROFT, J. M. COSTELLO, and P. J. SCOTT
*From Princess Mary Hospital and Auckland Hospital, Auckland, New Zealand*

(RECEIVED FOR PUBLICATION JUNE 24, 1964)

In 1950 Bassen and Kornzweig described a new syndrome when they reported the presence of irregular erythrocytes in an 18-year-old Jewish girl who had retinitis pigmentosa and a neurological disorder similar to Friedreich's ataxia. Several years later they described the same triad (abnormal erythrocytes, retinitis pigmentosa, and neuropathy) in the patient's brother (Kornzweig and Bassen, 1957). The parents of these sibs were first cousins.

In 1952 Singer, Fisher, and Perlstein described a similar case and suggested the term acanthrocytosis for the irregular red cells (Akantha = thorn). This patient had irregular red cells and neuropathy. Retinopathy, though not present at 13½ years, had developed by 19 years (Jampel and Falls, 1958). Druez (1959) later reported a case from Belgium and suggested that the correct term was acanthocytosis. Druez's patient had hypocholesterolaemia, a feature that had been noted in one of the previously reported cases (Jampel and Falls, 1958).

In 1960, Salt, Wolff, Lloyd, Fosbrooke, Cameron, and Hubble described a child suffering from acanthocytosis and demonstrated virtual absence of serum low-density lipoproteins (i.e. β-lipoproteins). This finding has been confirmed in other patients with this syndrome.

Twelve cases with this condition have now been reported. Steatorrhoea, hypocholesterolaemia, reduction of total serum lipids and serum phospholipids are now known to be features of the syndrome. Acanthocytosis and a-β-lipoproteinaemia occur in all cases, but neuropathy and retinopathy have not been present in all. Where biopsy of the small intestinal mucosa has been carried out the histological appearance has always been the same. The columnar cells covering the villi have unusually clear cytoplasm (Salt *et al.*, 1960; Mabry, Di George, and Auerbach, 1960; Lamy, Frézal, Polonovski, and Rey, 1961; Schwartz, Rowland, Eder, Marks, Osserman, Hirschberg, and Anderson, 1963; Ways, Reed, and Hanahan, 1963).

The patient to be described was diagnosed at the age of 10 months and showed some unusual features that led to his early death.

### Case Report

The patient, J.M., was born on April 19, 1962 following a 39-week pregnancy, his birth weight being 5 lb. 14 oz. (2,663 g.). At the age of 3 months he developed lobar pneumonia and was admitted to the Waikato Hospital under the care of Dr. D. H. H. Pullon. At the time of admission he was malnourished, his weight being 7 lb. 12 oz. (3,515 g.). Investigations at this time revealed Hb 9·2 g./100 ml. Microspherocytes, burr cells, and hypochromic macrocytes were described in the blood film. The erythrocytes showed decreased osmotic fragility. The serum non-protein nitrogen which was 31 mg./100 ml. on the first examination later rose to 64-74 mg./100 ml. The bowel motions were bulky and 53% of the dried weight was fat. A non-specific amino-aciduria was present. An intravenous pyelogram was normal. During his stay in hospital his motions were loose. No pathogens were isolated from the stools at first but later *Staphylococcus aureus* was isolated. A recurrence of pneumonia at the age of 8 months responded satisfactorily to antibiotics,

He was given a course of iron dextran intramuscularly, and folic acid, and his haemoglobin rose to 15·2 g./100 ml.

At the age of 9 months he weighed 10 lb. 12 oz. (4,875 g.) and was transferred to the Karitane Hospital, Auckland, for feeding management. At the age of 9½ months he developed basal bronchopneumonia and was transferred to the Princess Mary Hospital for Children under the care of Dr. R. H. Caughey.

**Family History.** The child's parents are Maoris who are second cousins. The father suffers from spinal tuberculosis. There are 8 living sibs, 3 of whom are adopted out. A ninth sib died at the age of 1 year from gastro-enteritis.

**Examination.** At the time of admission examination revealed a mentally retarded Maori child (mental age 4 months, chronological age 10 months). He weighed 11 lb. 5 oz. (5·2 kg.). His head appeared small and the occiput was flattened. Slight flexion contractures of the knees were present. The deep reflexes were diminished in the legs. Signs of bronchopneumonia with bronchospasm were present. There was no evidence of retinopathy.

TABLE 1

HAEMATOLOGICAL DATA

| | |
|---|---|
| Hb (g./100 ml.) | 11·6 |
| Haematocrit (%) | 36 |
| MCHC (%) | 32 |
| Acanthocytes | 35–40% of erythrocytes |
| Reticulocytes | 2/100 RBCs |
| WBC | 7,600/c.mm. |
| ESR (Westergren) | 3 mm. in 1 hour |
| Red cell osmotic fragility | Decreased |
| Direct Coombs test | Negative |
| Plasma bilirubin (mg./100 ml.) | 0·2 mg./100 ml. |

**Investigations.** Preliminary examination of the peripheral blood revealed a haemoglobin of 11·6 g./100 ml. Approximately 35% of red cells were conspicuously small and darkly staining. Irregularity of shape of the majority of these cells was at first dismissed as artefact and the cells identified as microspherocytes. Demonstration of decreased red cell fragility led to examination of further blood films and recognition of the consistency of the red cell irregularity (Fig. 1). This irregularity was present in wet preparations, on suspension of the cells in normal saline, and was particularly well seen by phase contrast microscopy (Fig. 2). Under phase contrast the abnormal cells showed intense golden yellow coloration, contrasting sharply both with normal red cells and with cells showing normal crenation, the latter being numerous in all preparations examined. Each abnormal cell had one or more spiculate projections which frequently branched or curved and often had a length greater than the diameter of the body of the cell, resulting in many bizarre shapes. There was no rouleaux formation.

TABLE 2

LIPID AND RELATED STUDIES

| | |
|---|---|
| Serum β-lipoprotein (mg./100 ml.) Turbidometric method* | 10, 20, 15 — 3 separate estimations (normal 130-500) |
| Immunological assay† | None detected |
| Ultracentrifugal analysis‡ | Low density (< 1·063) lipoproteins absent; chylomicra absent |
| Serum cholesterol (mg./100 ml.)§ | 23 (normal 120–220) |
| Serum fatty acid esters (mEq/l.) | 2·5 (normal 9–14) |
| Serum carotenoids (μg./100 ml.) | 12·5 (normal 60–260) |
| Faecal fat excretion (g./day) | 11·6 |
| D-xylose absorption | 24% excretion in urine |
| Sweat sodium (mEq/l.) | 33 |
| Sweat chloride (mEq/l.) | 38 |
| Total serum protein (g./100 ml.) | 6·3 |
| Electrophoretic analysis serum proteins | Slight increase γ-globulin |
| Barium meal and follow through | Moderate dilatation of small bowel; thickened jejunal mucosal folds; some clumping of barium |
| Radiological bone-age | Slightly retarded at 10 mth.; normal at 17 mth. |

* Method of Walton and Scott (1964).
† Method of Soothill (1962).
‡ Modification of method of Havel, Eder, and Bragdon (1955).
§ Method of Sackett (1925).

In view of the peculiar shape of the red cells, and the clinical picture, the possibility of the child having the Bassen-Kornzweig syndrome was entertained.

Further investigations (Table 2) revealed virtual absence of serum β-lipoproteins, profound hypocholesterolaemia, considerable reduction of serum fatty acid esters and serum carotenoids. Steatorrhoea was present.

These investigations confirmed that the child was suffering from the Bassen-Kornzweig syndrome.

Further investigation (Table 3) revealed a persistently raised blood urea. A generalized aminoaciduria was present but the serum amino acids were normal, indicating that the aminoaciduria was of a low renal threshold type.

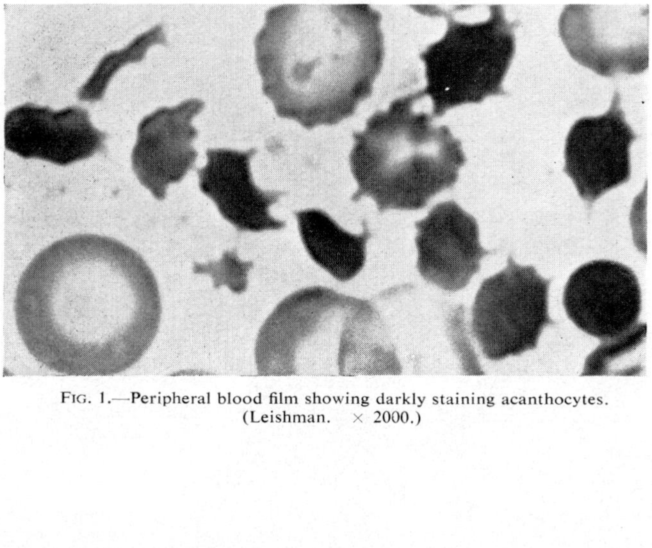

FIG. 1.—Peripheral blood film showing darkly staining acanthocytes. (Leishman. × 2000.)

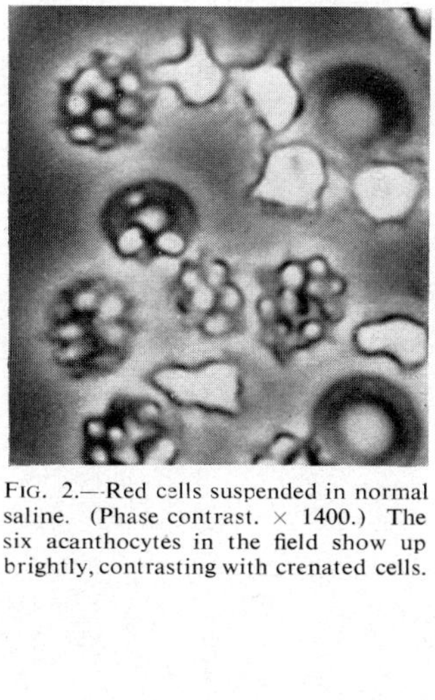

FIG. 2.—Red cells suspended in normal saline. (Phase contrast. × 1400.) The six acanthocytes in the field show up brightly, contrasting with crenated cells.

TABLE 3

ASSESSMENT OF RENAL FUNCTION

| | |
|---|---|
| Blood urea (mg./100 ml.) | 40–67 |
| Serum creatinine (mg./100 ml.) | 1·1 |
| Creatinine clearance (uncorrected) (ml./min.) | 15 |
| Creatinine clearance (corrected for surface area) (ml./min.) | 66 |
| Plasma $CO_2$-content (mEq/l.) | 21·9 |
| Serum phosphorus (mg./100 ml.) | 5·6 |
| Urine *p*H | 5·4 |
| Urine bacterial count/ml. | 10,000 |
| Urinary amino acids | Non-specific aminoaciduria |
| Serum amino acids | Normal |

No glycosuria was present and the urine was free from protein and infection.

**Investigation of Family.** The blood of both parents and five of the patient's sibs was examined for acanthocytes, serum β-lipoprotein, serum cholesterol, and serum carotenoids. No abnormality was detected (Table 4). The other three sibs have been adopted out of the family and were not available for testing.

**Progress.** During his stay in hospital the patient had several episodes of asthma which responded satisfactorily to treatment. No dietary treatment such as fat restriction was attempted (cf. Lamy, Frézal, Polonovski, Druez, and Rey, 1963), because it was considered that dietary management would not be continued following discharge from hospital. Vitamin supplements were given.

He was discharged from hospital at the age of 14½ months weighing 14 lb. 3 oz. (6·4 kg.). He was readmitted for reassessment of renal function at the age of 17 months. At the time of admission he was suffering from otorrhoea and basal bronchitis for which he received antibiotics. There was still no evidence of retinopathy. Further investigations revealed blood urea 40 mg./100 ml., creatinine clearance 15 ml./min.; serum phosphorus 5·6 mg./100 ml., Na 144 mEq/l.; K 5 mEq/l.; plasma $CO_2$-content 21·9 mEq/l.; *p*H of urine 5·4, urine bacterial count 10,000/ml.

Three weeks after readmission to hospital he developed an exacerbation of bronchitis and asthma which was associated with cardiac enlargement and left ventricular failure. He responded initially to digoxin but deteriorated again and died on the seventh day of the illness. Unfortunately consent for necropsy was not obtained.

## Discussion

The patient described was undoubtedly a case of the Bassen-Kornzweig syndrome.

*Retinopathy* was not present in our patient. Retinal changes have been observed in 6 of the 12 previously reported cases (Bassen and Kornzweig, 1950; Jampel and Falls, 1958; Kornzweig and Bassen, 1957; Druez, 1959; Friedman, Cohn, Zymaris, and Goldner, 1960; Mier, Schwartz, and Boshes, 1960) and electroretinography has been abnormal in one case in which the retinoscopy was normal (Lamy *et al.*, 1961). The 5 patients without retinopathy were all under the age of 14 years at the time of reporting (Salt *et al.*, 1960; Mabry *et al.*, 1960; Wolff and Bauman, 1961; Schwartz *et al.*, 1963; Ways *et al.*, 1963). The patient reported on by Singer *et al.* had no retinopathy at the age of 13 years, but at the age of 19 marked atypical retinitis pigmentosa was present (Jampel and Falls, 1958). It is probable therefore that all patients with this disorder will develop retinopathy as they become older.

*Neurological abnormalities*, particularly areflexia,

TABLE 4

SERUM CHOLESTEROL, CAROTENOIDS AND β-LIPOPROTEIN, AND ACANTHOCYTOSIS IN PATIENTS AND RELATIVES

| Subject | Age-group or Age | Serum Cholesterol | Serum Carotenoids | Serum β-Lipoprotein Determined as: Protein by Gel-diffusion Immuno-assay | Lipoprotein by Dextran Sulphate Precipitation | Low Density (< 1·063) Lipoprotein by Salt Density Method of Fractionation | Acanthocytes |
|---|---|---|---|---|---|---|---|
| Approximate normal range | 0 to 10 yr. | 120 to 220 mg./100 ml. | 60 to 260 μg./100 ml. | 50 to 150% of normal control | 120 to 570 mg./100 ml. | | None |
| | 30 to 40 yr. | | | | 250 to 780 mg./100 ml. | 300 to 750 mg./100 ml. | None |
| Patient J.M. | 10 mth. | 23 | 12·5 | 0 | 15 | 0 | Present |
| Mother | 37 yr. | 164 | 112 | 75 | 410 | — | Absent |
| Father | 38 yr. | 236 | 122 | 150 | 800 | — | Absent |
| Brother | 17 yr. | 164 | 132 | 75 | 375 | — | Absent |
| Brother | 15 yr. | 136 | 99 | 75 | 360 | — | Absent |
| Sister | 11 yr. | 141 | 167 | 75 | 360 | — | Absent |
| Sister | 8 yr. | 177 | 177 | 75 | 440 | — | Absent |
| Sister | 5 yr. | 180 | — | 50 | 240 | — | Absent |
| Patient of Salt *et al.* | 17 mth. | 22 | 0 | 0 | 20 | 0 | Present |
| Mother of Salt's patient | 30 yr. | 127 | 84 | 50 | — | — | Absent |
| Father of Salt's patient | 32 yr. | 107 | 68 | 50 | — | — | Absent |

have been present in most of the 12 reported cases (Schwartz *et al.*, 1963). Our patient showed diminished tendon reflexes, and this almost certainly represented the early stages of the neuropathy of this disease.

*Steatorrhoea*, which was present in our patient, appears to be a constant feature in this disease. Biopsy of the small intestinal mucosa was not carried out in our patient. In contrast to coeliac disease the glucose tolerance test in patients with the Bassen-Kornzweig syndrome is usually normal (Lamy *et al.*, 1963). In several cases with this disorder the D-xylose absorption test has been normal (Mier *et al.*, 1960; Mabry *et al.*, 1960; Lamy *et al.*, 1963), but in others it has been abnormal (Schwartz *et al.*, 1963). Two oral glucose tolerance tests were carried out on our patient. The first one at the age of 11 months showed apparent decreased tolerance with the blood sugar still above fasting levels at 2 hours. The second tolerance test at 17 months was normal. The D-xylose absorption was normal.

**Lipid Studies.** The low serum cholesterol level fell within the range of 20-50 mg./100 ml. previously reported for this syndrome. Ultracentrifugal analysis of our patient's serum using a density gradient method showed that the small amount of cholesterol present was associated with the high density lipoprotein (α-lipoprotein). This analysis showed no detectable low density lipoprotein (i.e. β-lipoprotein), and no chylomicra were present. The lipoprotein pattern was similar to that reported by Schwartz *et al.* (1963) and Salt *et al.* (1960). The density gradient used was identical to that employed by Dr. K. W. Walton in investigations on the case reported by Salt and his colleagues.

The dextran sulphate turbidometric method for assay of β-lipoprotein was developed after Salt *et al.* had published their paper. However, the turbidometric assay was later carried out by one of us (P.J.S.) on the serum from their patient and gave a result of 20 mg./100 ml. This result, and that of 15 mg./100 ml. in our own patient, indicate virtual absence of β-lipoprotein. The small amount of turbidity recorded represents a fixed error due to precipitation of some γ-globulin components other than low density lipoproteins.

Gel diffusion precipitin analysis (Soothill, 1962) showed no detectable protein component of β-lipoprotein. The antibody used was prepared by Dr. Soothill and reactions of identity had been undertaken previously to confirm that the antiserum was specifically directed against human β-lipoprotein. Employing this particular antiserum, the method was capable of detecting β-lipoprotein concentration of the order of 2 mg./100 ml. (whole lipoprotein molecule) or 0·4 mg./100 ml. of β-lipoprotein protein component. The results obtained in our patient were identical to those found by Dr. Soothill in Salt and Wolff's patient. Immunoelectrophoresis also failed to reveal any detectable β-lipoprotein in our patient's serum.

Conversely, we failed to produce protein precipitation lines on gel diffusion plates when we used our patient's serum as a potential source of precipitin against varying dilutions of purified β-lipoprotein in saline and against normal serum. Allotypes of human β-lipoprotein have been described (Blumberg, Bernanke, and Allison, 1962). Blumberg (1963) has observed, in the serum of two patients with the Bassen-Kornzweig syndrome, precipitins capable of reacting with β-lipoprotein of normal serum. It is not yet clear whether such precipitins are naturally occurring antibodies or the result of an immune phenomenon.

We did not undertake fatty acid or phospholipid analysis of serum or red cells (cf. Phillips, 1962). In normal people 70% of plasma cholesterol, 50% of phospholipid, and virtually all of the plasma carotenoids are carried by the β-lipoproteins. The immunological studies showing virtual absence of the protein components of β-lipoprotein in our patient are compatible with the hypothesis that one of the major defects was complete absence of this normal transport system. Schwartz *et al.* (1963), Mabry *et al.* (1960), and Ways *et al.* (1963) suggest that abnormalities in phosphatide distribution may be of more fundamental importance in this syndrome than defects in absorption or metabolism of particular lipid components such as linoleic acid.

**Acanthocytosis.** In young children without the ocular and neurological manifestations of the syndrome, recognition of acanthocytes in blood films is the most likely means by which the diagnosis will be reached. In our patient the red cells were recognized as abnormal in infancy, but at various times the use of the terms 'burr cell', 'pyknocyte', and 'microspherocyte' directed attention to other clinical syndromes and delayed the eventual diagnosis. For this reason some consideration of the definition of acanthocytes and their differentiation from other abnormal red cells is indicated, particularly their separation from crenated cells, 'burr cells', and 'pyknocytes', terms that, in the purely descriptive sense, might equally well be applied to the acanthocyte.

DEFINITION AND DIFFERENTIATION FROM CRENATION. The original description of the red cells by

Bassen and Kornzweig remains the most detailed and the most vivid.

'No two cells look exactly alike. In general they present a crenated appearance but of such degree that they took on bizarre shapes simulating small beetles, crabs and turtles. Others were star shaped. The variations depended on the number and length of what appeared to be appendages growing out of the cells. Some of the cells appeared small and deeply stained. They resembled spherocytes from which buds or pseudopods were protruding and these cells in particular varied from ordinary crenation.'

Singer *et al.* (1952) likewise noted that among the abnormally shaped erythrocytes many were 'relatively small and deeply stained, thus resembling crenated spherocytes'.

It is considered that the name acanthocyte is best restricted to these small deeply staining cells in which the thorny appearance is most marked. They can then be differentiated from cells identical in appearance to normal red cells crenated by hypertonic solutions. Such crenated cells, having normal size and staining intensity, appeared in considerable numbers in dry films and wet preparations of blood from our patient. The difference between acanthocytes and crenated cells was less obvious in the thinner parts of the film but was readily seen in saline suspension and was found to be accentuated using phase contrast microscopy. With phase contrast, 35 to 40% of red cells had the appearance of acanthocytes, and crenated cells were present in approximately equal numbers, proportions that are similar to those shown by illustrations accompanying other case reports. The description by Salt *et al.* of the acanthocyte as having a serrated margin with a cog-wheel appearance is more appropriate to crenation, and does not do justice to the striking variation in outline shown by the typical cells. The presence of acanthocytosis has been claimed in two cases of hereditary vitreo-retinal degeneration and one of Eales's disease (Kahán, Kahán, and Benkö, 1963a, b). The cells illustrated by these authors do not conform with the definition of the acanthocyte given above and appear to be showing crenation. Furthermore, in these cases the sedimentation rates were not depressed and serum lipid levels were not comparable with those found in the Bassen-Kornzweig syndrome.

Differentiation from Microspherocytosis. Confusion with microspherocytosis results from an artefact occurring in thinner parts of dry films in which the projections on the surface of the acanthocyte become less obvious and many cells appear small, darkly staining, and spherical. Examination of the thicker parts of the film is therefore essential.

Differentiation from 'Burr' Cells. Burr cell was a term introduced in 1949 by Schwartz and Motto to describe a cell '7·5 microns or less in diameter, having one to several spiny projections along its periphery'. These cells were associated with uraemia, carcinoma of the stomach, and bleeding peptic ulcers. Subsequently other authors (Dacie, Mollison, Richardson, Selwyn, and Shapiro, 1953; Allison, 1957; Aherne, 1957; Shumway and Miller, 1957; Lock and Dormandy, 1961) described similar cells and other bizarre types of poikilocyte in cases with renal failure of varied cause, but often in association with haemolytic anaemia and thrombocytopenia occurring in childhood.

Brain, Dacie, and Hourihane (1962) have suggested that the common pathogenesis is not uraemia *per se*, but disease in small blood vessels, and have suggested the term 'micro-angiopathic haemolytic anaemia' for the condition. The abnormal red cells described by Brain *et al.* included red cell fragments and various contracted and distorted microcytes of which triangular and helmet-shaped forms were common, plus crenated cells. Crenation occurring in cells already contracted and distorted was considered to give rise to cells corresponding exactly with the burr cells described by Schwartz and Motto (1949). Schwartz and Motto in fact made no mention of contraction of cells in their description; nevertheless it is quite clear that occasional cells indistinguishable from the acanthocyte will be seen in blood films in association with the 'burr cell phenomenon', 'microangiopathic haemolytic anaemia', or 'red cell fragmentation syndrome', whichever name is considered the most appropriate. No diagnostic difficulty should arise, because in the latter condition the characteristic cells will be only one of many abnormal cell types which together comprise only a minority of red cells. In contrast, in acanthocytosis, at least one-third of all red cells will have the typical appearance, and crenation will be the only other red cell abnormality.

Differentiation from 'Pyknocytosis'. The pyknocyte is a less well-defined entity. Tuffy, Brown, and Zuelzer (1959) gave the name to distorted and contracted erythrocytes which they found in the blood of many apparently normal full-term infants. These cells were more numerous in normal premature infants but, at most, comprised only 5·6% of all red cells whereas up to 50% of red cells had this appearance in 11 newborn babies with an unexplained haemolytic anaemia. This anaemia was severe enough in some cases to require transfusion, but then resolved spontaneously with disappearance of the abnormal cells. Tuffy *et al.* considered these cells to be morphologically identical to burr cells but proposed the term pyknocyte because the density of the cells was regarded as a fundamental feature and resembled that of spherocytes. The cells were also regarded as identical in appearance to acanthocytes. Lovric (1960), however, in reporting the occurrence of pyknocytosis in twins with haemolytic anaemia compared the appearances of the red cells with those from a case of acanthocytosis. He found that in pyknocytosis abnormal cells were fewer in number, but that almost all had the appearance of 'contracted spherocytes with pseudopodia', whereas in acanthocytosis out of 70% irregular cells only a proportion had this appearance.

To summarize, there are three conditions in which contracted, deeply-staining, highly irregular, spiny red cells occur, but consideration of the over-all appearance of the blood film will enable the correct clinical correlation to be made. In acanthocytosis the cells will comprise one-third to one-half of all cells and will be accompanied by many showing normal crenation. In the burr cell phenomenon, only a small proportion of abnormal cells will have this appearance, the remainder will show a wide variety of irregular shapes among which triangular, crescentic, and helmet-shaped cells will be prominent. In pyknocytosis it has been stated that one-third to one-half of cells will resemble the acanthocyte but there will be few if any other abnormal cell types.

Acanthocytes retain their abnormal shape when incubated in normal serum. Conversely the serum of patients with this disorder does not convert normal cells into acanthocytes. The abnormality would, therefore, appear to be inherent in the erythrocyte rather than in the serum. It has been shown that acanthocytes can be converted into the shape of normal erythrocytes by exposure *in vitro* to a non-ionic detergent (Switzer and Eder, 1962) and *in vivo* by administration of cotton-seed oil emulsion intravenously (Di George, Mabry, and Auerbach, 1961).

Other constant haematological features in acanthocytosis are absence of rouleaux formation and a low erythrocyte sedimentation rate. Our case had an erythrocyte sedimentation rate of 3 mm. (Westergren) at the height of a respiratory infection.

Anaemia is not a constant feature in this disorder. In three patients the half life of the erythrocytes has been shown to be shortened by the radioactive chromium method (Druez, 1959; Mier *et al.*, 1960; Ways *et al.*, 1963). The anaemia in our patient appeared to respond to intramuscular iron and folic acid and presumably was nutritional in origin.

**Unusual Features.** Our patient showed several unexplained features which have not been noted in previous cases, these features being recurrent pulmonary infections, impaired renal function, and aminoaciduria. The recurrent pulmonary infections suggested the possibility of mucoviscidosis but the sweat sodium and chloride concentrations were normal and the stools showed proteolytic activity to a titre of 1 : 300.

The nature of the renal lesions causing impaired renal function and aminoaciduria was not ascertained in our patient. We do not know whether the impaired renal function, renal aminoaciduria, and recurrent pulmonary infections were related to the Bassen-Kornzweig syndrome or not. As these features do not seem to have been present in the 12 previously reported cases with this disease, it is possible that they are unrelated.

A final puzzling feature in our patient was the development of cardiac failure with pulmonary oedema during an episode of bronchitis and asthma. This complication contributed to his death and is unexplained. Schwartz, Rowland, Eder, Marks, Osserman, Anderson, and Hirschberg (1961) in their review of Bassen and Kornzweig's second case mention the presence of cardiomyopathy. Their diagnosis of cardiomyopathy was based on the presence of a loud systolic murmur. Whether cardiomyopathy can occur as a complication of the Bassen-Kornzweig syndrome will only become apparent by study of a greater number of cases. Cardiomyopathy has been reported in other malabsorptive states (McGiven, 1962).

**Aetiology.** Di George *et al.* (1961) have suggested that the clinical and biochemical abnormalities are all secondary to a genetically determined inability to absorb and transport lipids. Salt *et al.* considered that the primary gene defect was inability to form the β-lipoprotein molecule. They found subnormal β-lipoprotein levels in both parents and the paternal grandfather of their patient. However, in the family of the patient we are describing and in several other families reported serum β-lipoprotein levels have been normal (Wolff and Bauman, 1961; Lamy *et al.*, 1963; Ways *et al.*, 1963; Schwartz *et al.*, 1963). These investigations do not confirm the presence of biochemical abnormality in the presumed heterozygous state, but the familial occurrence (Kornzweig and Bassen, 1957) and frequency of parental consanguinity remain as evidence for the disease being due to an autosomal recessive gene. Salt *et al.* also favoured Singer's view that the ocular and nervous disturbances were genetically determined, and speculated that a factor essential for the production of β-lipoprotein was also essential for the normal structure and function of nerve cells. However, they did not dismiss the possibility that these disturbances result from abnormal fat absorption and transport.

## Summary

A 17-month-old Maori child with Bassen-Kornzweig syndrome is described. As well as showing acanthocytosis, a-β-lipoproteinaemia, hypocholesterolaemia, and steatorrhoea, he had incipient neuropathy.

The child also had impairment of renal function, aminoaciduria, and suffered from recurrent pulmonary infections. None of these features appear to have been described in other patients with this disease and therefore they may be unrelated to the primary disorder.

We are most grateful to Dr. R. H. Caughey for permission to publish this case.

We are also grateful to Professor P. H. G. Gel and to Dr. J. F. Soothill, Birmingham Medical School, for generously supplying the specific antiserum used in the immunological studies. We wish to thank Dr. F. H. Sims and staff of the Biochemistry Department, Auckland Hospital, for estimations of carotenoids and serum fatty acid esters.

We are also grateful to Dr. J. A. Malloch, Deputy Superintendent of Waikato Hospital, for permission to publish material from Waikato Hospital records, and to Dr. W. E. Henley, Superintendent-in-Chief, Auckland Hospital Board, for permission to publish material from Auckland Hospital records. Dr. D. H. H. Pullon and Dr. M. Powell kindly supplied clinical information relating to the patient.

### References

Aherne, W. A. (1957). The 'Burr' red cell and azotaemia. *J. clin. Path.*, **10**, 252.

Allison, A. C. (1957). Acute haemolytic anaemia with distortion and fragmentation of erythrocytes in children. *Brit. J. Haemat.*, **3**, 1.

Bassen, F. A., and Kornzweig, A. L. (1950). Malformation of the erythrocytes in a case of atypical retinitis pigmentosa. *Blood*, **5**, 381.

Blumberg, B. S. (1963). Multiple inherited antigenic differences in serum beta-lipoproteins. *Clin. Res.*, **11**, 202.

——, Bernanke, D., and Allison, A. C. (1962). A human lipoprotein polymorphism. *J. clin. Invest.*, **41**, 1936.

Brain, M. C., Dacie, J. V., and Hourihane, D. O'B. (1962). Microangiopathic haemolytic anaemia: the possible role of vascular lesions in pathogenesis. *Brit. J. Haemat.*, **8**, 358.

Dacie, J. V, Mollison, P. L., Richardson, N., Selwyn, J. G., and Shapiro, L. (1953). Atypical congenital haemolytic anaemia. *Quart. J.Med.*, **22**, 79.

Di George, A. M., Mabry, C. C., and Auerbach, V. H. (1961). A specific disorder of lipid transport (acanthrocytosis): Treatment with intravenous lipids. *Amer. J. Dis. Child.*, **102**, 580.

Druez, G. (1959). Un nouveau cas d'acanthocytose. *Rev. Hémat.* **14**, 3.

Friedman, I. S., Cohn, H., Zymaris, M., and Goldner, M. G. (1960). Hypocholesteremia in idiopathic steatorrhea. *Arch. intern. Med.*, **105**, 112.

Havel, R. J., Eder, H. A., and Bragdon, J. H. (1955). The distribution and chemical composition of ultracentrifugally separated lipoproteins in human serum. *J. clin. Invest.*, **34**, 1345.

Jampel, R. S., and Falls, H. F. (1958). Atypical retinitis pigmentosa, acanthrocytosis, and heredodegenerative neuromuscular disease. *Arch. Ophthal.*, **59**, 818.

Kahán, A., Kahán, I. L., and Benkö, A. (1963a). Acquired acanthocytosis and myelophthisis in a case of Eales's disease. *Brit. J. Ophthal.*, **47**, 632.

——, ——, —— (1963b). Erythrocytic anomalies in hereditary vitreo-retinal degeneration (degeneratio hyaloideoretinalis). *ibid.*, **47**, 620.

Kornzweig, A. L., and Bassen, F. A. (1957). Retinitis pigmentosa, acanthrocytosis, and heredodegenerative neuromuscular disease. *Arch. Ophthal.*, **58**, 183.

Lamy, M., Frézal, J., Polonovski, J., Druez, G., and Rey, J. (1963). Congenital absence of beta-lipoproteins. *Pediatrics*, **31**, 277.

——, ——, ——, and Rey, J. (1961). L'absence congénitale de bêta-lipoprotéines. *Presse méd.*, **69**, 1511.

Lock, S. P., and Dormandy, K. M. (1961). Red cell fragmentation syndrome. A condition of multiple aetiology? *Lancet*, **1**, 1020.

Lovric, V. A. (1960). Infantile pyknocytosis occurring in dissimilar twins. *Med. J. Aust.*, **2**, 579.

Mabry, C. C., Di George, A. M., and Auerbach, V. H. (1960). Studies concerning the defect in a patient with acanthrocytosis. *Clin. Res.*, **8**, 371.

Mier, M., Schwartz, S. O., and Boshes, B. (1960). Acanthrocytosis, pigmentary degeneration of the retina and ataxic neuropathy: a genetically determined syndrome with associated metabolic disorder. *Blood*, **16**, 1586.

McGiven, A. R. (1962). Myocardial fibrosis in fibrocystic disease of the pancreas. *Arch. Dis. Childh.*, **37**, 656.

Phillips, G. B. (1962). Quantitative chromatographic analysis of plasma and red blood cell lipids in patients with acanthocytosis. *J. Lab. clin. Med.*, **59**, 357.

Sackett, G. E. (1925). Modification of Bloor's method for the determination of the cholesterol in whole blood or blood serum. *J. biol. Chem.*, **64**, 203.

Salt, H. B., Wolff, O. H., Lloyd, J. K., Fosbrooke, A. S., Cameron, A. H., and Hubble, D. V. (1960). On having no beta-lipoprotein. A syndrome comprising a-beta-lipoproteinaemia, acanthocytosis and steatorrhoea. *Lancet*, **2**, 325.

Schwartz, J. F., Rowland, L. P., Eder, H. A., Marks, P. A., Osserman, E., Anderson, H., and Hirschberg, E. (1961). Bassen-Kornzweig syndrome: neuromuscular disorder resembling Friedreich's ataxia. *Trans. Amer. neurol. Ass.*, **86**, 49.

——, ——, ——, ——, ——, Hirschberg, E., and Anderson, H. (1963). Bassen-Kornzweig syndrome: Deficiency of serum beta-lipoprotein. *Arch. Neurol. (Chic.)*, **8**, 438.

Schwartz, S. O., and Motto, S. A. (1949). The diagnostic signficance of 'burr' red blood cells. *Amer. J. med. Sci.*, **218**, 563.

Shumway, C. N., Jr., and Miller, G. (1957). An unusual syndrome of hemolytic anemia, thrombocytopenic purpura and renal disease. *Blood*, **12**, 1045.

Singer, K., Fisher, B., and Perlstein, M. A. (1952). Acanthrocytosis: a genetic erythrocytic malformation. *ibid.*, **7**, 577.

Soothill, J. F. (1962). Estimation of eight serum proteins by a gel diffusion precipitin technique. *J. Lab. clin. Med.*, **59**, 859.

Switzer, S., and Eder, H. A. (1962). Interconversion of acanthocytes and normal erythrocytes with detergents. *J. clin. Invest.*, **41**, 1404.

Tuffy, P., Brown, A. K., and Zuelzer, W. W. (1959). Infantile pyknocytosis. *Amer. J. Dis. Child.*, **98**, 227.

Walton, K. W., and Scott, P. J. (1964). Estimations of the low-density (beta) lipoproteins of serum in health and disease using large molecular weight dextran sulphate. *J. clin. Path.*, **17**, 627.

Ways, P., Reed, C. F., and Hanahan, D. J. (1963). Red cell and plasma lipids in acanthocytosis. *J. clin. Invest.*, **42**, 1248.

Wolff, J. A., and Bauman, W. A. (1961). Studies concerning acanthocytosis: A new genetic syndrome with absent beta lipoprotein. *Amer. J. Dis. Child.*, **102**, 478.

*Arch. Dis. Childh.*, 1965, **40**, 47.

# A-β-LIPOPROTEINAEMIA

BY

CONSTANCE C. FORSYTH, JUNE K. LLOYD, and AUDREY S. FOSBROOKE
*From the Department of Child Health, University of St. Andrews, Queen's College, Dundee, and the Department of Paediatrics and Child Health, University of Birmingham*

(RECEIVED FOR PUBLICATION SEPTEMBER 28, 1964)

Absence of β-lipoprotein from the serum was reported by Salt, Wolff, Lloyd, Fosbrooke, Cameron, and Hubble (1960) in a child who had steatorrhoea and acanthocytosis. Simultaneously and independently, Lamy, Frézal, Polonovski, and Rey (1960) and Mabry, Di George, and Auerbach (1960) made similar observations. Three of the earlier cases of steatorrhoea with acanthocytosis, retinopathy, and disease of the central nervous system (Bassen and Kornzweig, 1950; Kornzweig and Bassen, 1957; Druez, 1959) have subsequently been shown to have a-β-lipoproteinaemia (Phillips, 1962; Schwartz, Rowland, Eder, Marks, Osserman, Anderson, and Hirschberg, 1961; Schwartz, Rowland, Eder, Marks, Osserman, Hirschberg, and Anderson, 1963; Druez, Lamy, Frézal, Polonovski, and Rey, 1961), and the case reported by Singer, Fisher, and Perlstein (1952) was later found to have a serum cholesterol level of 37 mg./100 ml. and a very low level of β-globulin (Jampel and Falls, 1958) so that even in retrospect the diagnosis of a-β-lipoproteinaemia can be confidently made. Further cases have been reported by Friedman, Cohn, Zymaris, and Goldner (1960); Mier, Schwartz, and Boshes (1960); Wolff and Bauman (1961); Ways, Reed, and Hanahan (1961); Kuo and Bassett (1962); and Schwartz *et al.* (1963). This paper describes another example of this rare syndrome.

## Case Report

A.L., a boy, was born in Dundee, on April 8, 1956 after a normal pregnancy and labour and weighed 7 lb. 6 oz. (3,345 g.). He was breast fed for two weeks and then given half cream Ostermilk until the age of 4 months when full cream liquid cows' milk was introduced. At the age of 3 weeks he was noted to be passing four to five loose stools daily. The diarrhoea persisted and he failed to gain weight normally. At the age of 20 months he was referred to hospital when his weight was 14 lb. 7 oz. (6,548 g.) and his length 27 in. He could neither crawl nor stand and was wasted and hypotonic, with a distended abdomen (Fig. 1). In addition minor congenital abnormalities of the toes were noted. He passed two to three large, pale, offensive stools daily and vomited at least once daily. The tuberculin skin test, chest radiograph, sweat sodium and chloride concentrations, and tryptic activity of the duodenal juice were all normal. The serum cholesterol was 29 mg./100 ml., the serum albumin 4·7 g./100 ml. and globulin 1·5 g./100 ml. The serum

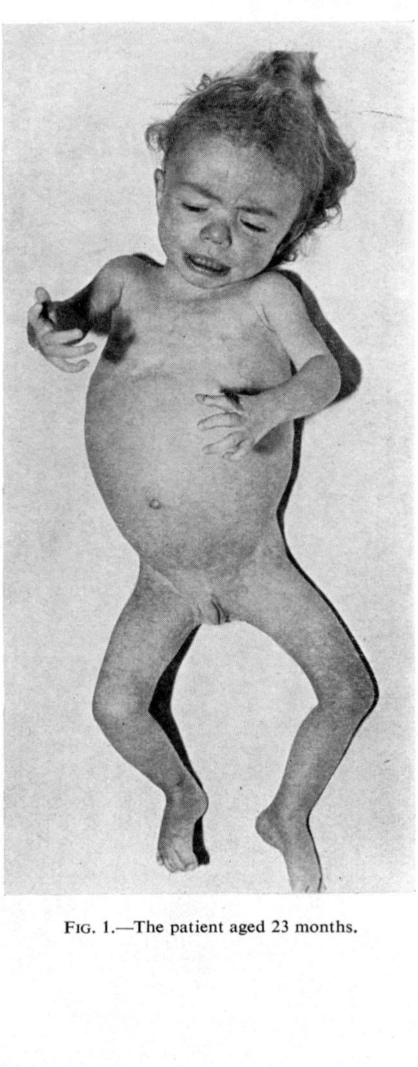

FIG. 1.—The patient aged 23 months.

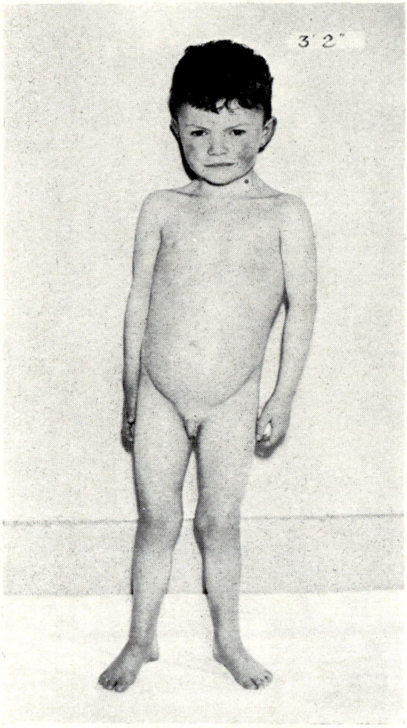


FIG. 2.—The patient aged 7 years.

sodium, chloride, potassium, $CO_2$ combining power, bilirubin, urea, and thymol turbidity were all normal. The haemoglobin was 11·1 g./100 ml., and the blood film showed anisocytosis with both microcytosis and macrocytosis, poikilocytosis, and hypochromia. It was impossible to perform a fat balance study owing to severe vomiting and diarrhoea and a clinical diagnosis of coeliac disease was made though the onset of diarrhoea in early infancy was considered to be unusual. He was treated with a gluten-free diet. During the next six months he had many intercurrent infections, failed to gain weight, and developed mild radiological rickets with a serum calcium of 7·9 mg./100 ml. and alkaline phosphatase of 47 King-Armstrong units/100 ml. The haemoglobin fell to 9·3 g./100 ml. The rickets responded to 4,000 i.u. of oral vitamin D (Abidec 2·4 ml.) daily, and the anaemia to intramuscular iron and folic acid. Subsequently oral iron (27·5 mg. elemental iron) and vitamin D 1,000 i.u. with vitamin A 5,000 i.u. daily (Abidec 0·6 ml.) were continued. His haemoglobin thereafter was above 13·0 g./100 ml. He did not, however, respond to a gluten-free diet, remaining physically retarded (Fig. 2) with a bone age of 4 years at the age of 7 years. In addition he was mentally retarded with an intelligence quotient of 65 when tested at 5 years and again at 7 years. An electroencephalogram was normal.

When, at the age of 7 years, the serum cholesterol level was again found to be very low—29 mg./100 ml.—the diagnosis of a-β-lipoproteinaemia was considered and confirmed by the failure to demonstrate β-lipoprotein in the serum by paper or immunoelectrophoresis. The

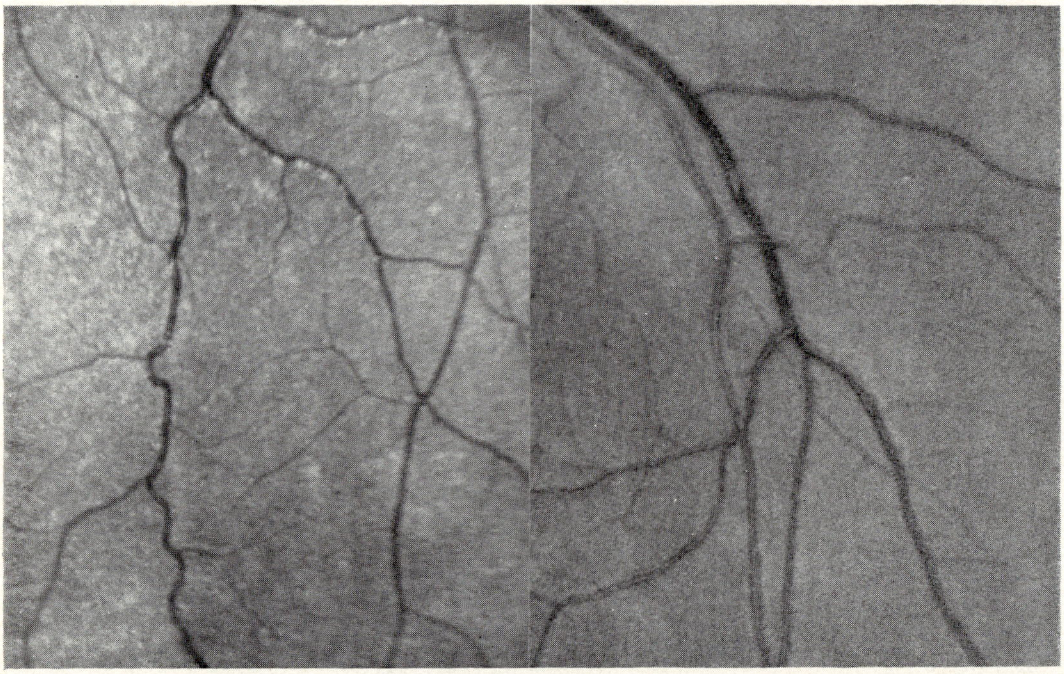

FIG. 3.—Retinal photograph at the age of 7 years showing, on the left, abnormality of choroidal pigment; the appearances are compared with a normal control on the right.

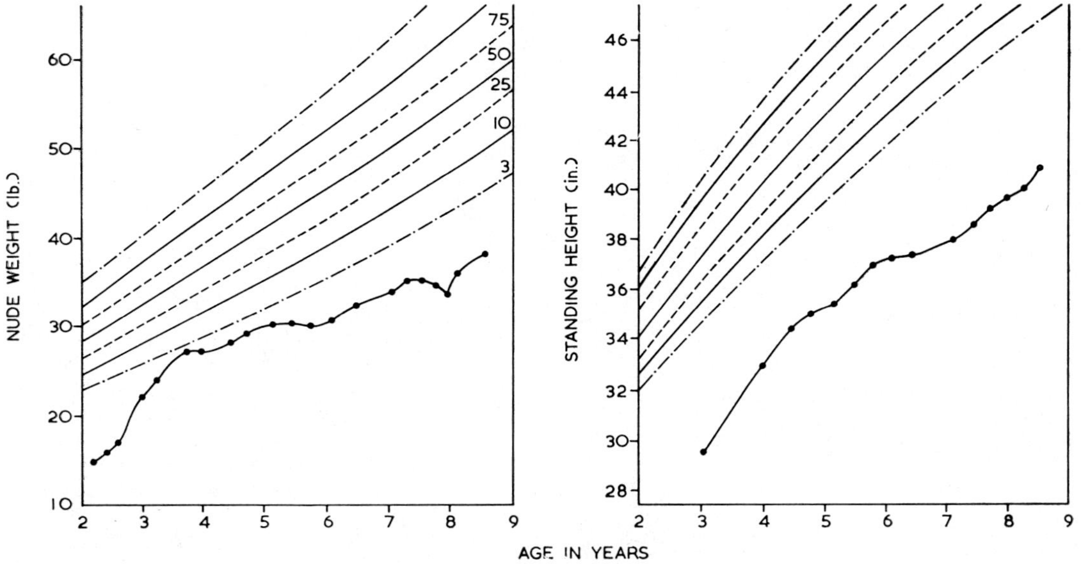


FIG. 4.—Height and weight charts.

analytical methods used were the same as those already described (Salt *et al.*, 1960), and the serum was obtained after an overnight fast. The total amount of lipid was very low and the composition of the lipid present was similar to that of α-lipoprotein, containing more phospholipid (53%) than cholesterol (26%). Immunoelectrophoresis confirmed the presence of α-lipoprotein. Carotenoids were absent, and the level of vitamin A depleted in spite of the fact that the patient was receiving additional vitamin A at the time of investigation. Details of the serum lipid investigations are given in the Table. A fresh wet preparation of blood showed the presence of acanthocytes and failure of rouleaux formation. The failure to form rouleaux was reflected in the erythrocyte sedimentation rate which failed to show any fall in the first hour. The faecal fat excretion averaged 5 g. daily over a 10-day period (84% absorption). An oral glucose tolerance test was normal, serum folate was slightly depleted (3 μg./ml.), vitamin $B_{12}$ was normal (420 μμg./ml.), and the prothrombin time was 20 seconds (control 15 seconds). Urinary 17-oxosteroids were 1·5 mg. in 24 hours and 17-hydroxycorticosteroids 4·5 mg. in 24 hours. The chromosomes of peripheral blood cells appeared normal. The retinae showed an abnormality of choroidal pigment in the equatorial region of the fundi (Fig. 3). Visual acuity was 6/9 in each eye and visual fields full. No gross abnormality in dark adaptation could be demonstrated. Neurological examination revealed no abnormalities apart from diminution of the knee and ankle-jerks and slight pes cavus of the right foot. During the following six months he developed further evidence of a neurological lesion in the legs: a slightly stepping gait, more marked pes cavus of the right foot, and the knee and ankle-jerks could no longer be elicited. There has been no further deterioration in his condition.

Following diagnosis at the age of 7 years and 3 months supplementary iron therapy was continued and vitamin A was increased to 20,000 units daily of a water miscible preparation (Abidec 2·4 ml.). After three months the gluten-free diet was replaced by a normal diet containing approximately 40 g. of fat daily. Neither of these measures influenced the clinical picture or rate of growth (Fig. 4). After a further three months a low fat diet (approximately 20 g. daily) was started and though the bulk of his stools has been reduced, his rate of growth has not increased to date. The serum vitamin A level after one year's treatment with 20,000 units of vitamin A daily was still below normal (72 i.u./100 ml.) and the dose of vitamin A has, therefore, been increased to 40,000 units daily.

**Family Study**

Fig. 5 shows the family tree. The parents, both aged 36 years, are first cousins, the paternal grandfather and maternal grandmother being sibs. We were able to examine serum from both parents, the maternal grandmother, three of the mother's sibs and one of the father's sisters. None of these relatives had visual, neurological, or alimentary symptoms, and the wet blood films of the parents were normal. In all cases the blood samples were obtained in the fasting state and the results of the investigations are summarized in the Table. In no instance was a low level of total lipid or β-lipoprotein found. In both parents, the maternal grandmother, and two of the mother's sibs increased concentrations of total lipid, cholesterol, and β-lipoprotein were found. α-lipoprotein in these individuals tended to be depleted and

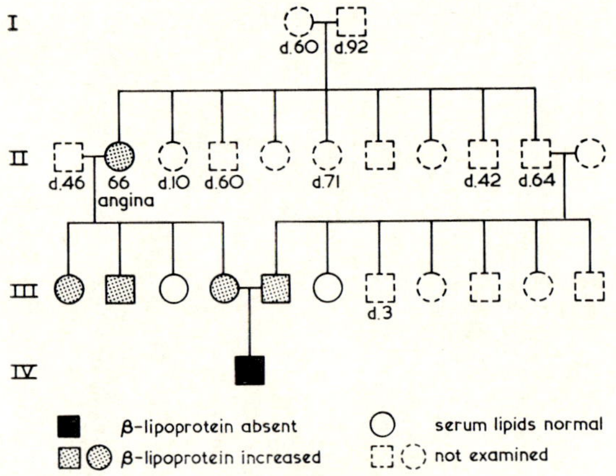


FIG. 5.—Family tree.

the β-α ratio raised. Separation of the mother's serum by density gradient ultracentrifuging (Cornwell, Kruger, Hamwi, and Brown, 1961) confirmed the increased concentration of $S_f$ 3-9 (β) lipoprotein. The one paternal aunt examined and a maternal aunt had a normal lipid pattern.

## Discussion

Symptoms due to steatorrhoea are one of the first manifestations of a-β-lipoproteinaemia and estimation of the serum cholesterol in all children with steatorrhoea is an important screening test. In most cases of a-β-lipoproteinaemia levels of 20-40 mg./100 ml. are found and such low levels are usually diagnostic. In a few patients, however, higher values up to 90 mg./100 ml. are reported (Schwartz *et al.*, 1961; Druez, 1959; Ways, Reed, and Hanahan, 1963; Schwartz *et al.*, 1963) and such levels may sometimes be found in coeliac disease and in cystic fibrosis. In both the latter conditions, however, β-lipoprotein can be demonstrated by paper and immunoelectrophoresis. The appearance of the intestinal mucosa is quite distinct from that seen in coeliac disease; the villi are clearly defined but the columnar cells have unusually clear cytoplasm, and frozen sections stained for fat show an accumulation of lipid in these cells (Mabry *et al.*, 1960; Lamy, Frézal, Polonovski, and Rey, 1961; Wolff, 1962). Mabry *et al.* suggest that this appearance is diagnostic. It has been shown that chylomicrons do not appear in the blood after the ingestion of fat (Salt *et al.*, 1960), and the accumulated lipid in the mucosal cells is unabsorbed triglyceride (Ways and Parmentier, 1963). Frézal, Rey, Polonovski, Lévy, and Lamy (1961) found no improvement in fat absorption when normal serum β-lipoprotein levels had been achieved by means of exchange transfusion, and the mechanism of the fat absorption defect remains obscure.

Acanthocytes may be missed in stained blood films, where they are usually mistaken for crenated red cells, but are easily identified in a fresh wet preparation. Phillips (1962) and Ways *et al.* (1963) have shown that though the total amount of lipid in the red cell membrane is normal, the lipid composition is altered, with a relative increase in sphingomyelin and a decrease in lecithin. These workers have also found similar alterations in the serum phospholipids. It has been shown that free exchange occurs between the phospholipids of the red cells and those in the serum (James, Lovelock, and Webb, 1957), and it is possible that the changes in the red cell membrane may be secondary to the serum lipid abnormalities. Di George, Mabry, and Auerbach (1961) showed that normally shaped red cells could be produced in a patient after prolonged intravenous fat infusion (Lipomul), acanthocytes being formed again on cessation of treatment, but Switzer and Eder (1962) have demonstrated that a detergent (Tween 80) is the

TABLE

SERUM LIPIDS AND LIPOPROTEINS IN THE PATIENT AND MEMBERS OF HIS FAMILY

| Subject | Patient | Mother | Father | Grand-mother (Maternal) | Aunt (Maternal) | Uncle (Maternal) | Aunt (Maternal) | Aunt (Paternal) | Normal Range |
|---|---|---|---|---|---|---|---|---|---|
| Age (yr.) | 7 | 36 | 36 | 65 | 43 | 39 | 30 | 28 | |
| *Serum lipids:* | | | | | | | | | |
| Total lipid (mg./100 ml.) .. | 110 | 900 | 1000 | 980 | 900 | 990 | 750 | 730 | 470–860 |
| Cholesterol (mg./100 ml.) .. | 29 | 328 | 318 | 308 | 275 | 282 | 254 | 214 | 120–250 |
| Phospholipid (mg./100 ml.) .. | 58 | 257 | 287 | | | | | | 160–310 |
| Vitamin A (i.u./100 ml.) .. | 55 | 125 | 200 | | | | | | 80–180 |
| Carotenoid (μg./100 ml.) .. | Nil | 41 | 71 | | | | | | 60–260 |
| *Serum lipoproteins** | | | | | | | | | |
| ω lipoprotein (mg./100 ml.) .. | Absent | 94 | 104 | 137 | 78 | 125 | 61 | 63 | 0–105 |
| β lipoprotein (mg./100 ml.) .. | Absent | 612 | 770 | 720 | 599 | 782 | 480 | 500 | 300–580 |
| α lipoprotein (mg./100 ml.) .. | 110 | 164 | 127 | 123 | 223 | 83 | 209 | 168 | 150–280 |
| β-α ratio .. .. .. .. | | 3·7 | 6·0 | 5·9 | 2·7 | 9·4 | 2·3 | 3·0 | 1·5–3·0 |

* As lipid by paper electrophoresis.

constituent of Lipomul which produces this change. Ways *et al.* (1963) discussing the aetiology of the red cell defect suggest that a primary abnormality of the red cell membrane, or a combination of a primary membrane abnormality and exchange between serum lipids and red cells, might be responsible for their abnormal shape. At present they prefer to use the term acanthocytosis rather than a-β-lipoproteinaemia to describe the condition.

It is only possible to speculate about the pathogenesis of the neurological lesions and the retinitis, as no direct examination of nervous tissue has been made. Most of the proteins of nervous tissue are present as lipoproteins, and it has been shown that they are metabolically active and not inert as previously assumed. Furthermore, the turnover rates of the different brain phospholipids vary and are probably slower for those in the myelin sheath Gaitonde, 1963). In two other rare syndromes in which retinitis pigmentosa is a feature (Refsum syndrome and Hooft syndrome) hypolipidaemia has been reported, though β-lipoprotein is present (Harders and Dieckmann, 1964; Hooft, De Laey, Herpol, De Loore, and Verbeeck, 1962), and we speculate that prolonged exposure of retinal and/or nerve cells to serum deficient in lipoproteins may result in impairment of cell function and ultimate degeneration. It is unlikely that the changes are due solely to low serum levels of vitamin A, since in one patient with a-β-lipoproteinaemia, in whom normal levels have been maintained since the age of 22 months, retinal changes appeared at the age of 5 years (Wolff, Lloyd, and Tonks, 1965). In our patient additional vitamin A had been given for several years before diagnosis at which time the serum level though low (55 i.u./100 ml.) was not grossly depleted, and yet by the age of 7 years he had developed retinitis and neurological signs. We cannot, however, exclude the possibility that low levels of vitamin A may contribute in part to retinal degeneration, as Campbell and Tonks (1962) have demonstrated reduced levels of vitamin A in the serum of some patients with retinitis pigmentosa.

Mental retardation has been reported in three other patients, (Druez *et al.*, 1961; Lamy *et al.*, 1960; Singer *et al.*, 1952), but in the majority of cases intelligence has remained normal. It is of interest that, like our patient, those with mental retardation come from families in which consanguinity has occurred. In those with normal intelligence only one has a history of consanguinity, the parents being fourth cousins (Schwartz *et al.*, 1963). The original report that the parents of Bassen and Kornzweig's cases were cousins has since been denied (Schwartz *et al.*, 1963).

Family studies have shown no clinical or haematological features in any of the presumed heterozygotes. Salt *et al.* (1960) found β-lipoprotein levels reduced to about half the normal value in both parents and a grandparent of their patient, but this abnormality has not been found in the relatives of the other patients. The finding of increased concentrations of β-lipoprotein in several of the relatives including both parents of our patient was unexpected, and we are unable to explain the relation between this finding and the absence of β-lipoprotein in the patient. Kuo and Bassett (1962) report slight increases in $S_f$ 0-12 (β) lipoproteins in the mother of an adult with hypo-β-lipoproteinaemia; fatty acid chromatography of the serum and red cell lipids showed a normal pattern.

Treatment remains symptomatic. A low fat diet has been successful in relieving the intestinal symptoms and in improving growth and development in the patients of Salt *et al.* (1960) and Lamy, Frézal, Palonovski, Druez, and Rey (1963). Kuo and Bassett (1962) report clinical improvement in their adult patient by elimination of dairy and meat fats from the diet and by the supplementation of 60 g. of corn oil daily, emulsified with Tween 80. Normal serum vitamin A levels can be maintained by giving large doses of a water miscible preparation (Wolff *et al.*, 1965).

## Summary

A 7-year-old boy who presented with diarrhoea in early infancy was found to have a-β-lipoproteinaemia. The typical features of the syndrome, i.e. steatorrhoea, acanthocytosis, retinal degenerative changes, and an ataxic neuropathy were all present. He was also mentally retarded, a finding reported in three other patients with this condition. His parents' marriage was consanguineous and the serum from several relatives including both parents showed increased concentrations of β-lipoprotein.

The pathogenesis of the various features is discussed and it is suggested that prolonged absence of β-lipoprotein from the serum may play a part in the changes found in the erythrocytes, retina, and central nervous system.

It is a pleasure to thank Dr. O. H. Wolff for his interest and encouragement, Dr. A. K. Tulloch for his assessment of visual function, Mr. F. M. Duncan for the retinal photographs, and Miss E. L. Tonks for the serum vitamin A and carotenoid estimations. We are grateful to the Medical Research Council for financial assistance.

References

Bassen, F. A., and Kornzweig, A. L. (1950). Malformation of the erythrocytes in a case of atypical retinitis pigmentosa. *Blood*, **5**, 381.

Campbell, D. A., and Tonks, E. L. (1962). Biochemical findings in human retinitis pigmentosa with particular relation to vitamin A deficiency. *Brit. J. Ophthal.*, **46**, 151.

Cornwell, D. G., Kruger, F. A., Hamwi, G. J., and Brown, J. B. (1961). Studies on the characterization of human serum lipoproteins separated by ultra-centrifugation in a density gradient. *Amer. J. clin. Nutr.*, **9**, 24.

Di George, A. M., Mabry, C. C., and Auerbach, V. H. (1961). A specific disorder of lipid transport (acanthrocytosis): treatment with intravenous lipids. *Amer. J. Dis. Child.*, **102**, 580.

Druez, G. (1959). Un nouveau cas d'acanthocytose: dysmorphie érythrocytaire congénitale avec rétinite, troubles nerveux et stigmates dégénératifs. *Rev. Hémat.*, **14**, 3.

——, Lamy, M., Frézal, J., Polonovski, J., and Rey, J. (1961). L'acanthocytose: ses rapports avec l'absence congénitale de bêtalipoprotéines. *Presse méd.*, **69**, 1546.

Frézal, J., Rey, J., Polonovski, J., Lévy, G., and Lamy, M. (1961). L'absence congénitale de β-lipoprotéines: étude de l'absorption des graisses après exsanguino-transfusion: mesure de la demi-vie des β-lipoprotéines injectées. *Rev. franç. Étud. clin. biol.*, **6**, 677.

Friedman, I. S., Cohn, H., Zymaris, M., and Goldner, M. G. (1960). Hypocholesterolemia in idiopathic steatorrhea. *Arch. intern. Med.*, **105**, 112.

Gaitonde, M. K. (1963). The turnover of proteolipids and phosphatido-peptides in the brain. In *Brain Lipids and Lipoproteins, and the Leucodystrophies*, ed. J. Folch-Pi, and H. Bauer, p. 42. Elsevier, Amsterdam.

Harders, H., and Dieckmann, H. (1964). Heredopathia atactica polyneuritiformis. *Dtsch. med. Wschr.*, **89**, 248.

Hooft, C., De Laey, P., Herpol, J., De Loore, F., and Verbeeck, J. (1962). Familial hypolipidaemia and retarded development without steatorrhoea. *Helv. paediat. Acta*, **17**, 1.

James, A. T., Lovelock, J. E., and Webb, J. (1957). The biosynthesis of fatty acids by human red blood cells. *Biochem. J.*, **66**, 60P.

Jampel, R. S., and Falls, H. F. (1958). Atypical retinitis pigmentosa, acanthrocytosis, and heredodegenerative neuromuscular disease. *Arch. Ophthal.*, **59**, 818.

Kornzweig, A. L., and Bassen, F. A. (1957). Retinitis pigmentosa, acanthrocytosis, and heredodegenerative neuromuscular disease. *ibid.*, **58**, 183.

Kuo, P. T., and Bassett, D. R. (1962). Blood and tissue lipids in a family with hypo-beta-lipoproteinemia. *Circulation*, **26**, 660.

Lamy, M., Frézal, J., Polonovski, J., Druez G., and Rey, J. (1963). Congenital absence of beta-lipoproteins. *Pediatrics*, 31, 277.

——, ——, ——, and Rey, J. (1960). L'absence congénitale de β-lipoprotéines. *C.R. Soc. Biol. (Paris)*, **154**, 1974.

——, ——, ——, —— (1961). L'absence congénitale de bêtalipoprotéines. *Presse méd.*, **69**, 1511.

Mabry, C. C., Di George, A. M., and Auerbach, V. H. (1960). Studies concerning the defect in a patient with acanthrocytosis. *Clin. Res.*, **8**, 371.

Mier, M., Schwartz, S. O., and Boshes, B. (1960). Acanthrocytosis, pigmentary degeneration of the retina and ataxic neuropathy: a genetically determined syndrome with associated metabolic disorder. *Blood*, **16**, 1586.

Phillips, G. B. (1962). Quantitative chromatographic analysis of plasma and red blood cell lipids in patients with acanthocytosis. *J. Lab. clin. Med.*, **59**, 357.

Salt, H. B., Wolff, O. H., Lloyd, J. K., Fosbrooke, A. S., Cameron, A. H., and Hubble, D. V. (1960). On having no beta-lipoprotein; a syndrome comprising a-beta-lipoproteinaemia, acanthocytosis, and steatorrhoea. *Lancet*, **2**, 325.

Schwartz, J. F., Rowland, L. P., Eder, H. A., Marks, P. M., Osserman, E., Anderson, H., and Hirschberg, E. (1961). Bassen-Kornzweig syndrome: Neuromuscular disorder resembling Friedreich's ataxia associated with retinitis pigmentosa, acanthocytosis, steatorrhoea, and an abnormality of lipid metabolism. *Trans. Amer. neurol. Ass.*, **86**, 49.

——, ——, ——, ——, ——, Hirschberg, E., and Anderson, H. (1963). Bassen-Kornzweig syndrome: deficiency of serum β-lipoprotein. *Arch. Neurol. (Chic.)*, **8**, 438.

Singer, K., Fisher, B., and Perlstein, M. A. (1952). Acanthrocytosis: a genetic erythrocyte malformation. *Blood*, 7, 577.

Switzer, S., and Eder, H. A. (1962). Interconversion of acanthocytes and normal erythrocytes with detergents. *J. clin. Invest.*, **41**, 1404.

Ways, P., and Parmentier, C. (1963). G.I. mucosal lipids in acanthocytosis. *Clin. Res.*, **11**, 77.

——, Reed, C. F., and Hanahan, D. J. (1961). Abnormalities of erythrocyte and plasma lipids in acanthocytosis. *J. clin. Invest.*, **40**, 1088.

——, ——, —— (1963). Red cell and plasma lipids in acanthocytosis. *ibid.*, **42**, 1248.

Wolff, J. A., and Bauman, W. A. (1961). Studies concerning acanthocytosis: a new genetic syndrome with absent beta lipoprotein. *Amer. J. Dis. Child.*, **102**, 478.

Wolff, O. H. (1962). A-beta-lipoproteinaemia. In *Erbliche Stoffwechsel-Drankheiten*, ed. F. Linneweh, p. 603. Urban and Schwarzenberg, Berlin.

——, Lloyd, J. K., and Tonks, E. L. (1965). A-β-lipoproteinaemia: with special reference to the visual defect. *Exp. Eye Res.* In the press.

*Arch. Dis. Childh.*, 1965, **40**, 53.

# MEGALOBLASTIC ANAEMIA IN PREMATURE INFANTS

BY

O. P. GRAY and E. BLANCHE BUTLER

*From the Departments of Child Health and Obstetrics, Welsh National School of Medicine*

(RECEIVED FOR PUBLICATION FEBRUARY 18, 1964)

The common anaemia in premature infants is iron deficiency anaemia, but megaloblastic anaemia can also occur and here we report three such cases. Our interest in megaloblastic anaemia was stimulated by a recent case in which megaloblastic anaemia developed when a low phenylalanine diet was being given for treatment of phenylketonuria (Royston and Parry, 1962). In the discussion of this paper Royston and Parry advocated the need for more frequent marrow biopsy in the unexplained anaemias of infancy. As a result of this policy we have discovered the following cases in premature infants.

## Case Reports

**Case 1.** A male infant weighing 850 g. was born on November 12, 1962, the third child in the family. The mother was aged 39 years and her pregnancy had ended prematurely at 29 weeks. During the pregnancy the mother herself had suffered from a severe iron deficiency anaemia. This was not diagnosed until November 6, 1962 when she presented with a haemoglobin level of 6·6 g./100 ml. Her diet had been adequate but she had received no supplementary iron during pregnancy. She was admitted on November 8, 1962 for a course of parenteral iron but she was already draining liquor and went into labour spontaneously three days later. By this time she had received 850 mg. of parenteral iron and 1,100 ml. blood were transfused when labour began. The foetal heart was not heard for an hour before birth and the chance of survival seemed slight, but a live child in a fairly good condition was born. As the mother's membranes had been ruptured for four days the infant was given oral erythromycin stearate 40 mg./day for the first week. During the first 36 hours he showed mild respiratory distress, and the maximum Silverman score (Silverman and Andersen, 1956) was 4. He became mildly jaundiced but the serum bilirubin did not rise above 14 mg./100 ml. On the fifth day he was noted to have developed some lower sternal retraction, and two days later crepitations were heard on the right side of the chest. He improved and progress was normal until the 14th day. Then his colour became a little dusky at times, the insuction increased, the respiratory rate rose to 60 a minute, and there were fine crepitations again on the right side. He was given intramuscular streptomycin sulphate and a further course of oral erythromycin stearate as he was thought to have a bronchopneumonia; but response to this treatment was poor and he was therefore given cloxacillin, and $\gamma$-globulin 250 mg. At this time coliform organisms were isolated from the umbilicus and from gastric washings. On the 24th day the haemoglobin level was 12·1 g./100 ml., but in the following week there was a rapid fall and at the age of 30 days the haemoglobin was 7·7 g., RBC 2,030,000/c.mm., haematocrit 24%, MCV 116 c.$\mu$, MCH 37·5 $\mu\mu$g., MCHC 32%. The white cell count was 8,000/c.mm. with 2 nucleated red cells per 100 white cells. The red cells in the blood film showed anisocytosis and poikilocytosis, and many macrocytes were present. Red cell precursors were seen in the blood film and in the buffy coat; these were mainly normoblastic in type but many were atypical with eccentric nuclei or double nuclei, and a few contained Howell Jolly bodies. A few cells showed nuclei transitional in type between the normoblast and megaloblast pattern. White cell changes were not prominent in this case.

The bone marrow was examined on the 33rd day, and erythropoiesis was found to be mainly megaloblastic in type. Occasional giant metamyelocytes were seen. Blood taken later the following day showed a serum folate level of 3·0 $\mu\mu$g./ml. and a serum vitamin B12 level of 134 $\mu\mu$g./ml. On the 33rd day the child was, therefore, given folic acid 10 mg. intramuscularly, and treatment was continued with folic acid 10 mg./day orally for the next three weeks. The maximum reticulocyte count was 32% and this was reached on the sixth day of treatment (the 39th day of life). This coincided with a marked improvement in the child's condition; a systolic murmur, previously heard, had gone, the insuction was no longer present, and the respiratory rate had dropped to 33 a minute. The haemoglobin rose initially and reached a level of 10·2 g./100 ml. on the 51st day, but there was a further slight fall, and by the 64th day the haemoglobin was stationary at 8·9 g. The reticulocyte count was 9·2%. A blood film examined at this time showed evidence of iron deficiency and this was treated with parenteral iron 25 mg. on alternate days to a total of 75 mg. The vitamin B12 level was again estimated and found to be 132 $\mu\mu$g./ml. This was still below the lower limit of normal as given by Boger, Bayne, Wright, and Beck (1957) and therefore vitamin B12 300 $\mu$g. intramuscularly was given over a period of one week. Fig. 1 shows the haemoglobin and reticulocyte response to folic acid.

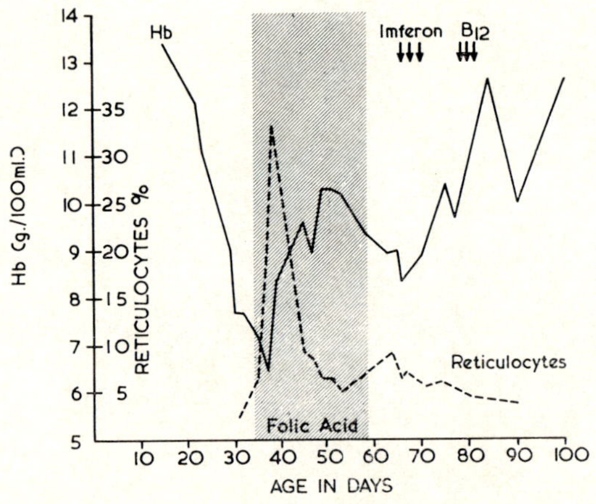


FIG. 1.—Case 1. The marked reticulocyte and haemoglobin response to folic acid, followed by a later haemoglobin rise after Imferon.

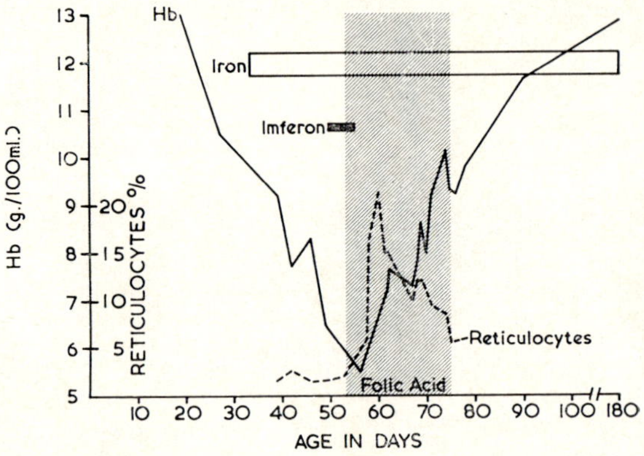


FIG. 2.—Case 2. Hb and reticulocyte response to folic acid.

**Case 2.** (This was the second case briefly mentioned by Parry, 1963). A male infant weighing 1,000 g. was born on December 1, 1961. The mother was 34 years and she had a severe pre-eclamptic toxaemia which necessitated delivery by caesarean section at the 33rd week. The infant's condition was good at birth and he progressed well until the 14th day. He then developed insuction, the respiratory rate rose to 60 a minute and at times his colour was dusky. He was treated as a chest infection with 'albamycin-T,' but the insuction became worse, though at this time there were no added sounds in the lungs. By the 40th day coarse râles were heard in the chest and coliform organisms were isolated from the nose and stomach washings. The temperature rose to 38° C., and a systolic murmur was heard. On the 48th day the haemoglobin level was found to have fallen to 6·5 g./100 ml. (44%), RBC 2,000,000/c.mm., haematocrit 22%, MCV 110 c.$\mu$, MCH 77 $\mu\mu$g., MCHC 29%, WBC 8,700/c.mm., platelets 500,000/c.mm. A number of nucleated red cells were seen in the blood film and, though the majority of these were normoblastic in type, some contained Howell Jolly bodies and a few showed a nuclear structure very similar to that seen in megaloblasts. In addition occasional multisegmented polymorphs were seen. The bone marrow was examined on the 50th day and this confirmed the presence of megaloblastic erythropoiesis, and many giant metamyelocytes were found. Blood taken at this time showed a serum vitamin B12 level of 334 $\mu\mu$g./ml. (facilities were not then available for serum folate estimations). Treatment with folic acid 20 mg./day was begun on the 54th day and continued for three weeks. The maximum reticulocyte count was 21·5% and was reached on the 7th day after starting treatment (the 61st day of life), but insuction was less by the fourth day and had disappeared entirely after two weeks. Further progress in this case was uneventful. The marrow examination was repeated 9 days after beginning folic acid and in this specimen normoblastic erythropoiesis was seen, though occasional giant metamyelocytes were still present. Fig. 2 shows the haemoglobin and reticulocyte response to folic acid.

**Case 3.** A boy weighing 1,150 g. was born on July 29, 1963. The mother had an antepartum haemorrhage at the 32nd week of her pregnancy and following this went into premature labour. The child's condition at birth was poor, the Apgar (1953) score being only 4, but he was resuscitated and had normal spontaneous respiratory movements at 5 minutes. He then developed the respiratory distress syndrome and within an hour of birth needed treatment with intravenous sodium bicarbonate for associated acidosis. He was also anaemic with a haemoglobin of 8·9 g./100 ml. There was no obvious cause for the anaemia, the mother's blood group was O Rh +ve, and no antibodies were found during pregnancy; the infant's blood group was O Rh +ve. It was thought that there had been a haemorrhage from the foetal side of the placenta at the time of the antepartum haemorrhage. The mother's liquor was draining for six days before delivery and so the child was given intramuscular streptomycin sulphate and oral erythromycin stearate for 5 days. He made a slow but satisfactory recovery from the respiratory distress syndrome, but for a fortnight he was hypotonic and lying in the frog position. During this time the haemoglobin level rose to 11·3 g., presumably a response to the anaemia at birth. It then began to fall again, and by the 19th day was 8·1 g. Insuction was also present and a few crepitations appeared over the left upper chest, and so the child was again given oral erythromycin stearate. He became more lethargic and on the 24th day he had the first of several severe apnoeic attacks which lasted for about 5 minutes. The blood picture on the 21st day was as follows: Hb 7·7 g./100 ml., RBC 1,970,000/c.mm., haematocrit 21%, MCV 107 c.$\mu$, MCH 39 $\mu\mu$g., MCHC 36%, reticulocytes 1·6%. Megaloblasts, transitional cells, and atypical normoblasts were seen in the blood film and in the buffy coat. Macrocytes and macro-ovalocytes were present but, as in

Case 1, white cell changes were minimal. Marrow biopsy was taken on the 25th day, and though this was a poor specimen, it was possible to confirm the presence of megaloblasts. Blood was taken for vitamin B12 and serum folate levels, but because of a technical error only the serum B12 level was estimated; this was 182 $\mu\mu$g./ml.

Treatment was started with folic acid on the 24th day, 4 mg./day. The maximum reticulocyte count was only 7·4% in this case, but the extent of the reticulocytosis was obscured as a blood transfusion was given. This became necessary because the apnoeic attacks were coincident with the increasing anaemia and threatened the child's life. It is our belief that cerebral hypoxia is one of the factors in apnoeic attacks in infants, and so the anaemia was thought to be largely responsible for these attacks. We felt unable to wait for the natural response to folic acid to relieve the situation, and so gave a small blood transfusion of 20 ml. on the 26th day; a further 35 ml. of blood was given on the 33rd day because of a further drop in haemoglobin level to 6·9 g. Further progress was uneventful with no more cyanotic attacks, and at the age of 36 days the haemoglobin was 13·6 g. Fig. 3 shows the haemoglobin and reticulocyte response to folic acid.

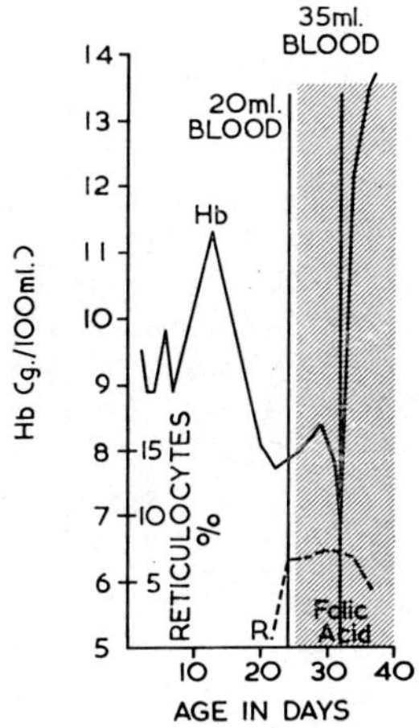


FIG. 3.—Case 3. The marked reticulocyte and haemoglobin rise follows folic acid and blood transfusions, the latter given because of the infant's deterioration.

## Discussion

These three premature infants had megaloblastic anaemia which responded well to folic acid. The anaemia was diagnosed at a very early age, the youngest child was 25 days and the oldest 50 days. The age incidence of megaloblastic anaemia in infancy is generally given as between 8 and 14 months, but Zuelzer and Rutzky (1953) found that cases of less than 4 months were not uncommon, while their own youngest case was 6 weeks old.

These cases had several features in common. Their birth weights were low, 850, 1,000, and 1,150 g. Before the development of the megaloblastic anaemia they each had an illness thought to be a chest infection. The respiratory rate was raised, they were listless and lethargic, hypotonic, and developed insuction. Radiographs showed an increase in bronchovascular markings. Each child was treated with antibiotics. In each case the megaloblastic anaemia was accompanied by an increase in insuction, and after the experience with the first child the diagnosis was suggested in the other two by this sign, together with progressive anaemia. It seems possible that an infant born prematurely has a low reserve of folic acid and that infection exhausts the small supplies available. It is also possible that the antibiotics used might interfere with folic acid metabolism to produce a relative deficiency.

According to the figures given by Boger *et al.* (1957) for normal infants at birth, the serum vitamin B12 level was well within the normal range in Case 2, at the lower level of the normal range in Case 3, and below that level in Case 1. In a series of paired sera from mothers and babies at one hospital Boger *et al.* found that the range in babies was 190-1,400 $\mu\mu$g./ml., with an average of 560 $\mu\mu$g./ml. It is possible that here we should take into account variations in results from different laboratories. In the series of Boger the average serum B12 level in women at term was 310 $\mu\mu$g./ml. with a range of 200-490. In the laboratory at this hospital the average serum B12 level in a group of women in the last four weeks of pregnancy was 218 $\mu\mu$g./ml. with a range of 85-520. This suggests that slightly lower levels are normally obtained in this laboratory, and that even Case 1 had a serum B12 level which can be considered to be within the normal range. In addition to this, Luhby, Cooperman, MacIver, and Montgomery (1960) state that, 'serum cyanocobalamin levels below 120 $\mu\mu$g./ml. in infants reflect cyanocobalamin deficiency'. Work is in progress at this hospital on serum vitamin B12 and serum folate levels in normal and premature infants paired with maternal levels at the time of delivery, but this is not sufficiently advanced to give a normal range for this laboratory.

In general the value is shown of careful examination of the blood film and buffy coat in premature infants who have a progressive anaemia that does not respond to iron. In one case (S.T.) megaloblasts were seen in the peripheral blood, and in the other two cases the appearances were highly suggestive of a megaloblastic anaemia. It is now our practice to examine the buffy coat of every premature infant with a haemoglobin below 9 g./100 ml., and when it is not conclusive to proceed to marrow biopsy. It is interesting to note that in these three infants white cell changes were only prominent in one (Case 2). It is suggested that in the treatment of established megaloblastic anaemia in premature infants the initial treatment should be folic acid 20 mg./day, given intramuscularly, but as a prophylactic, our present practice is to give folic acid 5 mg./day in addition to the routine vitamins A, D, and C and oral iron commencing at the end of the first week.

## Summary

Three premature babies developed megaloblastic anaemia in the early days of life. They responded well to folic acid. It is thought that the chest infection that each had before the anaemia exhausted the small folic acid reserves and was partly responsible for the anaemia.

We are grateful to Professors A. G. Watkins and A. S. Duncan for their help and advice in the preparation of this article; to Dr. T. E. Parry for advice and help with the bone marrow examinations; to Dr. J. L. Withey for estimating the Vitamin B12 and folate levels; to Mr. R. Marshall of the Department of Medical Illustration, Cardiff Royal Infirmary, and to Mr. P. Stinchcombe for the figures; and to Miss K. E. Heide and Miss A. S. Caldwell for their kind secretarial help.

### References

Apgar, V. (1953). A proposal for a new method of evaluation of the newborn infant. *Curr. Res. Anaesth.*, **32**, 260.

Boger, W. P., Bayne, G. M., Wright, L. D., and Beck, G. D. (1957). Differential serum vitamin B12 concentrations in mothers and infants. *New Engl. J. Med.*, **256**, 1085.

Luhby, A. L., Cooperman, J. M., MacIver, J. E., and Montgomery, R. D. (1960). Folic acid and cyanocobalamin (Vitamin B12) metabolism in kwashiorkor. *Amer. J. Dis. Child.*, **100**, 542.

Parry, T. E. (1963). Nutritional megaloblastic anaemia in infancy. In Paediatric Pathology Club. Proceedings of the Eighth Annual Meeting. *Arch. Dis. Childh.*, **38**, 95.

Royston, N. J. W., and Parry, T. E. (1962). Megaloblastic anaemia complicating dietary treatment of phenylketonuria in infancy. *ibid.*, **37**, 430.

Silverman, W. A., and Andersen, D. H. (1956). A controlled clinical trial of effects of water mist on obstructive respiratory signs, death rate and necropsy findings among premature infants. *Pediatrics*, **17**, 1.

Zuelzer, W. W., and Rutzky, J. (1953). Megaloblastic anemia in infancy. *Advanc. Pediat.*, **6**, 243.

*Arch. Dis. Childh.*, 1965, **40**, 57.

# DYSCEPHALIA MANDIBULO-OCULO-FACIALIS*

## (HALLERMANN-STREIFF SYNDROME)

BY

D. HOEFNAGEL and K. BENIRSCHKE

*From the Departments of Pathology and Pediatrics, Dartmouth Medical School, the Department of Pediatrics, Hitchcock Clinic, Hanover, New Hampshire, the Department of Pediatrics, Boston City Hospital, Boston, Massachusetts, and the Laconia State School, Laconia, New Hampshire, U.S.A.*

(RECEIVED FOR PUBLICATION APRIL 14, 1964)

The classification of the cranio-facial dysostoses is hampered by the great heterogeneity of the various developmental anomalies of face and skull. The purpose of this paper is to describe three cases of one of the rarer of these entities, dyscephalia mandibulo-oculo-facialis. Cases of this syndrome have been described under a variety of names: 'Vogelgesicht und Cataracta congenita' (Hallermann, 1948); 'Dysmorphie mandibulo-faciale (tête d'oiseau) et altérations oculaires' (Streiff, 1950); 'Dyskephalie mit Cataracta congenita und Hypotrichose' (Ullrich and Fremerey-Dohna, 1953); 'Hallermann-Streiff syndrome' (Falls and Schull, 1960); 'Syndrome dyscéphalique de François' (Carones, 1961); 'Dyscephalia mandibulo-oculo-facialis' (Waardenburg, Franceschetti, and Klein, 1961).

TABLE
RELEVANT DATA IN THE CASES

| Case No. | Age of Parents at Time of Birth of Child (yr.) | Pregnancy | Birth-weight (kg.) | Teeth Present at Birth |
|---|---|---|---|---|
| 1 | Fa: 36<br>Mo: 37 | Full-term | 2·4 | Yes |
| 2 | Fa: 35<br>Mo: 33 | Full-term | 2·6 | Yes |
| 3 | Fa: 39<br>Mo: 34 | 7 months | 1·91 | Yes |

### Case Reports

Some relevant data of the three cases have been summarized in the Table. In none of the families was there evidence of consanguinity or familial disorders. The pregnancies and deliveries had a normal course in all three cases. Tests for galactosaemia and congenital lues were negative in all 3 cases.

* This study was supported by Grant GM 10210 of the United States Public Health Service and a Grant from the Charles H. Hood Dairy Foundation.

**Case 1.** White female examined at the age of 1 year because of nystagmus. The child weighed 5·35 kg.; severe retardation of growth and development was evident. The head was small and flattened posteriorly (Fig. 1). The eyes were examined under anaesthesia: both globes were small, the corneae were clear, but small; the anterior chambers were of average depth, there were extensive posterior synechiae, no details of the ocular fundi were visible because of dense cataracts. The eyelids were lax and the tarsal plates missing or rudimentary; the lacrimal punctae were present. Tear secretion was normal. Eyebrows and eyelashes were absent. When examined at the age of 8 years (Fig. 2) her weight was 11 kg. and height 102 cm. The head was brachycephalic with a circumference of 47 cm. and prominent frontal and parietal eminences; there was sparse growth of fine blond hair restricted to the posterior part of the head; the

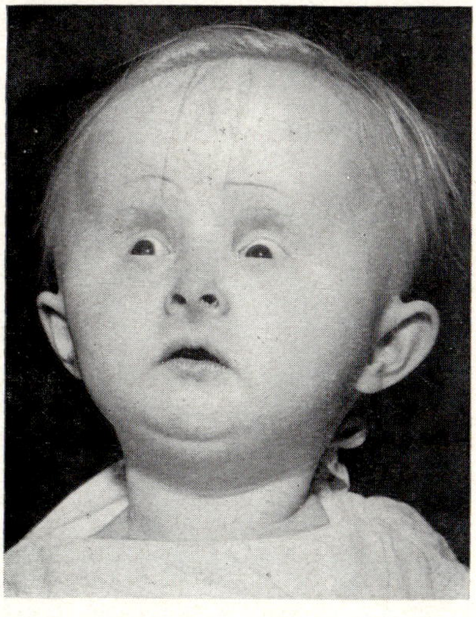

FIG. 1.—Appearance of Case 1 at the age of 1 year.

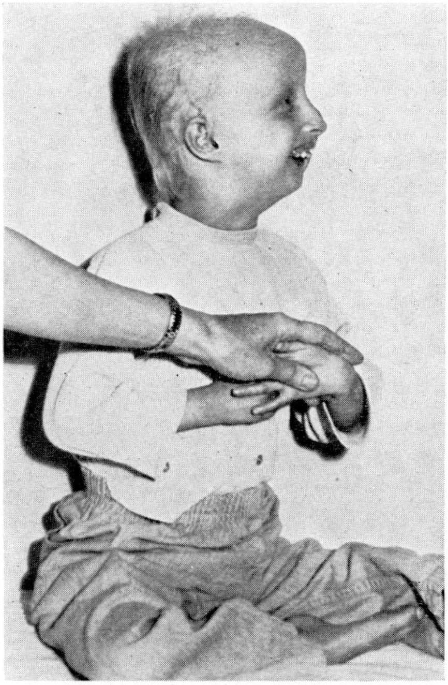

FIG. 2.—Case 1 at the age of 8 years.

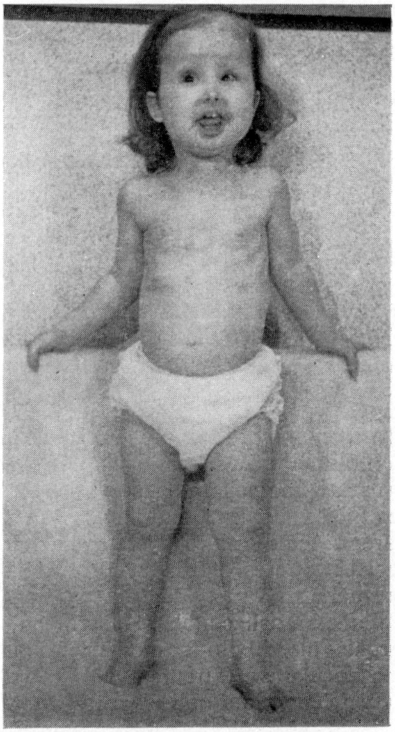

FIG. 5.—Case 3 at the age of 2½ years.

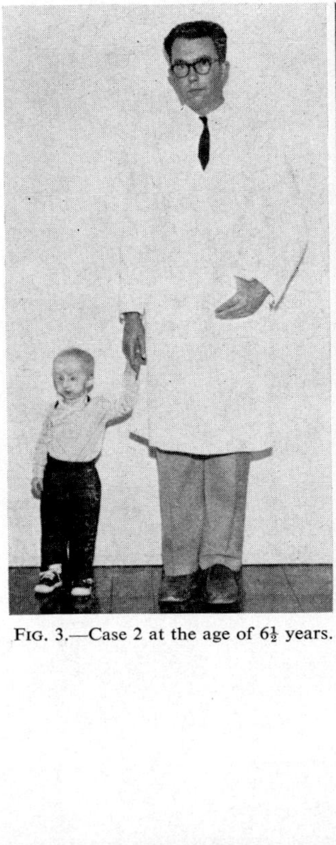

FIG. 3.—Case 2 at the age of 6½ years.

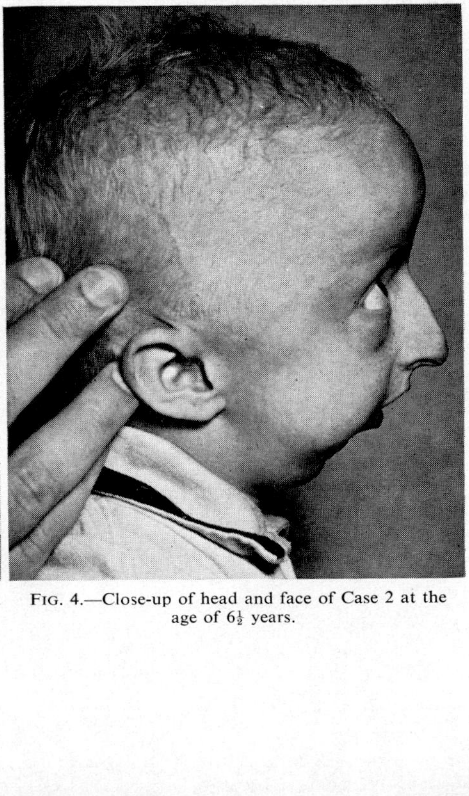

FIG. 4.—Close-up of head and face of Case 2 at the age of 6½ years.

fontanelles were closed to palpation, but radiologically the anterior and posterior fontanelle were still open. The ears were low set. There was severe micrognathia with marked limitation of movement in both temporo-mandibular joints. The nose was beaked with a deviation of the nasal septum. The mouth was small and the palate had a high arch; the tongue was very small, but it moved normally. Twelve teeth were present, irregular in shape and implantation; the right upper central incisor was missing. The joints were hyperextensible, particularly in the elbows and knees. The reflexes were normal. The external genitalia were hypoplastic. The child drooled excessively, had no intelligible speech, could not walk, was not toilet-trained, and could not feed herself.

General laboratory studies of blood and urine were normal. Sex chromatin bodies were present in 5% of buccal smear cells and drumsticks in 2% of leucocytes. Short-term cultures of peripheral blood on three separate occasions showed a modal number of 46 chromosomes. Karyotypes of numerous metaphases were prepared and all these were normal.

X-ray studies at the age of 7 years showed generalized osteoporosis of the skeleton. The anterior and posterior fontanelles were open, there was no platybasia, and the sella turcica and paranasal sinuses were normal. The orbits were small. The ascending ramus of the mandible was very small bilaterally and the temporo-mandibular joints were absent. Films of the wrists showed a bone age of 4 years.

There were four normal sibs, an older and a younger brother and sister; the mother had had one miscarriage between her first and second child.

**Case 2.** White male, examined at the age of 5 months because of slow growth and development. Bilateral cataracts were noted at that time and these were subsequently removed. Examination at the age of 6½ years showed a boy of diminutive proportions (Fig. 3) with a high-pitched, shrill voice and infantile behaviour; he was greatly handicapped by poor vision. He weighed 7·5 kg. and his height was 76 cm. The brachycephalic skull measured 46 cm. in circumference and showed prominent frontal bossing, while the anterior and posterior fontanelles were still open. There was sparse, thin blond hair limited to the posterior two-thirds of the skull. The nose was sharply hooked with a prominent deviation of the nasal septum. There was marked micrognathia (Fig. 4) and considerable symmetrical limitation of movement in the temporo-mandibular joints where no movement could be felt. The palate was highly arched and the tongue was thin and small. Many of the teeth, 16 in number, were irregular in shape. The following abnormalities were noted in the eyes: a constant searching, pendular nystagmus, blue sclerae, bilateral microphthalmus, and microcornea, absence of eyebrows, eyelashes, and lacrimal punctae; the tarsal plates could be felt and tears were present. Scrotum and penis were small, the latter showing a coronal hypospadias; no testes could be felt and there were no inguinal herniae. The joints were hyperextensible, particularly in the knees, leading to marked genu recurvatum. The reflexes were normal.

General laboratory studies of blood and urine were normal. At the age of 7 years the 24-hour output of 17-ketosteroids, determined on two separate occasions, was 810 μg. and 670 μg./24 hr. X-ray studies showed a generalized osteoporosis of the skeleton, and films of the wrists showed a bone age of 2 years and 3 months. The anterior and posterior fontanelles were open, there was no platybasia, the sella turcica and paranasal sinuses were normal, and the orbits were small. The ascending rami of the mandible and the temporo-mandibular joints were absent.

There were no sex chromatin bodies in the cells of a buccal smear and no drumsticks in 200 leucocytes of peripheral blood. There were two older normal sisters, and the mother denied having had miscarriages.

Minor respiratory infections often led to marked obstruction of the upper respiratory tract; in addition the patient suffered from grass and weed pollinosis; this allergy was present in several members of the immediate family. At the age of 8 years, in the course of an illness with fever and coryza, the child acutely developed severe respiratory distress and died soon after admission to the hospital.

Necropsy. The eyes were fixed with formalin immediately after death. Histological sections showed, in addition to the findings of post-operative aphakia, congenital focal tapeto-retinal adhesions in a region just nasal to the macula, characterized by proliferation of the pigment epithelium and focal gliosis of the outer layers of the retina. The optic nerves were normal. Pertinent findings of the general necropsy included a chronic bronchitis and oedema, and congestion and focal pneumonitis in the lungs. Both grossly and microscopically no testicular tissue could be found and only seminal vesicles and vasa differentia were identified with certainty. The lymphoid system, brain, endocrine glands, and the skin with appendages were normal.

**Case 3.** This girl was examined at the age of 3 months because of a pendular nystagmus in both eyes.

Examination showed bilateral cataracts, blue sclerae, microphthalmia and microcornea; the eyebrows were absent and the eyelashes sparse. Extracapsular cataract extractions were performed at the age of 10 months. Subsequent examination of the fundi showed the presence of punched-out areas of depigmentation with scalloped borders at the posterior poles of both eyes, involving the macular areas. There were numerous scattered hyaline dots within these areas of depigmentation, but there was no area of actual detachment.

The following additional findings were made at the age of 2½ years (Fig. 5): the skull was brachycephalic with a circumference of 37·5 cm. and prominent frontal bossing. There was absence of hair growth over the frontal part of the skull with the anterior hairline approximately at the level of the coronal sutures. The nose was small and beaked with small nostrils, the mandible was underdeveloped, but movement in the temporo-mandibular joints was normal. The palate was highly arched and the tongue was of normal size. The teeth had erupted in a disorderly fashion. X-ray studies at the age of 2 years and 3 months showed a normal sella turcica, thick and short ascending rami of the mandible and normal temporo-mandibular joints. The orbits were small.

Minor respiratory infections caused much difficulty with breathing, because of the underdeveloped nasal structures. In the course of such an infection at the age of 3 years and 3 months, the child unexpectedly died. The pertinent finding at necropsy was a massive haemorrhagic bronchopneumonia and dilatation of the right side of the heart. No histological abnormalities were noted in other organs, including the brain. The eyes were not examined.

There were two other brothers and one older sister, the mother had not had any known miscarriages.

## Discussion

An extensive review of the first 25 reported cases of dyscephalia mandibulo-oculo-facialis has been published by François (1958). Subsequently other cases have been described by Falls and Schull (1960), Calmettes, Déodati, Cadenat, and Béchac (1960), Bonamour and Léopold (1960), Carones (1961), van Balen (1961), Ponte (1962), and Manzitti and Alezzandrini (1963). It is evident from a survey of these reports that dyscephalia mandibulo-oculo-facialis is to be regarded as a separate entity and that a variation in degree of the deformity exists, which not only concerns the principal anomalies of head and eyes, but also pertains to other features such as dwarfism and the retardation of motor and mental development.

The outstanding features of the syndrome are as follows: (1) abnormalities of the skull; (2) malformations of the face; (3) dental anomalies; (4) localized hypotrichosis; (5) congenital abnormalities of the eyes; (6) dwarfism; and (7) motor and mental retardation. The skull is brachycephalic in most instances, with a discrepancy in size of the large cranial vault and the small facial skeleton. By measurement, the head circumference can be normal or at the lower limits of normal. Prominent frontal and parietal eminences are present. The posterior fontanelle is frequently open at birth and remains so for a long time. The anterior fontanelle is large and remains patent well into childhood, as in our cases, or even later; in Case 6 of Falls and Schull (1960) the anterior fontanelle was still open at the age of 20 years. The sutures are usually widely open. The skin of scalp and face, especially over the nose, is white, thin, and tense with many small blood vessels readily visible. A striking feature is the diminished hair growth on the scalp. The hair is thin and sparse with areas of complete baldness; the latter either consists of patches of alopecia along the lambdoid and coronal sutures or, more typically, there is a complete baldness over the frontal area with an anterior border at the level of the coronal sutures. Radiology of the cranial vault has shown in some cases the presence of a shallow sella turcica, platybasia or increased digital markings.

The ears are low set and, except for minor abnormalities of the ear-lobes, have a striking absence of deformities. In the majority of cases hearing is normal, but occasionally deafness is suspected (Bonamour and Léopold, 1960). The nose is small and beaked, with a sharp nasofrontal angle and often a deviation of the nasal septum. The narrow upper air passages lead to feeding difficulties in the newborn period and early infancy, and minor respiratory infections in later life cause obstruction, at times making tracheotomy necessary (van Balen, 1961; Falls and Schull, Case 3, 1960). The mouth is small with thin lips, and the palate is high arched. Fully erupted teeth at the time of birth are frequently present. The deciduous and permanent teeth erupt irregularly, are often malformed or sometimes absent altogether, especially one or more of the upper incisors. The zygomatic process is hypoplastic, but the most impressive change in the facial skeleton concerns the mandible and the temporomandibular joints. Clinically there is pronounced 'open bite', because of marked mandibular hypoplasia, while the deformities of the temporomandibular joints lead to limitation in opening the mouth. In some cases the temporo-mandibular joint is absent.

The most common anomalies of the eyes are bilateral microphthalmia, congenital cataract, ocular nystagmus, and strabismus. In several of the cases reported, spontaneous resorption of the cataracts occurred. In addition to these principal anomalies, many others have occurred in individual cases; these have been described by François (1960). In several cases in which the fundi have been inspected, degenerative disease of the retina has been noted such as chorioretinal atrophy or peripapillary choroid atrophy (Cases 2 and 3).

Bodily growth is severely retarded in most cases, resulting in a proportionate dwarfism with retarded bone age. Pubic and axillary hair are sparse to absent, the external genitalia under-developed and, in the males, the testes are commonly undescended or, when palpable, small in size. In Case 2 necropsy showed the testes to be absent. Hyperextensibility of joints, particularly in the knees, leading to genu recurvatum is commonly found. Motor, mental, and speech development are usually retarded, often profoundly so.

The family histories of most of the cases so far reported are incomplete. Consanguinity between parents has been reported in the first case of Manzitti and Alezzandrini (1963), but the degree of blood relationship is not mentioned. Familial occurrence has been reported by Larmande, as quoted by Manzitti and Alezzandrini (1963). Van Balen (1961) described the condition in two male twins, allegedly uniovular. With few exceptions, the pregnancies have been uncomplicated and full-term, and the birth weights have been in the normal range. Birth order within sibships has not shown any particular trend and there has not been an unusual number of abortions in the reproductive histories of the mothers. Male and female cases have been reported with equal frequency. The ages of the parents are too infrequently mentioned to be of use in the evaluation of this factor. The patient of Ponte (1962), a woman with the syndrome in an unusually mild form, had given birth to two normal children.

Normal sex chromatin findings were reported in Case 6 of Falls and Schull (1960) and in the case of Bonamour and Léopold (1960). Carones (1961) has reported the results of cytogenetic studies in his case; cultures of fascia lata showed a normal modal number of chromosomes and in the karyotypes some discrepancy in size of two members of a pair of the 13-15 (D) group was noted. In our first case there was no structural abnormality observed in the chromosomes of the 13-15 group.

At first sight dyscephalia mandibulo-oculo-facialis is commonly confused with progeria (Hutchinson-Gilford), but the presence in the latter of a generalized atrophy of the skin and muscles, arthritis, early arteriosclerotic changes, and the absence of cataracts are some points of difference. Other entities with a superficial resemblance to the condition under discussion are mandibulo-facial dysostosis and cleidocranial dysostosis; François (1958) has given an extensive differential diagnostic tabulation.

## Summary

Clinical and radiological findings are described in three cases of dyscephalia mandibulo-oculo-facialis (Hallermann-Streiff syndrome). This syndrome consists of abnormalities of the skull, malformations of the facial skeleton and jaws, dental anomalies, including the presence of erupted teeth at birth, localized hypotrichosis, congenital abnormalities of the eyes, dwarfism, and motor and mental retardation. The results of cytogenetic studies in one case and necropsy findings in two of the cases are reported.

We thank the following colleagues for clinical information and help in obtaining material for histopathological examination of Cases 2 and 3: Dr. E. Twible and Dr. W. Mosig, Springfield, Massachusetts; Dr. J. Giammalvo, Holyoke, Massachusetts; Dr. S. D. Liebman, Boston, Massachusetts; Dr. S. E. Wheelock, Hitchcock Clinic, Hanover, New Hampshire; Dr. H. Buckbee, Dolgeville, New York, Dr. W. R. Redline, Utica, New York, Dr. D. G. Cogan, Howe Laboratory of Ophthalmology, Boston, Massachusetts described the histopathology of the eye.

### References

Balen, A. Th. van (1961). Dyscephaly with microphthalmos, cataract and hypoplasia of the mandible. *Ophthalmologica (Basel)*, **141**, 53.

Bonamour, G., and Léopold, P. (1960). Syndrome dyscéphale avec tête d'oiseau (syndrome de François). *Bull. Soc. Ophtal. Fr.*, p. 85.

Calmettes, L., Déodati, P., Cadenat, H., and Béchac, G. (1960). La dysmorphie mandibulo-faciale type François (à propos d'un cas). *Rev. oto-neuro-Ophtal.*, **32**, 275.

Carones, A. V. (1961). Syndrome dyscéphalique de François. *Ophthalmologica (Basel)*, **142**, 510.

Falls, H. F., and Schull, W. J. (1960). Hallermann-Streiff syndrome. A dyscephaly with congenital cataracts and hypotrichosis. *A.M.A. Arch. Ophthal.*, **63**, 409.

François, J. (1958). A new syndrome. Dyscephalia with bird face and dental anomalies, nanism, hypotrichosis, cutaneous atrophy, microphthalmia, and congenital cataract. *ibid.*, **60**, 842.

—— (1960). Syndromes with congenital cataract (XVI Jackson Memorial Lecture). *Trans. Amer. Acad. Ophthal. Otolaryng.*, **64**, 433.

Hallermann, W. (1948). Vogelgesicht und Cataracta congenita. *Klin. Mbl. Augenheilk.*, **113**, 315.

Manzitti, E., and Alezzandrini, A. A. (1963). Syndrome dyscéphalique de François. *Ann. Oculist. (Paris)*, **196**, 456.

Ponte, F. (1962). Further contributions to the study of the syndrome of Hallermann and Streiff (Congenital cataract with 'Bird's Face'). *Ophthalmologica (Basel)*, **143**, 399.

Streiff, E. B. (1950). Dysmorphie mandibulo-faciale (tête d'oiseau) et altérations oculaires. *ibid.*, **120**, 79.

Ullrich, O., and Fremerey-Dohna, H. (1953). Dyskephalie mit Cataracta congenita und Hypotrichose als typischer Merkmalskomplex. *ibid.*, **125**, 73 and 144.

Waardenburg, P. J., Franceschetti, A., and Klein, D. (1961). *Genetics and Ophthalmology*, Vol. 1. Blackwell, Oxford.

*Arch. Dis. Childh.*, 1965, **40**, 62.

# THE RESPIRATORY DISTRESS SYNDROME OF THE NEWBORN: IMMATURITY VERSUS PREMATURITY

BY

PETER M. DUNN*

*From The Birmingham Maternity Hospital*

(RECEIVED FOR PUBLICATION MAY 4, 1964)

The respiratory distress syndrome (RDS) remains the most important cause of morbidity and mortality among anatomically normal infants during the first few days of life. There is no general agreement as to the aetiology or pathogenesis of this condition. However, its association with a number of maternal and foetal factors is well recognized; foremost among these is prematurity. While the definition of the premature infant is based on low birth weight (5 lb. 8 oz. (2·5 kg.) or less), the term is often used loosely to denote immaturity. This may lead to confusion, for immature infants may be heavier than the average full-term baby. At the same time, about one-third of all 'premature' infants born in this country have had a gestation of 38 weeks or more (Butler and Bonham, 1963).

In this paper, a study has been made of the relative importance of birth weight and length of gestation on the incidence of RDS and its mortality.

### Subjects and Method

All infants of 28 weeks gestation or more who were born alive in this hospital during 1961 were admitted to the study. Length of gestation was reckoned in terms of weeks completed since the first day of the last menstrual period. When this date was in doubt, the obstetrician's antenatal judgment was accepted. If, however, clinical examination of a newborn infant suggested that the estimated length of gestation was incorrect by at least a month, then a suitable adjustment was made. This was thought necessary for between 6 and 7% of all deliveries. Seven (9·5%) of the infants who developed RDS were involved; in each case radiological assessment of bone age was also obtained.

All babies were weighed and examined on the first day of life. Small or sick infants were usually seen at or soon after birth. Records on every baby were kept by the author who examined approximately 97% of those born alive. Information on the remainder was obtained from the case notes.

The diagnosis of RDS was based on the characteristic clinical picture and course of the disease, an excellent description of which has been given by Usher (1961a). All the affected infants showed oedema, diminished air entry on auscultation, and dyspnoea with inspiratory retraction. The great majority demonstrated expiratory grunting and tachypnoea after the first hour of life; many became cyanosed. Infants that also suffered from coexistent disease, such as Rh incompatibility, were not excluded. However, infants, usually fairly mature, showing transient signs of respiratory distress that subsided within six hours of birth, have not been included as cases of RDS. Four previable infants (less than 28 weeks gestation) who showed respiratory distress during life and complete primary atelectasis after death have also been excluded from this study.

With one exception, necropsy was performed on all infants born in this period that died during the first week of life. In the case of every infant thought to have suffered from RDS, post-mortem examination confirmed the presence of atelectasis and venous congestion; with the exception of two of the most immature infants, there was also pulmonary congestion, alveolar duct distension, and resorption atelectasis with or without hyaline membrane formation.

At the time of the study, RDS was treated in this hospital with oxygen, digoxin, and antibiotics.

### Results

During 1961, 2,051 infants were born alive after a gestation of 28 weeks or more; and 49 (2·4%) died during the neonatal period.

In Table 1, infants are grouped according to birth weight (± 2,500 g.) and length of gestation (± 37 weeks or 259 days). The distribution of the deaths is also shown. Thus, 11·6% of all infants weighed less than 2,500 g. at birth, while 10·5% were born before 37 weeks. The number of deaths in each group was the same, 77·5% of the total neonatal mortality.

Fig. 1 shows the distribution of all births and deaths according to length of gestation. The heavy toll among the most immature infants decreases sharply at first and then more slowly until it reaches an average low of 0·5% between 38 and 41 weeks.

* Present address: Royal Hospital for Sick Children, Bristol.

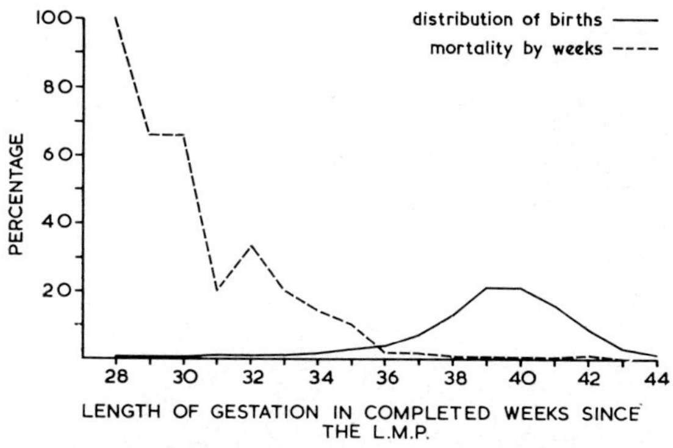


FIG. 1.—Distribution according to length of gestation of 2,051 infants born alive after the 28th week. The neonatal mortality at weekly intervals is also shown.

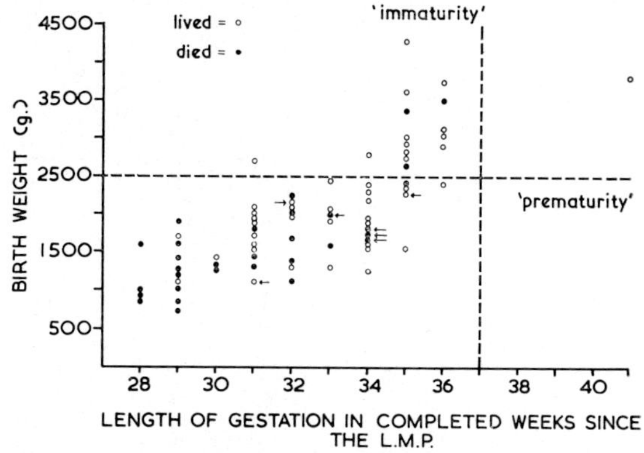


FIG. 2.—The birth weight, length of gestation, and fate of the 76 infants with the repiratory distress syndrome. Arrows mark the cases in which the antenatal estimate of length of gestation has been corrected after birth in the direction shown.

**Respiratory Distress Syndrome.** 76 infants were diagnosed as suffering from this disease and 31 (40·8%) of them died. A second diagnosis was present in 13 cases (non-traumatic intracranial haemorrhage in 8, Rh haemolytic disease in 2, infection in 2, and massive pulmonary haemorrhage in 1). These 31 deaths represent 63% of all the neonatal deaths, 81·5% of those among infants born before 37 weeks' gestation and 73·5% of those weighing 2,500 g. or less at birth.

Table 2 is similar to Table 1 except that only infants with RDS are represented. Fig. 2 shows the length of gestation, birth weight, and fate of these babies; 97·3% of them (and all that died) were of less than 37 weeks' gestation. Low birth weight was present in only 77·5% of cases and in 90% of deaths.

The incidence of RDS, according to length of gestation, is plotted in Fig. 3, as is also the mortality from this disease. It can be seen that RDS not

TABLE 1

LIVE BIRTHS AND NEONATAL DEATHS IN RELATION TO BIRTH WEIGHT AND LENGTH OF GESTATION

| Gestation | Birth Weight | | | | Total | |
|---|---|---|---|---|---|---|
| | < 2,500 g. | | > 2,500 g. | | | |
| | Infants | Deaths | Infants | Deaths | Infants | Deaths |
| < 37 weeks (259 days) .. | 135 (6·5) | 35 (71·5) | 81 (4·0) | 3 (6·1) | 216 (10·5) | 38 (77·5) |
| 37 weeks or more .. .. | 102 (5·0) | 3 (6·1) | 1,733 (84·5) | 8 (16·3) | 1,835 (89·5) | 11 (22·5) |
| Total .. .. .. .. | 237 (11·6) | 38 (77·5) | 1,814 (88·4) | 11 (22·5) | 2,051 (100) | 49 (100) |

Percentages of all infants and of all deaths are shown in brackets.

TABLE 2

INCIDENCE OF RDS AND MORTALITY FROM IT IN RELATION TO BIRTH WEIGHT AND LENGTH OF GESTATION

| Gestation | Birth Weight | | | | Total | |
|---|---|---|---|---|---|---|
| | < 2,500 g. | | > 2,500 g. | | | |
| | Infants | Deaths | Infants | Deaths | Infants | Deaths |
| < 37 weeks (259 days) .. | 59 (77·5) | 28 (90·3) | 15 (19·8) | 3 (9·7) | 74 (97·3) | 31 (100) |
| 37 weeks or more .. .. | 0 (0) | 0 (0) | 2 (2·7) | 0 (0) | 2 (2·7) | 0 (0) |
| Total .. .. .. .. | 59 (77·5) | 28 (90·3) | 17 (22·5) | 3 (9·7) | 76 (100) | 31 (100) |

Percentages are shown in brackets.

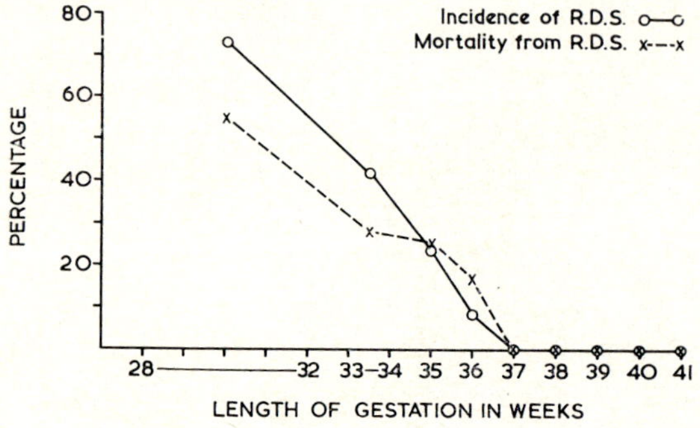


FIG. 3.—Incidence of the respiratory distress syndrome and the mortality from this disease in relation to length of gestation.

only becomes more common with decreasing maturity, but is also more liable to be fatal.

## Discussion

The Birmingham Maternity Hospital receives obstetric problems from a wide area. For example, the incidence of Rh haemolytic disease in this hospital during the period under study was over eight times as great as for the country as a whole. The incidence of prematurity was, however, only twice the national average. This was due to the deliberate policy of not admitting women in *uncomplicated* premature labour in order to conserve nursery space. As a result, the great majority of premature infants were born following an abnormal pregnancy or complicated delivery.

Thus, no less than 24·5% of the 'immature' infants in this series were delivered by caesarean section. These factors, which will be discussed in greater detail in a further communication, help to explain the very high incidence of RDS in this study; at 3·7% this was at least twice as high as that in any of the four other maternity units in which the author has worked. For the same reasons, the neonatal mortality rate was also high (1·7 × the national average), though in fact the lowest recorded for this hospital during a 15-year period.

The neonatal mortality among the 90% of infants who were born after the 37th week (259 days) was 0·6% or, if deaths due to gross congenital malformation are excluded, only 0·38%. The neonatal mortality for all births in England and Wales during 1961 was 1·5%. When it is recalled that virtually every pregnancy in this study was complicated in one way or another, it will be appreciated how tough the mature newborn infant is and how well equipped to adapt himself to extrauterine life.

In contrast, the mortality among the 10% of infants delivered before 37 weeks' gestation was nearly 29 times as great at 17·6%. RDS was the main cause of death in four-fifths of cases. Though this disease has been called one of prematurity, this description only appears to be accurate in so far as babies of low birth weight are usually also immature. Where, in this study, immature infants were relatively heavy at birth (usually in association with maternal diabetes), the risk from RDS remained. In fact, 22·5% of the infants having RDS weighed more than 2,500 g. at birth, while only 2·7% were of more than 37 weeks' gestation. This is in close agreement with the observations of Usher (1961b) and Usher, McLean, and Maughan (1964). Though 43% of 'premature' infants were delivered after the 37th week (Table 1), none developed RDS: it must be admitted, however, that five RDS infants have been removed from this group because it was felt reasonably certain that their maturity was less than had been expected (Fig. 2).

The very rapid decrease in mortality from the limits of viability at 28 weeks down to 1% at 37 weeks, only 63 days later, is shown in Fig. 1. Approximately, this implies that for every day less that the foetus remained *in utero* between the 31st and 37th weeks of gestation, its chances of dying in the neonatal period increased by 1%. Between 28 and 31 weeks, the chance of death increased at twice this rate. For this reason, when induction of labour or caesarean delivery is contemplated because of *foetal* indications, the dangers of a continued intrauterine existence must be balanced with great care against those of immaturity. *Every day is important.* Decisions may be difficult enough when the length of gestation can be estimated with confidence. Unfortunately, this confidence is frequently lacking. In this study, the author estimated that between 6 and 7% of infants were either a month less or more mature than had been expected. The size of this group is less surprising when it is remembered that half the pregnant women in this country attend their doctor for the first time *after* the first four months of pregnancy (Butler and Bonham, 1963) and another half rely completely on memory for the accuracy of their 'dates' (unpublished data). In addition, the menstrual history may mislead in many ways. The price of a misjudgment may be an unexpectedly immature infant that dies from RDS. This type of tragedy occurred on four occasions in this study. Postnatal examination showed that the bone age was about four weeks less than expected in every case. Bone development is making such huge strides during the last trimester of pregnancy that antenatal radiological assessment of maturity may be of great assistance (Hartley, 1957). At the worst, radiological interpretation is extremely unlikely to mislead by as much as four weeks. Unfortunately, this useful aid is sometimes withheld because of fear of damage to the foetus from irradiation (Brown, Doll, and Hill, 1960). Without denying this risk, its dangers seem to be much smaller and less immediate than those of immaturity and RDS.

**Summary**

The effect of birth weight and length of gestation on the occurrence of the respiratory distress syndrome of the newborn was studied in a maternity hospital.

The incidence of this disease was related to low birth weight only in so far as the latter was related to immaturity. RDS was rare after the 37th week of gestation (259 days), providing the mothers' dates were correct. Before this time, both the incidence of this disease and the mortality from it rose steeply with decreasing maturity. It was, in the main, responsible for four-fifths of the neonatal deaths among immature infants.

I would like to thank Dr. B. S. B. Wood both for his helpful criticism and for permission to publish this case material; also the Consultant Obstetricians of the Birmingham Maternity Hospital for allowing me access to their case records, and Dr. H. G. Kohler for his thorough post-mortem reports.

References

Brown, W. M. Court, Doll, R., and Hill, A. Bradford (1960). Incidence of leukaemia after exposure to diagnostic radiation *in utero*. *Brit. med. J.*, **2**, 1539.

Butler, N. R., and Bonham, D. G. (1963). *Perinatal Mortality. The First Report of the 1958 British Perinatal Mortality Survey*, pp. 62, 142. Livingstone, London.

Hartley, J. B. (1957). Radiological estimation of foetal maturity. *Brit. J. Radiol.*, **30**, 561.

Usher, R. H. (1961a). Clinical investigation of the respiratory distress syndrome of prematurity. *N.Y. St. J. Med.*, **61**, 1677.

—— (1961b). The respiratory distress syndrome of prematurity: Clinical and therapeutic aspects. *Pediat. Clin. N. Amer.*, **8**, 525.

——, McLean, F., and Maughan, G. B. (1964). Respiratory distress syndrome in infants delivered by cesarean section. *Amer. J. Obstet. Gynec.*, **88**, 806.

*Arch. Dis. Childh.*, 1965, **40**, 66.

# THE INFLUENCE OF ANDROGEN TREATMENT ON ULTIMATE HEIGHT IN MALES

BY

GEORGE L. FOSS

*From The United Bristol Hospitals*

(RECEIVED FOR PUBLICATION MAY 25, 1964)

For the past 25 years androgens have been used to accelerate growth, particularly in boys backward in development or of short stature. There has been considerable controversy whether such treatment would increase, decrease, or not affect, ultimate height.

In a group of 13 boys aged 5½ years to 10 years, Sobel, Raymond, Quinn, and Talbot (1956) found that methyl testosterone, 5-40 mg. daily, produced a greater average increase in skeletal age than in height age during the treatment period of two to six months. Skeletal maturation continued to advance at a rate greater than the control rate after treatment was finished, whereas growth increments reverted to average normal within the period of follow-up of two years.

However, Bayley, Gordan, and Lisser (1957) found that methyl testosterone 5 to 30 mg. daily (usually 10 mg. daily) for an undefined period led to no disproportionate skeletal maturation, and in 20 cases in which growth was followed to adult stature there was no reduction in ultimate height from that predicted before treatment.

During the past 18 years the growth of a series of boys has been observed, and an analysis has been made of the findings to help elucidate this problem.

### Method and Material

A total of 208 young males are included, and are divided into 120 controls and 88 treated with androgens. All were white, and came from the Bristol area.

The control cases were referred for apparent cryptorchism, gynaecomastia, or obesity. Dietetic restriction was prescribed for some of the latter.

The treated group is sub-divided into three groups: (A) 30 boys whose skeletal age was equivalent to their chronological age, or slightly advanced; (B) 37 boys whose skeletal age was a year or more retarded. (These two groups were treated for cryptorchism, inadequate development compared with their fellows, or for small stature.) (C) 21 cases who were all suffering from infantilism to complete eunuchoidism, and whose skeletal age averaged 6 years' retardation over their mean chronological age (19·57 years).

They were measured on a vertical metal height scale with vernier reading made to my own design (Fig. 1), to the nearest 1/16 in. (0·15 cm.) in their socks, at one to three-monthly intervals according to whether they were receiving treatment or not. Span was also measured with the same apparatus with the scale in the horizontal position. They were also weighed in trousers, socks, and shirt.

A postero-anterior radiograph was taken of their left hands and wrists at intervals of six months. In the past three years all these serial radiographs have been compared with the standards in Greulich's and Pyle's atlas (1959), and skeletal ages were obtained. Predicted heights have then been found in the appropriate tables of Bayley and Pinneau (1952), according to whether skeletal age was normal or advanced or retarded over a year. For calculation of the figures the initial radiograph of hand and wrist was used to obtain skeletal age and prediction of height. Though many of the growth records were complete, with radiological evidence of epiphysial union, it was necessary to attempt the follow-up of 177 of these cases in order to obtain their ultimate height. Unfortunately it was only possible to obtain this measurement in 54·8% of the whole series. The ages of these patients in the control and treated Groups A and B when followed up ranged from 24-33 years at final measurement, and with the knowledge of their last assessment of skeletal age it was concluded that growth was complete.

In Group C, 20 cases were the subject of more intensive study. The double check of span and height measurements was confirmed by serial radiographs of the left hand and wrist. The time taken until closure of the epiphyses after the onset of treatment, recorded to the nearest six months, is shown in Table 1. In Case Mo, though growth had ceased, epiphysial closure was not completed until 39 years of age, after a further intensive course of injections of testosterone esters: previously he had been disinclined to have further treatment.

Treatment in Groups A and B has varied from 5-30 mg. methyl testosterone for two to 14 months continuously, or in 5 cases intermittently, with doses up to 75 mg. daily for 30 months. This steroid was ingested in some cases and absorbed sub-labially in others.

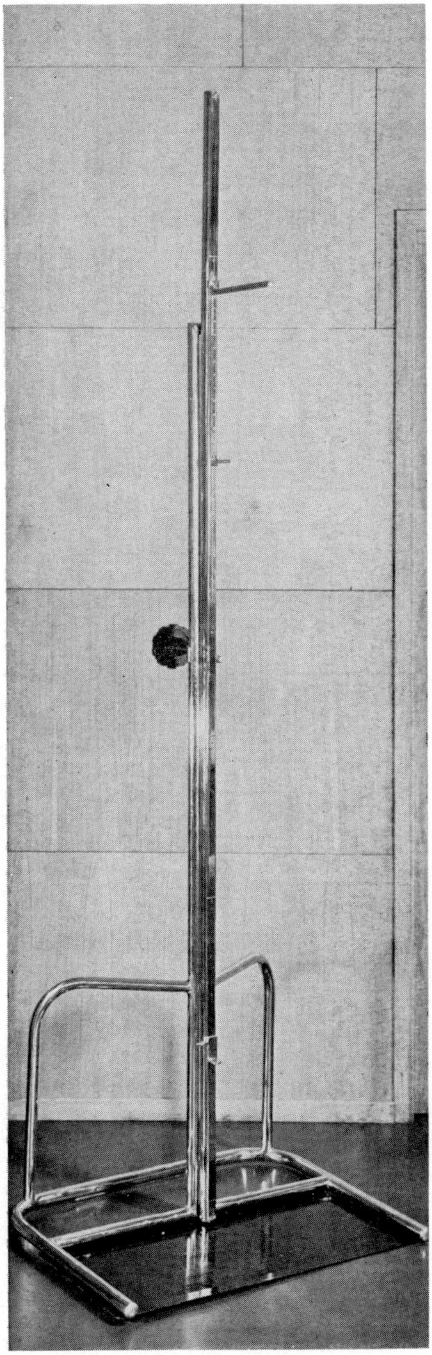

FIG. 1.

In Group C intensive androgen treatment was given, with implantations of testosterone at regular intervals of 6 months, continuous oral methyl testosterone or fluoxymesterone, or injections of testosterone in the form of short and/or long-acting esters, or combinations of these methods (Table 1), for 2-14 years.

## Results

**Controls.** In the whole group of 120 cases, when first seen the mean age was 12·13 years (range 9-17 years), mean skeletal age 11·81 years (range 8-18 years), and mean height was 58·72 in. (149 cm.). The mean predicted height was 70·16 in. (177 cm.) (S.D. 2·64). Of these, 50 were measured when growth had ceased, with a mean increment of 10·57 in. (26·7 cm.) and a mean ultimate height of 69·45 in. (176 cm.) (S.D. 2·54). The mean figures, when prediction was made for the 50 cases with a completed growth record, compare closely with those of the whole group of controls (Table 2).

**Treated.** (A) These boys of similar age to the controls had a similar mean skeletal age, initial height and prediction, and also a mean ultimate height within 0·2 in. (0·5 cm.) (S.D. 0·91), and a mean total increment of 10·69 in. (27·15 cm.) growth (Table 2).

(B) The mean age was a little higher, 14·46 years, in the completed growth studies with a mean skeletal age of 11·92, so that their skeletal ages were retarded by over 2 years. Mean initial height was an inch less and their mean prediction was nearly 2 inches less than in Group A. Their total growth increment had an average of 9·77 in. (24·8 cm.), and their mean ultimate height was within 0·5 in. (1·27 cm.) (S.D. 1·22) of the predicted mean (Table 2).

(C) In this series of cases of infantilism (Table 1), intensively treated with androgens for long periods of 2-8 years, the mean age was 19·57 years, and skeletal age 13·68. They were initially taller 63·88 in. (168·25 c.m.), and started treatment with a mean percentage of ultimate height of 93·43. Their mean predicted height was similar to that of the controls, but they only showed a mean increment of 4·42 in. (11·2 cm.), and mean ultimate height after fusion of the epiphyses was nearly 2 inches below that predicted (Table 2). Even with continuous large doses of androgens two of these cases of hypogonadism have become fertile (Foss, 1962).

A comparison of the predicted and ultimate heights in these four groups is shown in Fig. 2, and these figures were submitted to statistical analysis as shown in Table 3.

The only group which is significantly different from the controls is Group C. Group B could quite likely have occurred by chance from a normal

TREATED, INT

| Case | Condition | Age (yr.) | Skeletal Age (yr.) | Weight (lb.) | Height (in.) | Predicted Height (in.) | Ul Hei |
|---|---|---|---|---|---|---|---|
| Ha | Infantilism | 18·5 | 12·8 | 75 | 58·5 | 67·3 | |
| Je | Infantilism | 17·3 | 13·5 | 72 | 57·6 | 63·7 | |
| Bu | Eunuchoid | 17·5 | 13·0 | 138 | 67·5 | 77·0 | |
| Mo* | Testic. dysgen. and infantilism | 25·0 | 15·5 | 91 | 64·1 | 65·7 | |
| Th | Infantilism | 15·0 | 11·0 | 63 | 54·3 | 65·8 | |
| Wha† | Malabsorption syndrome | 18·8 | 13·0 | 97 | 61·5 | 70·0 | |
| Ba‡ | Testic. dysgen. | 24·5 | 16·5 | 146 | 68·3 | 69·1 | |
| Pl | Immature voice | 17·0 | 16·0 | 130 | 64·8 | 65·9 | |
| Sw | Testic. dysgen. and infantilism | 19·5 | 13·0 | 88 | 59·8 | 68·2 | |
| So | Eunuchoid | 24·0 | 15·0 | 143 | 70·5 | 72·8 | |
| Har | Eunuchoid | 19·8 | 13·6 | 128 | 64·3 | 71·3 | |
| Win | Anorchism | 23·0 | 14·6 | 118 | 70·0 | 73·8 | |
| Whish | Retarded puberty | 15·9 | 14·0 | 98 | 66·0 | 73·2 | |
| Ham | Eunuchoid | 22·0 | 14·0 | 103 | 65·0 | 70·1 | |
| Whit | Eunuchoid | 20·0 | 14·0 | 143 | 70·5 | 76·0 | |
| Tap§ | Retarded growth | 12·8 | 8·0 | 69 | 52·3 | 69·0 | |
| Lo | Testic. dysgen. and infantilism | 16·0 | 13·5 | 106 | 61·5 | 68·1 | |
| Da | Eunuchoid | 21·5 | 13·0 | 133 | 71·3 | 77·7 | |
| Co†** | Delayed puberty | 17·0 | 13·0 | 100 | 63·3 | 71·9 | |
| Geo | Eunuchoid | 28·0 | 15·5 | 112 | 68·1 | 69·8 | |
| Hear | Eunuchoid | 17·7 | 15·0 | 96 | 62·3 | 64·3 | |

* Epiphyses fused at 39 years after further treatment without further growth.
† These cases had children.
‡ Previously given M.T. 15 mg./day for 12 months elsewhere.
§ Follow-up age 26.
** Skeletal age 16 at 19, National Service, final follow-up age 30.

MEAN FIGURES IN CON

| Group | No. of Cases | | Mean Age (yr.) | Mean S.A. (yr.) | Mean Height at Prediction (in.) | Mean Pe Ult. F Predi |
|---|---|---|---|---|---|---|
| | Total | Complete | | | | |
| Controls .. .. .. | 120 | | 12·13 | 11·81 | 58·72 | |
| | | 50 | 12·0 | 11·87 | 58·88 | 84· |
| Treated (A) .. .. .. | 30 | | 12·06 | 12·13 | 59·12 | |
| S.A. ∝ C.A. .. .. .. | | 19 | 12·12 | 12·21 | 59·32 | 84· |
| Treated (B) .. .. .. .. | 37 | | 14·28 | 11·74 | 57·51 | |
| S.A. > C.A. .. .. .. | | 24 | 14·46 | 11·92 | 58·29 | 85· |
| Intensive treatment (C) .. .. | 21 | 21 | 19·57 | 13·68 | 63·88 | 93· |

S.A. = skeletal age; C.A. = chronological age.

population. Group A compared with the controls did not quite reach the 5% level of probability.

## Discussion

Sobel *et al.* (1956) suggest that oral methyl testosterone even in doses of 5 mg./day (which they state was as effective a growth promoter as 10-20 mg./day), was in fact a growth inhibitor, despite its immediate action of accelerating growth, as in more than half of their small series of young girls and boys there was disproportionately greater acceleration in skeletal age. They further suggest that there was a lag in development of x-ray evidence of maturation of ossification centres. All their conclusions were based on a short follow-up of two years.

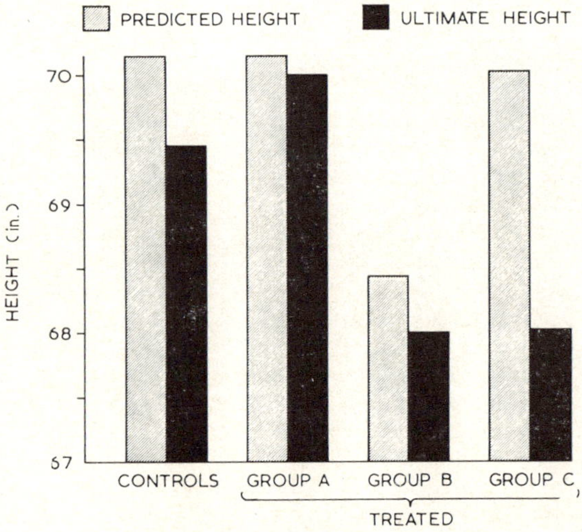


FIG. 2.—A comparison of predicted and ultimate heights in the four groups.

GENS, GROUP C

| (in.) | Time to Fusion of Epiphyses (mth.) | Treatment, MT or FM (mg./day) | Treatment Injection (mg.) | Treatment Implant (mg.) |
|---|---|---|---|---|
| | 30 | 40 for 18 months | | |
| | 62 | 15-30 for 36 months | TP 100 weekly for 24 months | |
| | | | TO 250 bi-weekly for 3 months | |
| | 82 | 30-60 for 10 months | Triol 1000 monthly for 3 months | T 1000 every 6 months for 7 years |
| | 168 | | TPP 100 weekly for 6 months | T 800 |
| | 62 | 15-30 for 60 months | TPP 100 weekly for 6 months | |
| | 54 | 30-60 for 72 months | TPP 100 weekly for 18 months | |
| | 15 | | | T 1000 every 6 months for 14 years |
| | 14 | | TIB 200 weekly for 12 months | |
| | 81 | 30 for 84 months | | |
| | 40 | 50 for 36 months | TIB 300 weekly for 12 months | |
| | 50 | | | T 1000 every 6 months for 14 years |
| | 36 | 75 for 36 months | TPP 100 weekly for 7 months | T 1000 every 6 months for 2 years |
| | 40 | 30-60 for 18 months | TPP 100 weekly for 10 months | |
| | 24 | 20-60 for 120 months | TIB 300 bi-weekly for 3 months | T 1000 every 6 months for 4 years |
| | 48 | 30-60 for 12 months | Triol 1000 monthly for 12 months | T 1000 every 6 months for 4 years |
| | >60 | 5-20 for 18 months | | |
| | 88 | 15 for 6 months | TP 100 weekly for 6 months | T 1000 every 6 months for 10 years |
| | 56 | 30 for 120 months intermittent | | |
| | >24 | | | T 600 every 6 months for 1 year |
| | 26 | 30 for 14 months | TIB 200 weekly for 6 months | T 1000 every 6 months for 10 years |
| | 38 | 25 for 36 months | | T 600 |

thyl testosterone
oxymesterone

TP = testosterone propionate
TO = ,, oenanthate
Triol = { ,, propionate + ,, valerianate + ,, undecenylate }
TPP = ,, phenyl propionate
TIB = ,, isobutyrate

T = testosterone implant

EATED GROUPS

| Predicted Height | | Ultimate Height | | Ultim. Ht. minus Pred. Ht. | | Growth (in.) | |
|---|---|---|---|---|---|---|---|
| an | S.D. | Mean | S.D. | Mean | S.D. | Mean | S.D. |
| 16 | 2·64 | | | | | | |
| 17 | 2·54 | 69·45 | 2·54 | −0·716 | 1·49 | 10·57 | 4·42 |
| 17 | 2·78 | | | | | | |
| 16 | 3·63 | 70·01 | 3·36 | −0·153 | 0·91 | 10·69 | 3·04 |
| 09 | 2·73 | | | | | | |
| 44 | 2·71 | 67·98 | 2·86 | −0·462 | 1·22 | 9·77 | 3·53 |
| 03 | 3·99 | 68·30 | 3·94 | −1·750 | 1·42 | 4·42 | 2·98 |

They did not state whether the oral methyl testosterone was merely swallowed or absorbed transmucosally under the tongue or in the buccal pouch. Theoretically absorption through the mucosa of the mouth should increase its efficacy, as some of it by-passes the portal circulation and is not detoxicated by the liver. It was shown that the ratio of effectiveness of transmucosal to orally ingested methyl testosterone in women was 1·38 : 1 (Foss, 1956).

The doses of methyl testosterone that they used for these young children were much too high, and produced virilization, and in some, given 40 mg./day, treatment was withdrawn after two and a half to

TABLE 3

ULTIMATE HEIGHT MINUS PREDICTED HEIGHT

| Group | No. of Cases | Mean Height (in.) | Standard Deviation | Comparison of Group Mean with Control Mean | |
|---|---|---|---|---|---|
| | | | | t | p |
| Controls .. .. .. .. | 50 | −0·716 | 1·49 | | |
| *Treated* (A) .. .. .. .. | 19 | −0·153 | 0·91 | 1·901 | Not significant |
| (B) .. .. .. .. | 24 | −0·462 | 1·22 | 0·726 | Not significant |
| (C) .. .. .. .. | 21 | −1·750 | 1·42 | 2·709 | <0·01 |

three months. Androgenic effect is dependent on the product of dose and duration of treatment; and whereas their maximum growth acceleration was no greater with doses of more than 5 mg./day, on their time/dose schedule of 20 mg./day for six months their figures showed a greater average increment in skeletal age. Over such a short follow-up of 2 years this presumably led them to the false assumption that ultimate height would be reduced.

Bayley *et al.* (1957) included in their study 25 controls for which there were predicted and ultimate heights, and 20 treated cases were similarly followed up. The mean difference for ultimate height minus predicted height was + 1 in. (2·54 cm.) for controls, and + 1·1 in. (2·8 cm.) for the treated group.

In the present study, which is about twice as large as that of Bayley *et al.* (1957), methyl testosterone in doses usually of 5-15 mg. daily for periods of 3-14 months, or 20-75 mg. intermittently for 30 months, did not significantly alter the mean ultimate height or the total mean growth. In two boys on the latter régime, one was 2 in. (5 cm.) shorter and the other 1 in. (2·54 cm.) taller than their predicted heights.

The group with gross retardation of skeletal age included 9 cases of eunuchoidism, 8 cases of testicular dysgenesis and infantilism, and the rest with delayed puberty. Eight of these cases were over the age of 20 when first seen.

Intensive treatment (Table 1) with large doses of androgens by implantation, injection, and/or by mouth significantly reduced their growth compared with the original prediction. However, these were mostly cases with androgen deficiency, and perhaps cannot be compared with boys with normal testes and of a lower age-group, with a greater expectancy of potential growth. With such gross retardation of skeletal age when first seen, predictions of their ultimate height from the tables of normal boys (Bayley and Pinneau, 1952) are probably open to considerable error.

It is interesting that the assessments of predicted height were slightly more than the ultimate heights in all groups in this series, whereas in Bayley's series it was the reverse. Nevertheless, these results confirm the finding of Bayley *et al.* (1957) that there is no deleterious effect of methyl testosterone on growth.

The indication for use of androgens in accelerating growth and development in boys without endocrine disorders is limited, and is only warranted when for psychological reasons it is necessary to adjust development to the normal for the chronological age of the boy. Methyl testosterone in doses of 5-10 mg. daily will achieve this purpose satisfactorily without any fear of reducing expected height, or inhibiting growth.

Whether the lesser virilizing anabolic steroids will increase ultimate height over predicted height is open to conjecture, and this point can only be settled when a sufficient number of cases have been followed up to adult stature. In a series of 35 boys (treated with various anabolic steroids) some of whom have been observed for 6 years, there appears to be no disproportionate epiphysial maturation during the period of treatment.

## Summary

Out of a series of 208 boys whose growth was studied during the past 18 years, final adult height was measured in 114. Of these, 50 were controls, and their growth and skeletal ages, with height prediction and ultimate heights, were compared with those measurements for 2 groups with normal or retarded skeletal age, treated with methyl testosterone in small to moderate doses for up to 30 months, and for a third group treated intensively with large doses of androgens for longer periods, until epiphysial closure and complete virilization.

In the first two treated groups ultimate growth was not affected, but in the third group ultimate height was reduced by 2 in. (5 cm.).

I am indebted to the Registrar of the Bristol Executive Council for considerable help in tracing many cases: to Miss Ethel Duncan, Lecturer in Medical Statistics, University of Bristol, for help and advice with the statistical analysis: to Professor A. V. Neale for permission to include results of some of his cases, and to Dr. J. M. Tanner for his very valuable criticism and comments.

### References

Bayley, N., Gordan, G. S., and Lisser, H. (1957). Long-term experiences with methyltestosterone as a growth stimulant in short immature boys. *Pediat. Clin. N. Amer.*, **4**, 819.

——, and Pinneau, S. R. (1952). Tables for predicting adult height from skeletal age: revised for use with the Greulich-Pyle hand standards. *J. Pediat.*, **40**, 432.

Foss, G. L. (1956). A comparison of the relative efficacy of methyltestosterone by the gastric and oral transmucosal routes. *J. Endocr.*, **13**, 269.

—— (1962). Infantilism to fatherhood in the malabsorption syndrome. *Brit. med. J.*, **2**, 368.

Greulich, W. W., and Pyle, S. I. (1959). *Radiographic Atlas of Skeletal Development of the Hand and Wrist*, 2nd ed. Stanford University Press, California; Oxford University Press, London.

Sobel, E. H., Raymond, C. S., Quinn, K. V., and Talbot, N. B. (1956). The use of methyltestosterone to stimulate growth: relative influence on skeletal maturation and linear growth. *J. clin. Endocr.*, **16**, 241.

*Arch. Dis. Childh.*, 1965, **40**, 71.

# THYROTOXICOSIS IN CHILDREN: A FOLLOW-UP STUDY

BY

T. McKENDRICK* and G. H. NEWNS

*From The Hospital for Sick Children, Great Ormond Street, London*

(RECEIVED FOR PUBLICATION APRIL 27, 1964)

Thyrotoxicosis in childhood is uncommon and there are few reports regarding either its treatment or prognosis. There is no agreement on whether medical or surgical therapy is better. Arnold, Talbot, and Cope (1958) summarized the choice as follows.

(a) *Surgical excision:* short in duration, but carrying a mortality risk and the possibilities of recurrence or hypothyroidism.

(b) *Medical therapy:* frequent and prolonged, with the need for supervision, the risk of toxic reactions, and the chance of eventual failure.

Surgical mortality may be small but is present in most of the recorded series (Hayles, Kennedy, Beahrs, and Woolner, 1959; Kunstadter and Stein, 1955; McClintock, Frawley, and Holden, 1956; Van Wyk, Grumbach, Shepard, and Wilkins, 1956) where a total of 7 children died after 275 operations. Arnold *et al.* (1958) and Root, Bongiovanni, Harvie, and Eberlein (1963) had no mortality in 28 patients. In all these series the recurrence rate was not less than 5%, while no less than 73 children operated on were subsequently found to be hypothyroid. On the other hand some patients were submitted to operation only because medical therapy had failed.

Medical therapy carries few risks. There are few reports of toxic drug reactions in children who seem to be at less risk than adults. Kunstadter and Stein (1955) had no reactions in 17 children treated with thiourea derivatives; Hung, Wilkins, and Blizzard (1962) reported maculo-papular rashes and fever in 2 of 9 children treated with perchlorate, urticarial rashes in 3 of 23 children who had propylthiouracil, and 'granulocytopenia accompanied by buccal ulceration and sore throat' in 1 of these children; Root *et al.* (1963) noted that 3 of their 17 children had mild leucopenia with fever and a skin rash.

With these 9 and one child in the present series who developed leucopenia while on a small dose of methylthiouracil, there were, therefore, 10 children out of 99 treated who developed toxic reactions. This figure is similar to the incidence (2-10%) reported in adults.

In some reported series medical therapy has had to be abandoned because of the lack of co-operation by patient or parents. Though this did not occur in the present study, it may have to be considered an important factor influencing the choice of therapy.

As nearly all patients respond to some antithyroid drug, the duration of medical therapy may be the main factor dictating the choice between medical or surgical therapy. There is little recorded experience of this yet. Hung *et al.* (1962) suggest that probably over one-third of thyrotoxic children are cured by therapy lasting for two years or more.

In the decade 1953-63, 26 children attended The Hospital for Sick Children with thyrotoxicosis. With the records of 7 other children seen before 1953, they are here reviewed in an attempt to assess the therapy of this condition in childhood.

Of the 33 children, 29 were girls and 4 were boys. Symptoms appeared before the age of 5 years in 10 patients, between 5 and 10 years in 14 patients, and between 10 and 14 years in 9. It is likely that the last figure is artificially low because some children with onset at this age are referred to adult units. The duration of symptoms before the diagnosis was made is shown in Table 1.

There was no relation between the age of the child and the delay in diagnosis. The shortest history was 2 weeks, the longest 19 months.

The long delay in diagnosis in nearly one-third of

TABLE 1

INTERVAL BETWEEN ONSET OF SYMPTOMS AND DIAGNOSIS

| Time in Months | Number of Children |
|---|---|
| 0–3 | 7 |
| 3–6 | 9 |
| 6–9 | 7 |
| 9–12 | 0 |
| > 12 | 10 |

* Present address: Department of Child Health, Alder Hey Children's Hospital, Liverpool.

the series reflects, as in adults, the difficulty of differentiating the insidious onset of thyrotoxicosis from longstanding behaviour, and emotional disturbances, and anxiety states. The occurrence of other thyroid disorders in the families did not always reduce this delay. Of 11 families, 17 members had thyroid abnormalities of some kind, i.e. either goitre or thyrotoxicosis; these included 6 parents, 3 grandparents, and 8 aunts or cousins.

TABLE 2

MAIN SYMPTOMS AT THE TIME OF DIAGNOSIS IN 33 CHILDREN

| Symptom | No. of Patients |
|---|---|
| Nervousness | 26 |
| Prominent eyes | 26 |
| Goitre | 21 |
| Excessive growth | 16 |
| Loss of weight | 16 |
| Excessive sweating | 12 |
| Diarrhoea | 8 |
| Restlessness | 7 |
| Choreiform movements | 5 |
| Insomnia | 4 |
| Excessive appetite | 3 |
| Other personality change | 3 |

## Symptoms and Signs

The *symptoms* are listed in Table 2. They are similar to those noted in adults though the choreiform movements are probably peculiar to children. Young patients do not evidently complain of feeling too hot. A thyrotoxic crisis occurred only once and was precipitated by an operation.

The symptom of personality change merits special attention. As a presenting feature it was uncommon. Closer inquiry, however, elicited that in 13 children abnormal behaviour had been noted for some years, often beginning long before any other symptom appeared. Only in retrospect did the parents recognize that such behaviour change had become more marked when other symptoms began. Since behaviour problems sufficiently marked to require medical advice occur in about 5 to 10% of children,* it is difficult to know how much of these features could be attributed to hyperthyroidism. There was no specific pattern. Misbehaviour, lack of concentration, bullying, 'not trying' and backwardness at school, perversity, wilfulness and temper tantrums at home, as well as enuresis, and other symptoms of being 'highly strung' were recorded. Recovery from them was sometimes dramatic when thyrotoxicosis was controlled but it was not always either rapid or complete. The first symptom of a relapse was usually behaviour disorder.

* Ministry of Education (1955). *Report of the Committee on Maladjusted Children.*

TABLE 3

HEIGHT AND WEIGHT BY PERCENTILE DISTRIBUTION

| Percentile | Height | | Weight | |
|---|---|---|---|---|
| | No. | % | No. | % |
| > 90 | 15 | 51 | 9 | 27 |
| 75–90 | 8 | 27 | 5 | 15 |
| 50–75 | 3 | 11 | 8 | 24 |
| < 50 | 3 | 11 | 10 | 30 |
| Not known | 4 | — | 1 | — |

In most patients *signs* were sufficiently clear to confirm the diagnosis suggested by the history. Most were similar to those seen in adults. Thus 30 patients had an abnormal tachycardia and 21 an unusually high pulse pressure; warm moist palms were noted in 26 patients. Prominent eyes, whether due to lid retraction or exophthalmos were obvious in 23 and present in another 4 patients but absent in 6. Lid lag and other ocular signs could be demonstrated in 14 patients, usually in the older age-groups. Only 2 patients had no abnormal movements. Though tremor was commonly recorded it was seldom of the classical thyrotoxic fine type. Choreiform movements were seen in 7 patients. Anxiety, nervousness, restlessness, and fidgeting were evident in 25.

The accelerated growth associated with hyperthyroidism is shown in Table 3. It will be noted that excessive height was common but that nearly half the children were able to eat enough to keep their weight approximately commensurate with height.

All the patients had an enlarged thyroid gland, but in 4 this was very slight and only in 2 was it described as large. All the glands were smooth, most were symmetrical, and over most a *bruit* was heard.

## Investigations

Estimation of the blood cholesterol was unhelpful. In 5 patients the level was over 200 mg./100 ml.; in 16 it was within the normal range of 100-200 mg./100 ml., and in 1 it was low.

The basal metabolic rate (BMR) was measured in 24 patients. In 8 it was unequivocally raised, i.e. over 140% of the normal levels related to surface area; in 8 it was less clearly raised, i.e. between 120 and 140% and in 8 it was hardly abnormal, i.e. 100 to 120%. In no child was it less than 100%. In one other child, lack of co-operation twice prevented any worth-while measurement. There was considerable discrepancy (over 30%) between duplicate measurements in three children.

The level of protein bound iodine (PBI) before treatment was obtained from only 12 patients. Of

TABLE 4

RELATION BETWEEN PROTEIN-BOUND IODINE AND BASAL METABOLIC RATE

| Basal Metabolic Rate (%) | Protein-bound Iodine (μg./100 ml.) | | |
|---|---|---|---|
| | < 4 | 4–8 | > 8 |
| 100–120 | | | 3 |
| 120–140 | | 1 | 2 |
| 140 | | 2 | 1 |

TABLE 5

SUMMARY OF THERAPY

| Therapy | Initially | Subsequently |
|---|---|---|
| Methyl thiouracil .. .. .. | 5 | 0 |
| Carbimazole .. .. .. | 12 | 3 |
| Perchlorate .. .. .. | 8 | 1 |
| Surgery .. .. .. | 4 | 5 |
| Other therapy .. .. | 4 | — |

these, 9 had high levels (greater than 8 μg./100 ml.), and 3 had normal levels (4-8 μg./100 ml.), the lowest level being 5·5 μg./100 ml. The correlation between BMR and PBI in the 9 patients in which both were estimated was not high (see Table 4).

## Diagnosis

In spite of the newer techniques, such as the study of radio-iodine uptake by the thyroid, measurement of BMR by diapherometry, and estimation of PBI, the diagnosis of thyrotoxicosis remains a clinical exercise. In none of the children in this series was the diagnosis suggested by any such investigation and the chief value of these tests was in confirming the diagnosis *vis-à-vis* psychological disorder more rapidly and certainly. They also enabled a more rational approach to the control of the condition by drug therapy; but they have not so far eased the problem of how long treatment should continue.

## Therapy

Therapy is summarized in Table 5.

The early patients in this series were either subjected to partial thyroidectomy or were treated with sedation and prolonged bed-rest. Of the 4 who were operated on, 3 were known to have remained well (and euthyroid) for 6½, 10½, and 20 years respectively, though one child developed an inactive thyroid adenoma. The fourth child was well 1½ years later, after which she was lost to follow-up. This apparently favourable outlook must be tempered by the fate of 2 of the 5 children who were operated on after apparent failure of medical therapy: one died suddenly on the day after an uneventful thyroidectomy; the other relapsed within a year of operation and is threatened with a further thyroidectomy. Two other children in this group have been operated on too recently to be able to comment on the result.

**Methyl Thiouracil.** The experience with methyl thiouracil is summarized in Table 6. This group of 5 cases is too small and the results too variable to allow of any generalization. The only child who showed any toxic reaction (P.N.) was in this group.

**Carbimazole.** Table 7 summarizes the results with this drug in 15 patients.

All the patients except one treated with carbimazole became euthyroid within 3 months, and over half of them within one month. There seemed little difficulty in maintaining this state for several years but even after nearly 6 years of therapy, relapse could still occur while on therapeutic doses.

Five patients have remained euthyroid for more than a year after cessation of one course of therapy. The duration of the course, however, has varied from 3 to 39 months. Only one patient has relapsed after having stopped treatment for more than a year; 7 others have relapsed either within 9 months of cessation or while still on maintenance therapy. There is no relation between liability of relapse and duration of therapy or rapidity of control of symptoms.

Of these 15 patients, 4 became hypothyroid during therapy. Though they all had low serum PBI levels, only one showed clinical signs. Serial estimation of PBI level undoubtedly facilitated smoother control in the other 3 as well as those who relapsed.

TABLE 6

THERAPY WITH METHYL THIOURACIL

| Patient | Age (yr.) | Initial Dose (mg./day) | Maintenance Dose (mg./day) | Duration of Therapy (mth.) | Result | Subsequent Therapy |
|---|---|---|---|---|---|---|
| C.A. | 10 | 300 | 50 | 9 | Euthyroid | |
| P.N. | 10 | 50 | — | 20 days | Leucopenia | Carbimazole |
| H.T. | 5½ | 200 | 50 | 9 | Erratic control | Surgery |
| L.W. | 4 | 300 | 25-50 | 142 | 2 mild relapses | |
| E.H. | 4 | 50 | — | 1 | No control | Surgery† |

† died.

TABLE 7

THERAPY WITH CARBIMAZOLE

| Patient | Age | Initial Dose (mg./day) | Maintenance Dose (mg./day) | Duration of Therapy (mth.) | Time Since Stopping Therapy (mth.) | Result |
|---|---|---|---|---|---|---|
| J.A. | 7½ | 15-20 | 10-15 | 28 | 15 | Relapsed |
| J.C.(1)* | 7 | 20 | 15 | 42 | 9 | Relapsed |
| (2) | 11¼ | 10-15 | 10 | 5 | Continues therapy | Euthyroid |
| S.C. | 4½ | 20 | 7·5 | 21 | Continues therapy | Euthyroid |
| C.D. | 9 | 20 | 5-15 | 70 | — | Relapsed (P) |
| J.F. | 4½ | 15 | 5 | 6 | 80 | Euthyroid |
| A.H.(1) | 8 | 15 | 10 | 12 | 6 | Relapsed |
| (2) | 9½ | 10 | 5 | 32 | 3 | Relapsed |
| (3) | 12½ | 2·5 | 2·5 | 20 | 12 | Euthyroid |
| J.M. | 10 | 20 | 5-15 | 39 | 16 | Euthyroid |
| D.N. | 12 | 20 | 10-15 | 27 | 24 | Euthyroid |
| P.N.† | 10 | 10 | 2·5 | 3 | 84 | Euthyroid |
| T.O. | 11½ | 30 | 10-15 | 45 | Continues therapy | Relapsed on maintenance dose |
| K.R. | 9½ | 20 | 10-45 | 99 | Continues therapy | Relapsed × 3 (S) |
| P.T. | 11¾ | 30 | 10-45 | 47 | — | Relapsed (S) |
| V.W.(1) | 10½ | 30 | 10 | 40 | 5 | Relapsed |
| (2) | 14 | 40 | 7·5 | 11 | Continues therapy | Euthyroid |
| S.B. | 4 | 15 | 10 | 12 | Continues therapy | Euthyroid |
| V.M.* | 11½ | | | 40 | — | Poor control (S) |

* Previously treated with perchlorate.
† Previously treated with methyl thiouracil.
(P) Subsequently treated with perchlorate.
(S) Subsequently treated by operation.

**Perchlorate.** This drug was introduced relatively recently and only 9 patients received sodium (or potassium) perchlorate (see Table 8). Though only one patient has so far been followed up for more than a year after treatment, this group suggests that perchlorate has little advantage over carbimazole. Of the 9 patients, one failed to respond to a moderate dose and subsequently responded quickly to carbimazole. All the others became euthyroid in less than 3 months (on average rather less than 2 months) irrespective of the dose given. So far 3 have relapsed, one while on perchlorate, the other 2 five months after stopping treatment.

Hypothyroidism as judged by serial PBI estimations has been commoner, occurring in 5 of the 9 patients.

## Discussion

Therapy with anti-thyroid drugs was given to 25 patients. All except 3 were brought under control within 3 months and of the exceptions, 2 (E.H., Table 6 and J.C., Table 8) were inadequately treated; 7 have completed one or more courses lasting in all between 3 and 39 months and subsequently remained euthyroid for more than a year; 7 relapsed after completing up to 42 months therapy; with one exception all relapsed within a year of cessation of therapy and all except 2 had been treated for more than 2 years; 6 have relapsed while still on maintenance therapy, 2 more than once, and these relapses have been as early as 5 months or as late as 11 years after beginning treatment; 8 patients (including some

TABLE 8

THERAPY WITH PERCHLORATE

| Patient | Age (yr.) | Initial Dose (mg./day) | Maintenance Dose (mg./day) | Duration of Therapy (mth.) | Time Since Stopping Therapy (mth.) | Result |
|---|---|---|---|---|---|---|
| J.C. | 7 | 400-600 | — | 3 wk. | — | No effect (C) |
| P.C. | 10¼ | 800 | | 27 | 1 | Euthyroid |
| C.D.* | 15 | 1,500 | 500 | 18 | Continues therapy | Euthyroid |
| J.E. | 11¾ | 400 | 200 | 17 | 5 | Relapsed |
| V.M.(1) | 11¾ | 400 | 300-600 | 16 | — | Relapsed |
| (2) | 13 | 500 | 500 | 20 | — | Unsatisfactory (C) (S) |
| C.M.† | 14½ | 1,000 | 200 | 5 | 12 | Euthyroid |
| L.R.(1) | 10¼ | 1,500 | 250 | 38 | 5 | Relapsed |
| (2) | | 1,000 | | | | |
| K.V. | 10 | 300 | 400 | 6 | 6 | Euthyroid |
| S.W. | 5¾ | 700 | 300 | 14 | Continues therapy | Euthyroid |

*N.B.* In 5 patients the PBI fell to hypothyroid levels.
* Previously treated with carbimazole.
† A mongol child in whom assessment was difficult.
(C) Subsequently treated with carbimazole.
(S) Subsequently treated by operation.

TABLE 9

DAILY DOSAGE OF DRUGS USED IN DIFFERENT PUBLISHED SERIES

| Drug | | Present Series | Hung *et al.* | Root *et al.* |
|---|---|---|---|---|
| Methyl or propyl thiouracil | Initial (m.g.) | 50-300 | 300 | 150-300* |
| | Maintenance (m.g.) | 25-50 | 100-150 | 50-150* |
| Carbimazole | Initial (mg.) | 15-40 | 40 | 15-30* |
| | Maintenance (mg.) | 5-20 | 10-20 | 5-15* |
| Sodium or potassium perchlorate | Initial (g.) | 0·3-1·5 | 3·0 | |
| | Maintenance (g.) | 0·2-0·6 | 0·5-0·75 | |

* Initial doses expressed as 6·7 mg./kg. and 0·6-0·8 mg./kg. respectively and maintenance as one-third to one-half of these doses.

who have previously relapsed) are at present euthyroid while on therapy having been treated for periods of up to 12 years.

It is difficult to compare the results of therapy in the series with those of other workers; numbers are small and other factors are too variable (e.g. duration of therapy and of follow-up after therapy has ceased). Nevertheless they differ probably only slightly from those reported by Hung *et al.* (1962) and Root *et al.* (1963). In the former 15 of 28, and in the latter 7 of 14, patients have so far remained euthyroid for more than a year after one or two completed courses of medical therapy. In the former series, only 5 of 33 patients were treated by operation; in the latter 7 of 17. In the present series, 7 of 17 adequately treated medically have remained euthyroid for over 1 year following cessation of therapy and 6 of 23* have come to operation. It is possible that smaller dosage of drugs may be responsible for the difference (Table 9).

The average initial doses of carbimazole and perchlorate used were about half those stated by Hung *et al.* and Root *et al.* The incidence of drug reactions, 1 in 33, was less than in either of these series. With the 2 patients in this series who were given clearly inadequate dosage this comparison suggests that dosage must be higher than the minimum needed to control symptoms. The risk of more frequent toxic reactions may be outweighed by the higher proportion of patients who do not require operation. Very few patients, provided co-operation is adequate and toxicity does not occur, require operation before puberty. In view of the high incidence of post-operative hypothyroidism this is an important advantage.

The optimum duration of therapy is even more difficult to assess. Three of the present series were apparently cured by one course of less than 6 months' duration. Three others have not responded permanently in 6, 8, and 12 years, respectively. Such prolonged therapy is undesirable, for there is always the risk of 'breaking through' control especially if after long periods administration of the drug becomes less regular.

The scheme suggested by Root *et al.* seems the best compromise. Drugs are used for two years and then stopped. One relapse is treated similarly but any subsequent relapse is an indication for operation as are toxic drug reactions and lack of co-operation. It also seems reasonable to treat pre-pubertal patients medically even if this means more than 2 years of therapy.

* E.H. and J.C. are omitted from this total.

## Summary

In an attempt to assess the value of medical therapy of thyrotoxicosis in children, the progress of 33 children was studied. Most were girls and the onset of symptoms occurred at all ages after 4 years. The more valuable diagnostic features were nervousness, proptosis, goitre, tachycardia, sweating, and abnormal movements. Excessive growth was common. Abnormal behaviour tended to delay the diagnosis. Special investigations were of relatively slight value in the initial diagnosis but facilitated the later supervision.

One of 9 children treated by operation died; one more has relapsed. All except 1 of 23 who were given adequate medical therapy were controlled without difficulty. About one-third have remained euthyroid for over a year after the cessation of therapy. Similar proportions have relapsed either on maintenance therapy or within a year or so of its cessation. The slightly lower dosage of drugs used (compared with other series) may have accounted for this less satisfactory result and for the lower incidence of drug toxicity.

On the basis of this and other series it is suggested that a two-year course of medical therapy should be given in the first place. A relapse should be followed by a second course also lasting two years. Any further relapse should be treated by operation.

Thanks are due to the Physicians of The Hospital for Sick Children for permission to include patients under their care in this series.

REFERENCES

Arnold, M. B., Talbot, N. B., and Cope, O. (1958). Concerning the choice of therapy for childhood hyperthyroidism. *Pediatrics*, **21**, 47.

Hayles, A. B., Kennedy, R. L. J., Beahrs, O. H., and Woolner, L. B. (1959). Exophthalmic goiter in children. *J. clin. Endocr.*, **19**, 138.

Hung, W., Wilkins, L., and Blizzard, R. (1962). Medical therapy of thyrotoxicosis in children. *Pediatrics*, **30**, 17.

Kunstadter, R. H., and Stein, A. F. (1955). Treatment of thyrotoxic children with thio-urea derivatives. *Amer. J. Dis. Child.*, **90**, 373.

McClintock, J. C., Frawley, T. F., and Holden, J. H. P. (1956). Hyperthyroidism in children: observations in 50 treated cases, including an evaluation of endocrine factors. *J. clin. Endocr.*, **16**, 62.

Ministry of Education (1955). *Report of the Committee on Maladjusted Children*, Chap. 8 and Appendix H. H.M.S.O., London.

Root, A. W., Bongiovanni, A. M., Harvie, F. H., and Eberlein, W. R. (1963). Treatment of juvenile thyrotoxicosis. *J. Pediat.*, **63**, 402.

Van Wyk, J. J., Grumbach, M. M., Shepard, T. H., II, and Wilkins, L. (1956). The treatment of hyperthyroidism in childhood with thiouracil drugs. *Pediatrics*, **17**, 221.

## Addendum

Since this paper was submitted, a review of 70 patients cared for over 20 years has been published by Saxena, Crawford, and Talbot (1964). 52 were treated surgically. Permanent hypothyroidism occurred in 18 (38%), and hypoparathyroidism with tetany in 10%. Three developed a recurrence of thyrotoxicosis. The remaining 18 patients had been treated with iodides and latterly antithyroid drugs. The follow-up of most of these was too brief to draw conclusions.

REFERENCE

Saxena, K. M., Crawford, J. D., and Talbot, N. B. (1964). Childhood thyrotoxicosis: A long-term perspective. *Brit. med. J.*, **2**, 1153.

*Arch. Dis. Childh.*, 1965, **40**, 77.

# AN ASSESSMENT OF GASTRIC ACID SECRETORY RESPONSE WITH 'MAXIMAL' AUGMENTED HISTAMINE STIMULATION IN CHILDREN WITH PEPTIC ULCER

BY

O. P. GHAI, MEHARBAN SINGH, B. N. S. WALIA, and N. G. GADEKAR

*From the Departments of Pediatrics and Radiology, All India Institute of Medical Sciences, New Delhi, India*

(RECEIVED FOR PUBLICATION JUNE 1, 1964)

Numerous recent reports have outlined the clinical profile of childhood peptic ulcer (Alexander, 1951; Fallstrom and Reinand, 1961; Gadiyar, Taneja, and Ghai, 1963; Girdany, 1953; Michener, Kennedy, and Du Shane, 1960; Muggia and Spiro, 1959; Ramirez Ramos, Kirsner, and Palmer, 1960). Investigation of its pathogenesis, however, has not received much attention. There is general agreement that peptic ulceration cannot persist in the absence of acid and pepsin (Grossman, 1951). The concept of a physiological balance between two sets of opposing forces, i.e. the hydrochloric acid and pepsin on the one hand and mucosal resistance on the other, have given a dynamic approach to the problem (Shay, 1959). The present study was undertaken to assess the role of gastric hydrochloric acid in the aetio-pathogenesis of childhood duodenal ulcer.

### Material and Method

Sixteen children with minor illnesses unrelated to the gastro-intestinal tract and 18 radiologically proved cases of duodenal ulcer with a crater were studied for gastric acid secretory capacity with the 'maximal' augmented histamine test (Kay, 1953, modified by Card and Marks, 1960). A triple sedative (pethidine 1·5 mg./kg., chlorpromazine 0·5 mg./kg., and promethazine 0·5 mg./kg.) was injected subcutaneously half an hour before intubation. The position of the tube was checked by fluoroscopy. Suction pressure was kept between 10-15 cm. of water. The results of total acidity were expressed as (i) basal acid output (BAO) or the first hour interdigestive secretion; (ii) the 'maximal' acid output (MAO) or the post histamine one-hour secretion.

### Results

The results of the investigation are summarized in Tables 1 and 2, and Fig. 1.

The test was repeated in two patients with duodenal ulcer after four to six months of relief from symptoms. Radiologically healing had taken place. There was no significant change in basal acid output, but MAO was reduced from the initial values of 15·71 and 11·82 to 7·31 (53% drop) and 4·82 (61% drop).

### Discussion

There are few published reports of gastric secretory pattern after a test meal or histamine stimulation in childhood peptic ulcer. It appears that the 'maximal' augmented histamine test has not so far been employed in children.

The mean basal and maximal acid outputs in our control subjects were 0·32 mEq./10 kg. hour and 2·02 mEq/10 kg. hour, respectively. A significant correlation between maximal acid output and the weight of the child was obtained (Fig. 1). This conforms to the belief that increase in the size of the

TABLE 1

COMPARATIVE DATA ON AGE, WEIGHT, HEIGHT, AND GASTRIC ACID SECRETION IN TWO GROUPS

| | Patients | Controls |
|---|---|---|
| No. of cases | 18 | 16 |
| Mean age (yr.) | 11·3 | 10·9 |
| Mean weight (kg.) | 28·2 | 25·3 |
| Mean height (cm.) | 134 | 130 |
| BAO (mEq/hour) | 1·04 ± 0·05 (0·38–2·10) | 0·83 ± 0·05 (0·24–2·09) |
| MAO (mEq/hour) | 8·39 ± 0·72 (4·15–15·70) | 5·25 ± 0·48 (2·82–9·85) |

TABLE 2

GASTRIC ACID SECRETORY PATTERN IN ACTIVE AND QUIESCENT ULCER CASES

| | Active Ulcer | Quiescent Ulcer |
|---|---|---|
| No. of cases | 10 | 8 |
| BAO (mEq/hour) | 1·16 ± 0·02 (0·38 – 2·10) | 0·89 ± 0·01 (0·52 – 1·50) |
| MAO (mEq/hour) | 10·10 ± 0·88 (7·05–15·70) | 6·25 ± 0·62 (4·15–9·40) |

$p < 0·001$ for control and active ulcers (MAO only).
$p < 0·01$ for active and quiescent ulcers (MAO only).
p insignificant for control and quiescent ulcers (MAO only).

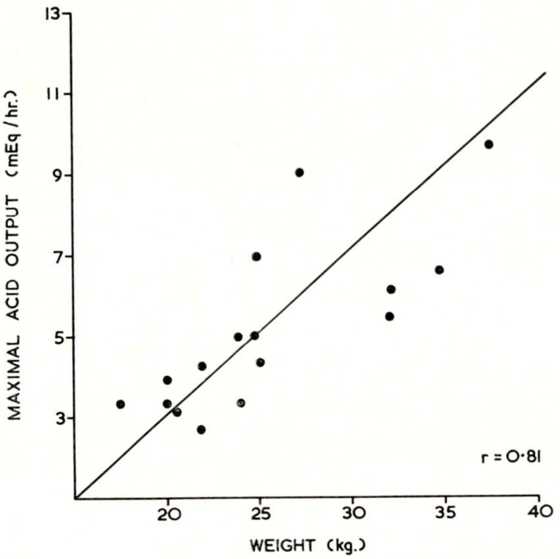


FIG. 1.—Relation between maximal acid output and body weight.

child is associated with growth of the stomach and hence an increase in the parietal cell mass (W. I. Card, 1963, personal communication).

The mean basal acid output in duodenal ulcer patients was 0·43 mEq/10 kg. hour. There was no significant difference in the basal acid ouput of the two groups. This is in contrast to the findings in the adults where mean basal acid output in duodenal ulcer patients is significantly higher than in the controls. The exact significance of these findings is unknown. It may be due partly to suppression of basal secretory mechanisms by large doses of pethidine, chlorpromazine, and promethazine, which were given to all these children.

Of the duodenal ulcer patients, 11 (61%) secreted maximal acid of more than 2·50 mEq/10 kg. hr., while only 3 controls (19%) secreted that amount. A correlation between high maximal acid output and activity of the ulcer at the time of the first test was observed. Serial estimations of MAO in 2 patients showed a fall during the quiescent phase of the ulcer. No such relation was seen with basal secretion (Table 2). Bolo, Palol, and Los Santos (1961), while studying basal gastric secretions in 199 adults with duodenal ulcer, reported that during activity while 86% of them showed hyperchlorhydria, during quiescence, only 36% showed hyperacidity. Littman (1962) showed a clear drop in basal secretion in 9 patients with duodenal ulcer during their first remission.

Maximal acid output obtained under the conditions of the original test is considered as a fairly good index of parietal cell mass (Card and Marks, 1960; Cox, 1952; Marks, 1956; Tongen, 1950). However, it does not represent the maximal secretory capacity of the stomach under all conditions. Ward, Gillespie, Passaro, and Grossman (1963), have shown that by the use of histalog in doses of 100 mg. subcutaneously, the gastric acid output is much higher than that obtained with the 'maximal' augmented histamine test. It is difficult to explain the exact significance of the positive correlation between MAO and the activity of the ulcer. It is possible that in the active phase the parietal cells are in a hyperexcitable state, so that heightened secretory response to exogenous stimulus is obtained. This 'end-organ excitatory tonus' may also exist for stimuli other than histamine, resulting in perpetuation of ulceration. However, more observations are needed to confirm these findings.

## Summary

The results of the 'maximal' augmented histamine test on 18 radiologically proven cases of duodenal ulcer in children and 16 control subjects are presented. All received triple sedative injection half an hour before the start of the test. The mean basal and the maximal acid output in control subjects were 0·32 mEq/10 kg. hour and 2·02 mEq/10 kg. hour, respectively. There was a significant correlation between body weight and 'maximal' acid output in control subjects. There was no significant difference between basal outputs in duodenal ulcer patients and control subjects. Eleven patients with duodenal ulcer (61%) secreted 'maximal' acid in amounts more than 2·50 mEq/10 kg. hour while only 3 control children (19%) did so. A direct correlation between the activity of the ulcer and maximal acid output was observed. The significance of these findings is discussed.

### REFERENCES

Alexander, F. K. (1951). Duodenal ulcer in children. *Radiology*, **56**, 799.

Bolo, P. O., Palol, J. de, and Los Santos, M. A. de (1961). Correlation of basal gastric secretion with peptic ulcer activity. *Amer. J. dig. Dis.*, **6**, 784.

Card, W. I., and Marks, I. N. (1960). The relationship between the acid output of the stomach following 'maximal' histamine stimulation and the parietal cell mass. *Clin. Sci.*, **19**, 147.

Cox, A. J., Jr. (1952). Stomach size and its relation to chronic peptic ulcer. *Arch. Path.*, **54**, 407.

Fallstrom, S. P., and Reinand, T. (1961). Peptic ulcer in children. *Acta paediat.* (*Uppsala*) **50**, 431.

Gadiyar, B. N., Taneja, P. N., and Ghai, O. P. (1963). Recurrent pain in abdomen in children. *Indian J. Child Hlth*, **12**, 289.

Girdany, B. R. (1953). Peptic ulcer in childhood. *Pediatrics*, **12**, 56.

Grossman, M. I. (1951). A critical analysis of various theories of the pathogenesis of peptic ulcer. In *Peptic Ulcer*, ed. D. J. Sandweiss. Saunders, Philadelphia.

Kay, A. W. (1953). Effect of large doses of histamine on gastric secretion of HC1 : an augmented histamine test. *Brit. med. J.*, **2**, 77.

Littman, A. (1962). Basal gastric secretion in patients with duodenal ulcer: a long term study of variations in relation to ulcer activity. *Gastroenterology*, **43**, 166.

Marks, I. N. (1956). The relationship of the acid output of the parietal cell population of the stomach. *Scot. med. J.*, **1**, 242.

Michener, W. M., Kennedy, R. L. J., and Du Shane, J. W. (1960). Duodenal ulcer in childhood. *Amer. J. Dis. Child.*, **100**, 814.

Muggia, A., and Spiro, H. M. (1959). Childhood peptic ulcer. *Gastroenterology*, **37**, 715.

Ramirez Ramos, A., Kirsner, J. B., and Palmer, W. L. (1960). Peptic ulcer in children. *Amer. J. Dis. Child.*, **99**, 135.

Shay, H. (1959). Emotional stress and parietal cell mass: their role in the aetiology of peptic ulcer. *Amer. J. dig. Dis.*, **4**, 846.

Tongen, L. A. (1950). The quantitative relationship between parietal cells and gastric acidity. *Surgery*, **28**, 1009.

Ward, S., Gillespie, I. E., Passaro, E. P., and Grossman, M. I. (1963). Comparison of histalog and histamine as stimulants for maximal gastric secretion in human subjects and in dogs. *Gastroenterology*, **44**, 620.

*Arch. Dis. Childh.*, 1965, **40**, 80.

# EXTERNAL INJURY CAUSING FOETAL DEFORMITY

BY

E. HINDEN

*From Whipps Cross Hospital, London*

(RECEIVED FOR PUBLICATION JUNE 16, 1964)

Mechanical injury to the mother's abdomen, causing damage to a *foetus in utero*, must be an extreme rarity; I can find but one reference. Sheldon (1962) quotes 'Gibb, 1858' (no other details supplied) as follows.

'Accidents and injuries to the mother's abdomen may sometimes damage the foetal brain—this was so in an infant who died at birth and was found to have an old haemorrhage in the right hemisphere which had resulted from a severe blow by a plank of wood on the mother's abdomen.'

This reference is over a century old. Neither Potter (1961) nor Willis (1962) in their exhaustive treatises on foetal pathology mention external trauma as a pathogen. In his long account of prenatal damage, Pliess (1962) says,

'While formerly mechanical influences (non-penetrating abdominal injuries) as a cause of deformity were considered the more important, nowadays radiation . . . and amniotic puncture. . . .'

and there leaves the subject. He gives but one reference out of a bibliography of 606 items. This reference (Wiedemann, 1955) is as follows.

'Mechanical factors causing damage may occasionally lead to the death and rejection of the foetus, but they have previously been very much exaggerated, to say the least, as causes for prenatal malformations or disease.'

Neither of these last two writers quotes any example. The following case history may therefore be of interest.

## Case Report

Marina X, the fifth child of Greek-Cypriot parents, was born at Forest Gate Hospital on October 12, 1958. The pregnancy and delivery were apparently quite normal, but it was noticed at birth that there was an unusual fresh scar across the bridge of the child's nose, which was depressed as though pushed in. There was speculation as to the cause of this, but no firm diagnosis was made. Mrs. X, who was concerned about the well-being of her other children, did not stay the usual 10 days (she left after 4) so I did not see the baby at my usual neonatal round.

The child grew and developed normally till June 1960. She then suffered from a swelling of her left eye, with fever; this soon got better. In July she sustained her first fit, a major convulsion. The fits persisted, and in October of that year she was admitted to St. Mary's Hospital, Plaistow. Treatment did not control the convulsions, so in December 1960 she was referred to Dr. Sandifer at The Hospital for Sick Children, Great Ormond Street. A radiograph at that time showed 'a midline bone defect on the right of the nose associated with a defective development of the nasal bones' (Fig.), but neurological examination was essentially negative. She was referred to the plastic surgeon for treatment of her nose.

Her condition did not change until July 11, 1961, when she was admitted to The Hospital for Sick Children for the first time because of a prolonged seizure which had started at 9.30 p.m. the previous evening, with a right hemiplegia. Intensive neurological and neurosurgical investigations were carried out, culminating in a craniotomy on August 25. This showed enlargement of the left lateral ventricle of the brain, which did not communicate with the rest of the ventricular system. The surgeon commented that he did not find the expected signs of increased intracranial tension. An opening was made through the septum pellucidum to restore circulation of the cerebrospinal fluid. The child made a good recovery, though the hemiplegia persisted.

There was no major change in her condition thereafter. She was admitted twice subsequently for intercurrent minor infections, and once for probing of her lachrymal ducts. This attempt was not successful, and further operation is under consideration. Her right foot was spastic and her right hand clumsy, but she had no great disability. In September 1963, when she was not yet 5, she was accepted by her local primary school. However, the head teacher soon saw that her physical and mental performances were not normal, thought she was 'spastic', and asked for an ascertainment of her educational needs. Accordingly she was examined at a conference at the West Ham Development Clinic.

At this conference (October 11, 1963) the above history

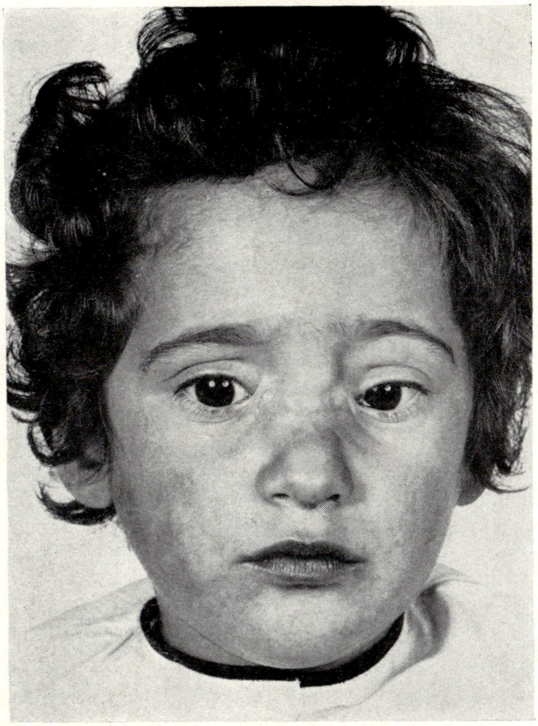

FIG.—Appearance of child.

was presented, together with an I.Q. test (revised Stanford-Binet, form L) of 65%. We found a pleasant, somewhat retarded child, with a mild residual hemiplegia. But a vital piece of evidence, hitherto unrevealed, was brought out. Mrs. X's mother-tongue is Greek and her knowledge of English poor, so she does not talk about herself much. However, over the years her health visitor has built up a warm relationship with her. Recently Mrs. X told this lady that when she was 6 months pregnant, she had fallen down some steps into a basement area, striking her abdomen, a little above the pubis, on a metal boot-scraper fixed at the foot of the steps. Her abdominal wall was badly bruised ('it was all black and blue') and very sore; at night she found it hard to get to sleep as she could not settle herself in comfort. She also noticed that the foetal movements, which had been vigorous till then, stopped abruptly. She was very upset and frightened by this accident, and deliberately delayed her next antenatal visit till all the bruising had gone: this took four weeks. By that time the foetus was moving again; she hoped all was well and did not report the occurrence.

When she saw the baby after birth, she at once connected the damaged nose with the blow on her abdomen, and tried to explain this to her attendants. But her English was quite inadequate; she saw she was not being understood, and gave up the attempt.

## Comment

Everyone who saw the baby at birth wondered at the scar; it did not conform with the usual developmental abnormalities; it looked like an injury. While it seems most likely that the foetus did sustain an intrauterine injury, crushing the bridge of her nose and causing gross damage to her brain, it is not possible to assert this dogmatically. Congenital deformity may take bizarre forms and could be responsible. This is the view of Prof. R. A. Willis (personal communication). Dr. Edith Potter (personal communication) also thinks that it is not proven that trauma caused the child's condition. However, bearing in mind the injury during pregnancy and its effect upon the foetus at the time, the obvious scar on the infant's face at birth, and the unusual damage to the nasal bones and the naso-lachrymal duct, it seems barely credible to assume that all this is simple coincidence with non-traumatic congenital malformation.

It remains to consider the nature of the neurological lesion. This may have been a haemorrhage blocking the foramen of Monro; but Dr. K. M. Laurence (personal communication) suggests that it may have been a porencephalic cyst, distorting the ventricular system.

I would like to thank Mr. D. N. Matthews, Mr. K. Till, and Dr. P. H. Sandifer, of the Children's Hospital, for their helpful comments and for permission to quote from their findings. I also gratefully acknowledge the help given by Dr. H. R. Dennison, M.O.H. of West Ham, and his team of health visitors.

### References

Pliess, G. (1962). Praenatale Schäden. *Ergebn. inn. Med. Kinderheilk.*, **17**, 264-384 (on page 362).

Potter, E. L. (1961). *Pathology of the Fetus and the Infant*, 2nd ed. Year Book Medical Publishers, Chicago.

Sheldon, W. (1962). *Diseases of Infancy and Childhood*, 8th ed., p. 477. Churchill, London.

Wiedemann, H. R. (1955). Schädigungen der Frucht in der Schwangerschaft. *Med. Mschr.*, **9**, 141.

Willis, R. A. (1962). *The Borderland of Embryology and Pathology*, 2nd ed. Butterworth, London.

*Arch. Dis. Childh.*, 1965, **40**, 82.

# PARTIAL DELETION OF THE SHORT ARMS OF A CHROMOSOME OF THE 4-5 GROUP (DENVER)

BY

H. V. DYGGVE and MARGARETA MIKKELSEN

*From the State Institution for Mentally Retarded, 'Andersvaenge', Slagelse, and the University Institute for Human Genetics, Copenhagen, Denmark*

(RECEIVED FOR PUBLICATION JUNE 22, 1964)

Whereas in man life is possible in the presence of an extra autosome (though not without considerable defects), absence of an autosome appears to be incompatible with life. Even absence of parts of an autosome appear, as a rule, to be lethal and may lead to spontaneous abortions (Jacobsen, Dupont, and Mikkelsen, 1963).

Grouchy, Lamy, Thieffry, Arthuis, and Salmon (1963) described a child with various malformations in addition to defective intelligence, who had absence of the short arms of a chromosome No. 17 or 18. Shortly after this, Lejeune, Lafourcade, Berger, Vialatte, Boeswillwald, Seringe, and Turpin (1963) described 3 patients all of whom presented the same cytological picture, in that part of the short arms of a chromosome in the 4-5 group were absent. All 3 patients were mentally retarded, their somatic development was retarded, they had microcephaly, hypertelorism, epicanthus, low-set ears, and cat-like mewing.

We have had the opportunity of examining a child with similar clinical symptoms who also presented deletion of the short arms of a chromosome in the 4-5 group.

## Case Report

L.M.C., a male, was born on June 5, 1960. There was no known disposition to mental retardation, dwarfing, or deformities in the family. The parents were healthy, normal, and were not blood relatives. The patient is the fifth of six children. The first three children were triplets (two boys and a girl) who were born two and a half months prematurely and died shortly after birth. They did not present any visible malformations but no necropsy

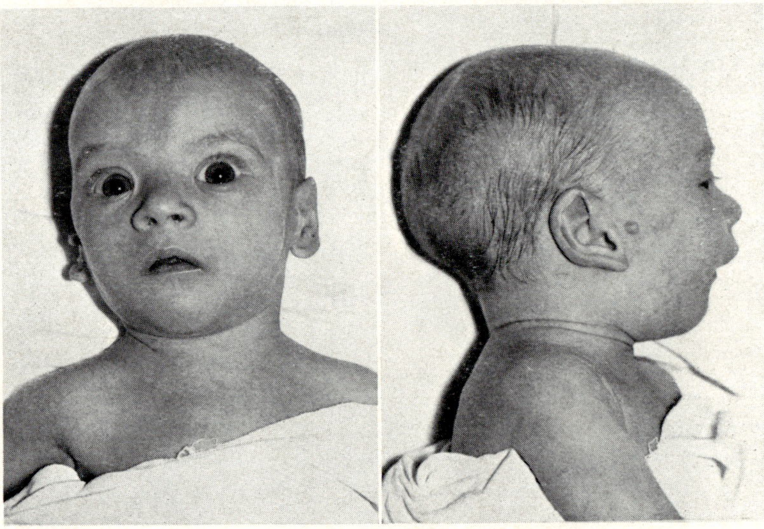

1a 1b

FIG. 1.—The appearance of patient at the age of 2 months. Note hypertelorism, epicanthus, retrognathia, low-set ears, and a dimple anterior to the right ear.

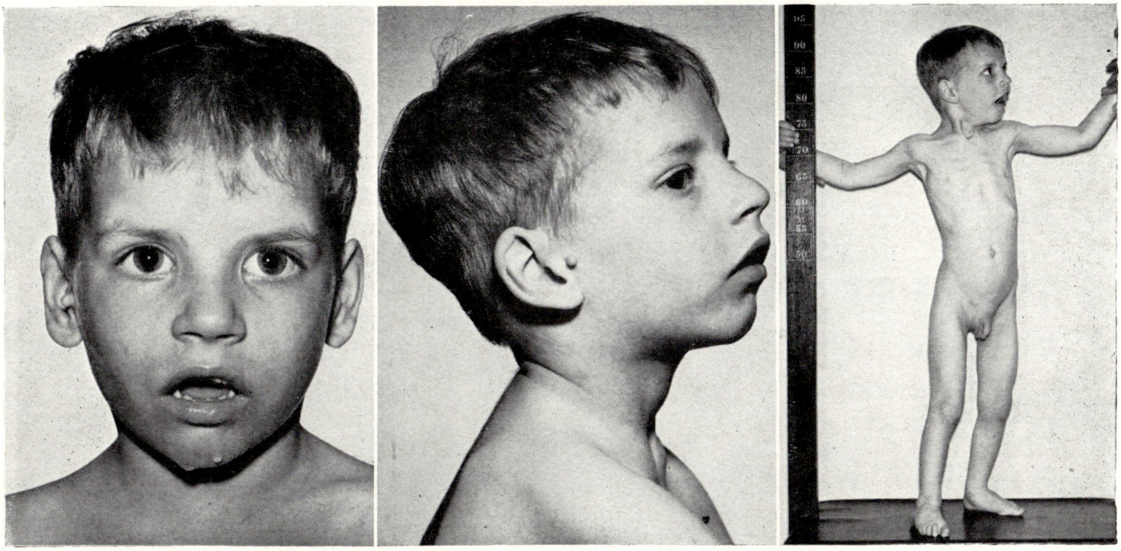

2a 2b 2c

FIG. 2a, b, and c.—The patient at 4 years.

was performed. The fourth and the sixth children are normal boys, born in 1957 and 1961.

Both parents were 33 years at the patient's birth. The pregnancy was uneventful. The delivery was normal and at term. Birth weight 3,200 g., length 51 cm. There was marked inspiratory stridor with a tendency to cyanosis from birth. Feeding difficulties occurred and the infant failed to thrive. He was admitted to hospital from the age of 1 month until the age of 2 years. At the age of 2 months, the circumference of the head was 35 cm. (normal 39 cm.) (Fig. 1).

At the age of 2 years, the boy weighed only 7·7 kg. and inspiratory stridor and feeding difficulties persisted. A marked tendency to respiratory infections was present. At the age of 4 years, he could walk only with support and could not speak. Slightly stridulous respiration on exertion persists. No epileptic seizures have occurred.

*Physical examination* at the age of 4 years showed his height to be 94 cm., his weight 11 kg.; head circumference 45 cm. Nuchal region was rather prominent. Epicanthus and hypertelorism were present but no other ocular changes. The ears were low set but otherwise normal. A dimple without cartilage was observed anterior to the right ear. The palate was high and formed an inverted V and the chin was small and retracted (Figs. 2a, b, c). There was no webbing of the neck. A moderate systolic murmur was heard inferiorly along the left sternal margin; no cyanosis or retraction occurred during inspiration. The external genitalia were normal. Transverse palmar creases were present in both palms (Fig. 3a, b). The extremities were otherwise normal with normal tone and tendon reflexes.

The child was able to walk with slight support in a rather bent position. The voice had a peculiar bleating character. He could say 'Ja' (yes) but no other intelligible words. His play and behaviour correspond to the normal for a child of approximately 1 year.

**Investigations.** Repeated thoracic radiographs have shown the heart to be normal in form and size. Screening revealed that the excursions of the diaphragm were limited but otherwise normal. Neither dislocation nor compression of the trachea were present. The position of the oesophagus was shown to be normal on contrast filling. Radiograph of the cranium revealed no abnormality.

Direct and indirect laryngoscopy (under anaesthesia) revealed no congenital malformations. 'The case is one of pronounced congenital inspiratory stridor.'

No abnormality was revealed on electroencephalography. The urine contained no sugar, albumin, or phenyl-pyruvic acid, and microscopic examination was normal. Serum calcium and phosphorus, and acid and alkaline phosphatases all showed normal values. Blood group studies are set out in the Table.

**Cytology.** The patient and his parents were examined. Sex chromatin was determined on Feulgen-stained

TABLE

BLOOD GROUP STUDIES

| | | | | | | | |
|---|---|---|---|---|---|---|---|
| The father .. .. | O | Ns | P + | $R_1 R^1$ | Le (a − b +) | Fy (a +) | K − |
| The mother .. .. | $A_1$ | Ns | P + | $R_2r$ | Le (a + b −) | Fy (a +) | K − |
| The patient .. .. | $A_1$ | Ns | P + | $R_1r$ | Le (a + b −) | Fy (a +) | K − |

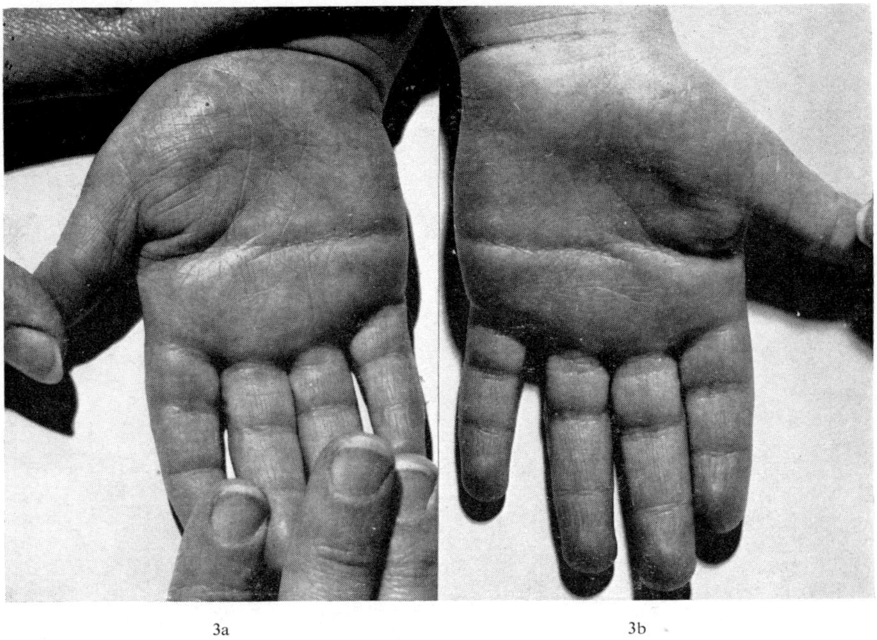


FIG. 3.—Right and left hand of the patient. Transverse palmar creases are evident in both palms.

buccal smears and was, in all cases, in agreement with the phenotypical sex. The patient's karyotype was studied in cells from peripheral blood, cultured according to the micromethod described by Frøland (1962) and in fibroblasts from skin culture according to Frøland (1961). In both blood and skin culture, the modal number was 46. In all 60 cells examined, one chromosome of the 4-5 group showed deletion of the short arms. The other chromosomes were as in a normal male (Fig. 4).

The parent's karyotypes were studied in blood cells cultured according to Moorhead, Nowell, Mellman, Battips, and Hungerford (1960). Both had normal karyotypes.

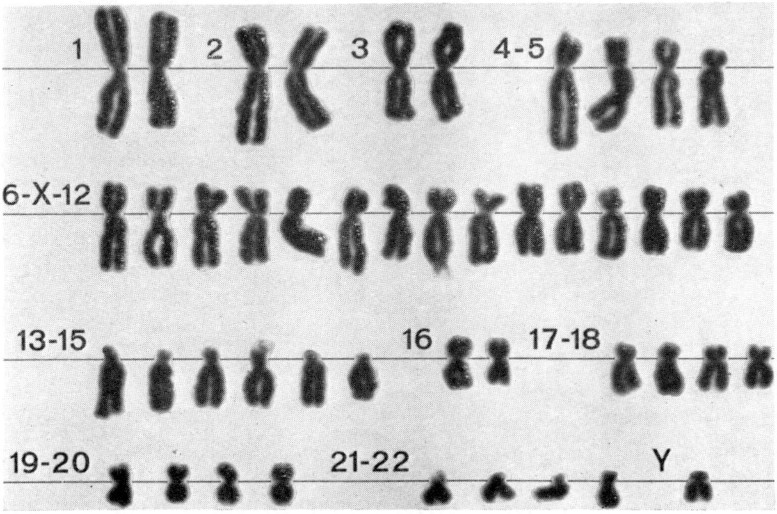


FIG. 4.—The karyotype of the patient. 46 chromosomes. Note the deletion of the short arms of one chromosome in the 4-5 groups. Blood culture. (Giemsa stain.)

## Discussion

Our cytological observations correspond to the findings made by Lejeune *et al.* The clinical picture presented by our patient also resembles the three patients previously described. According to a personal communication to Lejeune, a similar case was encountered by J. Böök.

This can scarcely be mere coincidence. Deletion of the short arms of a chromosome in the 4-5 group thus appears to produce a characteristic and quite definite clinical picture of which the main symptoms are somatic dwarfing, microcephaly, hypertelorism, epicanthus, low-set ears, transverse palmar creases, and severe mental retardation.

In the cases hitherto published there was no evidence to suggest that the condition was hereditary. Maternal age appeared to be of significance, since at the birth of two of the cases presented by Lejeune *et al.* the mothers were 40, and in their third case and in our case they were 33.

It is difficult to estimate whether the deleted chromosome is a chromosome No. 4 or 5. In normal subjects it is only possible to differentiate between chromosomes Nos. 4 and 5 in a fraction of the cases. Deletion produces, in addition, so much optical illusion that we prefer to consider the 4-5 groups as such.

It is doubtful whether we are justified in describing our patient as microcephalic, for though the circumference of the head was distinctly reduced for his age, it was reduced in proportion to the remainder of the body. The most marked symptom was the severe inspiratory stridor which was so pronounced during the first months of life that he required oxygen therapy and so inconveniencing that tracheostomy was considered. There was abnormal flaccidity of the epiglottis and possibly also of other parts of the larynx which might have contributed to this.

## Summary

In a boy aged 4 years, partial deletion of the short arms of a chromosome in the 4-5 groups was found in all the cells from skin and blood that we examined. The boy presented somatic dwarfing, microcephaly, micro-retrognathia, congenital stridor, hypertelorism, epicanthus, low-set ears, transverse palmar creases in both hands, and severe mental retardation.

Similar findings were described previously in three somewhat younger patients by Lejeune and his co-workers.

### References

Böök, J. A., Atkins, L., and Santesson, B. (1963). Some new data on autosomal aberrations in man. *Path. et Biol.*, **11**, 1159.

Frøland, A. (1961). A simplified method for making chromosome preparations from skin biopsies. *Acta path. microbiol. scand.*, **53**, 319.

—— (1962). A micromethod for chromosome analysis on peripheral blood-cultures. *Lancet*, **2**, 1281.

Grouchy, J. de, Arthuis, M., Salmon, C., Lamy, M., and Thieffry, S. (1964). Le syndrome du cri du chat. Une nouvelle observation. *Ann. Génét.*, **7**, No. 1.

——, Lamy, M., Thieffry, St., Arthuis, M., and Salmon, C. (1963). Dysmorphie complexe avec oligophrenie: délétion des bras courts d'un chromosome 17-18. *C.R. Acad. Sci.* (*Paris*), **256**, 1028.

Jacobsen, P., Dupont, A., and Mikkelsen, M. (1963). Translocation in the 13-15 group as a cause of partial trisomy and spontaneous abortion in the same family. *Lancet*, **2**, 584.

Lejeune, J., Lafourcade, J., Berger, R., Vialatte, J., Boeswillwald, M., Seringe, P., and Turpin, R. (1963). Trois cas de délétion partielle du bras court d'un chromosome 5. *C.R. Acad. Sci.* (*Paris*), **257**, 3098.

——, ——, Grouchy, J. de, Berger, R., Gautier, M., Salmon, C., and Turpin, R. (1964). Délétion partielle du bras court du chromosome 5. Individualisation d'un nouvel état morbide. *Sem. Hôp.* (*Paris*), **40**, 1069.

Moorhead, P. S., Nowell, P. C., Mellman, W. J., Battips, D. M., and Hungerford, D. A. (1960). Chromosome preparations of leukocytes cultured from human peripheral blood. *Exp. Cell Res.*, **20**, 613.

## Addendum

Since this paper was prepared at least four more cases have been described: Lejeune, Lafourcade, Grouchy, Berger, Gautier, Salmon, and Turpin (1964), Böök, Atkins, and Santesson (1963) and Grouchy, Arthuis, Salmon, Lamy, and Thieffrey (1964).

In addition one of us (M.M.) has examined a newborn girl with hypertelorism, round face, transverse palmar crease, and low-set ears. Again chromosome studies revealed a partial deletion of the short arms of a chromosome in the 4-5 group. The child was referred to cytological investigation on account of its cat-like cry by Dr. N. Hobolth, Pediatric Department, Copenhagen County Hospital, Gentofte.

A full report will be published elsewhere.

*Arch. Dis. Childh.*, 1965, **40**, 86.

# INTRATHORACIC KIDNEY IN A PREMATURE INFANT

BY

EMMANUEL SHAPIRA, EFRAIM FISHEL, and STANLEY LEVIN

*From the Departments of Paediatrics and Radiology, Kaplan Hospital, Rehovoth, Israel*

(RECEIVED FOR PUBLICATION JUNE 12, 1964)

Though ectopia of the kidney is a common anomaly (Campbell, 1951) displacement is usually downwards towards the pelvis, or medially. Upward displacement into the thoracic cavity is a much rarer finding. Ashley and Mostofi (1960), in a review of some quarter of a million necropsies, did not find a single case of thoracic kidney.

The present report is of interest because of the diagnosis of this condition in a living newborn premature baby.

## Case Report

A premature infant, weighing 2,400 g., was born to healthy parents following normal pregnancy and childbirth. There are two healthy sibs, but one previous premature infant died soon after birth.

At the age of 13 days, the infant was admitted to the paediatric department with an infection of the skin in the region of the sacrum. The weight at this time was 2,400 g. Breathing was normal. The facies was somewhat peculiar (Fig. 1), with a narrow forehead, flattened base of nose, and with eyes set wide apart. The mouth was smallish, with a narrow high-arched palate. The ears were low set. There were flexion deformities of the 3rd, 4th, and 5th fingers of the left hand, and 4th and 5th fingers of the right hand, which prevented normal extension at the finger joints. The thumbs were somewhat abnormally positioned, and flexion and abduction were slightly limited. These latter features were unlike arthrogryposis, in that on flexing the wrist and relaxing tension of the flexor tendons, full extension of the fingers could be obtained. Difficulty was entertained in abducting the hips, but there was no other evidence of subluxation at the hip joints.

Dullness was noted over the left lower chest, and air entry was diminished in this area. There were no abnormal adventitious sounds.

Laboratory examinations of the blood including blood count, urea, sugar, calcium, phosphorus, alkaline phosphatase, G.O. transaminase, and electrophoresis of proteins were within normal limits. Several examinations of urine were normal, as well as examination for total urinary amino acid excretion, and amino acid chromatography. Urinary calcium and phosphorus excretion were normal.

Chest radiographs showed a homogeneous density of the lower third of the left thorax, with no displacement of the heart or mediastinum. Radiographs of the spine, sacrum, and pelvis showed no evidence of abnormalities. Because of the skin infection and the abnormal chest findings, the infant was treated with antibiotics as a suspected case of cellulitis with pneumonia.

The skin infection responded to this therapy, and the infants condition improved. At no time was there any respiratory distress. Repeat radiographs of the chest showed no change, though it was noted that the posterior medial aspect of the left diaphragm appeared abnormal. Barium swallow was performed because of the suspicion of a diaphragmatic hernia, but the digestive system was found to be normal.

Because of the congenital deformities of the limbs, together with the peculiar facies and low-set ears, an abnormally placed kidney was suspected as the cause of the pathology in the left chest.

Intravenous pyelography with multi-section tomography demonstrated an ectopic left kidney occupying the left lower chest. The calyces were normal and were

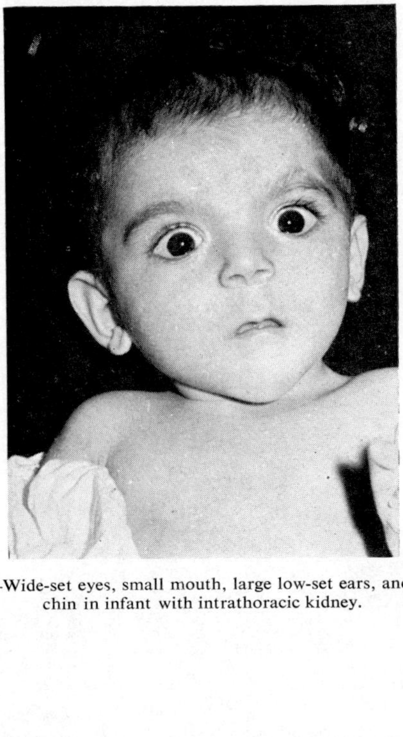

FIG. 1.—Wide-set eyes, small mouth, large low-set ears, and pointed chin in infant with intrathoracic kidney.

noted to be above the diaphragm. The pelvis seemed a little dilated. The right kidney and the bladder were normal (Fig. 2).

In an attempt to delineate further the kidney, intravenous pyelogram was performed together with pneumoperitoneum and pre-sacral air insufflation. The liver and spleen were found in their normal positions. The left kidney was noted to be retroperitoneal with the greater proportion above the diaphragm.

At the age of 1 year the infant is well, but small, and has had several respiratory infections requiring admission to hospital. At this time bilateral subluxation of the temporo-mandibular joints was found.

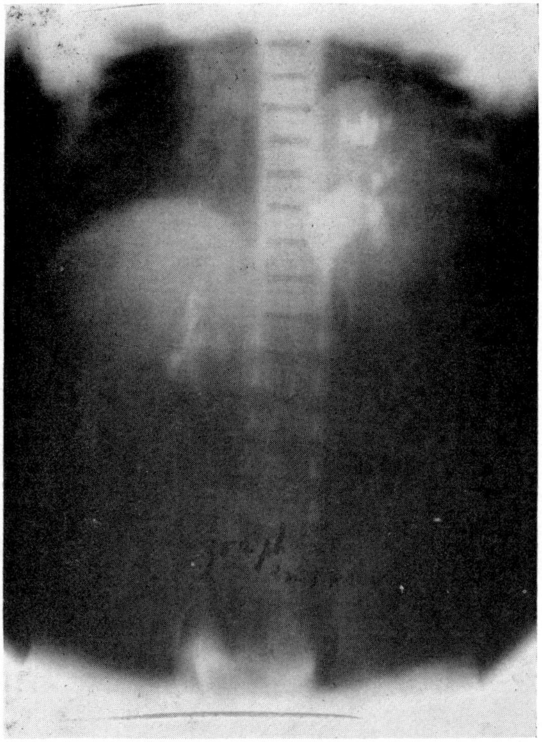

FIG. 2.—Intravenous pyelography with tomography showing left intrathoracic kidney.

## Discussion

A review of the published material indicates that cases of thoracic kidney are rarely diagnosed clinically because of lack of symptoms, and that the present case is the youngest in which such diagnosis has been made. Thoracic kidney in foetuses and stillborns has been reported (Gruber, 1927), as well as at necropsy in young children (Campbell, 1951). In the majority of necropsy reports, multiple congenital deformities have been noted, and in many cases, various other viscera have been found displaced into the chest. The first case diagnosed clinically was reported by Wolfromm (1940) who described a 40-year-old woman who was found on retrograde pyelography to have a thoracic kidney. Three reports during 1949-50 (Williams and Tillinghast, 1949; Spillane and Prather, 1949; Fleischner, Robins, and Abrams, 1950) purported to describe the first clinically diagnosed cases. Schwartz and Fränkel (1952) described a 65-year-old women, in which a left homogeneous basal density was noted on a routine chest radiograph, and which was proved to be an ectopic left kidney. Robbins and Lich (1954) reported a further case and reviewed the literature available to him, and found 6 cases in which the diagnosis was made clinically, and 4 others that were found at necropsy.

The present review considers cases diagnosed during life, and includes the literature up till 1961 (Gondos, 1955; Bulgrin and Holmes, 1955; Barloon, Goodwin, and Vermooten, 1957; Berlin, Stein, and Poppel, 1957; Laumonier, Verger, Fréour, Nicol, and Delormas, 1957; Herrenschmidt and Daumet, 1957; Pescione, 1957; Witz, Reys, and Wagner, 1958; Reboud and Bernard, 1958; Veran, Moigneteau, and Auvigne, 1958; Röhrig, 1958; Frančišković and Martinčić, 1959; Bernard, Reboud, and Maestraggi, 1959; Hill and Bunts, 1960; Paul, Uragoda, and Jayewardene, 1960; Nini, 1961). A further 8 reports (Pini, Newkirk, and Casal, 1954; Sypniewska, 1955; Herink and Jagdschian, 1960; Hayashi, 1961; Manfredi, 1961; Daroczy, 1959; De Langlade and Pelizza, 1958; Toole, Chrysopathis, and Papadimitriou, 1961) were not available for review.

In all, 28 cases of thoracic kidney diagnosed clinically have been reported; 14 were left-sided, 13 were right-sided, and one (Berlin *et al.*, 1957) was bilateral.

The greater proportion of them were discovered following investigation of abnormal basal densities in chest radiographs. Several cases were operated on because of the suspicion of lung neoplasm. The abnormality was found three times more often in males. The youngest reported case, until the present report, was in a child of 4 years of age, and the oldest in a 75-year-old person. The average age of reported cases was 41 years.

Embryologically, the explanation for the displacement of the kidney is not clear, and various possibilities have been suggested. Spillane and Prather (1952) and Barloon *et al.* (1957) felt that the cause of the abnormality was due to a maldevelopment of the pleuro-peritoneal membrane, causing the ascending process of the kidney to continue into the chest.

Others believed the cause to be a delay in the caudal migration of the mesonephron, leading to a defect in the diaphragm which allowed the kidney to be displaced cranially. Gondos (1955), on the other hand, believed that delay in the joining of the ureteric bud to the metanephron led to late differentiation of metanephronic tissue, which in turn caused accentuation of the ascending process. Frančišković and Martinčić (1959) thought the cause was primarily a high cephalic establishment of the renal germ.

Clinically, thoracic ectopic kidney is asymptomatic, there being no hydrodynamic changes in the urinary outflow tract, and it therefore does not require specific therapy. The majority of cases are diagnosed incidentally to fluoroscopy of the chest. On the other hand, pelvic or abdominal ectopy may lead to recurrent urinary tract infections, stone formation, and hydronephrosis. These latter cases are usually diagnosed during investigation of the genito-urinary tract.

## Summary

Ectopic displacement of the kidney into the left or right chest is a rare anomaly. A review of the literature revealed 28 cases in which this condition was diagnosed clinically. The great majority of cases were in adults and almost all were asymptomatic, and were diagnosed incidental to chest fluoroscopy. A case is reported of a left thoracic kidney diagnosed clinically in a premature newborn infant with peculiar facies, congenital abnormalities of the fingers, and subluxation of the temporo-mandibular joints.

### References

Ashley, D. J. B., and Mostofi, F. K. (1960). Renal agenesis and dysgenesis. *J. Urol. (Baltimore)*, **83**, 211.

Barloon, J. W., Goodwin, W. E., and Vermooten, V. (1957). Thoracic kidney: case reports. *ibid.*, **78**, 356.

Berlin, H. S., Stein, J., and Poppel, M., H. (1957). Congenital superior ectopia of the kidney. *Amer. J. Roentgenol.*, **78**, 508.

Bernard, R., Reboud, E., and Maestraggi, P. (1959). A propos d'une image en coucher de soleil de l'hémi-coupole diaphragmatique droite (ectopie rénale intra-thoracique). *Pédiatrie*, **14**, 293.

Bulgrin, J. G., and Holmes, F. H. (1955). Eventration of the diaphragm with high renal ectopia. *Radiology*, **64**, 249.

Campbell, M. (1951). *Clinical Pediatric Urology*, p. 195. Saunders, Philadelphia.

Daroczy, G. (1959). Intrathoracic kidney dystopia. *Magy. Sebész.*, **9**, 201.

De Langlade, E., and Pelizza, A. (1958). Su di un raro caso di ectopia toracica del rene destro. (An unusual case of thoracic ectopia of the right kidney.) *Minerva pediat.*, **10**, 981.

Fleischner, F. G., Robins, S. A., and Abrams, M. (1950). High renal ectopy and congenital diaphragmatic hernia. *Radiology*, **55**, 24.

Frančišković, V., and Martinčić, N. (1959). Intrathoracic kidney. *Brit. J. Urol.*, **31**, 156.

Gondos, B. (1955). High ectopy of the left kidney. *Amer. J. Roentgenol.*, **74**, 295.

Gruber, G. B. (1927). Die Missbildungen des Zwerchfells. In *Die Morphologie der Missbildungen des Menschen und der Tiere*, ed. E. Schwalbe and G. B. Gruber, Part III, Div. 3, Chapter 2. Fischer, Jena.

Hayashi, Y. (1961). Thoracic kidney. A case report. *Jap. J. Urol.*, **52**, 676.

Herink, M., and Jagdschian, V. (1960). Klinischer Beitrag zur partiellen rechtsseitigen Zwerchfellrelaxation mit dystoper Niere in der rechten Thoraxhöhle. *Thoraxchirurgie*, **8**, 463.

Herrenschmidt, M. M., and Daumet, P. (1957). Diagnostic radiologique d'un rein en ectopie thoracique. *Poumon*, **13**, 817.

Hill, J. E., and Bunts, R. C. (1960). Thoracic kidney: case reports. *J. Urol. (Baltimore)*, **84**, 460.

Laumonier, Verger, Fréour, Nicol, and Delormas (1957). Ectopie thoracique du rein droit. *Poumon*, **13**, 119.

Manfredi, L. (1961). On a case of Bochdalek's hernia in the adult with thoracic ectopy of the right kidney. *Acta chir. ital.*, **17**, 223.

Nini, W. (1961). Le rein intrathoracique. *Bull. Soc. int. Chir.*, **20**, 548.

Paul, A. T. S., Uragoda, C. G., and Jayewardene, F. L. W. (1960). Thoracic kidney with report of a case. *Brit. J. Surg.*, **47**, 395.

Pescione, E. (1957). High renal ectopy—A contribution to the knowledge of the so called 'thoracic kidney'. *Urol. int. (Basel)*, **4**, 142.

Pini, A. E., Newkirk, G., and Casal, J. (1954). Ectopía renal torácica. *Rev. argent. Urol.*, **23**, 111.

Reboud, E., and Bernard, R. (1958). Un nouveau cas d'ectopie rénale intrathoracique. *Poumon*, **14**, 597.

Robbins, J. J., and Lich, R., Jr. (1954). Thoracic kidney. *J. Urol. (Baltimore)*, **72**, 133.

Röhrig, H. (1958). Kongenitale thorakale Ektopie der rechten Niere. *Fortschr. Röntgenstr.*, **89**, 371.

Schwartz, A., and Fränkel, M. (1952). High renal ectopia, detected on routine chest examination: case report. *Acta radiol. (Stockh.)*, **37**, 583.

Spillane, R. J., and Prather, G. C. (1949). High renal ectopy: a case report. *J. Urol. (Baltimore)*, **62**, 441.

——, —— (1952). Right diaphragmatic eventration with renal displacement: case report. *ibid.*, **68**, 804.

Sypniewska, M. (1955). Wrodzone wysokie polozenie nerki. *Pol. Przegl. chir.*, **27**, 467.

Toole, H., Chrysopathis, P., and Papadimitriou, D. (1961). Über die thorakale Nierendystopie Mitteilung eines neuen Falles. *Z. Urol.*, **54**, 1.

Veran, P., Moigneteau, C. R., and Auvigne, J. (1958). Opacité de la base droite par malformation rénale. *Poumon*, **14**, 763.

Williams, R. G., and Tillinghast, A. J. (1949). Diaphragmatic herniation of kidney: case report. *Radiology*, **53**, 566.

Witz, J. P., Reys, P., and Wagner, J. P. (1958). Ectopie thoracique partielle du rein gauche. *Poumon* **14**, 595.

Wolfromm, G. (1940). Situation du rein dans l'éventration diaphragmatique droite. *Méd. Acad. Chir.*, **66**, 41.

## Addendum

After submitting this report, chromosome analysis was performed on leucocytes of this child by Dr. B. Pade, of the Chromosome Laboratories, Tel Hashomer Hospital, Tel Aviv. These studies showed a trisomy 16-18 pattern with translocation of one of the 6-12 X chromosomes to No. 2 chromosome, which was occasionally of giant size.

Details of these findings, including family studies, will be the subject of an additional report.

*Arch. Dis. Childh.*, 1965, **40**, 89.

# FANCONI'S ANAEMIA WITH HYDROCEPHALUS AND THYROID ABNORMALITY

BY

RUTH LONDON, AHARON DRUKKER, and URI SANDBANK
*From the Paediatric Department "A" and the Department of Pathology, Kaplan Hospital, Rehovoth, Israel*

(RECEIVED FOR PUBLICATION JUNE 23, 1964)

Since the first report of three cases of 'familial infantile pernicious-like anaemia' (Fanconi, 1927), more than 100 similar cases have been reported. The condition has been reviewed by Nilsson (1960), Gasser (1961), McDonald and Goldschmidt (1960). Until recently no effective treatment was known, and the pancytopenia was treated by repeated transfusions of fresh blood, and by splenectomy in those cases with evidence of hypersplenism. Shahidi and Diamond (1959) proposed combined corticosteroid and anabolic treatment, and some good results were reported on this regimen (McDonald, 1962; Shahidi and Diamond, 1961). In the following case, which presents some unusual clinical and pathological findings, the pancytopenia was resistant to this therapy.

## Case Report

A 10-month-old girl was referred to our out-patient clinic in August 1961 because of failure to thrive and suspected dwarfism. She was born after a normal confinement which followed an uneventful, slightly prolonged pregnancy, though her birth weight (2,220 g.), was below normal. The mother received no medication during this, the third of her four pregnancies.

Both parents of Ashkenasi origin were in good health. There was no consangui ity and no known evidence of hereditary or metabolic disease in the parents' families. The first pregnancy resulted in a stillbirth, and the second pregnancy in a third month spontaneous abortion. A younger sister of the patient, at present 1½ years of age, is in good general health and is developing normally.

Our patient's past history did not disclose anything out of the ordinary, apart from a retardation in physical development. There was no history of contact with a toxic chemical agent or ingestion of a toxic antibacterial drug.

On first examination, at the age of 10 months, she was a small underdeveloped, but fairly well-nourished girl. Her weight was 4,680 g., and her height 59 cm. (both corresponding to the 50th percentiles for the age of 3 months). The head was relatively large, with a circumference of 39 cm. compared with a chest circumference of 34 cm. Otherwise, she was well proportioned. There was marked microphthalmia, but no strabismus, and the greater fontanelle was small, not bulging. In addition, she had severe bilateral dislocation of the hips, bent little fingers, and pointed thin distal phalanges of both thumbs. There was no hepato-splenomegaly, lymphadenopathy, or cutaneous bleeding. The thyroid gland was not enlarged and the external genitalia were normal.

The blood picture at the first examination was normal. Haemoglobin 10·9 g./100 ml., haematocrit 32%, and leucocytes 7,250 c.mm., with normal differential count.

For 14 months the girl was observed at the out-patient clinic. As primordial dwarfism was thought to be the most likely diagnosis, no treatment was applied.

At the end of December 1962, at the age of 2 years and 3 months, the girl was admitted to hospital for further investigations. The physical examination on admission did not reveal any new pathological findings. Her weight was 6,450 g., and her height 64 cm. The initial blood count was again within normal limits. Sedimentation rate: 90/120 (Westergren). Total proteins: 5·7 g./100 ml., albumin 2·7 g./100 ml., globulin 3·0 g./100 ml. Electrophoresis showed marked hypoalbuminaemia and $\alpha_2$-hyperglobulinaemia. Other liver function tests were normal. The blood levels of urea, electrolytes, calcium, and phosphorus were all within normal limits. The alkaline phosphatase level was below normal. Radiographs of the chest and skull were normal, whereas those of the wrist showed a severely retarded bone-age, of 6 months (Greulich and Pyle). On intravenous pyelography the left kidney could not be visualized. Protein-bound iodine in the serum was determined in order to rule out a thyroid-dependant dwarfism and high levels were found on several occasions, i.e. more than 16 μg./100 ml. Further investigation in both the patient's mother and sister revealed the same high levels of PBI, but normal values were found in the father and maternal grandmother. The mother was euthyroid and her basal metabolic rate was normal.

A few days after admission, without any previous acute illness, petechiae appeared for the first time. From then and until death nine months later, the clinical course was dominated by haematological manifestations. There was no further practical possibility of determining her endocrine status, the origin of the dwarfism, nor of investigating the urinary tract.

The haemogram showed anaemia (Hb 8·2 g./100 ml.), leucopenia (3,700/c.mm.), and thrombocytopenia (40,000/c.mm.). In the peripheral blood smears anisocytosis, hypochromia, and macrocytosis were seen, and on several occasions normoblasts. Among the white blood cells myelocytes and metamyelocytes were evident. Differential count always showed a relative lymphocytosis. Red cells were between 2 and 3 million/c.mm. Bleeding time was 4·5 minutes, and the prothrombin consumption test showed a low value (55%). No thrombo-agglutinins could be detected, and no lupus erythematosis cells. The direct Coombs test was negative as were the Kahn and Wassermann tests. On one occasion a high level of foetal haemoglobin (5·7%) was determined, but no other haemoglobinopathy could be found on haemoglobin-electrophoresis.

*Bone marrow*, aspirated on different occasions from the iliac crest, the tibia, and the vertebral spine, revealed extreme hypoplasia. Almost no younger elements were seen, but there was a relatively high number of lymphocytes and a few megaloblasts; no megakaryoblasts were detected.

The radioactive $^{59}$Fe clearance test confirmed our diagnosis of aplastic anaemia and in addition showed signs of blood loss.

The blood picture during the last 9 months of the patient's life can be briefly summarized. The haemoglobin fell steadily, and repeated transfusions were required, 13 in all being given. Reticulocytes were below 1%, except for two isolated occasions when counts of about 3% were recorded. The leucocytes also tended to fall gradually, from an initial level of 3,700 to a preterminal level of 1,200/c.mm. Thrombocytes varied between 10,000 and 50,000/c.mm.

During the first weeks of her haemorrhagic illness—due to thrombocytopenia—45-20 mg. of prednisolone was given a day without benefit. The patient was therefore placed (three months after the first bleeding signs) on triamcinolone 8 mg. per day and methyltestosterone 10-20 mg. per day. During a 6-month period on this regimen no improvement was seen. The haemoglobin level continued to fall, there was no sustained reticulocytosis, and the bone-marrow remained aplastic. The child developed severe side-effects of the combined corticosteroid and anabolic therapy: moon face, generalized osteoporosis, oedema of both legs, hirsutism, and acne. For one month, folic acid (15 mg. a day), vitamin C (100 mg. a day), and oral iron (0·6 g. a day) were added.

The patient suffered several severe intercurrent febrile attacks caused by respiratory illnesses and by a urinary tract infection due to *Esch. coli*. In February-March 1963 there was a prolonged febrile period without any obvious cause, perhaps due to septicaemia. Blood cultures showed *Esch. coli* and *Staph. albus*. The patient received intensive antibiotic treatment.

Her general condition remained satisfactory until September 1963, when the bleeding tendency increased, and for the first time haematuria, melaena, and haematemesis appeared, and her condition deteriorated rapidly. Extreme apathy became evident and a tremor of both upper extremities, probably due to a central nervous system haemorrhage. Gradually dyspnoea, jaundice, uraemia, and signs of acute haemorrhagic enterocolitis appeared and the patient died in September 1963 at the age of 3 years, nine months after the first manifestations of the hypoplastic anaemia.

**Necropsy.** This revealed a well-nourished girl measuring 67 cm. in length and weighing 6,200 g. The skin showed a mild icteric tint and multiple petechiae and ecchymoses scattered over the body and extremities. Both eyes were smaller than normal.

On examination of the *thoracic cavity* multiple small haemorrhages were seen in the visceral pleurae. The *lungs* weighed 60 and 65 g. and showed severe congestion and focal bronchopneumonia. The *heart* was normal.

The *peritoneum*, *omentum*, and *mesentery* were dotted with multiple haemorrhages. Similar pin-point haemorrhages were found in the mucosa of the entire gastro-intestinal tract. The *liver* histologically showed Kupffer cells containing a moderate amount of haemosiderin. The *spleen* was hypoplastic (4 g.) as compared to a normal 37 g. for this age. There was a marked depletion of lymphatic tissue as well as severe haemosiderosis of the reticuloendothelial cells. A double fused *kidney* with double ureter was found on the right side, histologically showing acute pyelonephritis with a moderate amount of haemosiderin in the interstitial tissue.

Examination of the *endocrine system* showed that the right *adrenal* was absent; the left was small, 10 × 10 × 2 mm., with the cortex less than 1 mm. in width. Microscopically, the normal organization of the cortex was well preserved, though there was a depletion of lipids. The *thyroid* isthmus was missing, each lobe measured 10 × 5 × 4 mm., and showed follicles of varying diameter filled with colloid and lined by low cuboidal epithelium, without interstitial fibrosis. The *ovaries* were very small, 10 × 3 × 2 mm. and contained only a few ova within a fibrotic stroma. A small *pituitary gland*, 2 mm. in diameter, was situated in a small flat sella turcica and was covered by a thick layer of dura. Histologically no basophils could be identified with haematoxylin and eosin or PAS-orange G stains; eosinophils constituted about 40% and chromophobe cells about 60% of all cells of the anterior lobe.

The *thymus* weighed 8 g.; it was yellow and of soft consistency: histologically there were small groups of lymphocytes with few Hassal-bodies scattered in fatty and fibrous tissue.

The *brain* weighed 535 g. A subarachnoid haemorrhage was present above the right fronto-parietal lobe as well as a small cortical haemorrhage in the right parietal region. Cut sections of the brain revealed marked dilatation of all ventricles (Fig.), absence of the septum pellucidum, and extreme stenosis of the aqueduct of Sylvius at the mid-brain to a diameter of 0·5 mm.

The *bone-marrow* was aplastic and was composed of fatty tissue and young connective tissue fibres. It contained a few small groups of non-identifiable haematopoietic cells and large quantities of haemosiderin.

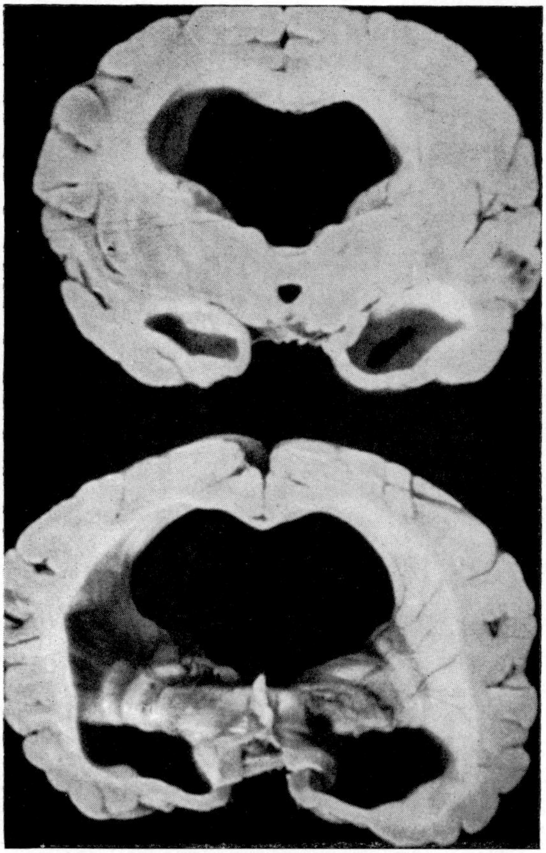

FIG.—Coronal sections of the brain, showing internal hydrocephalus and absence of septum pellucidum.

## Discussion

In this case, the diagnosis of Fanconi's anaemia was based on the severe pancytopenia, dwarfism, and multiple congenital malformations found. According to some authors (Gasser, 1961; Kopyść and Lehnert, 1962) this diagnosis cannot be established without the presence of abnormal pigmentation of the skin and/or mucous membranes, caused by an aberration of melanin metabolism (McDonald and Goldschmidt, 1960; Wintrobe, 1961), a criterion that was not fulfilled in this patient. The disease, however, manifested itself earlier than usual (at the age of 2 years) and its duration was short. Therefore, it may be that the pigmentation would have ultimately appeared, had the child remained alive longer.

Although microcephaly is a very frequent malformation in this syndrome (McDonald and Goldschmidt, 1960), no other case of hydrocephalus, to our knowledge, has been described. Kunz (1952) mentioned that the brother of his case of Fanconi's anaemia died at the age of 17 months from obstructive hydrocephalus without any haematological symptoms during life. In the present case the hydrocephalus was not recognized during life because it was symptomless, and the patient's head was of fairly normal size for her age, being enlarged only in relation to the size of her body.

The necropsy revealed severe hypoplasia of the spleen and of almost all endocrine glands; the pituitary, the thyroid, the left adrenal, the ovaries; and, in addition, the right adrenal was absent. These endocrinological findings may be regarded as congenital malformations, for they are found in Fanconi's anaemia, but they might have been the result of prolonged hormonal treatment. The presence of a small pituitary situated in a corresponding small sella turcica points towards a true congenital malformation of the pituitary and to a primary congenital hypopituitarism. Thus the dwarfism and the absence of pigmentation can be easily understood. Though in many cases of Fanconi's anaemia retarded growth is present (Kunz, 1952; Cowdell, Phizackerley, and Pyke, 1955), in only 2 reported cases has the pituitary been examined at necropsy, and in both these it was found to be hypoplastic as in our patient. Hypoplasia of the thyroid was found at necropsy in both cases of Cowdell *et al.* (1955), and hypoplasia of the spleen was described by Wintrobe (1961).

On several occasions high PBI-serum levels were found in our patient, and also in both her mother and her younger sister. All were euthyroid, without goitre. (The thyroid status of these relatives is at present being assessed.) Most probably we are dealing with either a hereditary enzymatic defect in hormone production, or a familial increase in thyroxine-binding-proteins (Beierwaltes and Robbins, 1959), both of which occur in rare instances. It remains therefore to be decided whether there is any pathogenetic connexion between these endocrine anomalies and the hypoplastic anaemia. Alternatively, the family might be affected by two independent hereditary traits.

The pancytopenia was resistant to a combined therapy of corticosteroids and testosterone in the advised dosages (triamcinolone 4 mg./day, methyltestosterone 1-2 mg./kg. day) during a period of 6 months. Because of technical reasons testosterone could not be given in the form of buccal linguets, and was therefore given orally in a higher dose (3 mg./kg. day) in order to cope with the inactivation of the drug in the liver when given orally.

The lack of erythropoietic response is perhaps not surprising in the light of the extreme bone marrow aplasia in this patient. The side-effects of the therapy were related in the first place to the action of the corticosteroids (moon face, oedema of the legs). Testosterone therapy led to acne and hirsutism. The jaundice in the final stage of the disease had an obstructive character and was perhaps due to prolonged testosterone administration. Of interest was the generalized osteoporosis in spite of the testosterone therapy, while the bone-age failed to advance during this therapy.

## Summary

A case is described of Fanconi's anaemia in a girl who suffered from dwarfism due to congenital hypoplasia of the pituitary and from other congenital malformations. The pancytopenia manifested itself at the age of 2 years and was resistant to a combined corticosteroid-testosterone treatment. Unusual findings in this case were congenital hydrocephalus, hypoplastic spleen, and hypoplasia of thyroid together with persistently high PBI serum levels but without apparent changes in thyroid function.

## References

Beierwaltes, W. H., and Robbins, J. (1959). Familial increase in the thyroxine-binding sites in serum alpha globulin. *J. clin. Invest.*, **38**, 1683.

Cowdell, R. H., Phizackerley, P. J. R., and Pyke, D. A. (1955). Constitutional anemia (Fanconi's syndrome) and leukemia in two brothers. *Blood*, **10**, 788.

Fanconi, G. (1927). Familiäre infantile perniziosaartige Anämie (perniziöses Blutbild und Konstitution). *Jb. Kinderheilk.*, **117**, 257.

Gasser, C. (1961). Panmyelopathien im Kindesalter. Beitrag zur Fanconi-Anämie. *Helv. paediat. Acta*, **16**, 752.

Kopyśč, Z., and Lehnert, A. (1962). Pancytopenia 3 licznymi wadami rozwojowymi typu Fanconiego. (Pancytopenia with numerous developmental defects of Fanconi type.) *Pediat. pol.*, **37**, 295.

Kunz, H. W. (1952). Hypoplastic anemia with multiple congenital defects (Fanconi syndrome). *Pediatrics*, **10**, 286.

McDonald, R. (1962). Drug-induced remission in hypoplastic anaemia (Fanconi type.) *S. Afr. med. J.*, **36**, 310.

——, and Goldschmidt, B. (1960). Pancytopenia with congenital defects (Fanconi's anaemia). *Arch. Dis. Childh.*, **35**, 367.

Nilsson, L. R. (1960). Chronic pancytopenia with multiple congenital abnormalities (Fanconi's anaemia). *Acta paediat. (Uppsala)*, **49**, 518.

Shahidi, N. T., and Diamond, L. K. (1959). Testosterone-induced remission in aplastic anemia. *Amer. J. Dis. Child.*, **98**, 293.

——, —— (1961). Testosterone-induced remission in aplastic anemia of both acquired and congenital types. *New Engl. J. Med.*, **264**, 953.

Wintrobe, M. M. (1961). *Clinical Hematology*, 5th ed., p. 561. Kimpton, London.

*Arch. Dis. Childh.*, 1965, **40**, 93.

# OBSTETRICAL PARALYSIS DUE TO ISCHAEMIA OF THE SPINAL CORD

BY

J. HUME ADAMS and HECTOR M. CAMERON*

*From the Department of Pathology, the University and Western Infirmary, Glasgow, and the Department of Pathology, Stobhill General Hospital, Glasgow*

(RECEIVED FOR PUBLICATION MAY 1, 1964)

Obstetrical paralysis after a difficult labour is usually attributed to tearing or stretching of the nerve trunks of the brachial plexus or to avulsion of nerve roots from the spinal cord. Injury to the cord itself, however, is not excessively rare (Ford, 1960), the principal findings at necropsy being subdural or extradural haemorrhage, laceration or rupture of the cord, or a haematomyelia. In the case described here, paralysis of both arms at birth was found to be due to necrosis of the grey matter in the cervical part of the spinal cord, a condition that does not appear to have been described previously.

## Case Report

**Clinical History.** The subject was a male infant whose birth was complicated by a face presentation. This was very easily converted to a vertex presentation by external version 4½ hours after the commencement of labour. The baby was then delivered without difficulty, the second stage lasting about 10 minutes. He was deeply cyanosed and responded to resuscitation only slowly. Both arms were flaccid and he was thought to have a bilateral Erb's palsy. In addition, it was noted that the head tended to flop forwards on to the chest. There was little change for a few days, but on the sixth day he was noted to be very pale and breathing rapidly. His colour improved when in an incubator but the respiration rate remained at about 100 a minute. Chest radiograph suggested that there might be some pulmonary collapse in the region of the lingula. On the next day, he became deeply cyanosed while being fed and the respirations became more rapid and strenuous. The diaphragm retracted with inspiration suggesting that it was paralysed, but this was not confirmed radiologically. The further chest radiographs showed that both lungs were consolidated and contained little air. The cerebrospinal fluid was normal, examination of the stools revealed no pathogenic organisms, and virological investigations were negative. The baby continued to be cyanosed when out of oxygen and when being handled, and died on the tenth day.

**Family History.** There are two sibs: one, aged 4 years, is said to have suffered from haemorrhagic disease of the newborn, and is now very backward mentally; the other, aged 2 years, is of normal mentality but has gross asymmetry of the head, scoliosis, and weakness of the muscles on one side of the body.

**Necropsy.** A normally developed male infant, weighing 8 lb. 4 oz. (3,741 g.). The only abnormalities noted in the *chest* and *abdomen* were marked congestion and collapse of the lungs, and aspiration of material from the stomach into the trachea. The scalp and skull were normal. There was slight bruising of both leaves of the tentorium cerebelli, but no overt haemorrhage. The *brain* was normal externally and on section. The *spinal cord in situ* appeared entirely normal; there was no blood in the epidural space, and no tearing of nerve roots. Examination after removal revealed no evidence of haemorrhage or of external damage to the cord or nerve roots, and transverse cuts through the cervical, dorsal, and lumbar segments appeared normal. There was no indication of any traumatic damage to the *vertebral column*.

Before being examined in greater detail, the spinal cord was fixed in 10% formal saline for three weeks. Multiple transverse sections now revealed brownish discoloration and softening of the anterior horns extending from the second to the seventh cervical segments. All other levels appeared normal.

**Histology.** Relevant histological abnormalities were confined to the spinal cord where the principal feature was necrosis of the grey matter. From the second to the seventh cervical segments there was an almost total loss of nerve cells from the dorsal and ventral horns. The central parts of both ventral horns were rarefied and cystic (Fig. 1) but elsewhere there was increased cellularity of the grey matter caused by gemistocytic astrocytes (Fig. 2), hypertrophied microglial cells, and moderate capillary

* Present address: Department of Pathology, Royal Infirmary, Glasgow, C.4.

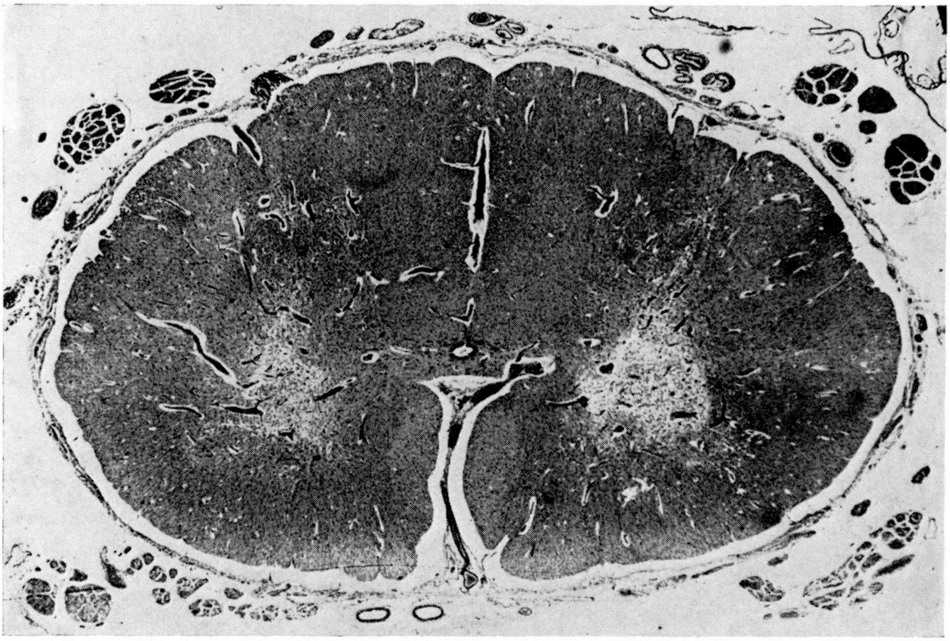

FIG. 1.—Cervical spinal cord (C.4 segment). Note the rarefaction and cystic change in the grey matter. (Haematoxylin and eosin. × 15.)

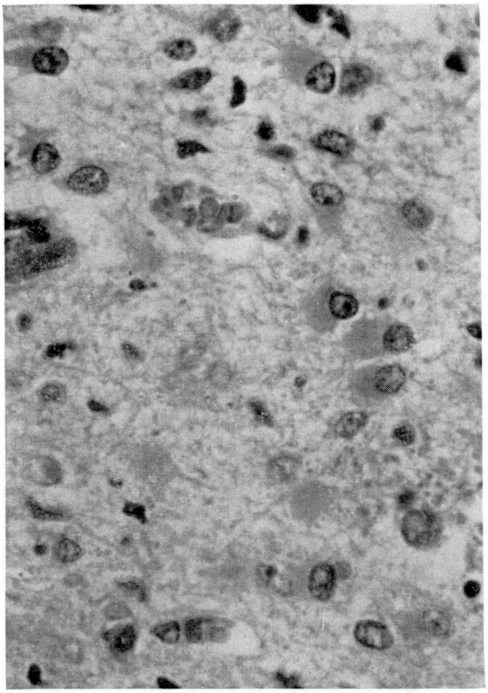

FIG. 2.—Same section as Fig. 1. Tip of dorsal grey horn. Note the numerous gemistocytic astrocytes and the absence of neurones. (Haematoxylin and eosin. × 500.)

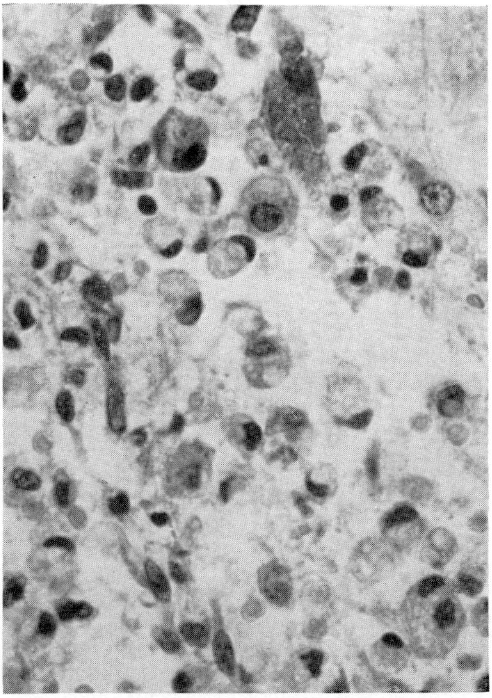

FIG. 3.—Same section as Fig. 1. Edge of cystic area in ventral grey horn. Note the numerous compound granular corpuscles. (Haematoxylin and eosin. × 500.)

endothelial hyperplasia. A very few large motor neurones could still be identified in the most anterior parts of the ventral horns. Adjacent to and within the cystic areas there were numerous compound granular corpuscles (Fig. 3) and many fragmented axis cylinders. In sections stained by Heidenhain's method for myelin and the Gros-Bielschowsky technique for axis cylinders, the white columns were normal but there was a fine fibrillary gliosis in the anterior and lateral white columns, most prominent adjacent to the grey matter, and in the grey matter. There was no infiltrate of inflammatory cells in the cord or in the leptomeninges, and in none of the numerous sections examined were there abnormal vessels or thrombi. The thoracic and lumbar segments of the cord were normal, and in sections stained by Marchi's method, no degenerating myelin was seen. Representative sections of cerebral hemispheres, cerebellum, and brain-stem were normal.

## Discussion

The abnormalities found *post mortem* in this case indicate that the bilateral paralysis of the arms which existed from birth until death 10 days later was due to selective necrosis of the grey matter in the cervical part of the spinal cord. An infective aetiology, such as an intrauterine or neonatal poliomyelitis, can be excluded by the absence of a typical inflammatory infiltrate in the affected region or elsewhere in the central nervous system, by the normal cerebrospinal fluid and by the circumscribed nature of the lesion. Direct trauma, which might have been produced by the manipulation of the foetus, is unlikely to have produced such extensive necrosis without also having caused laceration or haemorrhage. In the absence of vascular occlusion or of a vascular malformation, we suggest that the necrosis of the spinal grey matter resulted from severe impairment of the local circulation.

There is a considerable amount of experimental evidence in support of this hypothesis, as a very similar lesion was observed in the cat after the circulation through an isolated segment of spinal cord had been drastically reduced by increasing the intradural pressure (Van Harreveld, 1941; Van Harreveld and Schadé, 1962). Further, in the cat, the dog, and the rabbit, reduction of the circulation through the spinal cord by occluding the aorta leads to selective necrosis of neurones in the central parts of the dorsal and ventral horns (Tureen, 1938; Krogh, 1945; Gelfan and Tarlov, 1959). The most peripheral neurones characteristically survive and the appearances of the cord a fortnight after the ischaemic episode are very similar to those observed in the present case. Symmetrical necrosis of the central neurones of the ventral horns of the spinal cord is present in some naturally occurring diseases in sheep and pigs (Innes and Saunders, 1962) and, in the absence of any other obvious aetiological factors, the authors conclude that impaired circulation through the cord is the main pathogenic factor.

In the case described here it seems likely that some mechanism had caused severe impairment of the circulation through the cervical part of the spinal cord of sufficient duration to cause selective necrosis of the grey matter. The only apparent factor is severe hyperextension of the neck associated with the face presentation early in labour. Hyperextension of the neck in adults with cervical spondylosis can obstruct the blood flow through the vertebral arteries (Yates and Hutchinson, 1961), but there is no evidence to suggest that a similar mechanism is of importance when there is no bony damage. Particular care was taken to ascertain if there was any damage to the vertebral canal in the present case, but none was found. Further, if both vertebral arteries had been obstructed by the hyperextension, some evidence of ischaemia in the brain-stem or cerebellum might have been expected.

There are, however, two other possible mechanisms: one is that anterior displacement of the ligamenta flava, which is known to occur in association with hyperextension of the neck (Taylor, 1953), had so compressed the spinal arteries and the cord that the circulation through it was grossly impaired; alternatively, hyperextension may itself have interfered with the blood flow through the spinal branches of the vertebral arteries. The former mechanism is analogous to the experimental procedure used by Van Harreveld and Schadé (1962) to produce a closely similar lesion in the spinal cord of the cat.

As the abnormalities in the spinal cord in the present case were not seen until it had been fixed, it seems possible that similar cases have been overlooked and that selective necrosis of spinal grey matter may be a hitherto unrecognized cause of obstetrical paralysis in the upper limbs.

## Summary

A case of obstetrical paralysis which presented as a bilateral Erb's palsy was found at necropsy to be due to selective ischaemic necrosis of the grey matter in the cervical part of the spinal cord. It is suggested that this necrosis was caused by severe impairment of the circulation through the cord due to hyperextension of the neck.

We wish to thank Dr. E. G. Fox, Consultant Paediatrician, Stobhill Hospital, Glasgow, for permission to publish this case.

### References

Ford, F. R. (1960). *Diseases of the Nervous System in Infancy, Childhood and Adolescence*, 4th ed., Chapter 8. Thomas, Springfield, Illinois.

Gelfan, S., and Tarlov, I. M. (1959). Interneurones and rigidity of spinal origin. *J. Physiol.* (*Lond.*), **146**, 594.
Innes, J. R. M., and Saunders, L. Z. (1962). *Comparative Neuropathology*, Chapters 15 and 23. Academic Press, New York and London.
Krogh, E. (1945). Studies on the blood supply to certain regions in the lumbar part of the spinal cord. *Acta physiol. scand.*, **10**, 271.
Taylor, A. R. (1953). Mechanism and treatment of spinal-cord disorders associated with cervical spondylosis. *Lancet*, **1**, 717.
Tureen, L. L. (1938). Circulation of the spinal cord and the effect of vascular occlusion. *Res. Publ. Ass. nerv. ment. Dis.*, **18**, 394.
Van Harreveld, A. (1941). The resistance of central synaptic conduction to asphyxiation. *Amer. J. Physiol.*, **133**, 572.
——, and Schadé, J. P. (1962). Nerve cell destruction by asphyxiation of the spinal cord. *J. Neuropath. exp. Neurol.*, **21**, 410.
Yates, P. O., and Hutchinson, E. C. (1961). Cerebral infarction: the role of stenosis of the extracranial cerebral arteries. *Spec. Rep. Ser. med. Res. Coun.* (*Lond.*), No. 300.

*Arch. Dis. Childh.*, 1965, **40**, 97.

# CONJUGATION REACTIONS IN THE NEWBORN INFANT: THE METABOLISM OF PARA-AMINOBENZOIC ACID

BY

MARKUS F. VEST* and RENÉ SALZBERG

*From the Children's Hospital, University of Basel, Switzerland*

(RECEIVED FOR PUBLICATION JULY 8, 1964)

It has been shown that the liver of the newborn infant has a limited capacity to perform certain transformation or conjugation reactions when compared to older subjects (Driscoll and Hsia, 1958; Kretchmer, Levine, McNamara, and Barnett, 1956). This limitation is evident in the formation of glucuronides (Brown and Zuelzer, 1958; Vest, 1958) and plays an important role in the genesis of neonatal jaundice. There are indications that other conjugation or detoxification mechanisms are also carried out in a different way from that of later life. The observation that after administration of sodium benzoate the excretion as hippuric acid is incomplete and delayed during the first three to four months of life (Vest, 1959) prompted us to investigate hippurate formation and acetylation in this age period.

## Material and Methods

Para-aminobenzoic acid (PAB) in the form of the sodium salt (NaPAB)†, was injected intravenously in a dose of 100 mg. per kg. body weight into four children 8 to 11 years old, three newborn premature infants of 2 to 6 days, two newborn full-term infants, and two 5- and 8-week-old infants. All subjects were male. Fluid intake was not restricted during the test.

Blood, 1-2 ml., was collected 5, 15, and 30 minutes, 1, 2, 3, 4, and, if necessary, 6 and 8 hours after the administration of the test dose. Urine was collected over 24 hours, divided in three 4-hour and a final 12-hour period. The urine was kept at 4° C. when assayed within a few hours, otherwise it was frozen at minus 20° C.

The sodium-p-aminobenzoate solution for intravenous use was prepared as follows: 10% NaPAB was dissolved in distilled water (w/v). The water was boiled before use and nitrogen bubbled through to remove carbon dioxide; 10 ml. amounts were put into brown ampoules which were filled with nitrogen just before sealing. The ampoules were sterilized by autoclaving at 120° C. for a quarter of an hour.

The method of Deiss and Cohen (1950) was used for the estimation of PAB and para-aminohippuric acid (PAH). PAH was estimated after extraction of PAB with ether. After extracting mixtures of known composition, on the average 1% PAB and 98% PAH remained. For the estimation of acetylated PAB and PAH (acetamido-benzoic and acetamido-hippuric acid‡) in the serum aliquots of the deproteinized supernatant were hydrolysed by boiling with 0·05 volume of 4 N HCl for 20 minutes. In the case of urine better results were obtained by hydrolysing for 45 minutes. In some experiments the hydrolysis of acetylated compounds was carried out by heating at 96° C. for three and a half hours as suggested by Smith, Finkelstein, Aliminosa, Crawford, and Graber (1945). After addition of the diazo reagents, the samples were read against a reagent blank at 540 mμ in a Coleman junior spectrophotometer. The amounts were determined from a calibration curve made with various concentrations of PAH. All results are expressed in micromols (μM) of PAH.

The colour intensity obtained without hydrolysis is equal to the free PAB and PAH. By extracting PAB, PAH alone can be measured. After hydrolysis the colour development is equal to the sum of PAH, PAB, and acetylated compounds. From this value the amount of total acetyl-metabolites (acetylated PAB and PAH) can be calculated by subtracting free PAB and PAH. Acetylated PAH is found by extracting the hydrolysate with ether (which removes the free and the formerly acetylated PAB) and subtracting the value of free PAH.

In two infants and one child the urinary metabolites were separated by counter-current distribution techniques. With each plate 5 ml. ethyl acetate was used as organic, and 5 ml. 1·6 M acetate buffer *p*H 3·4, as aqueous phase (Way, Smith, Howie, Weiss, and Swanson, 1948; Tabor, Freeman, Baily, and Smith, 1951). 50 to 100 plate distributions were run and both layers analysed for PAB, PAH, acetylated PAB and PAH, and glucuronides. For analysis the organic layer was first taken to dryness. A drop of ethanol facilitated dissolving the residue in water. The acetate phase was analysed directly. Glucuronide was estimated by the carbazole method of Dische (1947).

* Address: Children's Hospital, Römergasse 8, Basel, Switzerland.

† Fluka, Buchs.

‡ Roche, Basel.

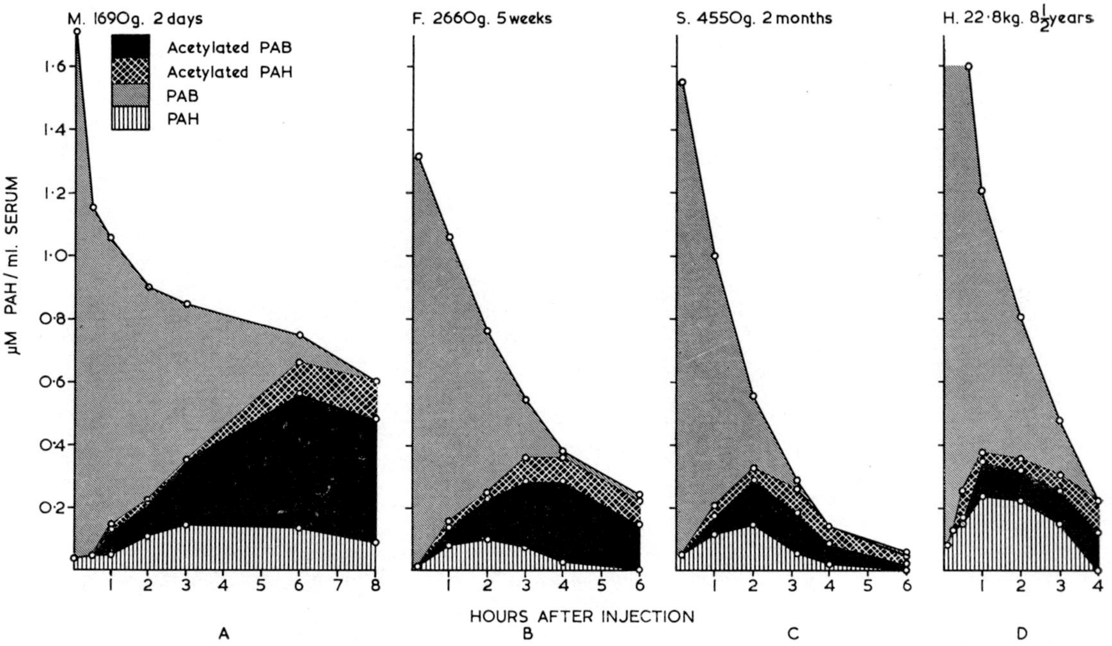


FIG. 1.—Concentration of p-aminobenzoic acid (PAB) metabolites in the serum after intravenous injection of 100 mg. sodium p-aminobenzoate per kg. body weight. All values are expressed as µM p-aminohippuric acid per 1 ml. serum. (A) newborn infant, (B) infant 5 weeks old, (C) infant 2 months old, (D) child 8½ years.

The identity of the urinary metabolites separated by counter-current distribution was studied by running aliquots on paper chromatograms. An ascending system of butanol-glacial acetic acid and water in the proportions 4 : 1 : 2 (v/v) was used with Whatman No. 1 paper. Standards of PAH, PAB, acetylated PAH, and acetylated PAB were run simultaneously. Ehrlich reagent (p-dimethylaminobenzaldehyde, 10% in concentrated HC1 solution (w/v) 1 vol., acetone 4 vol.) gave an immediate yellow colour with PAB, PAH, and PAB-glucuronide. With acetylated PAB and PAH the colour development was delayed. Compounds with a free amino group can also be distinguished from the acetylated metabolites by the Ekman reagent specific for diazotizable amines. Glucuronyl derivatives were identified by the napththoresorcinol and aniline-diphenylamine reagent (Smith, 1960).

## Results

**PAB Metabolites in the Serum.** Fig. 1 shows typical examples of the course of the various PAB acid metabolites in the serum in the different age-groups. In the 2-day-old premature infant (Fig. 1A) free PAB disappears slowly from the circulation. PAH is the first conjugate to appear. It reaches a peak of 0·12 µM per ml. serum 3 hours after injection of NaPAB. Acetylated PAB is the chief conjugate formed. It reaches a peak concentration of up to 0·6 µM per ml. at 6 hours. Besides PAH and acetyl-PAB small amounts of acetylated p-aminohippuric acid are formed. This conjugate is the last to appear in significant amounts.

Compared to the newborn infants, free PAB decreases quicker in the 5-week-old and more so in the 2-month-old infant (1B and C). At an age of 5 weeks acetyl-PAB is still the major conjugate formed (Fig. 1B). In the 2-month-old infant PAH formation is more prominent, though it is still less than that found in older children (Fig. 1C). Acetylated PAB is present to a greater degree than in older children, but much less than at 5 weeks. Some acetylated PAH is also present. In the 8½-year-old child (Fig. 1D) there is a rapid decrease of free PAB. The major conjugate now is PAH which reaches a peak of 0·25 µM per ml. at 1 hour. Acetyl-PAB appears later and its concentration remains lower than that of PAH. Some acetyl-PAH is also present. Both acetylated metabolic products are still present 4 hours after injection, when PAB and PAH have already disappeared. No attempt has been made to investigate glucuronide conjugation in the serum.

Fig. 2 shows the average plasma disappearance curves of total PAB metabolites at different ages. In the newborn period it is rather flat; at 8 weeks it reaches the slope found in older children. The 5-week-old infant takes an intermediate position.

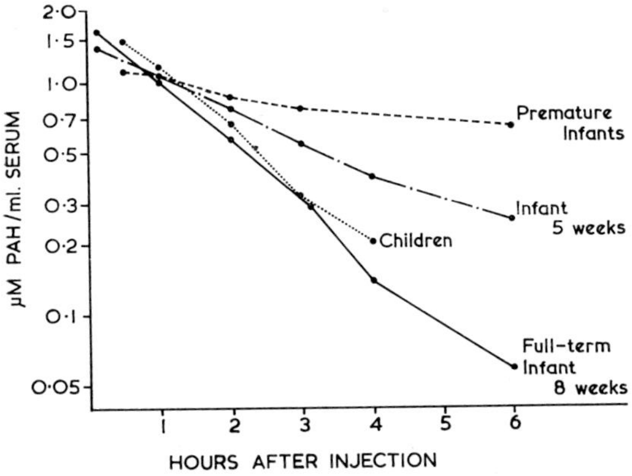


FIG. 2.—Rate of disappearance of total PAB from plasma in the newborn period, in infants and in children after intravenous injection of sodium p-aminobenzoate.

The time elapsing until the plasma concentration of total PAB has fallen to 50% of the initial level, is about 6 hours for the newborns, 3 hours 40 minutes in the 5-week-old infant, and 1 hour and 40 minutes in the 8-week-old infant and in the children.

**PAB Metabolites in the Urine.** The excretion of PAB derivates in the urine reflects the situation in the serum. In Fig. 3 the cumulative urinary excretion of the 4 metabolites is given as a percentage of the injected dose of sodium PAB for the same children whose serum concentrations are shown in Fig. 1. In the newborn infant (Fig. 3A), the metabolites appear slowly. After 4 hours only about 10% of the given PAB is excreted. In the serum (Fig. 1A) the PAH formed has been largely excreted after 6 to 8 hours. The same is evident in the cumulative urinary excretion, i.e. after 8 to 12 hours the amount excreted as PAH hardly increases any further. The chief metabolites, acetylated PAB and PAH on the other hand, appear more slowly and are excreted predominantly between 8 to 24 hours. Free PAB accounts for less than 7% of the total excreted.

Fig. 3B and C show the transition from the pattern prevailing in the newborn period to the one later in childhood. Not only does the total 24-hour recovery increase but the excretion accelerates. In the 5-week-old infant the chief metabolites are still acetyl-PAB and -PAH, but at 8 weeks PAH is the major conjugate. Even at this age however, much more acetyl-PAB is excreted than later in life.

In the child (Fig. 3D), the excretion is much more rapid, so that 70 to 85% is recovered within 4 hours after injection. The chief conjugate is p-amino-hippuric acid, which accounts for about 50% of the total PAB recovered. Free p-aminobenzoic acid generally takes the second place. Acetylated p-aminohippuric acid accounts for less than 10% of the recovered PAB.

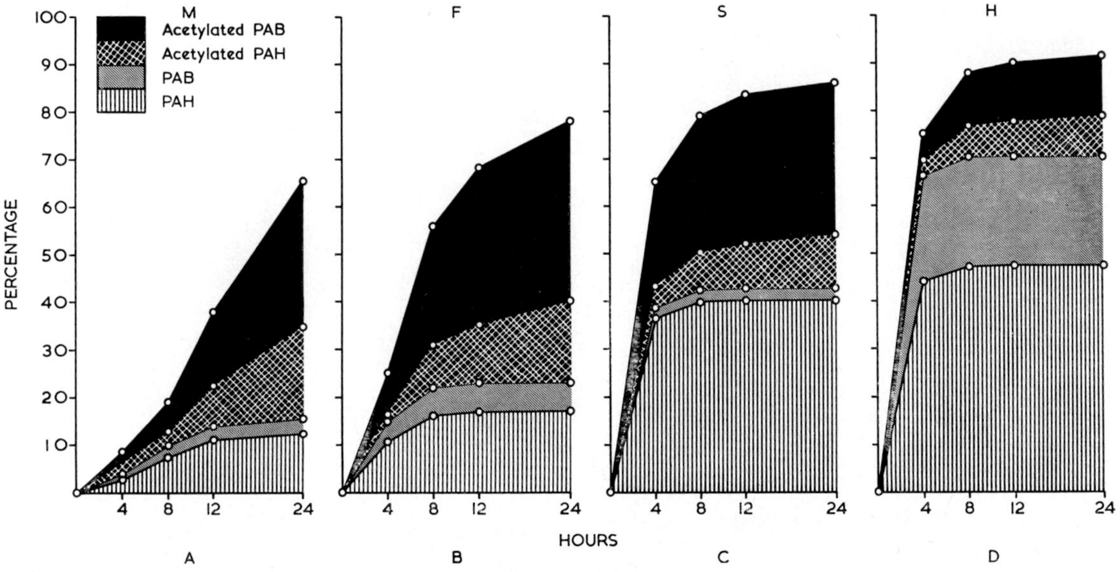


FIG. 3.—Cumulative 24-hour urinary excretion of the various PAB metabolites in percentage of the given dose of PAB. (A) newborn infant, (B) infant 5 weeks old, (C) infant 2 months old, (D) child 8½ years.

TABLE 1

PERCENTAGE DISTRIBUTION OF THE DIFFERENT PAB DERIVATIVES IN THE URINE IN RELATION TO AGE-GROUPS

| Name | Age | Total 24-hour Recovery (%) | PAH (%) | PAB (%) | Acetyl PAH (%) | Acetyl PAB (%) | Glucuronides (%) |
|---|---|---|---|---|---|---|---|
| Premature new-borns | | | | | | | |
| M.P. | 2 days | 65·2 | 12·8 | 2·5 | 19·2 | 30·7 | 7·9 |
| Sch. A. | 4 days | 47·7 | 14·6 | 1·4 | 15·5 | 16·2 | 7·7 |
| L.R. | 6 days | 70·6 | 10·2 | 5·9 | 21·1 | 33·4 | 6·2 |
| Mean | | 61·1 | 12·5 | 3·2 | 18·6 | 26·7 | 7·2 |
| Full-term new-borns | | | | | | | |
| M.R. | 3 days | 72·8 | 29·0 | 2·2 | 20·5 | 21·1 | 23·5 |
| A.D. | 5 days | 62·3 | 24·5 | 2·3 | 12·2 | 23·3 | 13·7 |
| Infants | | | | | | | |
| F.R. | 5 wk. | 78·4 | 16·9 | 6·0 | 17·0 | 38·5 | 16·9 |
| S.J. | 8 wk. | 85·6 | 39·4 | 1·9 | 11·7 | 32·6 | 21·9 |
| Children | | | | | | | |
| H.B. | 8½ yr. | 90·9 | 47·1 | 22·3 | 8·8 | 12·7 | 15·7 |
| P.C. | 9 yr. | 76·0 | 42·0 | 17·0 | 4·0 | 13·0 | 19·4 |
| E.J. | 10 yr. | 88·4 | 49·8 | 15·8 | 11·1 | 11·7 | 14·2 |
| C.J. | 11 yr. | 93·6 | 50·0 | 7·9 | 8·9 | 26·8 | 17·9 |
| Mean | | 87·2 | 47·2 | 15·7 | 8·2 | 16·0 | 16·8 |

**Glucuronic Acid Conjugates.** Because glucuronic acid conjugates are present in the urine even without PAB administration, it is difficult to estimate the percentage of PAB glucuronides accurately. If the quantity of glucuronic acid found in a 24-hour urine sample before the test is subtracted from the amount found after PAB injection, it is possible to get an estimate of the percentage of PAB excreted as a glucuronyl conjugate. As will be shown later two glucuronyl conjugates, p-aminobenzoyl- and p-acetamido-benzoyl glucuronide, are present in various proportions depending on age. Because their solubility is not very different from that of the glycine conjugates, they stay behind when PAB is extracted. In the colorimetric assay these conjugates are therefore estimated along with PAH and acetyl-PAH respectively. They can, however, be measured separately by the Dische (1947) method. Analysis of the consecutive urine samples shows that in the newborn the glucuronides follow the same course as

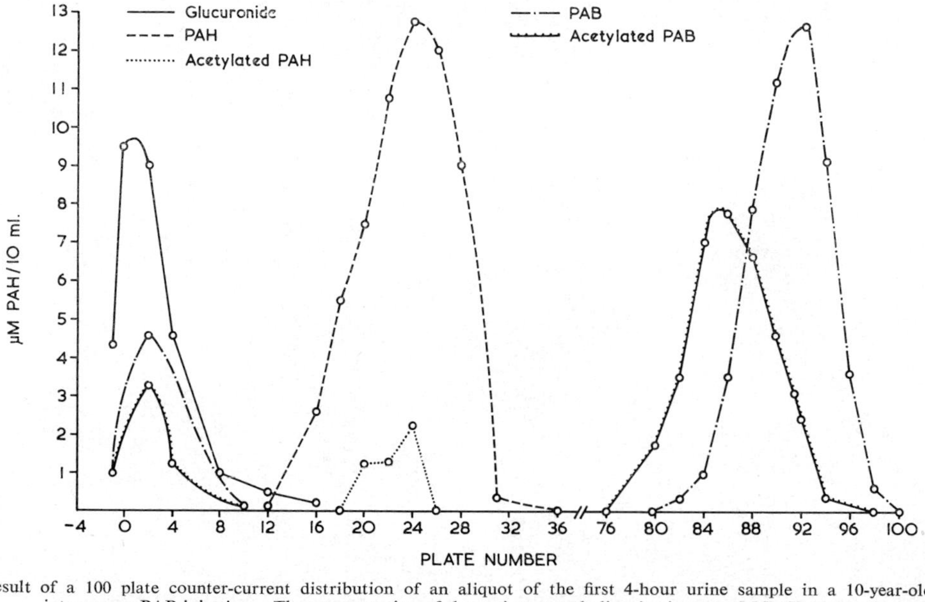


FIG. 4.—Result of a 100 plate counter-current distribution of an aliquot of the first 4-hour urine sample in a 10-year-old child after intravenous PAB injection. The concentration of the various metabolites is given as µM PAH per plate.

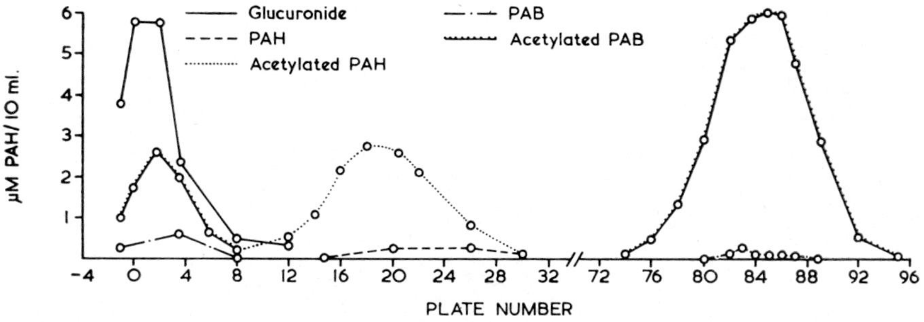


FIG. 5.—Newborn infant. Result of a 95-plate counter-current distribution of a urine sample collected from 8 to 24 hours after intravenous PAB injection.

the other PAB conjugates, i.e. they appear much slower than in the group of children.

In Table 1 the percentage of the various PAB derivatives in the urine is given for the different age-groups. The value for the glucuronides is given separately but is already included in the column headed Total 24-hour Recovery, because, as mentioned above, they form a part of PAH and acetyl-PAH.

**Separation of PAB Metabolites by Counter-current Distribution.** Fig. 4 shows the results of the counter-current distribution in a 10-year-old child. A distribution of an aliquot of the first four-hour urine sample was run. A complete separation of PAH from acetyl-PAH and of PAB from acetyl-PAB could not be achieved, but the glucuronides were clearly separated from PAH and acetyl-PAH respectively and the latter from PAB and acetyl-PAB. The results agree with those obtained by colorimetric estimation. The chief metabolite present is PAH, with free PAB, acetylated PAB, and acetylated PAH following in decreasing order. There are two glucuronic acid conjugates: PAB- and acetyl-PAB-glucuronide. These do not quite account for all the glucuronic acid in the first plates. This is to be expected as other glucuronides are present in the urine. Planimetry of the curve results in the following percentage distribution: PAH 36·7, acetyl-PAH 2·7, PAB 28·8, acetyl-PAB 19·4, p-aminobenzoyl glucuronide 7·7, and acetamidobenzoyl glucuronide 4·7.

The result in a newborn infant is shown in Fig. 5. It was obtained from an aliquot of the urine collected from 8 to 24 hours and confirms the predominance of acetylated PAB and acetylated PAH over PAH, and the presence of PAB-glucuronides. In contrast to older children, p-acetamidobenzoyl glucuronide, not p-aminobenzoyl glucuronide is the main glucuronic acid conjugate in infants. The percentage distribution is as follows: PAH 3·7, acetyl-PAH 26·7, PAB 0·7, acetyl-PAB 54·8, p-aminobenzoyl glucuronide 2·2, acetamidobenzoyl glucuronide 11·9.

In Table 2 the ratio of distribution of the four standard compounds between ethyl acetate and buffer is compared to that calculated from the counter-current distribution. They agree only to a limited extent.

**Chromatography of PAB Metabolites.** Fig. 6 shows a chromatogram of the main peaks obtained by counter-current distribution in child E. J. Plate No. 24 has the same value (Rf 0·62) as PAH, 81 as acetyl-PAB (Rf 0·89), and 97 as PAB (Rf 0·83). In No. 2, which gives the highest reading for glucuronic acid, there are two spots the Rf values of which are

TABLE 2

RATIO OF DISTRIBUTION BETWEEN ETHYL ACETATE AND ACETATE BUFFER OF PAB AND DERIVATIVES COMPARED WITH DISTRIBUTION CONSTANTS OBSERVED IN COUNTER-CURRENT DISTRIBUTION

| PAB-derivative | Constant | Child E. | | Infant M. | |
|---|---|---|---|---|---|
| | | Plate No.* | Constant | Plate No.† | Constant |
| PAH | 0·29 | 24 | 0·31 | 22 | 0·30 |
| PAB | 11·5 | 92 | 11·5 | PAB too low for calculation | |
| Acetyl-PAH | 0·31 | 24 | 0·31 | 19 | 0·25 |
| Acetyl-PAB | 7·85 | 86 | 6·15 | 85 | 8·5 |

* 100 plates. † 95 plates.

below that of the standards used. The lower one is diazotizable and gives an immediate Ehrlich reaction, i.e. it has a free amino group. Both react with naphthoresorcinol and aniline-diphenylamine. It is likely therefore that the lower spot (Rf 0·28) is PAB glucuronide, whereas the second from the base-line (Rf 0·45), which gives a delayed reaction with Ehrlich reagent, is acetyl PAB-glucuronide.

the standards. In child E.J., starting from the front-line there are two spots for acetyl-PAB (Rf 0·92) and free PAB (Rf 0·83). There is no acetyl-PAH present, only PAH (Rf 0·63). Two spots for the glucuronyl conjugates are clearly visible (Rf 0·46 and 0·38). The two newborn infants show a different pattern. Acetyl-PAB is nearest to the front (Rf 0·92). PAB is missing or very feeble. But in both infants there is a spot for acetyl-PAH (Rf 0·76) beside the one for PAH (Rf 0·63). From the PAH glucuronides only the upper spot corresponding to acetyl-PAB glucuronide (Rf 0·46) is present.

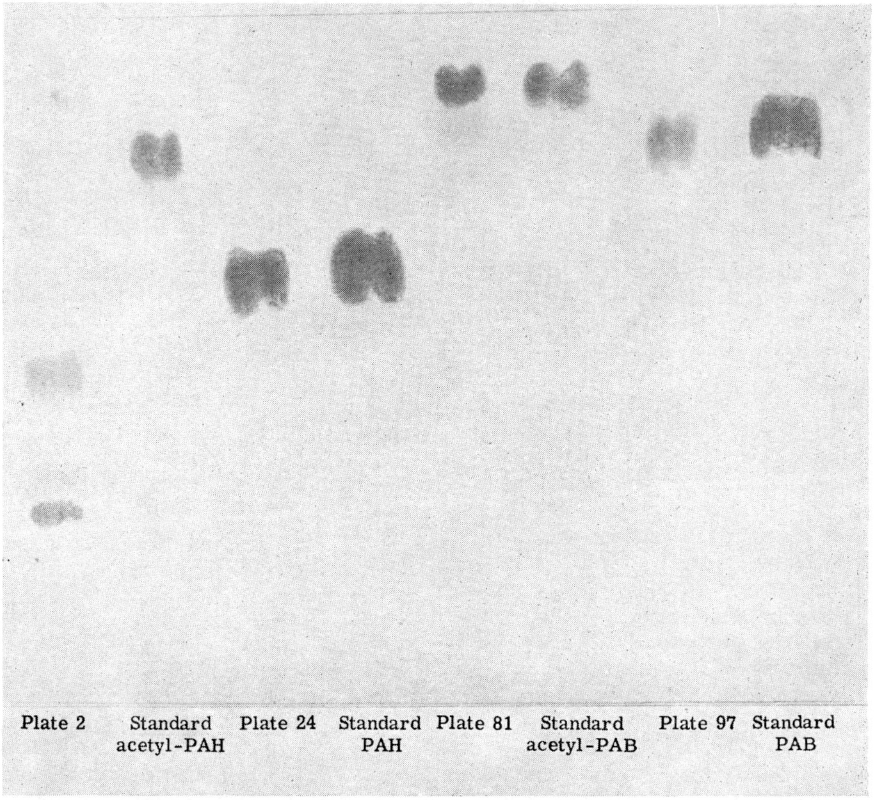


FIG. 6.—Chromatogram of the PAB metabolites separated by counter-current distribution in a child. Below the base-line the plate numbers and the different standard compounds are indicated.

In Fig. 7 the same is shown for the newborn, M.P. Here, in plate No. 2, the upper spot, acetamido-benzoyl glucuronide (Rf 0·46) is much more prominent than PAB-glucuronide (Rf 0·30). Plate No. 17 corresponds to acetyl-PAH (Rf 0·79) and 84 to acetyl-PAB (Rf 0·89). As the counter-current distribution was done on the 8- to 24-hour urine sample no detectable PAH is present.

Direct chromatography of the urine shows the same metabolites (see Fig. 8). The 0-4 hour urine sample of child, E.J., and the 4 to 8 hour sample of the infants, M.P. and L.R., are shown together with the standards.

## Discussion

In children, intravenously administered NaPAB is rapidly cleared from the plasma mainly by conjugation with glycine, and to some extent by acetylation and glucuronidation. Nearly 50% of the administered dose is excreted as p-aminohippuric acid.

Other important metabolites are free and acetylated PAB (about 15% each) and the glucuronides of PAB and acetyl-PAB (about 16%). Little is excreted as acetylated PAH. This agrees with the results in human adults (Deiss and Cohen, 1950; Tabor *et al.*, 1951), whereas in animals different proportions of the various metabolites have been found (Riggs and Christensen, 1951; Williams, 1959).

In newborn infants PAB disappears, more slowly from the circulation. There is diminished and delayed conjugation with glycine. This confirms the observation of Brandt (1960) who found that the activity of the hippurate synthesizing system of the liver in foetal and newborn rats is diminished. Instead of hippurate formation, acetylation at the amino group is much more prominent than in the children. This is to a certain extent at variance with the report of a limited acetylation of sulphonamides in the newborn period (Fichter and Curtis, 1955). With PAB there is, however, not only a predominance of acetyl-PAB over free PAB, but also of acetyl-PAH over PAH and acetamidobenzoyl glucuronide over p-aminobenzoyl glucuronide. In accordance with previous results (Brown and Zuelzer, 1958; Vest, 1958), the extent of glucuronide formation is also lower in the newborn premature infants than later in life.

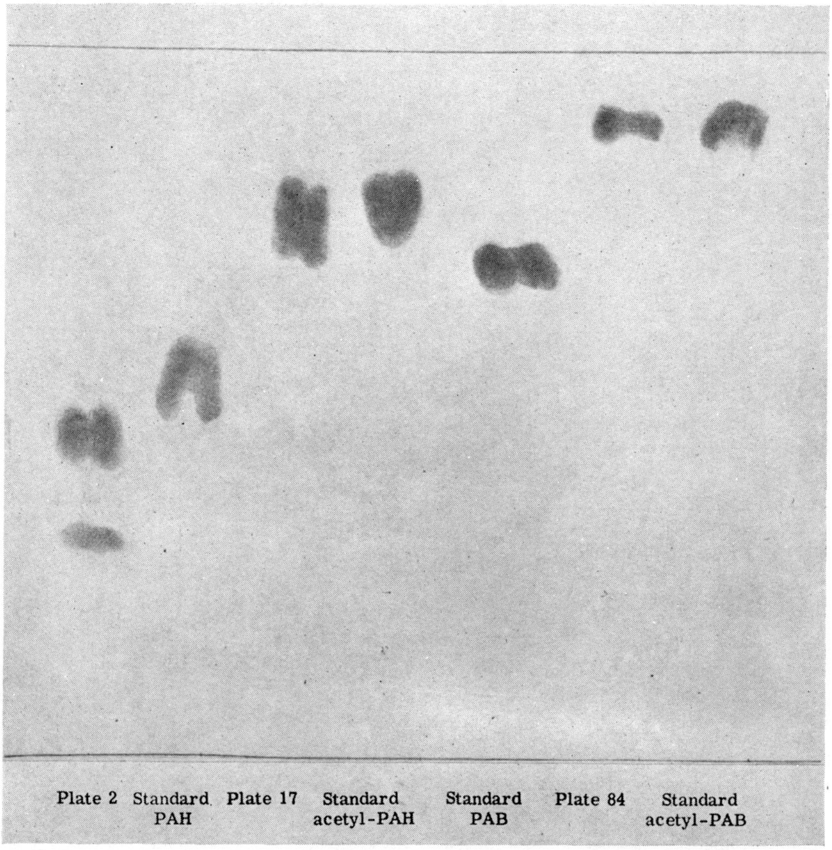


FIG. 7.—Newborn infant. Chromatogram of the PAB metabolites separated by counter-current distribution and of the standard compounds.

It is difficult to establish to what extent a diminished renal clearance of the different metabolites contributes to the lower plasma disappearance rate and the slower urinary excretion in the newborns. Clearance of the various metabolites during constant infusion of NaPAB was done in 3 full-term newborn infants, 3 to 8 days old and in one 12-year-old child (L. Strebel and M. Vest: unpublished results). Inulin clearance in the newborns ranged from 22 to 49 ml./min./1·73 sq. m. It was not influenced by the infusion of NaPAB. PAH clearance amounted to 45 to 267 ml./min./1·73 sq. m., PAB 0·8 to 23·4 ml., acetyl-PAH 34 to 154 ml., and acetyl PAB 8·4 to

105 ml. In the child the inulin clearance was 111, PAH 535, PAB 80, acetyl PAH 260, and acetyl PAB 430 ml./min./1·73 sq. m. The low PAB clearance accounts for the small amount of free PAB excreted by the newborn infants. The predominance of the acetylated metabolites cannot, however, be explained by the clearance studies.

Every alteration of these reactions or their rate could influence the extent of hippurate formation. So it is conceivable that the glycine-condensing enzyme matures more slowly than the acetylase.

Lack of available glycine could contribute to the decreased PAH formation. Administration of 1 g. glycine to newborn infants one hour before the

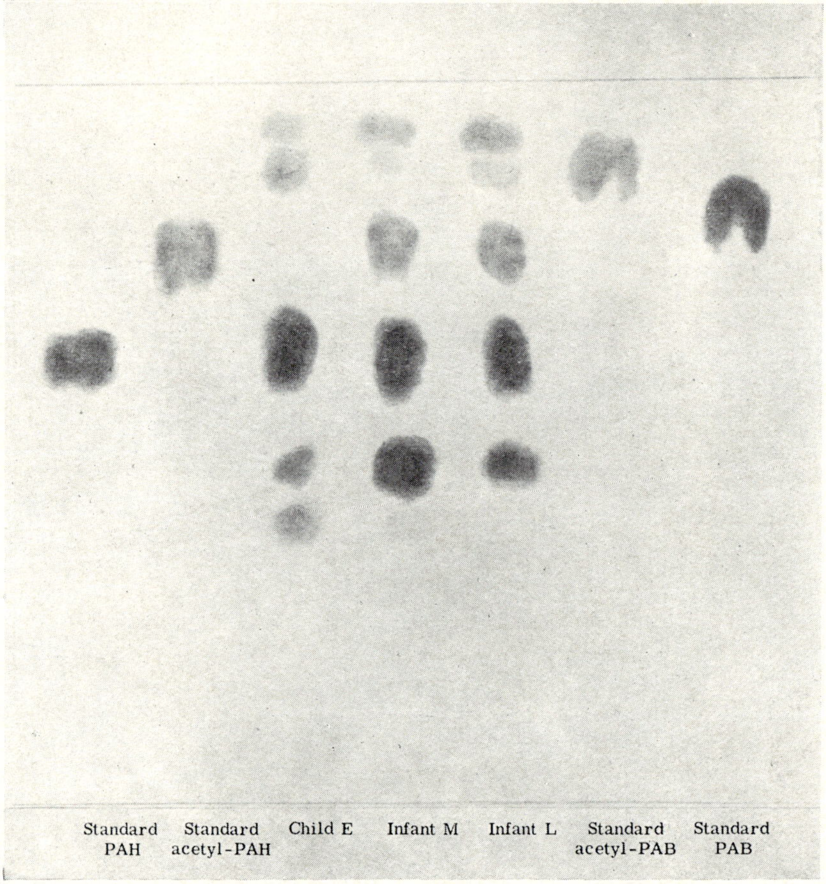


FIG. 8.—Chromatogram of urine and standard compounds in a child and two newborn infants showing the different PAB metabolites present.

The reason why acetylation is enhanced in the newborn at the expense of hippurate formation is not clear. Hippuric acid and PAH synthesis requires an activated form of benzoic acid, benzoyl co-enzyme A. The later is then able to acylate glycine (Schachter and Taggart, 1953). This reaction is catalysed by the enzyme glycine-N-acylase (Schachter and Taggart, 1954). Similarly acetylation requires the previous formation of 'active acetate', i.e. acetyl co-enzyme A. In the case of aromatic amines the acetylating enzyme is called arylamine acetylase.

PAB injection actually leads to increased PAH concentration in the plasma and to a rise in the PAH excretion in the urine as it does in adults, but PAH formation is still much inferior to that found in children (Vest and Rossier, 1963).

## Summary

The metabolism of p-aminobenzoic acid (PAB) was studied by injecting a dose of 100 mg. per kg. of the sodium salt into 3 newborn premature infants, 2 full-term newborns, 2 infants 5 and 8 weeks old, and 4 children 8½ to 11 years old. In the children PAB is rapidly cleared from the serum, chiefly by formation of p-aminohippuric acid (PAH). The 24-hour recovery in the urine lies between 76 and 93%, of which 68 to 85% are excreted within the first 4 hours. The chief conjugate in the urine is PAH, which accounts for nearly half of the total. Other metabolites are acetyl-PAB, free PAB, acetyl-PAH, PAB- and acetyl-PAB-glucuronides. In the newborn infants PAB is eliminated tardily from the circulation. The main conjugate formed is acetyl-PAB. PAH, acetyl-PAH, and free PAB are other metabolic products. The excretion in the urine is also delayed so that only about 10% of the given dose appears within the first 4 hours. The 24-hour recovery amounts to between 48 and 70%. Again the major metabolite is acetylated PAB with acetyl-PAH, PAH, and free PAB following in decreasing order. Glucuronides account for only about 7%, acetamidobenzoyl glucuronide prevailing over p-aminobenzoyl glucuronide. As the two older infants show, the transition from the pattern in the newborn period to that in children takes place around the 8th week of life.

## References


Brandt, I. K. (1960). Hippurate synthesis in the newborn rat. *Amer. J. Dis. Child.*, **100**, 538.

Brown, A. K., and Zuelzer, W. W. (1958). Studies on the neonatal development of the glucuronide conjugating system. *J. clin. Invest.*, **37**, 332.

Deiss, W. P., and Cohen, P. P. (1950). Studies in para-aminohippuric acid synthesis in the human: its application as a liver function test. *ibid.*, **29**, 1014.

Dische, Z. (1947). A new specific color reaction of hexuronic acids. *J. biol. Chem.*, **167**, 189.

Driscoll, S. G., and Hsia, D. Y. (1958). The development of enzyme systems during early infancy. *Pediatrics*, **22**, 785.

Fichter, E. G., and Curtis, J. A. (1955). Sulfonamide administration in newborn and premature infants (abstract). *Amer. J. Dis. Child.*, **90**, 596.

Kretchmer, N., Levine, S. Z., McNamara, H., and Barnett, H. L. (1956). Certain aspects of tyrosine metabolism in the young. I. The development of the tyrosine oxidizing system in human liver. *J. clin. Invest.* **35**, 236.

Riggs, T. R., and Christensen, H. N. (1951). Metabolic conjugations of *p*-aminobenzoic acid in the rat. *J. biol. Chem.*, **193**, 675.

Schachter, D., and Taggart, J. V. (1953). Benzoyl coenzyme A and hippurate synthesis. *ibid.*, **203**, 925.

——, —— (1954). Glycine *N*-acylase: purification and properties. *ibid.*, **208**, 263.

Smith, H. W., Finkelstein, N., Aliminosa, L., Crawford, B., and Graber, M. (1945). The renal clearances of substituted hippuric acid derivatives and other aromatic acids in dog and man. *J. clin. Invest.*, **24**, 388.

Smith, I. (1960). *Chromatographic and Electrophoretic Techniques*, 2nd ed., Vol. 1. *Chromatography*. Heinemann, London.

Tabor, C. W., Freeman, M. V., Baily, J., and Smith, P. K. (1951). Studies on the metabolism of para-aminobenzoic acid. *J. Pharmacol.*, **102**, 98.

Vest, M. (1958). Insufficient glucuronide formation in the newborn and its relationship to the pathogenesis of icterus neonatorum. *Arch. Dis. Childh.*, **33**, 473.

—— (1959). *Physiologie und Pathologie des Neugeborenenicterus*. S. Karger, Basel.

——, and Rossier, R. (1963). Detoxification in the newborn. *Ann. N.Y. Acad. Sci.*, **111**, 183.

Way, E. L., Smith, P. K., Howie, D. L., Weiss, R., and Swanson, R. (1948). The absorption, distribution, excretion and fate of para-aminosalicylic acid. *J. Pharmacol.*, **93**, 368.

Williams, R. T. (1959). *Detoxication Mechanisms*, 2nd ed. Chapman and Hall, London.

*Arch. Dis. Childh.*, 1965, **40**, 106.

# OSTEOCHONDRODYSTROPHIA DEFORMANS WITH MUCOPOLYSACCHARIDOSIS

BY

S. VESTERMARK

*From the Queen Louise's Children's Hospital, Copenhagen, Denmark*

(RECEIVED FOR PUBLICATION JULY 8, 1964)

In 1929, Morquio described a peculiar skeletal disease, which he called familial osseous dystrophy. The disease develops gradually after the first year of life and is characterized by dwarfism with short neck, deformed chest with protruding sternum, deformed legs with pronounced genu valgum, and broad flat feet. The skull and face are normal and the intelligence is normal. The disease is often accompanied by muscular weakness. Radiologically, in Morquio's patients the epiphyses of the long bones were deformed with irregular calcifications, and the development of the ossification centres of the carpal and tarsal bones was defective. Only slight changes were found in the spine. The same year Brailsford (1929) described a similar entity, which he called chondro-osteodystrophy, but in his patient radiography showed distinct changes also in the spine, the vertebral bodies being of irregular shape and size with blurred edges and a tongued anterior surface. The disease is now called osteochondrodystrophia deformans, Morquio's disease, or Morquio-Brailsford's disease. In 1926 Silfverskiöld described a disorder with similar radiological changes in the epiphyses and in the spinal column, but the clinical picture was much less peculiar, the patients exhibiting only moderate retardation of growth, moderate thoracic kyphosis, and pronounced varus position of the feet.

The characteristic skeletal changes may vary from very slight lesions which can only be detected radiologically, to gross changes with dwarfism and deformed spinal column (Brailsford, 1948). The most pronounced forms of Morquio-Brailsford's disease offer many points of resemblance to gargoylism (Robinow, 1958), and the question whether Morquio-Brailsford's disease and gargoylism are variants of the same disorder or whether they are two different entities remains to be solved. Some authors state that the radiological skeletal changes in Morquio-Brailsford's disease and gargoylism are indistinguishable (Eichenberger, 1954), and clinically there exist transitional forms, i.e. Morquio-Ullrich's disease, between the two entities (Wiedemann, 1954); hence it has been suggested that the various entities be united under the name of gargoylism (Eichenberger, 1954). However, this term seems inapposite, since gargoylism refers to the grotesque appearance seen only in the most severe case. Others maintain that gargoylism and Morquio-Brailsford's disease are two different disorders and that Morquio-Ullrich's disease comes under neither (Zellweger, Ponseti, Pedrini, Stamler, and von Noorden, 1961). In gargoylism, accumulation of acid mucopolysaccharides with a high content of hexosamines in brain, liver, bones, and other organs, and increased urinary excretion of acid mucopolysaccharides has been demonstrated. In Morquio-Ullrich's disease deposits of acid mucopolysaccharides in bone tissue and increased urinary excretion of acid mucopolysaccharides were also found, but the excreted mucopolysaccharides were different from those excreted in gargoylism (Zellweger *et al.*, 1961; Dyggve, Melchior, and Clausen, 1962).

Such biochemical differences as have hitherto been demonstrated between gargoylism, Morquio-Brailsford's disease, and Morquio-Ullrich's disease are hardly sufficient to decide that they are three different entities.

This paper reports a study of a family consisting of five members, all of whom had increased urinary excretion of mucopolysaccharides, two out of three children furthermore having a slight degree of osteochondrodystrophia deformans.

### Method

The technique used for demonstrating acid mucopolysaccharides has previously been described by Dyggve *et al.* (1962). The urine is collected for 24 hours and concentrated 100 times by vacuum dialysis. After electrophoresis on filter paper the patterns are stained with Alcian blue and compared with the patterns obtained from standard preparations of hyaluronic acid, chondroitin sulphate, and heparin.

**Case Reports**

The father was born in 1907. About 20 years ago he was admitted to hospital for examination because of muscle weakness. He now walks heavily and with difficulty and has to lean on the furniture. Radiography of chest shows an arcuate thoracic kyphosis with slightly wedge-shaped vertebral bodies (Fig. 1), while that of the knees shows slightly irregular joint surfaces and formation

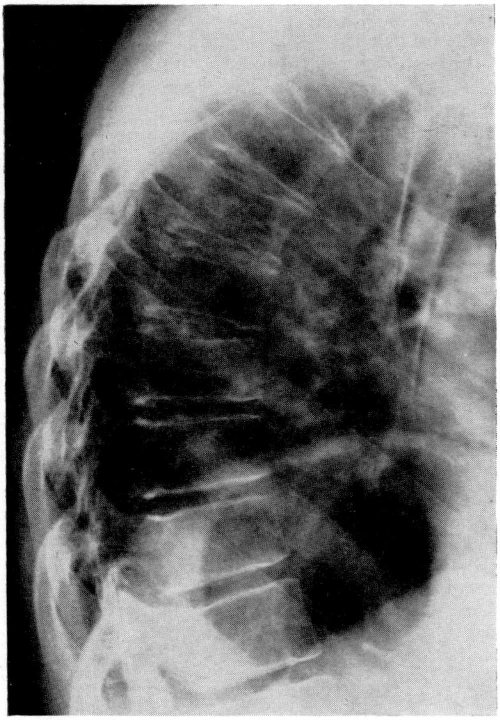

FIG. 1.—The spine of the father, aged 56. There is kyphosis with small osteophytes in the upper part.

of osteophytes. The urine contains acid mucopolysaccharides which by electrophoresis appear to consist of one fraction with a rate of migration similar to that of chondroitin sulphate and one fraction with a lower rate of migration.

The mother was born in 1925. She has no symptoms. Her height and appearance are normal. Radiological examination of the spine, wrists, hips, and pelvis shows nothing abnormal. The serum levels of calcium, phosphorus, and alkaline phosphatase are normal. In the urine, acid mucopolysaccharides are present, electrophoresis revealing also in this case one fraction with a rate of migration similar to that of chondroitin sulphate, and one fraction with a lower rate of migration.

**Case 1.** The first child is a boy who was born in 1949. Since the age of 2 years his gait has been poor, with varus feet. On examination in 1963 he was 17 cm. below the

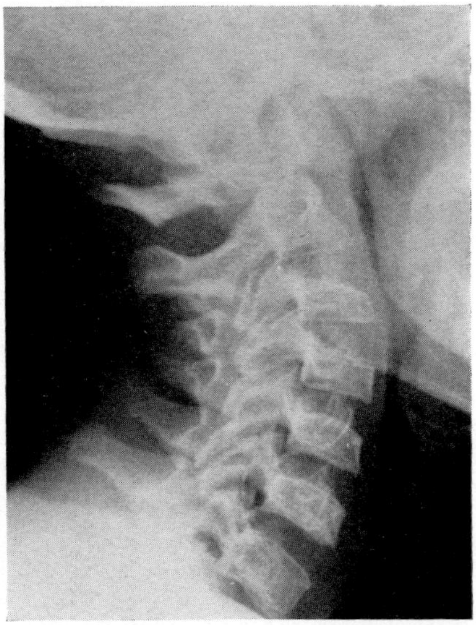

FIG. 2.—Case 1. The cervical part of the spine with flattened bodies.

expected height. He is not short necked and his face is normal. The chest is slightly deformed with a prominence of the right side but no protrusion of the sternum. There is increased lumbar lordosis and a moderate arcuate thoracic kyphosis. The upper limbs show hyperextension of the terminal phalangeal joints and Heberden's nodes. The lower limbs show moderate atrophy of the femoral muscles, but no pareses. The feet show pronounced cavovarus deformity and prominence of the lateral malleoli. Knee and ankle reflexes are absent.

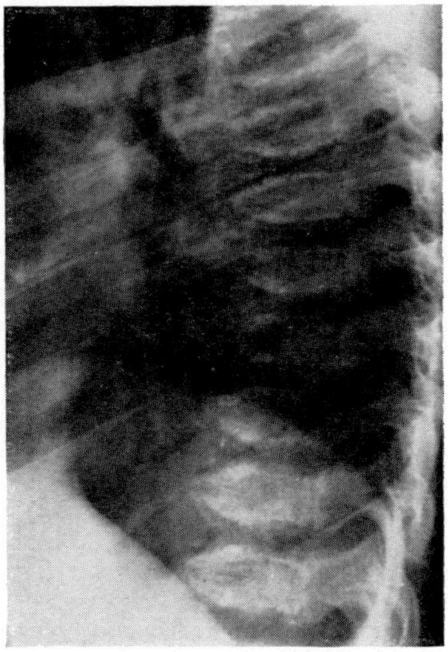

FIG. 3.—Case 1. The thoracic corpora are flattened with blurred edges and wedge-shaped anterior surfaces.

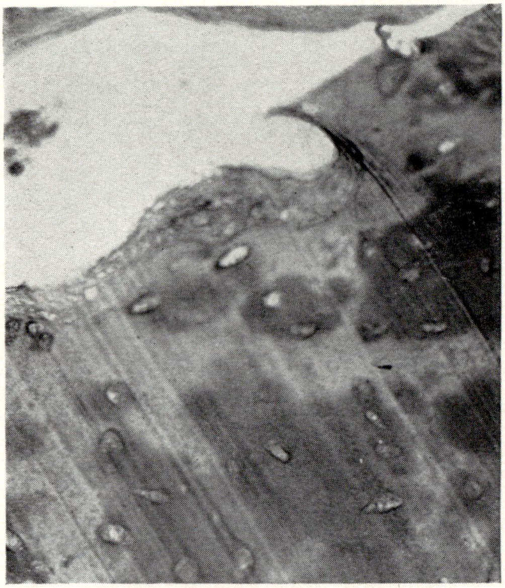

FIG. 4.—Case 1. Biopsy from the iliac crest. The darkly stained areas indicate a high content of acid mucopolysaccharides. (Alcian blue and periodic acid-Schiff. × 100.)

The gait is somewhat clumsy but not ataxic. Plantar reflexes normal. The skin of fingers and toes is thick and rough. Radiological examination of the spine reveals pronounced changes in almost all vertebral bodies which are flat with irregular blurred edges and wedge-shaped anterior surfaces (Figs. 2 and 3). Radiological examination of hip joints and pelvis reveals increase in width of the femoral neck and irregular skeletal structure. Radiological examination of skull, chest, upper limbs, and lower limbs shows nothing abnormal. Bone age, 11 years at chronological age 14. Intelligence and hearing are normal. Eye examination shows slight hypermetropia and red-green colour blindness, but no corneal opacities. Electromyography shows degeneration of motor units in tibialis anterior, while the rate of conduction is normal. Skin biopsy reveals nothing abnormal. Biopsy from tibialis anterior muscle shows partially atrophied muscle fibres in some regions and completely atrophied fibres in others, with abundant interstitial fatty tissue, i.e. neurogenic muscular atrophy. Bone biopsy from the iliac crest shows cartilaginous fragments with irregularly proliferating small islands of normal cartilage cells, bordering on regions with scarce and irregular calcification and with few osteoblasts. Cartilage matrix shows areas of pronounced Alcian blue staining, indicating the presence of mucopolysaccharide (Fig. 4). Protein-bound iodine and tri-iodothyronine in blood, serum proteins, electrolytes, GO-transaminases, and GP-transaminases, lactic acid dehydrogenase, creatine phosphokinase, and serum citric acid are normal. Serum calcium is normal, but serum phosphorus is low (2·6 mEq/l.), and alkaline phosphatase slightly increased (32·6 K.A. units). Serum immunoelectrophoresis is normal. Wasserman reaction negative. Urinary excretion of 17-ketosteroids normal. Excretion of amino acids normal. Creatine/creatinine index 131%. In the urine there is increased excretion of acid mucopolysaccharides with a rate of migration similar to that of chondroitin sulphate.

**Case 2.** The second child is a girl, born in 1951. She has no symptoms and her height and appearance are normal. Tendon reflexes normal. Fractional serum protein, serum citric acid, serum calcium, and creatine phosphokinase normal. Serum phosphorus slightly decreased (2·7 mEq/l.); alkaline phosphatase slightly increased (27 K.A. units). Radiological examination of skull, spine, and limbs shows nothing abnormal. In the urine there is increased excretion of acid mucopolysaccharides, which by electrophoresis are identified as one fraction with a rate of migration similar to that of chondroitin sulphate and one fraction with a slower rate of migration.

**Case 3.** The third child is a girl who was born in 1954. She is 13 cm. shorter than normal for her age. Her face is normal and she is not short necked. There is an increased lumbar lordosis but no kyphosis, and her chest is not deformed. There is hyperextension of the terminal phalangeal joints, and Heberden's nodes are present. The skin of her fingers is somewhat thick and rough. No muscular atrophy or pareses are present. The knee and ankle reflexes cannot be elicited. Plantar reflexes are normal. Her feet show rather pronounced cavovarus deformity with protrusion of the lateral malleoli. Eye examination reveals a slight hypermetropia, but no corneal opacities. Hearing and intelligence are normal. Electromyography of tibialis anterior, normal. Radiological examination of the skull and the limbs, normal. Radiological examination of the spine shows flattened vertebral bodies with irregular bone structure and irregular edges (Figs. 5 and 6). Wassermann reaction, negative. Serum proteins, GO-transaminases, GP-transaminases, creatine phosphokinase, lactic acid dehydrogenase, serum amino acids, and citric acid are normal. Serum calcium, normal, phosphorus somewhat low (2·7 mEq/l.), and alkaline phosphatase slightly increased (29 K.A. units). Serum immunoelectrophoresis normal. Creatine/creatinine index 133%. Examination of urine shows increased excretion of acid mucopolysaccharides with a rate of migration similar to that of chondroitin sulphate.

Summarizing the urinary mucopolysaccharide findings: in urine from the father, the healthy mother, and the healthy sister, an electrophoretic fraction with the same rate of migration as chondroitin sulphate, together with an unidentified fraction with a somewhat lower rate of migration are present, while urine from the two children with skeletal affection contains chondroitin sulphate only. In all five cases the acid mucopolysaccharide fractions are weak, but distinctly pathological by comparison with normal urine. No quantitative determination of the acid mucopolysaccharides has been possible.

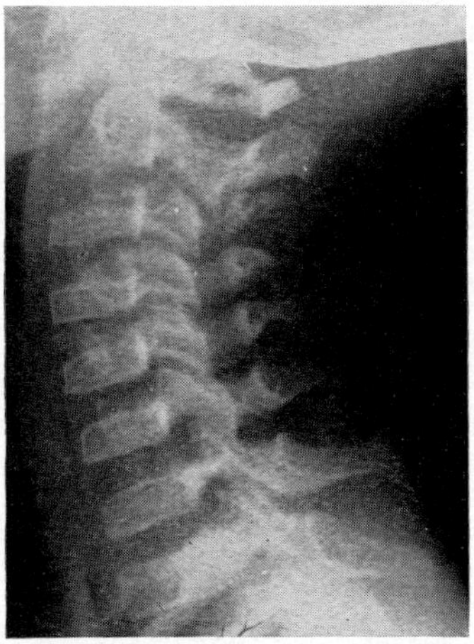

FIG. 5.—Case 3. The bodies of the cervical vertebrae are flattened.

## Discussion

The radiological changes of the spine in our two patients are characteristic of osteochondrodystrophia deformans (Brailsford, 1948). The father has an arthrosis deformans. Whether he has previously had osteochondrodystrophy is not known, but in some familial cases of osteochondrodystrophy the parents have sometimes had arthrosis deformans (Guldager, 1945; Silfverskiöld, 1926). Both our patients are somewhat smaller than normal for their ages, with slender extremities and increased lumbar lordosis, but their faces are normal and they are of normal intelligence. The neck is not shortened and there are no corneal opacities. These findings are consistent with the difficulty of detecting the slighter cases clinically. In our two patients the creatine/creatinine index is slightly raised, but the enzymatic activity in the serum is normal. In the elder patient there is a moderate symmetrical muscular atrophy of the thighs. It is not clear whether the muscle disorder is myogenic or neurogenic, since the younger patient has a normal electromyogram, while muscle biopsy and electromyogram in the elder patient point towards a neurogenic affection. Both patients have symmetrical areflexia on their lower limbs, favouring a neurogenic affection, though it is strange that no other neurological degeneration symptoms can be detected. Osteochondrodystrophia deformans, however, seems only occasionally to be accompanied by neurological degeneration; Einhorn, Moore, Ostrum, and Rowntree (1941) described 3 patients with pronounced neurological symptoms and ascribed these to cord compression in the spinal canal, which was confirmed in one of the patients coming to necropsy (Einhorn, Moore, and Rowntree, 1946).

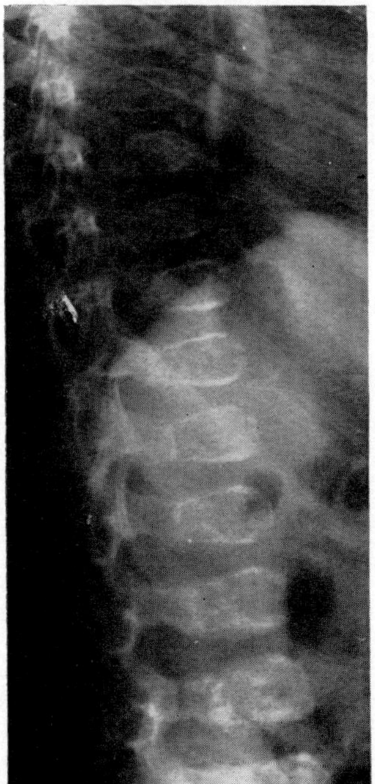

FIG. 6.—Case 3. The bodies of the thoracic vertebrae are flattened with slightly wedge-shaped anterior surfaces. The lumbar vertebrae show irregular edges.

The elder of our patients exhibits delayed development of ossification centres, but in neither patient do the blood analyses give any evidence of endocrine, renal, or hepatic disorder. Alkaline phosphatase is slightly raised and serum phosphorus reduced both in the two patients and in their healthy sister. A few other authors have previously demonstrated raised alkaline phosphatase in osteochondrodystrophia deformans (Andersen, 1937; Crawford, 1939; Whiteside and Cholmeley, 1952), but in most cases serum calcium, phosphorus, and alkaline phosphatase were normal.

Bone biopsy from the elder patient shows irregular arrangement of cartilagenous cells. The basic substance stains strongly, but irregularly with Alcian blue. Similar changes have been described previously in Morquio-Brailsford's disease (Shelling, 1957). In Morquio-Ullrich's disease Zellweger *et al.* (1961) found changes which partly correspond to those described above and partly resemble the changes seen in gargoylism.

The mucopolysaccharides found in our patients are not quite identical with those found in patients with Morquio-Ullrich's disease (Clausen, Dyggve, and Melchior, 1963; Zellweger *et al.*, 1961), but since few quantitative and qualitative studies into the excretion of acid mucopolysaccharides in Morquio-Brailsford's disease and Morquio-Ullrich's disease have been published, the importance of this finding cannot be assessed. Increased urinary excretion of acid mucopolysaccharides is a non-specific mesenchymal reaction (Hauss, Junge-Hülsing, and König, 1962), but when it is associated with an accumulation of acid mucopolysaccharides in the bone tissue, as in one of our patients, it must be presumed that the disease is due to an inborn error of metabolism as in gargoylism and Morquio-Ullrich's disease.

Robinow (1958) states that the heredity in osteochondrodystrophy may be autosomal recessive or autosomal dominant, and that these two forms of heredity represent two different diseases. Looking at the clinical symptoms alone the pattern of disease in our family implies an autosomal dominant inheritance, but if we take the pathological excretion of acid mucopolysaccharides into consideration the pattern implies a recessive autosomal inheritance with the mother and the normal daughter as carriers. This latter conclusion seems not unjustified; a recessive autosomal inheritance would provide a link with gargoylism and with Morquio-Ullrich's disease.

## Summary

A family with increased urinary excretion of acid mucopolysaccharides is described. In two of the cases radiological changes in the spine were found, like those of Morquio-Brailsford's disease, though the clinical appearances of the patients are normal. Bone biopsy from one of the two patients showed increased content of acid mucopolysaccharides. It is concluded that even mild forms of Morquio-Brailsford's disease are due to an inborn error of metabolism as in Morquio-Ullrich's disease and gargoylism.

## References

Andersen, T. (1937). Et tilfælde af typisk chondrodystrofi. *Ugeskr. Laeg.*, **99**, 169.

Brailsford, J. F. (1929). Chondro-osteo-dystrophy. *Amer. J. Surg.*, 7, 404.

—— (1948). *The Radiology of Bones and Joints.* Churchill, London.

Clausen, J., Dyggve, H. V., and Melchior, J. C. (1963). Mucopolysaccharidosis. Paper electrophoretic and infra-red analysis of the urine in gargoylism and Morquio-Ullrich's disease. *Arch. Dis. Childh.*, **38**, 364.

Crawford, T. (1939). A case of Morquio's disease. *ibid.*, **14**, 70.

Dyggve, H. V., Melchior, J. C., and Clausen, J. (1962). Morquio-Ullrich's disease. An inborn error of metabolism? *ibid.*, **37**, 525.

Eichenberger, K. (1954). Kann die Dysostosis Morquio als selbständiges Krankheitsbild vom Gargoylismus abgetrennt werden? *Ann. paediat.* (*Basel*), **182**, 107.

Einhorn, N. H., Moore, J. R., Ostrum, H. W., and Rowntree, L. G. (1941). Osteochondrodystrophia deformans (Morquio's disease). *Amer. J. Dis. Child.*, **61**, 776.

——, ——, and Rowntree, L. G. (1946). Osteochondrodystrophia deformans (Morquio's disease). *ibid.*, **72**, 536.

Guldager, A. (1945). Osteochondrodystrophia deformans. Silfverskiöld-Morquio's sygdom. *Ugeskr. Laeg.*, **107**, 327.

Hauss, W. H., Junge-Hülsing, G., and König, F. (1962). Über das Vorkommen von Veränderungen des Mucopolysaccharidstoffwechsels in der Klinik. 1. Klinische Beobachtungen zur unspezifischen Mesenchymreaktion. *Med. Welt* (*Berl.*), **2**, 2371.

Morquio, L. (1929). Sur une forme de dystrophie osseuse familiale. *Arch. Méd. Enf.*, **32**, 129.

Robinow, M. (1958). Morquio's disease. *Clin. Orthop.*, **11**, 138.

Shelling, D. H. (1957). Osteochondrodystrophia deformans. In Brenneman's *Practice of Pediatrics*, Vol. 4, Chap. 29. Prior, Hagerstown, Maryland.

Silfverskiöld, N. (1926). Sur la question de l'achondroplasie atypique et de sa forme périphérique. *Acta radiol.* (*Stockh.*), **5**, 223.

Whiteside, J. D., and Cholmeley, J. A. (1952). Morquio's disease. A review of the literature with a description of four cases. *Arch. Dis. Childh.*, **27**, 487.

Wiedemann, H.-R. (1954). Ausgedehnte und allgemeine erblich bedingte Bildungs- und Wachstumsfehler. *Mschr. Kinderheilk.*, **102**, 136.

Zellweger, H., Ponseti, I. V., Pedrini, V., Stamler, F. S., and von Noorden, G. K. (1961). Morquio-Ullrich's disease. *J. Pediat.*, **59**, 549.

## Editorial Notice

In March 1965 the Australian Paediatric Association will begin publication of a quarterly journal entitled *Australian Paediatric Journal.*

The members of the Publication Board of the journal are Stanley Bellmaine (New South Wales), John Rendle-Short (Queensland), Peter Masters (Western Australia), John Alexander (Secretary, Australian Paediatric Association), Norman Wettenhall (Victoria), Eric Sims (South Australia), and Robert Wall (Tasmania).

The members of the Editorial Committee are Charlotte M. Anderson, Peter G. Jones, Howard E. Williams, and Bernard W. Neal.

The Editorial Committee of the *Archives of Disease in Childhood* extend a warm welcome to the new journal and wish the Australian Paediatric Association, the Publication Board, and the Editors every success in their new venture.

# BOOK REVIEWS

**A Handbook on Diseases of Children Including Dietetics and the Common Fevers.** 9th ed. By BRUCE WILLIAMSON and R. M. MAYON-WHITE. (Pp. xi + 524; 133 figures + tables. 42s.) Edinburgh and London: Livingstone. 1964.

It is difficult to say when a 'handbook' becomes a 'textbook', but though this one still only measures about 7 by 5 inches, the increase of material through the addition of Dr. Mayon-White to the authorship has almost brought about this metamorphosis.

The 524 pages are closely packed with information the range of which equals most of the other commonly used small textbooks on this subject, yet the style remains a somewhat discursive one and the book is in no way a 'synopsis'. In the past it has been relatively popular with medical students because its size seemed to promise a rapid grasp of the subject without involving too much hard work; this may always have been a delusion and it is even more likely to be one now.

This is the first new edition for six years, but the changes in the text are clearly attributable more to Dr. Mayon-White's reappraisal than to any advances in paediatrics which have taken place in this time. Perhaps because it has only been partially rewritten the book leaves an impression of lack of balance, with much space given to subjects that seem to merit only a few paragraphs while others of more importance are dismissed too quickly. Compare, for instance, the detailed section of 12 pages in small print on food values with the single page on dwarfism and the causes of growth failure, which reads as if it must have remained unchanged since the first edition of 1933.

The introductory chapter setting out figures for changes in mortality rates and causes of death in the past decade is most valuable, and it is unfortunate that this standard is not consistently maintained throughout. There are too many statements which are out of tune with generally accepted current views and which may, therefore, be misleading to the undergraduate reader. Examples of this are the reference to use of the umbilical vein for injection of respiratory stimulants like nikethamide, the assertion that 75% of cyanotic congenital heart disease is Fallot's tetralogy, the inadequate paragraph on 'septal defects' which makes no distinction between atrial and ventricular ones, the mention of Eisenmenger's complex as a separate anatomical malformation, and the revival of the myth of 'the adenoid facies' by an illustration. The indications for exchange transfusion in haemolytic disease of the newborn are not given clearly and it is implied that the umbilical vein may not be used after the second day. Are daily haemoglobin estimations necessary for the first week after transfusion? Is it really true that infant mortality in breast-fed babies is still much below that of the artificially fed in this country?

While passages such as these are open to criticism, much of the rest of the book is excellent and has been greatly improved in this most recent edition. The sections on acute infections of the respiratory tract, the description of the common fevers, and the early diagnosis of congenital dislocation of the hip joints are especially worthy of praise. There is a good appendix on the subject of practical procedures and a useful drug dosage table.

Illustrations are plentiful though some are too small to make their point clear, and the volume is well produced.

It seems fair comment to say that since this is really no longer a short cut to learning paediatrics, the book now has to compete with several other possible choices for the medical student's reading. It has some way to go in future editions before it comes near to leading the field.

**Die Pflege des gesunden und des kranken Kindes. Zugleich ein Lehrbuch der Ausbildung, zur Säuglings-und Kinderkrankenschwester.** By WERNER CATEL. (Pp. xxiv + 702; 353 figures + 11 tables. DM.42.) Stuttgart: Georg Thieme. 1964.

This book is magnificent. Dare one use the word 'colossal'? 700 pages (all glossy) on paediatric nursing. How the Germans can produce a book of this quality for roughly £3 10s. 0d. is a mystery. There are 353 photographs—the black and white ones good, the coloured often indifferent. As this is the eighth edition since 1939 this book clearly is the standard text, and rightly so. Its scope is astonishing. Not only is the nursing care of the healthy and the ill child covered, but there are also clearly written chapters on anatomy and physiology, genetics, diseases of childhood, a chapter on surgical emergencies and aftercare, chapters on anaesthesia, pharmacology, and dietetics, and even a chapter on legal questions as they apply to mother and child.

This is a splendid book and no major criticism is called for. There are, however, a number of minor points and omissions which, one hopes, will be corrected in the next edition. Does anyone still use a woollen truss to control an inguinal hernia? Why three photographs showing the strapping of an umbilical hernia when the author has already agreed that these hernias disappear spontaneously? Why five pages on counter-irritants and poultices—in 1964? Don't the Germans use hyaluronidase or scalp vein needles? Do they really still administer oxygen by funnel? Do they really use that Heath Robinson contraption on p. 515 when a modern aerosol dispenser is described on p. 516? Why an ulcer diet but no mention of phenylketonuria? Is the 'standard' artificial feed of German babies really half milk, half pap, and 5% sugar merely because Czerny described Milchnährschaden in 1919? Can German babies really not digest an egg-yolk before 6 months, nor meat before 10 months? How odd! Why no mention of mother regard and the social smile? And why ever no mention of the fact that children in hospital like to be visited by their parents? One last, rather snide remark: in the section dealing with the nurse's duties when a child has died, why no mention of the correct procedure when the child was Jewish?

**Paediatric Nursing Procedures.** By R. M. SACHARIN and M. H. S. HUNTER. (Pp. viii + 299; 85 figures + 3 tables. 30s.) Edinburgh and London: Livingstone. 1964.

*Paediatric Nursing Procedures* covers the whole range of work encountered by the nurse working in a paediatric ward. The information is thoughtfully explained and systematically covered with a realistic approach.

Illustrations and diagrams give a clear picture where words are inadequate. The simplest procedures, which may yet be understood with difficulty by the student, are included.

The inclusion of dietetics and simple explanations of drug dosages are of value, especially when these subjects are mostly dealt with by a special department. Equipment and methods used may not be universal, but the basic reasons for their use give adequate guidance to any nurse, student, or otherwise. We look forward to adding this book to our shelves, and we especially value the references at the end of each chapter, many of them being to the *Nursing Times* and other nursing periodicals.

**The Surgery of Childhood for Nurses.** 2nd ed. By RAYMOND FARROW and DUNCAN FORREST. (Pp. xi + 292; 146 figures. 32s. 6d.) Edinburgh and London: E. and S. Livingstone. 1964.

A second edition of this book is welcome at a time when the rapid advance in paediatric surgery can only succeed with the help of the well-trained paediatric nurse. Extensive revision has eliminated many faults of the first edition but the chapters on general topics are still not quite so successful as those on specific disorders. The conversational style and attempts to simplify tend sometimes to result in verbosity and even ambiguity. In the important new chapter on neonatal surgery, measurement of blood loss 'by colour' presumably means haemoglobin estimation, a term with which every reader of this book is surely familiar.

Valuable new sections on intestinal obstruction, cardiac surgery, and locomotor disorders concisely cover an adequate range of conditions, and the very high standard of illustration is maintained. More practical guidance on details of nursing care might profitably be included in the next edition, especially where the nurse might expect to benefit from these authors' special experience, e.g. the pre-operative care of the membranous sac in exomphalos and meningomyelocele.

Despite these criticisms the authors have fulfilled their stated intention, 'to direct the nurse's attention to the fundamental features of those surgical conditions of childhood with which she will most commonly deal' and the very good printing and general lay-out add greatly to the attraction of this book.

*Arch. Dis. Childh.*, 1965, **40**, 113.



# REVIEW ARTICLE

## THE UNDESCENDED TESTIS

BY

J. H. JOHNSTON

*From Alder Hey Children's Hospital and the Department of Child Health, University of Liverpool*

(RECEIVED FOR PUBLICATION NOVEMBER 20, 1964)

There can be few subjects in surgery where the published material contains so many divergent and even directly contradictory statements and expressions of opinion as that of the undescended testis and its management. The reasons lie in our incomplete knowledge of some of the very fundamentals of the matter. We are well informed concerning the anatomy of cryptorchidism and the effects of persisting undescent on testicular structure and function, but we know little about the late results of treatment, and much of the available information relating to the natural history of the condition and the frequency of complications is suspect since it is the outcome, not of the observation of boys and men with undescended testes, but of deductions made from the numbers of such individuals occurring in statistical surveys of the general population and of series of patients with testicular diseases. Moreover, throughout large areas of this sea of only indirectly relevant figures swim the twin red herrings, observer error and the retractile testis.

### Anatomy

The first comprehensive account of the surgical anatomy of testicular retention was that of Sir Denis Browne (1938), and most of the views expressed in his classic article concerning the types of undescent, their clinical and operative features, and their prognostic implications are now universally accepted. Browne classified the retained testis into the *truly undescended* or *incompletely descended* organ which halts somewhere along its normal route of descent, and the *ectopic* or *maldescended* testis which, having traversed the inguinal canal, is diverted from its course to an abnormal position. The incompletely descended variety is further subdivided, according to the lower extremity of its range of movement, into *abdominal*, *inguinal* or *canalicular*, and *emergent* types, the last two and sometimes also the first being associated with a patent processus vaginalis which often extends considerably further towards the scrotal fundus than does the testis. The ectopic testis, with which a complete hernial sac is rare, may occupy a *pubic*, *penile*, *femoral*, *perineal* or, most commonly, *superficial inguinal* position, in which it is contained in the *superficial inguinal pouch*, a recess lying between the fascia of Scarpa and the external oblique aponeurosis, lateral to the superficial inguinal ring.

Browne also drew attention to the phenomenon of testicular retraction or pseudocryptorchidism, that important variant of the normal in which the testes of small boys may be elevated by the brisk cremasteric contractions of childhood to reside for lengthy periods in the groin. In the great majority of cases the testis retracts, as Browne described, into the superficial inguinal pouch, but on occasion it moves to an impalpable position within the inguinal canal, apparently because the inguinal ring is, in such instances, of sufficient size to allow its passage whereas ordinarily it is not. The retracted testis can readily be manipulated to the bottom of the scrotum where, after puberty, it will reside permanently and function normally but, particularly in fat boys, it is not infrequently mistaken by the inexperienced observer for true cryptorchidism. This error remains the bugbear of large clinical surveys and invalidates much of the statistics relating to the incidence of testicular undescent during childhood, the frequency of late spontaneous descent, and the response to non-operative therapy.

The unilateral undescended testis is, at all stages of its development, smaller than its normally sited fellow, though, as Williams (1958) points out, the discrepancy may be apparent only when the two testes are viewed side by side. When the processus vaginalis is patent, the testis and its vessels are suspended within it by a peritoneal mesentery and the Wolffian derivatives are usually abnormally disposed. The epididymis may be widely separated from the testis and its globus minor may be elongated towards the scrotum. Not infrequently the vas and its accompanying artery extend to the fundus of the hernial sac and then loop back to the incompletely descended epididymis. On occasion the abnormalities are more gross: Badenoch (1946) recorded 3 cases of testicular undescent in which the epididymis was malformed and the vasa efferentia absent on histological scrutiny, and Devens (1964) described 2 cases where the vas deferens was atretic proximal to the epididymis. Such interruptions of ductal continuity may readily remain undetected at orchidopexy; it is likely that they are more common than would appear from the numbers recorded, and they may contribute significantly to the incidence of infertility associated with testicular retention.

As the development of the testis and its ductal system is closely associated with that of the urinary tract, urological malformations might be expected to occur frequently in cases of testicular undescent. Abdominally retained testes form part of the 'prune belly' syndrome of deficient abdominal musculature and bilateral megaureters, but, apart from this constant association, the over-all incidence of urinary tract abnormalities is unknown since, in most centres, few patients with undescended testes have undergone urological investigation in the absence of suggestive symptoms. Felton (1959), however, performed intravenous urography in 61 unselected cryptorchids and found major abnormalities of the urinary tract to be present in 8 of them. This is a considerably greater proportion than would be expected, from post-mortem statistics, to occur by chance, and Felton's findings support his contention that a larger scale investigation of the subject is warranted.

**Embryology**

The intra-abdominal position of the foetal testis was known to Galen (Frankl, 1895), but it was von Haller (1755) and John Hunter (1762) who drew attention to the descent of the testis during late intrauterine life and who recognized and described the gubernaculum as a fibromuscular cord connecting the testis to the scrotum. While the precise role played by the gubernaculum during testicular descent remains uncertain, the present concept of its structure and mode of action is that of an undifferentiated mesenchymal band (Backhouse and Butler, 1960) which prepares the way for the testis and guides it to its destination, rather than, as was formerly thought (Eberth, 1904), a smooth muscle which by its contraction and retraction pulls the testis to the scrotum. Embryological anatomical studies and animal experiments suggest that the descent of the testis is controlled by its own production of testosterone under the influence of gonadotrophins of chorionic and possibly of foetal pituitary origin. In the female foetus the gubernaculum develops as in the male until the gonad differentiates to an ovary (Backhouse, 1964); Rost (1933) prevented testicular descent in rodents by hypophysectomy and Raynaud (1958) and Backhouse (1964) caused the cessation of gubernacular development by the administration of oestrogen to developing male animals *in utero*.

Since our knowledge of the normal mechanism of testicular descent is scanty, it is not surprising that our comprehension of the pathogenesis of non-descent is also limited. Testicular retention has been attributed to prenatal hormonal imbalance (Lombard, 1934), but such influences are likely to be significant only in bilateral cases with other evidence of endocrinopathy. With the great majority of undescended testes the descensive stimulus must be regarded as normal, but the testis fails to descend completely either because of an intrinsic fault that prevents its response or because of some anatomical hindrance to its movement. The former concept originated with Hunter (1762) who, noting the small size of the undescended organ, stated that he was inclined to suspect that the reason for its undescent lay in the testis itself. Later histological studies have shown that primarily and irreversibly abnormal testes do exist (Sohval, 1954; Charny and Wolgin, 1957), but operative results (Gross and Jewett, 1956) suggest that they form only a small proportion of all retained testes. Some of the mechanical factors described as causative of incomplete descent, such as inadequate length of the spermatic vessels (Büdinger, 1907) or of the vas deferens (Basilico, 1950), or an insufficiently large inguinal canal (Campbell, 1951), or superficial inguinal ring (Wells and State, 1947) are obviously as likely to be the result as the cause of the condition. In those not uncommon instances where the epididymis or the vas deferens is elongated beyond the level of the testis, Scorer (1962) found abnormalities in the proximal gubernacular insertion and considered that this faulty attachment caused the Wolffian structures rather than the testis to migrate towards the scrotum. An ectopic position of the testis was thought by Lockwood (1888) to be the result of the organ following one of four secondary distal gubernacular attachments to the pubic, perineal, femoral, or inguinal regions instead of the main one leading to the scrotal terminus. Others (Sonneland, 1924; McGregor, 1929) have failed, on dissections, to find the gubernacular tails of Lockwood, but Backhouse (1964) described fibrous encroachment on the gubernaculum, which may similarly divert it partly and the testis entirely from the scrotum. McGregor (1929) and Scorer (1962) thought that a fascial barrier at the scrotal entrance constituted an obstruction to descent and was the factor responsible for the testis assuming a pubic or superficial inguinal position. There is no doubt of the existence of this barrier, as it is invariably encountered at operation in the case of the superficial inguinal ectopic testis, but again it is impossible to determine whether it is the cause or the result of the abnormal testicular situation.

Genetic influences appear, at least in certain instances, to be of importance in the aetiology of cryptorchidism. The occurrence of undescended testes in brothers is not uncommon: Corbus and O'Conor (1922) described a family in which six were affected. Examples of hereditary cryptorchidism, affecting father and sons, were recorded by Caucci (1951) and by Charny and Wolgin (1957), and testicular undescent in three generations was described by Wiles (1934).

Comparative anatomical studies suggest that incompletely descended and ectopic situations of the testis may have an atavistic significance since they have counterparts in lower animals (Wakeley, 1953). In the otter and the camel the testes are inguinal, in swine and wild boars they are perineal, and in the kangaroo they occupy a pubo-penile position. The most interesting but unanswered question is the teleological one of why the testes of man and some of his fellow mammals descend at all. It is inconceivable that a vulnerable external position confers any advantage as regards individual or species survival. Badenoch (1945) saw an analogy with the migration of certain fishes and birds to cooler climes for breeding and thought that the testes descend in search of a lower temperature. It seems more reasonable, however, to regard the thermal influence on the testis as an adaptation to, rather than the cause of its descent; in some mammals, for example the elephant and the whale, the testes remain permanently inside the abdomen without loss of fertility.

### The Natural History of Testicular Undescent: Late Spontaneous Descent

Many testes that are undescended at birth reach the scrotum during the first few months of life. Scorer (1956, 1957) examined 2,700 newborn boys and found that in 108 (4%) of them one or both testes had failed to descend; as would be expected, the incidence of undescent was much higher in premature (30·3%) than in full-term (3·4%) babies. In 60 (58%) of the affected infants the testes were fully descended at the age of 1 month and in 89 (82%) they were in the scrotum within one year of birth. Later observations (Scorer, 1964) revealed that if descent occurred within six weeks of birth in a full-term infant or within three months in a premature, an anatomically normal testis resulted. With later descent, the testis failed to reach the bottom of the scrotum and remained smaller than a normal fellow on the opposite side.

There has been considerable disagreement as to the incidence of spontaneous descent during later childhood and adolescence. Some observers (Bevan, 1929; Turner, 1937; Scorer, 1957) have regarded descent after infancy as being extremely rare while others (Johnson, 1939; Smith, 1941) have considered that a very high proportion of undescended testes reach the scrotum at puberty. The opinion of further authors has lain between these extremes. Hunter (1762), awaiting the appropriate moment to apply a truss to the accompanying inguinal hernia, found that testicular descent occurred frequently between the ages of 2 and 10 years; it is likely, however, that the enlarging hernia was the descensive agent in these cases. Gross and Jewett (1956) believed that spontaneous descent was possible up to the age of 9 or 10 years, and Browne (1938) was of the opinion that the high retractile testis, which has a range of movement extending from the superficial inguinal pouch to the upper scrotum, took up a scrotal position at puberty.

The results of clinical surveys relating to the frequency of occurrence of cryptorchidism before and after puberty appear, from the reported differences between the two age-groups, to support the conclusion that spontaneous pubertal descent is extremely common. Drake (1934) found the incidence of testicular undescent in pre-pubertal as compared with post-pubertal males to be in the proportion of 4·2% : 0·76%, and the comparable figures recorded by McCutcheon (1938), by the Society of Medical Officers of Health, East Anglian Branch (1958), and by Ward and Hunter (1960) in their two series were 9·4% : 0·8%, 6% : 0·7%, 5·2% : 0·4%, and 4·1% : 0·23%. The authors of the series in which several observers were involved confess, however, to diagnostic difficulties and to wide variations in the clinical findings of the different examiners, and there can be little doubt that there was lack of recognition of the retractile testis in pre-pubertal boys so that the figures obtained are invalid in respect of true cryptorchidism.

The present majority view and the basis of the modern management of testicular retention is that an undescended testis will, because of its increased bulk and because of diminished cremasteric activity, take up at puberty the lowest position in its range of movement, but that spontaneous complete descent after infancy is very uncommon and, if it does occur, the testis will have suffered degenerative changes proportionate in their severity to its delay in reaching the scrotum. Late spontaneous testicular descent is, therefore, neither to be expected nor desired.

**The Effect of Testicular Undescent: Spermatogenic Insufficiency**

In cases of unilateral undescent, the descended testis is, in the majority of cases, a normally functioning organ, and the fertility and the endocrine status of the patient are assured. Hansen (1949) estimated that such men produce, on the average, only about half as many spermatozoa as normal men, but Charny and Wolgin (1957) and McLeod (personal communication to Charny and Wolgin, 1957) found the incidence of unilateral cryptorchids in their series of infertile males to approximate to that in the general population. The untreated bilateral cryptorchid on the other hand, though he achieves normal maturity as regards sexual potency and the development of secondary male characteristics in spite of a subnormal androgen excretion (Engberg, 1949), will almost certainly be sterile. Since Hunter's (1762) original observations, there has been conjecture as to whether the spermatogenic insufficiency of the retained testis is due to an inherent and irreversible inadequacy or dysgenesis, or is the result of a potentially normal organ being adversely affected by an inimical environment. In recent years, both this question, which is of obvious therapeutic importance, and also that of the effects of undescent on the structure of the testis, have been extensively investigated by the microscopic examination of testicular specimens and biopsies. Histologists are unanimous that the tubules of the retained testis degenerate rapidly at and after puberty but, apart from this, their opinions on the subject of testicular undescent unfortunately vary almost as widely as those of clinicians. Sniffen (1952) could detect little or no difference between the undescended and the normal testis before puberty. Robinson and Engle (1954), on the other hand, concluded that the unilateral undescended testis was rarely completely normal, as compared with its fellow, at any age, but that the changes became more obvious after the age of 5 years. Cooper (1929) and Nelson (1951) were of similar opinion but put the age at which the undescended testis begins to lag behind at 3 years and at 6 to 7 years, respectively. Sohval (1954) recorded that over one-half of the undescended testes he examined showed evidence of primary maldevelopment or dysgenesis, but de la Balze, Mancini, Arrillaga, Andrada, Vilar, Gurtman, and Davidson (1960) thought that the degenerative changes they observed were due solely to the abnormal position of the testis. Charny and Wolgin (1957) stated that dysgenesis, which they considered to be evident in early childhood and to be characterized mainly by tubules that were smaller than normal and filled with undifferentiated cells, occurred in 20% of their cases. In the remaining 80% they found that histological abnormalities were detectable only after the age of 10 years, at which age the testis normally begins to mature under the influence of pituitary gonadotrophins. The initial tubular changes described are those of delayed development, but subsequently cellular retrogression and peritubular fibrosis are observed so that when puberty is well established only Sertoli cells remain. In the adult, the tubules may become fibrotic and hyalinized. At all ages the Leydig cells remain intact and, with the shrinkage of the tubules, they often appear prominent and give an impression of an increase in their number.

It is not possible to reconcile the differing histological views that exist concerning the age at which tubular degenerative changes commence in the undescended testis, but the satisfactory results that can follow orchidopexy in bilateral cases (MacCollum, 1935; Gross and Jewett, 1956) support the views of de la Balze *et al.* (1960) and of Charny and Wolgin (1957) that the majority of undescended testes are not dysgenetic but of normal, or at least functionally adequate, spermatogenic potential.

The testis is capable of normal spermatogenesis only within a relatively small environmental temperature range which is regulated by the dartos and cremasteric musculature, and it is generally accepted that, when the testis is undescended, the deterrent to structural and functional development is the abnormally high temperature to which it is exposed. Badenoch (1945) found the average difference between the intra-abdominal and intrascrotal temperatures in man to be 2·2° C. In animal experiments, Moore (1924), Moore and Quick (1924), and Moore and Oslund (1924) noted the occurrence of degenerative changes in a testis that was replaced within the abdomen or, alternatively, was warmed by the application of external heat, and found also that the changes could be reversed when thermal normality was restored. Acquired testicular retention during childhood, as may occur when a normal testis becomes adherent to an inguinal herniotomy scar, produces a similar structural deterioration (Williams, 1958). McLeod and Hotchkiss (1941) raised the body and environmental temperatures for some hours in human volunteers and recorded a pronounced decrease in the production of spermatozoa, which began three weeks later and lasted for about seven weeks.

Little information is available concerning the correlation between the position of an undescended testis and its developmental potential. Southam and Cooper (1927) stated that the more fully descended the testis, the more it approached normal size, but Charny and Wolgin (1957) found that the degree of histological degeneration varied with the age rather than with the site of the testis. It is common clinical and operative experience that the superficial inguinal ectopic testis approximates more nearly to the normal as regards size and consistency than the testis that is emergent or that lies in the inguinal canal or higher, and Mack, Scott, Ferguson-Smith, and Lennox (1961) found that while germ cell defects appeared histologically in both types, they were more marked in the true undescended organ than in the ectopic one. This observation may be related to the smaller temperature differential involved in the latter case; Badenoch (1945) found the difference between the scrotum and the inguinal region to average 0·8 °C.

## Complications

**Inguinal Hernia.** In the majority of cases of true testicular undescent, as distinct from testicular ectopia, there is a patent processus vaginalis, but very often the sac is too narrow to allow the entry of abdominal viscera. A clinical hernia is therefore the exception rather than the rule; when it does occur it usually appears in the first year or two of life.

**Psychological Effects.** Unless parental anxiety is transmitted to the child, a pre-pubertal boy is rarely worried about, or even interested in, the position of his testicles. In the adult, however, cryptorchidism, even if unilateral, can on occasion lead to emotional disturbances by inducing feelings of sexual inadequacy and inferiority (Snyder and Greaney, 1962).

**Trauma.** The testis that lies in a superficial inguinal or pubic position is commonly stated to be more liable to and more susceptible to the effects of external trauma than the normally-sited organ which is cushioned by its mobility in the scrotum. While this hazard is probably significant in certain occupations in the adult, one cannot recollect a child cryptorchid complaining of it. A canalicular or emergent testis may, however, be traumatized by abdominal muscular activity, and it is possible that this is responsible for the local pain that is occasionally associated with testicular undescent. The perineal ectopic testis is likely to be injured when a sitting posture is assumed and for this reason its early placement in the scrotum is indicated.

**Torsion.** Because of its usually abnormal mesorchial attachments the undescended testis is more prone to undergo torsion than the normally-sited organ, but the incidence of the complication appears, from the available statistics, to have lessened appreciably in recent years. The collected series of O'Conor (1919), Wallenstein (1929), and Abeshouse (1936) totalled 430 cases of testicular torsion of which 234 (54%) involved a retained testis. In only 5 of Smith's (1957) 31 cases, 7 of Jones's (1962) 55 cases, and 3 of Barker and Raper's (1964) 38 cases of torsion, however, was an undescended testis affected, while of 65 testicular torsions admitted to Alder Hey Hospital in the past 10 years, 15 were in undescended testes, and 9 of these occurred in children under the age of 1 year. Since these figures are not matched against the numbers of undescended testes in the same series of cases they are no more than presumptive evidence of a diminished incidence of torsion in association with testicular retention, but it is likely that the greater numbers of orchidopexy operations performed now as compared with former years have indeed reduced the over-all frequency of the complication and led to it occurring most commonly in early childhood.

**Malignancy.** Testicular malignancy during childhood is an extremely rare disease and its occurrence in an undescended organ is even more rare. Gordon-Taylor and Wyndham (1947) recorded an example in a boy of 5 months who developed a malignant tumour in a retained testis, but in each of the 26 cases of malignancy of the testis in boys reviewed by Doyle (1955) a scrotal testis was affected. In the adult, on the other hand, there can be no doubt from the recorded data that the undescended testis has a greater liability to malignant change than has the normally-situated organ. Gilbert and Hamilton (1940) found 11% of 7,000 testicular tumours to be associated with undescent and in the series of Hinman (1924), Dean (1935), Gordon-Taylor and Wyndham (1947), and Collins and Pugh (1964) the incidence was 12·2% of 649 cases, 14·3% of 292 cases, 11·8% of 629 cases, and 5·9% of 995 cases, respectively. The undescended testis has been estimated to be up to 50 times as likely as a scrotal testis to develop a malignant tumour, with the intra-abdominal testis at greatest risk (Rea, 1939). The bilateral cryptorchid is particularly unfortunate; if he develops a tumour in one testis, the chance of malignancy occurring in the other is 1 in 4 (Gilbert and Hamilton, 1940).

While testicular undescent increases the likelihood of a tumour forming, it does not hasten its development. The average age of onset is, in fact, some years later in the undescended as compared with the scrotal testis; the latter undergoes malignant change most frequently between the ages of 35 and 39 years (Gilbert and Hamilton, 1940).

The retained testis may be affected by any of the pathological types of testicular tumour, but in the series of Gilbert and Hamilton (1940) and in that of Collins and Pugh (1964) the teratoma was relatively less common and the seminoma relatively more common in the undescended than in the scrotal organ.

We do not know if the performance of orchidopexy lessens the risk of testicular malignancy developing but the operation does not prevent its occurrence. Gilbert and Hamilton's (1940) series contained 77 examples of tumour following orchidopexy and nearly one-quarter of Collins and Pugh's (1964) 58 patients with neoplasm associated with undescent had previously undergone operation. The time interval between orchidopexy and the onset of malignancy has varied from 3 months (Gordon-Taylor and Wyndham, 1947) to 29 years (Sumner, 1959). The development of a tumour shortly after operation suggests the possibility of there being a causal traumatic relationship, and Coley (1919) believed that trauma was a most important factor in the causation of tumour in the retained testis. This hypothesis appears, however, to be invalidated by the fact that the well-protected abdominal testis carries the highest incidence of malignancy.

The failure of orchidopexy to prevent tumour formation indicates that the factor that is carcinogenic to the undescended testis is not merely its abnormal position. Sohval (1956) found undifferentiated seminiferous tubules, similar to those he encountered in undescended testes, to be often present in scrotal testes affected by both seminomata and teratomata, and concluded that the same congenital defect which contributed to undescent of a testis also rendered it more prone to tumour development. The complexity of the relation between cryptorchidism and malignancy is demonstrated by the not infrequent occurrence, in series of testicular neoplasm associated with unilateral undescent, of the tumour arising in the scrotal testis and not in the undescended one. This was the case in 23 of 840 testicular tumours associated with undescent in the series of Gilbert and Hamilton (1940) and in no less than 9 of 58 cases in the series of Collins and Pugh (1964). The figures suggest that the coincidence of scrotal testicular neoplasm and contralateral undescent is unlikely to be purely fortuitous, but the implications of the combination as regards the pathogenesis of the tumour can only be guessed at.

The survival rates for men with testicular tumours are considerably less when undescended than when scrotal testes are affected (Gilbert and Hamilton, 1940), and it is often stated that orchidopexy, while it does not prevent malignancy, is nevertheless of benefit in that it permits an earlier diagnosis if and when a neoplasm develops. Prompt diagnosis may be an advantage if the tumour is a seminoma which, with modern therapy, has a 79% 5-year survival rate when a scrotal testis is affected (Pugh and Cameron, 1964), but if it is a teratoma or a combined tumour, which have a 4-year survival rate of only 36% and 43% respectively (Pugh and Cameron, 1964), early diagnosis obviously does not necessarily infer a good prognosis. A particular hazard of testicular malignancy after orchidopexy is that the tumour may metastasize to the inguinal lymph glands (Witus, Sloss, and Valk, 1959).

The increased liability of the undescended testis to neoplasia, the failure of orchidopexy to prevent it, and the rather poor outlook for the patient if a mixed or teratomatous tumour develops, appear at first sight to indicate the need for the wholesale removal of undescended testes. It must be remembered, however, that the statistics relating to the association of malignancy and cryptorchidism have been obtained from the study of cases of testicular tumour and not from the observation of individuals with undescended testes, and the most important statistical detail, i.e. the incidence of tumour formation in cryptorchid males, treated or untreated, consequently remains unknown.

Gross and Jewett (1956) were sceptical of the conclusions that have been drawn from the statistics and were of the opinion that the available figures did not justify any stronger statement than that an undescended testis might possibly be more prone to malignancy than a normal one. Carroll (1949), never having encountered a malignant undescended testis, also questioned the validity of the figures and circulated fellow urologists concerning their experiences. From the 662 replies received he concluded that the incidence of malignancy in cryptorchids was so minute that the potential of an undescended testis for neoplastic change could not be used as an indication either for orchidopexy or orchidectomy.

Tumour of the testis, retained or scrotal, is a rare condition. The recorded frequency of the disease in different communities in England and the United States ranges from 2·1 to 2·3 cases per 100,000 males per annum (Collins and Pugh, 1964), and testicular neoplasm is responsible for only 1 of 15,000 annual male deaths from all malignant tumours (Kark, 1962). It follows that even if the undescended testis is accepted to have a much greater liability to malignancy than the normal, the chance of a cryptorchid male developing a testicular tumour is still small. The undescended testis cannot, therefore, be regarded as a pre-cancerous lesion, and orchidectomy solely with the object of preventing tumour formation is unjustified.

**Treatment**

The child with bilateral cryptorchidism is threatened with sterility as an adult and the object of therapy is to secure a scrotal position of the testes at a sufficiently early age to allow them to reach their maximal functional potential. When only one testis is undescended, the fertility of the patient is, in the majority of cases, already assured and the possibility of complications arising then assumes greater importance. The most serious of these, malignant degeneration, can, however, be prevented only by orchidectomy and the risk of its development is not sufficiently great to warrant this measure. The other complications, psychic as well as physical, can be averted by obtaining a scrotally situated testis and it is logical, as an insurance against possible subsequent disease of or injury to the normal organ, that this, as in the bilateral case, should be achieved at such an age as to permit normal testicular development.

**Hormone Treatment.** The use of gonadotrophin in the management of testicular undescent was introduced by Schapiro in 1931 and for some years hormone was administered enthusiastically, extravagant claims being made for its efficacy. In a collected survey of 579 reported cases, Thompson and Heckel (1938) noted that hormone therapy was stated to have been successful in inducing testicular descent in 65% of bilateral and 47% of unilateral cases. Later, it became apparent that the selection of patients had been indiscriminate and Rea (1940) concluded that the good results reported were largely due to the inclusion, in those treated, of boys with retractile testes.

Gonadotrophin may produce undesirable precocity in young boys and there have been reports of it causing damage to the testis. Maddock and Nelson (1952) and Charny and Wolgin (1957), in studies of testicular biopsies performed before and after treatment, found that tubular degeneration with impaired spermatogenesis had resulted. Robinson and Engle (1954) and Anderson, Andreassen, and Quaade (1955), on the other hand, found no such histological changes, and Brunet, de Mowbray, and Bishop (1958) believed that they occurred only when hormone was given in excessive dosage.

Except in the rare case of testicular undescent associated with pituitary insufficiency, when its use is obviously indicated, gonadotrophic hormone now plays little part in the management of cryptorchidism, either unilateral or bilateral. Williams (1958) pointed out its value as a therapeutic test in distinguishing the high retractile testis, with its potentiality for the assumption of a scrotal position at puberty, from the superficial inguinal ectopic testis which requires surgical intervention. Deming (1952) considered that a course of hormone therapy prior to operation lengthened the cord and facilitated the performance of orchidopexy, an opinion the truth of which is equally difficult to prove or to disprove.

**Orchidopexy.** The time for operative intervention is occasionally determined by the development of a complication such as testicular torsion or, more often, a hernia, but as a rule it is a matter of choice.

There is general agreement that if orchidopexy is not carried out until puberty is well advanced it is scarcely worth performing from the point of view of subsequent spermatogenesis, but opinions vary widely as to the precise age at which the operation should be recommended, because they are based mainly on divergent histological observations and beliefs. Scorer (1957) thought that the sooner the abnormality was corrected the better and advocated operation in infancy for the superficial inguinal ectopic testis. Minor (1959) believed it important to correct the abnormality before the child went to school so that he would not be subjected to the scorn and derision of his normally developed, and apparently highly observant fellows in the kindergarten jungle; he found that the cord often required less mobilization to allow full testicular descent in the younger than in the older boy. Gross and Jewett (1956), who alone amongst the holders of various opinions are in a position to support their views with post-operative functional results, recommend orchidopexy between the ages of 9 and 11 years. They accept that some histological observations suggest that operation should be undertaken earlier but believe that the technique is sufficiently easier, and therefore safer for the testis, in later childhood to warrant the delay. In bilateral cases, where it is vital to give the testes every chance of attaining normal spermatogenic function, earlier operation is advisable; Williams (1958) favours the age of 5 years. When intervention is required bilaterally it is preferable, unless orchidopexy is particularly easily accomplished, to allow an interval of several months to elapse between the operations because the result obtained from the first may modify the nature of the second.

The essential feature of orchidopexy is the dissection of the spermatic cord from its adherence to its surroundings so that it may lengthen sufficiently to allow the testis to be brought to the scrotum. Care is required during separation of gubernacular remnants below the testis to avoid injury to an elongated epididymis or a prolapsed vas deferens. When a complete hernial sac is present it must be divided immediately proximal to the testis, separated from the cord, ligated at its neck, and removed. The facility of performance of this manoeuvre, which often requires some dexterity and considerable patience, varies with the age of the patient; the younger the child the more easily does tiresome tearing of the sac occur and the more readily can damage be inflicted upon the testicular and vasal vessels. The laterally convex curve described by the intra-abdominal part of the spermatic vessels is straightened and very considerable lengthening obtained by division of the firm band of fibres, described by Browne (1933) as forming the lower end of the suspensory ligament of the testis, which radiates upwards and laterally from the cord at the deep inguinal ring. Further descension, if necessary, is achieved by division of the sharp medial edge of the deep ring and the fascia transversalis forming the posterior wall of the inguinal canal. The cord can then move medially with the result that its angulation at the deep inguinal ring is eliminated; the inferior epigastric vessels are readily displaced inwards and do not usually need to be divided. In the majority of cases these procedures are sufficient to allow the testis to come to the scrotum. If they are not, the exposure may be extended by division of the fibres forming the curved lower margins of the internal oblique and transversus muscles and, with adequate retraction, the spermatic vessels may be mobilized almost to their origin and the vas deferens to the base of the bladder. One usually finds, however, that this extensive intra-abdominal dissection achieves little more length than that obtained by the full mobilization of the cord from within the operative confines of the inguinal canal.

If, in spite of complete mobilization, the testis will not reach the scrotum it may be fixed by suture at the lowest point attained and re-explored after an interval of about one year. The second instalment of this two-stage operation is often difficult, since the testis and cord are intimately involved in scar tissue but, if the testis has been brought through the superficial ring at the first stage, it is usually possible to lengthen the cord sufficiently to allow it to descend fully.

In an important recent contribution to the technique of orchidopexy, Fowler and Stephens (1963) reaffirmed the experience of Bevan (1903) and others that the vasal vessels alone might be adequate for the vascularization of the testis, so that division of the spermatic vessels was often permissible provided it was carried out at a sufficiently high level to preserve the anastomotic communications between the two vascular supplies. Fowler and Stephens' method has its main application in those cases in which the vas and its accompanying vessels extend as a recurrent loop below a high-sited testis. Division of the short spermatic vessels and, if necessary, of one or two of the vascular arcades which cross the loop from one limb to the other, then allows the vas to be straightened and the testis to swing down to the scrotum without tension. It is, of course, important to avoid injury to the vasal vessels during separation of the hernial sac, and the adequacy of the testicular blood supply must be assured before the spermatic pedicle is finally divided by applying a light vascular clamp to the latter for some minutes and noting the persistence of arterial bleeding from an incision in the tunica albuginea.

All the eponyms applied to the operation of orchidopexy relate to its least important aspect, the fixation of the testis. It is sufficient to attach the testis to the scrotal skin with one suture, care being taken when picking up the tunica albuginena to avoid injury to one or other of the main arterial branches which are visible immediately beneath it. If the scrotum is thoroughly stretched digitally from within, dartos contraction in the early post-operative days is prevented and, since the cremasteric attachments have been removed, the testis will not recoil unless it is drawn up by the tension of the spermatic cord. Any pull on the testis by the application of elastic bands or by its fixation to the thigh is best avoided. When the testis reaches the bottom of the scrotum such traction is unnecessary, and when it does not the spermatic cord will be stretched thereby and the testicular vascularity jeopardized. It is preferable to have an adequately vascularized testis in the upper scrotum than an ischaemic one at the fundus.

When all manoeuvres and stratagems fail and the testis cannot be made to reach the scrotum, orchidectomy is indicated if the normality of the opposite organ is not in doubt; if it is, abdominal replacement of the testis should be performed so that its internal secretory function will be retained.

Certain aspects of orchidopexy, particularly the division of the posterior wall of the inguinal canal which allows the cord to come directly rather than obliquely through the abdominal wall, must destroy the normal inguinal mechanism and it is possible that, even though the fascia and musculature are carefully resutured, there remains a predisposition to the later development of a direct inguinal hernia. The writer has not, however, observed such a post-operative hernia during childhood nor has a case appeared as yet in the Liverpool Register of Inguinal Hernia, which relates to adults (A. J. Marsden, 1964, personal communication).

**Results**

Since the main object of orchidopexy is the achievement of useful spermatogenesis, the results of the operation must be judged by this criterion. A bad result, the outcome of a gross error in surgical technique, may be obvious clinically when the testis atrophies; the incidence of this complication has varied in reported series from over 50% (Aird, 1949) to 2% (Eisenstaedt, 1950: Snyder and Chaffin, 1955). Gross and Jewett (1956) stated that over 90% of orchidopexies could give a good result as assessed by the post-operative position, size, consistency, contour, and sensitivity of the testis, but Charny and Wolgin (1957) have shown that clinical excellence can coincide with functional inadequacy. The latter authors, having studied testicular biopsies before and after a modified Torek (1909) thigh fixation operation, take such a dismal view of the results achieved that they consider orchidopexy unjustified in unilateral cases and, when the condition is bilateral, only to be undertaken with little prospect of success when all else fails.

Apart from the examination of biopsies, the functional efficacy of orchidopexy can be determined only in bilateral cases by the patient's paternity and/or by his spermatozoa counts. Few series of bilateral operations have been recorded and the results obtained in these have been either extremely bad or extremely good. Hansen (1949), in whose cases the operative technique was not stated, found only 2 of 25 men to be of normal fertility. Each of Rea's (1951) 8 patients, all treated by the Torek method, was sterile. MacCollum (1935) and Gross and Jewett (1956) on the other hand, reporting the results obtained in Boston Children's Hospital, found 30 of 38 men who had undergone bilateral orchidopexy during childhood to be fertile. The Boston authors, who strongly condemned the Torek technique, did not, unfortunately state the position of the testes in their cases before operation, but their results must be regarded as approximating to the best possible, since a certain proportion of the patients can be assumed to have had intrinsically abnormal testes incapable of responding to a normal environment.

Apart from the Boston series, the present widespread popularity of orchidopexy rests much more on selected theoretical concepts than on the cold facts of late results. The anatomical classification of cryptorchidism and the optimal technique of orchidopexy, with the necessity for gentle, thorough mobilization of the cord and the avoidance of strong post-operative traction on the testis or its fixation to the thigh have, however, now been generally recognized for a sufficient number of years to encourage the hope that many series of orchidopexy results, fully classified as to the initial position and condition of the testes and their post-operative anatomical and functional status, will shortly be available. Until they are, accurate pre-operative prognostication will remain impossible and doubt will continue to exist as to whether, in many or even most instances, orchidopexy is anything more than a cosmetic operation.

REFERENCES


Abeshouse, B. S. (1936). Torsion of the spermatic cord; report of 3 cases and review of the literature. *Urol. cutan. Rev.*, **40**, 699.

Aird, I. (1949). *A Companion in Surgical Studies.* E. and S. Livingstone, Edinburgh.

Anderson, H., Andreassen, M., and Quaade, F. (1955). Testicular biopsies in cryptorchidism. *Acta endocr. (Kbh.)*, **18**, 567.

Backhouse, K. M. (1964). The gubernaculum testis Hunteri; testicular descent and maldescent. *Ann. roy. Coll. Surg. Engl.*, **35**, 15.

——, and Butler, H. (1960). The gubernaculum testis of the pig. *J. Anat. (Lond.)*, **94**, 107.

Badenoch, A. W. (1945). Descent of the testis in relation to temperature. *Brit. med. J.*, **2**, 601.

—— (1946). Failure of the urogenital union. *Surg. Gynec. Obstet.*, **82**, 471.

Barker, K. and Raper, F. P. (1964). Torsion of the testis. *Brit. J. Urol.*, **36**, 35.

Basilico, M. V. (1950). Ectopia testicular. *Bol. Soc. argent. Ciruj.* **34**, 738.

Bevan, A. D. (1903). The surgical treatment of undescended testicle: a further contribution. *J. Amer. med. Ass.*, **41**, 718.

—— (1929). The operation for undescended testis. *Ann. Surg.*, **90**, 847.

Browne, D. (1933). Some anatomical points in the operation for undescended testicle. *Lancet*, **1**, 460.

—— (1938). The diagnosis of undescended testicle. *Brit. med. J.*, **2**, 168.

Brunet, J., de Mowbray, R. R., and Bishop, P. M. F. (1958). Management of the undescended testis. *ibid.*, **1**, 1367.

Büdinger, K. (1907). Die Aetiologie der Hodenretention. *Dtsch. Z. Chir.*, **90**, 532.

Campbell, M. (1951). Undescended testicle and hypospadias. *Amer. J. Surg.*, **82**, 8.

Carroll, W. A. (1949). Malignancy in cryptorchidism. *J. Urol (Baltimore)*, **61**, 396.

Caucci, A. (1951). Contro la terapia ormonica dell'ectopia testicolare. *Accad. med.*, **66**, 90.

Charny, C. W., and Wolgin, W. (1957). *Cryptorchism.* Cassel, London.

Coley, W. B. (1919). Operative treatment of undescended or maldescended testis with especial reference to end-results. *Surg. Gynec. Obstet.*, **28**, 452.

Collins, D. H., and Pugh, R. C. B. (1964). Classification and frequency of testicular tumours. In *The Pathology of Testicular Tumours. Brit. J. Urol.*, **36**, Suppl. 1.

Cooper, E. R. A. (1929). The histology of the retained testis in the human subject at different ages, and its comparison with the scrotal testis. *J. Anat. (Lond.)*, **64**, 5.

Corbus, B. C., and O'Conor, V. J. (1922). The familial occurrence of undescended testes. *Surg. Gynec. Obstet.*, **34**, 237.

Dean, A. L. (1935). Teratoid tumors of the testis. *J. Amer. med. Ass.*, **105**, 1965.

de la Balze, F. A., Mancini, R. A., Arrillaga, F., Andrada, J. A., Vilar, O., Gurtman, A. I., and Davidson, O. W. (1960). Puberal maturation of the normal human testis: a histologic study. *J. clin. Endocr.*, **20**, 266.

Deming, C. L. (1952). The evaluation of hormonal therapy in cryptorchidism. *J. Urol.* (*Baltimore*), **68**, 354.
Devens, K. (1964). Atresia of the vas deferens. Paper read at British Association of Paediatric Surgeons Annual Meeting, Rotterdam.
Doyle, G. B. (1955). Embryonal carcinoma of the testis in an infant. *Brit. J. Urol.*, **27**, 287.
Drake, C. B. (1934). Spontaneous late descent of the testis. *J. Amer. med. Ass.*, **102**, 759.
Eberth, C. J. (1904). *Die mannlichen Geschlechtsorgane*. (Handbuch der Anatomie der Menschen hrsg. K. v. Bardeleben, 12.) Fischer, Jena.
Eisenstaedt, J. S. (1950). Imperfect descent of the testis and its management. *Surg. Clin. N. Amer.*, **30**, 141.
Engberg, H. (1949). Investigations on the endocrine function of the testicle in cryptorchidism. *Proc. roy. Soc. Med.*, **42**, 652.
Felton, L. M. (1959). Should intravenous pyelography be a routine procedure for children with cryptorchism or hypospadias? *J. Urol.* (*Baltimore*), **81**, 335.
Fowler, R., and Stephens, F. D. (1963). The role of testicular vascular anatomy in the salvage of high undescended testes. In *Congenital Malformations of the Rectum, Anus and Genito-urinary Tracts*, by F. D. Stephens, p. 306. Livingstone, Edinburgh.
Frankl, O. (1895). Einiges über die, Involution des Scheidenfortsatzes und die Hüllen des Hodens. *Arch. Anat. Physiol.* (*anat. Abt.*), 339.
Gilbert, J. B., and Hamilton, J. B. (1940). Studies in malignant testis tumours. III. Incidence and nature of tumors in ectopic testes. *Surg. Gynec. Obstet.*, **71**, 731.
Gordon-Taylor, G., and Wyndham, N. R. (1947). On malignant tumours of the testicle. *Brit. J. Surg.*, **35**, 6.
Gross, R. E., and Jewett, T. C. (1956). Surgical experiences from 1,222 operations for undescended testis. *J. Amer. med. Ass.*, **160**, 634.
von Haller, A. (1755). *Opuscula Pathologica*. Bousquet, Lausanne.
Hansen, T. S. (1949). Fertility in operatively treated and untreated cryptorchidism. *Proc. roy. Soc. Med.*, **42**, 645.
Hinman, F. (1924). Tumors of the testicle. In *Modern Urology*, ed. H. Cabot, vol. 1, p. 580. Lea and Febiger, Philadelphia.
Hunter, J. (1762). Observations on the state of the testis in the foetus and on the hernia congenita. In Hunter, W. *Medical Commentaries*, Part 1, p. 75. A. Millar, London.
Johnson, W. W. (1939). Cryptorchidism. *J. Amer. med. Ass.*, **113**, 25.
Jones, P. (1962). Torsion of the testis and its appendages during childhood. *Arch. Dis. Childh.*, **37**, 214.
Kark, W. (1962). The problem of cryptorchidism and malignancy. *Med. Proc.*, **8**, 83.
Lockwood, C. B. (1888). Development and transition of the testis, normal and abnormal. Lecture III. *J. Anat. Physiol.*, **22**, 505.
Lombard, P. (1934). La migration testiculaire est un phénomèna hormonal. *Bull. Mém. Soc. natn. Chir.*, **60**, 878.
MacCollum, D. W. (1935). Clinical study of the spermatogenesis of undescended testicles. *Arch. Surg.*, **31**, 290.
McCutcheon, A. B. (1938). Further observations on delayed testis. *Med. J. Aust.*, **1**, 654.
McGregor, A. L. (1929). The third inguinal ring. *Surg. Gynec. Obstet.*, **49**, 273.
Mack, W. S., Scott, L. S., Ferguson-Smith, M. A., and Lennox, B. (1961). Ectopic testis and true undescended testis: a histological comparison. *J. Path. Bact.*, **82**, 439.
McLeod, J. Personal communication to Charny and Wolgin (1957).
——, and Hotchkiss, R. S. (1941). The effect of hyperpyrexia upon spermatozoa counts in men. *Endocrinology*, **28**, 780.
Maddock, W. O., and Nelson, W. O. (1952). The effects of chorionic gonadotropin in adult men: increased estrogen and 17-ketosteroid excretion, gynecomastia, leydig cell stimulation and seminiferous tubule damage. *J. clin. Endocr.*, **12**, 985.
Minor, C. L. (1959). The empty scrotum. *Pediat. Clin. N. Amer.*, **6**, 1137.
Moore, C. R. (1924). Properties of the gonads as controllers of somatic and physical characteristics. VI. Testicular reactions in experimental cryptorchidism. *Amer. J. Anat.*, **33**, 269.
——, and Quick, W. J. (1924). The scrotum as a temperature regulator for the testes. *Amer. J. Physiol.*, **68**, 70.
——, and Oslund, R. (1924). Experiments on the sheep testis; cryptorchidism, vasectomy and scrotal insulation. *ibid.*, **67**, 595.
Nelson, W. O. (1951). Mammalian spermatogenesis: Effect of experimental cryptorchidism in the rat and non-descent of the testis in man. *Recent Progr. Hormone Res.*, **6**, 29.
O'Conor, V. J. (1919). Torsion of the spermatic cord; report of 2 cases and review of the literature. *Surg. Gynec. Obstet.*, **29**, 580.
Pugh, R. C. B., and Cameron, K. M. (1964). Relative malignancy of testicular tumours. In *The Pathology of Testicular Tumours. Brit. J. Urol.*, **36**, Suppl. 107.
Raynaud, A. (1958). Inhibition, sous l'effet d'une hormone oestrogène, du développement du gubernaculum du foetus mâle de souris. *C.R. Acad. Sci.* (*Paris*), **246**, 176.
Rea, C. E. (1939). Functional capacity of the undescended testis. *Arch. Surg.*, **38**, 1054.
—— (1940). Further report on the treatment of the undescended testes by hormonal therapy at the University of Minnesota Hospitals; a discussion of spontaneous descent of the testis and an evaluation of endocrine therapy in cryptorchidism. *Surgery*, **7**, 828.
—— (1951). Fertility in cryptorchids. *Minn. Med.*, **34**, 216.
Robinson, J. N., and Engle, E. T. (1954). Some observations on the cryptorchid testis. *J. Urol.* (*Baltimore*), **71**, 726.
Rost, F. (1933). Versuche zum Descensus testiculorum. *Langenbecks Arch. klin. Chir.*, **177**, 680.
Schapiro, B. (1931). Ist der Kryptorchismus chirurgisch oder hormonal zu behandeln? *Dtsch. med. Wschr.*, **57**, 718.
Scorer, C. G. (1956). The incidence of incomplete descent of the testicle at birth. *Arch. Dis. Childh.*, **31**, 198.
—— (1957). A treatment of undescended testicle in infancy. *ibid.*, **32**, 520.
—— (1962). The anatomy of testicular descent—normal and incomplete. *Brit. J. Surg.*, **49**, 357.
—— (1964). The descent of the testis. *Arch. Dis. Childh.*, **39**, 605.
Smith, K. H. (1957). Torsion of the spermatic cord. *Brit. J. Surg.*, **45**, 280.
Smith, R. E. (1941). The undescended testicle. *Lancet*, **1**, 747.
Sniffen, R. C. (1952). Histology of the normal and abnormal testis at puberty. *Ann. N.Y. Acad. Sci.*, **55**, 609.
Snyder, W. H., and Chaffin, L. (1955). Surgical management of undescended testes; report of 363 cases. *J. Amer. med. Ass.*, **157**, 129.
——, and Greaney, E. M. (1962). Undescended testes. In *Pediatric Surgery*, ed. C. D. Benson, M. M. Ravitch, W. H. Snyder, Jr., and K. J. Welch. Year Book Medical Publishers, Chicago.
Society of Medical Officers of Health, East Anglian Branch (1958). The significance of the empty scrotum. *Med. Offr*, **100**, 379.
Sohval, A. R. (1954). Testicular dysgenesis as an etiologic factor in cryptorchidism. *J. Urol.* (*Baltimore*), **72**, 693.
—— (1956). Testicular dysgenesis in relation to neoplasm of the testicle. *ibid.*, **75**, 285.
Sonneland, S. G. (1924). Congenital perineal testicle. *Ann. Surg.*, **80**, 716.
Southam, A. H., and Cooper, E. R. A. (1927). Hunterian Lecture on the pathology and treatment of the retained testis in childhood. *Lancet*, **1**, 805.
Sumner, W. A. (1959). Malignant tumor of testis occurring 29 years after orchiopexy. *J. Urol.* (*Baltimore*), **81**, 150.
Thompson, W. O., and Heckel, N. J. (1938). Precocious sexual development from an anterior pituitary-like principle. *J. Amer. med. Ass.*, **110**, 1813.
Torek, F. (1909). The technique of orcheopexy. *N.Y. med. J.*, **90**, 948.
Turner, G. G. (1937). Imperfect migration of the testicle: the surgical problem. *Proc. roy. Soc. Med.*, **30**, 1319.
Wakeley, J. C. N. (1953). Perineal testis. *Lancet*, **1**, 1025.
Wallenstein, S. (1929). Torsion of an intra-abdominal testis. *J. Urol.* (*Baltimore*), **21**, 279.
Ward, B., and Hunter, W. M. (1960). The absent testicle. A report on a survey carried out among schoolboys in Nottingham. *Brit. med. J.*, **1**, 1110.
Wells, L. J., and State, D. (1947). Misconception of the gubernaculum testis. *Surgery*, **22**, 502.
Wiles, P. (1934). Family tree, showing hereditary undescended right testis and associated deformities. *Proc. roy. Soc. Med.*, **28**, 157.
Williams, D. I. (1958). *Urology in Childhood.* (Handbuch der Urologie, ed. C. E. Alken *et al.*, XV). Springer, Berlin.
Witus, W. S., Sloss, J. H., and Valk, W. L. (1959). Inguinal node metastases from testicular tumors developing after orchiopexy. *J. Urol.* (*Baltimore*), **81**, 669.

*Arch. Dis. Childh.*, 1965, **40**, 123.

# THE DEVELOPMENT OF HEART SURGERY IN CHILDREN

BY

SIR RUSSELL BROCK*

I must thank you for inviting me to be one of your guests of honour and to speak to you on the development of heart surgery in children. This is a big task but one of special interest to me because I have been fortunate in having watched much of this development and even participated in some small part.

I start with a story. In 1930 I had the privilege of spending a year in St. Louis with Dr. Evarts Graham as a Rockefeller Research Fellow. Pulmonary surgery was about to unfold and heart surgery was almost non-existent and entirely non-existent in children. Professor Graham, who as you know was a great surgical pioneer, was interested in the possibilities of heart surgery and had begun some work on the surgical relief of mitral stenosis. He told me that in the early 1920's he became convinced that it was desirable and feasible to close the persistent ductus arteriosus. He therefore approached the professor of paediatrics at the St. Louis Children's Hospital, explained his thoughts and plans, and asked if a patient could be sent to him with a view to operation. The paediatric professor without further comment sent along a man aged 53 years.

I have no doubt that he thought this was a clever act, powerful enough to stop once and for all this imaginative but troublesome surgeon. It was, of course, a cruel and stupid thing to do and, as Graham said, delayed the advent of cardiovascular surgery in children for some 15 years until Robert Gross, encouraged and stimulated by a physician wiser than the professor at St. Louis, achieved the first successful closure of a ductus and ushered in the cardiovascular surgery of childhood. This great paediatric surgeon, in addition to making many other contributions, shared also the establishment of the surgery of aortic coarctation.

While I was in St. Louis the leading thoracic surgical problems lay in connexion with lung surgery and especially with lung resection, both in children and in adults. The development of heart surgery was scarcely possible before familiarity with intrathoracic techniques had been established, including that of the parallel disciplines of anaesthesia, blood transfusion, chemotherapy, radiology etc. The path to this achievement was fated to lie in the surgery of the lungs and again I was fortunate to be a ringside observer. In this year while I was in St. Louis, Shenstone and Janes of Toronto announced their success with one-stage lobectomy for bronchiectasis in the development of the tourniquet technique pioneered by Brun of San Francisco. Their report of 11 patients operated on with only 2 deaths was epoch-making because it not only proclaimed the ability to cure the loathsome disease of bronchiectasis but showed the way by which familiarity and success could be achieved in operating within the thorax. The eight years that remained of the 1930's before the second war came to disrupt normal progress were the golden years of lung surgery and of thoracic surgery and culminated in 1938 in the success of Robert Gross to which I have already referred. I emphasize to you again how, in my opinion, the establishment of safe thoracotomy for non-cardiac intrathoracic disease was the essential preliminary to the advent of cardiac surgery.

Dwight Harken's splendid work during the war on the successful removal of foreign bodies from within the chambers of the heart showed that the heart could tolerate direct intervention, and when the war ended the stage was set for the exciting development of heart surgery that we have since witnessed.

It seems convenient to divide progress into that of closed operations and of open operations for heart disease.

### Closed-heart Surgery

Many of the closed procedures are now of chiefly historical interest because they have been replaced by open technique, but a place still remains for closed operations. This is often so in infants and small children who do not well tolerate open operations done with present techniques of total body perfusion. It may be that newer techniques will be better tolerated, but at present this intolerance of very young children for open procedures must be recognized.

I need not expand upon the surgery of persistent ductus and of aortic coarctation because most of you are familiar with these two conditions. I merely

* President of the Royal College of Surgeons, and guest Lecturer at a meeting of the British Association of Paediatric Surgeons in Rotterdam, September 1964.

mention the complex and difficult problems that arise when either is associated with other congenital heart lesions; especially congenital mitral stenosis, ventricular septal defect, and aortic stenosis. With such combinations we are faced with grave problems to which I can do no more than refer in this short address.

Of the closed procedures I must mention closed pulmonary valvotomy and closed operations on the outflow tract of the right ventricle.

Closed pulmonary valvotomy for pure valve stenosis or associated with reversed flow through an atrial communication has been largely displaced by open valvotomy; a development that all must welcome. I would not like you to think, however, that there is no place for closed pulmonary valvotomy. It is still an excellent and safe operation in poor risk cases; some of these are in older patients, especially over 20 years of age, who are severely cyanosed; another group consists of very young children or infants and especially those who are deeply cyanosed. A quick closed valvotomy can be not only life saving but can give a brilliant and long-lasting result. Many of you may not agree with this and will prefer an open valvotomy on all occasions. I must tell you that I have many patients who remain in excellent health and with complete relief of their pulmonary stenosis, having been operated on as children ten or more years ago. Cyanosis is usually completely relieved even when the atrial communication is not closed. In only a few cases has it proved necessary to close the septal defect by a second operation.

We have, in connexion with pulmonary valvotomy, the problem of coincident secondary infundibular stenosis due to hypertrophic muscular changes. Most of you are familiar with this but some may not be, and I must explain briefly that even after an open valvotomy in which there can be no doubt about the complete relief of the valve stenosis the pressure in the right ventricle may still be as high as before, or even higher. The explanation lies in the fact that as soon as the ventricle is decompressed by the valvotomy the grossly hypertrophied walls of the infundibulum approximate during systole and constitute another obstruction. This obstruction can be relieved by resection of the infundibulum and the right ventricular hypertension may be immediately converted. In case you think the problem is thus easily solved I will show you examples in which this is not so; in fact the hypertension may be made worse. Nature in time can correct this state over the course of one to two years, and with the spontaneous regression of the right ventricular hypertrophy the pressure in the right ventricle returns to normal.

In spite of this observation that a natural cure can occur, it is still dogmatically stated that if hypertension is present after valvotomy, infundibular resection is obligatory. I warn you against accepting this advice and practice without deeper study of the facts. I specially warn you of this in young children who, of course, are your chief concern.

In children the muscular hypertrophy in response to valve obstruction may be florid and excessive and this is especially significant when one considers the absolute smallness of the right ventricular cavity and how it may be much more severely obstructed than in an adult. It is particularly dangerous to do an open infundibular resection on little children in such circumstances, because you will find that it is difficult or impossible to perform a satisfactory resection of the very thick muscle and it may be quite impossible to relieve the right ventricular hypertension. The net result is that in addition to carrying the burden of the unrelieved ventricular hypertension the patient has suffered a major damage to the efficiency of the right ventricle by virtue of the incision and resection. It is small wonder that the mortality is high. There may still be an argument for infundibular resection in older children, but I strongly advise you against doing this in young children and especially when the right ventricular pressure is as high as 200 or 250 mm. Hg. The temptation is then great; so is the risk of failure and the risk of death; and so is the ability of the ventricular hypertrophy to recede spontaneously. Be patient and wait. You are much more likely to have a live patient, and if the right ventricular hypertension does not resolve spontaneously you can always do a secondary operation.

The management of hypertrophic infundibular stenosis illustrates the great difference between simple operating and true surgery; between cutting and thinking. In heart surgery, as in all other branches, it is not enough to be able to do a particular operation. The significance of every procedure must be understood by a full knowledge of the underlying problems presented.

I now come to closed operations on the outflow tract of the right ventricle in Fallot's tetralogy. This grave condition consists essentially of a varying degree of pulmonary stenosis and a ventricular septal defect. The pulmonary stenosis is caused by valvar stenosis or infundibular stenosis or by a combination of the two.

The brilliant contribution of Blalock and Taussig demonstrated that the obstruction to the outflow of blood from the right ventricle could be by-passed by a systemic-pulmonary anastomosis; the Potts' operation follows the same principle. These operations have been and still are widely accepted, and rightly so. I notice, however, that among the published papers of this meeting is an article on the surgical palliative treatment of the tetralogy of Fallot in children, in which it is rightly pointed out that complete correction, using extracorporeal circulation, is often not possible in children, and it mentions the need for some preliminary procedure or first stage operation. It is stated, 'the only surgical treatment in this group of children is to improve the pulmonary flow by means of a Blalock or Potts anastomosis'.

I must point out, with some sorrow, that this statement is just not true. Excellent palliation is possible by relief of the outflow tract obstruction either by valvotomy or by infundibular resection or by both combined. This is in accord with sound surgical principles and achieves more than a short-circuiting procedure, which a systemic-pulmonary anastomosis essentially is. Increasing the blood flow through the right ventricular outflow tract encourages the growth and development of the tract so that the haemodynamic conditions are more favourable when the time comes to close the septal defect. I cannot enlarge upon this subject here but must refer you to my many writings on it and also to the supporting writings of others. By all means reject palliative operations on the outflow tract or say you do not like them, but please do not ignore them. This indicates either ignorance of their existence or contempt for them. They can be very useful in infants or young children who are gravely ill and deeply cyanosed. A quick closed operation on the outflow tract can give results as good as an anastomotic procedure and often with less disturbance. You should follow the example of many cardiac and paediatric surgeons and try them.

### Open-heart Surgery

I now come to the vast field of open-heart surgery and can only deal with it in rather general terms aided by references to a few specific problems.

We all recognize the very high mortality in newborn babies and infants during the first 6-12 months of life from congenital heart lesions. Many of these are incurable, but even when an anatomically curable condition is present the infant will usually not tolerate a radical operation. Hence, whenever feasible, the preference is for some palliative procedure that will carry the infant on until he can tolerate a fully corrective operation. One of the most difficult problems is that of transposition of the great vessels and my friend Dr. Brom will deal with this in a separate lecture.

At present these young patients do not tolerate total body perfusion well. A special heart-lung machine is essential for them, but even then the margins of haemodynamic inbalance are easily transgressed and this is badly tolerated. This does not mean, however, that we must admit defeat. It remains a challenge to surgery, and sooner or later the grave problems of open-heart surgery in babies and small infants will be largely overcome.

The reluctance to operate on very small infants is obligatory, but it is often quite wrong to show the same reluctance in older children. A decision not to operate or to delay operation often springs from prejudice or fear, or from ignorance of the factors involved. The heart of a child of 5 years or more with an atrial septal defect and even more so with a ventricular septal defect is exposed to unnecessary and undesirable overwork all day and every day, exactly as with a persistent ductus, and closure is indicated to relieve the cardiovascular burden alone. But there is another strong reason for correcting the abnormality; one that I am sure that an audience of paediatric surgeons is acquainted with as it plays an important part in many other diseases, namely general retardation of growth and the development of severe thoracic skeletal deformities. I notice a paper is in fact being presented at this congress on the physical development of children with congenital heart disease, and I need only emphasize this important consideration and how the years that the locusts have eaten can never be regained, as the skeletal deformity or retardation of growth cannot be fully corrected.

A straightforward atrial septal defect of secundum type should present no problem in a child. Various techniques can be used to expose the lesion; conventional hypothermia, total body perfusion with a standard pump oxygenator or the disposable oxygenator primed with 5% dextrose as popularized particularly by Denton Cooley. This latter technique has certain advantages for a short procedure in children, including easing the demand on the supply of blood, now so important with open-heart surgery. Much more caution is necessary in an atrial septal defect of primum type; the technical difficulties in these can be very great and the mortality and morbidity can be high. It is often wiser to delay operation in children.

Uncomplicated ventricular septal defect is also a relatively straightforward procedure and my policy is to recommend routine closure even when the lesion is a small one, though usually not before the age of 5 to 7 years.

When the defect is large or when it is complicated by a rise in pulmonary arterial resistance, the risk and problems of operation increase. I can only refer to the problems of heart block; the best treatment is avoidance, and the technique of closure must be directed to this. If heart block occurs, it must always be controlled either temporarily or permanently by a pacemaker. It is no good hoping for the best and doing nothing or relying upon medical means.

The problems of raised pulmonary artery resistance are also difficult and complex. We know that this is often present in infants, and operation below the age of 2 years is followed by a very high mortality. Temporizing is necessary; perhaps in newborn babies with a palliative procedure, such as banding the pulmonary artery. I am convinced that the changes in the lung vessels in children are not permanent and certainly are not progressive. I have observed regression over the years and feel that it is wrong to operate on an infant simply because of fear that the pulmonary resistance will worsen or will become permanently raised. Many infants and young children have lost their lives because of too early operation.

Congenital mitral stenosis and regurgitation are serious lesions. My experience with the former has been particularly disappointing and even with an open operation it is difficult or impossible to correct the severely mal-developed valve.

The present results of operation for congenital aortic valve stenosis are good and the mortality is low. In the early days, especially when hurried operations were done under hypothermia, serious regurgitation was often inflicted. Experience has shown the need for great care in cutting the valve, and that serious complication is now less common. I feel, however, that the long-term results of aortic valvotomy for congenital stenosis in children will be disappointing and certainly so with a bicuspid valve. Calcification and recurrence of stenosis seem inevitable and the same must occur when the valve cusps contain large myxomatous nodules. In many such cases valve excision and replacement will be needed later in life, and a guarded prognosis must be given.

I have already made a brief reference to Fallot's tetralogy and the place for palliative operations. I now turn to its radical cure or so-called total correction.

The most difficult common congenital heart lesion we have to deal with is transposition of the great vessels, and the second most difficult is Fallot's tetralogy. I emphasize that Fallot's tetralogy is *always* a serious lesion; even when the clinical state is not severe the actual cardiac lesion is always severe. All treatment and management must be based on this fact.

I am against performing a total corrective operation in young children below the age of 7 years. I am aware that success is possible in younger children but the mortality is so much higher that it is not wise to expose the child to the extra risk. The younger the child the more does this apply. Total correction of Fallot's tetralogy is a severe physical strain for a child to undergo and many are just not strong enough nor have sufficient reserve to tolerate it. A preliminary operation such as an anastomosis or an outflow tract operation is desirable to carry the child along until he is older and stronger.

I have great reservations about the use of an outflow patch and particularly one that extends across the pulmonary valve into the pulmonary trunk, thus causing severe pulmonary regurgitation. It is disturbing, even distressing, to read reports of outflow patches being used in some two-thirds of patients submitted to 'total correction'. This is not total correction because the heart is still far from normal. If the outflow tract is too small to carry the correct amount of blood, it is better to give Nature a chance to enlarge it by doing a preliminary relief of outflow tract obstruction rather than rushing things by artificially enlarging the outflow by sewing in a gusset. The years ahead are likely to disclose disappointments after this so-called total correction.

## Conclusions

I have barely touched on the problems of heart surgery in children, but I wish to refer to some of the problems of organization which have appeared now that success has been achieved and now that paediatric surgery has come so much into its own as a specialty.

Everyone must surely accept that the problems of operating on and caring for newly born and young infants demand the organization, resources, and skills of special paediatric units. I need not, before this audience, enlarge upon the requirements of special knowledge, of nursing skills, and of special equipment and ward design and organization. The surgeon who wishes to undertake these difficult and anxious cardiac operations in very young patients must either be a paediatric surgeon who has chosen cardiovascular surgery as an extra specialty within his specialty or a cardiac surgeon who elects to make a special study of these infant problems and works closely with a paediatric colleague in a properly organized unit or hospital. Without this I can see little prospect of good work being achieved.

In older children this need is not so urgent. Older children of course derive great benefit from being in a special paediatric environment, but the operating and after-care do not demand the same highly specialized paediatric knowledge and experience as in the case of young infants. The essential requisite is experience and ability in cardiac surgical techniques. If these are possessed by a paediatric surgeon then a very happy position exists. I think you will agree that there is no justification for a paediatric surgeon, just because he is a paediatric surgeon, to attempt these very difficult cardiac procedures in children. The road to specialization lies with the necessary techniques and special clinical knowledge and not in the age of the patient.

Advance in this very difficult field of surgery has come and will continue to come both from non-paediatric surgeons and from paediatric surgeons. I have, for example, mentioned the great contributions of Robert Gross. We all look forward with eagerness to progress in the field of newborns and infants. Here lie the true problems, the very great difficulties and the present high death rate. But in this field brilliant advances can emerge to save the lives of many more babies suffering from congenital heart disease. Success can only come from close co-operation between paediatrics and cardiac surgery, whether the surgeon be primarily paediatric or cardiac in training.

The problems presented are immense but the joys of success are equally great. Let us hope that it will not be long before a meeting of your Association listens to papers being presented that record the success in cardiac surgery in young infants that we all realize is so desirable.

*Arch. Dis. Childh.*, 1965, **40**, 128.

# THE SURGERY OF TRANSPOSITION OF THE GREAT VESSELS*

BY

A. G. BROM, H. V. D. SCHAAR, and J. NAUTA

*From the Academisch Ziekenhuis, Leiden, the Netherlands*

In transposition of the great vessels the aorta gets its blood from the right side of the heart into which the caval veins enter, and the pulmonary artery arises from the left side of the heart, getting its blood from the lungs. The normal crossed circulation has changed into two parallel circulations, and the patient can live only if there are shunts between the two circulations. The interior of the heart may also be grossly deformed, but fortunately in this respect most of these hearts are nearly normal, and it is these that will be discussed.

The diagnosis of transposition is suspected in babies who are blue from birth. Murmurs and ECG are not characteristic. X-ray pictures show the degree of filling of the pulmonary vessels. Angiocardiography shows the aorta arising from the right heart, and is at the same time important as showing the anatomy of the interior of the heart, especially the formation of the ventricular septum. Heart catheterization is extremely valuable *if* the pressure in the left ventricle is recorded.

According to Noonan, Nadas, Rudolph, and Harris (1960) patients with transposition are of four types.

*Group I.* Patients in whom transposition is combined with a *ventricular septal defect* (a) with pulmonary stenosis (b) with pulmonic vascular obstruction, and (c) with large pulmonary blood flow.

(a) Ventricular septal defect and pulmonary stenosis. In the absence of an angiocardiogram a diagnosis of 'a severe case of Fallot's tetralogy' will be made. This does not make much difference, as a shunt, according to Blalock or Potts, is indicated, because a total correction is difficult if not impossible, since the overlying left coronary artery does not allow the stenotic area of the pulmonary outflow to be enlarged. The results of a shunt, however, are gratifying, and here we find the first interesting fact in the study of transposition. Compared to the relatively large number of 17 patients with a shunt who were operated on, we find only *one* with this anomaly in our anatomical collection of un-operated transpositions (Fig. 1). This means that the combination of transposition with pulmonary stenosis is favourable for long survival (Fig. 2).

(b) The patients with ventricular septal defect and high pulmonary resistance are quite a different group. In the cyanotic child the loud single second sound implies pulmonary hypertension. Radiographs show increased central lung fields. Angiocardiography confirms the diagnosis, and if one succeeds in taking the pressure in the left ventricle this will be high—as in the first group with pulmonary stenosis.

Until about a year ago we treated these patients with a partial transposition of the venous return according to Baffes, but lately we have changed our policy. The Baffes operation renders a patient less cyanotic and sometimes very much improved, *but* the high pulmonary resistance is not changed, and ultimately the patient dies from heart failure. Because the patients with transposition and pulmonary stenosis have done well (Fig. 2), we decided to 'band' the pulmonary artery, combining this—when the shunting from left to right is insufficient—with the creation of an atrial septal defect. Follow-up is too short to evaluate this approach, but we are impressed by the good results in 3 patients in whom banding plus atrial septal defect was carried out; the results in 7 patients where only banding was performed are far less gratifying. So we think the combined operation is better, and as the possibility of curing high pulmonary resistance is slight after the age of 3 years, the operation should be done in early childhood in the hope of preparing the children for a total correction in the future.

(c) This group comprises patients with a ventricular septal defect and an increased pulmonary

* A paper read at a meeting of the British Association of Paediatric Surgeons in Rotterdam, September 1964.

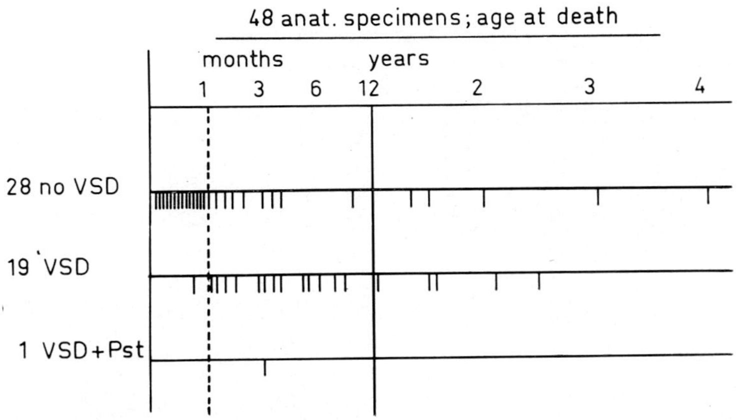


FIG. 1.—Age at death in 48 cases of transposition. Note the tendency for longer survival if a VSD is present.

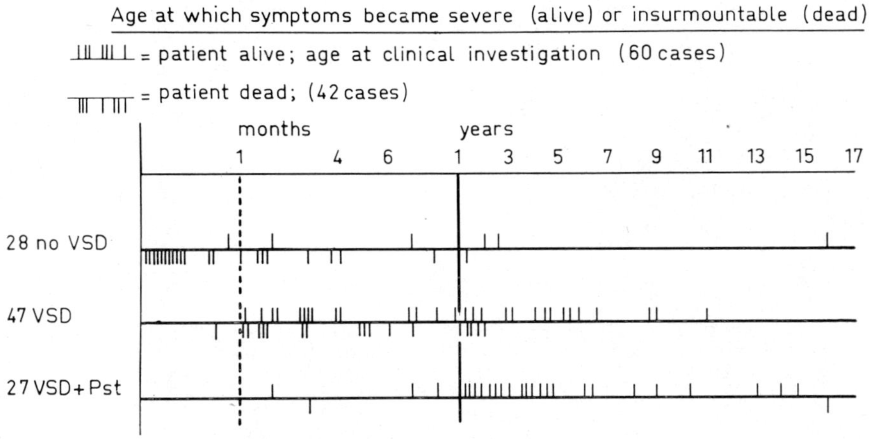


FIG. 2.—Fate of 102 cases of transposition. Note (1) predominantly early death if there is no VSD, and (2) predominantly long survival if VSD and pulmonary stenosis (Pst) are present.

flow. This is rare and the diagnosis is difficult, but again the important point is the pressure in the left ventricle. If this pressure is low or slightly raised in a patient with increased lung fields on radiography, the presence of a (usually) small ventricular septal defect should be suspected. As regards treatment, this group presents the same possibilities as Group 4.

*Group II.* Patients in whom *no ventricular septal defect* is present: they survive by virtue of a patent ductus or an atrial septal defect, both of which are seldom adequate, and the children die very soon. Our anatomical collection (Fig. 1) shows 28 amongst 48, nearly all of them having died early. This is a pity as these are just the patients most suitable for a total correction. Thus if one finds a newborn baby, deeply cyanosed, in heart failure, and going rapidly downhill, think of this diagnosis: transposition with no (or small) ventricular septal defect. For the very ill patients in this group an emergency operation is needed to keep them alive, because the available shunts are small. Making a large atrial septal defect will help them to survive and give them a chance to be cured later in life.

For many years anatomists and cardiologists have been 'flirting' with transposition—according to the definition of flirting, paying a lot of *attention* without real *intention* of doing something about it. But lately surgeons like Albert, Kay, Merendino, Senning, and Mustard have developed methods of correcting transposition by switching the venous return. These operations have been tried many times, but only a few—I think about 15—successes are known. We are convinced this is because the success of the

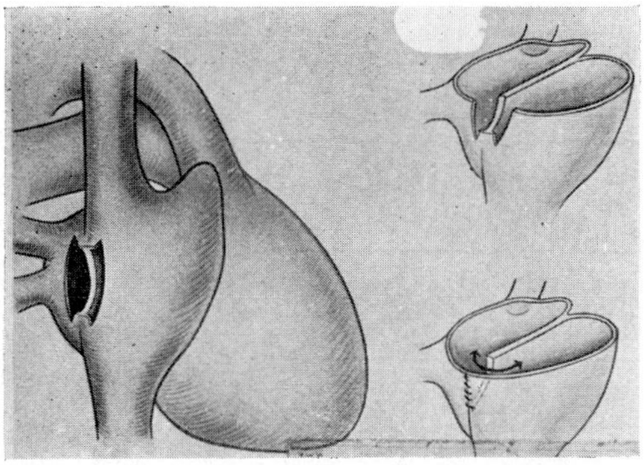

FIG. 3.—Transposition of the great vessels. Creation of an ASD by the Hanlon-Blalock operation. Incision of the right and left atrium on both sides of the septum. Resection of a graft of the interatrial septum, which is withdrawn from the circulation by means of a Satinsky clamp.

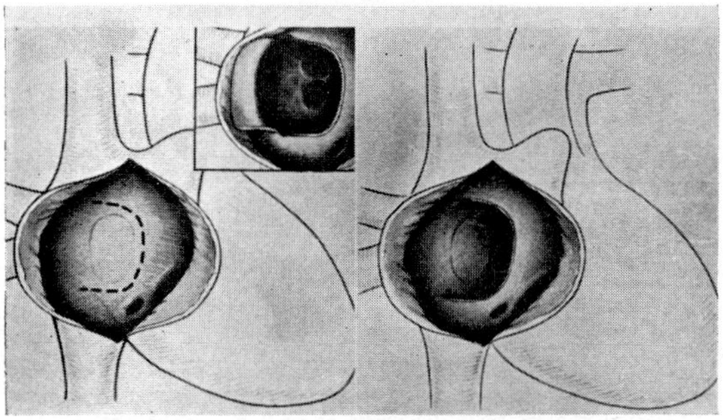

(a) (b)

FIG. 4.—Transposition of the great vessels. Total correction by the Senning procedure. (a) An incision is made in the atrial septum. Inset: The atrial septal flap formed is lifted, showing the orifices of the pulmonary veins. (b) Suturing this flap in front of the veins.

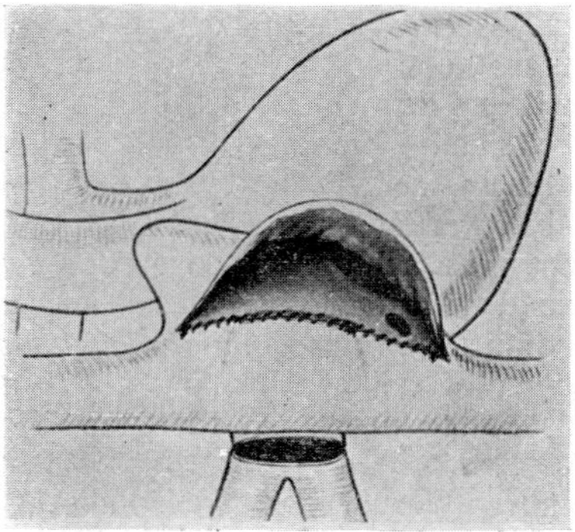

FIG. 5.—The right flap of the atrial incision is sutured to the left border of the atrial septum.

operation depends upon the degree of pulmonary vascular resistance. If this is high, success is impossible; but results should be good in cases with normal or only moderately raised pressure in the left ventricle (the ventricle from which the pulmonary artery arises). We take pressure readings at the left side before or during operation, Mustard takes lung biopsies in dubious cases and if the pulmonary resistance is not raised, he proceeds with the correction.

Figs. 3-5 illustrate variations of the Senning operation. The atrial septum is resected and the switching of the veins is accomplished by the use of an interatrial prosthesis of a plastic material or pericardium (Mustard). I believe it is better for the total correction to be done after the preliminary creation of an atrial septal defect, but so far we have not done this.

### Results of Surgery

The results of operation in 11 cases of transposition are set out in Table 1.

The shunt operations give good palliation in transpositions with pulmonary stenosis. The Hanlon-Blalock procedure is done in all transpositions without pulmonary stenosis, mostly as an emergency operation in extremely ill children, which gives rise to a high mortality. To do the operation under hyperbaric oxygen may perhaps be an advantage.

The essential part of this communication is to give our results for total correction by Senning's technique. A study of the few repaired cases that have been successfully operated on shows that they have one thing in common—*there is no high pulmonary resistance and no pulmonary stenosis.*

We have tried the Senning operation 7 times (Table 2) with a successful outcome in 2; 2 other patients lived for some time after correction: one died the day before she should have returned home, from a haemoptysis after pleural puncture, and the second after 3 months from brain damage due to excessive (more than 1 hour) total circulatory arrest at low temperature. (We no longer use circulatory arrest.) However, both these patients remained free of cyanosis between operation and death. Two died from mistakes in perfusion technique, which is difficult in these small infants, and in the last patient we missed an atresia of the isthmus of aorta and so, while on perfusion, no blood reached the brain.

### Summary and Conclusions

In patients with transposition and pulmonary stenosis the Blalock and Potts procedures give good

TABLE 1

RESULTS IN SIX DIFFERENT TYPES OF OPERATION IN 71 CASES OF TRANSPOSITION

| Procedure | No. | Operative Mortality | Late Mortality | Survival |
|---|---|---|---|---|
| Senning | 7 | 3 | 1 died after 1 mth.<br>1 died after 3 mth. | 2 |
| Blalock-Hanlon | 22 | 9 | 2 died after 1 mth. | 11 |
| Baffes | 15 | 5 | 0 | 10 |
| Anastomosis | 17 | 0 | 2 had too big a shunt: and died 3 and 6 mth. after operation | 15 |
| Banding PA | 7 | 0 | 0 | 7 |
| Creation of ASD + banding PA | 3 | 0 | 0 | 3 |
| Total .. .. .. | 71 | 17 | 6 | 48 |

TABLE 2

RESULTS OF SENNING OPERATION FOR TOTAL CORRECTION IN 7 CASES OF TRANSPOSITION

| Case No. | Age | Pre-operative Pressures (mm. Hg) | | Anatomy | Corrections | Post-operative Condition |
|---|---|---|---|---|---|---|
| | | RV | LV | | | |
| 1 | 3 mth. | — | — | PFO, PDA, VSD atretic, aortic isthmus | Closure PDA and VSD, Senning operation | Died |
| 2 | 11 mth. | 80/0 | 25/0 | PFO | Senning operation | Died 3 mth. later neurological complications |
| 3 | 3½ mth. | 70/0 | 50/0 | PFO | Senning operation | Died |
| 4 | 8 mth. | 140/5 | 42/0 | PFO, PDA, coarctation | Resection coarctation, closure PDA, Senning operation | Died |
| 5 | 2½ yr. | 70/0 | 32/0 | PFO | Senning operation | Good |
| 6 | 16 yr. | 100/0 | 27/0 | PFO | Senning operation | Died after 1 mth. |
| 7 | 5 yr. | 100/5 | 45/0 | PFO | Senning operation | Good |

PFO = patent foramen ovale; PDA = patent ductus arteriosus; VSD = ventricular septal defect.

palliation, and will keep the patients alive until a way is found to deal with the coronary artery which crosses the stenotic pulmonary artery.

The creation of an atrial septal defect can be highly effective as an emergency operation and may prepare the patient for a total correction. The same is true for the treatment of high pulmonary resistance by 'banding', combined with the creation of an atrial septal defect.

The shunt, the banding, and the atrial septal defect prepare for the final answer—total correction. And here the Senning procedure (or its modifications) is proving to be valuable in carefully selected patients.

REFERENCE

Noonan, J. A., Nadas, A. S., Rudolph, A. M., and Harris, G. B. C. (1960). Transposition of the great arteries. *New Engl. J. Med.*, **263**, 592.

*Arch. Dis. Childh.*, 1965, **40**, 132.

# PANCREATITIS IN CHILDHOOD: EXPERIENCE WITH 15 CASES*

BY

W. HARDY HENDREN, JACOBUS M. GREEP, and ANTHONY S. PATTON

*From the Children's Service, Massachusetts General Hospital, and the Departments of Surgery at Massachusetts General Hospital, Children's Hospital Medical Center and Harvard Medical School, Boston, Mass., U.S.A.*

Pancreatitis is considered generally to be an unusual condition during infancy and childhood; much of the literature on this subject is confined to single case reports and post-mortem studies (Anderson, 1923; Blumenthal and Probstein, 1961; Collins, 1958; Gibson and Gibson, 1956; Gruenwald, 1950; Haigh, 1956; O'Brien, 1961; Pender, 1957; Plechas, 1960; Power, 1961; Steiner and Tracy, 1943; Stickler and Yonemoto, 1958; Warwick and Leavitt, 1960). In the first report on pancreatitis, Fitz (1889) had no children in his series from the Massachusetts General Hospital; in 1935 Dobbs called attention to the occurrence of pancreatitis in childhood.

During the past 9 years we have encountered 15 children with pancreatitis, and these cases are the subject of this report. They do not represent material drawn from hospital files, but living patients whom we have seen during this period. From this experience we believe that pancreatitis in children, if looked for, is probably more common than previously supposed.

TABLE 1

PRESENTING PICTURE IN 15 CASES OF PANCREATITIS IN CHILDREN

| No. of Cases | Presenting Symptoms |
|---|---|
| 5 | Intermittent abdominal pain (1 with jaundice) |
| 4 | Acute 'surgical abdomen' |
| 3 | Acute onset of ascites with fever |
| 1 | Abdominal mass following trauma |
| 1 | Contusion with ruptured spleen |
| 1 | Pancreatitis with mumps |

## Clinical Presentation

As outlined in Table 1, the presenting clinical picture was variable: 5 patients had intermittent abdominal pain, 1 with jaundice (Cases 3, 8, 10, 12, and 14); 4 presented as acute abdominal emergencies (Cases 1, 2, 7, and 13); 3 had acute onset of ascites with fever (Cases 4, 6, and 11); in one a large abdominal mass developed a month after removal of a ruptured spleen (Case 9); in another explored two days after rupture of the spleen, the distal part of the tail of the pancreas was found to be acutely inflamed from trauma and was removed (Case 15); in one mild pancreatitis was found in association with mumps (Case 5).

TABLE 2

AETIOLOGY IN 15 CASES OF PANCREATITIS IN CHILDREN

| No. of Cases | Aetiology |
|---|---|
| 6 | Unknown aetiology (2 with pseudocysts) |
| 3 | Obstruction at ampulla of Vater |
| 2 | Trauma (1 with pseudocyst) |
| 1 | Gastric duplication in accessory pancreatic lobe |
| 1 | Gall-stone in ampulla (with pseudocyst) |
| 1 | Sepsis |
| 1 | Mumps |

## Aetiology

The causes of pancreatitis in this series are summarized in Table 2. In 6 cases, 2 with pseudocysts, we are uncertain as to the cause of pancreatitis (Cases 1, 3, 4, 6, 12, and 14); in 3 we think there was evidence of obstruction at the ampulla of Vater (Cases 8, 10, and 11); 2 occurred after abdominal trauma, one with pseudocyst formation (Cases 9 and 15); in one a small gastric duplication communicating with an accessory lobe of pancreas was the cause (Case 13); one child had gall-stones, with acute fulminating pancreatitis caused presumably by passage of a common duct stone with temporary obstruction of the ampulla (Case 2); in another, a small infant, pancreatitis appeared secondary to overwhelming sepsis in association with malnutrition

* A paper read at a meeting of the British Association of Paediatric Surgeons in Rotterdam, September 1964.

and dehydration brought on by a hiatus hernia (Case 7); another had mumps (Case 5).

It is intriguing to speculate about the 6 patients with pancreatitis of unknown aetiology. Only one of them, Case 14, had exploration and pancreatography; the sphincter of Oddi was normal, but the pancreatogram was inconclusive; this case may possibly represent a duct anomaly. Case 1 has had no further trouble in 8½ years since exploration and simple drainage; with no recurrence it appears unlikely that she had obstructive pancreatitis. Case 3 had sphincterotomy which excluded stenosis of the ampulla, but pancreatography was not performed, thus a duct anomaly has not been disproved. Case 4, treated by enteric drainage of a pseudocyst, had neither exploration of the ampulla nor pancreatography; this could be a case of obstruction relieved by proximal drainage via the pseudocyst. Case 6 is one of obscure aetiology; the background of this youngster raised the suspicion of maltreatment. Case 12 has not been operated on; with his history of recurring pain, and a repeatedly positive morphine-prostigmine provocative test, he may have obstructive pancreatitis.

We have not recognized a case of pancreatitis in children on steroid therapy as has been reported (Baar and Wolff, 1957; Marczynska-Robowska, 1957; Oppenheimer and Boitnott, 1960) or from hydrochlorothiazide (Shanklin, 1962). Similarly we have not had a patient with pancreatitis secondary to *Ascaris* obstruction of a pancreatic duct, undoubtedly due to the low prevalence of round worm infestation in New England. Successful operative relief of pancreatitis due to acute duct obstruction by this worm was recorded many years ago by Novis (1923). In a recent series of 17 children with pancreatitis J. H. Louw (personal communication) had 12 children with pancreatitis secondary to *Ascaris* in a region where there is a high prevalence of the parasite. He has also treated two children with congenital stenosis of the ampulla of Vater. Pancreatitis has been reported in association with choledochal cysts (Gibson and Haller, 1959) and other anomalies such as annular pancreas (Frey and Redo, 1963), but we have not seen this association. The hereditary occurrence of pancreatitis has been noted (Gross and Comfort, 1957), and Case 11 in this series may be such an example: there was obstruction at the ampulla. Gerber (1963) reported hereditary pancreatitis in childhood treated by direct operation on the duct system of the pancreas. Oeconomopoulos and Lee (1960) reported 3 cases of pancreatic pseudocyst in childhood and found an additional 8 case reports; they concluded that many such cases were unrecognized. Our own experience with 4 pseudocysts tends to support that view.

In reviewing the published reports relating to obstruction of the pancreatic duct outflow we have found 16 cases; 4 additional examples can be recorded from this series (Cases 2, 8, 10, and 11). We think it likely that more would be brought to light by exploration of the sphincter of Oddi and pancreatography in selected patients. The points of obstruction are shown in Fig. 1.

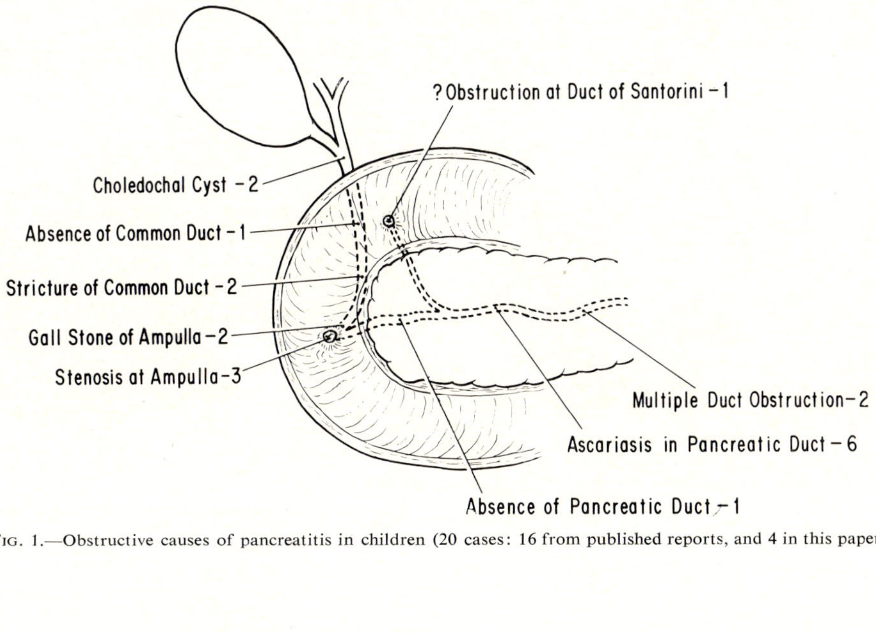


FIG. 1.—Obstructive causes of pancreatitis in children (20 cases: 16 from published reports, and 4 in this paper).

### Treatment

Operation was carried out in 12 of these 15 cases as shown in Table 3. Transduodenal sphincterotomy was done in 4 (Cases 3, 8, 10, and 11). In 3 of these the sphincter was found to be abnormal; operation relieved the problem. In one (Case 3) the sphincter was not stenotic and further difficulty has ensued; later subtotal gastrectomy was done to decrease pancreatic stimulation. Simple drainage of the lesser peritoneal sac was done in 2 patients (Cases 1 and 7). Sphincterotomy and cyst gastrostomy was performed in one patient (Case 14); the sphincter was normal. Sphincterotomy (normal) and later partial pancreatectomy was performed in one (Case 13) in whom the underlying problem was found later to be an unusual cystic duplication of the stomach attached to an accessory lobe of pancreas. One patient (Case 2) was treated initially by cholecystostomy, removing gall-stones, and later marsupialization of a pseudocyst. One patient had a Roux-en-Y cyst jejunostomy (Case 4). One patient had simple transgastric cyst gastrostomy for a pseudocyst (Case 9) four weeks following removal of a ruptured spleen. One had partial caudal pancreatectomy with removal of a ruptured spleen (Case 15). No operation was undertaken in 3 (Cases 5, 6, and 12); these children were not severely ill, and conservative treatment seemed advisable. One of these children (Case 12) is having recurrent mild symptoms and may eventually require exploration.

TABLE 3

TREATMENT IN 15 CASES OF PANCREATITIS IN CHILDREN

| No. of Cases | Treatment |
|---|---|
| 4 | Sphincterotomy and cholecystectomy (1 later had subtotal gastrectomy) |
| 2 | Drainage of lesser sac |
| 1 | Sphincterotomy and cyst gastrostomy |
| 1 | Sphincterotomy and cholecystectomy; later partial pancreatectomy |
| 1 | Cholecystostomy, removal of gall-stones; later cyst marsupialization |
| 1 | Roux-en-Y cyst jejunostomy |
| 1 | Cyst gastrostomy |
| 1 | Resection of tail with ruptured spleen |
| 3 | No operation |

### Case Reports

The following case reports are presented in order of occurrence from 1956 to 1964. Cases 1, 2, 4, 5, and 7 were treated at the Children's Hospital, Boston; Cases 6, 8, 9, 10, 11, 12, 13, 14, and 15 were treated on the Children's Service of the Massachusetts General Hospital; Case 3 was treated as a child at the Children's Hospital, and later as a young adult at the Massachusetts General Hospital.

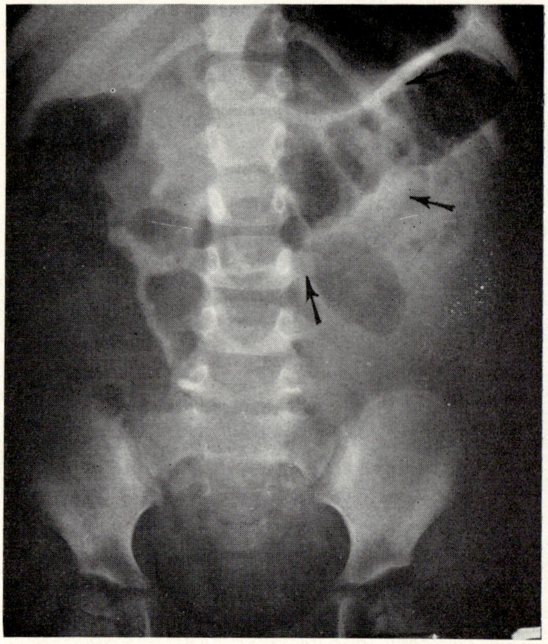

FIG. 2.—Abdominal film from Case 1, before operation, showing dilated loops of intestine and a suggestion of an epigastric mass that proved to be an enlarged, inflamed pancreas.

**Case 1.** S.W., a 6-year-old white girl, was admitted on January 3, 1956 with a three-day history of pain in the upper abdomen, nausea, and vomiting. Past history was negative except for a known congenital hip dislocation and coarctation of the aorta. There was diffuse upper abdominal tenderness and spasm; palpation suggested a mid-epigastric mass of considerable size. Temperature 102° F. (38·9° C.); pulse 140 min.; blood pressure 140/40 mm. Hg in left arm. Leucocyte count, 26,000. Abdominal film (Fig. 2) suggested a mass in the upper abdomen. After preliminary hydration, exploratory laparotomy (W.H.H.) revealed typical acute haemorrhagic pancreatitis with fat necrosis. There were 300 ml. of serous fluid in the abdominal cavity; amylase determination on this fluid 1,729 Somogyi units. There was discoloration, induration, and oedema of the entire pancreas. The gall-bladder was small, easily compressible; no stones were felt. Two large drains were placed in the lesser omental bursa; they were removed 10 days later. The serum amylase was 166 Somogyi units (normal value under 150) the day after the operation and was 192 one week later. After the operation the patient made an uneventful recovery and was discharged two weeks later with no further drainage. She was readmitted to the hospital in December 1956 for resection of coarctation of the thoracic aorta (W.H.H.). She is at present alive and well; there have been no further episodes of abdominal pain.

**Case 2.** W.C., a 13-year-old white boy, was admitted on September 4, 1956 with severe upper abdominal pain,

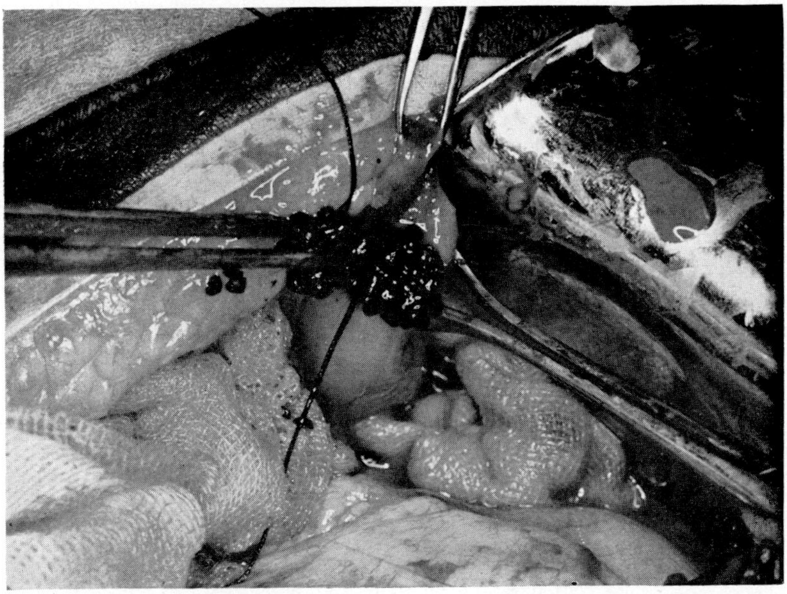

FIG. 3.—Multiple pigmented stones being removed from the gall-bladder in Case 2 at initial emergency operation. The patient had congenital hereditary spherocytosis. Pancreatitis was caused, presumably, by temporary impaction of a stone in the ampulla.

vomiting, and diarrhoea of three days' duration. His past history included congenital haemolytic anaemia, for which his father and sister had undergone splenectomy; operation had been refused for this child. He was in shock; there was diffuse tenderness of the upper abdomen; jaundice was evident; the spleen was palpable 6 cm. below the costal margin. Leucocyte count of 40,000; haematocrit 63%; serum amylase 605 Somogyi units; bilirubin 5 mg./100 ml. direct (0·4 normal) and 21·5 mg./100 ml. indirect (0·4 normal). After treatment of shock by hydration and transfusion, exploratory laparotomy (Dr. Lester Martin) revealed 1,500 ml. of serous fluid in the peritoneal cavity; the pancreas was diffusely inflamed and swollen. Two large drains were placed in the lesser sac. The gall-bladder was opened, removing numerous pigment stones (Fig. 3) and inserting a cholecystostomy tube. The patient's condition was thought too precarious to explore the common bile-duct for a stone in the ampulla. After the operation his course was very stormy with a large amount of necrotic debris in the drainage from the lesser sac. Two weeks later dye was instilled into the biliary tree through the cholecystostomy tube, and flowed freely into the duodenum with no evidence of a common duct stone; it was thought that a stone had probably been present but that it had passed into the duodenum. The cholecystostomy tube was clamped three weeks later and then removed. Gastro-intestinal series four weeks later showed widening of the duodenal loop and displacement of the stomach consistent with a pseudocyst (Fig. 4). On October 3, 1956 he was again operated on and the spleen was removed; the pseudocyst wall was thin, not suitable for anastomosis to the gastro-intestinal tract, and it was treated by

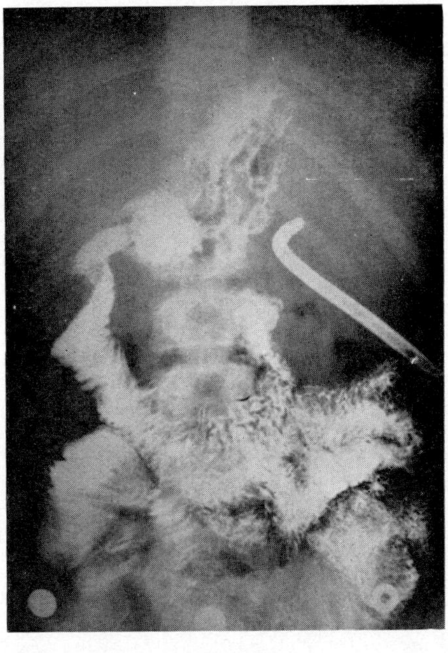

FIG. 4.—Gastro-intestinal series in Case 2 four weeks after initial laparotomy. The duodenal loop is wide and there is a pseudocyst in the lesser sac displacing the stomach anteriorly and to the right. A rubber tube lies in the lesser sac, replacing one of the simple drains placed at first operation. Cyst was subsequently marsupialized to surface.

marsupialization with large drains to the surface. Drainage continued for 9 months and then ceased spontaneously. He is at present a college student and free of abdominal complaints.

This boy was precariously ill with severe pancreatitis. It was felt that lesser sac drainage and biliary decompression were probably life saving, and that conservative, non-operative treatment would probably have ended fatally. It is difficult to know in retrospect whether expeditious duodenotomy and gentle exploration of the ampulla for a stone might have been wise at initial exploration. It seemed to be unwise under the circumstances to perform classical common duct exploration with blind probing of the ampulla from above with dilators and stone forceps in the face of severe pancreatitis.

**Case 3.** R.P., a 12-year-old white boy, was admitted on October 2, 1956 with a history of several months' duration of anorexia, fever, weight loss, and recurrent upper abdominal pain radiating to the back and between the scapulae. There was slight tenderness in the upper abdomen; bowel sounds were diminished, the abdomen was distended. During two weeks of observation symptoms improved. Gastro-intestinal series was negative. Serum amylase determination was 194 Somogyi units. Bilirubin, alkaline phosphatase, and leucocyte count were normal. Laparotomy on October 17, 1956 (Dr. Nicholas M. Stahl) disclosed that the gall-bladder was large but emptied on compression; that the pancreas was enlarged and nodular; and that there were inflammatory adhesions at the foramen of Winslow. Three days later serum amylase was 358. The patient was treated with a bland diet, antispasmodics, and sedation, but abdominal pain continued. He was admitted to the Massachusetts General Hospital on July 15, 1961. Exploration (Dr. Marshall K. Bartlett) showed that the entire pancreas was enlarged and oedematous, especially the head; there was adjacent fat necrosis; large varices up to 1 cm. in diameter were found near the common bile-duct; pressure in a varix was measured at 15 cm. of saline. The bile-duct, ampulla, and main pancreatic duct orifice were explored and found to be normal. Cholecystectomy and sphincterotomy were performed; pancreatography was thought to be unwise in the presence of active chronic pancreatitis. The patient's symptoms did not change and he was re-explored January 31, 1962. The pancreas was large and nodular. Pressure in the right gastro-epiploic vein was 30 cm. of saline; the spleen was four times enlarged. Subtotal gastrectomy with vagotomy was performed, restoring continuity with an anticolic Hofmeister gastrojejunostomy. Though improved, the patient continues to have brief attacks of abdominal pain which improve with temporary fasting.

It is contemplated that he will need further pancreatic surgery and probably a decompressive shunt operation for portal hypertension in the future. Pancreatography might prove useful in this case to exclude ductile obstruction amenable to caudal pancreatico-jejunostomy.

**Case 4.** K.G., a 6-month-old white girl with fever and ascites of three days' duration was admitted by Dr. Robert Haggerty on June 5, 1959. Although previously well, she developed a temperature of 102° F. (38·9° C.) and irritability 8 days before. Paracentesis revealed serous fluid with a specific gravity of 1·015, containing many erythrocytes and leucocytes; a cell block for microscopy was negative for tumour cells. On rigid dietary sodium restriction she lost ground steadily; exploration June 26 (W.H.H.) revealed 800 ml. of serous fluid in the peritoneal cavity; amylase determination was 182 Somogyi units on this fluid (normal under 150). There was diffuse inflammation throughout the upper abdomen, especially at the base of the transverse mesocolon and in the porta hepatis, all consistent with pancreatitis. Pressure in the portal vein was normal (8 cm. of saline). After exploration the patient was treated with antibiotics and a diet low in sodium and fat, but she deteriorated, and was readmitted two months later with massive abdominal distension and wasting (Fig. 5 and 6). There was pitting oedema of the anterior abdominal wall. Neck veins were distended and there was pulsus paradoxicus. It was felt that the child would soon expire and that the over-all diagnosis was still unclear. Constrictive pericarditis in association with a systemic disorder was considered. On August 12, 1956 she was operated on again (W.H.H.). A small left anterior thoracotomy was made to exclude pericarditis; the pericardium was normal. There was no free fluid in the abdomen but there was a tremendous pseudocyst containing 1,000 ml. of murky brown fluid. Roux-en-Y cyst jejunostomy was carried out, followed by rapid convalescence. The patient is now a normal youngster with no apparent gastro-intestinal problems (Fig. 7).

Pancreatitis was not even considered originally in this child, and even after the findings at first operation we did

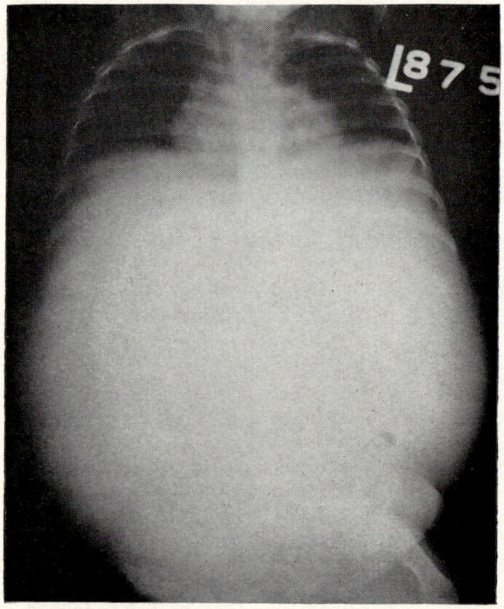


FIG. 5.—Plain film of abdomen in Case 4 before second operation, interpreted as ascites. At second operation no free fluid was found in abdomen; this was fluid in a huge pseudocyst.

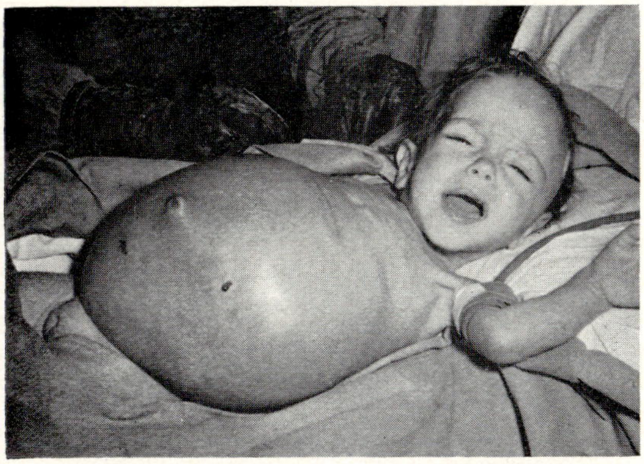

Fig. 6.—Case 4 just before second operation. The child was very wasted and had enormous abdominal distension caused by a pseudocyst; it was drained by Roux-en-Y cyst jejunostomy.

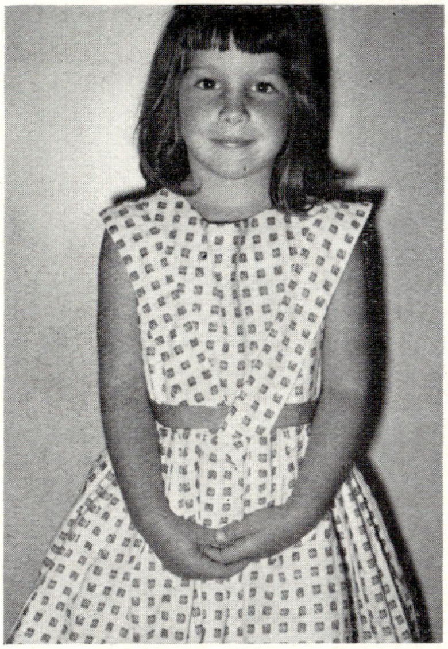

Fig. 7.—Case 4 five years after cyst jejunostomy. She is a healthy child with no pancreatic problems. The aetiology of her pancreatitis is not known.

not suspect development of a pseudocyst. In retrospect common duct exploration, transduodenal sphincterotomy, and pancreatography might have proved quite helpful at initial exploration. This may be a case with obstructive pancreatitis relieved by retrograde drainage via the pseudocyst into the gastro-intestinal tract.

**Case 5.** C.K., a 4-year-old white girl, was admitted on March 20, 1960, with vomiting and severe upper abdominal pain for one day; mumps appeared three days previously. There was pronounced upper abdominal tenderness with spasm; bowel sounds were diminished. The serum amylase was 344 Somogyi units. Two serum lipase determinations were normal. Leucocyte count 12,000. The patient's tenderness subsided gradually; she was discharged four days later perfectly well, and has had no further difficulty.

Though mild pancreatitis is not rare in association with mumps (Bole and Thompson, 1958), this is the only case we have seen in the past 9 years.

**Case 6.** L.A., a 3-year-old negro boy, entered the hospital on August 6, 1961 with swelling of the abdomen, hands, and feet for one day. These abnormalities were noted when he was received by his third set of foster parents. There was a history of serious family problems and possible maltreatment. His abdomen was protuberant, but he was not in acute distress (Fig. 8). There was a palpable fluid wave and minimal tenderness to deep palpation of the epigastrium. Normal values were obtained for alkaline phosphatase, transaminase, blood sugar, blood urea nitrogen, prothrombin time, serum electrolytes, cephalin flocculation, serum electrophoresis, bromsulphalein retention test, intravenous pyelogram, barium enema, and upper gastro-intestinal series. Leucocyte count 12,150. Paracentesis revealed serous fluid on which amylase determination was 2,480 Russell units (normal 4-25), and lipase determination 41·2 units per ml. (normal less than 2 units per ml.). The serum amylase and lipase values were normal. Morphine-prostigmine provocative test was normal. During 4 weeks of observation the abdominal protuberance subsided, tenderness disappeared, and there has been no recurrence.

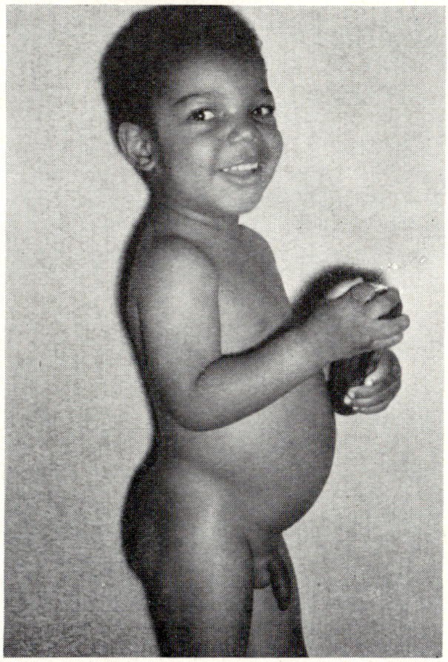

Fig. 8.—Case 6 two weeks after admission showing abdomen filled with fluid, but the child was not ill. The fluid disappeared spontaneously and he has done well during continued observation.

It is not certain that this child had pancreatitis, though this diagnosis seems reasonable with upper abdominal tenderness and ascites containing high levels of pancreatic enzymes. The aetiology is unknown; maltreatment is possible, but this is speculative.

**Case 7.** D.M., a 3-month-old white infant boy, was admitted June 26, 1961 for vomiting since 1 month of age. He was premature and while being fed by gavage there was no problem. When he reached 5 lb. (2,267 g.) weight he began having oral feeds, and vomiting occurred and continued. Two gastro-intestinal x-ray series were negative but the third demonstrated a sliding hiatus hernia. Conservative treatment was poorly tolerated; prolonged vomiting resulted in lethargy and hypoglycaemia (blood sugar 13 mg./100 ml.). After rehydration transabdominal hiatus herniorrhaphy was performed 5 days after admission (W.H.H.). The fundus of the stomach was incarcerated in the hiatus; it was reduced and repair was accomplished. The liver was abnormal, with greenish discoloration suggesting neonatal hepatitis; a biopsy was taken, which suggested cholangiolitis, possibly of bacterial origin. Two days after operation the infant became deeply jaundiced, distended, and finally moribund. Abdominal exploration was performed under local anaesthesia (W.H.H.), revealing murky abdominal fluid which contained Gram-positive cocci. There was fat necrosis at the root of the transverse mesocolon. The pancreas was oedematous and indurated; the gall-bladder was tense, and was decompressed with a tube. The lesser omental bursa was drained widely; a decompressive gastrostomy tube was placed in the stomach. Serum amylase 106 Somogyi units; peritoneal fluid amylase was 26·4. After an initially precarious post-operative course the child recovered and has thrived subsequently with no further illness and no vomiting.

In retrospect we believe that this child may have been at the onset of septicaemia when he was first operated on, complicating dehydration and starvation, and that pancreatitis may have been just a part of a generalized infection. Trauma to the tail of the pancreas during hiatus hernia repair may have been a factor, but with the liver biopsy report and the over-all clinical picture together with bacteria in the peritoneal fluid we favoured sepsis.

**Case 8.** R.H., a 2½-year-old white girl, was admitted on November 5, 1961 with recurrent upper abdominal pain and jaundice for 3 months. Leucocyte count 13,700; alkaline phosphatase 36·3 Bodansky units (5-14 normal); transaminase 143 (10-40 normal); bilirubin 5·4 mg./100 ml. (0·7 normal); serum amylase 72 Russell units (4-25 normal). Oral and intravenous cholangiography showed non-filling of the gall-bladder. An upper gastro-intestinal series showed indentation of the duodenal bulb, presumably by a distended gall-bladder (Fig. 9). Exploration was performed (W.H.H.). The gall-bladder was distended and the common duct was very dilated. On opening the duodenum a prominent ampulla of Vater (Fig. 10) was found in which there appeared to be no opening. The common bile-duct was opened, and a probe was passed down into the ampulla demonstrating a pin-point orifice through which the smallest probe would not pass. Sphincterotomy was performed. The orifice of the duct of Wirsung was normal; pancreatography was not carried out because there was induration and oedema of the pancreas suggesting active pancreatitis. The patient has had no further abdominal pain or jaundice and is completely well now 2½ years after operation.

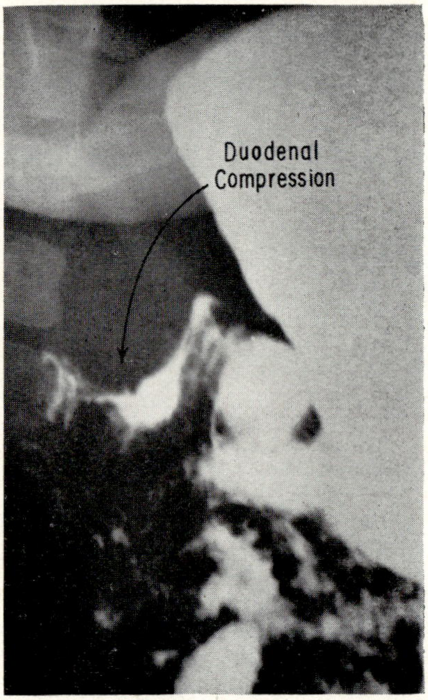

FIG. 9.—Gastro-intestinal x-ray in Case 8 showing compression of the duodenum by the gall-bladder. At operation the gall-bladder was large and the common bile-duct was quite dilated. Obstruction was found in the ampulla of Vater.

Congenital malformation of the sphincter of Oddi appears responsible in this case for both obstructive jaundice and pancreatitis.

**Case 9.** S.D., a 15-year-old white boy, was admitted on December 9, 1961 one hour after a blow to the left upper abdomen playing football. At operation (Dr. Chester J. Dexter) a ruptured spleen was removed. There was no other intra-abdominal injury . The post-operative course was complicated with vomiting and fever; serum amylase rose to 240 Russell units. No abdominal mass appeared and the patient was discharged three weeks later to be observed for the possibility of a post-traumatic pseudocyst. Shortly after discharge severe upper abdominal pain developed and he was readmitted; serum amylase determination was 610 Russell units. Gastro-intestinal x-ray one week later showed a large mass displacing the stomach anteriorly (Fig. 11). At re-exploration on January 13, 1962 (C.J.D.) a pseudocyst containing 4,000 ml. of clear yellow fluid was anastomosed to the posterior wall of the stomach. The patient made an uneventful recovery and has done well since.

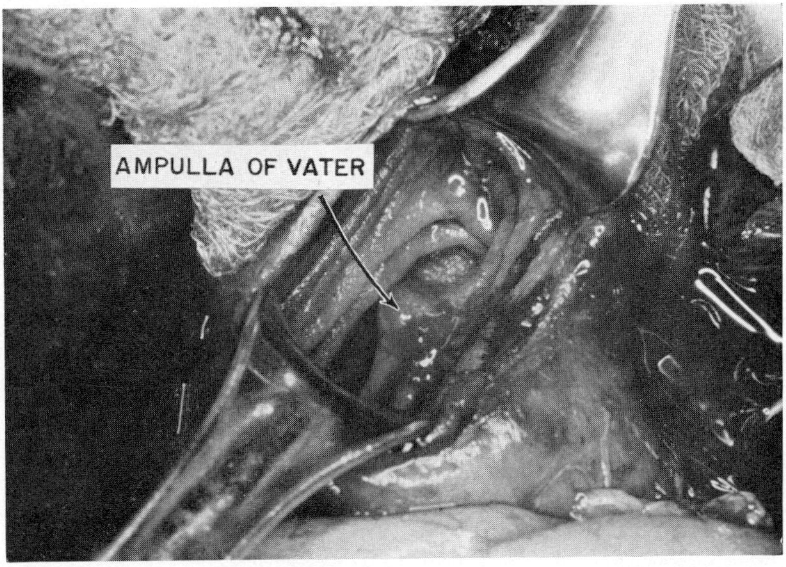


FIG. 10.—Operative view in Case 8 showing the enlarged, polypoid ampulla of Vater; the drainage orifice was found to be a pin-point opening. There was also pancreatitis, probably secondary to obstruction of the ampulla into which the duct of Wirsung drained. Sphincterotomy was performed; the child has had no further jaundice or abdominal pain.

This case is a clear-cut example of pancreatic trauma resulting in pseudocyst formation and serves to emphasize that delayed pancreatic complications should be considered following upper abdominal trauma in any age-group. A baseline amylase determination is desirable in children with upper abdominal trauma; the pancreas should be inspected routinely if exploration is performed (see also Case 15).

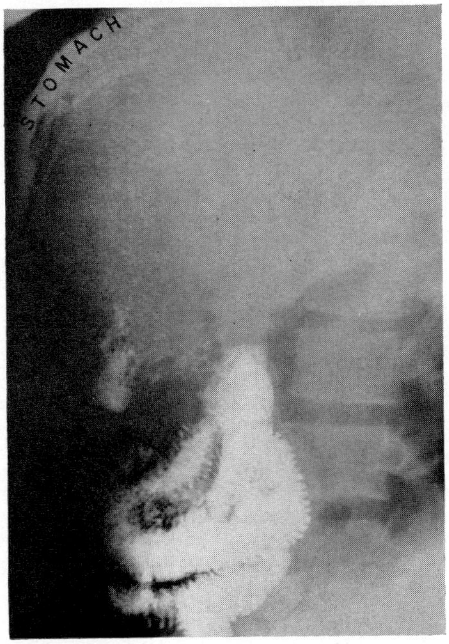


FIG. 11.—Gastro-intestinal x-ray from Case 9 four weeks after removal of traumatically ruptured spleen. This large pseudocyst was anastomosed to the back wall of the stomach.

**Case 10.** N.S., a 7-year-old white girl, was admitted on February 23, 1962 with upper abdominal pain and vomiting for one day. There had been several similar attacks in the previous two years. Past history included resection of a coarctation of the thoracic aorta at the age of 4. There was tenderness in the epigastrium and right upper quadrant. Normal values were obtained for the leucocyte count, serum amylase, bilirubin, and alkaline phosphatase. Gastro-intestinal x-rays showed slight displacement of the duodenum by the gall-bladder. Intravenous cholangiogram showed satisfactory function of the gall-bladder, though it appeared slightly enlarged. The child's pain and tenderness disappeared and she was discharged a week after admission. One week later she re-entered with the same complaints, and on this occasion a morphine-prostigmine provocative test was performed (5 mg. morphine and 0·3 mg. prostigmine) with abnormal findings: fasting amylase 17 Russell units; 1 hour, 96; 3 hours, 275; 5 hours, 208. Lipase values were also raised. The test produced the pain noted by the patient on admission. Repeat cholangiography showed an enlarged gall-bladder with dye remaining at 48 hours. It was felt that the clinical picture was consistent with mild recurrent pancreatitis with ampullary obstruction and exploration was performed on March 12, 1962 (W.H.H.). There was oedema adjacent to the head of the pancreas which was indurated. There were adhesions surrounding the gall-bladder. The common bile-duct was thought slightly

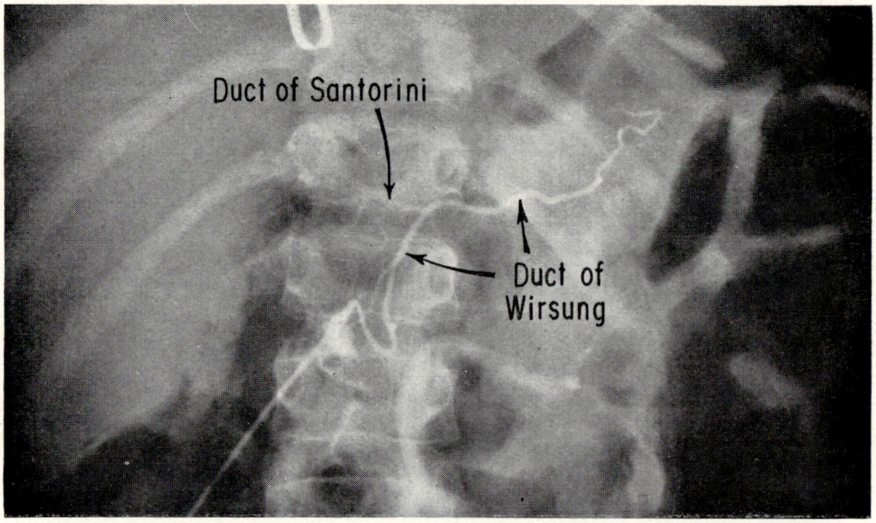


FIG. 12.—Pancreatogram obtained after transduodenal sphincterotomy in Case 10. The ducts are normal. The ampulla was stenotic.

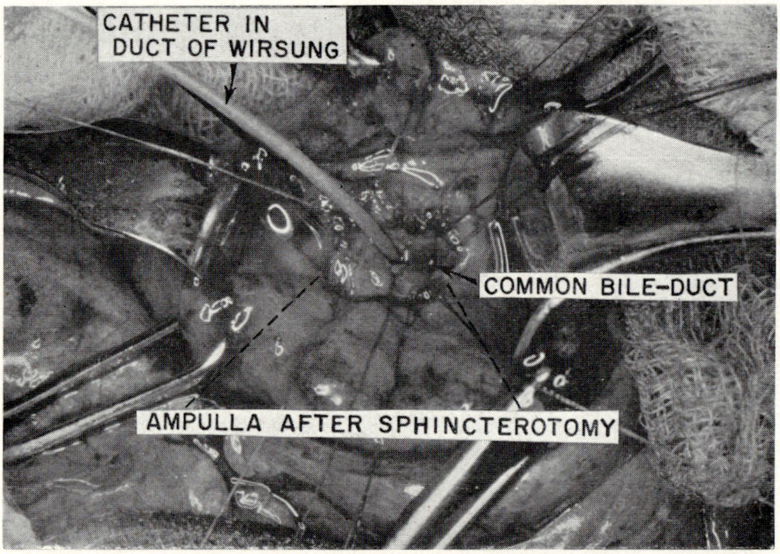


FIG. 13.—Case 10 showing operative findings during a typical transduodenal sphincterotomy. The ampulla has been incised upwards from the drainage orifice, suturing mucosa of the ampulla to mucosa of duodenum. (These sutures have been left long for traction to facilitate exposure.) A small catheter is seen in the duct of Wirsung for pancreatography. The lower common bile-duct is visible just craniad to the pancreatic duct orifice.

dilated for this age, measuring 8 mm. in diameter. The duodenum was opened and a 1 mm. probe was found to be very tight in the orifice of the sphincter of Oddi. Sphincterotomy was performed and bile gushed from the ampulla. The orifice of the duct of Wirsung was situated 3 mm. from the lower rim of the ampulla. The orifice was enlarged by operation, a ureteral catheter was inserted; a pancreatogram (Figs. 12 and 13) was normal. The gall-bladder was removed. Microscopical examination of the ampulla showed chronic inflammation with fibrosis. A post-operative morphine-prostigmine test revealed a flat curve with no rise in amylase levels in contrast to two pre-operative tests (Fig. 14). A week after discharge the patient developed acute intestinal obstruction which proved to be due to a small bowel intussusception which was reduced at laparotomy. There were two brief admissions 2 months and 8 months later for alleged abdominal pain, but there were no

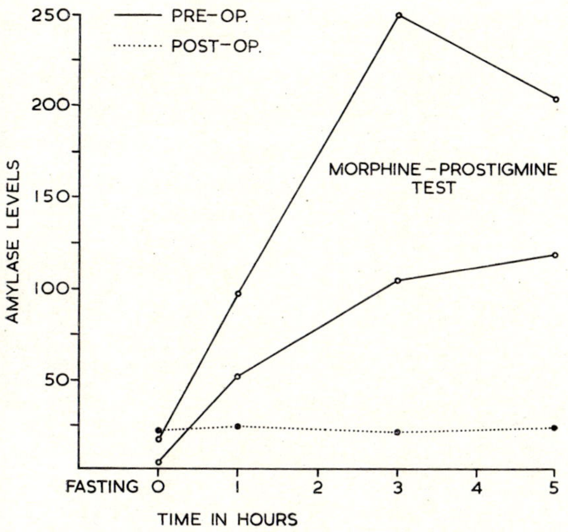


FIG. 14.—Morphine-prostigmine provocative test in Case 10. The two high curves were obtained before operation, showing a marked rise in serum amylase values. The flat curve was obtained following transduodenal sphincterotomy of the stenotic ampulla of Vater.

abnormal physical findings or laboratory determinations, and it was felt by all observers that this was a psychological attention-seeking reaction to the birth of a new sib. During the past year and a half there has been no further trouble.

We believe that this child had mild recurring pancreatitis caused by obstruction at the ampulla of Vater. The pre-operative and post-operative morphine-prostigmine provocative tests, together with the operative findings, and the pathology report, as well as the subsequent clinical course, tend to support this contention.

**Case 11.** E.P., an 11-month-old white infant boy, was admitted by Dr. John Robey on April 25, 1962 with fever and ascites. Two weeks before, the child had developed diarrhoea, abdominal pain, and then abdominal swelling three days before admission. He was irritable and febrile. There was impressive abdominal distension with a palpable fluid wave. The liver and spleen were not felt. Leucocyte count was 6,800; haematocrit 23%. Blood urea nitrogen, serum electrolytes, transaminase, alkaline phosphatase, and total protein showed normal values. The serum amylase was 280 Russell units. Paracentesis yielded bloody fluid (haematocrit 13%) with an amylase value of 1,560 Russell units. Two days later exploration (W.H.H.) revealed about 1,000 ml. of bloody fluid which was removed from the peritoneal cavity. There was abundant fat necrosis in the greater omentum and at the root of the transverse mesocolon. There was oedema of the structures at the porta hepatis. No gall-stones were felt. The pancreas was only slightly enlarged and slightly oedematous, much less impressive than anticipated. Fat necrosis was maximal near the tail of the pancreas. Two large drains were placed in the lesser sac. The serum amylase determination was 62 two days later. The patient convalesced uneventfully and was discharged 11 days after exploration, only to be readmitted 10 days later with acute intestinal obstruction which did not improve with gastro-intestinal intubation. At laparotomy (W.H.H.) a single stout band was found obstructing the terminal ileum; there was considerable fat necrosis at the site of this peritoneal band. The patient was readmitted on June 18, 1962 at the age of 13 months for elective reinvestigation. Morphine-prostigmine provocative test (2·4 mg. morphine and 0·24 mg. prostigmine) was abnormal: fasting amylase 21 Russell units; 2 hours, 172; 4 hours, 130. An intravenous cholangiogram was normal. It was decided to re-explore the patient to exclude obstruction as the cause for pancreatitis (W.H.H.). The pancreas was firm and enlarged to at least twice its normal size; the gall-bladder was surrounded by adhesions. On opening the duodenum the orifice of the ampulla appeared normal, but a probe met a point of obstruction 6 mm. from the tip of the ampulla; sphincterotomy revealed marked fibrotic narrowing of the midportion of the ampulla. The main pancreatic duct opening was located exactly at this point of fibrotic narrowing. The pancreatic duct orifice was enlarged by operation, releasing clear pancreatic juice. Pancreatogram was attempted, but the film appeared to show extravasation of dye, and so a second injection was not performed at that site. The accessory duct of Santorini orifice was located 3 cm. proximal in the duodenum, and a pancreatogram of this duct revealed a normal duct system out into the tail of the pancreas. The gall-bladder was removed. Morphine-prostigmine provocative test was performed one week after operation: fasting, 37 Russell units; 2 hours, 232; 3 hours, 248. This test was repeated one month later: fasting, 15; 1 hour, 130; 2 hours, 136. This patient has done well since discharge.

This appears to be a case in which an anomaly of the ampulla caused the pancreatitis. In retrospect the first exploration might have been avoided, since the diagnosis seemed fairly certain and the patient was not deteriorating. The two post-operative morphine-prostigmine tests were abnormal but they were obtained in the early post-operative period. Further study of this child is contemplated. It is of considerable interest that this boy's paternal grandfather has recently undergone exploration for obstructive jaundice, found to be due to pancreatitis. Additional delving into the family history has revealed an uncle with pancreatic calcification discovered incidentally during radiological examination, and that the father has post-prandial epigastric pain. This boy may be an example of hereditary pancreatitis.

**Case 12.** J.M., an 11-year-old white boy, was admitted on September 5, 1962 with vomiting and abdominal pain radiating to the back for two days. There was upper abdominal tenderness. He had had splenectomy three years before for hereditary spherocytosis. Leucocyte count 12,200. Normal values were obtained for serum amylase, bilirubin, transaminase, alkaline phosphatase, cephalin flocculation, and thymol turbidity. Gastro-intestinal series and oral cholecystogram were normal.

A morphine-prostigmine provocative test was abnormal: fasting amylase, 16 Russell units; 45 minutes, 100; 1½ hours, 360; 2½ hours, 580; a repeat test was confirmatory; the tests provoked his abdominal pain. This child was not clinically ill and it was decided to follow his course. He has continued to have mild episodes of mid-epigastric pain radiating to the back and further study is contemplated. We suspect that he may have obstructive pancreatitis of mild degree.

**Case 13.** W.C., a 5-year-old white boy, was admitted on March 19, 1963 with abdominal pain and a mid-epigastric mass. He had been well until three months before when he developed recurrent dull upper abdominal pain. Exploratory laparotomy three weeks before had revealed subsiding acute haemorrhagic pancreatitis. Three days before admission pain had recurred, a mass was discovered, and he was referred for further evaluation. There was a large, slightly tender upper abdominal mass. Normal values were obtained for Van den Bergh, alkaline phosphatase, cephalin flocculation, bromsulphalein retention, transaminase, and leucocyte count. The fasting serum amylase determination was normal (24 Russell units), but morphine-prostigmine provocation resulted in an abnormal rise: 1 hour, 61; 2 hours, 138; 3 hours, 142; no pain was evoked by the test. Exploration was planned but the patient developed an upper respiratory infection and was discharged to be readmitted six weeks later. The mass had diminished, remaining as a small sausage-shaped mass. A repeat morphine-prostigmine provocative test was again abnormal: fasting serum amylase, 18 Russell units; 1 hour, 204; 2 hours, 700; 3 hours, 690; 5 hours, 520. Exploration on May 18 (Dr. Stephen E. Hedberg) revealed a cystic structure 5 cm. in diameter adjacent to the body of the pancreas. Probing of the ampulla of Vater revealed no stenosis. Sphincterotomy was performed to obtain a pancreatogram which showed a cystic structure communicating with the duct system. The gall-bladder was removed. The patient continued to have abdominal pain and was readmitted four months later; again a small upper abdominal mass was palpable. At operation on October 14, 1963 (S.E.H.) the cystic mass adjacent to the body of the pancreas was mobilized and found to be located at the tip of an accessory lobe of pancreas arising from the mid-portion of the tail of the pancreas (Fig. 15). Resection was easily accomplished; microscopic examination revealed a muscular wall lined with gastric epithelium with peptic ulceration. The patient has had no further difficulty since operation. This case has been reported previously in greater detail (Case Records of the Massachusetts General Hospital, 1964).

In retrospect it might have been better to attempt excision of this cystic gastric duplication at the second laparotomy, in view of the finding of a normal ampulla and lack of obstruction in the pancreatic duct system to account for recurring pancreatitis. There was no way to suspect that this was not a cyst of the pancreas proper, and it had been hoped to avoid excessive manipulation of the pancreas lest further inflammation be caused by operative trauma.

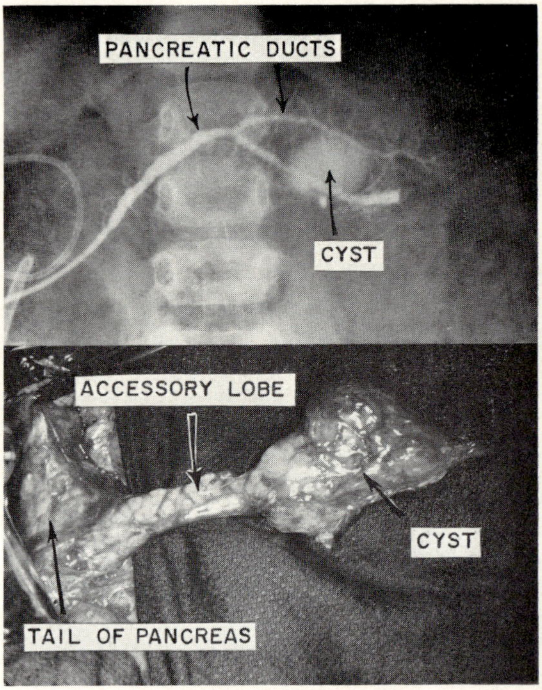


FIG. 15.—Operative findings in Case 13. A pancreatogram, showing a cyst-like structure communicating with the ducts in the tail of the pancreas. Though this 'cyst' communicated freely with the ducts, and sphincterotomy was performed, symptoms and the mass persisted. Lower half of figure shows findings at second operation. There was an accessory lobe arising from the tail of the pancreas. At the end of the accessory lobe lay a cyst-like structure which was lined with gastric mucosa; excision cured the patient.

**Case 14.** R.S., a 12-year-old white girl, was admitted on August 27, 1963 for severe weight loss and vomiting. Four months previously she had developed abdominal pain with vomiting and was explored elsewhere, with the finding of acute haemorrhagic pancreatitis. The serum amylase was reported at that time to be 625. After doing well for a short time, she developed recurrent abdominal pain, anorexia, vomiting, and severe weight loss. Leucocyte count, total protein, cholesterol, and bilirubin were all normal. The stool was strongly guiac positive. Fasting serum amylase determination was increased (204 Russell units). No pseudocyst was palpable; gastro-intestinal series suggested slight anterior displacement of the stomach. The patient was discharged after a week of observation, but was readmitted 2 months later because of further deterioration. She was very cachectic, weighing only 39 lb. (17·7 kg.) (Fig. 16); there was a palpable upper abdominal mass consistent with a pseudocyst. A morphine-prostigmine provocative test was performed: fasting amylase, 84 Russell units; ½ hour, 94; 1 hour, 92; 1½ hours, 94; 2 hours, 110; 3 hours, 90. Gastro-intestinal series showed a large mass behind the stomach. On March 22, 1963 exploration (W.H.H.) revealed a large pseudocyst in the lesser sac which was decompressed by

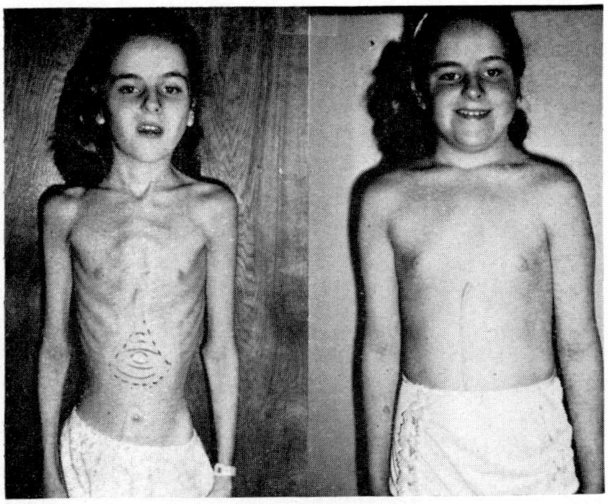

FIG. 16.—Pre- and post-operative photographs of Case 14, a 12-year-old girl. She weighed only 39 lb. (17·7 kg.), was emaciated, and the large epigastric mass outlined was palpable. Six months after transgastric anastomosis of her pseudocyst to the back of the stomach, her weight had doubled and she was well.

transgastric anastomosis to the posterior wall of the stomach, making a very large longitudinal opening between the cyst and the stomach. Sphincterotomy revealed a normal ampulla of Vater; the orifice of the duct of Wirsung was normal. Attempted pancreatogram showed apparent extravasation into the head of the pancreas, though it was thought that the dye could be in a dilated, distorted duct. The accessory pancreatic duct orifice was injected, demonstrating a normal duct of Santorini. The gall-bladder was removed. A Meckel's diverticulum was removed (thought to be the cause for the strongly guiac positive stool), and Ladd's procedure was performed for malrotation of the intestine. The child has done extremely well since operation, with impressive weight gain, and she is now perfectly well.

The aetiology of pancreatitis in this case is not known. The ampulla of Vater and both pancreatic duct orifices were normal. Pancreatography suggested that there might be an abnormality of the pancreatic duct system but we could not be certain that the dye shadow did not represent extravasation.

**Case 15.** L.J., a 9-year-old white boy, was admitted by Dr. Murrary Rosenthal on June 16, 1964 for observation after abdominal trauma from an automobile accident. There was slight upper abdominal tenderness; blood pressure was 110/70 mm. Hg, pulse 88/min. Haematocrit 35%; leucocyte count 10,100. Serum amylase, 7 Russell units. A plain abdominal film suggested slight displacement of the stomach. Though rupture of the spleen was considered possible, it was decided to observe the patient because his condition was completely stable and his tenderness was minimal. During the next 24 hours the haematocrit decreased to 29%, the leucocyte count rose to 12,000, and left upper abdominal tenderness became more marked. Exploration (W.H.H.) revealed 500 ml. of free intra-abdominal blood; there was a small laceration through the hilum of the spleen, filled with blood clot and not actively bleeding. There was considerable swelling and induration of the distal 2 in. of the tail of the pancreas adjacent to the spleen, with marked surrounding inflammatory reaction. The spleen was removed together with the contused part of the tail of the pancreas; the rest of the pancreas was completely normal. Amylase determination four days later was normal. The patient made an uneventful recovery.

Partial distal pancreatectomy appeared to be a reasonable manoeuvre in this patient, for it could be done with little additional risk and it may have prevented formation of a post-traumatic pseudocyst such as that encountered in Case 9.

## Discussion

Pancreatitis is a disease of variable aetiology and should be considered in children with either acute or chronic upper abdominal pain, in ascites of obscure aetiology, and following upper abdominal trauma. The serum amylase determination is helpful if raised, but the amylase value may fall rapidly to normal levels even in severe pancreatitis. Upper gastro-intestinal x-rays can be helpful in certain instances by showing deformity of the duodenum or compression of the stomach by a pseudocyst.

We believe that the morphine-prostigmine provocative test merits further trial in children. The physiological basis of this test rests on morphine-induced contraction of the sphincter of Oddi with concomitant stimulation of pancreatic secretion by prostigmine, causing a rise in the serum amylase value if the sphincter is abnormal. As shown in Case 13, the test can be positive under other circumstances. An increase of over three times the fasting amylase value is considered significant in adults; the test has not been used to our knowledge in childhood and we do not know what normal values should be in children. We have performed the test in a small number of children not suspected of having pancreatitis with no significant rise in amylase values. This test was performed in six patients in this series (Cases 6, 10, 11, 12, 13, and 14). In Case 6 the test was normal, and this child has had no further trouble. In Case 10 (Fig. 14) there was a marked rise in amylase levels before sphincterotomy, with a completely flat curve after sphincterotomy. The test was abnormal in Case 11 before operation, and also after it to a lesser extent, but the determination was made only shortly after the operation. A subsequent study is planned and it will be of interest to see whether it is different. The test was abnormal on three occasions in Case 12; this lad is continuing to have mild clinical difficulty; the test reproduces his pain which is suggestive of obstructive pancreatitis. The test was abnormal in Case 13 in which the pathology lay not at the ampulla but in a cystic duplication arising from an accessory lobe of the pancreas. The duplication had a muscular wall which may have contracted with morphine stimulation, producing a temporary rise in pancreatic duct pressures causing an increase in serum amylase values. It is of interest that the fasting amylase determination in Case 14, where no ampullary stenosis was found, was raised both before and after operation, but provocation did not result in a significant rise in the amylase value.

The role of surgical intervention in pancreatitis is variable. In mild cases where the diagnosis is certain and the patient is not dangerously ill emergency laparotomy is not necessary; initial treatment should be supportive, including stopping oral alimentation, nasogastric suction, antibiotics, an anticholinergic drug to suppress pancreatic secretion, a drug to relieve pain (not morphine), intravenous fluids and electrolytes, and occasionally calcium. Contrary to popular opinion, we believe that surgical exploration is indicated in certain cases of severely ill children; in some, laparotomy is necessary to confirm the diagnosis, because other conditions such as intestinal perforation can cause a marked rise in serum amylase values. If there is strong reason to suspect acute duct obstruction from a gall-stone, such as in Case 2, or by a worm, exploration of the common bile-duct, ampulla of Vater, and even pancreatic duct should be considered even in a very ill child to relieve total duct obstruction rather than treating such a patient supportively and risking a fatal outcome. In any patient who is severely ill we favour drainage of the lesser sac to remove the highly irritative enzymes which come forth from the inflamed pancreas; drainage may avert pseudocyst formation by evacuating such a collection (this did not prove to be true however in Case 2). Possible pseudocyst formation should be anticipated in any child after pancreatitis or after upper abdominal trauma. A thin-walled pseudocyst is probably treated best by marsupialization to the surface, though this has the disadvantage of pancreatic cutaneous fistula formation in some instances. Rarely, a cyst of the pancreas may be amenable to excision. Most pseudocysts are best drained into the adjacent stomach or by means of a Roux-en-Y loop of jejunum; it is important to make the anastomotic opening as large as possible to prevent spontaneous closure with reformation of the cyst. We believe that more attention should be focused on the ampulla of Vater and on the ductile system of the pancreas as visualized by pancreatography. Three children in this series have undergone elective exploration of the ampulla with relief following sphincterotomy. Finally, in surgical exploration for upper abdominal trauma, we think that the pancreas should be inspected routinely for lacerations or contusions. In an occasional case partial pancreatectomy may be indicated, such as Case 15. In rare instances suturing is necessary to stop bleeding or to reapproximate severed duct structures. All cases of pancreatic injury should be drained in anticipation of leakage of necrotizing digestive enzymes.

The clinical course following a severe attack of pancreatitis in childhood is variable. Case 1 has had no further trouble during 8½ years of follow-up. Blumenstock, Mithoefer, and Santulli (1957) reported a similar case with normal follow-up into adult life. In contrast we have in this series several children in whom there were serious sequelae requiring operation. We feel that a child should be watched carefully after an episode of acute pancreatitis; studies should include upper gastro-intestinal series, cholecystography and choledochography, and the morphine-prostigmine provocative test. In some cases transduodenal exploration of the ampulla and common bile-duct together with pancreatography will be rewarding. Sphincterotomy is not difficult. The duodenum is mobilized and opened through a vertical incision, exposing the ampulla; if a small probe cannot be passed into the ampulla from below, it is passed down into the ampulla from an opening in the common bile-duct. With a probe in the ampulla incision is made upward from the orifice, a little bit at a time, sewing the mucosa of the ampulla to the mucosa of the duodenum. Interrupted fine chromic cat gut sutures are used, placing gentle traction on the sutures to afford better exposure. No sutures are placed in the medial aspect of the ampulla or near the orifice of the ampulla until the opening of the duct of Wirsung is identified for certain, lest a suture be placed inadvertently through it. Administration of 'secretin' can stimulate pancreatic secretion as an aid in locating the duct orifices. If the incision in the ampulla is extended too far upward, there is danger of cutting through the back wall of the duodenum. Probing and manipulation of pancreatic ducts should be done very gently; pancreatography should be performed with great care; forceful injection is dangerous and can produce pancreatitis. Duodenal closure is done transversely to avert narrowing at the site. The gall-bladder is removed with sphincterotomy in the belief that opening the sphincter disturbs the physiological mechanism of gall-bladder emptying, which can result in stasis and stone formation.

## Summary

15 children with pancreatitis have been observed during the past 9 years, and the diverse aetiology,

variable course, and possible surgical sequelae of this condition have been outlined. All patients survived. It is concluded that pancreatitis may be more common in childhood than previously suspected, and that this condition should be considered in children with upper abdominal pain, ascites of acute onset, and after trauma.

We would like to express appreciation to the following for permission to report certain of these cases: Dr. Robert E. Gross, Cases 1 and 2 from the ward service of the Children's Hospital; Drs. Nicholas M. Stahl, J. Roswell Gallagher, Warren W. Point, and Marshall K. Bartlett, Case 3; Dr. Chester J. Dexter, Case 9; Drs. Anne P. Forbes and George L. Nardi, Case 14.

## References

Anderson, H. B. (1923). Acute pancreatitis in children: report of a case with cirrhosis of liver. *J. Amer. med. Ass.*, **80**, 1139.
Baar, H. S., and Wolff, O. H. (1957). Pancreatic necrosis in cortisone-treated children. *Lancet*, **1**, 812.
Blumenstock, D. A., Mithoefer, J., and Santulli, T. V. (1957). Acute pancreatitis in children. *Pediatrics*, **19**, 1002.
Blumenthal, H. T., and Probstein, J. G. (1961). Acute pancreatitis in the newborn, in infancy and in childhood. *Amer. Surgn*, **27**, 533.
Bole, G. G., Jr., and Thompson, O. W. (1958). Acute mumps pancreatitis. *Univ. Mich. med. Bull.*, **24**, 442.
Case Records of the Massachusetts General Hospital (1964). *New Engl. J. Med.*, **270**, 736.
Collins, J. (1958). Pancreatitis in young children. *Arch. Dis. Childh.*, **33**, 432.
Dobbs, R. H. (1935). Acute pancreatitis in childhood. *Lancet*, **2**, 989.
Fitz, R. H. (1889). Acute pancreatitis. *Med. Rec. (N.Y.)*, **35**, 197.
Frey, C., and Redo, S. F. (1963). Inflammatory lesions of the pancreas in infancy and childhood. *Pediatrics*, **32**, 93.
Gerber, B. C. (1963). Hereditary pancreatitis. *Arch. Surg.*, **87**, 70.
Gibson, J. M., and Gibson, J. M., Jr. (1956). Acute hemorrhagic pancreatitis in childhood. *J. Pediat.*, **48**, 486.
Gibson, L. E., and Haller, J. A. (1959). Acute pancreatitis associated with congenital cyst of the common bile duct. *ibid.*, **55**, 650.
Gross, J. B., and Comfort, M. W. (1957). Hereditary pancreatitis: report on two additional families. *Gastroenterology*, **32**, 829.
Gruenwald, P. (1950). Asphyxia, trauma, and shock at birth. *Arch. Pediat.*, **67**, 103.
Haigh, E. (1956). Acute pancreatitis in childhood. *Arch. Dis. Childh.*, **31**, 273.
Marczynska-Robowska, M. (1957). Pancreatic necrosis in a case of Still's disease. *Lancet*, **1**, 815.
Novis, T. S. (1923). Partial obstruction of the pancreatic duct by round-worms. *Brit. J. Surg.*, **10**, 421.
O'Brien, S. E. (1961). Adult surgical disorders encountered in children. *Canad. med. Ass. J.*, **84**, 530.
Oeconomopoulos, C. T., and Lee, C. M., Jr. (1960). Pseudocysts of the pancreas in infants and young children. *Surgery*, **47**, 836.
Oppenheimer, E. H., and Boitnott, J. K. (1960). Pancreatitis in children following adrenal cortico-steroid therapy. *Bull. Johns Hopk. Hosp.*, **107**, 297.
Pender, B. W. T. (1957). Acute pancreatitis in a child aged 3 years. *Lancet*, **1**, 409.
Plechas, N. P. (1960). Chronic recurrent pancreatitis in childhood. *Arch. Surg.*, **81**, 883.
Power, W. H. (1961). Pancreatic cyst in infancy: Recovery after marsupialization. *Brit. med. J.*, **2**, 625.
Shanklin, D. R. (1962). Pancreatic atrophy apparently secondary to hydrochlorothiazide. *New Engl. J. Med.*, **266**, 1097.
Steiner, M. M., and Tracy, P. C. (1943). Diabetic coma and pancreatitis and *Bacillus Welchii* peritonitis. *Amer. J. Dis. Child.*, **65**, 36.
Stickler, G. B., and Yonemoto, R. H. (1958). Acute pancreatitis in children. *Amer. J. Dis. Child.*, **95**, 206.
Warwick, W. J., and Leavitt, S. R. (1960). Chronic relapsing pancreatitis in childhood. *ibid.*, **99**, 648.

*Arch. Dis. Childh.*, 1965, **40**, 146.

# THE ROLE OF VENTRAL HERNIA IN THE CORRECTION OF DIAPHRAGMATIC DEFECTS IN THE NEWBORN*

BY

IRVING A. MEEKER, JR. and WILLIAM N. KINCANNON

*From the Department of Surgery, School of Medicine, University of Southern California, the Children's Hospital and the Los Angeles County Hospital, Los Angeles, California, and the Huntington Memorial Hospital, Pasadena, California, U.S.A.*

A disconcerting rise in mortality following surgical repair of a congenital diaphragmatic hernia in the newborn has been encountered in many centres in recent years and has prompted this study. Paradoxically this rise in surgical mortality has occurred despite greater surgical knowledge and experience in the correction of such diaphragmatic defects. The rise may be attributable to the increasing number of infants with congenital diaphragmatic defects being correctly diagnosed and undergoing surgery within hours after birth (Bonham Carter, Waterston, and Aberdeen, 1962).

This study concerns the value of ventral hernia in the successful surgical management of infants under 24 hours of age undergoing correction of their diaphragmatic defects.

In the past, following surgical correction of a diaphragmatic defect in a newborn infant, regardless of the age of the child, primary closure of all layers of the abdominal wall has been advocated and carried out wherever possible. Primary closure of the abdominal wall increases intra-abdominal tension (Ladd and Gross, 1940) and limits free excursion and movement of the diaphragm, thus perpetuating the impaired respiratory exchange that existed before operation. Increased intra-abdominal tension incident to primary wound closure may compress the inferior vena cava, reducing venous return to the right heart, causing inadequate tissue perfusion, potentiating tissue anoxia and acidosis (lactic acid accumulation) already established, further lowering arterial oxygen saturation and blood *p*H to lethal levels.

It was postulated that the increased mortality following surgical repair of diaphragmatic defects in infants under 24 hours of age might well be related to such increases in intra-abdominal tension following primary wound closure, and that the lethal physiological derangements that might ensue could be consistently and effectively combated by arbitrarily employing ventral hernia in such cases.

In addition to our experiences with ventral hernia after closure of a diaphragmatic defect, this report will include current adjunctive therapeutic considerations as regards pre- and post-operative management, with particular emphasis on the value of chest drainage and gastrostomy in such infants.

## Clinical Material

There are 38 consecutive, unselected infants in this study representing—regardless of associated congenital anomalies or other considerations—all cases accurately diagnosed or undergoing surgical repair of their congenital diaphragmatic defects during the first 24 hours of life from 1957 to 1963 at the Children's Hospital of Los Angeles, the Los Angeles County General Hospital, and the Huntington Memorial Hospital of Pasadena. These patients are divided into four main groups. *Group I:* 11 infants who died en route to the hospital, on admission, or shortly thereafter before an operation could be performed. *Group II:* 11 infants who had standard correction (Gross, 1953) of a diaphragmatic defect through a divided rectus muscle incision and a skin-covered ventral hernia created. *Group III:* 6 infants who had standard correction of the diaphragmatic defect through a paramedian incision and creation of ventral hernia with temporary closure. *Group IV:* 10 infants who had standard correction of the diaphragmatic defect followed by primary closure of all layers of the abdominal incision.

Table 1 documents the pertinent clinical data in the 27 surgical cases in Groups II, III, and IV.

In the 27 infants whose diaphragmatic defects were repaired, the type of abdominal wall closure selected in each instance was determined solely by the practice of the surgical service to which the child was admitted.

* A paper read at a meeting of the British Association of Paediatric Surgeons in Rotterdam, September 1964.

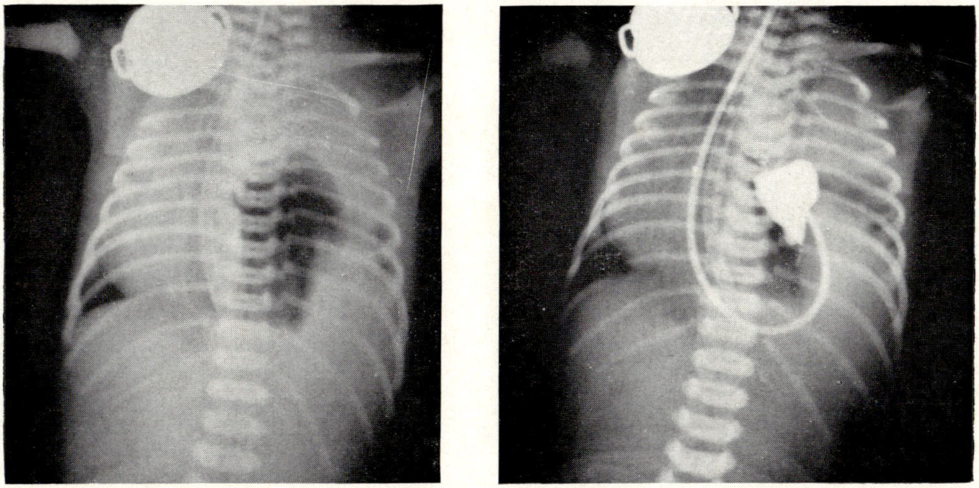

FIG. 1.—Portable radiographs of Case 5 showing the thorax (left) before instillation of 'dionosil oily' into the stomach and (right) 5 minutes after insertion of the oily media into the stomach.

No infant who had a heart beat and was still breathing was denied surgical repair, no matter how desperate the risk or the gravity of apparent central nervous system damage from prolonged anoxia. Of the 27 cases, 26 were full-term infants: the lone premature infant weighed 4 lb. 9 oz. (2,069 g.).

### Pre-operative Management

The impressively large number of infants dying or moribund during the first day of life and before correction indicates that any delay in diagnosis and surgical intervention may permit natural selection by 'survival of the fittest', and this may well have favourably affected over-all mortality statistics in the past when related to the present. To give as many infants as possible a chance for survival, surgical correction of the diaphragmatic defect must be done as soon as the child can be transported to an area where experienced anaesthetic and surgical personnel are available and appropriate operating facilities can be made ready.

A nasogastric tube is inserted into the stomach as soon as the diagnosis is made to prevent dilatation of the intestinal tract by swallowed air, which causes further compression of the lungs and impairment of pulmonary function. At all times this tube should be on continuous suction—or clamped during transport—to prevent the 'sucking' of large volumes of air into the stomach and intestine in the thorax with each respiratory movement.

If there is difficulty in differentiating a congenital diaphragmatic defect from other conditions affecting the lung and/or causing cyanosis, 5 to 10 ml. of 'lipiodol' or 'dionosil oily'* may be instilled through the tube into the stomach. With a diaphragmatic defect the contrast media will appear within 10 to 15 minutes in the gastro-intestinal tract within the thorax and can be noted easily on portable radiograph of the chest (Fig. 1), thus confirming the diagnosis in the deeply cyanotic infant with a sometimes equivocal chest film.

During the brief interim before surgical correction, the head and chest of such infants should be raised 30 degrees and the baby placed on the side of the diaphragmatic defect in an effort to improve function of the contralateral lung. If the infant's condition deteriorates rapidly before operating facilities are available, an anaesthetist should administer oxygen by mask or through an endotracheal tube, assisting respirations gently, assiduously avoiding increases in positive pressure that might cause spontaneous rupture of a bleb on the lung. If no improvement results, emergency reduction of the viscera from the chest through a 10 cm. divided rectus muscle incision may have to be carried out without waiting for more favourable circumstances. If cardiac arrest should occur, external compression of the thorax as described by Mathews, Avery, and Jude (1963) is most effective in managing this complication, once an adequate airway and supply of oxygen have been provided.

The intravenous administration of sodium bicarbonate or amine buffers (Tris, THAM) suggested by the studies of Kaplan (1962) and Kaplan, Fox, and

* Glaxo Laboratories, Ltd., Greenford, Middlesex, England.

TABLE 1
DATA ON 27 SURGICAL CASES

| Case No. | Age at Operation (hr.) | Viscera in Chest | Lung Aplasia | Major Assoc. Anomaly | Ladd's Bands | Gastros-tomy | Post-operative Result |
|---|---|---|---|---|---|---|---|
| | | | *Divided Rectus Incision, Ventral Hernia (Group II)* | | | | |
| 1 | 6 | GI, Sp, L | Agenesis | + | 0 | 0 | Died at 3 hr. |
| 2 | 18 | GI, Sp, L | 0 | 0 | + | + | Cured |
| 3 | 9 | GI | 0 | 0 | 0 | + | Cured |
| 4 | 7 | GI | 0 | 0 | + | + | Cured |
| 5 | 6 | GI, Sp, S, L | 0 | 0 | 0 | + | Cured |
| 6 | 12 | GI, Sp | X-ray | + | + | + | Cured |
| 7 | 6 | GI, Sp | Lt.-13 g. Rt.-8 g. | + | + | + | Died at 12 hr. |
| 8 | 7 | GI, Sp, S | 0 | 0 | + | + | Cured |
| 9 | 15 | GI, Sp, S | 0 | 0 | 0 | 0 | Cured |
| 10 | 23 | GI, L | Lt.-12 g. Rt.-4 g. | + | + | + | Died at 18 hr. |
| 11 | 4 | GI, Sp, L | X-ray | 0 | + | + | Cured |
| | | | *Paramedian Incision, Ventral Hernia (Group III)* | | | | |
| 12 | 12 | GI | 0 | 0 | 0 | 0 | Cured |
| 13 | 14 | GI, Sp, S | 0 | 0 | + | 0 | Cured |
| 14 | 12 | GI, Sp, S | 0 | 0 | 0 | 0 | Died at 1 hr. |
| 15 | 4 | GI, Sp, S | 0 | 0 | 0 | 0 | Died at 50 hr. |
| 16 | 10 | GI, Sp | Small bronchus | 0 | 0 | + | Died at 12 hr. |
| 17 | 13 | GI, Sp, S | X-ray | + | 0 | + | Died at 36 hr. |
| | | | *Primary Abdominal Wall Closure, No Hernia (Group IV)* | | | | |
| 18 | 8 | GI, Sp, S | 0 | 0 | 0 | 0 | Died at 40 hr. |
| 19 | 14 | GI, Sp | 0 | 0 | 0 | 0 | Died at 50 hr. |
| 20 | 10 | GI, L | Rt.-12 g. | 0 | + | + | Died at 1 hr. |
| 21 | 8 | GI, Sp, S | Lt.-12 g. | 0 | 0 | 0 | Died at 60 hr. |
| 22 | 13 | GI, Sp, S | Lt.-14 g. | 0 | 0 | 0 | Died at 36 hr. |
| 23 | 11 | GI, Sp, S | 0 | 0 | + | 0 | Died at 3 hr. |
| 24 | 4 | GI, L | 0 | 0 | + | + | Died at 36 hr. |
| 25 | 15 | GI | Lt.-13 g. | + | 0 | 0 | Died at 24 hr. |
| 26 | 4 | GI, Sp | 0 | 0 | + | 0 | Lived |
| 27 | 7 | GI, Sp | 0 | 0 | + | 0 | Died at 17 hr. |

GI = small bowel and colon; Sp = spleen; S = stomach; L = liver; g. = gram.

Clark (1962) to correct a low blood *p*H at the time of admission, should be deferred until assisted respiration has been given an adequate opportunity to reduce the $Pco_2$. Sodium bicarbonate, though initially helpful in raising a low blood *p*H, may subsequently contribute to a rise in the $Pco_2$ and deepening of the acidosis as in Cases 15 and 16 (Table 1). For this reason amine buffers are preferred when available.

### Surgical Considerations

Most surgeons agree that the abdominal surgical approach advocated originally by Ladd and Gross (1940) is far more satisfactory than the thoracic approach for correction of these defects. With the thoracic approach, malrotation of the small intestine and partial obstruction of the duodenum by bands, —which occurs in slightly more than 50% of the cases (Table 1)—cannot be visualized. Reducing the viscera into the diminutive abdominal cavity is often extremely difficult; according to Potts, it is 'akin to forcing spaghetti into a soda pop bottle', and may result in a marked increase in intra-abdominal tension which cannot be relieved simply by creation of an incisional hernia at the time of abdominal wound closure.

In the authors' experience, a 10 cm. long abdominal incision as depicted in Fig. 2a, completely dividing the ipsilateral rectus muscle, should be utilized rather than a paramedian incision (Fig. 2b) for the following reasons: (1) a 10 cm. divided rectus muscle incision permits construction of the most capacious ventral hernia in such newborn, (2) the gaping rectus muscle does not limit the hernia size and promotes free effective excursions of the diaphragm, i.e. more normal infant abdominal respiration after operation, (3) it provides optimal exposure of the diaphragmatic defect and facilitates closure of particularly large diaphragmatic defects by an 'overhead-sliding-door' technique (Meeker, to be published).

Once repair of the diaphragmatic defect has been accomplished, a chest tube should be inserted through the corner of the diaphragmatic closure, brought out through the corner of the abdominal wound and attached to water-seal drainage. Subsequently examination for Ladd's bands and their division

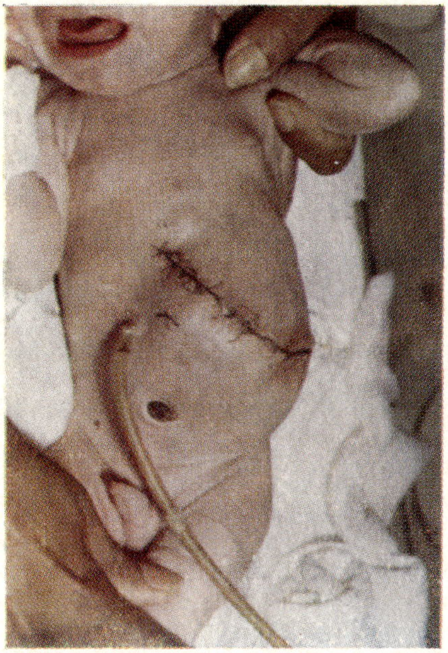

FIG. 2a.—Case 11, 10th day. Note the left 10 cm. divided rectus ventral hernia still filled to capacity, precluding primary abdominal wound closure.

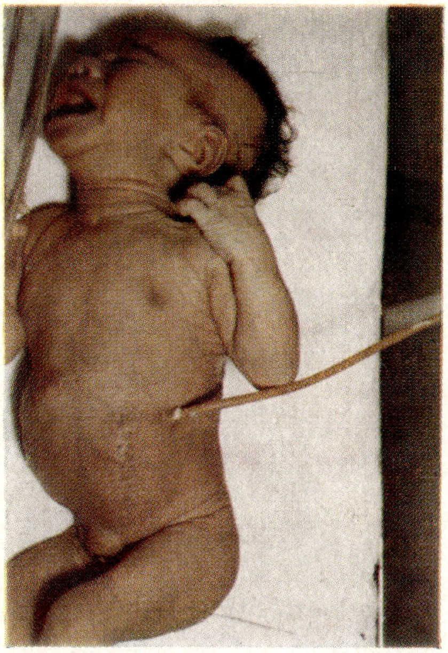

FIG. 2b.—A 2-week old infant following surgical correction of a massive eventration of the right diaphragm, gastrostomy, and construction of two intentional skin-covered ventral hernia, i.e. right 10 cm. divided rectus, and left paramedian incision. Note the divided rectus incisional hernia is full and bulging and the paramedian incisional hernia flat and empty.

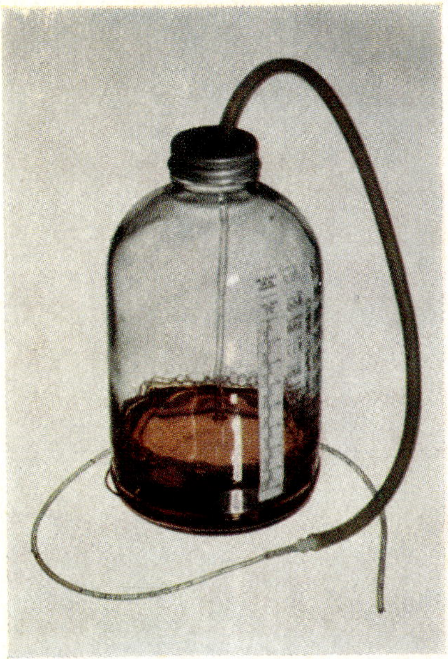

FIG. 2c.—A photograph of a 1,000 ml. parenteral fluid flask adapted for water-seal chest drainage. Note there is only 1-2 cm. of fluid in the bottle so that water-seal of the chest is insured, yet the level of fluid is sufficiently low so that any appreciable increase in positive pressure following a spontaneous pneumothorax can be decompressed and will 'bubble out'.

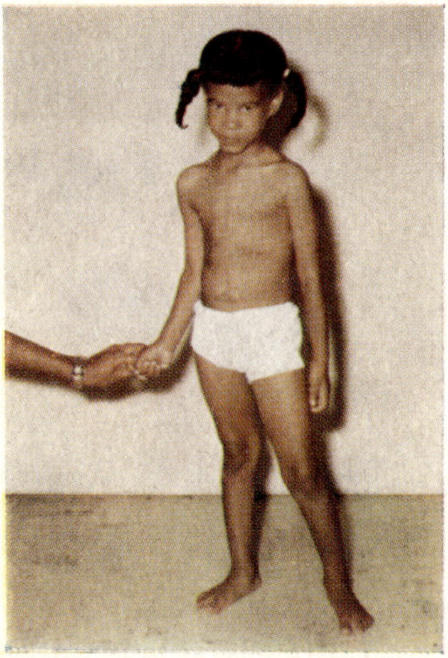

FIG. 2d.—A photograph of the same child as Fig. 2b at 5 years of age showing that the 10 cm. divided rectus ventral hernia had undergone spontaneous closure and the paramedian incision had healed well.

should be carried out, followed by establishment of a gastrostomy (Meeker and Snyder, 1962a). Finally the divided rectus ventral hernia should be constructed and primary abdominal wall closure deferred.

### Construction of Ventral Hernia

In approximately half of the cases in this study (Group II) the abdominal cavity was underdeveloped, diminutive, and of inadequate capacity to accept the viscera reduced from the thorax. Thus the surgeon had no choice but to undermine the subcutaneous tissue peripheral to the cut edges of the incision (preferably not superiorly over the thorax) to create a 'skin pouch' or ventral hernia of sufficient size to contain the viscera reduced from the thorax.

Before skin closure of a ventral hernia, if the patient's condition permits, the parietal peritoneum should be mobilized and sutured over the divided rectus and abdominal wall musculature and approximated to the anterior abdominal wall fascia around the entire periphery of the wound, to reduce formation of dense adhesions between the cut edges of the muscle and herniating loops of bowel. Thus a 'peritonealized surface' may be created up to the level of the subcutaneous tissue (Meeker and Snyder, 1962b). Drugs, to be effective, should be given parenterally during the first 3 days after operation. The skin edges alone are approximated as in a skin closure of an omphalocele (Gross, 1953) using interrupted 4-0 black silk sutures for the subcutaneous fascia and interrupted 5-0 black silk vertical mattress sutures for apposition of the skin edges. Particular attention is needed not to pierce the bowel loops that are lying directly below the surface of the skin.

Not infrequently (10 cases, Group IV) the capacity of the abdominal cavity may seem adequate to accommodate the reduced abdominal viscera, particularly when there is little air in the gastro-intestinal tract, without undue increases in intra-abdominal tension, and it becomes readily apparent that primary abdominal wall closure can be accomplished. The temptation to close the wound primarily in such infants less than 1 day of age, even when deceptively easy, should be resisted, and empirically a skin closure alone done and primary wound closure deferred. This clinical situation, where primary wound closure could be and was accomplished with ease, was encountered by experienced surgeons in 3 (Cases 24, 25, and 27) out of 10 patients in Group IV, and each of the infants died within 36 hours following apparently uneventful, successful correction of their diaphragmatic defects. In contrast the favourable outcome and clinical course of 2 (Cases 11 and 5 in Group II) with a 10 cm. divided rectus ventral hernia are documented by the blood-gas studies in Table 2 and Table 3, respectively. It should be added that haste to shorten the anaesthesia and operating time may be less of a virtue than a hazard since, within reason, prolonged gentle assisted respirations benefit these infants very materially. Although significant numbers of survivors have been

TABLE 2

BLOOD STUDIES OF *p*H, $P_{CO_2}$, AND BASE EXCESS AFTER OPERATION IN CASE 11, SHOWING MIXED ACIDOSIS WITH RESPIRATORY DEPRESSION

| | *p*H | $P_{CO_2}$ (mm. Hg) | Base Excess (mEq/l.) | Left Lung Expansion | Respiratory Rate |
|---|---|---|---|---|---|
| Before operation .. .. .. .. | 6·990 | 105·2 | −20·5 | 0 | 52 |
| Operation + assisted respiration 2 hr. .. | 7·110 | 70·4 | −13·2 | 0 | 72 spont. |
| Spontaneous respiration 6 hr. post-op. .. | 7·145 | 41·0 | −13·6 | 20% | 120 |
| Spontaneous respiration 18 hr. after operation | 7·198 | 55·0 | − 8·5 | 75% | 90 |
| Tracheal suction 24 hr. after operation .. | 7·330 | 38·0 | − 4·4 | 90% | 110 |
| 48 hr. after operation .. .. .. .. | 7·320 | 41·5 | − 4·0 | 100% | 70 |

TABLE 3

BLOOD STUDIES OF *p*H, $P_{CO_2}$, AND BASE EXCESS AFTER OPERATION IN CASE 5, SHOWING MIXED ACIDOSIS WITH $CO_2$ NARCOSIS AND RESPIRATORY DEPRESSION

| | *p*H | $P_{CO_2}$ (mm. Hg) | Base Excess (mEq/l.) | Left Lung Expansion | Respiratory Rate |
|---|---|---|---|---|---|
| Before operation .. .. .. .. | 6·900 | 112·0 | −13·6 | 0 | 48 |
| Operation + assisted respiration 2 hr. .. | 6·960 | 95·0 | −11·0 | 0 | 50 spont. |
| Assisted respiration 4 hr. .. .. .. | 7·125 | 57·5 | −13·0 | 0 | 65 spont. |
| Spontaneous respiration 2 hr. after operation | 6·910 | 110·0 | −20·8 | 50% | 44 |
| Tracheostomy, Tris 4 hr. after operation .. | 7·105 | 69·0 | −14·0 | 70% | 66 |
| 20 hr. after operation .. .. .. .. | 7·228 | 33·5 | −12·5 | 80% | 85 |

reported (Cerilli, 1964) following correction of a diaphragmatic defect and primary abdominal wall closure in infants less than 24 hours after birth, the over-all mortality has approached 50%.

### Post-operative Management

**Clinical Appraisal of Status.** In the first 48 hours after operation, expansion of the lung, the respiratory rate, and the state of alertness and responsiveness of the infant are the most significant clinical guides, and reflect changes in the blood-gas levels which are of greatest therapeutic significance.

During this period serial portable chest radiographs showed that in 14 of the 27 surgical cases 50 to 75% expansion of the lung occurred on water-seal drainage in the first 48 hours following operation. If this does not occur, hypoplasia of the lung should be suspected.

If during the first 48 hours after operation the respiratory rate falls to 40 to 50 breaths a minute regardless of the expansion of the lung, it should be interpreted not as a favourable sign but an ominous one portending or representing a falling blood *p*H and incipient respiratory depression due to a rising blood $P_{CO_2}$. Concomitant development of lethargy and the need to stimulate the baby to breathe generally indicates $CO_2$ narcosis. Cyanosis often develops slowly, almost imperceptibly, and is a late or the last feature of the clinical picture which changes insidiously. This clinical situation, when coupled with cyanosis and irregular respirations, initially suggests strongly that some major central nervous system catastrophe has occurred. However, it can be differentiated from a central nervous system abnormality by noting that the pupils are equal and react to light; and the child, on vigorous stimulation, can be roused momentarily to react and manifest reflexes like a normal newborn infant with an intact normal central nervous system.

To be safe, one should anticipate and suspect a transient fall in the blood *p*H and a rise in the $P_{CO_2}$ in the first 24 to 36 hours after operation. Regardless of the apparently favourable clinical course of the patient and whenever possible, appropriate blood-gas studies should be performed at least every 12 hours, in order to anticipate the need for additional therapy.

During the first 36 hours after operation, when well-documented evidence of falling blood *p*H and rising $P_{CO_2}$ are obtained, tracheostomy and gentle manually assisted respirations, and the administration of amine buffers may have to be considered. Fortunately this is rarely necessary when a 10 cm. divided rectus incision and ventral hernia has been employed (in this series only Case 5, Table 1).

**Management of 'Shallow' Water-seal Chest Drainage.** 'Shallow' water-seal chest drainage employing preferably a Baxter K-61 plastic catheter is the safest and most effective method of gradually removing air and fluid from the infant's chest, yet protecting against a spontaneous tension pneumothorax. Creation of a vacuum, or suction on the chest catheter, should be avoided assiduously and supplanted effectively by water seal only.

A plastic catheter is ideal for 'shallow' water-seal chest drainage in these particular infants because it has a relatively larger lumen than does a comparable rubber catheter and because it rarely becomes plugged with blood clots. This latter fact is particularly important because *shallow* water-seal chest drainage, *only 1 to 2 cm. of fluid in the bottle*, protects against the sudden development of a spontaneous pneumothorax by permitting immediate 'blow off' of accumulated air (Fig. 2c).

At first the column of water in the tube in the water-seal bottle fluctuates with each breath. When fluctuation ceases after the first day or two, the lung is usually expanded and this can be confirmed radiologically. If bubbles appear continuously in the water-seal bottle, a spontaneous tension pneumothorax has developed, but this will seal itself as a rule without resorting to chest suction which promotes air leakage and is usually contraindicated. Of the 27 surgical patients, 20 had chest drainage with water seal: 2 (Cases 14 and 20) of the remaining 7 without chest drainage died immediately after operation from spontaneous tension pneumothorax.

**Management of Gastrostomy.** Gastrostomy is an important adjunct in preventing vomiting with pulmonary aspiration, particularly in cases where malrotation with duodenal obstruction has been corrected. It was employed in 9 out of 11 cases in Group II, 2 of 6 cases in Group III, and 2 of 10 cases in Group IV. A further advantage of gastrostomy in such infants is that air normally swallowed by a crying baby is vented continuously through an open gastrostomy tube (Meeker and Snyder, 1962a), preventing distension of the intestinal tract. In conjunction with ventral hernia, it reduces to a minimum post-operative intra-abdominal tension and the space required by the loops of intestine, distended with air, that have been returned to the abdomen.

Though effective in this latter regard, in no case to date has gastrostomy resulted in a noticeable reduction in the size of the ventral hernia in the immediate post-operative period (Fig. 2a) sufficient to permit primary closure of the abdominal wall in the first two weeks of life.

**Management of Ventral Hernia.** Generally, growth or increase in the capacity of the abdominal cavity occurs slowly and the ventral hernia may be needed and filled to capacity, as shown in Fig. 2a, during the first days and weeks following correction of the diaphragmatic defect. The necessary delay in closure permits the abdominal cavity to enlarge and the fascial defect to become progressively smaller with diminution in the size of the ventral hernia. Complete closure occurred spontaneously in one patient, as shown in Fig. 2d. Mothers report that the ventral hernia is small or empty in the morning before the child has been fed and that the abdominal contour is relatively normal. In this study, closure of the fascia and rectus muscle to correct the ventral hernia (Group II cases) during the neonatal period has had to be deferred, but has been carried out electively at 1 to 3 years of age when no further spontaneous closure of the fascial defect is noted.

Dense adhesions will form as a result of construction of a temporary ventral hernia, and it must be recognized that families of such patients have had time to know and love their child, which makes ventral herniorrhaphy after the neonatal period a most formidable surgical undertaking.

Ventral herniorrhaphy should be preceeded by effective gastro-intestinal suction 24 hours before operation. There have been no deaths in any case in this study (Group II or III, Table 1) following ventral herniorrhaphy, but the calculated risk of repair and the inherent disadvantages of a ventral hernia are acknowledged and accepted because of what is believed to be its life-saving importance following repair of diaphragmatic defects in infants during the first 24 hours of life.

## Results in Surgical Cases

During the period of this study, 1957 to 1963, as shown in Table 1, 10 infants (Group IV) had surgical repair of a diaphragmatic defect with primary closure of all layers of the abdominal wall, and there was only one survivor. Aplasia of the lung was documented in 4 (Cases 20, 21, 22, and 25) and each infant died. One major associated anomaly was noted in one child (Case 25) who developed hyaline membrane disease.

Diaphragmatic defects in 6 infants (Group III) were corrected by the standard technique employing a paramedian incision and creating a ventral hernia, and 2 survived. Aplasia of the lung was described in 2 in this group (Cases 16 and 17) and both patients died. There was one major associated anomaly (Case 17) with congenital heart disease and one death (Case 14) that might have been averted by water-seal chest drainage.

Finally in 11 entirely comparable, unselected infants (Group II) a 10 cm. divided rectus muscle incision was employed and only a skin-covered ventral hernia was constructed. There were 8 survivors in this group, and significantly 2 (Cases 6 and 11) subsequently manifested aplasia of the ipsilateral lung on chest film. There were 3 deaths, 2 (Cases 7 and 10) occurring in children moribund with irreversible central nervous system damage due to anoxia before operation, and the third (Case 1) who had absence of the diaphragm and ipsilateral lung. There were 4 instances of aplasia of the lung in the entire group and 4 instances of a major associated congenital anomaly.

## Conclusions

The lower mortality in Group II suggests that reducing intra-abdominal tension by creating an intentional ventral hernia, utilizing a 10 cm. incision that divides the rectus musculature, is of real benefit and is preferred to a paramedian approach because of the greater capacity of the ventral hernia. Gastrostomy is also a valuable adjunct.

The decision to create a temporary ventral hernia should be made primarily on the basis of the infant's age and not on clinical appraisal of the infant's condition and the adequacy of the capacity of the abdominal cavity.

A separate study made by the authors of full-term and premature infants with diaphragmatic defects between 2 and 7 days of age (not included in this report) indicates that creation of an intentional ventral hernia may be extremely valuable in this group also. A further study of 33 cases with diaphragmatic defects, repaired after the age of 1 week, showed that there were only 2 deaths following surgical correction of the defect and in no instance was a ventral hernia created, so that in older children who represent the 'survival of the fittest' temporary ventral hernia has little to offer.

Procrastination regarding surgical repair in infants under 1 day of age is to be condemned, since without prompt surgical intervention, relatively few such infants will survive the first day of life (Butler and Claireaux, 1962).

## Summary

Increasing the capacity of the abdomen by creating a 10 cm. divided rectus ventral hernia, after repair of a diaphragmatic defect in infants during the first day of life, improves ventilation and leads to early correction of the respiratory and circulatory disturbances present. Reduction of abdominal viscera from the thorax to an underdeveloped, diminutive abdominal cavity, followed by primary abdominal wall closure, increases intra-abdominal tension, limits excursion of the diaphragm, and compresses the inferior vena cava.

The resulting respiratory, circulatory, and physiological derangements consist of severe acidosis, $CO_2$-retention, respiratory depression from $CO_2$ narcosis, and tissue anoxia.

The ventral hernia created can be corrected most appropriately at the time when the abdominal cavity has enlarged sufficiently to accommodate all the abdominal viscera without undue tension.

The authors wish to acknowledge their indebtedness to Dr. Frederick Leix, Chief of the Pediatric Surgical Service, Los Angeles County Hospital, and his staff for many contributions and co-operation in this study.

References

Bonham Carter, R. E., Waterston, D. J., and Aberdeen, E. (1962). Hernia and eventration of the diaphragm in childhood. *Lancet*, **1**, 656.

Butler, N., and Claireaux, A. E. (1962). Congenital diaphragmatic hernia as a cause of perinatal mortality. *ibid.*, **1**, 659.

Cerilli, G. J. (1964). Foramen of Bochdalek hernia: a review of the experience at Children's Hospital of Denver, Colorado. *Ann. Surg.*, **159**, 385.

Gross, R. E. (1953). *The Surgery of Infancy and Childhood.* Saunders, Philadelphia.

Kaplan, S. A. (1962). Tris (hydroxymethyl) aminomethane (THAM) —a new buffer for therapeutic use. *Amer. J. Dis. Child.*, **103**, 1.

——, Fox, R. P., and Clark, L. C., Jr. (1962). Amine buffers in the management of acidosis: study of respiratory and mixed acidosis. *ibid.*, **103**, 4.

Ladd, W. E., and Gross, R. E. (1940). Congenital diaphragmatic hernia. *New Engl. J. Med.*, **223**, 922.

Mathews D. H., Avery, M. E., and Jude, J. R. (1963). Closed-chest cardiac massage in the newborn infant. *J. Amer. med. Ass.*, **183**, 964.

Meeker, I. A., and Snyder, W. H. (1962a). Gastrostomy for the newborn surgical patient. A report of 140 cases. *Arch. Dis. Childh.*, **37**, 159.

——, and —— (1962b). Surgical management of diaphragmatic defects in the newborn infant. *Amer. J. Surg.*, **104**, 196.

*Arch. Dis. Childh.*, 1965, **40**, 154.

# THALIDOMIDE EMBRYOPATHY AND LIMB DEFECTS

## EXPERIENCES IN HABILITATION OF CHILDREN WITH ECTROMELIAS*

BY

WOLFGANG A. MAIER

*From Universität Kinderklinik, Münich, Germany*

Abnormalities of limbs have been seen occasionally at all times. Thalidomide-embryopathy, however, has produced special types of defects of the extremities, which in variety and above all in numbers has made necessary the provision of special centres for treatment.

At the Dept. of Paediatric Surgery and Orthopaedics of the University Children's Hospital, Münich, we observed from January 1959 to December 1963 approximately 141 children with severe limb deformities, of which 135 children were diagnosed as the 'dysmelia syndrome' as defined by Wiedemann (1961), Lenz (1961), McBride (1961), Weicker and others (1962).

Retrospectively 79% of the mothers were certain they had taken thalidomide during the critical phase of pregnancy, that is between the 32nd and the 50th day after the first day of the last menstruation. With another 16% we found that either thalidomide had been in the house or had been used by a member of the family, or that the mother had taken analgesic, hypnotic, or sedative drugs during the critical time. In only 5% of the mothers could we discover no reason for the abnormalities.

Exactly 8 months after the voluntary withdrawal of all thalidomide-containing drugs by the firm concerned the wave of dysmelia cases suddenly retreated.

During the following 16 months only 3 newborn babies with extremity defects were seen at the hospital, and these could all be distinguished from the dysmelia syndrome.

In 1960 at this hospital we made our first efforts to treat dysmelic children. A treatment centre has now been established, working as an outpatient clinic for limb deformities.

The cases are divided up as shown in the Table.

The Dysmelia Centre was intentionally separated from the general hospital and was installed in an apartment nearby. From the beginning the infants were not to have the feeling that they were ill and had to come for treatment. In the neutral surroundings of a normal house they feel themselves more at home and soon regard the therapy as an ordinary part of their day. Physiotherapists and occupational therapist work in separate rooms. A psychologist has proved especially useful and is an important help in adapting the handicapped child to the use of technical aids, as well as in assisting the parents in educating their children. The parents leave their children at the centre, according to a time-table. If necessary, they themselves attend in order to go on with the exercises at home. The regular contact with the parents provides a good opportunity for influencing the home situation and therefore of preventing the child with limb defects from becoming spoilt by a misguided love and helpfulness. Unfortunately we also meet with the contrary; it is equally wrong for parents to try with exaggerated perseverance to get a highly differentiated skill out of their dysmelic children and to ask too much of them.

Apart from the traditional methods of examination, we make certain special inquiries, which need be mentioned only briefly.

With the aid of a modern constant current impulse apparatus we test the excitability of the muscles.

Arteriograms showed that even in those children with the severest deformities, i.e. with very short ectromelias of the axial type and with one-finger phocomelias, the regular topography and division of

TABLE

| Deformity | No. of Cases |
|---|---|
| Bilateral amelia | 2 |
| Unilateral amelia with phocomelia at the opposite side | 6 |
| Unilateral amelia with phocomelia of the 3 remaining limbs | 1 |
| Bilateral one-finger phocomelia | 2 |
| Tetra-ectromelia | 20 |
| Bilateral ectromelia (axial type) | 36 |
| Bilateral ectromelia (combined type, axial with distal) | 6 |
| Bilateral ectromelia (only distal type) | 35 |
| Malformations of the thumb | 27 |

* A paper read at a meeting of the British Association of Paediatric Surgeons in Rotterdam, September 1964.

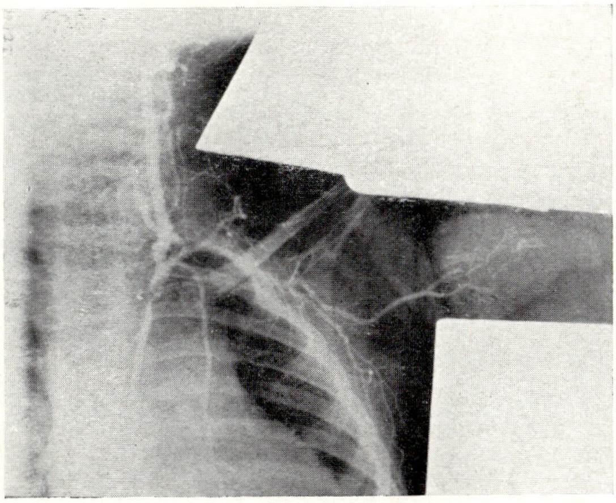

FIG. 1.—Arteriogram of a 2½-year-old boy with one-finger phocomelia.

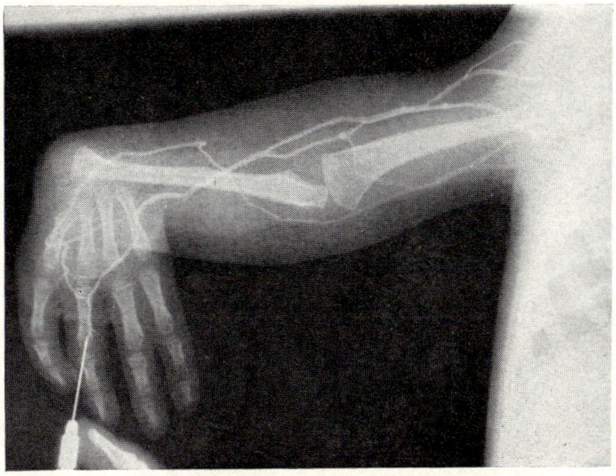

FIG. 3.—Venography of a 3-year-old girl. The cephalic vein divides into three branches.

the brachial artery and its branches was only reduced in proportion to the entire length of the arm. Even with one-finger phocomelias the arterial system is still normally developed, so that regular division of the brachial artery into radial and ulnar can be observed (Fig. 1). All existing fingers are supplied by the ulnar artery: the radial artery does not extend beyond the wrist (Fig. 2).

The picture of the venous system revealed by venography is different. It is characterized by the frequent hypoplasia or anomaly of the cephalic vein; for instance its division into three branches, the first of which joins the brachial vein (Fig. 3), or its direct junction with the jugular vein.

Such considerations are not without importance later on, in attempting operation at the shoulder in order to correct the frequent subluxation, and at the wrist to correct the radial deviation. For the therapy of ectromelic lower extremities (Fig. 4) the early correction of the club-foot which otherwise resists treatment has shown good results. We operate according to the method of Blauth (1963); the fibula is shortened by an osteotomy, and the distal end of the fibula is put on to the talus. In this way it will be easier later on to apply technical aids (Fig. 5a and b).

Surgery of the upper extremities during early infancy ought to be approached with the utmost caution. Children with bilateral amelia, one-finger phocomelia, and very short ectromelias of the axial type receive their first pneumatic prosthesis at the age of 18 months.

The main interest goes to the amelias, one-finger phocomelias, and severe ectromelias, of which, up to now, 17 patients have been fitted with powered prostheses of the Heidelberg type. Liquid carbon dioxide serves as a source of energy and is stored in a steel bottle. By means of this prostheses we can either move 'pat-hands' or a children's hook. For bilateral amelia and phocomelia we at first constructed 'pat-hands' (Fig. 6). With these only a

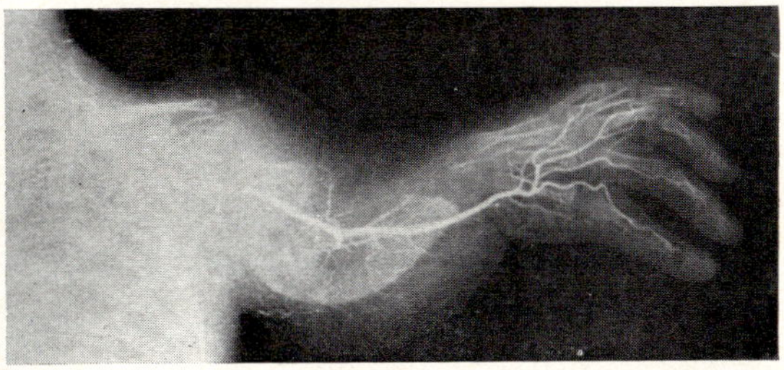

FIG. 2.—Arteriogram of a 3-year-old boy. All fingers are supplied by the ulnar artery.

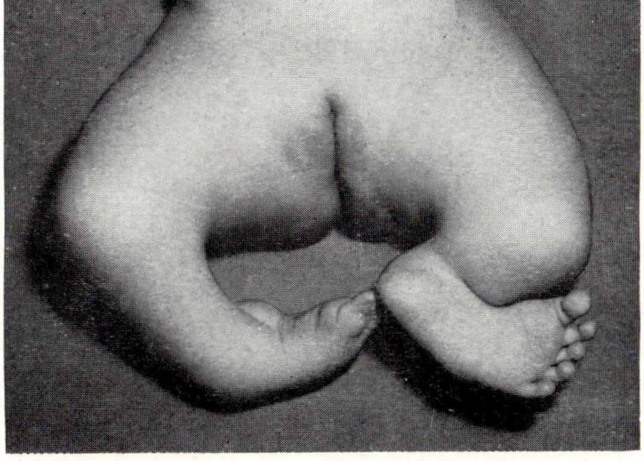

FIG. 4.—Lower extremity ectromelia before treatment.

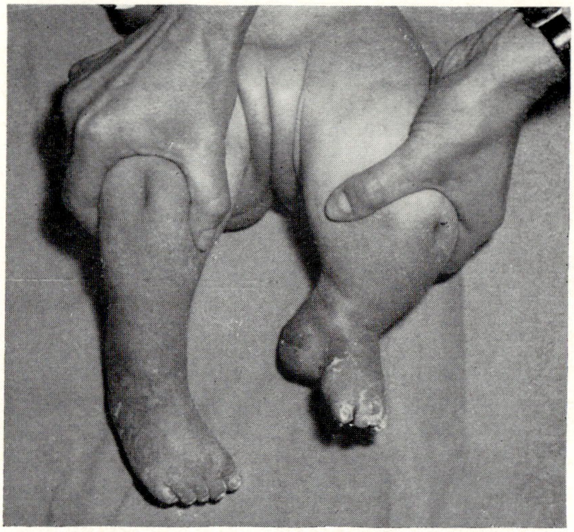

(a)

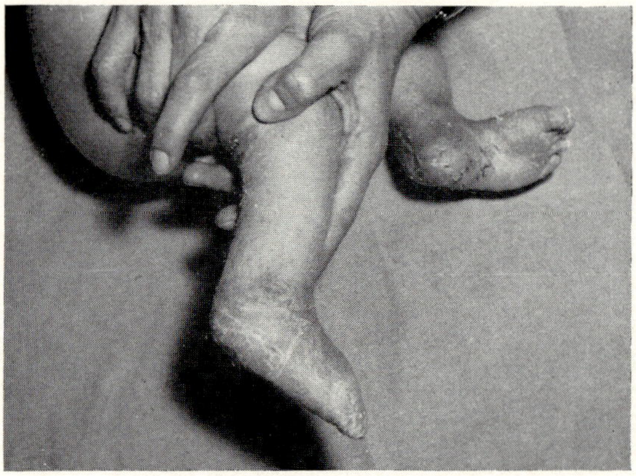

(b)

FIG. 5a and b.—The same child shown in Fig. 4 after operation.

movement in the form of a sickle is possible, through an adduction of the artificial forearms. One year later the babies have received powered hook prostheses instead of the 'pat-hand'. Short ectromelias were fitted with a hook from the beginning.

By the third year of life the children are skilled enough to perform correctly a turning movement of the hand like a pronation-supination (Fig. 7). This is effected either by additional key valves for the finger in the case of ectromelias, or for the chin with amelias (Fig. 8).

The children get used very quickly to the prostheses, with the assistance of an occupational therapist and a physiotherapist. They are obviously happy when able to play, and they resist when the prostheses have to be taken off for a while.

If they manage to reach their mouths with their short arms or to cross them over the breast, the fitting of technical aids can be delayed. All other deformities need training and guidance (Fig. 9 and 10).

In a centre for treatment of limb-deficient children

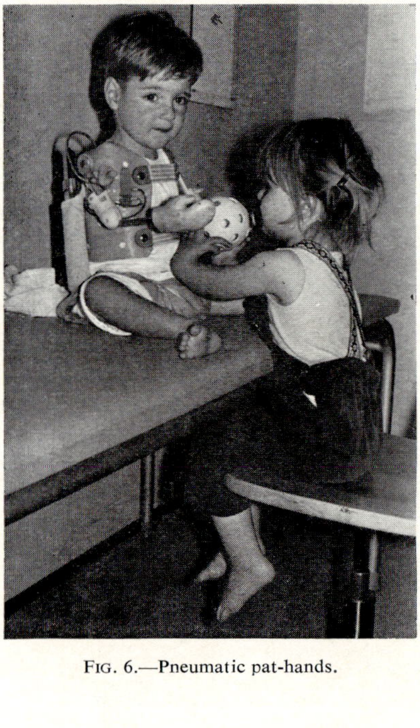

FIG. 6.—Pneumatic pat-hands.

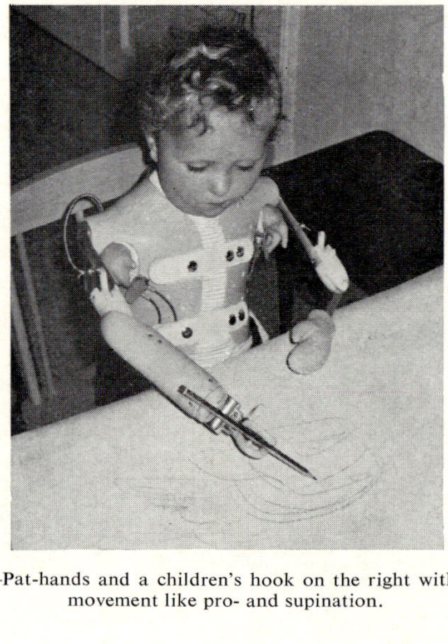

FIG. 7.—Pat-hands and a children's hook on the right with turning movement like pro- and supination.

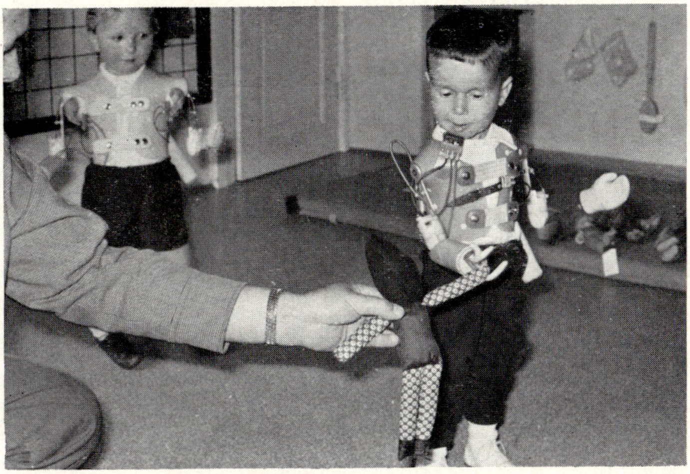

FIG. 8.—A key valve for the chin with bilateral amelia.

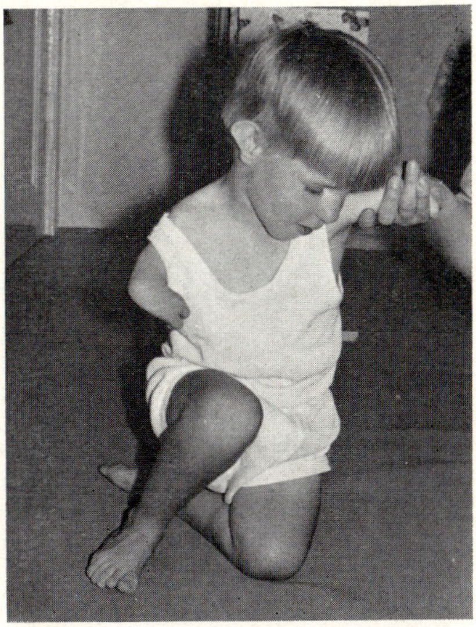

FIG. 10.—Physiotherapist gives instructions to a boy with ectromelic arms to get up without losing his balance.

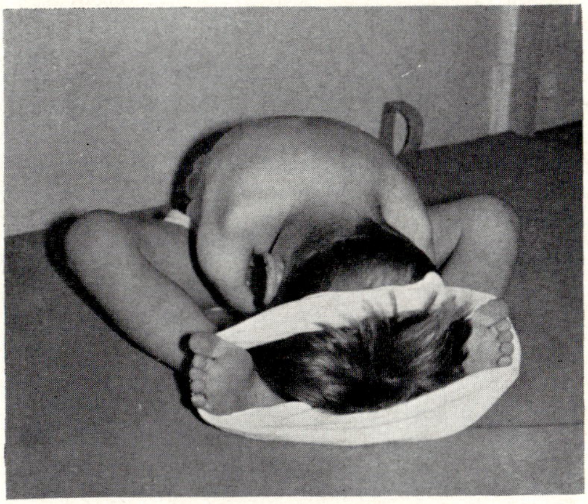

FIG. 9.—The daily training: a child with short ectromelic arms is learning to dress himself.

all those taking part, the physician, the orthopaedic mechanic, the physiotherapist, the occupational therapist, the psychologist, and the teacher have to work together closely. We plan to habilitate the children as effectively as possible for a normal life. How far we succeed will be apparent in the years to come when the first victims of thalidomide-embryopathy are admitted to regular schools.

BIBLIOGRAPHY


Blauth, W. (1963). Beitrag zur operativen Behandlung schwerer Mißbildungen der Unterschenkelknochen. *Arch. orthop. Unfall-Chir.*, **55**, 345.

——, and Willert, H. G. (1963). Klinik und Therapie ektromeler Mißbildungen der unteren Extremität. *ibid.*, **55**, 521.

Lenz, W. (1961). Discussion at the Congress of the 'Rheinisch-Westfälische Kinderärzte-Vereinigung' Düsseldorf, Germany, 19.11.1961.

—— (1963). Das Thalidomid-Syndrom. *Fortschr. Med.*, **81**, 148.

——, and Knapp, K. (1962). Die Thalidomid-Embryopathie. *Dtsch. med. Wschr.*, **87**, 1232.

Maier, W. (1963a). Early treatment of dysmelia. *Germ. med. Mth.*, **8**, 45. Shortened translation of the article in the *Dtsch. med. Wschr.*, **88**, 69.

—— (1963b). Die Thalidomid-Embryopathie aus kinderchirurgischer Sicht Bisherige Ergebnisse mit einer frühzeitigen prothetischen Versorgung. *Zbl. Chir.*, **88**, 1551.

—— (1964). Thalidomid-Embryopathie und Gliedmassenfehlbildungen. Erfahrungen bei der Versorgung von Kindern mit Ektromelien. *Bayer. Ärztebl.*, **19**, 201.

McBride, W. G. (1961). Thalidomide and congenital abnormalities. *Lancet*, **2**, 1358.

Weicker, H., Bachmann, K. D., Pfeiffer, R. A., and Gleiss, J. (1962). Thalidomid-Embryopathie. II. Ergebnisse individueller anamnestischer Erhebungen in den Einzugsgebieten der Universitäts-Kinderkliniken Bonn, Köln, Münster und Düsseldorf. *Dtsch. med. Wschr.*, **87**, 1597.

——, and Hungerland, H. (1962). Thalidomid-Embryopathie. I. Vorkommen inner- und außerhalb Deutschlands. *ibid.*, **87**, 992.

Wiedemann, H. R. (1961). Hinweis auf eine derzeitige Häufung hypo- und aplastischer Fehlbildungen der Gliedmaßben. *Med. Welt (Stuttg.)*, 37, 1863.

*Arch. Dis. Childh.*, 1965, **40**, 158.

# THE SURGERY OF INFANTILE OBSTRUCTIVE JAUNDICE*

BY

KEIJIRO SURUGA, ZENYA YAMAZAKI, SEIZO IWAI, KINJI NAGASHIMA, and WATARU MORI

*From the Department of Surgery, San-Iku-Kai Hospital and Tokyo University, and the Department of Surgery and Pathology, Tokyo Medical and Dental University, Japan*

Various diseases are responsible for infantile obstructive jaundice. But congenital biliary atresia is considered one of the most interesting diseases from the point of view of surgical treatment. There are many unsolved problems in its embryology, diagnosis, and therapy.

We collected 169 cases of infantile obstructive jaundice from clinics and hospitals in the area as well as from our own hospital. In 39 of them (23%), extrahepatic ducts were clearly visualized. In the remaining 130 (77%), no extrahepatic ducts were found.

For the cases in which extrahepatic ducts were visualized, the following operations were performed: choledocoduodenostomy, choledocojejunostomy, cholecystoduodeno- or jejunostomy, hepaticogastro-, duodeno-, or -jejunostomy, external fistula of hepatic ducts. The results were not good, however, because of complications such as infection, pulmonary complication, or liver failure. The post-operative mortality rate was 62%. There are few surviving cases.

On the other hand, for the cases in which no extrahepatic ducts were found, probe laparotomies were performed in the majority, and also anastomosis between porta hepatis and duodenum or jejunum, anastomosis between liver and stomach, duodenum or jejunum, external biliary fistula by partial hepatectomy, Sterling external fistula and Sterling internal fistula etc. were tried. The majority of the cases died after operation. The results of surgical treatment for this disease are unsatisfactory at present, not only in our country but in paediatric hospitals in other countries too.

## Relation between Hepatic Biliary Duct System and Lymphatic System

In searching for a solution to this difficult problem, we have, since 1962, studied the relation between the hepatic biliary duct system and the lymphatic system from a slightly different view-point. Johnson and Mann (1950) proved histologically the existence of a close relation between the intrahepatic biliary duct and the lymphatic duct. Bollman (1950) also stated that the lymphatic system took bile that was diffused from the biliary duct. Azuma (1963) pointed out the close relationship of the two systems in his experimental study on 'Excretion and absorption of ascites in ascitic dog'. He stated that the measured pressures of the intrahepatic lymphatic duct and the biliary duct were nearly identical in the same dog. Nishimaru and Yata (1956) also reported the existence of close communication between the two duct systems. Dumont and Mulholland (1962) stated that the excess bilirubin in blood regurgitated into the thoracic duct through the intrahepatic lymphatic system. Alican and Hardy (1962) created experimentally an obstruction in the common bile-duct of a dog and studied the bilirubin level of the thoracic duct lymph and of serum: they came to the conclusion that an intrahepatic lymphatic system was an important exit for bile regurgitation. According to the results of our own experiments on an icteric dog (Table 1) following a ligation of the common bile-duct, the bilirubin levels of the thoracic duct lymph and of the serum were much higher than normal. Also, when the thoracic duct lymph was conducted outside the body, the raised serum bilirubin level tended to fall (Fig. 1).

## Operative Method

From the results of our experiments, we thought some way of conducting the thoracic duct lymph into the upper alimentary tract might be applicable to the cases in which so-called probe laparotomies only were usually performed. The operative method is as follows. An incision is made along the anterior border of the sternocleidomastoid muscle. The latter is divided near the sternal and the clavicular insertion. The clavicle is then divided close to the sternoclavicular joint. The next step is to recognize the thoracic duct. We think that the thoracic duct itself

* A paper read at a meeting of the British Association of Paediatric Surgeons in Rotterdam, September 1964.

TABLE 1

BILIRUBIN LEVELS OF SERUM AND LYMPH IN DOGS AFTER LIGATION OF COMMON BILE-DUCT

| Dog No. | Weight (kg.) | Serum and Lymph | Time Interval After Ligation (days) | Bilirubin (mg./100 ml.) | Flow Rate (ml./min.) |
|---|---|---|---|---|---|
| 1 | 12·0 | S | 15 | 1·6 | |
| | | L | 15 | 2·0 | 0·5 |
| 2 | 13·0 | S | 14 | 2·8 | |
| | | L | 14 | 1·08 | 0·7 |
| 3 | 1·0 | S | 8 | 2·58 | |
| | | L | 8 | 1·15 | 0·3 |
| 4 | 12·0 | S | 6 | 5·5 | |
| | | L | 6 | 2·7 | 0·25 |
| 5 | 11·5 | S | 6 | 2·2 | |
| | | L | 6 | 1·68 | |
| 6 | 9·5 | S | 5 | 4·4 | |
| | | L | 5 | 3·6 | 0·28 |
| 7 | 8·0 | S | 5 | 5·0 | |
| | | L | 5 | 7·6 | |
| 8 | 11·0 | S | 5 | 10·3 | |
| | | L | 5 | 3·7 | |
| Normal Control | | S | | 0·2 | |
| | | L | | 0·2 | |

cannot be anastomosed directly to the alimentary tract owing to its smallness and the friability of the duct. Both the subclavian vein which is distal, and the brachiocephalic vein which is proximal to the venous angle where the thoracic duct joins, are ligated. The internal jugular vein is dissected and divided near the distal end so that it can be used for anastomoses. Therefore, only the thoracic duct lymph flows into the venous angle. In performing this procedure the following points should be noted: in cases where the cirrhosis has progressed to a certain degree, the lymphatic system around the venous angle is abnormally distended. One should avoid injuring the lymphatic system. Secondly, when the brachiocephalic vein is ligated, the dissection should be carried out carefully in order not to injure the thin pleura. Thirdly, there are tributary veins near the thoracic duct, which flow into the brachiocephalic vein. It is important to ligate these tributary veins so that only the thoracic duct lymph flows into the venous angle.

The first method we tried in 1962 was to conduct the thoracic duct lymph to the oesophagus, utilizing the venous angle and the internal jugular vein. In the majority of patients where this method was applied, it was past the optimum operative time and their general condition was unfavourable: 2 out of 3 had an anastomotic insufficiency and the other had pneumothorax and a

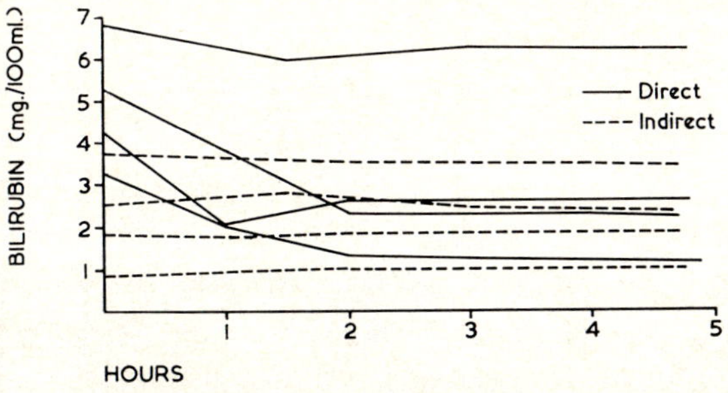


FIG. 1.—Serum bilirubin levels after diversion of thoracic lymph flow in dogs by ligation of common bile-duct.

complication that was probably due to anaesthesia. There were no long-term survivors. The survival periods were short and no fall in the bilirubin level was seen. MacKneally, Carey, Rogers, and Absolon (1963) also reported anastomotic insufficiency, thrombosis at the anastomotic site, and inflammatory stenosis as the complications.

We next tried experimentally and clinically the following method. First, the external fistula of the thoracic duct was created and then the fistula was anastomosed to the oesophagus using polyethylene tubing or natural rubber tubing.

Since 1962 we have used a method by which the thoracic duct lymph is conducted to the subglossal portion of the oral cavity, utilizing the venous angle and the internal jugular vein (Suruga-Yamazaki procedure) (Figs. 2 and 3). The details of the operative procedure are almost the same as in our original operation, but in order to utilize a long internal jugular vein, it was dissected well above the facial vein and divided (Fig. 3). However, if the internal jugular vein is divided too distally, the diameter of the stump may be too small for the subglossal opening. Before the anastomosis is made, the internal jugular vein is sutured to the adjacent tissue utilizing the previous tributary veins and thus the anastomosis is performed without tension. Usually, it is done by 6 to 8 simple sutures. The fewer the sutures used for anastomosis, the better the lymph flow to be expected. In this method, though there is no real danger of anastomotic insufficiency, prevention of post-operative infection becomes important. Even slight infection of the operative wound affects lymph flow. Therefore we finished the neck portion first and then operated in the mouth. After operation, we use a drain in order to avoid accumulation of lymph or blood.

## Results

Operations were carried out on 14 patients (Table 2). In 4, anastomosis between the thoracic duct and the oesophagus was performed: 3 in one stage, and 1

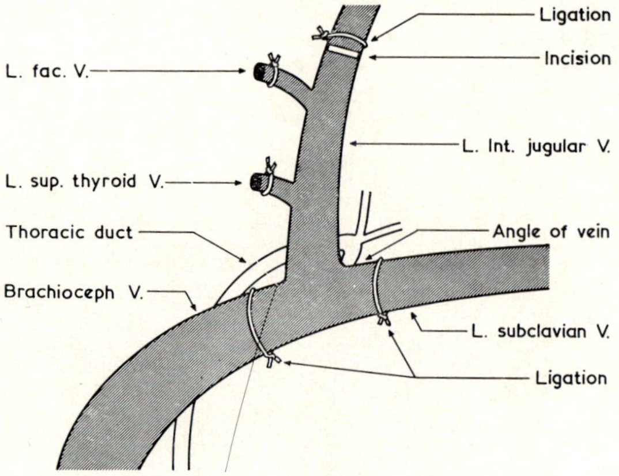


FIG. 2.—Suruga-Yamazaki procedure 1.

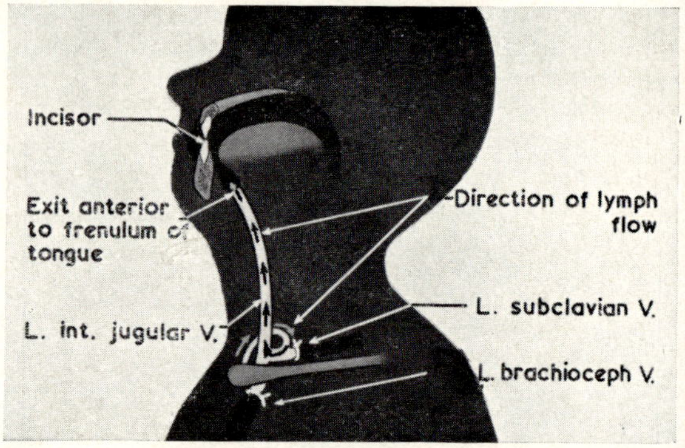


FIG. 3.—Suruga-Yamazaki procedure 2.

TABLE 2

DIVSERSION OF THORACIC LYMPH FLOW FOR TREATMENT OF CONGENITAL BILIARY ATRESIA

| Method | No. |
|---|---|
| 1: Oesophago-thoracic duct anastomosis . . . . | 3 |
| 2: Oesophago-thoracic duct anastomosis (two-stage procedure) . . . . . . . . . . . . | 1 |
| 3: Suruga-Yamazaki method . . . . . . . . | 10 |
| Total . . . . . . . . . . . . . . | 14 |

in two stages. In the remaining 10 cases the thoracic duct lymph was conducted to the subglossal areas using the internal jugular vein (Suruga-Yamazaki's method). The results of 4 thoracic duct oesophagus anastomoses have already been mentioned. The results of a further 10 cases in which Suruga-Yamazaki's method was used are as follows: one was 2 months old, 5 were between 2 and 3 months, and 4 were older than 4 months when the operation was performed. 8 cases were followed up after operation for a limited period and a fall in serum bilirubin level was seen in all. The direct bilirubin level was particularly lowered (Table 3). Kolmen (1961) experimentally revealed that a fall in the serum protein occurred when the thoracic duct lymph was led outside the body. In our cases, no fall in serum protein value was found.

Post-operative complications included 3 wound

TABLE 3

DIVERSION OF THORACIC LYMPH FLOW (SURUGA-YAMAZAKI METHOD)

| Case No. | Age (mth.) | Serum Protein (g./100 ml.) | Bilirubin (mg./100 ml.) | | | Result |
|---|---|---|---|---|---|---|
| | | | Direct | Indirect | Total | |
| 1 | 2 | 6·7 | 1·73 | 0·5 | 2·23 | Alive |
| | Op. → 3 | 6·5 | 0·8 | 0·03 | 0·84 | |
| | 10 | | 0·6 | 1·7 | 2·3 | |
| | 10 | | 0·8 | 0·4 | 1·2 | |
| 2 | 3 | 6·4 | 10·5 | 1·0 | 11·5 | Dead |
| | 4 | 5·4 | 10·0 | 2·0 | 12·0 | |
| | Op. → 4 | 5·0 | 9·5 | 0·9 | 10·4 | |
| | 5 | | 3·6 | 1·0 | 4·6 | |
| | 6 | | 3·6 | 0·21 | 3·81 | |
| 3 | 2 | 6·8 | 6·7 | 0·4 | 7·1 | Alive |
| | Op. → 3 | 7·1 | 5·5 | 1·5 | 7·0 | |
| | 4 | 8·1 | 1·66 | 0·47 | 2·13 | |
| 4 | 2 | 6·0 | 6·5 | 0·6 | 7·1 | Alive |
| | Op. → 2 | 5·4 | 6·6 | 0·5 | 7·1 | |
| | 3 | | 4·2 | 0·3 | 4·5 | |
| | 4 | 7·0 | 2·5 | 0·82 | 3·32 | |
| 5 | Op. → 2 | 6·6 | 5·35 | 7·63 | 13·0 | Dead |
| | 3 | 7·5 | 2·54 | 1·76 | 4·3 | |
| 6 | Op. → 4 | 6·7 | 3·1 | 2·4 | 5·5 | Dead |
| 7 | Op. → 9 | 6·9 | 9·4 | 5·1 | 14·5 | Dead |
| | 9 | | 4·7 | 4·3 | 9·0 | |
| 8 | Op. → 2 | 7·1 | 11·1 | 0·4 | 11·5 | Dead |
| | 3 | | | | | |
| 9 | Op. → 2 | 5·9 | 12·7 | 3·8 | 16·5 | Alive |
| | 3 | 7·3 | 11·1 | 2·4 | 12·5 | |
| 10 | Op. → 3 | 6·0 | 7·0 | 1·6 | 8·6 | Alive |
| | 4 | 6·6 | 4·4 | 1·1 | 5·6 | |

infections, and one air-way obstruction due to an excessive amount of thoracic duct lymph flowing into the oral cavity. In this case the operation was performed at a late stage, and cirrhosis was advanced. One pulmonary complication was seen. It is important to avoid infection of the operative wound when this method is performed. Also in order to avoid an excessive amount of lymph flowing into the oral cavity, the patient should be in a prone position in the immediate post-operative period. In 2 out of the 5 cases that died, liver cirrhosis was identified macroscopically at operation and serum bilirubin level fell, but death was finally caused by hepatic coma. One was operated on at 4 months and the other at 9 months. Other causes of death were as follows: one died within 24 hours due to air-way obstruction, one died from pulmonary complications and one from complications unrelated to operation.

Post-operative liver function tests and histological findings were studied. The post-operative liver function is gauged by serum cholinesterase levels, which can be measured with 0·05 ml. serum, correlated with B.S.P. test. The serum cholinesterase was raised in all. In general, a raised level of serum cholinesterase did not fall in cases older than 2 months.

Histologically, the biopsy from the right liver lobe was studied for cell infiltration, cell necrosis, fibrosis, giant cell transformation, hepatic duct hyperplasia, and bile stagnation.

Histological findings varied in individual cases. Prognosis seemed unfavourable in 4 cases in which marked fibrosis, cell necrosis, and hyperplasia of the hepatic duct were seen. This finding corroborates the results of previous liver function tests. On the other hand, in cases less than 2 months old, although marked bile congestion may be seen, other pathological findings tend to be slight and the prognosis is consequently better.

In congenital biliary duct atresia, according to our results, if the optimum operative time is missed, prognosis is unfavourable even if the thoracic duct lymph is led into the alimentary tract. MacKneally *et al.* (1963) produced experimentally in this way a decrease in ascites in a case with advanced cirrhosis. In one of our congenital biliary duct atresia cases, we produced the same decrease in ascites after this procedure.

## Conclusion

The results of Suruga-Yamazaki's procedure in congenital biliary duct atresia are reported. We have not found post-operative anorexia, diarrhoea, or oedema due to circulatory disturbance in the upper extremity after this operation.

The operation is technically difficult. Post-operative fat, protein, and electrolyte metabolism is a problem. In order to obtain better results this disease should be differentiated at an early period.

A long-term follow-up and continued study of this problem is required.

### References


Alican, F., and Hardy, J. D. (1962). Lymphatic transport of bile pigments and alkaline phosphatase in experimental common duct obstruction. *Surgery*, **52**, 366.

Azuma, K. (1963). Studies on production and absorption of ascites. *Jap. J. Gastroent.*, **60**, 183.

Bollman, J. L. (1950). Liver injury. 9th conference.

Dumont, A. E., and Mulholland, J. H. (1962), Alterations in thoracic duct lymph flow in hepatic cirrhosis. *Ann. Surg.*, **156**, 668.

Johnson, L. E., and Mann, F. C. (1950). Intrahepatic lymphatics. *Amer. J. Physiol.*, **163**, 723.

Kolmen, S. N. (1961). Chronic thoracic duct-esophageal shunt preparation in protein studies. *J. appl. Physiol.*, **16**, 369.

MacKneally, M., Carey, J. B., Rogers, W., and Absolon, K. B. (1963). Technique of thoracic duct-esophagus fistula and its potential application. *Surg. Forum*, **14**, 187.

Nishimaru, K., and Yata, H. (1956). Liver, hepatic lymph vessel, lymph flow and lymphatic fluid. *Saishin Igaku*, **11**, 377.

*Arch. Dis. Childh.*, 1965, **40**, 162.

# INTRAHEPATIC VASCULAR AND BILE-DUCT SYSTEMS AS RELATED TO OPERATIVE TREATMENT OF BILE-DUCT ATRESIA*

BY

WOLFGANG HASSE

*From the Department of Surgery, Free University, Westend Hospital, West-Berlin, Germany*

More than 80% of infants suffering from congenital biliary atresia are found to be inoperable at laparotomy (Grewe and Arius, 1961; Grewe and Pape, 1962; Grob, 1957; Gross, 1953; Hasse, 1963, 1964a, b; Hecker and Daum, 1964; Ladd, 1935; Rehbein and Neumann, 1957). The attempts to relieve the bile stasis by hepatogastrostomy (Gohrbandt, 1957), or cholangiojejunostomy (Longmire and Sanford, 1948, 1949) have been unsuccessful, nor has Sterling's (1961) method of establishing internal hepatic fistulae by using artificial bile-duct reduced the mortality rate.

In order to find a basis for treatment in inoperable extrahepatic biliary atresia, the intrahepatic vascular and bile-duct systems of 40 normal livers of newborns and infants have been studied. These studies began in May 1962 independently of the work of Healey and Sterling published in December 1963 in their monograph: 'Segmental Anatomy of the Newborn Liver'.

The livers were removed from the body 10 to 48 hours after death and the vascular and bile-duct systems were injected with 'plastoid' by Schummer's (1951) method. In addition, the intrahepatic bile-ducts were studied (a) radiographically by injecting barium, and (b) by the use of $^{131}$I-labelled hippuric acid solution.

As in adults (Rex, 1888; Cantlie, 1898; Healey and Schroy, 1953; Hjortsjö, 1948; Couinaud, 1954;

* A paper read at a meeting of the British Association of Paediatric Surgeons in Rotterdam, September 1964.

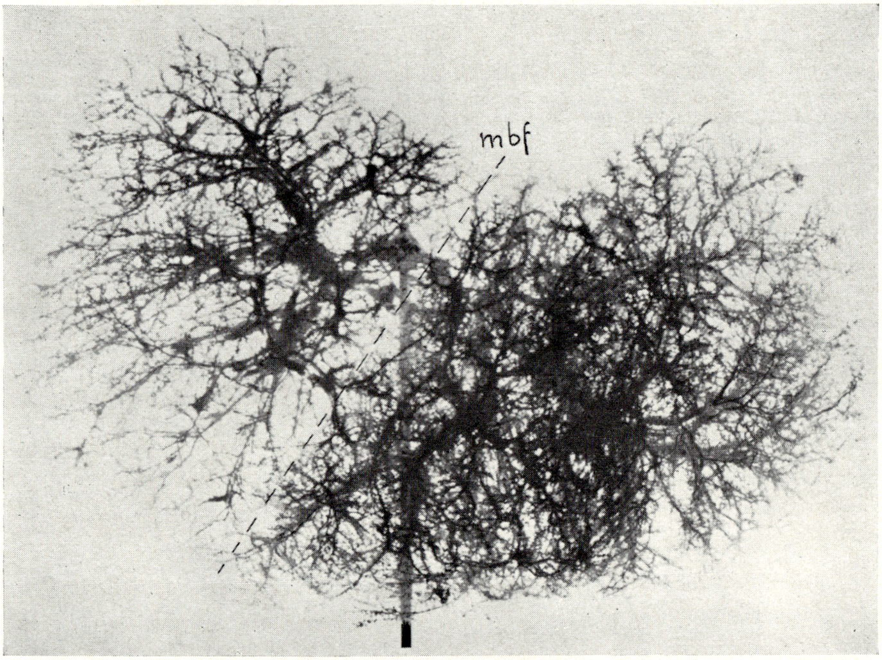


FIG. 1.—A liver cast of a 1-day-old infant, anterior view. Hepatic artery injected with 'plastoid' (mbf = main boundary fissure).

Stucke, 1959; Reifferscheid, 1957; Nettelblad, 1954; Røjel, 1958), the liver of the newborn infant is divided into a functional right and left lobe. Fig. 1 demonstrates the branches of the hepatic artery. The main boundary fissure is to be seen exactly between the two functional lobes. This fissure continues as a plane of connective tissue from the gall-bladder to the inferior vena cava.

The isolated injected right hepatic artery (Fig. 2) reveals the main boundary line very distinctly. No anastomoses are seen between the two functional lobes.

The intrahepatic branches of the portal vein demonstrate precisely the segments of the newborn and infant liver (Fig. 3).

To the right branch of the portal vein belong: (1) the right portion of the caudate lobe; (2) the processus caudatus; (3) a ventral segment; and (4) a dorsal segment.

The left branch of the portal vein provides: (1) the left portion of the caudate lobe; (2) the quadrate lobe; (3) a ventro-lateral segment; and (4) a dorso-lateral segment.

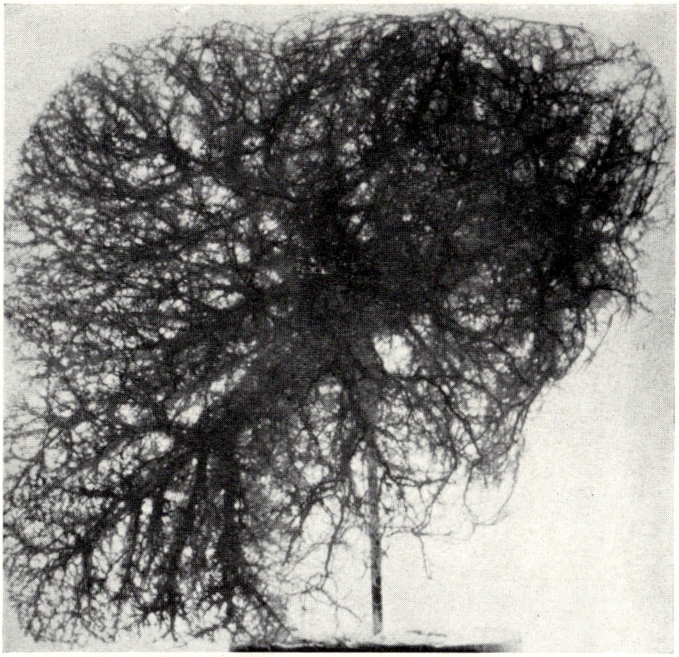

FIG. 2.—Isolated, injected right hepatic artery of a 4-day-old infant, anterior view. The absence of anastomoses between the two functional lobes has prevented any of the medium passing into the left functional lobe.

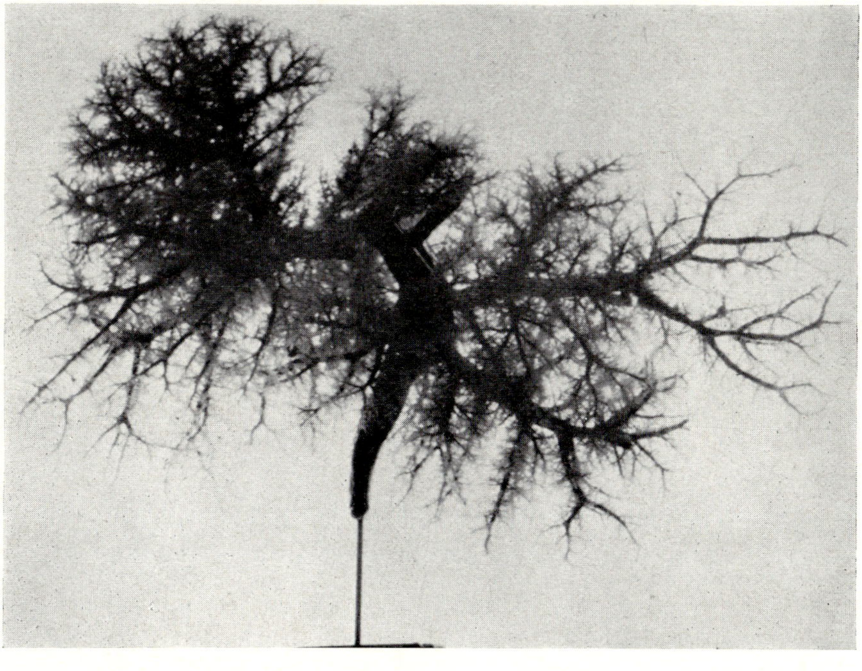

FIG. 3.—Segmental branches of the portal vein of a 3-day-old infant, anterior view. The ductus venosus and umbilical vein were patent.

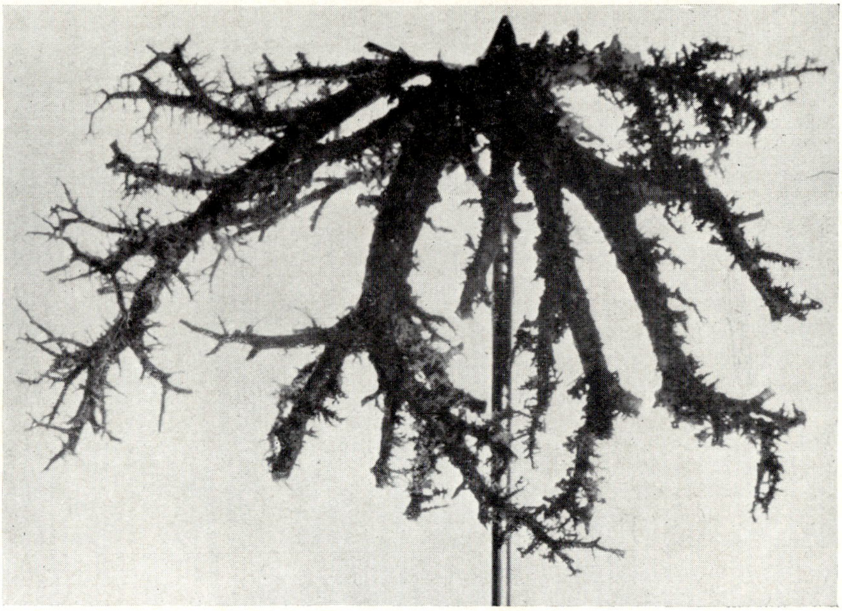

FIG. 4.—Hepatic veins of a 2-day-old infant, anterior view.

The hepatic vein receives a supply by a right, middle, and left hepatic vein (Fig. 4).

The intrahepatic bile-duct system of the infant is extremely delicate, as is shown in Fig. 5. Even the intrahepatic cholangiogram illustrates the fineness of the bile-duct system (Fig. 6). The segmental branches have a diameter of only 1 mm. Intrahepatic anastomoses of the bile-ducts between the two functional lobes are never seen, though Hartmann (1960) described such anastomoses in the adult liver.

Neither by injection of barium into the left

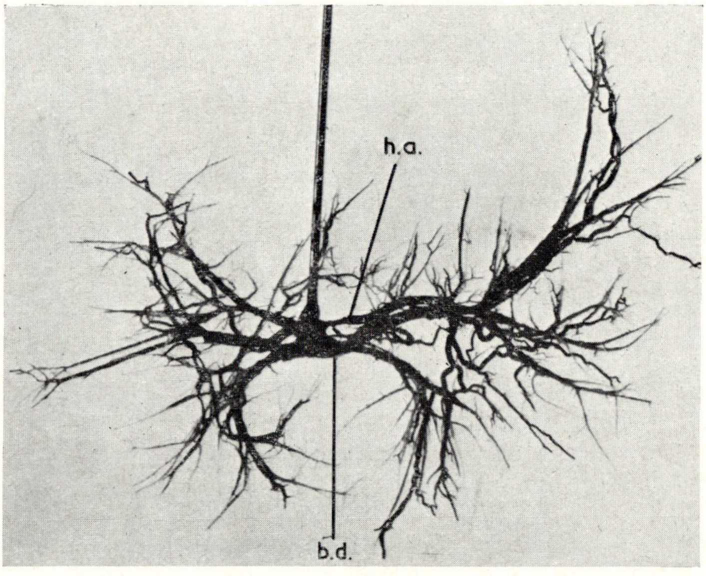


FIG. 5.—Segmental branches of the hepatic artery (h.a.) and bile-ducts (b.d.) of a 6-month-old infant, anterior view.

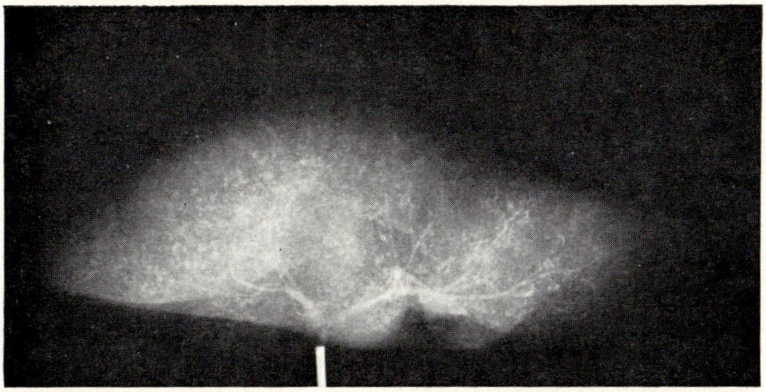

FIG. 6.—Intrahepatic cholangiogram of a 3-day-old infant. Caudo-cranial x-ray examination.

hepatic duct (Fig. 7), nor by injection of $^{131}$I-labelled hippuric acid solution into the right hepatic duct (Fig. 8), could the agents be detected in the contralateral lobes.

On the basis of these studies, the liver of the newborn infant can be divided into 6 segments (see Fig. 10): (1) caudate lobe with processus caudatus; (2) a right ventral segment; (3) a right dorsal segment; (4) quadrate lobe; (5) a left ventro-lateral segment; and (6) a left dorso-lateral segment.

As far as surgical treatment of the so-called inoperable extrahepatic biliary atresia is concerned, we concluded the following.

(a) To achieve a sufficient bile flow and a functioning anastomosis between the intrahepatic bile-ducts and the intestinal tract, the largest possible bile-ducts have to be identified. Only the hepatic ducts are sufficient in this sense, the peripheral segment branches being too small.

(b) These hepatic ducts may end blindly or with a confluence within the liver, as is shown in Fig. 9. This schematic drawing demonstrates a personal classification of the 10 possible types of biliary atresia. To identify these intrahepatic ducts in types 7 or 8, it seems to be necessary to resect the central portion of the quadrate lobe.

(c) The peripheral wedge excision of the quadrate lobe according to Nixon (1964) and Grewe (1964) seems not to be the treatment of choice, because the liver hilum, where the intrahepatic hepatic ducts should be found, cannot be opened widely enough.

(d) With type 8 biliary atresia, both functional lobes of the liver could be drained of bile only by resection of the central portion of the quadrate lobe.

(e) The procedures of hepatogastrostomy (Gohrbandt, 1957) and cholangiojejunostomy (Longmire and Sanford, 1948, 1949) must be inadequate on the basis of the present findings: whether or not a normal intrahepatic bile-duct system has developed must be unknown, and in the case of an atresia type 8 the biliary system of the right functional lobe would not be drained, because

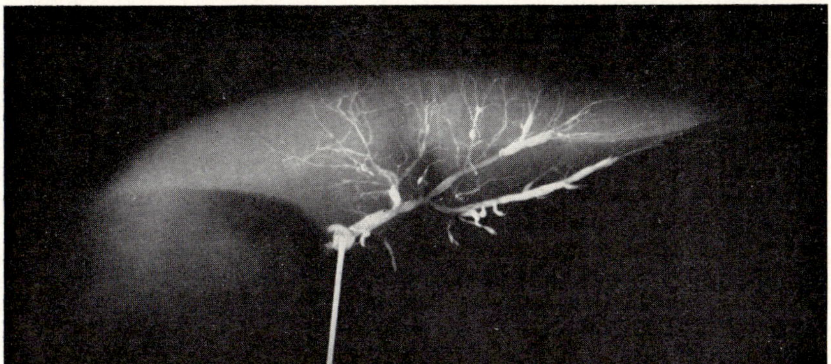

FIG. 7.—Isolated, injected left hepatic duct with barium. No anastomoses between the two functional lobes.

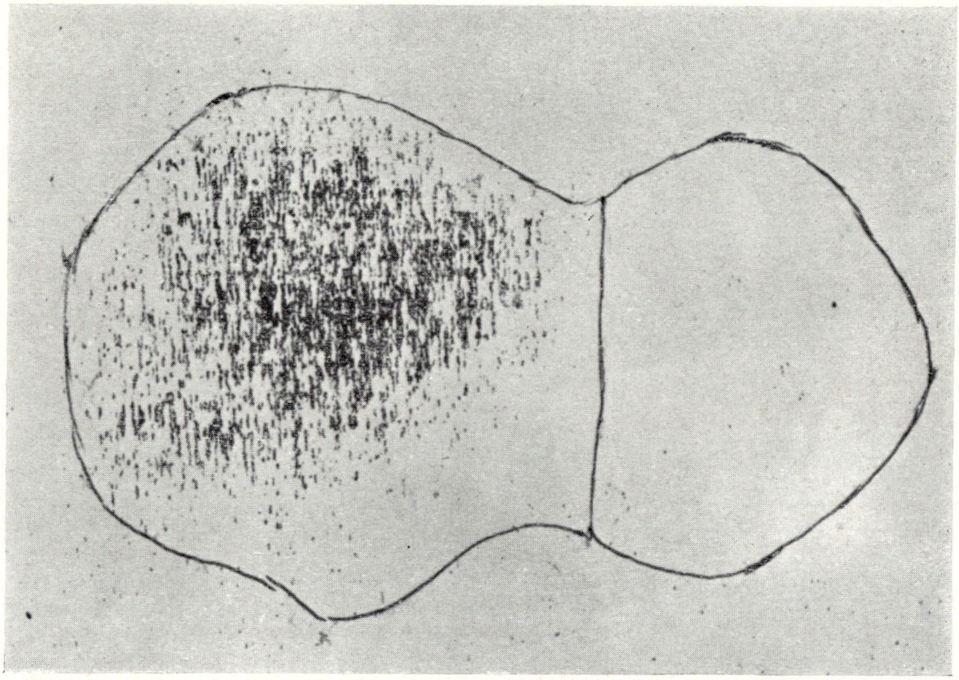

FIG. 8.—Scintigraph of a liver cast of a 6-day-old infant. Right hepatic duct injected with $^{131}$I labelled hippuric acid solution. Absence of anastomoses to the left functional lobe.

intrahepatic anastomoses of the bile-ducts are absent.

(f) Bile-duct atresias of type 9 and 10 cannot be corrected by resection of the quadrate lobe.

With these conclusions in mind, a resection of the central portion of the quadrate lobe was carried out in 3 infants suffering from an inoperable bile-duct atresia. The topographical relation of the quadrate

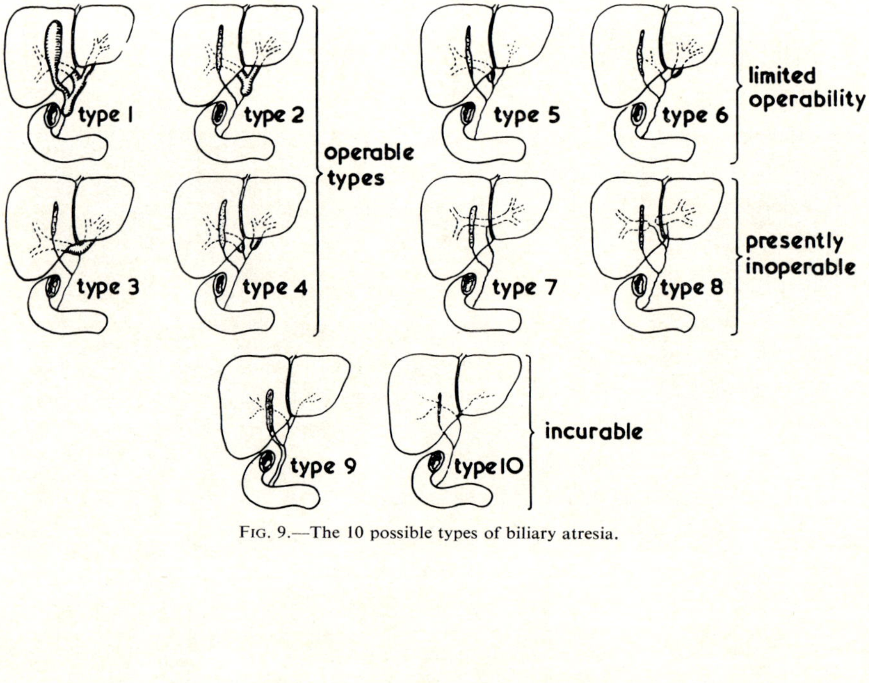


FIG. 9.—The 10 possible types of biliary atresia.

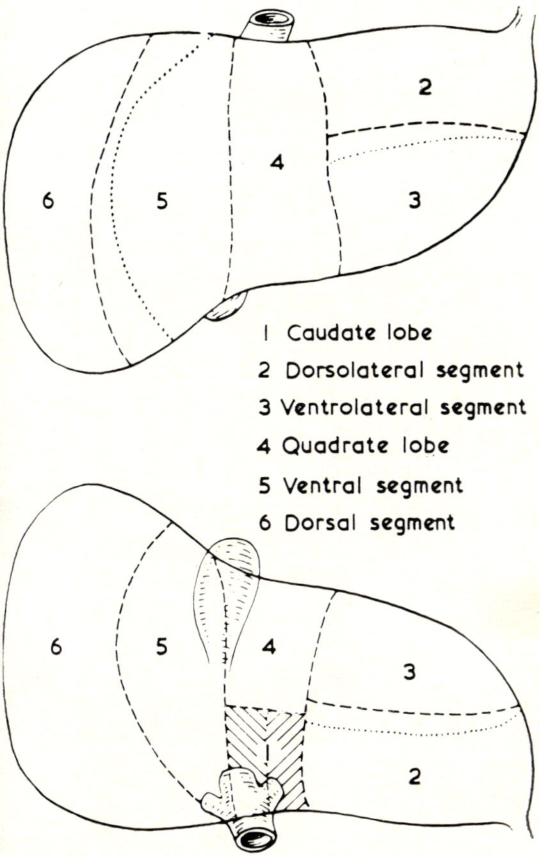


FIG. 10 (*left*).—The six segments of the newborn and infant liver.

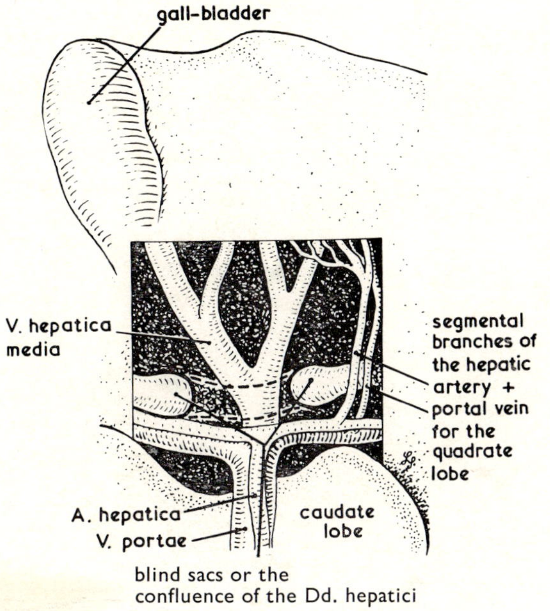


FIG. 11.—Schematic drawing of the quadrate lobe after resection of the central portion.

lobe is shown in Fig. 11. In no cases could blindly-ending hepatic ducts within the liver be found. In one an atresia of type 9 was seen and in the other two a type 10. The two cases of type 10 atresia were confirmed by necropsy; the other child is still alive.

## Summary

The normal anatomy of the vascular and bile-duct systems of the liver in the newborn infant has been studied.

The biliary systems of the right and left functional lobes do not anastomose with one another.

This fact provides a basis for the surgical treatment of those cases of extrahepatic biliary atresia that are generally considered as inoperable.

### REFERENCES

Cantlie, J. (1898). On a new arrangement of the right and left lobes of the liver. *J. Anat. Physiol.*, **32**, iv.

Couinaud, C. (1954). Étude des voies biliaires intra-hépatiques. *J. Chir. (Paris)*, **70**, 310.

Gohrbandt, E. (1957). Hepato-gastrostomie. *Zbl. Chir.*, **82**, 641.

Grewe, H. E. (1964). Zur operativen Behandlung von Gallengang-satresien. *ibid.*, **89**, 145.

——, and Arius, G. (1961). In *Die chir. Behandlung der angeborenen Fehlbildungen*, ed. K. Kremer. Thieme, Stuttgart.

——, and Pape, M. (1962). Zur Diagnostik und Therapie des Verschlussikterus im Säuglingsalter. *Mschr. Kinderheilk.*, **110**, 381.

Grob, M. (1957). *Lehrbuch der Kinderchirurgie*. Georg Thieme, Stuttgart,

Gross, R. E. (1953). *The Surgery of Infancy and Childhood.* Saunders, Philadelphia and London.

Hartmann, H. (1960). Beitrag zur Chirurgie der Gallenwegs-verschlüsse. *Langenbecks Arch. klin. Chir.*, **296**, 1.

Hasse, W. (1963). Inoperable Gallengangsatresie und Relaparotomie. *Chirurg*, **34**, 254.

—— (1964a). Gefässtopographische Studien als Grundlage zur Chirurgie der Säuglingsleber. Kinderchir. Symposion Wien.

—— (1964b). Gefässtopographische Studien an der Säuglingsleber als Grundlage für die Chirurgie der sog. inoperablen extra hepatischen Gallengangsatresie. *Lagenbecks Arch. klin. Chir.*, **308**, 766.

Healey, J. E., and Schroy, P. C. (1953). Anatomy of the biliary ducts within the human liver. *Arch. Surg.*, **66**, 599.

——, and Sterling, J. A. (1963). Segmental anatomy of the newborn liver. *Ann. N. Y. Acad. Sci.*, **111**, 25.

Hecker, W. Ch., and Daum, R. (1964). Beitrag zum Problem der sog. inoperablen Gallengangsatresie. *Zbl. Chir.*, **89**, 150.

Hjortsjö, C. H. J. (1948). Die Anatomie der intrahepatischen Gallengänge beim Menschen, mittels Röntgen- und Injektionstechnik studiert, nebst Beiträgen zur Kenntnis der inneren Lebertopographie. Gleerup, Lund.

Ladd, W. E. (1935). Congenital obstruction of the bile ducts. *Ann. Surg.*, **102**, 742.

Longmire, W. P., Jr., and Sanford, M. C. (1948). Intrahepatic cholangiojejunostomy with partial hepatectomy for biliary obstruction. *Surgery*, **24**, 264.

——, —— (1949). Intrahepatic cholangiojejunostomy for biliary obstruction—further studies. *Ann. Surg.*, **130**, 455.

Nettelblad, S. C. (1954). Die Lobierung und innere Topographie der Säugerleber. *Acta. anat.* (*Basel*), Supp. 20, 21.

Nixon, H. H. (1964). Leberchirurgie im Kindesalter. Kinderchir. Symposion Vienna,

Rehbein F., and Neumann, G. (1957). Angeborene Gallengangsatresie. *Kinderärztl. Prax.*, **25**, 78.

Reifferscheid, M. (1957). *Chirurgie der Leber*. Thieme, Stuttgart.

Rex, H. (1888). Beiträge zur Morphologie der Säugerleber. *Morph. Jb.*, **14**, 517.

Røjel, K. (1958). Surgical anatomy of the liver. *Acta chir. scand.*, **114**, 277.

Schummer, A. (1951). Vereinfachtes Plastoid-Korrosionsverfahren. *Anat. Anz.*, **98**, 288.

Sterling, J. A. (1961). Artificial bile ducts in the management of congenital biliary atresia. *J. int. Coll. Surg.*, **36**, 293.

Stucke, K. (1959). *Leberchirurgie*. Springer, Berlin.

*Arch. Dis. Childh.*, 1965, **40**, 169.

# HEPATIC TUMOURS IN CHILDHOOD AND THEIR TREATMENT BY MAJOR HEPATIC RESECTION*

BY

H. H. NIXON

*From The Hospital for Sick Children, Great Ormond Street, London*

Hepatic tumours in childhood are not common, and when seven cases were seen within a short time it seemed worth while to report them (see Table *overleaf*).

### Pathology

Five were described as hepatoblastomas. These are usually considered as embryomas analogous to the nephroblastoma. Though only the epithelial elements of the liver arise from the hepatic diverticulum of the primitive gut, the derivatives of the mass of mesenchyme into which it grows may take part in the neoplasia. Case 3 had an appearance suggestive of gargoylism, and punch biopsies were suggestive of storage disease as were some bone changes. Open biopsy and later examination of the operative specimen did not confirm this, the liver cells showing abundant fatty degeneration but no evidence of storage disease.

Case 6 was described as a hepatic carcinoma arising in an otherwise normal liver (Fig. 1). The tumour consisted of pleomorphic cells having some of the characteristics and arrangement of liver parenchyma. No embryonic mesenchyme was seen.

* A paper read at a meeting of the British Association of Paediatric Surgeons in Rotterdam, September 1964.

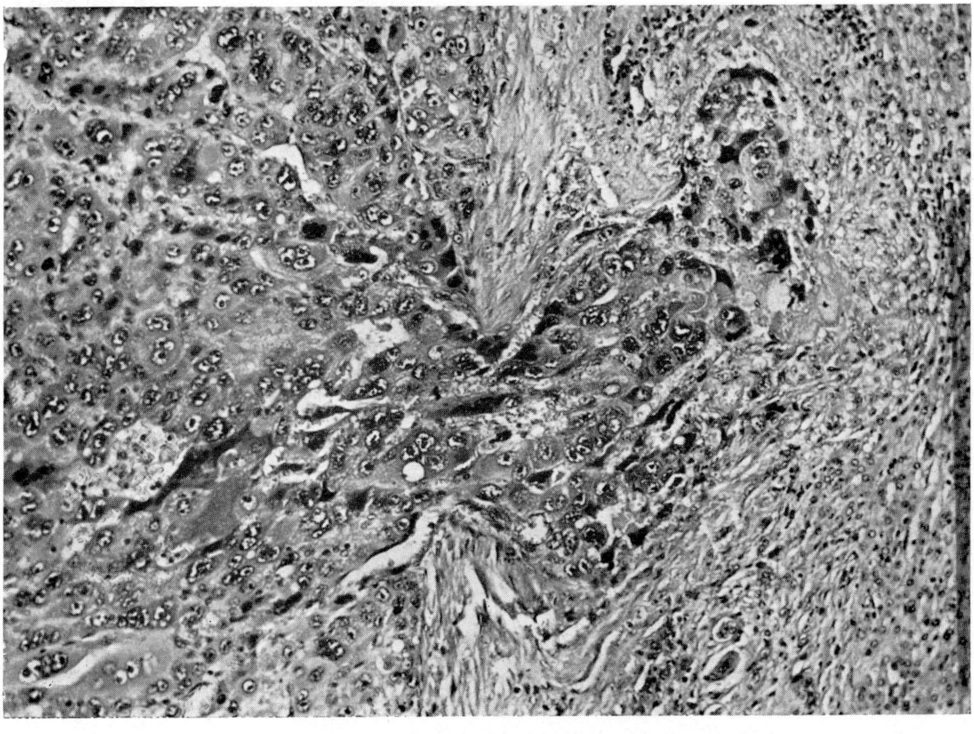

FIG. 1.—Case 1: carcinoma arising in normal liver. (× 130.)

AGE, PRESENTING SYMPTOMS, RESU

| Case No., Age, and Sex | | | Tumour | Presenting Symptoms | Duratio |
|---|---|---|---|---|---|
| 1 | 9 yr. | M | Hepatoblastoma | Malaise; palpable tumour | 1 mth. |
| 2 | 7 mth. | F | Hepatoblastoma | Palpable tumour | ? |
| 3 | 2 yr. | M | Hepatoblastoma | Hepatosplenomegaly (appearance like gargoylism) | 18 mth. |
| 4 | 5 mth. | M | Hepatoblastoma | Palpable tumour | 10 dy. |
| 5 | 1½ yr. | M | Hepatoblastoma | Irritable; pale; palpable mass | 10 wk. 6 wk. 1 wk. |
| 6 | 7 yr. | M | Carcinoma in normal liver | Loss of weight; palpable mass | 2 mth. |
| 7 | 1 wk. | M | Hamartoma | Palpable mass at birth | 1 wk. |

This must be very unusual, for the commonest age of appearance of carcinoma of the liver is in the sixth decade and it is usually associated with cirrhosis.

However, the difference in histological pattern may be one of degree, and Willis (1948) points out 'that the distinction between truly embryonic liver cell tumours and ordinary hepatomas arising in childhood may be neither histologically possible nor theoretically valid', and goes on to say 'suffice it to recognize that there are tumours of liver tissue of unquestionable embryonic qualities'.

The remaining case was a hamartoma, containing much vascular tissue.

### Presentation

In two cases vague malaise and in one weight loss had led to examination revealing the palpable tumour. In the others the palpation of the mass was the first sign of trouble. Six of the seven were boys.

### Treatment

**Operation.** The first boy presented with a large abdominal swelling. Laparotomy and frozen section biopsy confirmed this to be a hepatoblastoma filling the right lobe of the liver. 1,666 g. of soft tumour were scooped out of the cavity to relieve abdominal distension and the child returned home. He died four months later.

Reconsidering this case, it was felt that the mere size of the tumour should have been no justification for such a palliative approach, for hepatoblastomas grow locally but metastasize late (Steiner, 1938). The next six liver tumours were therefore treated by the following major resections: 2 right hemihepatectomies, 2 right hepatic lobectomies, 1 left hepatic lobectomy, and 1 left hemihepatectomy with partial right lobectomy.

The liver has joined those organs whose vascular hila have been charted so that major resections can be performed in a planned manner. I have found Hobsley's re-evaluation of the anatomy invaluable (Hobsley, 1958; Hobsley and Lloyd-Davies, 1959). The main divisions are into right and left halves along the principal plane from gall-bladder fossa to the right side of the inferior vena cava, or into right and left lobes along the falciform ligament (Fig. 2). The liver is unusual in having two hila, the bile-ducts, hepatic arteries, and portal veins all in the porta hepatis, and the hepatic veins separately leaving the liver near the upper border posteriorly. Unfortunately their drainage areas do not correspond. The Glissonian system fundamentally forms right and left halves, whereas the hepatic veins divide the liver into three areas with the central vein territory draining part of the right and left halves (Fig. 3). In this overlap and in the inaccessibility of the hepatic veins to demonstration by dissection lie the main technical problems of hepatic resection.

For right-sided resections the preferred incision is an oblique thoraco-abdominal one. The abdominal part is made first. Exploration of the abdomen and dissection of the porta hepatis to confirm operability precede opening of the chest and division of the diaphragm right into the opening for the inferior vena cava. Slings to control the cava should then be placed above the diaphragm and below the liver. It is usual to rotate the liver to the left to expose the right hepatic vein, and if necessary the central vein. Mercadier approaches the veins from the front, retracting the liver downwards and dissecting into the liver tissue. The latter may be easier depending on the distortion produced by the particular tumour, but the stout fascial investment of the vena cava in this region may be troublesome. I found the correct perivascular plane more easily by starting the dissection above the diaphragm and working down.

The left lobectomy (in a 1-week-old baby) proved a simple procedure and was completed from the abdomen and without control of the vena cava.

ION, AND PROGRESS IN 7 CASES

| Operation* | Result | Progress |
|---|---|---|
| Piecemeal evacuation of tumour | Survival | Tumour discharge from wound; died 4 mth. later |
| Right hepatic lobectomy | Died (thrombosis IVC) | |
| Right hemihepatectomy | Survival | Well 1 yr. later |
| Right hemihepatectomy | Died (pulmonary infarcts) | |
| (1) Right hemihepatectomy (2) Relief of adhesion obstruction | Survival | Methotrexate; died 3 mth. later (pulmonary metastases and local recurrence) |
| Left hemihepatectomy with partial right lobectomy | Survival | Methotrexate; well 6 mth. later |
| Left lobectomy | Survival | Well 6 mth. later |

* See Fig. 4.

The 'extended left hemihepatectomy' removed all but half of the right lobe with the gall-bladder attached. It was possible to divide the right lobe in a curved line so as to preserve the divisions of the right hepatic vein, which drained the remaining part of the lobe, and yet keep clear of the tumour. The right thoraco-abdominal approach was used, with control of the inferior vena cava.

In each of the resections the liver substance was divided with the diathermy, a few individual vessels being caught and undersewn as necessary. The biliary duct system was not drained. A tube drain into Morison's pouch only drained a little blood. Biliary leakage has not been noticeable.

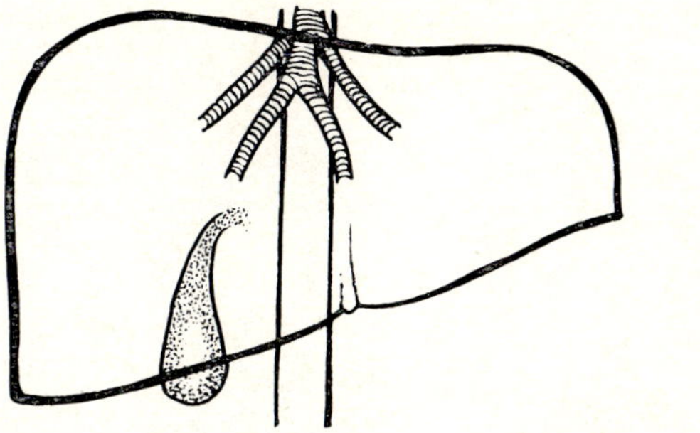

FIG. 3.—Hepatic venous drainage from three sectors—the middle hepatic vein draining an area supplied by right and left branches of the Glissonian system and hence complicating the technique of resection.

**Complications.** The first post-operative death was due to thrombosis of the inferior vena cava following trauma in attempting to control bleeding from the hepatic veins. Serious bleeding also arose during clearing of the central hepatic vein in the extended left hemihepatectomy, though it was successfully controlled. Both these episodes could have been avoided by adequate control of the vena cava by a sling placed above the diaphragm as mentioned above.

The other death occurred 3 days after operation

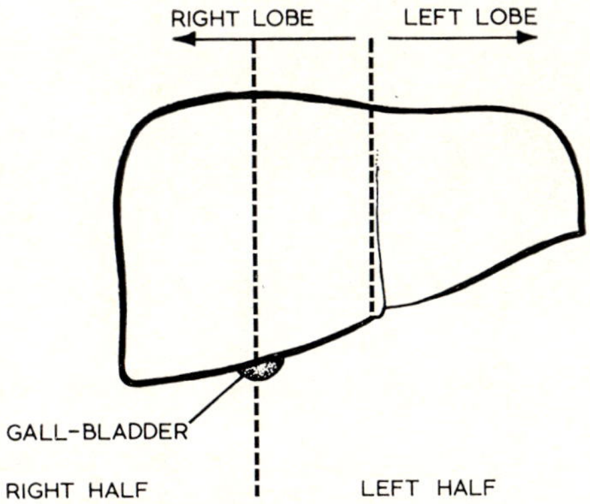


FIG. 2.—Classical division into right and left lobes through plane of falciform ligament and functional division into right and left halves as supplied by right and left branches of Glissonion system (arteries, portal veins, and bile-ducts) through gall-bladder fossa.

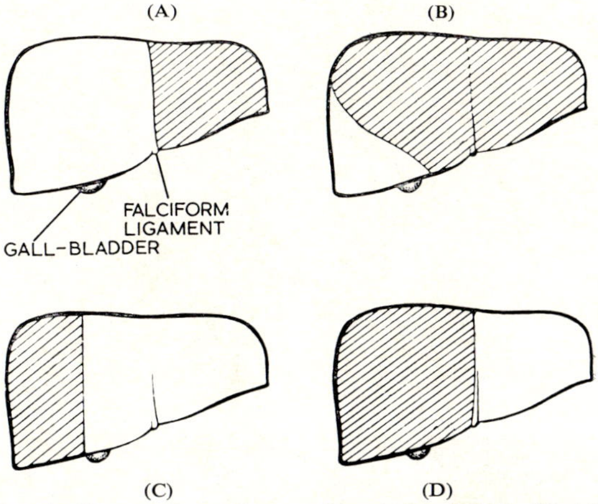


FIG. 4.—Extent of resections performed (see Table): (A) left lobectomy; (B) left hemihepatectomy; (C) right hemihepatectomy (D) right lobectomy plus partial right hemihepatectomy.

and was due to infarction of the upper lobes of both lungs. The veins within the abdomen were quite healthy and free of thrombi. It appears that the origin of the pulmonary thrombi was in emboli from the haemorrhagic and necrotic centre of the tumour disturbed during manipulation of the liver.

One right hemihepatectomy developed intestinal obstruction from adherence of a loop of ileum to the raw surface of the liver three weeks after the operation. An attempt had been made to cover the raw area with the mobilized falciform ligament as is usually advised. I have found this somewhat inadequate and have since sutured omentum over the surface instead.

Only one patient in the series (Case 3) showed post-operative signs of liver failure, and in this case the disturbance was temporary.

Two cases have been given methotrexate. Case 5 received 2·5 mg. daily for two months after operation; he then developed granulopenia and the drug was discontinued. He died with pulmonary metastases and local recurrence one month later. Case 6 has had the drug for the six months since removal of his hepatic carcinoma and remains well.

## Summary

Four children out of six survived major hepatic resection for tumour. Three remain well for periods of 6 to 12 months after operation. One was an unusual tumour, a hepatic carcinoma in the otherwise normal liver of a child. Comments are made on points of operative technique. Although the bile-ducts were not drained, significant leakage of bile did not occur, possibly because the liver was divided with diathermy. An aggressive attitude to these tumours seems justified.

My thanks are due to those colleagues who referred the cases to me, and to the late Dr. Martin Bodian and to Drs. Barraclough, Crome, and Ockenden, for the pathological reports. I am indebted to the Department of Medical Illustration at The Hospital for Sick Children, Great Ormond Street, for the photographs and diagrams.

### References

Hobsley, M. (1958). Intra-hepatic anatomy: a surgical evaluation. *Brit. J. Surg.*, **45**, 635.

——, and Lloyd-Davies, O. V. (1959). Survey on partial hepatectomy with especial reference to liver anatomy. In *British Surgical Practice*, ed. E. R. Carling and J. P. Ross. *Surgical Progress*, p. 40. Butterworth, London.

Steiner, M. M. (1938). Primary carcinoma of the liver in childhood; report of 2 cases with critical review of literature. *Amer. J. Dis. Child.*, **55**, 807.

Willis, R. A. (1948). *Pathology of Tumours*, p. 933. Butterworth, London.

*Arch. Dis. Childh.*, 1965, **40**, 173.

# POLYPS OF THE COLON BEYOND THE REACH OF THE SIGMOIDOSCOPE*

BY

JEAN DUHAMEL and PIERRE BAUCHE

*From Hôpitaux de Paris, France, and Université de Liège, Belgium*

Amongst 350 children treated for recto-colonic polyps at the Hôpital des Enfants-Malades, we have seen 11 cases of polyps of the colon out of reach of the sigmoidoscope (remote polyps). A further 4 cases from the Hôpital de Bavière de Liège (Belgium) have been added, making in all 15 out of a total of 400 cases of recto-colonic polyps.

Are remote polyps in children much less common than recto-sigmoidal polyps? In the adult, this disproportion is only apparent, systematic necropsies showing clearly that the localization of adenomas in the different segments of the large intestine (rectum included) is fairly regular (Chapman, 1963; Feyrter, 1931) (Fig. 1a).

The studies on adults show that the frequency increases with age, with 20% in the third and the fourth decades, 31% in the fifth, 61% in the sixth, and more than 75% after 80 years. Children's polyps are quite different. Helwig (1946) found that amongst 449 necropsies of children and young adults under 21 years of age, there were only 5 subjects suffering from polyps: 1 polyp of the rectum in a 4-year-old boy; 8 polyps of the rectum in an 8-year-old boy; 1 polyp of the rectum in a 12-year-old girl; 1 polyp of the ascending colon in a 7-year-old girl; and 1 polyp of the caecum in a 15-year-old girl. In all, there were 10 polyps of the rectum, 1 of the ascending colon, and 1 of the caecum (Fig. 1b). The incidence must be higher in small children on account of the extreme scarcity of these polyps in adolescents. It is well known that they are quite exceptional before the age of 1 year; their frequency increases very quickly after 2 years, to reach a maximum between 4 and 5 years (Duhamel, 1958). After this age, polyps become uncommon (possibly on account of self-destruction), and are very rare after 14 years. Between 15 and 20, adenomas are uncommon, though we have personally observed 5 cases. During the period that we shall call the 'adolescent gap', our observations have shown the persistence of infantile polyps after the age of 15. From this fact some very important problems emerge concerning the fate of polyps of childhood and the relation between these and adult polyps. This persistence into adolescence is very rare (only 3 such cases out of 350 polyps of the recto-colon were observed by Duhamel (1964)).

The histology has been amply described. These adenomas are of a particular type, with enormous hyperplasia and inflammation of the chorion; the glandular part is less affected but shows a peculiar irregularity in the size of the glands, some being hypertrophied and some cystic. The epithelial covering may desquamate giving the polyp the appearance of a fleshy bud. Some authors do not accept these as adenomas, but we believe, as Helwig does, that they are adenomas of a special type, for the following reasons: (1) predominance in males, as in adult adenomas and recto-colonic cancers; (2) the frequency of multiple polyps is the same for children and for adults; (3) the existence of forms resembling adult adenomas but only showing slight inflammation initially; and (4) the existence of adult adenomas

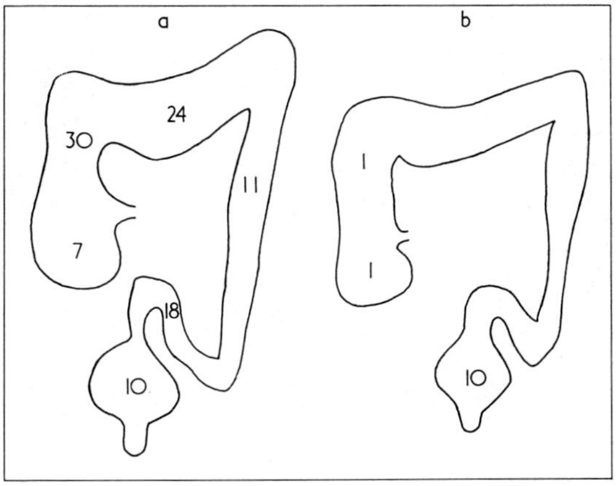


FIG. 1a and 1b.—(a) Distribution of adenomas in adults (after Chapman, 1963; Feyrter, 1931). (b) Distribution of adenomas in children, 449 subjects (after Helwig, 1946).

* A paper read at a meeting of the British Association of Paediatric Surgeons in Rotterdam, September 1964.

TABLE 1

DETAILS OF 'REMOTE' COLONIC POLYPS IN 15 CASES AGED 3 TO 11 YEARS

| Case No. | Sex | Age (yr.) | Number of Remote Polyps | Site | Diameter (cm.) | Pedicle (cm.) | Treatment | Polyps Also in Recto-sigmoid |
|---|---|---|---|---|---|---|---|---|
| 1 | F | 9 | 1 | Descending colon | 3 | 6 | Polypectomy | |
| 2 | M | 8 | 1 | Iliac colon | 2 | 2 | Polypectomy | |
| 3 | M | 3 | 1 | Descending colon | 3 | 6 | Polypectomy | |
| 4 | F | 11 | 2 | Descending colon<br>Sigmoid colon | 2<br>3 | 3 | Polypectomy | 2 rectal polyps |
| 5 | F | 7 | 1 | Transverse colon | 3 | 1 | Polypectomy | 1 rectal polyp |
| 6 | M | 5 | 1 | Descending colon | 4 | ? | Polypectomy | |
| 7 | F | 5 | 1 | Descending colon | 4 | 3 | Polypectomy | 1 rectal polyp |
| 8 | M | 5 | 1 | Sigmoid colon | 2 | 'Long' | Polypectomy | |
| 9 | M | 5 | 1 | Descending colon | 2 | 'Long' | Left *in situ* | |
| 10 | F | 3 | 1 | Descending colon | 3 | ? | | |
| 11 | F | 7 | 2 | Descending colon<br>Sigmoid colon | 2<br>2 | | Polypectomy | |
| 12 | F | 6 | 5 | 2 angles, transv., sigm., desc. | 0·5–3 | | Polypectomy | |
| 13 | M | 3½ | 2 | 2 sigmoid colons | 1·5<br>0·5 | | Polypectomy | 1 rectal polyp |
| 14 | F | 3½ | 3 | 2 transverse colons<br>1 sigmoid colon | <br>2 | | <br>Polypectomy | |
| 15 | M | 3½ | 2 | 2 descending colons | | | Spontaneous shedding | 1 rectal polyp |

of inflammatory type, histologically resembling those of the child.

In comparing the appearances of remote polyps, we are faced with the problem that they cannot be viewed by sigmoidoscopy, nor are biopsies or endoscopic operations possible.

### Clinical Features

These are summarized in the Table. The average age is between 3 and 5 years as with recto-sigmoidal polyps. Recto-sigmoidal polyps in the child nearly always declare themselves by the appearance of fresh blood in the stools. A polyp of the colon which may bleed slightly, or because of its distance produces only coagulated blood in the faeces, may go unnoticed. A valuable indirect sign of a polyp out of reach of the sigmoidoscope is the presence of traces of fresh blood higher up when a polyp of the recto-sigmoid region has already been removed. This is an indication for barium examination of the colon.

### Radiography

All cases require a radiological examination. A special technique is necessary: purge, enema, finely particulate and adhesive barium, moderate filling, pictures taken after evacuation and insufflation, double contrast, patient horizontal and erect. From the study of our x-ray material we have noted three characteristic appearances.

(1) Bowel filled or half filled: a transparency (lacuna) more or less circular (14 instances).

(2) Bowel inflated: polyp coated with barium, appearing opaque on a translucent background (8 instances).

(3) After evacuation: polyp expanding the collapsed lumen, the 'bead on a string' appearance (3 instances).

The figures show that the 'half-filled' picture more often gives the characteristic appearance, but these results must be completed and confirmed by other technical means. The pedicle has been correctly observed 8 times: 4 times in the 'half-filled' state, once in evacuation, and on 3 occasions during insufflation, each time with the help of compression. Even if the image of the polyp is characteristic, radiological control before operation is absolutely necessary, as it is a check on false images that may be extremely puzzling and even simulate a pedicle.

### Anatomy

The polyp of the colon was single in 9 out of 15 cases. There were multiple (up to 4) polyps in 6 cases. In the collection as a whole there were 5 instances of a remote colonic polyp associated with a recto-sigmoid polyp.

The average size for all remote polyps was from 2 to 4 cm. This shows that even with perfect techniques, small polyps remain unseen. The polyps were situated in 10 instances on the descending colon, in 8 on the iliac colon and high sigmoid, and in 6 on the transverse colon. The predominance of the left colon may be explained by the fact that this portion is of a slight diameter, is tubular and easily compressible, making the contrast between polyp and barium more demonstrable. The pedicle was nearly always long, generally being more than 5 cm.

The *histology* was the same as that of recto-sigmoidal polyps, with inflammatory changes, intrapolypoid haemorrhage, some suppurating areas, and surface ulceration.

### Spontaneous Evolution

It appears that evolution proceeds the same way as the recto-sigmoidal polyps, with spontaneous shedding of the polyp due to progressive ischaemia, haemorrhage, and suppuration, leading to a partial or total amputation of the polyp itself or of its pedicle. This seems to happen less often in the colon because here there is no trauma from defaecation or extrusion. The longer life of the polyps in the colon explains why its pedicle is also longer than that of its fellow in the recto-sigmoid. It also implies that views about the prognosis of these polyps must be reserved.

### Problems of Recurrence *in situ*

Is this spontaneous separation the sign of final healing? Or, on the contrary, is a recurrence on the stump of the pedicle a danger? This is an important question because these polyps cannot be watched by means of endoscopy.

Concerning this spontaneous separation of remote polyps, we have observed a polyp in the upper sigmoid with a long pedicle that was out of sight at a previous examination. Two polyps in the same child (Case 15) were also thought to be behaving in this way. In two other cases (Nos. 9 and 10) in children aged 3 and 5 years, the shedding of the polyps has still not occurred.

If we cannot as yet answer the question for colonic polyps, we have a much larger experience of the recto-sigmoidal polyps, which are of the same nature. We have often observed that after spontaneous detachment of the polyp the pedicle remains, and we have noted its position with accuracy. Two changes may follow. (1) Sometimes the pedicle is absorbed in a few days or a few weeks leaving no trace. (2) More rarely the pedicle remains and grows into a new polyp: such a recurrence may also be seen after an incomplete removal of the polyp by the use of biopsy forceps, insufficient electrocoagulation, or snare. We have tried to reproduce this phenomenon in the following way.

We selected a few cases of low-sited polyps and cut the pedicle at its distal part by means of scissors or biopsy forceps or ligature, deliberately leaving *in situ* a large segment of the pedicle. A recurrence on the pedicle was observed in several cases in the ensuing months. The end became club-shaped and red, and within a few weeks or months a new polyp had formed.

When the root of the pedicle is resected there is no recurrence.

**Histology of the Pedicle.** The samples showing the pedicle are scarce, as the polyp is generally removed by the diathermy loop, with fulguration of the pedicle. Lengthwise section of the pedicle is necessary, when three distinct areas may be observed: (1) a proximal area, where glands are compressed one against the other, of small size, regularly shaped, having the same appearance as normal mucous membrane; (2) an intermediate area, with dilated glands with flattened epithelium next to normal glands in a chorion, showing some hypertrophy but little inflammation, and with vascular spaces; (3) a distal area, with all the characteristics of the infantile polyp, but with less marked inflammation, haemorrhage, or suppuration.

We conclude that the propensity for polyp formation resides especially in the middle and distal areas. Resection at the base of the pedicle, or better still in the sound mucous membrane, will not be followed by recurrence, as we have confirmed experimentally. A section in the middle or distal part will favour relapse. Since we do not know where the polypogenous area begins, a fairly deep fulguration is required, while avoiding the risk of a scar. In the recto-sigmoidal area we try to limit the parietal cautery scar to an average of 5 mm. diameter.

### Surgical Treatment

For *rectal polyps* this presents few problems, though it may be somewhat difficult to regulate which part is to be left to fulguration and which to section when the diathermy loop is used. If coagulation is followed by even slight bleeding, it proves that it has been insufficient, and in that case it must be completed by a fulguration of the remaining stump by means of the ball-shaped electrode or of the diathermic tag. In certain cases it would be simpler to cut the polyp with biopsy tongs and to coagulate the pedicle.

The problems of treating *polyps of the colon* are more complex. Because of (a) the frequent continuation of bleeding, (b) the persistence in certain cases of rectal polyps from infancy to beyond 15 years (of which we have a few examples), and the impossibility of asserting, from our present standpoint, that a benign adenoma will not in the long run become malignant, we advise surgical intervention without waiting for a spontaneous separation which may turn out to be a false cure. Abdominal incision is sited in relation to the polyp and the latter is then localized by palpation, transparietal traction to note the implantation, and above all endoscopy before removal, using a sterile proctoscope introduced through a colostomy. By inspection above and below, not only may the exact site of implantation of the pedicle be located, but other polyps not seen on a radiograph may be found. Segmental resection, which we advise for such polyps in the adult, is not appropriate here; simple polypectomy suffices, but must be performed with particular care, either by excision of the root of the pedicle and its base (*colerette d'implantation*) or by fulguration of the base of the pedicle. In the latter case, the risk of haemorrhage is small, for in 150 cases in which we removed polyps in the recto-sigmoid by the diathermy noose we only had one instance of haemorrhage following the sloughing of a scar 8 days later.

## Summary

In 400 recto-sigmoidal polyps in children observed at the Hôpital des Enfants-Malades, we have only found 15 colonic polyps. Even with modern radiological techniques small polyps in the colon are rarely detected. Colonic polyps have the same histological pattern as recto-sigmoidal polyps. They are generally spontaneously shed, but not so frequently as recto-sigmoid polyps. This shedding is not proof of healing, as regrowth from the pedicle is possible.

Total destruction is advised, by excision of the root of the pedicle and its base, or by fulguration after colostomy.

### References

Chapman, I. (1963). Adenomatous polypi of the large intestine: incidence and distribution. *Ann. Surg.*, **157**, 223.

Feyrter, F. (1931). Zur Geschwulstlehre (nach Untersuchungen am menschlichen Darm). I. Polypen und Krebs. *Beitr. path. Anat.*, **86**, 664.

Helwig, E. B. (1946). Adenomas of the large intestine in children. *Amer. J. Dis. Child.*, **72**, 289.

Duhamel J. (1958). *Affections Non-Congénitales de l'Anus et du Rectum Chez l'Enfant*, p. 260. Masson, Paris.

—— (1964). Les polypes recto-sigmoïdiens de l'adolescent. *Arch. Mal. Appar. dig.*, **53**, 1122.

*Arch. Dis. Childh.*, 1965, **40**, 177.

# PSEUDO-HIRSCHSPRUNG'S DISEASE*

BY

TH. EHRENPREIS

*From the Children's Clinic, Karolinska Sjukhuset, Stockholm, Sweden*

Largely thanks to the work of Swenson and Bill (1948), Whitehouse and Kernohan (1948), and Bodian, Stephens, and Ward (1949), the definition of Hirschsprung's disease and its differentiation from idiopathic and symptomatic megacolon has become a clear-cut diagnostic procedure which is now part of the daily routine in every paediatric surgical unit.

Occasionally a short-segment aganglionosis may present as an idiopathic megacolon, and complete aganglionosis of the colon may be difficult to distinguish from other types of low intestinal obstruction in the newborn. Rectal biopsy will always settle the diagnosis. Diagnostic difficulties in patients with a narrow segment of the usual length are rare. I have recently treated a child, presenting with an unusual type of megacolon which does not fit into the usual classification of this syndrome.

## Case Report

A 10-month-old girl was admitted with a history of severe constipation and abdominal distension, starting at the age of 8 months, when she was weaned. Before this time she had emptied her bowels only once a week, without, however, showing evidence of discomfort or abdominal distension. The anus was normal and the rectum was empty. Radiological examination had been performed in another hospital (Fig. 1), showing a normal-sized rectum and distal sigmoid colon and marked distension and faecal impaction proximal to this. The radiographs were typical of Hirschsprung's disease. After an unusually long period of difficult bowel cleansing, laparotomy was performed. Inspection of the colon seemed to confirm the diagnosis of Hirschsprung's disease. A narrow segment extending to the apex of the sigmoid flexure, with a funnel-shaped zone of transition into the grossly dilated proximal sigmoid, was seen. Two atypical features were soon disclosed, however. There was no hypertrophy of the bowel wall, and the gaseous contents of the dilated bowel could be propelled down through the narrow segment without the typical resistance. No mechanical obstruction could be demonstrated. Proximally, the dilatation gradually decreased. A Duhamel type of recto-sigmoidectomy was performed.

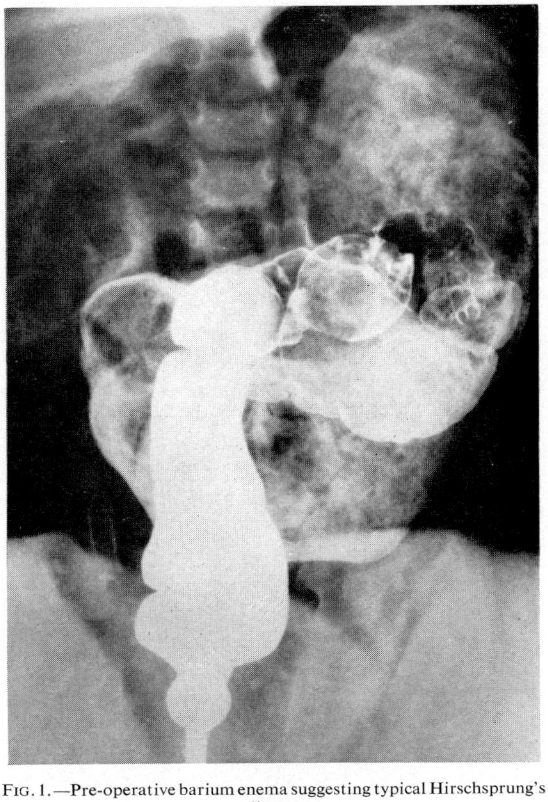

FIG. 1.—Pre-operative barium enema suggesting typical Hirschsprung's disease.

Histological examination revealed no abnormality of the intramural plexuses or other abnormality. The post-operative course was uneventful. The child recovered but a slight constipation persisted, which has been easily managed with a mild aperient. At a recent follow-up, 7 months after operation, the child was in an excellent condition and had no abdominal distension. Rectal examination revealed an adequate Duhamel anastomosis without faecal retention in the rectal pouch. Barium enema showed a moderate persistence of colon dilatation.

This is obviously not a case of Hirschsprung's disease, nor does the distal narrow segment belong to the ordinary criteria for a diagnosis of idiopathic

* A paper read at a meeting of the British Association of Paediatric Surgeons in Rotterdam, September 1964.

megacolon. There were no signs of gross mechanical obstruction nor of any other disease that might have caused a symptomatic megacolon. The intramural plexuses showed no degenerative changes, suggestive of the South American type of acquired megacolon. This seems to exhaust our diagnostic alternatives without, however, solving our diagnostic problem.

I would like to call the disease picture presented by this patient 'pseudo-Hirschsprung'. This term has been used as a synonym for idiopathic megacolon, especially by Ravitch (1958); idiopathic megacolon, however, as a rule has little in common with Hirschsprung's disease. Besides, idiopathic megacolon is a well-established term and a very good one, when properly used. It thus seems unwarranted to abandon an adequate name for one less appropriate. At the present time, 'pseudo-Hirschsprung' seems to be an adequate name for a chronic constipation with essentially the same clinical, radiological, and gross pathological changes as in Hirschsprung's disease but without the pathognomonic congenital aganglionosis.

Before entering into a discussion of the type of disturbance presented by our patient, a few reports of similar cases should be reviewed. Bill, Creighton, and Stevenson (1957) operated on 2 patients with constipation since birth, who fulfilled the clinical and radiological criteria for a diagnosis of Hirschsprung's disease. Both of the resected specimens showed normal ganglion cells in all areas. Both patients were relieved of obstruction following rectosigmoidectomy.

Swenson and Rathauser (1959) reported on 3 patients with a new disease entity entitled 'segmental dilatation of the colon'. All 3 patients had had constipation since birth. One child had a fusiform dilatation of the sigmoid colon which made it indistinguishable from aganglionic megacolon. In the second child, the lesion was in the proximal transverse colon and was thought to represent dilatation proximal to a long aganglionic segment extending from the anus to the mid-transverse colon. In the third patient the dilatation involved the entire sigmoid colon. At operation, the dilatation was found to start and end abruptly at its proximal and distal bowel attachments in all three patients. There was uniform hypertrophy of the muscle layer of the dilated segment. Normal ganglion cells and nerve fibres were found in the dilated segment as well as in the colon proximal and distal to it in all three patients.

Nixon (1961) described 2 patients with severe constipation and marked abdominal distension. Barium enema showed distension of the colon proximally with an undilated distal segment. There was no hypertrophy of the bowel wall. In both cases a colostomy was performed. The first infant died with faecal masses persisting in the right colon. At necropsy, cerebral atrophy was found. In the second child the colostomy discharged excessive fluid. After treatment of the electrolyte disturbance the colostomy was closed and the child recovered. In both of these patients normal ganglion cells were found in the bowel wall.

The first question to be answered is whether discussion of these 8 patients (including our own patient) as a homogeneous group is justified or not. There are obvious similarities between all the case reports: the patients presented with symptoms and signs of partial intestinal obstruction; barium enema studies revealed proximal megacolon with an undilated distal segment; and finally and most remarkably, the histological findings were perfectly normal in all of the specimens examined.

In other respects, however, some more or less essential dissimilarities exist. The three patients reported by Swenson and Rathauser presented a gross pathology of a specific type, which is clearly divergent from that of the remaining cases, from the ordinary findings in Hirschsprung's disease, and from those of idiopathic and symptomatic megacolon. The suggestion of these authors that 'segmental dilatation of the colon' is a new entity seems justified, and these three patients should be excluded from further discussion on the 'pseudo-Hirschsprung' group.

One of Nixon's patients died. At necropsy, the brain showed cerebral atrophy. Dr. M. Bodian suggested the possibility of a central origin for the bowel abnormality. Megacolon with a distal narrow segment has been described in patients with myxoedema (Salmi and Lahesmaa, 1956; Ravitch, 1958). These cases are not included in this review, because they are considered to belong to the group of symptomatic megacolon. The same may be true with regard to Nixon's case.

In the remaining 4 patients, no obviously essential dissimilarities were found. Absence of hypertrophy of the wall of the dilated bowel was a striking feature in Nixon's remaining patient as well as in our own. Bill *et al.* do not furnish any evidence in this respect. This feature is possibly related to the lack of resistance to propulsion of intestinal contents through the narrow segment, noted in our patient but not mentioned by Bill *et al.* or by Nixon. Normal intramural plexuses were found throughout the entire segments resected in the present case and in the 2 patients of Bill *et al.*, which should eliminate the diagnosis of segmental aganglionosis.

It seems, therefore, that at least 4 of the original 8 patients belong to a homogeneous disease entity, tentatively called pseudo-Hirschsprung's disease. The pathology and the aetiology of this entity remain obscure. The possibility of a neurogenic disturbance of unknown origin, located more centrally than in the intramural plexuses of the colon may be postulated. This is, however, a purely theoretical and hypothetical suggestion. The course of the disease in Nixon's surviving patient is most interesting from the pathogenetic point of view: this patient recovered after a temporary colostomy and was progressing nicely after closure of the colostomy. But the length of the follow-up period is not stated. Nixon suggests that the obstruction was due to a temporary functional paralysis of the colon. It is regrettable that our patient, as well as the 2 patients of Bill *et al.*, were treated by recto-sigmoidectomy, thus depriving us of the chance to confirm or exclude the temporary nature of the disorder in our patients.

## Summary

A case with many of the clinical features of Hirschsprung's disease, but without any abnormality of the intramural plexuses, is described. Similar cases have been reported previously by other authors, and the term pseudo-Hirschsprung's disease is suggested to describe the entity, the aetiology of which is obscure.

### References

Bill, A. H., Jr., Creighton, S. A., and Stevenson, J. K. (1957). The selection of infants and children for the surgical treatment of Hirschsprung's disease. *Surg. Gynec. Obstet.*, **104**, 151.

Bodian, M., Stephens, F. D., and Ward, B. C. H. (1949). Hirschsprung's disease and idiopathic megacolon. *Lancet*, **1**, 6.

Nixon, H. H. (1961). In Discussion on megacolon and megarectum with the emphasis on conditions other than Hirschsprung's disease. *Proc. roy. Soc. Med.*, **54**, 1037.

Ravitch, M. M. (1958). Pseudo Hirschsprung's disease. *Ann. Surg.*, **147**, 781.

Salmi, T., and Lahesmaa, P. (1956). Pseudo-Hirschsprung'sche Erkrankung bei einem Myxödem-Säugling. *Acta paediat.* (*Uppsala*), **45**, 428.

Swenson, O., and Bill, A. H., Jr. (1948). Resection of rectum and rectosigmoid with preservation of the sphincter for benign spastic lesions producing megacolon. *Surgery*, **24**, 212.

——, and Rathauser, F. (1959). Segmental dilatation of the colon. *Amer. J. Surg.*, **97**, 734.

Whitehouse, F. R., and Kernohan, J. W. (1948). Myenteric plexus in congenital megacolon. *Arch. intern. Med.*, **82**, 75.

*Arch. Dis. Childh.*, 1965, **40**, 180.

# ACQUIRED MEGACOLON AS A COMPLICATION OF RECTO-SIGMOIDECTOMY FOR HIRSCHSPRUNG'S DISEASE*

BY

TH. EHRENPREIS

*From the Children's Clinic, Karolinska Sjukhuset, Stockholm, Sweden*

Acquired megacolon, or aperistalsis of the colon and/or rectum, is a common disease in adults in certain rural areas of South America. It is often associated with mega-oesophagus. At times other parts of the digestive tract, the urinary tract, or the heart are involved. These are advanced phases of a systemic disease (Chagas' disease), caused by *Trypanosoma cruzi*. The underlying pathology is a lesion of the intramural ganglion cells, which results in degeneration (Hurst, 1925; Etzel, 1937) and a reduction in number of ganglion cells (Köberle, 1956).

Acquired megacolon is practically unknown outside South America. A recent observation of a Swedish case that fulfils the clinical and histological criteria for a diagnosis of 'acquired megacolon' seems to be of interest, though the aetiology is obviously different from the South American type of aperistalsis.

## Case Report

A 2½-year-old girl was admitted in 1959 with typical symptoms and signs of a short-segment Hirschsprung's disease (Fig. 1). A Swenson procedure was performed, the resection including 6-7 cm. of dilated bowel proximal to the transition zone and leaving 2-3 cm. of the anal canal behind. The length of the resected narrow segment was 7 cm. The specimen showed aganglionosis distally and normal findings proximally. The post-operative course was uneventful but no improvement of the patient's constipation occurred. After 6 weeks, a sphincterotomy was performed. A slight improvement was noted that soon proved to be temporary. Constipation continued and the bowels had to be cleared by an enema every second or third day. Moderate abdominal distension persisted and the child failed to thrive. She was re-admitted in March 1964 at the age of 6 years. Barium enema (Fig. 2) revealed a magnificent megacolon with a narrow segment extending to the level of the promontory. The anastomosis performed at the first operation was barely palpable 4 cm. from the anal opening. A secondary resection was performed with a subsequent oblique anastomosis according to Grob's latest modification of the Swenson and Duhamel procedures. The length of the resected narrow segment was 15 cm. The post-operative course was uneventful. The patient has been completely relieved of her constipation so far, though the follow-up period has been only three months.

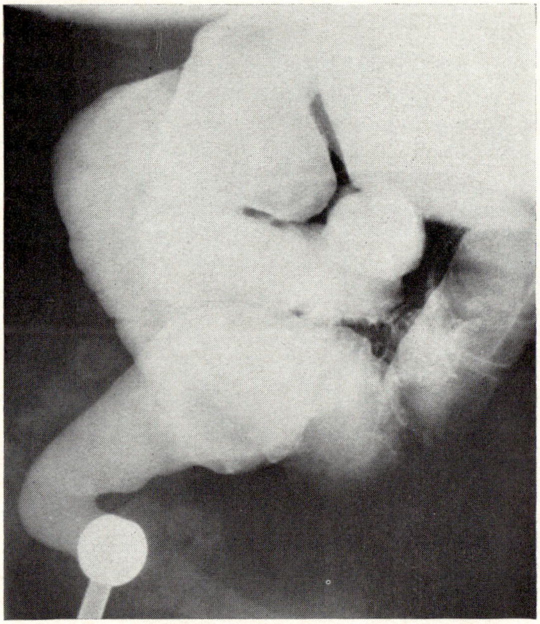

FIG. 1.—Pre-operative barium enema, showing short-segment Hirschsprung's disease.

Microscopic examination of the resected specimen showed normal findings proximally. Throughout the entire narrow segment ganglion cells were sparse and showed degenerative changes (Fig. 3). The blood vessels showed inclusions of hyaline material in their walls (Fig. 4).

* A paper read at a meeting of the British Association of Paediatric Surgeons in Rotterdam, September 1964.

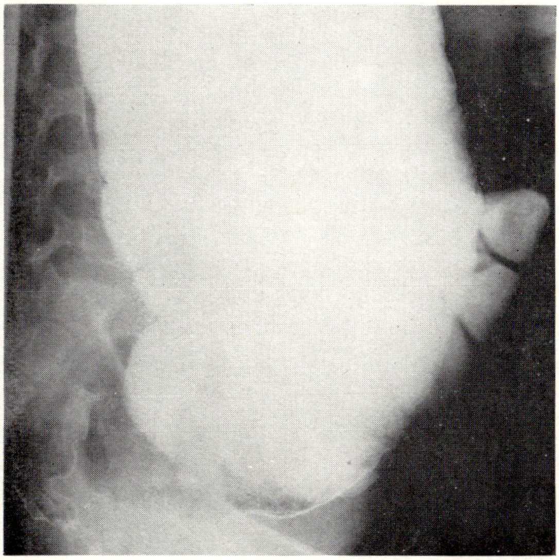

FIG. 2.—Barium enema 3½ years after recto-sigmoidectomy, showing pronounced megacolon with a recurrent narrow segment.

The interesting feature in this case is the persistence of constipation and the recurrence of a narrow segment after radical excision of the original aganglionic segment. The secondary narrow segment was much longer than that seen originally and could obviously not have been the result of growth of the 2-3 cm. of the anal canal that were left at the first operation. The primary anastomosis could be identified within the distal part of the secondary narrow segment.

The clue to the pathogenesis of the secondary narrow segment lies in the histological findings in the specimen removed at the second 'recto-sigmoidectomy'. As far as can be judged without personal experience of the South American type of acquired megacolon, the histological findings in this specimen are in good agreement with the description given by South American authors. It is, however, highly improbable that the aetiology could be similar. It would seem more likely that the degenerative changes in the myenteric plexus, as well as the hyaline vascular inclusions found in the present case, were caused by some unnoticed impairment to the vascular supply of the bowel segment which had been mobilized and pulled through at the primary recto-sigmoidectomy. If so, this vascular disturbance had been just severe enough to cause degeneration of the ganglion cells (which are probably more sensitive to such disturbances than other elements of the bowel wall) without compromising the vitality of the bowel itself. These assumptions are borne out by reports of experimentally-produced megacolon with degeneration or total destruction (depending on experimental conditions) of the intracolonic plexuses after injection of Urokon into the left colic artery (McElhannon, 1960) and after temporary occlusion

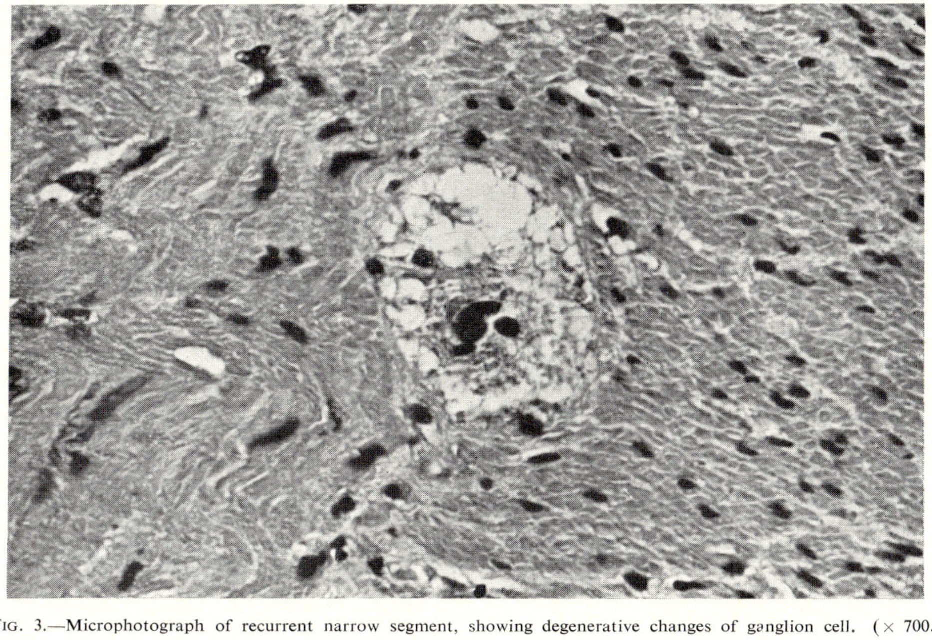

FIG. 3.—Microphotograph of recurrent narrow segment, showing degenerative changes of ganglion cell. (× 700.)

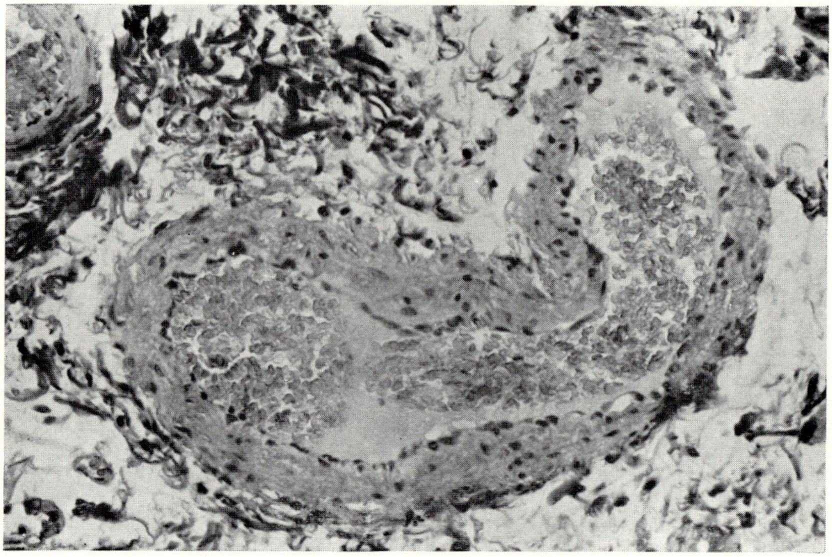

FIG. 4.—Microphotograph of recurrent narrow segment, showing hyaline inclusions in the wall of the blood vessel. (×50.)

of the inferior mesenteric artery (Hukuhara, Kotani, and Sato, 1961).

This type of complication has not been encountered previously in more than 100 recto-sigmoidectomies, performed personally, nor have any published reports on similar complications been found. This is remarkable considering the large number of recto-sigmoidectomies that have been done during the past 15 years.

## Summary

The case is described of a 2½-year-old child with Hirschsprung's disease, who, following a recto-sigmoidectomy, developed a severe degree of megacolon. This was considered to have resulted from impairment of the vascular supply to the colon at the time of operation, causing degeneration of the ganglion cells.

REFERENCES

Etzel, E. (1937). Megaoesophagus and its neuropathology: a clinical and anatomo-pathological research. *Guy's Hosp. Rep.*, **87**, 158.

Hukuhara, T., Kotani, S., and Sato, G. (1961). Effects of destruction of intramural ganglion cells on colon motility: possible genesis of congenital megacolon. *Jap. J. Physiol.*, **11**, 635.

Hurst, A. F. (1925). The sphincters of the alimentary canal and their clinical significance. *Brit med. J.*, **1**, 145.

Köberle, F. (1956). Zur Frage der Entstehung sog. "idiopathischer Dilatationen" muskulärer Hohlorgane. *Virchows Arch. path. Anat.*, **329**, 337.

McElhannon, F. M. (1960). Experimental production of megacolon resembling Hirschsprung's disease. *Surg. Forum*, **10**, 218.

*Arch. Dis. Childh.*, 1965, **40**, 183.

# SERUM LACTIC DEHYDROGENASE AND RIBONUCLEASE IN THE DIAGNOSIS OF MALIGNANT TUMOURS IN CHILDREN*

BY

ALOJZY MACIEJEWSKI and HENRYK BOBIŃSKI

*From the Departments of Paediatric Surgery and Physiological Chemistry, Medical Academy, Lodz, Poland*

In recent years increasing attention has been given to the fluctuations of serum enzymes in neoplastic disease. It is thought that increased activity of certain enzymes in cancer cells and in damaged tissues results in the release of enzymes into the serum. Among many enzymes that have recently received interest, in relation to malignant neoplasia, are *lactic dehydrogenase* (SLD) (Wróblewski, 1957, 1959; Blanchaer, Green, Maclean, and Hollenberg, 1958) and *ribonuclease* (RN-ase) (Wróblewski, 1961).

In 1930 Warburg, while investigating the metabolism of neoplastic tissue, showed that in carcinomatous cells respiration was irreversibly impaired, with the consequence that there was increased anaerobic glycolysis. In spite of Warburg's discovery it was not until 1954 that Hill and Levi showed that the activity of lactate dehydrogenase, the end-enzyme of anaerobic glycolysis, rose in the serum of some patients with neoplastic disease.

At present SLD activity seems to be a factor of some importance in the biochemical diagnosis of malignant neoplasia in adults (Wróblewski, 1961). Unfortunately, SLD can also be influenced by disease states other than malignant neoplasia, nor is its activity always increased in cancer (Zimmerman and Weinstein, 1956).

No data are available on SLD activity in children with malignant tumours, though the problem merits special attention since lactic dehydrogenase activity in tissues of the foetus and newborn is much higher than in adults. LD is a soluble enzyme located primarily in cytoplasm, so it would enter the blood more readily than would the insoluble enzymes located in mitochondria. Taking into consideration the high LD activity in young cells, one would expect SLD to be a much more sensitive index of neoplastic processes in newborns and very young children than in adults.

Available data on serum RN-ase activity mainly concern different forms of leukaemia in adults, and the results are contradictory (Wróblewski, 1961; Aleksandrowicz, Urbanczyk, Ostrowska, and Sierko, 1958). Since this enzyme is connected with cellular nuclei, the enhanced activity in serum should reflect a tissue breakdown and might be of importance in cancer detection.

In this paper an attempt is made to find out how far changes in serum activity of these two enzymes may be useful in the early diagnosis of congenital neoplasia.

## Material and Methods

As there are many conflicting reports of normal values for SLD (Rapp and Bell, 1961), we have established normal values for healthy children. The control group of healthy children was divided into three age-groups: 0-2, 2-7, and 7-14 years. Normal values for RN-ase activity in serum were determined for the same age-groups.

As well as cases with malignant neoplasia, a small group of benign tumours comprising cases of haemangiomata was studied.

The blood for SLD and RN-ase activity determinations was drawn by venepuncture and the serum separated. For SLD determination sera were stored frozen for periods not exceeding 3 days. RN-ase activity assays were performed only in fresh sera. The method used for SLD determination was that of Cabaud and Wróblewski (1958). RN-ase activity was determined according to Métais and Mandel (1955).

## Results

The values obtained for SLD and RN-ase activity in healthy children are listed in Table 1.

The highest SLD activity was observed in the age-group 0-2 years, the mean value for this group being significantly higher than those for older children and for adults. By contrast, serum activity of RN-ase rises with the child's age, the differences in mean values for each age-group being significant.

The activity of the two enzymes in cases of malignant neoplasia is shown in Table 2. Except

* A paper read at a meeting of the British Association of Paediatric Surgeons in Rotterdam, September 1964.

TABLE 1

NORMAL RANGES FOR LEVELS OF SERUM LACTIC DEHYDROGENASE AND RIBONUCLEASE IN CHILDREN

| Age-group (yr.) | Lactic Dehydrogenase | | | Ribonuclease | | |
|---|---|---|---|---|---|---|
| | Number | Range (units) | Mean Value (units) | Number | Range (units) | Mean Value (units) |
| 0–2 | 14 | 290–540 | 431 | 8 | 54–206 | 139 |
| 2–7 | 25 | 250–515 | 392 | 15 | 74–260 | 163 |
| 7–14 | 18 | 240–460 | 380 | 24 | 97–244 | 190 |
| Adults | 21 | 212–423 | 320 | | | |

TABLE 2

SERUM LACTIC DEHYDROGENASE (SLD) AND RIBONUCLEASE (RN-ASE) ACTIVITY IN 20 CASES OF MALIGNANT NEOPLASIA IN CHILDREN

| Case No. | Diagnosis | Age (yr.) | SLD Level (units) | RN-ase Level (units) |
|---|---|---|---|---|
| 1 | Malignant hepatic tumour | 1 | | 175 |
| 2 | Wilms' tumour | 1 | | 191 |
| 3 | Eosinophilic granuloma of skull and clavicle: multiple metastases | 2 | | 190 |
| 4 | Nephroblastoma | 6 | | 148 |
| 5 | Agranulocytosis | 13 | | 134 |
| 6 | Glioma | 4 | 660 | |
| 7 | Nephroblastoma | 4 | 950 | |
| 8 | Nephroblastoma | 5 | 690 | |
| 9 | Nephroblastoma | 5 | 1040 | |
| 10 | Nephroblastoma | 2 | 800 | |
| 11 | Ovarian tumour | 4 | 1220 | |
| 12 | Nephroblastoma | 6 | 860 | |
| 13 | Thyroid carcinoma | 7 | 980 | |
| 14 | Nephroblastoma | 9 | 830 | |
| 15 | Sarcoma | 3 | 1120 | |
| 16 | Glioma | 5 | 815 | |
| 17 | Malignant bone tumour | 8 | 880 | |
| 18 | Hepatoblastoma | 14 | 460 | |
| 19 | Neuroblastoma | 2 | 1015 | |
| 20 | Thyroid carcinoma | 3 | 634 | |

in one case of hepatoblastoma, SLD activity is higher than in controls. RN-ase level shows no such trend.

In a group of 7 (benign) haemangiomata the mean values for SLD amounted to 455 units, which does not differ statistically from the control group.

## Discussion

SLD was found to be raised in almost all cases of malignant neoplasia in this study. This result differs from those reported for neoplastic diseases in adults (Wróblewski, 1957, 1959; Blanchaer *et al.*, 1958; Zimmerman and Weinstein, 1956), where SLD is increased in only about 50% of cases of various neoplasia. Wróblewski (1961) states that SLD activity in adults may contribute to the diagnosis of neoplasia in three clinical situations—disseminated cancer, lymphoma, and myelogenous leukaemia. Our results show that in children SLD activity increased in malignant neoplasia, independently of the origin of the tumour in almost 100% of cases. In the only case, that of a hepatoblastoma, with a normal value for SLD, bilirubin may have interfered with the estimation of enzyme activity, as in this case jaundice was severe. The more consistent increase in SLD in neoplasia in children, when compared with findings in adults, is presumably the result of the increased metabolism in children. This is especially evident when comparing normal values for SLD at different age-groups. The highest mean value is for newborns, where some residue of foetal anaerobic metabolism is still present. Increased glycolytic activity of tumours seems to be more prominent in children than in adults, resulting in leaking of the enzyme into the serum. Due to the cytoplasmic, extra-mitochondrial site of LD, such leakage can take place before the breakdown of tissues, which is a factor of importance in the early diagnosis of neoplastic disease.

The absence of any increase in SLD in the benign neoplasia (haemangiomata) that we tested supports the significance of raised SLD levels in malignant neoplasia.

There are also certain non-neoplastic states associated with increased SLD, e.g. myocardial infarction, hepatitis, some haemolytic states, dermatomyositis, and muscle trauma.

Serum RN-ase activity appeared to be slightly raised only in a few cases of malignant neoplasm in children. This increase might be due to the tissue damage that takes place in advanced neoplastic disease. If so, an increased activity of RN-ase in serum might be an index of necrotic changes during the development of malignant tumours.

## Summary and Conclusions

Serum lactic dehydrogenase activity rises up to three times normal values in almost 100% of cases of malignant tumours in children. SLD level increases in every case of disseminated cancer. Hence it can be a factor of importance in the prognosis and diagnosis of neoplastic diseases in children, especially in the age-group 0-2 years. Ribonuclease activity in serum does not give as distinct a picture of neoplastic disease as SLD does.

REFERENCES

Aleksandrowicz, J., Urbanczyk, J., Ostrowska, A., and Sierko, J. (1958). Further research on the activity of ribonucleases in the blood and urine of patients suffering from proliferative hemocytopathia. *Blood*, **13**, 653.

Blanchaer, M. C., Green, P. T., Maclean, J. P., and Hollenberg, M. J. (1958). Plasma lactic dehydrogenase and phosphohexose isomerase in leukemia. *ibid.*, **13**, 245.

Cabaud, P. G., and Wróblewski, F. (1958). Colorimetric measurement of lactic dehydrogenase activity of body fluids. *Amer. J. clin. Path.*, **30**, 234.

Hill, B. R., and Levi, C. (1954). Elevation of serum component in neoplastic disease. *Cancer Res.*, **14**, 513.

Métais, P., and Mandel, P. (1955). Activité ribonucléasique du sérum humain. *Bull. Soc. Chim. biol. (Paris)*, **37**, 999.

Rapp, R. D., and Bell, E. R. (1961). Normal values for serum lactic dehydrogenase. *Amer. J. clin. Path.*, **35**, 116.

Warburg, O. (1930). *The Metabolism of Tumours*. Constable, London.

Wróblewski, F. (1957). The clinical significance of alterations in lactic dehydrogenase activity of body fluids. *Amer. J. med. Sci.*, **234**, 301.

—— (1959). The significance of alterations in lactic dehydrogenase activity of body fluids in the diagnosis of malignant tumors. *Cancer (Philad.)*, **12**, 27.

—— (1961). Lactic dehydrogenase activity in cancer diagnosis. *Med. Clin. N. Amer.*, **45**, 513.

Zimmerman, H. J., and Weinstein, H. G. (1956). Lactic dehydrogenase activity in human serum. *J. Lab. clin. Med.*, **48**, 607.

*Arch. Dis. Childh.*, 1965, **40**, 186.

# CHYLOTHORAX IN INFANCY AND CHILDHOOD

## A METHOD OF TREATMENT*

BY

IAN KIRKLAND

*Department of Surgical Paediatrics, Western General Hospital, Edinburgh, Scotland*

Chylothorax is a rare condition at any age, but especially so in childhood. It has been recognized as a clinical entity since the first report by Asellius in 1627-1628. Accumulations of chyle in the thorax occur at three periods in life: the neonatal, in childhood, and in adult life.

(1) In the *neonatal* period, what has been called 'spontaneous chylothorax' has probably rightly been referred to as congenital chylothorax in an excellent review by Randolph and Gross (1957). In very few instances can any aetiological factor be found, though possible birth trauma, convulsions, or respiratory obstruction may play a part It is possible, however, as less than 20 cases have so far been recorded, that some underlying abnormality of the lymphatic system must predispose to the development of chylothorax. I would therefore support the terminology of congenital chylothorax. The majority of reported cases have a right-sided effusion, there are a few on the left side, and only one bilateral case so far.

(2) In *childhood*, the most common aetiological factor is trauma, as a result of penetrating injuries or following operations on the heart and great vessels. Reports of spontaneous chylothorax in this group are exceedingly rare, and I have only been able to find references to three cases—two at just over 2 months of age and one at 2½ years. The case report following therefore now adds one more to this group. It appears that these rare cases could be called congenital, as it is likely that the underlying cause is a congenital abnormality of the lymphatic system.

(3) In *adult* life, trauma, neoplasm, and inflammatory obstruction to the lymphatic system all play their part.

At all ages trauma to the thoracic duct is the principal cause of chylous effusions. The traumatic agent in childhood is fairly clear cut, whether it be accidental or operative. Detailed study of the lymphatic system and its possible anomalies offer the best hope of defining precisely the other most common cause of chylothorax at this age period. Experimental chylothorax has been produced in a number of experimental animals by occlusion of the superior vena cava (Blalock, Cunningham, and Robinson, 1936). It is convenient, therefore, to summarize the aetiological factors.

### Aetiological Factors

A. **Traumatic.** (a) Operative. (b) Non-operative, i.e. penetrating wounds; crushing wounds; blast injuries; coughing; and spinal hyperextension—falls, diving, convulsions.

B. **Non-traumatic.** (a) Mediastinal malignancy —primary or metastatic of the thoracic duct or lymph glands. (b) Mediastinal infection, e.g. tuberculosis, filariasis. (c) Occasional erosions from aneurysms etc. or superior vena cava thrombosis. (d) Congenital abnormalities of the lymphatic ducts.

### Embryology and Anatomy

The lymphatic system is closely related to, and develops concurrently with, the venous system and, like it, acts as a channel for the return of fluid from the tissues.

Two conflicting concepts of the origin of the lymphatic system are as follows.

(1) All lymphatic channels are developed as outgrowths of the venous endothelium in 6 areas: 2 jugular lymph sacs; 2 iliac lymph sacs; 1 retroperitoneal lymph sac; and cisterna chyli. They invade the tissues by continuous growth and branching. The original connexions with veins may or may not remain as channels in the adult system (Sabin, 1902).

(2) Kampmeier (1912-13) and Huntington (1914) believe that the lymphatic system arises by confluence of perivenous mesenchymal spaces to form larger spaces, and these in turn become confluent to form

---

* A paper read at a meeting of the British Association of Paediatric Surgeons in Rotterdam, September 1964.

continuous vessels, opening eventually into the venous system.

Whichever is true, in the human embryo lymphatic spaces, the jugular lymph sacs in particular are seen at the 10-11 mm. stage. Two channels, right and left, with numerous cross anastomoses form a plexus of lymphatic vessels along the course of the aorta. Sabin reports the first appearance of the cisterna chyli in 23 mm. human embryos. The thoracic duct is first found in human embryos of 24 mm. and by 30 mm. is complete.

In a carefully documented study, Davis (1914-15) divides the 'adult pattern' of thoracic ducts into 9 potential groups and has found evidence of all but 2 of these in dissected specimens. There are many variations in pattern, and what the anatomists consider the normal description was only present in 63% of his series of 22 dissections, and a cisterna chyli in only 50%.

Further anatomical studies by Van Pernis (1949) and Anson (1950), and investigation of the free lymphatic venous collateral circulation by Lee (1922), emphasize the many variations in the structure of the lymphatic system in humans.

The thoracic duct is responsible for transferring chyle to the venous system, particularly is it the route through which unsplit fat travels (Frazer, 1943). CoTui, Barcham, and Shafiroff (1944) demonstrated that it was an important route for the transfer of mobilized protein from body depots after haemorrhage. Vitamin K transfer from the intestine is by this route, and lymphocytes are carried to the bloodstream by the thoracic duct.

Reports of anomalies of the lymphatic system in childhood are few. There are 4 necropsy reports in infants who died as a result of congenital chylothorax: in none of these was a thoracic duct demonstrated (Stewart and Linner, 1926; Hilgenberg, 1929; Everhart and Jacobs, 1939; Forbes 1944).

## Clinical Features

The clinical picture is fairly clear cut in the majority of patients. There is respiratory distress, evidence of pleural effusion, usually unilateral, and a possible history of trauma, either operative or non-operative. In the newborn there are symptoms and signs of respiratory distress which is associated with a pleural effusion. In patients with other evidence of lymphatic anomalies the possibility of chylous extravasation must be always kept in mind. Again respiratory symptoms, unassociated with pyrexia and possibly accompanied by nutritional inadequacy, should lead one to the diagnosis. The diagnosis is confirmed by aspiration of the chylous effusion, characterized by its milky appearance, sterility on culture, lack of odour, alkaline reaction, S.G. greater than 1·012, high protein content usually 1-6 g./100 ml., high fat content (0·4-40 g./ 100 ml.), lymphocytic predominance in leucocyte count, and separation into two distinct layers on standing.

## Treatment

Treatment can be summarized as conservative or operative. Conservative treatment consists of regular emptying of the pleural cavity by aspiration, with supportive general treatment with a high protein, high split-fat diet, with the fat soluble vitamin supplements especially vitamin K. Because of the bacteriostatic properties of chyle (Lampson, 1948; Whitcomb and Scoville, 1942), infection in the pleural cavity as a result of repeated aspiration is most unlikely. Plasma infusions may be necessary if large quantities of effusion continue to be aspirated.

Intravenous reinfusion of aspirated chyle was introduced by Oeken (1908) and has been tried subsequently by Bauersfeld (1937), Little, Harrison, and Blalock (1942), Peet and Campbell (1943), and Schnug and Ransohoff (1943), but this has been associated with unexplained sudden death.

There have been numerous reported survivors, both in neonatal patients and in those with post-operative chylothorax, as a result of vigorous conservative treatment, the chylous effusion suddenly ceasing and the patients remaining well (Maloney and Spencer, 1956; Boles and Izant, 1960).

Operative treatment consists of controlling, by direct suture or thoracic duct ligation above and below, the points of leakage after identifying the fistulae. Cauterization or irritation of the mediastinal pleura to produce post-operative viscero-parietal adhesions is often added. Opinion is divided sharply between those who advocate early or delayed operative treatment, but when there is obvious deterioration in the patient, particularly from a nutritional point of view, in spite of adequate supportive therapy, then operation becomes imperative. There has been little mortality and considerable success with operative treatment during the past few years (Burdette, 1959; Shumacker and Moore, 1951; Randolph and Gross, 1957).

As a result of experience with CSF drainage in hydrocephalus using a Holter valve, and with a similar procedure in treating ascites (Smith, Preshaw, and Bisset, 1962), it seemed worth considering this method of treatment in a patient with progressive bilateral chylothorax, in whom nutritional and respiratory problems were becoming acute. If continuous pleuro-venous drainage could be achieved instead of repeated thoracentesis, then the patient

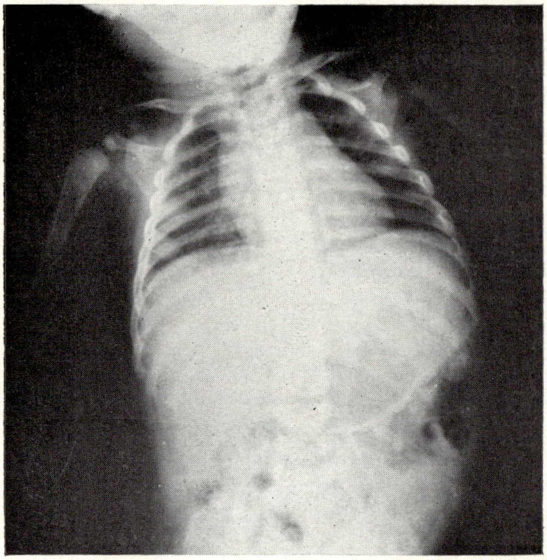

FIG. 1.—Patient aged 4 months. Chest radiograph normal.

could possibly be made fit for more definitive surgery later.

Before operation the aspirated chylous effusion was set up in a burette and allowed to drain continuously through a Holter valve, the maximum height of fluid being 18 in. (46 cm.) above the valve. Over a period of 3 days there was no evidence of clot formation or blockage of the valve in spite of the high protein content of the effusion.

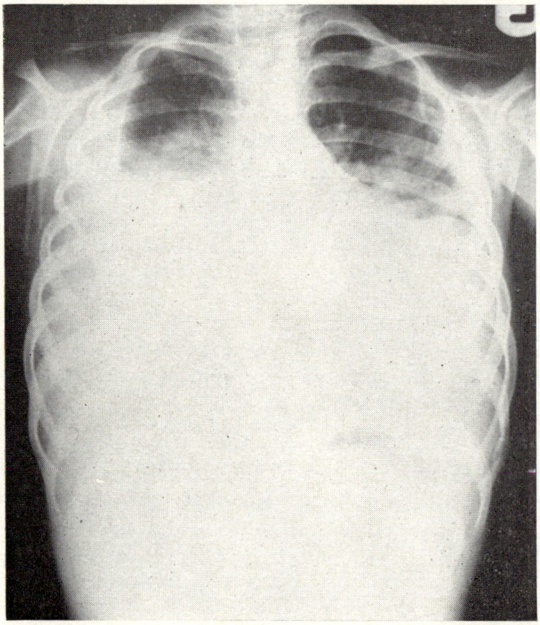

FIG. 2.—Patient aged 3 years and 11 months. Chest radiograph showing right-sided pleural effusion and apparent abdominal swelling.

The operation consisted essentially of exposing the right eighth and ninth ribs through a small curved mid axillary incision. A moulded 'ventricular' catheter was inserted through the eighth intercostal space by means of an introducer, and attached to a low pressure Holter valve which was anchored to the ninth rib by silk sutures along its length, so that the valve could be compressed against the rib. Chyle drained through the catheter and valve. A separate subinguinal incision exposed the right long saphenous vein. After ligature of its tributaries and the main trunk itself, a silicone rubber tube, previously attached to the distal end of the Holter valve and led to the inguinal region through a subcutaneous tunnel, was introduced through the long saphenous vein into the femoral vein, external iliac vein, and finally into the inferior vena cava. Its position was checked radiologically. Thus a continuous pleuro-venous shunt incorporating a Holter valve to allow flow in only one direction was achieved.

**Case Report**

A 7 lb. 12 oz. (3,515 g.) girl was born on May 15, 1957 after an assisted forceps delivery for delay in the second stage of labour. The mother was under treatment for pulmonary tuberculosis. At birth the baby was found to be normal except for a swelling on the medial aspect of the right thigh, diagnosed as a lymphangioma with some lymphoedema of the right leg, its bulk being 50% greater than the left. At the age of 1 month lymphangiograms of the right leg were undertaken with patent blue. These indicated a delay in lymph drainage from the toes of the right foot, with generalized spread of dye throughout the body before filling of the lymphangioma of the thigh. Removal of the lymphangioma was therefore undertaken at the age of 6 weeks. BCG vaccination was given before the baby went home, and thereafter the Heaf test was positive. The baby was under constant surveillance over the next 3½ years (Fig. 1), and had to be admitted to hospital on numerous occasions for control of the lymphoedema, for episodes of infection, and for fractures of the right leg. Throughout this time her general health was excellent. At the age of 4 years she was admitted to hospital suffering from respiratory symptoms, loss of weight, and general unwellness, and, because of the family history, pulmonary tuberculosis was suspected. A right-sided pleural effusion (Fig. 2) was found, which on aspiration proved to be chylous. On admission to the Surgical Paediatric Unit at the Western General Hospital for further investigation, she was a pale, thin, undernourished child, with an irritant non-productive cough, and variable breathlessness particularly at night. She could only sleep when kept upright on pillows. Her appetite was poor, but she had no other general symptoms. She had been confined to bed for several weeks.

On examination she was apyrexial with no evidence of lymphadenopathy, finger clubbing, or koilonychia. There was gross lymphoedematous swelling of the right leg extending suprapubically and into the vulva. There was some degree of protuberance of the abdomen without prominent veins and a soft fluctuant mass in the right renal area subcutaneously. The fluid in the limb was compressible and could be shifted from compartment to compartment along its length. There was evidence of pleural effusion on both sides, the right side being more extensive than the left.

Radiographs confirmed the presence of bilateral pleural effusions (Fig. 3).

**Laboratory findings.** Blood count normal. Plasma proteins 6·75 g./100 ml., albumin 4·20; globulin 2·55. Serum cholesterol 250 mg./100 ml.

*Urinalysis*, normal, no chyle.

*Aspirate from right pleural cavity*, 500 ml. Total protein 4·25 g./100 ml.; cholesterol 425 mg./100 ml.; total fat 710 mg./100 ml. Electrophoretic pattern, virtually that of plasma except for absence of fibrinogen. Culture sterile. Cells, occasional WBC, RBC, and debris; S.G. 1·014; *p*H, 8-9; sugar, negative.

**Progress.** Owing to respiratory distress, chest aspiration was necessary at intervals of a few days and amounts of chylous effusion from 500 ml. to 1,300 ml. were obtained, with a composition similar to the original specimen. Larger and larger aspirates were necessary to relieve the respiratory distress. It was noted both clinically and radiologically that aspiration of the right pleural cavity reduced the effusion on the left side (Fig. 4).

During this time a high protein supplemented diet with 'complan' was administered, but in spite of this the child's condition did not improve and the plasma proteins fell to a total of 4·25 g./100 ml., albumin 2·60 g./100 ml., and globulin 1·65 g./100 ml., necessitating a plasma transfusion.

Spontaneous cutaneous fistulae were noted at the vulva when large quantities of chylous fluid leaked for some hours intermittently.

Treatment to relieve the respiratory embarrassment and to improve her general condition seemed imperative, and operation was undertaken 6 weeks after admission. This consisted of a continuous pleuro-venous anastomosis incorporating a low pressure Holter valve (Fig. 5). The child withstood the operative procedure well, and the Holter valve continued to function. Drainage of the chylous effusion was assisted by regular 'pumping' of the valve.

Air entry into both lung fields remained adequate, but continued reaccumulation of chylous effusion required aspiration of the right pleural cavity (1,350 ml.) on the eighth post-operative day. She was able to get up in a chair for short periods without respiratory distress. Further aspiration of 1,200 ml. from the right pleural cavity was necessary a few days later, and regular 'pumping' of the valve was continued.

There was some improvement in her general condition, and air entry to both lungs remained adequate. Twenty days after operation, while she was having attention to the skin of her buttocks, she died suddenly.

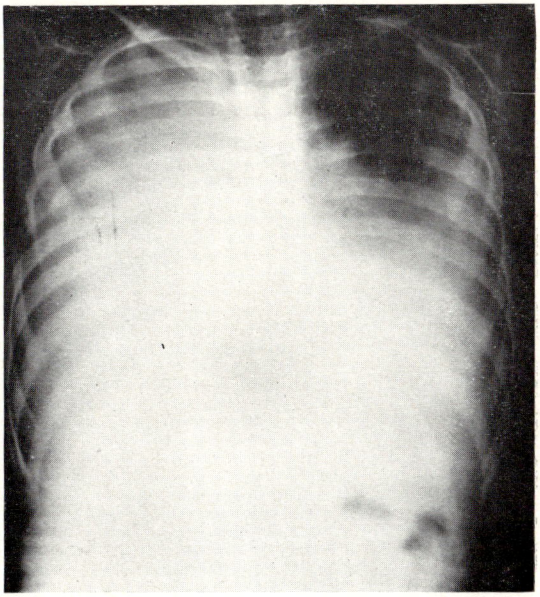

FIG. 3.—Patient aged 4 years and 1 month. Bilateral pleural effusion.

Necropsy the following day confirmed the presence of chylous effusion in both pleural cavities. This came from multiple fistulae along the lower half of the mediastinal pleura and along the attachments of the diaphragm to the lateral aspects of the vertebral bodies. These fistulae

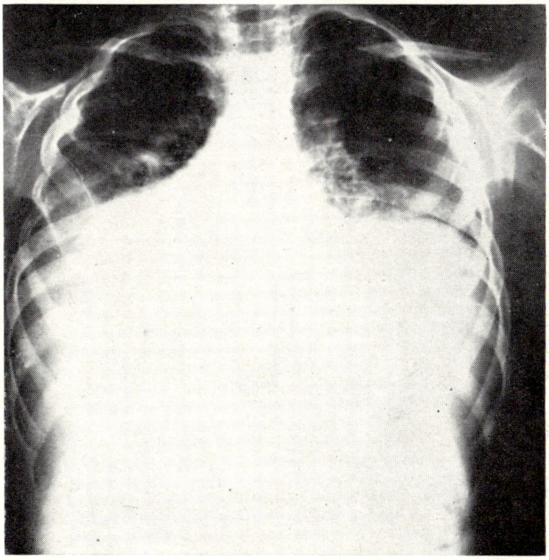

FIG. 4.—Patient two weeks after Fig. 3. Aspiration of right pleural cavity only, showing bilateral improvement.

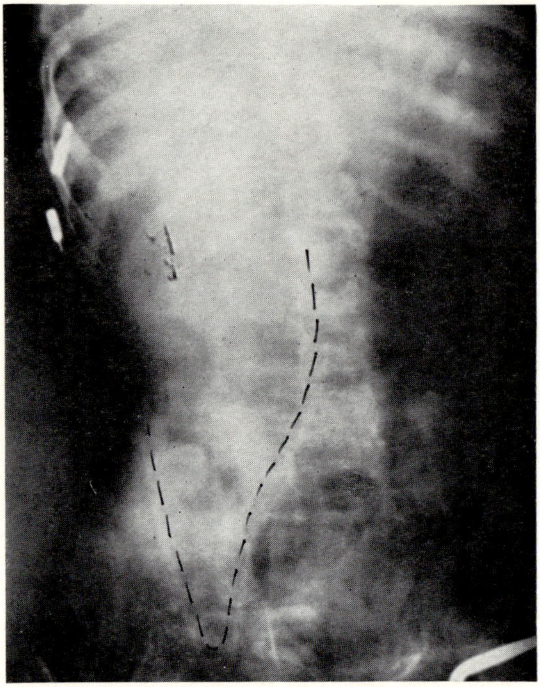

FIG. 5.—Shows Holter valve in position and siliconed rubber tube leading into inferior vena cava to the level of L1.

communicated with large mediastinal lymph spaces which in turn communicated with large dilated retroperitoneal lymphatic channels. There was no chylopericardium or dilated mesenteric lacteals. The amount of chyloperitoneum was minimal and could have been produced at necropsy. The other abdominal organs were unaffected. The large dilated lymphatics in both lower limbs and perineum were confirmed.

No thoracic duct was identified at first, but later multiple mediastinal lymph channels were identified. Dye injected shortly after death into a large lymphatic space in the inguinal region filled the large retroperitoneal lymph spaces and passed through the multiple fistulae into both pleural cavities.

## Comments

Chylothorax may occur in infancy and childhood as an entity on its own or in conjunction with other gross lymphatic abnormalities (Kinmonth and Taylor, 1964). The prognosis in patients with widespread lymphatic abnormalities appears to be more grave than in those with an isolated lesion. With the improvement in conservative and operative treatment of chylothorax on its own, the mortality from this condition has been considerably reduced.

There are still patients whose general health continues to deteriorate in spite of adequate conservative treatment, and others in whom gross congenital abnormalities of the rest of the lymphatic system preclude the usual operative measures to control the chylous fistulae. It is for this reason that a new attempt at treatment has been undertaken employing new materials and appliances, and utilizing the pressure differential between the pleural cavity (from 5 mm. Hg to atmospheric pressure or more) and the pressure in the inferior vena cava near its entry to the heart (which varies from 0 to − 5 mm. Hg).

The incorporation of a valve of the Holter type prevents the reflux of blood into the drainage system. The diminished content of fibrinogen in chyle appears to prevent clotting of the chylous effusion in the drainage system.

## Summary

A brief review of chylothorax is presented with comments on its occurrence, aetiology, clinical features, and treatment.

The embryology and anatomy of the lymphatic system as far as it is known is summarized. Scarcity of available published material detailing congenital anomalies is apparent and further investigation in this field is very necessary.

### REFERENCES

Anson, B. J. (1950). *An Atlas of Anatomy*. W. B. Saunders, Philadelphia and London.

Asellius, G. (1627-1628). De lactibus, sive lacteis venis, quarto vasorum mesarai coruum genere, novo invento, dissertation, Milan. Leydon, 1640, University Library.

Bauersfeld, E. H. (1937). Traumatic chylothorax from ruptured thoracic duct treated by intravenous injection of aspirated chyle. *J. Amer. med. Ass.*, **109**, 16.

Blalock, A., Cunningham, R. S., and Robinson, C. S. (1936). Experimental production of chylothorax by occlusion of the superior vena cava. *Ann. Surg.*, **104**, 359.

Boles, E. T., Jr., and Izant, R. J., Jr. (1960). Spontaneous chylothorax in the neonatal period. *Amer. J. Surg.*, **99**, 870.

Burdette, W. J. (1959). Management of chylous extravasation. *Arch. Surg.*, **78**, 815.

CoTui, Barcham, I. S., and Shafiroff, B. G. P. (1944). Ligation of the thoracic duct and the posthemorrhage plasma protein level. *Surg. Gynec. Obstet.*, **79**, 37.

Davis, H. K. (1914-15). A statistical study of the thoracic duct in man. *Amer. J. Anat.*, **17**, 211

Everhart, J. K., and Jacobs, A. H. (1939). Chylothorax: a review of the literature and report of case in newborn infant. *J. Pediat.*, **15**, 558.

Forbes, G. B. (1944). Chylothorax in infancy: observations on the absorption of vitamins A and D and on the intravenous replacement of aspirated chyle. *ibid.*, **25**, 191.

Frazer, A. C. (1943). Differentiation in the absorption of olive oil and oleic acid in the rat. *J. Physiol.* (*Lond.*), **102**, 306.

Hilgenberg, F. C. (1929). Ein Fall von Chylothorax beim Neugeborenen. *Mschr. Geburtsh. Gynäk.*, **83**, 225.

Huntington, G. S. (1914). The development of the mammalian jugular lymph sac, of the tributary primitive ulnar lymphatic and of the thoracic ducts. *Amer. J. Anat.*, **16**, 259.

Kampmeier, O. F. (1912-13). The development of the thoracic duct in the pig. *ibid.*, **13**, 401.

Kinmonth, J. B., and Taylor, G. W. (1964). Chylous reflux. *Brit. med. J.*, **1**, 529.

Lampson, R. S. (1948). Traumatic chylothorax: a review of the literature and report of a case treated by mediastinal ligation of the thoracic duct. *J. thorac. Surg.*, **17**, 778.

Lee, F. C. (1922). The establishment of collateral circulation following ligation of the thoracic duct. *Bull. Johns Hopk. Hosp.*, **33**, **21**.

Little, J. M., Harrison, C., and Blalock, A. (1942). Chylothorax and chyloperitoneum: Effects of reintroduction of aspirated chyle. *Surgery*, **11**, 392.

Maloney, J. V., Jr., and Spencer, F. C. (1956). The nonoperative treatment of traumatic chylothorax. *ibid.*, **40**, 121.

Oeken, H. (1908). Ein Fall von Zerreissung des Ductus thoracicus infolge Brustquetschung. *Munch. med. Wschr.*, **55**, 1182.

Peet, M. M., and Campbell, K. N. (1943). Massive chylothorax following splanchnicectomy: treatment with intravenous and intrasternal transfusions of chyle. *Univ. Hosp. Bull. mich.*, **9**, 2.

Randolph, J. G., and Gross, R. E. (1957). Congenital chylothorax. *Arch. Surg.*, **74**, 405.

Sabin, F. R. (1902). On the origin of the lymphatic system from the veins and the development of the lymph hearts and thoracic duct in the pig. *Amer. J. Anat.*, **1**, 367.

Schnug, E., and Ransohoff, J. (1943). Traumatic chylothorax—a case treated with intravenous chyle. *Surgery*, **14**, 278.

Shumacker, H. B., Jr., and Moore, T. C. (1951). Surgical management of traumatic chylothorax. *Surg. Gynec. Obstet.*, **93**, 46.

Smith, A. N., Preshaw, R. M., and Bisset, W. H. (1962). The drainage of resistant ascites, by a modification of the Spitz-Holter valve technique. *J. roy. Coll. Surg. Edinb.*, **7**, 289.

Stewart, C. A., and Linner, H. P. (1926). Chylothorax in the newborn infant—report of a case. *Amer. J. Dis. Child.*, **31**, 654.

Van Pernis, P. A. (1949). Variations of the thoracic duct. *Surgery*, **26**, 806.

Whitcomb, B. B., and Scoville, W. B. (1942). Postoperative chylothorax: sudden death following the infusion of aspirated chyle. *Arch. Surg.*, **45**, 747.

*Arch. Dis. Childh.*, 1965, **40**, 192.

# LATE RESULTS OF THE OPERATION FOR COARCTATION IN THE GROWING CHILD*

BY

J. A. NOORDIJK, F. T. I. OEY, and H. M. P. VAN DEN BOOGAARD

*From the Department of Thoracic Surgery, Leyden University, the Netherlands*

There are only incidental published reports on the late results of operations for aortic coarctation in growing children, since the first operations for this anomaly were not performed until 1944.

Animal experiments have shown that an anastomosis in the aorta, if established with knotted sutures, increases in size with the remainder of the aorta as the animal grows (Johnson and Kirby, 1950). These experiments, however, were carried out with a normal healthy aorta, and warrant no conclusions concerning the growth of the anastomosis following resection of a coarctation in an infant.

Now that the trend is more and more in favour of operating on very young children with imminent cardiac decompensation as a result of a coarctation (Waterston, 1961; Morris, Cooley, de Bakey, and Crawford, 1960; Kempton and Waterston, 1957), it seems important to follow up the results of resection of the stenotic part of the aorta with end-to-end anastomosis (Moss, Adams, O'Loughlin, and Dixon, 1959).

## Subjects and Methods

For inclusion in the follow-up series we decided that the patient's operation should have taken place six years ago or earlier, and that at the time of operation the patient should have been no older than 12 years.

Among a total of over 500 operations for coarctation, 45 met this requirement. Of these 45 patients, 36 were seen for follow-up, 4 are at present living abroad, and 5 failed to report.

The interval between operation and follow-up varied from 6 to 11 years.

Of the patients seen for follow-up the youngest was a year old and the oldest was aged 12 at the time of operation. There were 3 patients between 0 and 2 years, 5 between 2 and 6 years, and 28 between 6 and 12 years. The weight gain averaged 20·8 kg. (minimum 5·7 kg. and maximum 40·2 kg.). The gain in height averaged 33·6 cm. (minimum 13 cm. and maximum 58 cm.).

## Results

The object of resecting an aortic stenosis is (1) to abolish the stenosis; (2) to reduce the brachial systolic blood pressure; and (3) to reduce the brachial diastolic blood pressure.

**Abolition of Stenosis.** The causes of death in coarctation not surgically treated are known to be: rupture of an aneurysm in an intercostal artery; sepsis as a result of aortitis; rupture of the aorta; cardiac decompensation; and rupture of an aneurysm in one of the basilar arteries (Reifenstein, Levine, and Gross, 1947).

Resection of the stenosis prevents formation of aneurysms and reduces the risk of aortitis.

At the operation photographs were taken, first of the stenosis and then of the anastomosis; and the circumference of the anastomosis and that of the aortic arch was measured.

We thought it unjustifiable to obtain aortograms merely for the sake of a follow-up, so consequently we have no exact data on the size of the anastomosis at the time of the follow-up. The blood pressure was determined in the arms and in the legs in all follow-up patients. In 33 patients, an external femoral artery curve was plotted. In normal subjects the duration of the ascent is less than 0·14 second. In patients with coarctation this is increased (over 0·16 sec.) or cannot be registered.

In 33 patients a femoral artery curve was registered. Only one of these showed unmistakable retardation (ascent 0·25 sec.) (Fig. 1), while one showed dubious retardation (0·14-0·18 sec.).

In 34 of the 36 patients examined, the systolic blood pressure in the legs proved to be equal to or higher than that in the arms. Only in the 2 patients already mentioned was the systolic blood pressure in the leg lower than that in the arm, namely, Case A, whose arm pressure was 130/60, and leg 95/60 mm. Hg, and ascent femoral artery curve 0·25 sec., and Case B, whose arm pressure was 160/90, and leg

* A paper read at a meeting of the British Association of Paediatric Surgeons in Rotterdam, September 1964.

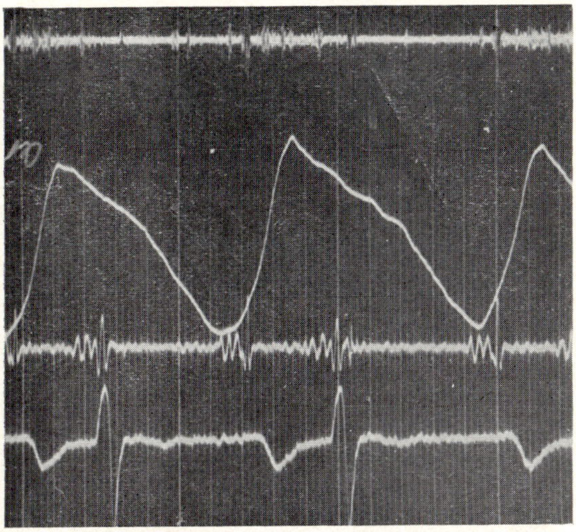

FIG. 1.—Femoral artery curve. The interval between two fine lines is 0·02 sec. Normal values for duration of ascent are 0·14 sec. Here it is clearly retarded (0·25 sec.).

130/115 mm. Hg, and ascent femoral artery curve 0·14-0·18 sec.

Case A is a boy who was operated on in 1954, at the age of 2 years. The pre-operative brachial blood pressure was 200/110 mm. Hg. The femoral artery was not palpable. He was completely asymptomatic at the time of follow-up; his performance was normal. An aortogram disclosed a slight stenosis (Fig. 2) at the anastomotic site. At the operation the circumference of the anastomosis had been 2·8 cm. and that of the arch 3·4 cm. Anatomical restoration of the aorta was less than ideal, and the picture taken at the operation shows unmistakable 'kinking' of the aorta (Fig. 3). Perhaps this kinking is partly responsible for the unsatisfactory result. In Leyden, therefore, efforts are made not only towards establishing the widest possible anastomosis but also towards optimal restoration of the normal shape of the aortic arch and isthmus.

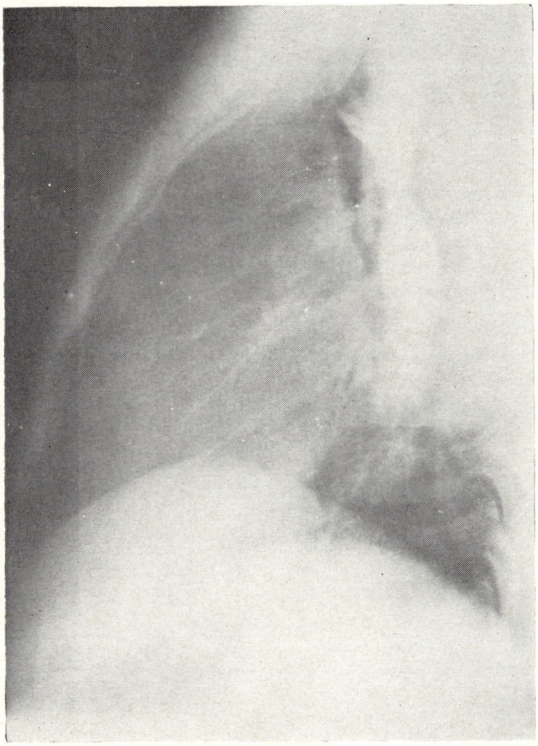

FIG. 2.—Aortogram shows stenosis at the site of the anastomosis.

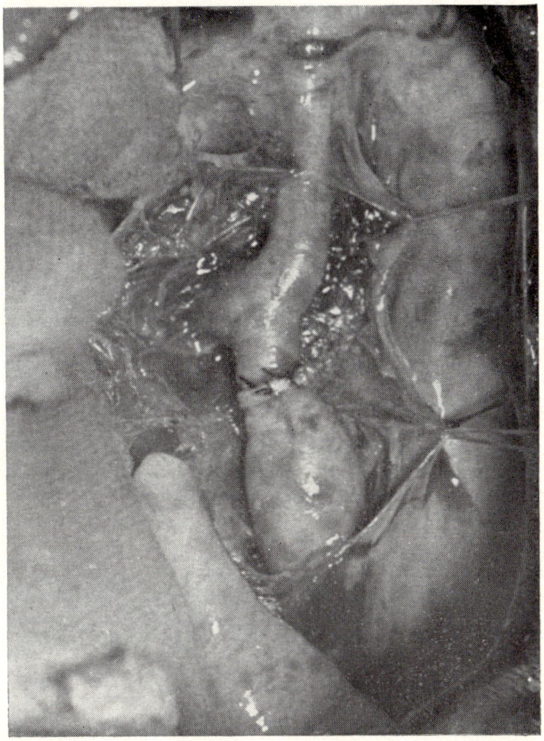

FIG. 3.—The anatomical restoration shown here is not ideal.

Case B was operated on in 1957 as a boy of 8 years. At the operation it was found that the aorta between the subclavian artery and the ligamentum arteriosum was hypoplastic (Fig. 4). The collateral arteries were more strongly developed and gave some trouble. The hypoplastic part and the coarctation were resected and a latero-terminal anastomosis was made in which the aortic arch, subclavian artery, and

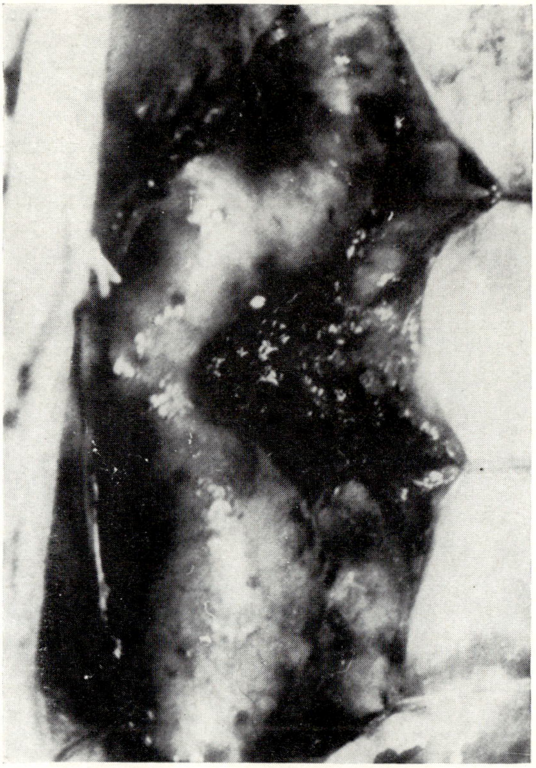

FIG. 4.—Hypoplastic aorta between subclavian artery and ligamentum arteriosum.

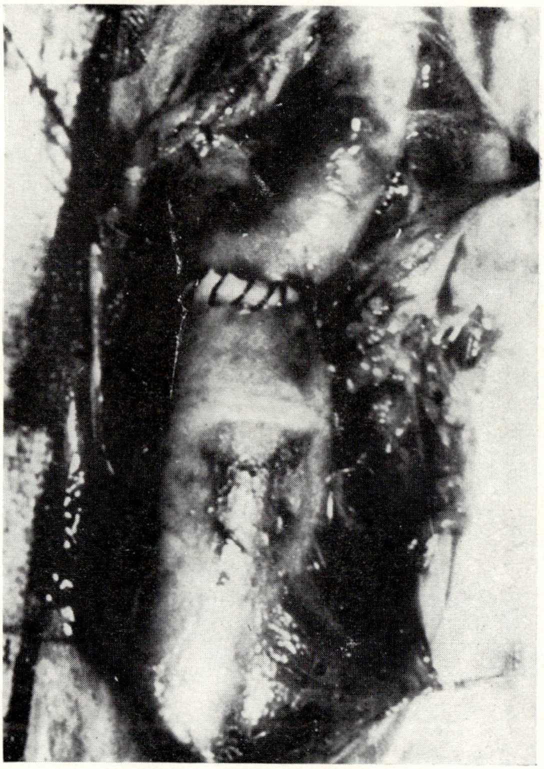

FIG. 5.—Reconstruction of aorta: subclavian artery and decending aorta together form a Y.

descending aorta together form a Y (Fig. 5). The circumference of the arch was 3 cm., of the subclavian artery 3·9 cm., and of the anastomosis 3·4 cm.

At follow-up the patient shows increasing symptoms of left ventricular hypertrophy, and the electrocardiogram and vectorcardiography indicate a valvular aortic stenosis with a slight insufficiency. He swims and used to play football but fatigues easily.

**Reduction of Brachial Systolic Blood Pressure.** If the brachial systolic blood pressure diminishes after resection of an aortic coarctation, the patient's expectation of life improves. The reduced brachial systolic blood pressure reduces the risk of a subarachnoid haemorrhage resulting from rupture of an aneurysm in one of the basilar arteries; and systolic blood pressure on effort is reduced (Taylor and Donald, 1960).

The pre-operative and post-operative brachial systolic blood pressure values are shown in Fig. 6, which indicates a post-operative decrease in all cases where this pressure was greatly increased.

A striking feature is, however, that in 5 cases it still remained higher than 140 mm. Hg. We have no explanation for this. Gelissen (1959) previously also observed that the decrease in systolic blood pressure in children was less pronounced than that in adults. The diastolic blood pressure in our patients was below 95 mm. Hg.

**Reduction of Brachial Diastolic Blood Pressure.** An increase in average blood pressure implies stress on the left ventricle. A high diastolic pressure means a high average blood pressure. Reduction of the diastolic blood pressure, therefore, improves the prognosis in these patients. The level of the diastolic blood pressure is shown in Fig. 7, which shows a post-operative decrease to 95 mm. Hg or lower in all patients.

**Subjective symptoms.** Only a few patients had pre-operative complaints, such as pain in the legs on effort or frequent headaches. One patient was

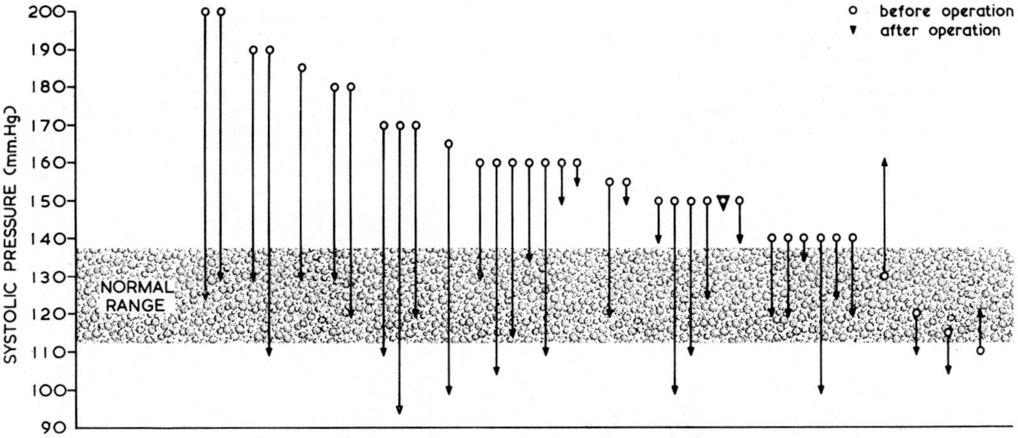


FIG. 6.—Decrease of systolic blood pressure after operation.

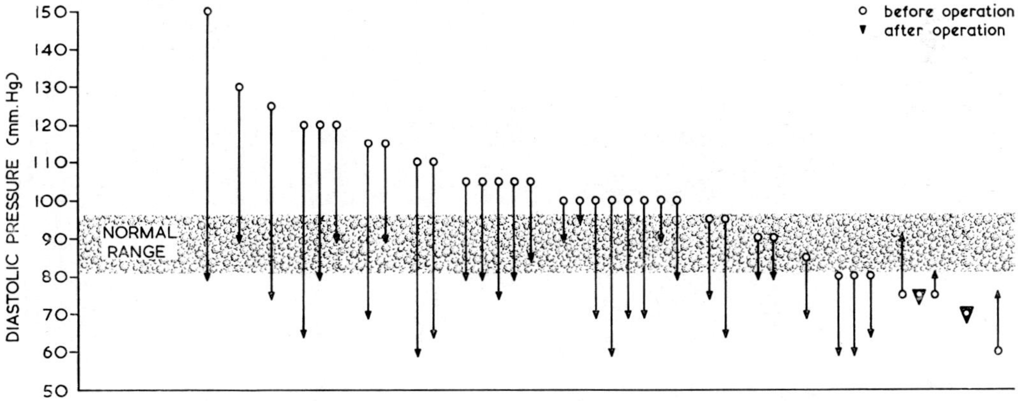


FIG. 7.—Decrease of diastolic blood pressure after operation.

unable to run. All patients were asymptomatic at the time of follow-up, except Case B already described.

These findings, however satisfactory, do not warrant the conclusion that the anastomosis does in fact participate in growth. To establish this, another follow-up on these patients after reaching adulthood is required.

## Summary and Conclusions

A follow-up study was made of patients submitted to resection for coarctation of the aorta more than six years previously, and aged 12 or younger at the time of the operation. The object was to establish whether results remained good after completion of the growth period. The results proved to be satisfactory.

Only in 2 patients of 36 seen for follow-up was the systolic blood pressure in the leg lower than that in the arm. Both these patients also had a prolonged rising time of the femoral artery curve.

### REFERENCES

Gelissen, J. (1959) Coarctatio aortae. Results of 258 operations. Thesis, Leiden.

Johnson, J., and Kirby, C. K. (1950). The relationship of the method of suture to the growth of end-to-end arterial anastomoses. *Surgery*, **27**, 17.

Kempton, J. J., and Waterston, D. J. (1957). Coarctation of aorta presenting as cardiac failure in early infancy. *Brit. med. J.*, **2**, 442.

Morris, G. C., Jr., Cooley, D. A., de Bakey, M. E., and Crawford, E. S. (1960). Coarctation of the aorta with particular emphasis upon improved techniques of surgical repair. *J. thorac. cardiovasc. Surg.*, **40**, 705.

Moss, A. J., Adams, F. H., O'Loughlin, B. J., and Dixon, W. J. (1959). The growth of the normal aorta and of the anastomotic site in infants following surgical resection of coarctation of the aorta. *Circulation*, **19**, 338.

Reifenstein, G. H., Levine, S. A., and Gross, R. E. (1947). Coarctation of the aorta: a review of 104 autopsied cases of the "adult type", two years of age or older. *Amer. Heart J.*, 33, 146.

Taylor, S. H., and Donald, K. W. (1960). Circulatory studies at rest and during exercise in coarctation of the aorta before and after operation. *Brit. Heart J.*, **22**, 117.

Waterston, D. J. (1961). Communication Annual Meeting Society o Thoracic Surgeons of Great Britain and Ireland, London.

*Arch. Dis. Childh.*, 1965, **40**, 197.

# OESOPHAGEAL STENOSIS DUE TO REFLUX OESOPHAGITIS*

BY

JOSÉ BOIX-OCHOA and FRITZ REHBEIN

*From The Surgical Department of the Children's Hospital, Bremen, Germany*

During childhood the majority of acquired oesophageal strictures are due to gastro-oesophageal reflux (Willich, 1963). Usually this reflux is caused by a hiatal hernia. Minor forms of hernia and cardiac achalasia may cause a reflux that is so severe that oesophagitis and subsequent stricture formation result. One-quarter of our operated cases had more or less well-formed strictures. Our routine is to try conservative treatment first, and this was successful in the majority of the minor forms of hernia. But in view of the high incidence of strictures among our cases, early operative treatment is recommended if conservative treatment fails.

### Subjects and Methods of Treatment

Between 1954 and 1964, 226 hiatal hernias were operated on in the surgical department of the Children's Hospital, Bremen. Included in this number are children with minor forms of hernias and cardiac achalasia in which conservative treatment failed. Of these, 54 were complicated by stenosis, an incidence of 24%. Bettex, Stillhart, and Nusslé's (1961) statistics showed an average of 17% strictures secondary to hiatal hernias. The incidence of the strictures increases with age (Fig. 1). While the number of hiatal hernias decreases from the first to the fifth year of age, the total number of stricture cases remains about the same.

The treatment of the strictures depends on their severity. In the minority gastrostomy and bouginage are sufficient. The gastrostomy makes the dilatation easier and diminishes its danger. The child is discharged home with the thread passing through the nose, oesophagus, and gastrostomy (Fig. 2a). The dilator is passed through the oesophagus by aid of this thread and a filiform bougie (Fig. 2b). Following this method very thick bougies may be used without any danger.

Six children in this series were dealt with successfully by operating on the hiatal hernia only. These stenoses were most probably mainly due to spasm with only minor organic changes (Table 1).

In Group C (Table 1), which includes the cases where

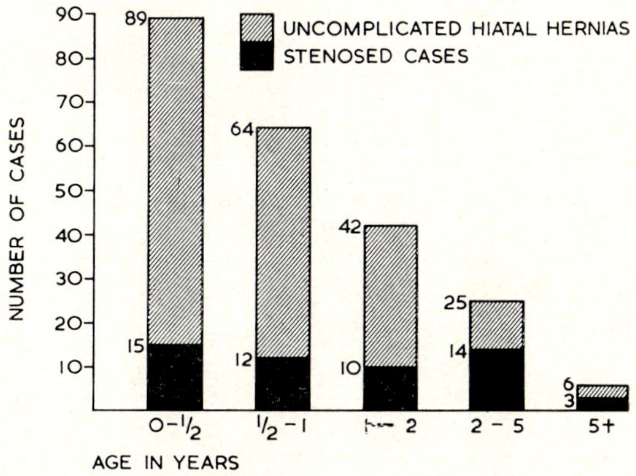


FIG. 1.—Incidence of oesophageal stenoses in 226 cases of hiata hernia.

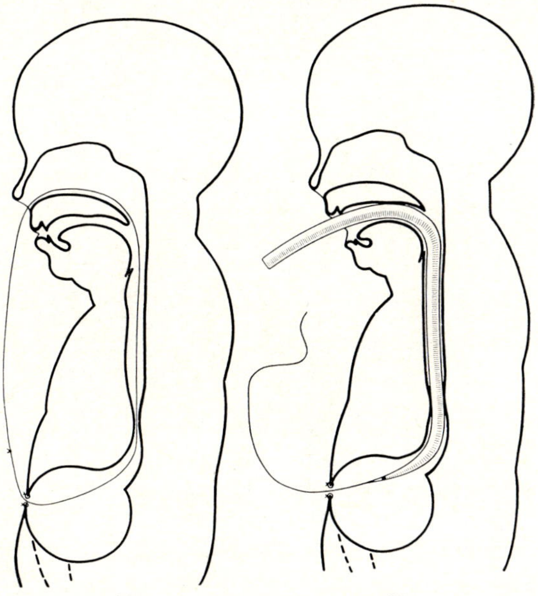

(a) (b)

FIG. 2.—Dilatation of oesophageal stricture in a child with gastrostomy (see text).

* A paper read at a meeting of the British Association of Paediatric Surgeons in Rotterdam September 1964.

TABLE 1
METHODS OF TREATMENT IN 54 CASES OF OESOPHAGEAL STRICTURE

| Groups | Methods of Treatment | No. of Cases |
|---|---|---|
| A | Gastrostomy, then bouginage | 3 |
| B | Operation on the hiatal hernia only | 6 |
| C | Operation on the hiatal hernia plus gastrostomy, then bouginage | 16 |
| D | Gastrostomy, then bouginage, then operation on the hiatal hernia, then bouginage again | 28 |
| E | Resection plus colon transplantation | 1 |
| | Total .. .. .. | 54 |

children are able to swallow liquid and semi-solid food, gastrostomy was performed in the same stage of operation for hiatal hernia. The gastrostomy is used for post-operative bouginage.

In Group D gastrostomy was first performed for feeding and for bouginage. Repeated dilatation is continued for a period of two to three months, after which in a second stage the operation for hiatal hernia is done. This is followed by further bouginage. Most of the operations were performed by a combined thoraco-abdominal approach (Rehbein and Röpke, 1962). The aim of this operation is to mobilize the oesophagus, to bring the cardia below the diaphragm, and to fix the lesser curvature of the stomach to the anterior abdominal wall.

Successful results are obtained from this method in non-complicated cases of hiatal hernias because normal anatomical conditions of the cardio-oesophageal region are achieved.

In advanced cases with severe strictures and short oesophagus, surgical repair of hiatal hernia cannot be complete and a clinical cure is not always to be expected. Colonic transplantation is then recommended. Our series includes one case (Table 1) with colonic transplantation: two years after the operation the child is in good condition.

## Results of Treatment

The results of treatment are shown in Table 2, which includes follow-up till March 31, 1964. The high percentage of successful results is due to the fact that many of the stenoses were mild and could easily be dilated, so that after operating on the hernia the reflux disappeared.

The result was poor in two children, one presenting with recurrence of the stricture many years after the operation. This child will need colonic transplantation, showing that in severe cases a relapse of the stenosis should always be expected.

TABLE 2
RESULTS OF TREATMENT

| Results | No. |
|---|---|
| Good | 44 |
| Still under treatment | 6 |
| Poor | 2 (colonic transplantation is indicated) |
| Died | 3 |
| Total .. .. .. | 55 |

## Discussion

Dilatation alone rarely produces successful results. Mere dilatation without operation for hiatal hernia leads to persistence of the reflux and subsequent oesophagitis with further stricture formation (Barrett, 1950; Bettex *et al.*, 1961). In early and mild cases of stenosis operation on the hiatal hernia alone may be successful. But in the majority, operation plus bouginage should be performed. We have found that in only a proportion of cases are there marked pathological changes in the oesophagus. In the remainder operative correction of the hernia alone may be successful, and only a few dilatations may be necessary for permanent cure. Waterston (1962) achieved satisfactory results by a single retrograde dilatation during the repair of the hernia. Bettex *et al.* successfully performed oesophago-gastropexy in those stenosed cases.

In some cases, however, the oesophagus is shortened and narrowed by severe stricture formation, in which case repair can only be incomplete, and prolonged bouginage is essential. It is surprising that in spite of incomplete surgical correction in this way a fairly good result may be achieved. Of course, observation has not yet continued long enough for final judgement. There were 3 failures in our series, and in view of the severity of the condition further recurrences must be expected. A resection will have to be performed. A direct anastomosis will usually not be possible (Franklin and Henderson, 1955), and at present intrathoracic colonic transplantation seems to be the best method (Johansson and Silander, 1963; Waterston, 1962). As vagotomy is connected with the performance of this operation, pyloroplasty must be done in the same stage. This diminishes the risk of reflux into the transplanted colon.

Although there are a few cases that require primary colonic transplantation, the easier method of correcting the hernia followed by bouginage is worth trying first.

## Summary

Fifty-five cases of oesophageal strictures due to reflux were analysed. The result of treatment depends on the severity of the stricture. In the great majority of cases operative correction of the hiatal hernia and prolonged bouginage lead to successful results. In cases of recurrence colonic transplantation is performed.

REFERENCES

Barrett, N. R. (1950). Chronic peptic ulcer of the oesophagus and oesophagitis. *Brit. J. Surg.*, **38**, 175.

Bettex, M., Stillhart, H., and Nusslé, D. (1961). Über peptische Oesophagusstenosen bei Hiatushernien im Kindesalter. *Helv. chir. Acta*, **28**, 594.

Franklin, R. H., and Henderson, I. D. (1955). Two cases of oesophageal stricture in childhood requiring resection. *Arch. Dis. Childh.*, **30**, 55.

Johansson, L., and Silander, T. (1963). Esophageal reconstruction for benign strictures. *Acta chir. scand.*, **125**, 329.

Rehbein, F., and Röpke, T. (1962). Abdomino-thorakale Operation der Hiatushernie beim Säugling und Kleinkind. *Chir. Praxis*, **6**, 291.

Waterston, D. (1962). In *Pediatric Surgery*, ed. C. D. Benson, W. T. Mustard, M. M. Ravitch, W. N. Snyder, and K. J. Welch. Year Book Medical Publishers, Chicago.

Willich, E. (1963). Die angeborenen und erworbenen Verengungen der Speiseröhre im Kindesalter. *Pädiat. Praxis*, **2**, 51.

*Arch. Dis. Childh.*, 1965, **40**, 200.

# ACTINOMYCIN D IN WILMS' TUMOUR: TREATMENT OF LUNG METASTASES*

BY

RUSSELL HOWARD

*From the Royal Children's Hospital, Melbourne, Australia*

This paper discusses recent world trends in the treatment of Wilms' tumour, particularly as exemplified by their impact on practice at the Royal Children's Hospital, Melbourne.

Following the use of actinomycin D in the therapy of lung metastases of Wilms' tumour (see below), it became apparent that this drug was able, at times, to inhibit their growth and, more rarely, to cause their complete regression.

In order to examine the merits of putting the drug to more general use in the treatment of this malignancy, a meeting of those interested was held at the Royal Children's Hospital on April 15, 1959.

Examination of records indicated that, since the introduction of post-operative irradiation of the tumour bed, death from Wilms' tumour was largely the result of blood-stream dissemination. Nevertheless, as adduced by the author in 1957, in a review of 26 consecutive cases, the recovery rate was still only 11·5%.

In view of the proved effect of actinomycin D on established lung metastases it was considered that if nephrectomy were performed under its cover haematogenous dissemination might be eliminated and any minimal undetectable metastases already present be suppressed.

Accordingly the following three decisions were taken.

(1) That actinomycin D be introduced into the treatment sequence; (2) that the drug be pushed to the limits of tolerance; and (3) that tumour bed irradiation be deferred for a limited period in order to avoid the simultaneous action of two bone marrow depressants.

The following plan was conceived and enunciated in terms of days of treatment.

Actinomycin D was administered in a total dosage of 120 μg./kg., divided into 8 equal injections to be given on Days 1, 2, 3, 4, 5, 7, 9, and 12. Nephrectomy was performed on Day 3.

Irradiation was commenced on Day 26 and continued daily to a dosage of 3,000 rads delivered over approximately 28 days.

The results of a series of 18 consecutive cases treated thus are here recorded and annotated in the accompanying Table. 11 of the 18 have survived without evidence of recurrence for periods of from 24 to 58 months—a recovery rate of 62% with a minimum survival time of 2 years.

TABLE

| Place in Series | Age at Time of Nephrectomy (mth.) | Sex | Result | Survival from Time of Nephrectomy (mth.) |
|---|---|---|---|---|
| 1 | 12 | F | Dead | 7 |
| 2 | 10 | M | Alive | 58 |
| 3 | 36 | M | Dead | 13 |
| 4 | 16 | F | Alive | 57 |
| 5 | 36 | M | Dead | 15 |
| 6 | 17 | M | Alive | 41 |
| 7 | 60 | F | Dead | 6 |
| 8 | 13 | M | Alive | 41 |
| 9 | 84 | F | Dead | 4 |
| 10 | 46 | F | Alive | 40 |
| 11 | 42 | F | Alive | 40 |
| 12 | 27 | F | Alive | 35 |
| 13 | 42 | F | Alive | 29 |
| 14 | 3 | M | Alive | 28 |
| 15 | 39 | F | Alive | 28 |
| 16 | 33 | F | Alive | 27 |
| 17 | 44 | M | Dead | 7 |
| 18 | 15 | F | Dead | 0·25 |

While one realizes that these patients are not yet assured of ultimate recovery it is still true to say that the usual experience of Wilms' tumour is that cases remaining completely well for 2 years after nephrectomy are likely to be permanent cures. The comparison with the previous recovery rate of 11·5%, recorded in 1957, is striking. Of the 7 deaths, 2 were cases of most unfavourable initial prognosis in so far as metastases were present before the start of treatment (in one case involving the liver, in the other the scalp) and a third died on the sixth post-operative day from septicaemia. The remaining 4

* A paper read at a meeting of the British Association of Paediatric Surgeons in Rotterdam, September 1964.

pursued a course that appeared to be uninfluenced by actinomycin D.

The only significant change in the treatment used in the present series has been the introduction of actinomycin D, and it is concluded that this drug is responsible for the improvement in results.

### Toxic Effects of Actinomycin D

Actinomycin D is a toxic antibiotic that appears to have a selective effect on Wilms' tumour.

The toxic effects are manifest in relation to (a) the bone marrow, where the activity is depressed even to the point of aplastic anaemia; (b) the skin and its appendages, causing macular rashes and epilation of the hair of the scalp; and (c) the gastro-intestinal tract, as instanced by anorexia, vomiting, ulcerative stomatitis, and diarrhoea (often blood-stained).

There have been two instances (Case 15 and a subsequent case too recent for inclusion in this series) of the development, 2 weeks after cessation of radiotherapy, of oedema of the extremities and ascites with marked liver and splenic enlargement: in both the tumour was in the right kidney. It is suggested that the effect of irradiation on the liver was potentiated by the previous action of actinomycin D with resultant swelling and portal obstruction. Investigations on Case 15 showed that there was no obstruction of inferior vena cava or hepatic veins (as determined by catheterization) but that the serum protein level had fallen to 5 g./100 ml., with decrease in the albumin fraction, accounting for the generalized oedema. The ascitic fluid was milky in appearance but proved unsatisfactory for cell examination owing to precipitation of lipid material. The second case (a recent one) presented a similar picture. Both recovered on supportive treatment only, liver and spleen returning to normal size over a period of 4 months.

In an even more recent case (still undergoing irradiation), on the eighth day after starting treatment, acute intussusception occurred in the lower ileum, demanding bowel resection. The bowel in the region of the apex of the intussusception displayed several swollen areas with central ulceration. Though specific pathological proof is lacking, it seems logical to place this occurrence in sequence with the well-known manifestation of blood-stained diarrhoea, and to class it as a further complication, hitherto unlisted, of actinomycin D administration (the child also exhibited skin lesions and stomatitis). The findings, recorded by Philips, Schwartz, Sternberg, and Tan in 1960, of extensive damage to small and large intestines of rats, with swelling of cells and submucosal oedema and congestion as a result of actinomycin D therapy, are an indication of what could occur in the human and could well be the basis of an intussusception.

It should be noted that toxic features may vary in nature and in degree from patient to patient and perhaps from one batch of actinomycin D to another. Treatment must be carefully monitored by both clinical and laboratory observations. Though no modification of dosage was necessary in any of the cases recorded here, in two recent cases it was thought wise to omit the final dose.

### Management of Established Lung Metastases

Cases of established lung metastases may be divided into two categories according to whether actinomycin D has or has not previously been administered.

Cases in the first category (i.e. in which actinomycin D has previously been administered) are in our experience resistant to further actinomycin D and should be treated initially by irradiation, supplemented by a modified course of actinomycin D (this combination is recommended in view of the probable potentiation of the effect of irradiation by the drug as suggested by D'Angio, Farber, and Maddock (1959), and by Farber, D'Angio, Evans, and Mitus (1960)). If these measures fail to procure radiographic disappearance of metastases, or if initial regression is not maintained, operative measures should be instituted unless the dissemination is obviously too extensive to attempt salvage. Other chemotherapeutic agents may be of use as adjuncts to operation, but our experience of these is inadequate to form a definitive opinion of their value.

Cases in the second category should be given initially a full course of actinomycin D (see above). Anything short of complete radiographic regression is an indication for irradiation. Thereafter management is along similar lines to those of the first category.

Surgical extirpation may be by wedge resection, segmental resection, lobectomy, or perhaps, pneumonectomy. Segmental resection or lobectomy is the procedure of choice if warranted by a favourable distribution of metastases. Numerous scattered deposits may indicate multiple wedge resections or, if limited to one lung, perhaps pneumonectomy. Bilateral deposits are not *per se* a contraindication to operation.

Seven cases have been operated on for lung metastases: 3 are still alive and free from metastases and have now been well for periods of from 4½ to 5 years. The fourth, and the sole case in which pneumonectomy was performed, died 6 months after this operation from liver secondaries. The fifth died of nephritis 4 years after bilateral wedge resection, and necropsy revealed no evidence of malignancy. The sixth died from a solitary cerebral metastasis with no other malignant deposits detectable at necropsy, and the seventh succumbed to his pulmonary metastases.

The first case treated along these lines is noted in some detail as an example of the routine adopted: V.C., a girl of 5 years, developed two metastases in the upper lobe of the right lung 17 months after left nephrectomy. In response to actinomycin D one of these disappeared radiographically and the other decreased in size, then remained stationary. A second course of actinomycin D, 6 months later, produced no further change. Right upper lobectomy was performed on August 1, 1959. One metastasis was found to have been completely replaced by macrophages and appeared as a yellow plaque under the pleura and the other presented as a whitish nodule which microscopically showed a very attenuated picture of a secondary Wilms' tumour. This child has remained well up to the time of writing.

Were a similar case to be treated now, irradiation would be used after the first course of actinomycin D and, if inadequate, this would be followed by lobectomy.

The salvage rate in this group has thus proved considerable and the agressive attitude to pulmonary dissemination seems to be justified. The treatment, however, is essentially a matter of combined therapy, using in their correct sequence chemotherapy, irradiation, and ablative surgery.

Lung metastases that show no response to chemotherapy or irradiation are probably unsuitable for surgery. Early massive lung secondaries are unlikely to respond to any therapy.

**Other Metastases.** Metastases in the liver are not suitable for irradiation, and we have had no success at all with actinomycin D. Bone metastases may show temporary regression with irradiation but recurrence seems to be the invariable rule. Actinomycin D was used in one case only and without effect.

Peritoneal recurrence has again been completely resistant to actinomycin D and has, in our hands, shown no noticeable response to irradiation. By the time these latter recurrences are manifest, of course, multiple organs tend to be involved.

## Summary

A series of 18 successive cases of Wilms' tumour, treated by a régime of actinomycin D, nephrectomy, and irradiation, is recorded.

The recovery rate over a minimal two-year period was 62% as compared with 11·5% recorded in a previous series in which actinomycin D was not used.

The toxic effects of actinomycin D are discussed.

Treatment of pulmonary metastases is discussed in detail, and that of other metastases is mentioned.

My thanks are due to my colleagues, medical and surgical, at the Royal Children's Hospital and to the representatives of the Peter MacCallum Institute at which the radiotherapy régime was devised and conducted.

### References

D'Angio, G J., Farber, S., and Maddock, C. L. (1959). Potentiation of x-ray effects by actinomycin D. *Radiology*, 73, 175.

Farber, S., D'Angio, G., Evans, A., and Mitus, A. (1960). Clinical studies of actinomycin D with special reference to Wilms' tumor in children. *Ann. N.Y. Acad. Sci.*, **89**, 421

Howard, R. (1957). Nephroblastoma: Wilms' tumour. *Med. J. Aust.*, **1**, 200.

Philips, F. S., Schwartz, H S., Sternberg, S. S., and Tan, C. T. C. (1960). The toxicity of actinomycin D. *Ann. N.Y. Acad. Sci.*, **89**, 348.

*Arch. Dis. Childh.*, 1965, **40**, 203.

# FUNCTIONAL STENOSIS AS A CAUSE OF PELVI-URETERIC OBSTRUCTION AND HYDRONEPHROSIS*

BY

L. BÄCKLUND, G. GROTTE, and A. REUTERSKIÖLD

*From the Department of Clinical Physiology and the Department of Paediatric Surgery, University of Uppsala, Uppsala, Sweden*

The operative findings in cases of hydronephrosis often do not suggest any obvious cause of obstruction, and as Innes Williams (1958) has recently emphasized the pathology of hydronephrosis cannot be discussed solely in terms of anatomy. When by pyelography the diagnosis of hydronephrosis in a child has been established, the cause of the hydronephrosis can be one out of many. From the surgical point of view the common problem at operation is to find out if an aberrant vessel might cause the obstruction, or if there is an obstruction at the pelvi-ureteric junction, usually then a 'congenital stenosis'. In many cases, no cause of obstruction is found in the tissues surrounding the pelvis and the pelvi-ureteric junction. When the pelvi-ureteric junction is opened it looks narrow, though it is possible to pass a fine ureteric catheter; by definition the urologist would not call this a stenosis, and hydrodynamic flow would be considered free in such cases. In the present investigation four cases of pelvi-ureteric obstruction have been studied during continuous infusion into the pelves at various rates of flow. During this infusion pressures have been continuously recorded in the pelvis and at two different levels of the ureter. A fifth case having calyceal dilatation but normal pelvi-ureteric junction was also studied. The data from this small series suggest the existence of a 'functional stenosis', in spite of the passage of ureteral catheters.

## Material and Methods

At operation the kidney and the proximal ureter were exposed through a flank incision. Two catheters, infant feeding tubes size 5†, were inserted into the part of the dilated pelvis that was to be resected (Fig. 1). One of these was then used for infusion of Salidex (Pharmacia Ltd., Uppsala, Sweden) at arbitrary flows. The rates of flow used varied between 0·10-10·0 ml./min. The other pelvic catheter was attached to the pressure recording apparatus. For this study a pressure recording device consisting of three pressure transducers (EMT 490 a) and electromanometers (EMT 469) and a direct writing recorder (Mingograf 42) was used. According to the manufacturer* the transducers work linearly from 0 to + 300 mm. Hg. They had a volume displacement of 0·07 c.mm. when exposed to 100 mm. Hg. The two pelvic catheters were tied in by water-tight ligatures. Two other catheters† were then introduced into the ureter by puncture, one into the upper and the other into the lower ureter (Fig. 1). These two ureteric catheters were also connected to the pressure recording device. Leakage from any of the catheters was controlled after each experiment. Continuous infusion was obtained by a machine built by Mr. B. Clementz at the Institute of Physiology, University of Lund.

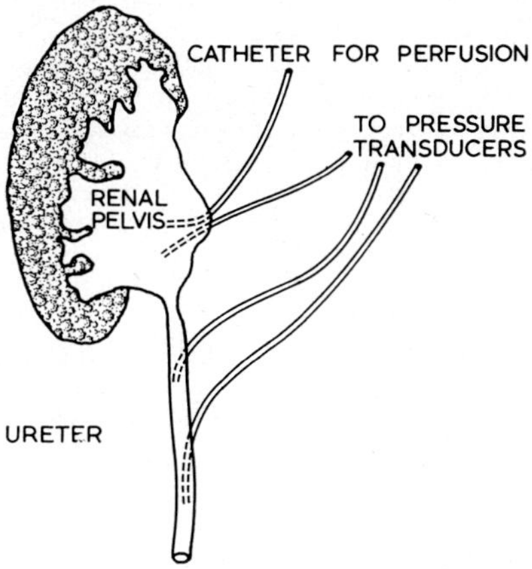


FIG. 1.—Arrangement of catheters during experiment.

* A paper read at a meeting of the British Association of Paediatric Surgeons in Rotterdam, September 1964.

† Bardic Inc. N.J., U.S.A.

* Elema-Schönander Ltd. Stockholm, Sweden.

† Intracath, Desereth, needle size 17 Bardic Inc., N.J., U.S.A.

TABLE 1
PRINCIPAL DATA CONCERNING PATIENTS

| Case No. | Diagnosis | Age at Onset of Symptoms (yr.) | Age at Operation (yr.) | Maximum Infusion Rate Without Pronounced Rise in Intrapelvic Pressure (ml./min.) | Infusion Time (min.) | Correspond-ing Diuresis (ml./hr./kidney) |
|---|---|---|---|---|---|---|
| 1 M | Hydronephrosis due to pelvi-ureteric obstruction | 2/12 | 4/12 | ≤0·56 | 10 | 34 |
| 2 F | ,, | 6/12 | 4 | 1·10 | 9·5 | 6 |
| 3 M | ,, | 9 2/12 | 9 3/12 | 3·2 | 6 | 192 |
| 4 F | ,, | 14 | 20 | 3·2 | 2·5 | 192 |
| 5 M | Pyelonephritis with normal pelvi-ureteric junction | 3/12 | 1·5 | >5·6 | 5 | >312 |

### Present Series

Five patients have been studied. Their ages at the onset of symptoms and at the operation are shown in Table 1.

The symptoms in Cases 1-3 were recurrent urinary infections. Case 4 had had diffuse pains in her right side from 14 years of age, but no diagnosis was made until she had a right-sided pyelonephritis at the age of 20. Pyelography in these four cases showed hydronephrosis with stenosis of the pelvi-ureteric junction. Operation revealed a so-called stenosis in all cases, but it was possible in every instance to pass a catheter Charr 2-3 from the renal pelvis through the stenosis into the ureter. After the flow-pressure studies were completed a Hyne-Anderson type of plastic operation was done (Anderson, 1963). The post-operative course was uneventful in every case.

Case 5 may be regarded as a control case. He had multiple malformations, high rectal atresia, agenesis of four sacral vertebrae, and bilateral congenital dislocation of the hips. At the age of 3 months he acquired his first urinary infection. Repeated intravenous pyelography showed dilatation of the calyces, but no significant dilatation of the renal pelvis of the right kidney. Because of recurrent infections, an exploration of the right kidney was made, but no hydronephrosis or pelvi-ureteric stenosis was confirmed. The calyceal dilatation was apparently due to severe pyelonephritic scarring.

### Results

The intrapelvic pressure was measured before the perfusion started and was found to vary between 0 and 10 mm. Hg (Table 2).

TABLE 2
RESTING PELVIC PRESSURE BEFORE AND MAXIMUM PELVIC PRESSURE DURING INFUSION

| Case No. | Initial Intrapelvic Pressure (mm. Hg) | Maximum Recorded Pelvic Pressure (mm. Hg) | Perfusion Rate at Maximum Recorded Pelvic Pressure (mm. Hg) |
|---|---|---|---|
| 1 | 0 | 25 | 0·56 ml./min. |
| 2 | 10 | 38 | 0·56 |
| 3 | 0 | 20 | 10·0 |
| 4 | 2 | 20 | 10·0 |
| 5 | 1–2 | 2·5 | 5·6 |

The infusion was then started and the pressures in the pelvis and ureter were continuously recorded. We tried to find the maximum perfusion rate not inducing a marked increase in pelvic pressure. The infusion time at that pressure is, together with other data, shown in Table 1. Higher rates of perfusion always gave a rapid increase in pelvic pressure. As can be seen the patients who started showing symptoms during the first year of life (Cases 1-2) did not tolerate as high a perfusion rate as those with a later onset of symptoms (Cases 3 and 4). As a contrast Case 5 is shown who, in spite of being very young, tolerated more than the 20-year-old girl (Case 4). The relation between the maximum recorded pelvic pressure and the corresponding infusion rate in the five cases is shown in Table 2. The recordings from a typical case (No. 2) are illustrated in Fig. 2a-c. The frequency of ureteric contractions was also studied. There was no change in contraction frequency with increasing perfusion rates in Cases 1, 3, and 4, whereas Case 2 showed a slight increase. In Case 5, however, the frequency of ureteric contractions was doubled during an increase of rates of perfusion used from minimum to maximum.

### Discussion

It is well known from the works of Underwood (1937), Davis (1954) Melick, Karellos, and Naryka (1961), and Kiil (1963) that the resting pressure in the hydronephrotic sac is not very high. This is confirmed here. In our series, however, the patient was dehydrated and anaesthetized and probably had a very small flow of urine, so it would have been possible for the hydronephrotic sac to empty itself and lower the pelvic pressure during the start of the operation before the catheters were put in place. This is in agreement with the fact that after stopping the infusion, intrapelvic pressure decreased in our series within a few minutes. Why pressure in the hydronephrotic sac is so low has been discussed by many authors (Hinman, 1963). No doubt the

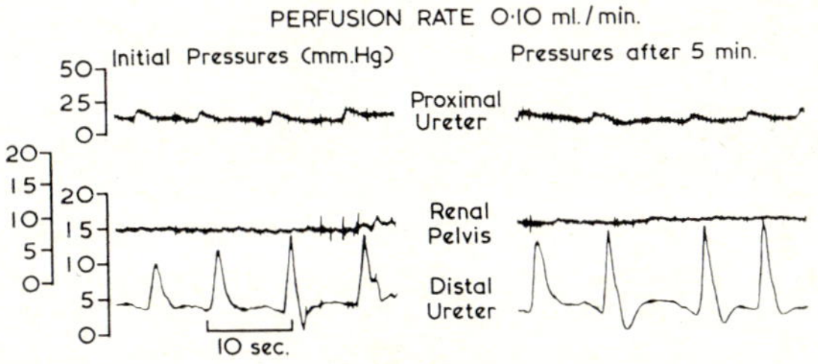


FIG. 2a.

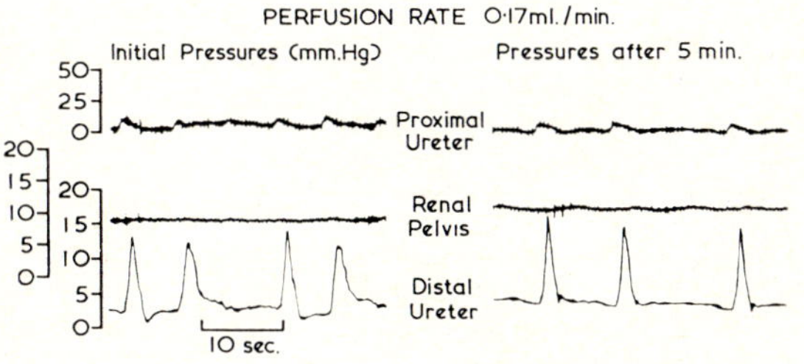


FIG. 2b.

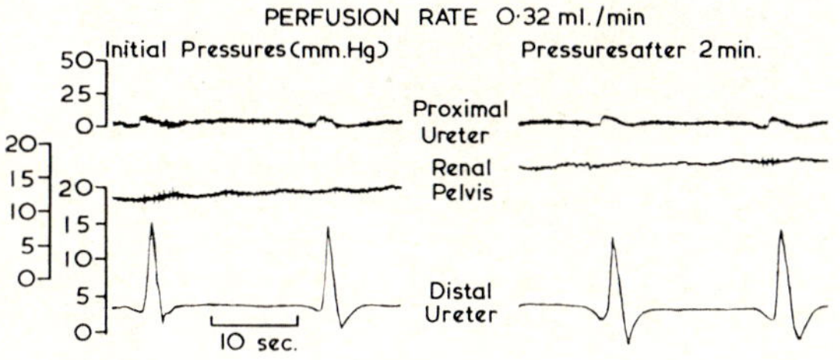


FIG. 2c.

Pressure recordings in renal pelvis, upper and lower ureter in Case 2, at three different flow-rates. Note increasing pelvic pressure at flow-rates over 0·10 ml./min.

pyelo-lymphatic, the pyelo-venous, and the pyelo-tubular backflow is involved in this mechanism.

For pelvic pressure recordings and infusion, most earlier investigators have used a catheter through the pelvi-ureteric junction inserted from below. These catheters no doubt disturb the outflow through the pelvi-ureteric junction. This is circumvented in our studies. With different perfusion rates we tried to mimic a diuresis within physiological limits. Within these flows we found a threshold value of interest, i.e. the maximum flow not inducing an increase in intrapelvic pressure during prolonged perfusion. According to Kiil (1957) the normal renal pelvis and ureter can tolerate a flow of 8-10 ml./min. per ureter without increasing pelvic pressure. The threshold values in Cases 1 to 4 are therefore considered to be quite low. On the other hand Case 5 showed a transport capacity of more than 5·6 ml./min., i.e. within the range for adults. No similar studies on children seem to have been reported.

Those patients having functional stenosis of the pelvi-ureteric junction are prone to get episodes of pelvic hypertension during moderate diuresis. This pelvic hypertension may promote pyelonephritis (Beeson, 1963).

May a pelvi-ureteric obstruction be explained by any structural deviation from the normal? Murnaghan (1958a, b) found a lack of circular muscles in the pelvi-ureteric junction in cases of pelvi-ureteric stenosis. However, no obvious anatomical stricture can be found at operation, and the abnormal histology must in some way interfere with the function. An explanation could be that when the urine enters the ureteral cone insufficient stretch reflex is elicited in the circular muscle and there is inadequate stimulus for the ureter to propel the urine. The importance of mechanical stimulation to the ureter was pointed out by Bäcklund (1963) among others; he studied the conduction mechanism of the ureter in dogs. A certain minimum distension of the smooth muscle is necessary to promote propagation. The orientation of the muscle fibres may be of importance in this connexion. It seems logical to assume that circular fibres become more distended and are therefore more easily excited than longitudinal muscles at increasing pressure in the ureteral cone. If the intraluminal pressure is not high enough to produce an adequate muscular distension in the abnormal region (lacking circular layer), the urine may merely be pressed through the abnormal segment without causing any peristalsis until it reaches a lower segment of the ureter. In Cases 1 to 4 it was found that in spite of increasing perfusion rates the ureteric activity remained fairly constant. In contrast to this the ureteric activity was doubled during increased perfusion in Case 5 who had a normal pelvi-ureteric junction. This may indicate that the flow through the ureteral cone is of the same magnitude in cases of functional pelvi-ureteric stenosis but varies with diuresis in the normal.

**Summary**

Four cases of hydronephrosis with evidence of pelvi-ureteric obstruction have been studied. A functional rather than an anatomical stenosis of the pelvi-ureteral junction is suggested.

This investigation was supported by generous grants from 'Ollie och Elof Ericssons Stiftelse för Vetenskaplig Forskning', Atvidaberg, Sweden.

REFERENCES

Anderson, J. C. (1963). *Hydronephrosis*. Heinemann, London.

Bäcklund, L. (1963). Experimental studies on pressure and contractility in the ureter. *Acta. physiol. scand.*, **59**, suppl. 212.

Beeson, P. B. (1963). Pyelonephritis and renal infections. In *Yearbook of Urology 1962-1963*, ed. W. W. Scott, p. 121. Year Book Medical Publishers, Chicago.

Davis, D. M. (1954). The hydrodynamics of the upper urinary tract (urodynamics). *Ann. Surg.*, **140**, 839.

Hinman, F., Jr. (1963). The pathophysiology of urinary obstruction. In *Urology*, ed. M. F. Campbell, vol. 1, p. 323. Saunders, Philadelphia and London.

Kiil, F. (1957). *The Function of the Ureter and Renal Pelvis*. Saunders, Philadelphia and London.

—— (1963). Physiology of the renal pelvis and ureter. In *Urology*, ed. M. F. Campbell, vol. 1, p. 81. Saunders, Philadelphia and London.

Melick, W. F., Karellos, D., and Naryka. J. J. (1961). Pressure studies of hydronephrosis in children by means of the strain gauge. *J. Urol.* (*Baltimore*), **85**, 703.

Murnaghan, G. F. (1958a). The dynamics of the renal pelvis and ureter with reference to congenital hydronephrosis. *Brit. J. Urol.*, **30**, 321.

—— (1958b). The mechanism of congenital hydronephrosis with reference to the factors influencing surgical treatment. *Ann. roy. Coll. Surg. Engl.*, **23**, 25.

Underwood, W. E. (1937). Recent observations on the pathology of hydronephrosis. *Proc. roy. Soc. Med.*, **30**, 817.

Williams, D. Innes (1958). *Urology in Childhood* (*Handbuch der Urologie*, ed. C. E. Alken *et al.*, XV), p.26. Springer, Berlin.

*Arch. Dis. Childh.*, 1965, **40**, 207.

# LIPOMA OF THE CAUDA EQUINA*

BY

V. DUBOWITZ, J. LORBER, and R. B. ZACHARY

*From the Department of Child Health, University of Sheffield and the Children's Hospital, Sheffield*

Although intradural lipomas of the cauda equina with extradural extension have been recognized for over a century, their importance is not widely known. The subcutaneous swelling is easily mistaken for a meningocele and since there is normal skin cover and no neurological involvement in the early stages, a conservative approach is usually advised. It is not generally appreciated that the subcutaneous lipoma is in fact a mushroom-like structure with a stalk which passes intradurally and is firmly adherent to the cauda equina, the filum terminale, and the conus medullaris.

In due course most of these lipomas cause neurological symptoms. The onset of neurological involvement may be early or late. It may be sudden and severe, and for this reason we now recommend early exploration, even in the absence of any neurological abnormality.

## Review of the Literature

Johnson (1857a, b) gave the first accurate description of this condition. A subcutaneous swelling in the sacral region, first noted at 3 weeks, gradually increased in size, but the child was symptom-free until 9 months of age when he developed twitching and convulsive movements of the right leg. At operation a month later there was a subcutaneous fatty tumour the size of a small orange, with a stalk protruding through a small opening in the sacral canal. It was continuous above with the membranes of the spinal cord from which it was dissected free without opening the membranes. The child improved after operation, the abnormal movements of the leg disappeared, and he was able to stand and to take a few steps. Six weeks later he died of peritonitis. At necropsy a fatty mass was found within the dura extending upwards and pressing on the spinal cord and involving the roots of origin of the lowest spinal nerves, which seemed to be embedded in its substance. There was an associated malformation of the lower sacral vertebrae.

In spite of Johnson's very detailed description there have been surprisingly few reports in subsequent papers. Ingraham and Swan (1943) commented on the frequent association of an overgrowth of fatty tissue with spina bifida and meningeal defects, and noted that where a meningeal defect was present, the lipomatous tumour might extend intradurally for some distance and even cause intrinsic compression of the nerves or the cord. Ingraham and Lowrey (1943) reviewed 65 patients with spina bifida occulta in whom symptoms were present: 31 had abnormality of gait or other orthopaedic symptoms; 22 had a local abnormality of the lower spine, either a swelling or an overgrowth of hair or a scoliosis; 7 had incontinence of urine; and in the remaining 9 patients the presenting symptoms were unrelated and the spina bifida was an incidental finding. In 13 of these 65 there was an associated lipoma. They observed that the lipoma might be at any tissue level, from the cord itself to the subcutaneous tissue, and might extend directly from one layer to another, binding the various tissues together and preventing the normal movement of the cauda equina and the spinal cord with growth. In 5 patients they found a combined intradural and extradural lipoma.

Groff and Yaskin (1947) described a 12-year-old boy who had had a congenital lumbosacral meningomyelocele operated on at 3 years, without improvement in his urinary incontinence. A second operation at 12 years of age revealed a fatty tumour extending from the end of the spinal cord down the sacral canal, with the roots of the cauda equina firmly adherent to it. There was thought to be some improvement after operation, but the bladder still needed manual expression.

Bassett (1950) presented the first detailed study of lipoma of the cauda equina as an entity and stressed the importance of early diagnosis and operative treatment. He reviewed 9 patients, all female, including 2 sibs. One of his patients (Case 4), operated on at 2 months of age, remained symptom-free. Another (Case 8), also seen initially at 2 months of age without neurological deficit, had operation deferred; at 16 months there was gross

* A paper read in part at a meeting of the British Association of Paediatric Surgeons in Rotterdam, September 1964.

weakness of the legs and inability to stand, with sensory and sphincter loss. Operation at that stage did not result in any marked improvement in motor power or bladder control. Of the remaining patients, 3 appeared to show some improvement in their neurological signs post-operatively, one was symptom-free at operation and remained so, one deteriorated markedly before operation and died in the post-operative period, one showed no change, and in the remaining one there was no follow-up.

A number of subsequent case reports also illustrate the progressive nature of the condition, and the poor results of late operation. Rand and Rand's (1960) book on intraspinal tumours in childhood contains two typical examples. The first, a boy, had progressive weakness of the legs from the age of 1 year and loss of sphincter control at the age of 4 years. Operation at the age of 7 years was not followed by any neurological improvement. The second, a girl, with motor and sensory changes as well as loss of sphincter control, was not benefited by surgery at the age of 8 years. Another case of interest was a 9-week-old infant, who had a sacral swelling since birth and two associated dermal sinuses. An intradural lipoma attached to the conus medullaris was continuous with the upper dermal sinus. The roots of the cauda equina were not involved. The lipoma was resected and no neurological deficit developed after operation.

Recently, Swanson and Barnett (1962) reviewed 9 cases of intradural lipomas in childhood. Four of these conform to lipoma of the cauda equina. In one child (Case 3) there were no associated signs at the age of 8 weeks, but by 4 years she had motor and bladder involvement. Another (Case 7) presented with a lumbosacral meningocele at the age of 5 months; because of the absence of neurological abnormality no operation was recommended. At the age of 10 years she had motor and urinary involvement. At operation in both these patients there was an extradural lipoma with an intradural extension involving the cauda equina.

As might be expected with a congenital lesion, lipomas of the cauda equina are essentially a paediatric problem. An unexpected contrast, however, is the interesting case of Di Biagio (1959). A 61-year-old woman had a swelling in the lumbar region since birth. It was not until the age of 53 that she developed weakness and sensory loss in the left leg, which become progressively worse. Subsequently the right leg was also affected and there was associated loss of bladder control. The lumbar swelling began to enlarge. The tendon jerks were pathologically brisk and there was a bilateral Babinski response. At operation the subcutaneous lipoma had an intradural extension and was firmly bound up with the cauda equina. It was removed as far as possible. After operation there was a considerable improvement in her motor power, the sensory changes almost completely regressed, the abnormal tendon jerks became less brisk but the plantar response remained extensor.

### Clinical Data

Twelve personal cases with typical features of lipoma of the cauda equina form the basis of this report. All have had detailed pre-operative neurological assessment and at least three months' post-operative follow-up. Three additional cases have been omitted because of inadequate post-operative follow-up and several others are still awaiting operation.

The first patient (Case 1), who drew our attention to this condition in September 1962, was a child previously thought to have a straightforward meningocele. However, there was a recent history of deterioration of bladder function and on examination she had an extensor plantar response and anaesthesia in the sacral distribution. Lipoma of the cauda equina was suspected and confirmed at operation.

The main clinical features of this and the subsequent 11 patients are summarized in Tables 1 and 2, and detailed clinical histories of three patients (Cases 1, 3, and 5) are given in the Appendix.*

Eight patients were male and four were female. There were no affected sibs nor was there any previous family history of a similar condition or of hydrocephalus or meningocele.

A swelling was present at birth in each case. An associated dermal sinus or a deep dimple was noted in four and a skin tag in an additional one. No neurological abnormality was noted at birth in any of the patients, and none developed hydrocephalus.

**Onset of Symptoms.** In infants it is often difficult to assess the exact age of onset of symptoms such as loss of sphincter control or sensory changes.

The earliest onset was in Case 3, who was examined in detail at birth and found to be normal. At the age of 3 weeks he had gross weakness of one leg. In contrast, Case 5 was symptom-free until the age of 3 years. Two patients (Cases 8 and 11) were still symptom-free at the time of operation.

**Neurological Signs.** The commonest neurological complications were motor weakness (9 patients) and

* Clinical histories of the remaining 9 cases are available from the author.

TABLE 1

| Case No. | Sex | Age at Onset of Neurological Symptoms(yr.) | Age at Operation (yr.) | Duration of Follow-up (mth.) |
|---|---|---|---|---|
| 1 | F | 2½ | 3 | 19 |
| 2 | F | 2 | 2 yr. 1 mth. | 15 |
| 3 | M | 3 wk. | 5 wk. | 11 |
| 4 (Fig. 1) | F | 2½ | 9 yr. 10 mth. | 8 |
| 5 | F | 3½ | 3 yr. 7 mth. | 7 |
| 6 | F | 1 yr. 9 mth. | 11 yr. 9 mth. | 5 |
| 7 | M | 1 yr. 6 mth. | 5 yr. 8 mth. | 4 |
| 8 (Fig. 2) | M | ? | 2 yr. 3 mth. | 7 |
| 9 | F | 1 | 3 yr. 3 mth. | 5 |
| 10 | F | 3 mth. | 5 yr. 2 mth. | 3 |
| 11 | M | — | 2 yr. 10 mth. | 3 |
| 12 | F | 6 mth. | 3 yr. 7 mth. | 3 |

loss of bladder control (9 patients). The latter usually presented as dribbling incontinence, but 2 patients presented with retention with overflow and a number of others had excessive residual urine on catheterization. Difficulty with defaecation affected only 3 patients.

Sensory loss in the sacral distribution was observed in 8 patients. The tendon reflexes in the lower limbs were diminished in 7, and an abnormal plantar response, either extensor or absent, was noted in 8 children.

**Urinary Tract Infection.** There was evidence of infection in 8 patients and 4 of these had hydronephrosis on intravenous pyelography. The infection usually required prolonged antibiotic therapy for adequate control.

**Skeletal Abnormality.** Asymmetry of the sacrum or agenesis of some of the sacral vertebrae occurred in 6 patients. It could usually be detected on rectal examination and confirmed on radiography. In addition all the patients had a spina bifida of varying extent.

**Observations at Operation.** The subcutaneous lipoma varied in size and overlay the sacrum or lower lumbar region. In each case there was a deep stalk-like extension which passed intradurally through the gap of the spina bifida. It was continuous with the

TABLE 2
NEUROLOGICAL INVOLVEMENT

| Neurological Involvement | No. Affected | No. Improved by Operation | |
|---|---|---|---|
| | | Definite | Doubtful |
| Motor paralysis | 9 | 5 | 1 |
| Depressed tendon reflexes | 7 | 2 | |
| Abnormal plantar responses | 8 | 1 | |
| Sensory loss | 8 | | 1 |
| Loss of bladder control | 9 | 2 | 2 |
| Loss of rectal control | 3 | 1 | |

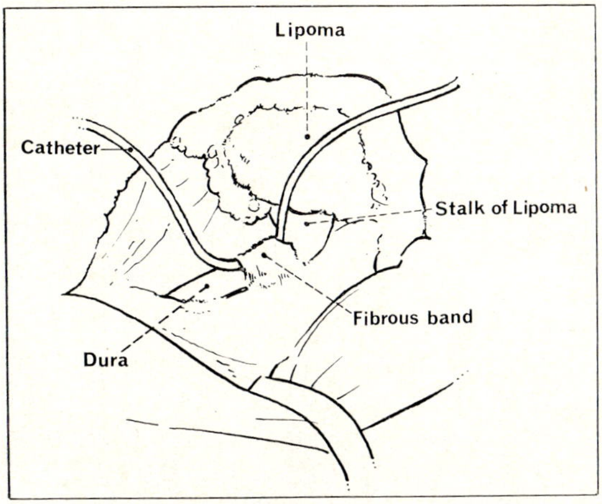


FIG. 1.—Case 4. Operative details. Child prone with head end to left. Shows lipoma attached to conus medullaris by stalk, which is angulated around a fibrous arch. A catheter has been passed under the arch. The dura is exposed after laminectomy.

conus medullaris and intimately connected with the nerves of the cauda equina. The lower end of the cord was never in its normal position but frequently as low as the first or second sacral vertebra. The roots of the cauda equina ran upwards from the conus medullaris and, after a variable course of up to 2 cm. or more, angled acutely downwards to their respective foramina.

At the upper limit of the spina bifida there was a firm fibrous or cartilaginous transverse arch around which the cord was acutely angulated. The liability to pressure on the cord at this site could be demon-

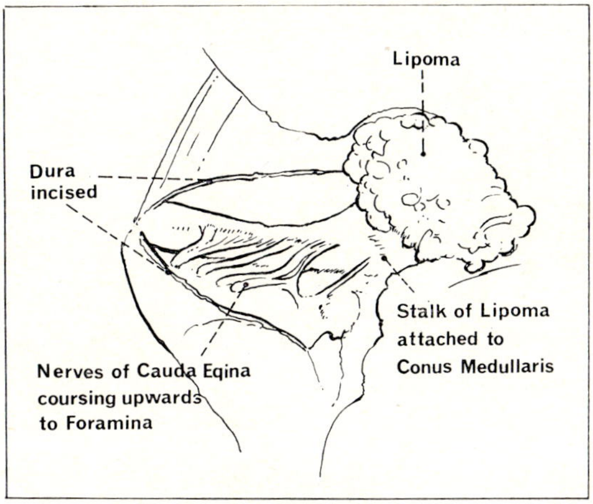


FIG. 2.—Case 8. Operative details. Child in prone position with head end to the left. Shows lipoma attached by stalk to conus medullaris. Cauda equina nerves run in an upward (cephalad) direction.

strated by traction on the lipoma. Complete resection of the lipoma was usually not practicable because of the danger of damage to the cauda equina, but a fairly extensive removal was usually achieved. In addition a laminectomy of two or three vertebrae above the spina bifida, and a vertical incision of the underlying dura were found to be essential to abolish the acute angulation of the cord and to allow it to retract up the spinal canal towards its normal position. After this the cauda equina roots had a more normal downward or transverse course.

**Post-operative Course.** During the first post-operative week a temporary deterioration in bladder control was frequently observed, but this invariably recovered within a few days. Apart from a tendency for the subcutaneous collection of CSF, which needed aspiration, there were no other post-operative complications.

*The follow-up* period is in many instances still relatively short for full appraisal of improvement or deterioration. However, an improvement in motor function has occurred in 5 patients and possibly also in a sixth. In one patient (Case 5), the response was dramatic and she regained the ability to walk within a week of operation and subsequently progressed to complete normality of motor function. It is also of interest that though Case 8 was thought to be neurologically normal, there was a definite improvement in motor function after operation. In retrospect, however, his early history does suggest some delay in motor milestones. Depressed tendon jerks became normal in two children, and an extensor plantar response reverted to flexor in Case 1.

Bladder function was improved in only two instances and a temporary improvement occurred in two others. One patient had improvement in rectal control after operation, while another (Case 2) showed deterioration which was very slow to resolve.

**Histology.** The lipoma consisted of normal adipose tissue, with additional connective tissue and frequently small nerve trunks. There was no sinus tract apparent in any of the specimens, and no teratomatous elements were found.

## Discussion

The dangers of this apparently benign lipoma are amply illustrated by the cases from the literature as well as the cases we have described. The chief condition from which one has to distinguish it is lumbar or sacral meningocele. A lipoma of the cauda equina should be suspected in any lumbo-sacral swelling with normal skin cover and no associated hydrocephalus.

In the majority of cases the onset of motor or sphincter disturbances is fairly gradual and insidious. It may, however, be quite sudden and dramatic, as in two of our patients. One child (Case 3), who was normal at birth, developed severe weakness of one leg at 3 weeks of age. The other (Case 5), a 3-year-old girl, lost the ability to walk in the course of 24 hours.

Once neurological involvement has occurred there is no guarantee that even immediate operation will give complete resolution. The dramatic recovery in Case 5 may well be exceptional. Certainly in Case 3 the improvement was slow and is still not complete. The outlook for bladder function seems worse than for motor function and only two patients have shown a long-term improvement.

The precise cause of the neurological disturbances is not easily determined. There are several possibilities.

(a) A traction lesion due to the cauda equina and the conus being densely adherent to the fat, which in turn is firmly fixed to lumbar or sacral skin.

(b) Compression of the cord, the conus, or the cauda equina by an extension of the lipoma within the canal.

(c) Pressure due to angulation of the terminal spinal cord around a cartilaginous or fibrous arch at the upper end of the spina bifida.

(d) A type of recurrent trauma due to the cord being dragged around this arch in movements of the trunk, comparable to traumatic ulnar neuritis.

Direct downward traction of the cord is, in our view, unlikely to be the only important factor; nor is the amount of lipoma within the canal sufficiently great in most cases to cause direct compression. Direct pressure or recurrent trauma due to movement of the cord at the site of angulation seems to us an important aetiological factor.

There are two important aspects of the operation; removal of the lipoma and laminectomy above the lesion. Of the two, the former is the more dangerous and possibly less important. As much lipoma as possible is removed without damage to the cord, the conus, or the cauda equina. A large part of the fatty tissue can be excised without risk, but the central portion is so closely intermingled with neural elements that complete removal is not possible.

In addition to this fatty tissue invading the lowermost neural elements, there is sometimes an upward extension of the lipoma within the canal around the cord, either outside or within the dura. This might be a factor causing compression and it can be removed without difficulty. In fact, the only part of the fatty tissue that is difficult to remove and particularly susceptible to damage is the deep central portion of the mass which is so densely bound to the lower part of the cord.

The purpose of removing two or three laminae is to release the cord from compression by the lowermost arch of fibrous tissue or cartilage at the upper end of the spina bifida, and to allow plenty of space for the cord to move upwards.

In each case the dura was incised the full length of the laminectomy, allowing the residual prominence of neural and lipomatous elements to lie at the top of the dural opening before closing the dura as far as possible around the remaining mass of tissue.

Clearly there is the possibility of damaging normally functioning nerve elements, and operation is not to be undertaken lightly. It would indeed be tragic to convert a normal child into one with some motor or sphincter weakness and it is certainly not much consolation to know that this paralysis might in due course have occurred spontaneously. Should the operation be deferred, however, the child must be examined at short intervals to detect the slightest neurological impairment. In addition, the parents must be given the strictest instructions to report any muscular weakness of the lower limbs, any tendency to trip or fall, any sign of abnormal gait, and any variation from normal bladder function.

We are convinced that in our hands it is wise to explore these lesions even before there are any signs of neurological involvement. In cases with established neurological abnormality the results of surgery may appear disappointing. However, it must be remembered that this is a progressive lesion. In these circumstances even an arrest of neurological deterioration would in itself justify operation.

We hope that the recognition of the potential dangers of leaving alone these apparently benign lesions will avert in others some of the tragic consequences that we have met in our own cases.

## Summary

Twelve cases of lipoma of the cauda equina are described with detailed neurological assessment and post-operative follow-up ranging from 3 to 19 months.

The benign-looking subcutaneous lipoma is readily mistaken for a lumbosacral meningocele with normal skin cover. However, the stalk-like intradural extension of the lipoma is firmly adherent to the cauda equina and conus medullaris, and neurological complications are common. These affect mainly motor and bladder function.

Early diagnosis is imperative and careful operative treatment before the onset of neurological signs may prevent the development of neurological complications. In cases with established neurological involvement, operation may in some instances produce improvement, while in others it may at least arrest the progression of the neurological deficit.

We wish to thank Mr. W. J. W. Sharrard and Mr. J. Lister for their help in the management of some patients; Dr. J. L. Emery for the pathological studies and Mr. A. T. Tunstill and Mr. A. S. Foster for the illustrations.

### References

Bassett, R. C. (1950). The neurologic deficit associated with lipomas of the cauda equina. *Ann. Surg.*, **131**, 109.

Di Biagio, F. (1959). Malformazioni rachidee multiple con lipoma della cauda. *Riv. Neurol.*, **29**. 401.

Groff, R. A., and Yaskin, J. C. (1947). Late occurrence of sphincter and other neurological disturbances associated with congenital malformations of the vertebral column. *Trans. Amer. neurol. Ass.*, **72**, 218.

Ingraham, F. D., and Lowrey, J. J. (1943). Spina bifida and cranium bifidum. III. Occult spinal disorders. *New Engl. J. Med.*, **228**, 745.

——, and Swan, H. (1943). Spina bifida and cranium bifidum. I. A survey of five hundred and forty-six cases. *ibid.*, **228**, 559.

Johnson, A. (1857a). Fatty tumour from the sacrum of a child, connected with the spinal membranes. *Trans. path. Soc. Lond.*, **8**, 16.

—— (1857b). Fatty tumour connected with the interior of the spinal canal of the sacrum. *ibid.*, **8**, 28.

Rand, R. W., and Rand, C. W. (1960). *Intraspinal Tumors of Childhood.* Thomas, Springfield, Illinois.

Swanson, H. S., and Barnett, J. C. (1962). Intradural lipomas in children *Pediatrics*, **29**, 911.

## Appendix

### Case Summaries

**Case 1.** Trudy T. (born October 24, 1959). A swelling in the lumbosacral region had been present since birth. At 6 weeks of age the swelling was about 12 cm. in diameter and there was no neurological abnormality or hydrocephalus. She was operated on at 9 months of age, and a large lipoma was found in association with a meningocele. About two-thirds of the lipoma was removed. The post-operative course was uneventful, and motor development progressed normally. She was walking and climbing stairs by 14 months.

She was referred to the Children's Hospital, Sheffield, in September 1962 aged 2 years 11 months, with a three months' history of deterioration of urinary control, which had previously been considered completely normal. She had become incontinent and lost bladder sensation. In addition the swelling over the sacrum had recurred and slowly increased.

Examination. There was a large lipomatous swelling in the sacral region, with an overlying scar. The urinary bladder was grossly distended. Her gait and motor power were normal, but the plantar response was extensor on both sides. Anaesthesia was present over the saddle area. The anal reflex was negative.

After manual expression of her bladder there was still 150 ml. of residual urine on catheterization. Cystoscopy revealed a large trabeculated bladder with wide ureteric orifices. Retrograde pyelography on the right side showed gross hydronephrosis and ureteric reflux. The left side was not catheterized.

On the basis of the sensory loss, the extensor plantar response and the deterioration in bladder function, a diagnosis of lipoma of the cauda equina was made.

Operation. October 29, 1962. A large lipomatous mass extended intradurally and was continuous with the conus medullaris. The subcutaneous part was adherent to the adjoining bone. The roots of the cauda equina were running in an upward direction before angling down towards their foramina. The lipoma was resected as far as possible.

Post-operative Course. Eighteen days after operation the child asked for her potty and passed urine spontaneously. She repeated this next day and four times in the course of the following 24 hours, and no manual expression was necessary. Following that she developed dribbling incontinence again and only used the potty intermittently. She was only able to pass about 50 to 100 ml. spontaneously, and a further 200 ml. could be expressed. By the time of her discharge (December 3) she only needed expression every four to five hours. She was kept on maintenance sulphadimidine therapy for her persistent urinary tract infection.

Follow-up. Her motor power remained normal, and the plantar response became flexor. However, there was no real improvement in her urinary control. She was again requiring two-hourly expression. The urinary infection persisted in spite of courses of various antibiotics. She was readmitted in March 1963 for bladder washouts and the urinary infection was again brought under control.

In July 1963, a Y-V plasty of the bladderneck was performed. This did not prove successful but resulted in continuous incontinence. In November 1963, the left ureter was joined to the right and a ureterostomy was performed. In March 1964 the urine was normal for the first time. Prophylactic sulphadimidine was again given. At her last visit in May 1964, 19 months after the spinal operation, she had not developed any further neurological abnormality and her urine was still free of infection.

Comment. A lipoma, present since birth, was partially removed at 9 months. Bladder symptoms appeared at 2½ years. Hydronephrosis was present, probably of longer duration than the symptoms suggest.

Resection of the lipoma led to only temporary improvement in bladder function and she subsequently needed ureterostomy.

**Case 3.** Michael P. (born August 1, 1963). A sacral swelling was noted at birth. A surgeon advised against operation because of the absence of neurological signs. At the age of 3 weeks his mother noted weakness of the left leg.

Examination. He was an active alert baby, with a subcutaneous lipomatous swelling over the sacrum (Fig. 3), approximately 7 cm. in diameter. There was a flaccid paralysis of the left leg with almost no active movement. The reflexes were asymmetrical. The withdrawal reflex was normal on the right but absent on the left. The knee-jerk was brisk on the right but absent on the left; the ankle-jerks were absent on both sides. The plantar response was extensor (normal) on the right, and absent on the left. The right leg appeared normal apart from intermittent spasm of the quadriceps and hip flexors, with associated increase in tone.

The tone in the anal sphincter was reduced and the anal reflex was negative. The bladder was not distended. He passed urine intermittently with a good stream, and there was no dribbling incontinence. It was difficult to assess his sensory function.

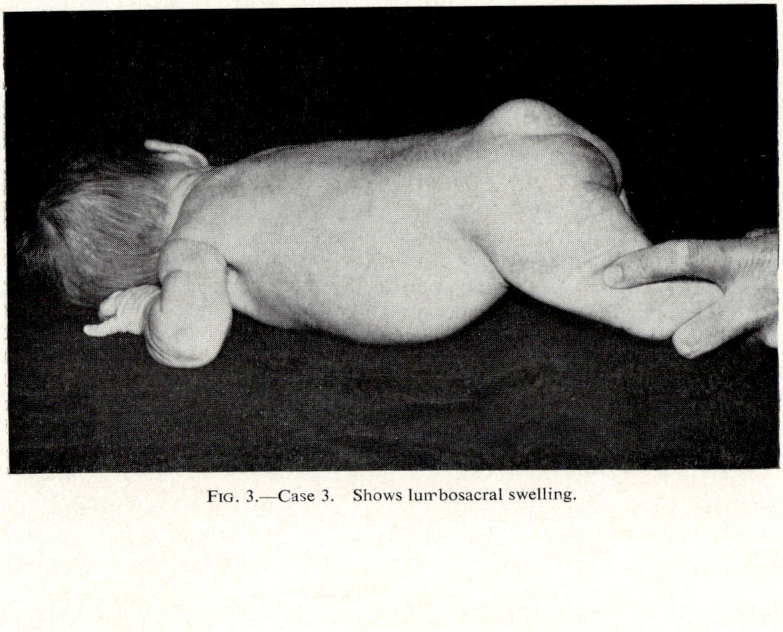

Fig. 3.—Case 3. Shows lumbosacral swelling.

Operation. September 4, 1963. The lipoma was continuous with the lower end of cord which was at the level of the second sacral vertebra. The cauda equina nerves ran upwards for about 2 cm. before angling down to their foramina. Laminectomy of L3 and L4 was performed and the lipoma dissected away as completely as possible. This allowed the cord to ride back up the canal.

Post-operative Course. When reassessed two months later there was a marked improvement in his left leg. He was able to move the leg as a whole and to bend the knee. The foot, however, was still completely paralysed. Abduction of the hips was limited beyond 60°. The withdrawal reflex on the left was present but still sluggish compared to the right. His general neurological development was normal.

Eleven months after operation there was further improvement in the power of his left leg, but he still had marked paralysis below the knee and an inversion deformity of the left foot. There was no weakness of the right leg and sphincter control appeared normal.

Comment. A sacral lipoma was present at birth with no neurological involvement. Severe paralysis of the left leg was present by the third week. An improvement in motor function followed operation.

**Case 5.** Mary P. (born April 21, 1960). A swelling over the sacrum was noted at birth, with no associated abnormalities.

She was first seen at the Children's Hospital aged 1 month. The sacral swelling, slightly to the left of the midline, was diagnosed as a meningocele. No weakness was noted in her legs. The anal sphincter had normal tone and the urinary stream was said to be good. There was no evidence of hydrocephalus. In view of the absence of any complication operation was not recommended.

Reassessment at 1, 2, and 3 years of age revealed no abnormality apart from some increase in the size of the swelling, and operation was deferred.

She continued well until October 1963, aged 3½, when she quite suddenly lost the ability to walk, though she was still able to stand. Apart from a slight limp the previous day, no abnormality had been noted. She was admitted to the Children's Hospital, Sheffield, three days later.

There appeared to have been some further deterioration and she could only just stand with support. It was difficult to assess individual muscles but there was a bilateral foot drop and also weakness of the hip extensors, and possibly other hip and knee muscles. There was no loss of sphincter control.

A diagnosis of lipoma of the cauda equina was made and urgent operation recommended.

Operation. November 6, 1963. A large subcutaneous lipoma (9 × 5 × 4 cm.) was found, with a stalk passing through a spina bifida defect of L5 and S1 vertebrae. A small meningocele was present in the depths of the lipoma. The lipoma passed through the meninges and was continuous with the lower end of the cord which was tethered down and reached practically to S1 level. The cauda equina nerves were passing upwards before turning acutely down again. After resection of the lipoma and a laminectomy of L4 vertebra, the cord could be freed and moved up at least 2 cm.

Post-Operative Progress. Neurological examination on the first post-operative day revealed spontaneous movements of both legs. She was able to flex the knees and hips, in response to painful stimulation of her soles. No sensory loss was apparent but the perineal region was difficult to assess. The knee-jerks were absent, the ankle-jerks present but sluggish, and the plantar response flexor.

A week after operation there was a striking improvement. She was able to walk around holding onto things and could also walk with one hand held. She was still unable to stand without support. The reflexes were unchanged. Sphincter control was normal. One week later she was walking well without support, and was discharged.

At follow-up assessment three months later there was further improvement. She walked well for up to 100 to 150 yards before tiring. There was slight inversion of the right foot but no obvious limp. She was able to go up steps and to climb on and off a bed. The knee-jerks were present and fairly brisk, the ankle-jerks were more active than before, and the plantar response still flexor. Sphincter control was completely normal.

Seven months after operation her gait was normal and she was able to run, to climb stairs, and to ride a tricycle. She could stand on one leg without support. The tendon jerks were normal and the plantar response flexor. There was no sensory loss and sphincter control was normal.

Comment. A child, unable to walk or to stand without support, returned to normal after operation.

*Arch. Dis. Childh.*, 1965, **40**, 214.

# RENAL VEIN THROMBOSIS IN INFANTS*

BY

ARIE D. VERHAGEN, JAMES P. HAMILTON, and MYRON GENEL

*From the Surgical Clinic of the Children's Hospital of Philadelphia, Bainbridge Street, Philadelphia 46, Pa, U.S.A.*

Renal vein thrombosis in children is an uncommon but not a rare condition that carries a grave prognosis unless recognized early and properly treated. Over 300 cases of various ages have been reported. About two-thirds of these occur in the paediatric age-group with a majority seen in the neonatal period. In young infants, renal vein thrombosis is often accompanied by haemorrhagic infarction of the involved kidney (Williams, 1958).

Renal vein thrombosis has been diagnosed in this clinic in 12 patients in the past six years. Half of the cases were unilateral and half bilateral; 10 of the 12 were under 3 months of age. Only one patient with unilateral thrombosis and one with bilateral involvement survived. In as much as these were the only patients surgically treated in each group it seemed worth while to record our experience in these two cases.

## Pathogenesis

Though the pathogenesis of renal vein thrombosis in infants is still obscure, severe gastro-intestinal symptoms are often noted as initial or accompanying symptoms; less frequently, the condition develops suddenly in a previously healthy infant. In older children, renal vein thrombosis may develop in a clinical history dominated by severe illness with toxaemia and sepsis. In the latter variety, the diagnosis is often made only at necropsy with the pathologist finding signs of incipient renal vein thrombosis which is attributed to marasmus. These two distinct clinical entities led Sandblom (1948) to separate a primary 'idiopathic' from the more common secondary variety.

From the time of its original description in an adult patient 125 years ago until 1932 when Grüneberg reported a nephrectomy for an infarcted kidney in a 3-month-old infant, renal vein thrombosis remained a post-mortem diagnosis. The successful outcome of this case resulted in an increased clinical interest in a condition previously considered to be hopeless. It soon became evident that the acute unilateral form of renal vein thrombosis lent itself to successful surgical management, and that early recognition was an important part of effective treatment (Campbell and Matthews, 1942). Several reports (Clatworthy, Dickens, and McClave, 1953; Kaplan, Straus, Grumbach, Dubois, Blondel, and Drapeau, 1958; Milburn, 1952; de la Torre, Villalpando, Esparza, and Olarte, 1958; Tveterås and Rudström, 1956) of children treated for renal vein thrombosis have been published, chiefly as scattered case reports. The youngest successful nephrectomy for unilateral renal vein thrombosis was in a 4-day-old infant (Miller and Benjamin, 1962).

## Case Reports

**Case 1.** A white male infant weighing 2,150 g. was born prematurely on August 17, 1959 to an 18-year-old toxaemic primipara. Urine passed on the first day was brick red in colour, and tetany-like tremors of the upper extremities were observed. General condition was considered only fair. A large, smooth globular mass was felt in the right upper quadrant. Serum electrolytes, including calcium, were normal. Blood urea nitrogen (BUN) was 45 mg./100 ml., a moderate leucocytosis existed and urinalysis showed haematuria. Blood culture was negative. Intravenous urogram showed a normal functioning left kidney but no visualization of the right. Pre-operative diagnosis was polycystic kidney.

At operation on August 24, the right kidney was three times normal size, and red-brown in colour as was the right adrenal. The left kidney was of normal size and consistency. The right kidney and adrenal were removed, the right renal vein being filled with a thrombus that involved the entire inferior vena cava below the renal vein. The suprarenal segment of the inferior vena cava was free of thrombosis and dilated. No attempt was made to remove the thrombus from the vena cava and no ligation of the vena cava was carried out.

After operation the child was treated with heparin. Histological sections revealed renal vein thrombosis and infarction of the right kidney and autolysis of the right adrenal. Except for a minor wound infection, the child made a satisfactory recovery with no oedema of the lower extremities, and no haematuria. BUN came down to 21 mg./100 ml. He left hospital on September 17, 1959,

* A paper read at a meeting of the British Association of Paediatric Surgeons in Rotterdam, September 1964.

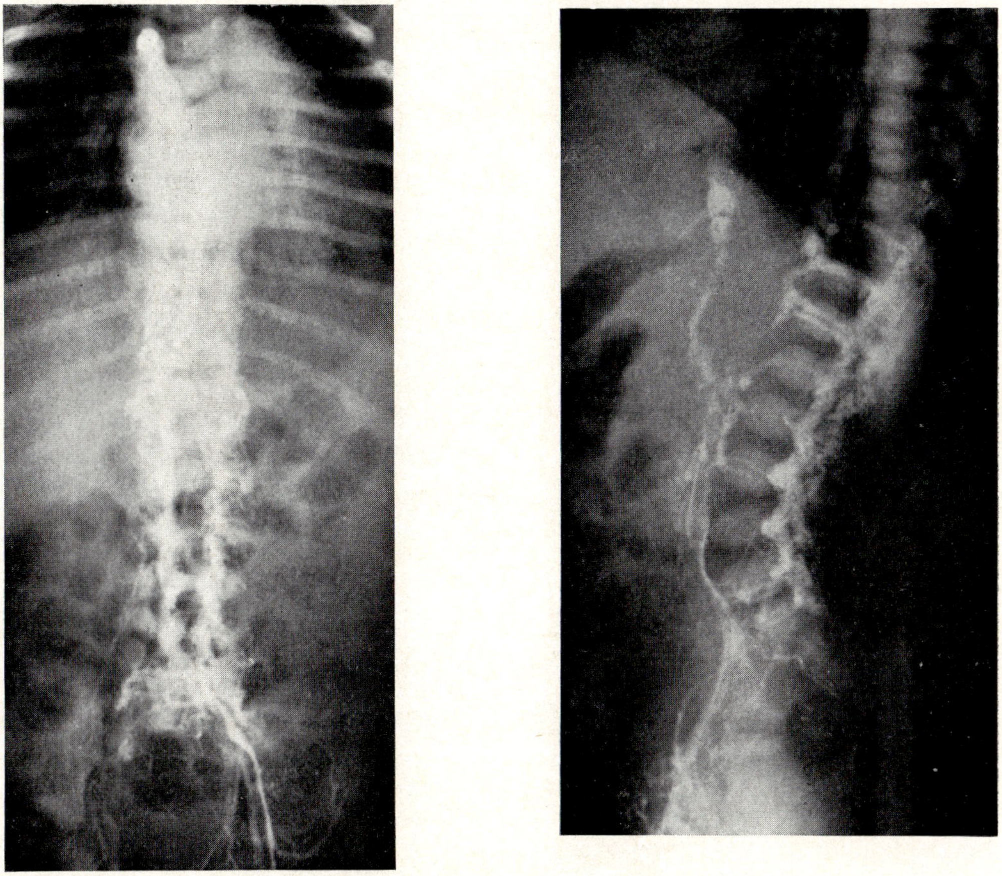

FIG. 1a and b.—Inferior vena cavagram revealing obliteration of IVC, with collateral flow through the azygos veins.

and a follow-up five years later showed a normal child without evidence of abnormal renal function.

**Case 2.** A 2-week-old negro male infant, born October 15, 1963, to a 17-year-old primipara of a full-term pregnancy, weighed 3,750 g. He refused feedings and then began to vomit and to have loose stools on the day before admission. Except for malnutrition and moderate dehydration he was alert and responsive. An abdominal mass was felt in the right upper quadrant and 'sclerema' of the legs was noted. Haematuria was present and electrolytes showed evidence of marked acidosis with a low serum calcium. Haemoglobin was 15·4 g./100 ml., platelets 24,000, leucocytes 23,100/c.mm. Anuria developed on the day of admission and the child had a convulsion.

On October 31 hydration was somewhat improved, but the 'sclerema' had extended to the trunk. Bilateral abdominal masses were now palpated. BUN was 160 mg./100 ml. The electrolyte imbalance was corrected, the fluid regimen was regulated for renal failure, and calcium and anticonvulsive therapy was started. On November 1 the abdominal masses seemed to be larger and until that time only a few ml. bloody urine had been produced. The diagnosis of bilateral renal vein thrombosis was made. An inferior vena cavagram was made via a saphenous vein (Fig. 1a and b), showing obliteration of the lower inferior vena cava with extensive collateral circulation connecting with the azygos system. Platelets rose to 64,000, BUN was still 150 mg./100 ml.

Operation was undertaken on November 1 with a tentative diagnosis of combined thrombosis of inferior vena cava and both renal veins. Both kidneys were found to be three to four times as large as normal, brown in colour, with diffuse haemorrhage and covered with dilated lymphatics that contained bloody lymph. The renal segment of the inferior vena cava was dilated and contained a thrombus that extended for 2 cm. proximally into the suprarenal segment of the vena cava and also for a short distance into both renal veins, occluding them both. The entire infrarenal segment of the inferior vena cava was irregularly narrowed and obviously obliterated with advanced thrombosis.

The inferior vena cava was transected 1 cm. distal to the take-off of the renal vein and the distal part was ligated. Through the proximal stump, thrombus material was removed both from the inferior vena cava and from the central part of the renal veins by extraction and saline irrigation until bleeding occurred. No heparin was used in view of the persistent thrombocytopenia. Histology showed beginning of organization of the thrombus. After operation a diuresis occurred and urine output returned gradually to normal as the haematuria disappeared. Continued low calcium levels required supplementary treatment and anticonvulsive therapy was continued. BUN came down to 17 mg./100 ml.

Intravenous urogram just before discharge showed kidneys of normal size with good function on both sides. The convulsions had subsided and calcium therapy was discontinued. Follow-up 9 months later showed, except for a low serum calcium, no other evidence of abnormal renal function. The BUN was 11 mg. Platelet count and urinalysis were also normal. There was no evidence of hypertension, but the child seemed developmentally slow.

## Discussion

Although one had unilateral and the other bilateral involvement, there is a striking similarity in the clinical picture of the two patients in the urinary symptoms, operative findings, and in the favourable outcome after surgery. On the basis of the clinical course both cases could probably be considered compatible with the primary type of renal vein thrombosis, according to Sandblom's classification.

Of the 8 infants who died, 6 were found to have a pre-existing congenital lesion, the importance of which may be questioned. They were noted to have toxoplasmosis, sickle cell disease, cyanotic heart disease, inclusion body disease, hydronephrotic kidney, and polycystic kidney. All these deaths occurred in patients with marked dehydration, shock, or sepsis without exhibiting obvious renal symptoms. In them the renal vein thrombosis was found only at necropsy and in the majority the diagnosis was based only on microscopic findings. Massive infarctions were not encountered in this group, and we are inclined to classify them in the second category of renal vein thrombosis in accordance with Sandblom's description.

In both surviving patients, the thrombosis also involved the lower segment of the inferior vena cava. This observation made in two living patients with renal vein thrombosis led us to consider angiography of the inferior vena cava as a promising method in the study of similar patients. As an addition to routine intravenous urography, inferior vena cava visualization can give valuable information, especially in patients presenting with renal tumours (Allen, Morse, Frye, and Clatworthy, 1964).

When both kidneys are involved in a thrombotic process, a fatal outcome is almost certain. According to Kaufmann (1958), in an analysis of the published reports, more than 45% of 91 childhood cases occurred bilaterally. Campbell (1951) also mentioned equal distribution in the incidence of unilateral and bilateral cases. Few reports of surgical cure of an adult patient with the proven diagnosis of bilateral renal vein thrombosis have appeared (Austen, 1961). Isolated reports claim recovery of bilateral renal vein thrombosis with conservative methods only, but in none of these was the diagnosis unequivocal (Fallon, 1949; Gaillard, Delphin, Cajfinger, and Brugiere, 1960; Michon, Aubertin, Jagerschmidt, and Valleteau de Moulliac, 1962).

Since the therapeutic effect of anticoagulants on established thrombosis is uncertain, we prefer to consider renal vein thrombosis in its acute stage as an urgent surgical problem. Though we prefer nephrectomy in strict unilateral renal vein thrombosis with a normal contralateral kidney, restoration of the renal venous return by removal of thrombus may also be effective. This is demonstrated in our second case in which we were forced to rely on this method because of bilateral involvement. Contrary to reports of cure with heparin alone (Fournier and Pauli, 1955; Gaillard *et al.*, 1960; Michon *et al.*, 1962), we are inclined to consider anticoagulant treatment mainly complementary to nephrectomy or thrombectomy. In situations where surgical intervention might be contraindicated, heparin therapy should be used. Reports suggesting renal vein thrombosis as the underlying cause of hypertension (Perry and Taylor, 1940; Schönenberg and Staemmler, 1960) or the nephrotic syndrome (Feinerman, Burke, and Bahn, 1957; Torres, 1962) in some patients seem to underline our views on the management of patients with renal vein thrombosis.

## Summary

Two cases of renal vein thrombosis, one unilateral and one bilateral, are reported. Both patients survived following operation. The importance of early diagnosis, the use of the vena cavagram as a pre-operative study, and the rationale of treatment are discussed.

### References

Allen, J. E., Morse, T. S., Frye, T. R., and Clatworthy, H. W. (1964). Vena cavagrams in infants and children. *Trans. Amer. Surg. Ass.*, **82**, 236.

Austen, F. K., ed. (1961). Cases from the medical grand rounds. Inferior vena cava thrombosis with renal vein occlusion. Mass. Gen. Hosp. case 496. *Amer. Practit.*, **12**, 370.

Campbell, M. (1951). *Clinical Pediatric Urology*, p. 443. Saunders, Philadelphia.

Campbell, M. F., and Matthews, W. F. (1942). Renal thrombosis in infancy. *J. Pediat.*, **20**, 604.

Clatworthy, H. W., Jr., Dickens, D. R., and McClave, C. R. (1953). Renal thrombosis complicating epidemic diarrhea of the newborn. *New Engl. J. Med.*, **248**, 628.

Fallon, M. L. (1949). Renal venous thrombosis in the newborn. *Arch. Dis. Childh.*, **24**, 125.

Feinerman, B., Burke, E. C., and Bahn, R. C. (1957). The nephrotic syndrome associated with renal vein thrombosis. *J. Pediat.*, **51**, 385.

Fournier, A., and Pauli, A. (1955). Les infarctus rénaux par thrombose des veines rénales chez le nouveau-né et le nourisson. *Nourrisson* **43**, 229.

Gaillard, L., Delphin, D., Cajfinger, M., and Brugiere, P. (1960). Thrombose bilatérale primitive probable des veines rénales chez un nouveau-né. *Pédiatrie*, **15**, 910.

Grüneberg, B., Sr. (1932). Nierenvenenthrombose linkerseits. *Münch. med. Wschr.*, **79**, 1054.

Kaplan, M., Straus, P., Grumbach, R., Dubois, F., Blondel, C., and Drapeau, P. (1958). Infarctus rénal unilatéral primitif chez un nouveau-né. *Arch. franç. Pédiat.*, **15**, 1238.

Kaufmann, H. J. (1958). Renal vein thrombosis. *Amer. J. Dis. Child.*, **95**, 377.

Michon, L., Aubertin, D., Jagerschmidt, G., and Valleteau de Moulliac, G. (1962). Deux cas de thromboses primitives de la veine rénale du nouveau-né. *Sem. thér.*, **38**, 401.

Milburn, C. L., Jr. (1952). Hemorrhagic infarction of the kidneys in infants. *J. Pediat.*, **41**, 133.

Miller, H. C., and Benjamin, J. A. (1962). Acute idiopathic renal vein thrombosis in infants. *Pediatrics*, **30**, 247.

Perry, C. B., and Taylor, A. L. (1940). Hypertension following thrombosis of the renal veins. *J. Path. Bact.*, **51**, 369.

Sandblom, P. (1948). Renal thrombosis with infarction in the newborn. *Acta Paediat.* (*Uppsala*), **35**, 160.

Schönenberg, H., and Staemmler, M. (1960). Maligne Hypertonie infolge einseitiger Nierenvenenthrombose beim Kleinkind. *Z. Kinderheilk.*, **83**, 259.

de la Torre, J. A. Villalpando, E., Esparza, H., and Olarte, J. (1958). Unilateral renal vein thrombosis in an infant with sepsis due to salmonella choleraesuis: nephrectomy with recovery. *J. Pediat.*, **52**, 206.

Torres, E. R. (1962). Nephrotic syndrome in an infant secondary to renal vein thrombosis. *Harper Hosp. Bull.*, **20**, 172.

Tveterås, E., and Rudström, P. (1956). Renal thrombosis in the newborn. *Acta Paediat.* (*Uppsala*), **45**, 545.

Williams, D. L. (1958). *Urology in Childhood*, (Handbuch der Urologie, ed. C. E. Alken *et al.*, XV), p. 230. Springer, Berlin.

*Arch. Dis. Childh.*, 1965, **40**, 218.

# CERVICO-AURICULAR FISTULAE

## A REVIEW OF PUBLISHED CASES WITH A REPORT

BY

J. C. R. LINCOLN*

*From the Department of Surgery, Hammersmith Hospital, Postgraduate Medical School of London*

(RECEIVED FOR PUBLICATION JUNE 4, 1964)

Congenital anomalies of the first branchial cleft are rare. Approximately 32 cases of cervico-auricular fistulae have been reported in the past hundred years: this includes the writer's own case in this review. The majority of sinuses and fistulae derived from the lateral cervical vestiges are concerned with the second pharyngeal pouch and its corresponding cleft.

Auricular and pre-auricular fistulae are not excessively rare, but cervico-auricular fistulae are still infrequently recorded. In some cases reported as cervico-auricular fistulae, there is little doubt from the description that these are auricular or pre-auricular fistulae.

Harding (1890) and König (1896) both recorded cases, but it was not until 1908 that Flint published a well-documented case report on this condition. Frazer (1923) postulated defects of closure of the first branchial cleft, though up to that time he thought that none had been reported. He stated that, 'If a cyst of such a vestige were present it would lie below the tube, behind (at any rate in part) the tensor palati and in front of the carotid and stylopharyngeus and if by any chance it opened in to the pharynx it would do so through the sinus of Morgagni.'

In the following review only those cases that are well documented have been considered.

### Embryology

The branchial apparatus appears as but a transient stage in the development of the human embryo, appearing between the 3 mm. and 14 mm. stage. The embryology of these cases is concerned with the branchial or lateral cervical vestiges.

At the fifth week, when the human embryo is about 5 mm. in length, five ridges are visible on the outer surface in the region of the primitive pharynx (Fig. 1a). The walls of the pharynx are lined by five bars or arches with four intervening clefts, the internal clefts being lined by foregut endoderm and the external clefts by ectoderm, but divided by a thin layer of mesoderm. Though there is confusion in the nomenclature, the general consensus of opinion names the pharyngeal clefts *pharyngeal pouches*, and the corresponding external clefts *branchial clefts*. Each arch has a central core of cartilage, a main blood vessel, and nerve.

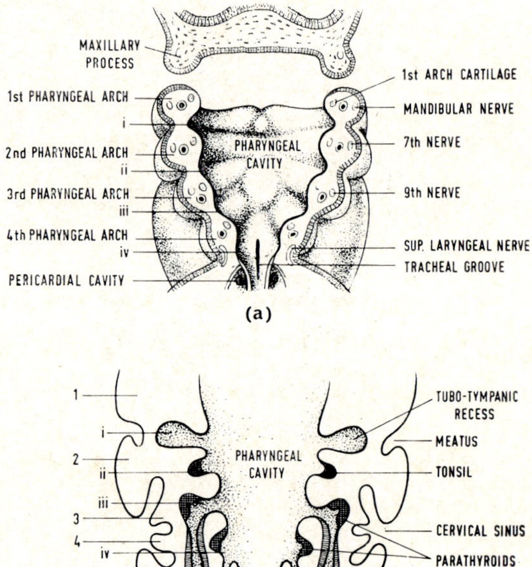


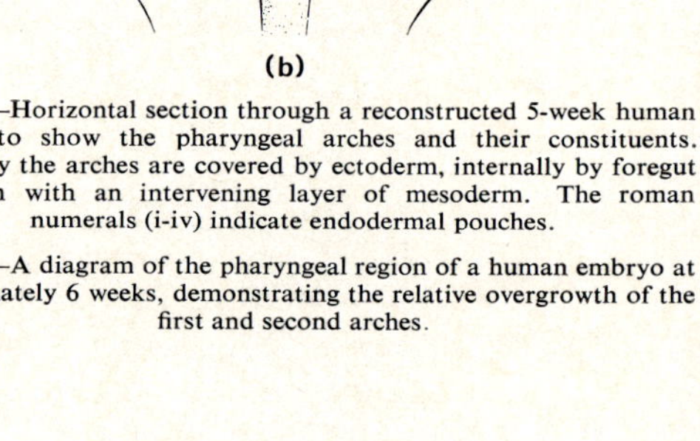


FIG. 1a.—Horizontal section through a reconstructed 5-week human embryo to show the pharyngeal arches and their constituents. Externally the arches are covered by ectoderm, internally by foregut endoderm with an intervening layer of mesoderm. The roman numerals (i-iv) indicate endodermal pouches.

FIG. 1b.—A diagram of the pharyngeal region of a human embryo at approximately 6 weeks, demonstrating the relative overgrowth of the first and second arches.

* Present address: Surgical Unit, University College Hospital Medical School, London W.C.1.

The muscular derivatives of each arch are supplied by the nerve of that arch. The nerve of the first arch is the mandibular division of the trigeminal nerve and supplies the muscles of mastication, the tensor palati, the tensor tympani, the mylohyoid, and the anterior belly of the digastric. The muscles of the second arch are supplied by the facial nerve, these muscles being those concerned with facial expression, the posterior belly of the digastric, the stapedius, and the stylohyoid. The third arch muscles make up part of the soft palate and the stylopharyngeus muscle, the nerve of supply being the glossopharyngeal. The constrictors of the pharynx and part of the soft palate are derived from the fourth arch and the nerve is the superior laryngeal. The fifth arch nerve, which is the recurrent laryngeal, supplies the intrinsic muscles of the larynx.

The vascular derivatives of each arch are modified, and there is a reduction in the number of arch vessels to facilitate pulmonary respiration and suit the new conditions of life. The original arteries of the first and second arches persist as the mandibular and stapedial arteries. The third arch arteries remain; the right third arch artery contributes to the development of the right common carotid artery and the commencement of the right internal carotid artery. The left third arch artery forms the left common carotid artery and distally the proximal part of the left internal carotid artery. The right fourth arch artery becomes the right subclavian artery and part of the arch of the aorta, and the left fourth arch artery forms the arch of the definitive aorta. The fifth arch arteries are present for only a short time and the sixth arch arteries persist as the pulmonary arteries.

The cartilaginous part of the first arch gives rise to the malleus, incus, the spleno-mandibular ligament, and the central core of the body of the mandible. The second arch cartilage forms the stapes, the lesser cornu of the hyoid bone, the styloid process, the stylohyoid ligament persisting as the intervening portion. The greater cornu and the lower part of the body of the hyoid bone is formed from third arch cartilage, and the cartilage of the fourth and fifth arches make up the skeleton of the larynx.

The glandular derivatives of the pharyngeal arches form parathyroid and thymic tissue, and the palatine tonsils. The palatine tonsils develop from the endodermal elements of the second pouch. The thymus, together with the inferior parathyroid gland, is developed from the third pouch, the parathyroid gland in this case being drawn caudally by the thymic rudiment. The superior parathyroid gland is derived from the fourth pouch.

The external ear is developed from a series of six tubercles which develop on the first and second arches on the dorsal end of the first groove which lies between. By growth and fusion, the tubercles and the immediately surrounding area give rise to the primitive pinna. This is situated around the end of the developing external auditory meatus. The tragus and its immediate area is derived from the first arch, and the greater contribution to the formation of the pinna comes from the second arch (Wood-Jones and I-Chuan, 1934; Streeter, 1922). The external auditory meatus is formed from two elements: the dorsal end of the first groove and an ingrowth of epithelium from this groove, the ventral end becoming flattened then disappearing. The endodermal derivatives of the first pouch are concerned with the epithelium of the internal part of the tympanic membrane, the tympanic cavity, mastoid air cells, the eustachian tube, and epithelium of much of the mouth and body of the tongue.

By the end of the sixth week, the growth of the first and second arches has exceeded that of the third and fourth and a sinus is formed, the pre-cervical sinus of His (Fig. 1b). The third arch still contributes in part to the skin over the anterior triangle of the neck; the fourth arch is completely overgrown. Two deep recesses are formed, and these are the cervical vesicles: meanwhile, the first pouch fills up ventrally to become part of the tongue, and the dorsal end, together with the dorsal end of the second pouch, forms the tubo-tympanic recess, this recess forming the eustachian tube and the middle ear; the mesodermic membrane forms the tympanic membrane.

Ectodermal remains may persist from the ventral part of the first groove, from any part of the second groove, and from the cervical vesicles. Endodermal remains may persist as cysts or sinuses and accessory glands.

The following anomalies of the branchial apparatus are recorded: branchial cysts, external sinuses, internal sinuses, complete pharyngo-cutaneous fistulae, cervico-aural fistulae, branchial cartilages, and cervical auricles.

### Case Report

A girl aged 2 years was admitted with a tender swelling in the left submandibular region. This had been present for three days and the child had been pyrexial. Since birth there had always been a 'dimple' in the region of the swelling.

Physical examination revealed a tender cystic swelling approximately 5 × 2 cm. in the left submandibular region anterior to the sternocleidomastoid muscle, at the junction of the upper and middle third. No other abnormality was noted. Radiographs of the chest and mandible were normal. The swelling was incised and brownish pultaceous material was evacuated. This was sterile on culture.

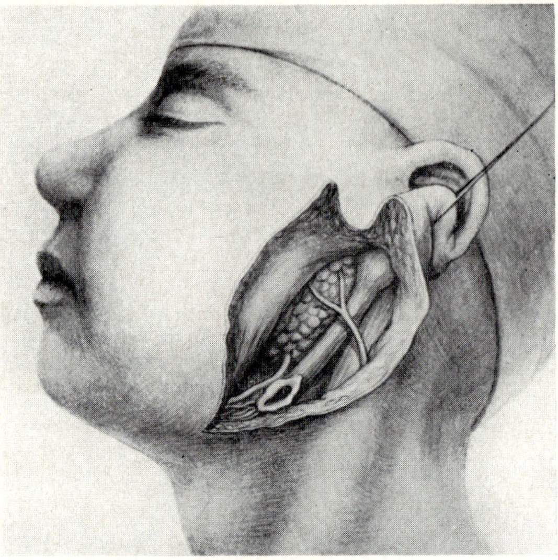

FIG. 2.—Artist's impression of operative area.

In the ensuing three months there was a continuous discharge from the site of the incision and for the first time it was noted that the left external auditory meatus was moist with a 'mucus like' discharge. No opening was seen in the external ear and the tympanic membrane was normal.

The child was readmitted for curettage of the sinus, and histopathological examination of the curettings demonstrated brownish granulation tissue, heavily infiltrated with polymorph plasma cells, lymphocytes, and macrophages, and one or two foreign body giant cells. There was no evidence of acid-alcohol fast bacilli, mycelia, or other specific aetiology. Amylase content of the exudate was 250 Somogyi units; this low level suggested tissue fluid or plasma rather than salivary gland excretion. A sinogram using 45% Hypaque demonstrated a small cavity below the left angle of the mandible. There was no evidence of deep extension.

It was decided to explore the sinus and dissect out the tract. Methylene blue, when injected into the sinus in the neck, emerged from a small pit in the floor of the external auditory meatus about 1 cm. from the external surface of the ear.

An elipse of skin was excised around the sinus opening in the plane of Langers lines, and two tracts were seen, one running posteriorly up to the region of the external ear and the other running anteriorly beneath the mandible. The incision was then extended similar to that used in parotid gland surgery. The posterior tract was dissected out and appeared to be cylindrical, 5 mm. in diameter and with a fibro-muscular wall. This tract admitted a silver wire probe 1 mm. in diameter. The tract passed deep to the inferior part of the parotid gland and the greater auricular nerve, posterior to the mandibular division of the facial nerve but superficial to the posterior belly of the digastric muscle. The main trunk of the facial nerve was not seen. The tract ended in a vestibule 1·0 cm. in diameter, lined by epithelium with hairs clearly visible and surrounded by its own wall of cartilage, the cartilage being continuous with that of the external ear.

The anterior 'tract' was 2 cm. long and fanned out in the sub-mandibular region as a series of tails that ran superficial to the sub-mandibular structures. There was some doubt as to the nature of this 'tract' and its extensions, as it was thought that it might be a branch of the facial nerve. Faradic stimulation of these structures provoked no response: the mandibular division of the facial nerve was positively identified using this technique (Fig. 2).

The two tracts and the vestibule were excised. After operation there was slight weakness of the corner of the mouth but this quickly resolved.

**Histopathology.** The specimen consisted of a 5 cm. fistula of varying diameter. Blocks were taken through the entire length, and over a length of 1·5 cm. at the cephalic end, serial sections were cut and every tenth section was examined.

The superior or cephalic end, 1 cm. long, was the widest portion of the tract, forming an ampulla 1 cm. in diameter. Here a ring of cartilage was included in the anterior three-quarters of the wall, the posterior wall consisting of fibrous tissue only. The ring of cartilage was partly continuous and partly formed by discrete curved plates. The cartilage consisted of mature hyaline cartilage, the central rounded cells becoming flattened peripherally and showing transition to the cells of the perichondrium. The cartilage stopped abruptly at the lower end of the ampulla.

The lumen of the fistula was 5 mm. in diameter in the ampullary region and 2-3 mm. elsewhere. The wall was lined by stratified squamous epithelium showing numerous pilo-sebaceous follicles and islands of cartilage; many short fair hairs projected into the ampullary lumen. The characteristic four layers of normal epidermis were present in the lining. A few melanoblasts were scattered through the basal layer and a moderate number of apocrine sweat glands were present in the deeper dermis (Fig. 3).

About the middle of the tract, the epithelium was partially replaced by granulation tissue and a moderate inflammatory infiltrate was present in the adjacent dermis. The ampullary region was free of inflammation.

Bundles of voluntary muscle formed the cords tethering the inferior end of the fistula to the submental tissues.

## Discussion

In reviewing the published case reports of cervico-aural fistulae, the ages ranged from 8 months to 45 years. There were 23 female and 9 male cases; in 14 it occurred on the left and in 18 on the right side of the head and neck.

In the 32 cases, the presenting signs and symptoms were as follows: 11 had a cystic swelling, either quiescent or inflamed below the angle of the jaw and concomitant with a chronic discharge from the

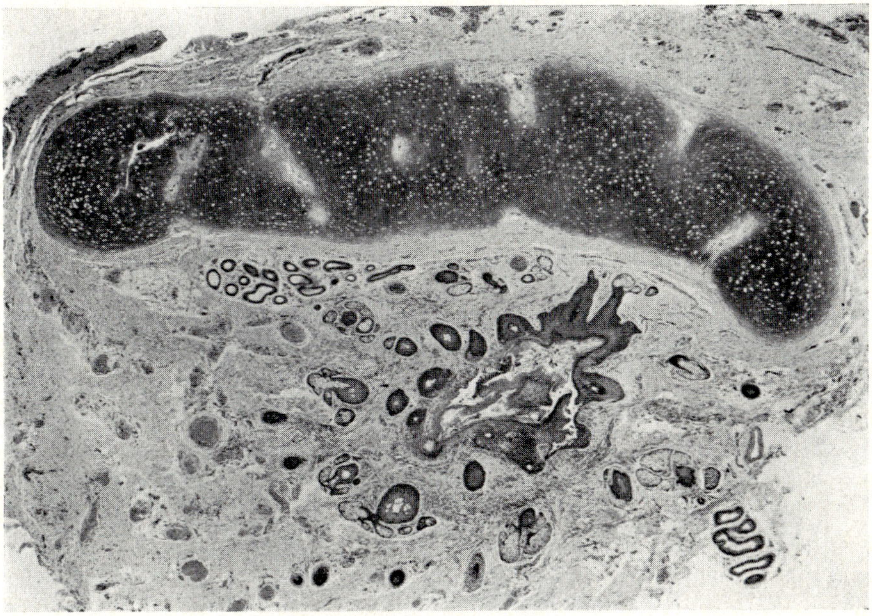

FIG. 3.—Photomicrograph of transverse section of middle of fistula. (H. and E. × 25.)

external ear; 10 presented with a cystic swelling in the same site; and 11 presented as a chronic draining sinus below the angle of the jaw, chronic ear discharge being present in 7, and no ear discharge evident in 4.

**Topography.** In the majority of cases the site of the lower end of the fistulae was in an area inferior to the angle of the mandible and anterior to the upper and middle third of the sternocleidomastoid muscle. The tracts ran cephalad, inclining dorsally to the external ear and in all cases running superficial to the posterior belly of the digastric muscle. The anatomical relation to the parotid gland varied, in 2 cases running deep (Caldera, 1922; De Bord, 1960 and own case), in 3 within (Aimi and Takino, 1962; De Bord, 1960; Lallemant and Poncet, 1961), and in 4 superficial to the gland (Gore and Masson, 1959; Ladd and Gross, 1937; Pagano, 1955; Stark, 1959). The opening of the tract in the external ear varied from deep in the fundus of the external ear, to superficial between the tragus and antetragus. In 4 cases, though the tract was attached to the external ear cartilage, there was no opening of communication.

**Facial Nerve.** It is well established that nerves grow to muscles and follow their subsequent migrations, but why a particular nerve filament reaches the muscle of supply is still uncertain. Once established, this connexion between nerve and myotome is permanent.

The position of the facial nerve in relation to the tract varies. In some cases the nerve is reported as being deep and in other cases superficial to the tract. Exploration and positive identification of the nerve were considered unwarranted in certain cases and the exact anatomical position was not recorded.

In one case the tract was medial to the zygomatic and mandibular branches of the nerve (De Bord, 1960). Following paresis of the facial muscles in another case, the facial nerve was explored from the stylomastoid foramen to the partoid gland; it was found that the nerve had been displaced by the cartilaginous bulb, posteriorly and inferiorly; it had then passed along the anterior surface of the mastoid process of the temporal bone, then forward and superficial to the cartilaginous bulb before entering the gland (Rankow and Hanford, 1953)

The nerve is that of the second arch, but terminates in part of the area derived from the first arch and, as the muscles of facial expression spread out to cover part of the first arch territory, one might expect to find the nerve superficial as it passes forward to reach the facial muscles. Conversely, if there is overgrowth of the first and second arches over the third and fourth, then the nerve should lie deep to the tract.

When the nerve passes superficial, the tract must be running fairly deep and the possibility arises of involvement of the endodermal pouch. If this is so, the tract should not communicate with the external ear.

In the 15 patients in whom the facial nerve was positively identified, 8 had the nerve running superficial and 7 had the nerve running deep to the tract.

The time of onset of the anomaly in relation to the change in character of the lateral surface of the foetal pharynx may well be an important factor in determining the final course of the seventh nerve. When interference with the normal process of growth in the region of the branchial cleft is early, then the tract may well be deep to the nerve and maintain this position; conversely, if the time of interference is late the nerve could be deep to the tract.

**Radiology.** Investigation of these anomalies by radiological methods proved unreliable. Use of radio-opaque media demonstrated the tract fully in only 4 cases (Lyall and Stahl, 1956; Oppikofer, 1946; Pagano, 1955; Stark, 1959). In 2 (Aimi and Takino, 1962 and our case), a localized cystic space was demonstrated, there being no evidence of extension, and in one (De Bord, 1960) a tract running deep to the parotid gland was noted.

**Operative Technique.** Nearly all the tracts were excised through an incision similar to that used in parotid gland surgery. 'Step ladder' incisions in Langers lines were occasionally used.

A useful adjunct to the operative technique was the use of methylene blue, which was injected into the lower end of the fistula either as a 0·5% solution, or as a mixture of hydrogen peroxide and methylene blue 5 : 1.

Faradic stimulation was used to identify the facial nerve in 2 cases.

**Histopathology.** Macroscopic examination of the tracts showed some as thin threads of tissue and others as cylindrical fibro-muscular structures, up to 5 mm. in diameter and 9 cm. in length. At the upper end of some of the tracts, cartilaginous structures were seen. These were noted in 4 cases as partly semicircular vestibules (Alvarez and Jacobson, 1961; Flint, 1908; Rankow and Hanford, 1953, own case), and in one as a well-developed cartilaginous sheath 4 cm. long and up to half the length of the tract: all were proximal to but communicating with the auricular cartilage.

Microscopic examination of the tracts showed stratified squamous epithelium lining the inner surface with the characteristic four layers of the epidermis present in the lining. Sweat glands, hair follicles, and focal lymphocytic infiltration were also present. The cartilage consisted of mature hyaline cartilage.

**Embryology.** The fate of the branchial clefts in the human embryo is still extremely vague. Growth is so complex that the anomalies must be even more complex.

It is reasonable to suggest that a cervico-auricular fistula represents part of the ectoderm of the first cleft which has been pulled dorsally as the ear migrates backwards; this ectoderm may be manifest as a solid tract, or hollow tube, the first ectodermal cleft not having been closed. Necrosis plays an essential part in the development of the human embryo and the fistula may be a result of a breakdown in a solid ectodermal tract. This may be due to a poor blood supply. The term 'failure of closure' of the first ectodermal cleft is misleading, because this presupposes that there is a gap between the first and second; this is not so.

The presence of a cartilaginous bulb or sheath in 4 cases may be explained as part of a misplaced auricular tubercle, or as part of some inductive action of the ectodermal tract on the surrounding mesenchyme.

Until further evidence is available concerning the fate of the external clefts in the human embryo, it is convenient to define a cervico-auricular fistula as a fistula derived from a persistence of part of the first ectodermal cleft, the skin roofing in the middle portion of the tract.

## Summary

A series of 31 reported examples of cervico-auricular fistulae have been collected and one further case added.

The diagnosis is made more certain by noting two physical signs, namely a chronic discharging sinus in the neck and a discharge from the external ear when other aural pathology has been excluded. There is little doubt that this anomaly is more common than previously realized, and that cases are missed.

Radiological investigation may well prove more satisfactory if a less viscous radio-opaque solution is used.

At operation the facial nerve may lie superficial or deep to the tract. The exposure of the main trunk of the facial nerve is unwarranted if it is not readily visualized. There has been a low incidence of paresis of the facial muscles.

I wish to thank Mr. Selwyn Taylor, under whose care the patient was admitted; Mr. David Hogg, Surgical

Registrar whom I assisted at the operation; and Dr. Anita Herdan of the Department of Pathology.

I would also like to thank Miss Olive Higdon for secretarial services, Mr. Brackenbury of the Photographic Department, and Mr. David Banks, Medical Artist.

BIBLIOGRAPHY

Aimi, K., and Takino, K. (1962). Anomaly of the first branchial cleft. Report of a case. *Arch. Otolaryng.*, **75**, 397.

Alvarez, E., and Jacobson, J. S. (1961). Anomalias del primo seno branquial: caso ilustrativo. *Med. esp.*, **46**, 33.

Bill, A. H., Jr. (1959). Cysts and sinuses of neck of thyroglossal and branchial origin. *Surg. Clin. N. Amer.*, **39**, 1599.

——, and Vadheim, J. L. (1955). Cysts, sinuses and fistulae of the neck arising from 1st and 2nd branchial clefts. *Ann. Surg.*, **142**, 904.

Byars, L. T., and Anderson, R. (1951). Anomalies of the first branchial cleft. *Surg. Gynec. Obstet.*, **93**, 755.

Caldera, C. (1922). Nuova varieta di fistula anris congenita e contemporaneo sdoppiamento del condotto uditivo esterno. *Arch. ital. Otol.*, **33**, 55.

De Bord, R. A. (1960). First branchial cleft sinus. *Arch. Surg.*, **81**, 228.

Flint, C. P. (1908). Sinus of first branchial cleft. *Ann. Surg.*, **48**, 165.

Frazer, J. E. (1923). The nomenclature of diseased states caused by certain vestigial structures in the neck. *Brit. J. Surg.*, **11**, 131.

—— (1953). *Manual of Embryology*, 3rd ed. by J. S. Baxter. Baillière, Tindall and Cox, London.

Gore, D., and Masson, A. (1959). Anomaly of first branchial cleft. *Ann. Surg.*, **150**, 309.

Hamilton, W. J., Boyd, J. D., and Mossman, H. W. (1962). *Human Embryology. (Pre Natal Development of Form and Function,)* 3rd ed. W. Heffer, Cambridge.

Harding, W. (1890). Ein Beitrag zur Kenntniss der congenitalen Halsfisteln. Dissertation, Fiencke, Kiel.

Keith, A. (1948). *Human Embryology and Morphology*, 6th ed. Edward Arnold, London.

König, F. (1896). Ueber Fistula colli congenita. *Langenbecks Arch. klin. Chir.*, **51**, 578.

Ladd, W. E., and Gross, R. E. (1937). Congenital branchiogenic anomalies. *Amer. J. Surg.*, **39**, 766.

Lallemant, Y., and Poncet, E. (1961). Fistule latérale congénitale du cou (Un cas de fistule auriculo-branchiale.) *Ann. Oto-laryng. (Paris)*, **78**, 623.

Lyall, D., and Stahl, W. M., Jr. (1956). Lateral cervical cysts, sinuses, and fistulas of congenital origin. *Int. Abstr. Surg.*, **102**, 417.

Oppikofer, E. K. (1946). Hals-Ohrfistel (Fistula collo-auralis congenita) und Trommelfellmissbildung. *Pract. oto-rhino-laryng. (Basel)*, **8**, 515.

Pagano, A. (1955). Fistola congenita laterale del collo comunicanta con il condotto auditivo esterno. *Arch ital. laryng.*, **63**, 193.

Randall, P., and Royster, H. P. (1963). First branchial cleft anomalies. *Plast. reconstr. Surg.*, **31**, 497.

Rankow, R. M., and Hanford, J. M. (1953). Congenital anomalies of the first branchial cleft. *Surg. Gynec. Obstet.*, **96**, 102.

Seebohm, I. D. (1938). Uber einen seltenen Fall einer Fistula auris et colli congenita. Dissertation, Reichenberg, Berlin.

Stark, D. B. (1959). Congenital tract of neck and ear. *Plast. reconstr. Surg.*, **23**, 621.

Streeter, G. L. (1922). Development of the auricle in the human embryo. *Contr. Embryol. Carneg. Instn*, **14**, 111.

Van den Wildenberg (1926). Fistules congenitales du cou. *Ann. Mal. Oreil. Larynx*, **45**, 677.

Willis, R. A. (1958). *The Borderland of Embryology and Pathology*. Butterworth, London.

—— (1960). *Pathology of Tumours*, 3rd ed. Butterworth, London.

Wood-Jones, F., and I-Chuan, W. (1934). The development of the external ear. *J. Anat. (Lond.)*, **68**, 525.

Wyt, L. (1955). Ein Fall von kongenitaler Hals-Ohren-Fistel (Küttner). *Mschr. Ohrenheilk.*, **89**, 164.

*Arch. Dis. Childh.*, 1965, **40**, 224.

# INTERNAL CAROTID ARTERY OCCLUSION IN A CHILD

BY

S. A. MELLICK and P. D. PHELAN*

*From the Princess Alexandra Hospital, Brisbane, and Department of Child Health, University of Queensland, and Brisbane Children's Hospital, Brisbane, Australia*

(RECEIVED FOR PUBLICATION SEPTEMBER 10, 1964)

Occlusion of the internal carotid artery is a rare condition in children. Mymin (1960) and Wisoff and Rothballer (1961) reviewed a total of 24 cases in children under the age of 10 years. Till and Hoare (1962) published carotid arteriograms of 3 children who presented with acute hemiplegia but they gave no additional clinical details. Brandt (1962) also mentioned a case of acute infantile hemiplegia due to internal carotid stenosis. Faris, Guth, Youmans, and Poser (1964) reported the case of a 7-year-old girl who presented with a left hemiplegia due to occlusion of the right internal carotid artery.

The following case is reported because of the comparative rarity of the condition, and in addition because it seems to be the first in which the pathology was demonstrated surgically and found to be amenable in part to corrective surgery.

### Case Report

L.K. was born in 1957 following a normal pregnancy and uncomplicated confinement, birth weight being 7 lb. 2 oz. (3·2 kg.). He was the seventh child in a family of eight. His parents and sibs are perfectly well and there is no family history of febrile convulsions or epilepsy.

The child was well until August 1961 when he was found unconscious in bed. He recovered consciousness fully within a few minutes. His parents did not notice any twitching and there was no incontinence. He was admitted to the Brisbane Children's Hospital and was found to have an upper respiratory tract infection with an associated fever. Physical examination at that stage did not reveal any abnormalities. Carotid artery pulses were not commented upon at that admission.

He remained well until December 1962 when, following a minor disagreement with his mother, without warning he fell to the floor and was found to be unable to move his left arm or left leg. He could not speak but he did not lose consciousness and he seemed to understand what was said to him. No twitching was observed. The weakness lasted about ten minutes and then disappeared spontaneously, and speech returned. Twenty-four hours later there was an identical episode again following minor conflict with parental discipline.

Over the next two months the child had about 10 further similar episodes. He seemed to have some indication that they were coming on as he would run to his parents and indicate that he was afraid just before the onset of the paresis. In at least some of the attacks there was a degree of weakness of the left facial muscles. During this period, the child began to complain of right frontal headache of sufficient severity to make him cry; the headaches did not appear to be associated with the attacks of weakness. Otherwise he enjoyed good health and indulged in normal activities for his age. He started school in January 1963.

He was first seen in the Neurology Department of the Brisbane Children's Hospital in February 1963. At this stage his right carotid pulse was noted to be considerably weaker than his left and a bruit could be heard over his right carotid artery and in his right frontal and temporal regions. There was a minor degree of weakness of the left leg and the left Babinski response was positive. No other neurological abnormalities were detected.

Further review of his past history at this stage revealed the fact that at the age of 3 months a superficial furuncle had been incised over his right mastoid region. In August 1960, he had fallen seven feet onto a concrete floor as a result of which he received minor abrasions to the face. There were no abrasions to the right side of the neck. The child was not subject to tonsillitis or cervical lymph node inflammation.

Further investigations were carried out at that stage. Skull radiographs showed slight underdevelopment of the right side. A right carotid angiogram demonstrated good filling of the external carotid artery and its branches but the intracranial branches of the right internal carotid artery did not fill and the cervical portion gradually tapered off (Fig. 1). In the left carotid angiogram there was reasonable cross-filling of the right anterior and middle cerebral arteries. An electroencephalograph showed some focal disturbance towards the posterior pole of the left cerebral hemisphere but no other local abnormality. No significant asymmetry or focal abnormality of the wave pattern developed during barbiturate-induced sleep. Other investigations were normal. In particular, serum cholesterol was 186 mg./

* Present address: Royal Children's Hospital, Melbourne, Victoria, Australia.

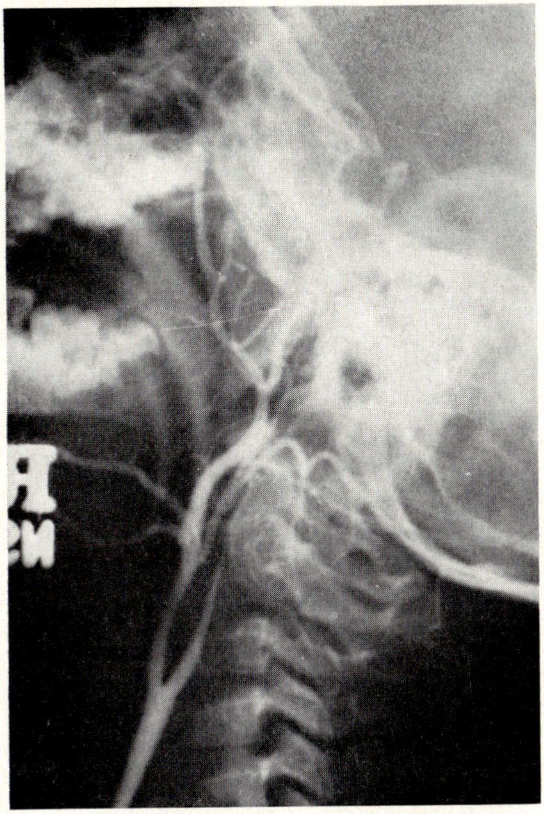

FIG. 1.—Right carotid angiogram.

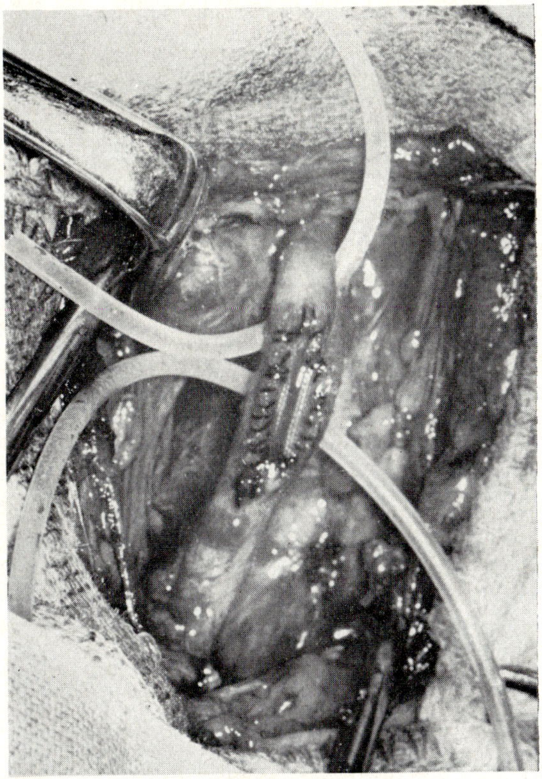

FIG. 2.—The internal carotid artery widened with 'dacron' cloth.

100 ml., cerebrospinal fluid was normal, and serological tests for syphilis were negative on blood and CSF.

Despite the confirmation of right internal carotid artery occlusion, it was decided to observe the child and treat him with anticonvulsants, as it was considered that the attacks of hemiparesis might have been dysrhythmic in origin. During this time his left Babinski response became negative but minimal weakness persisted in his left leg. However, he did have further attacks of left hemiparesis of short duration.

Four months later he was readmitted to hospital following a period of left hemiparesis lasting half an hour. On this admission he had weakness and hypotonia of his left upper and lower limbs and his left Babinski response was again positive. While in hospital he continued to suffer from severe right frontal headaches and had almost daily periods of hemiparesis. Because of the fear of further deterioration with the possibility of permanent hemiplegia, it was decided to explore surgically his right internal carotid artery.

An operation was performed in June 1963 under general anaesthesia administered through a cuffed endotracheal tube. The right carotid bifurcation was exposed. The right common carotid artery seemed slightly smaller than expected and an atheromatous plaque was palpable and visible within the wall of the proximal centimetre of the internal carotid artery. Beyond this, the internal carotid artery was about 2 mm. in external diameter. The leash of vessels and nerves joining the carotid crutch was displayed, and after infiltration with 1% xylocaine, these were divided in order to produce carotid sinus and carotid body denervation.

An arteriotomy was performed through the region of the plaque and the lesion was inspected from within the lumen. The yellowish white plaque showed up clearly through the overlying intima and could be distinguished readily from the adjacent normal tissue. Endarterectomy was not performed because of the very thin state of the adjacent vessel wall and the absence of a well-marked plane of cleavage outside the atheromatous plaque. The plaque itself extended for about 1 cm. in a longitudinal direction in the vessel and caused considerable narrowing of the lumen at that site. The back-flow from the distal internal carotid artery was poor. The arteriotomy wound was closed with a patch graft of 'dacron' cloth 10 × 2 mm. (Fig. 2), and this produced an immediate widening of the vessel beyond this site when the clamps were removed and it was felt that an increased blood flow had been achieved.

After the operation, the child continued to have transient attacks of left hemiplegia, but these have been much less frequent and of shorter duration than immediately before operation. About five months later, he started to have occasional clonic movements of the left arm and left leg, and about this stage it was noted that the tendon reflexes on his left side were more active than on his right. The headaches have not recurred. The bruit over the right carotid artery persists but it is not as marked and there has been improvement in the strength of pulsation of the right carotid artery but it is still weaker than the left. The electroencephalograph has remained unchanged.

Phenytoin started before operation has been continued and sulthiame (Ospolot) added as it was considered that there was permanent cortical damage as a result of ischaemia, and that the periods of hemiplegia and clonic movements might in part have arisen from an epileptic focus in the damaged area. The frequency of the attacks decreased following the addition of sulthiame.

## Discussion

This child differs from all previously reported cases of childhood carotid artery occlusion. In no other case has an apparently typical atheromatous patch been the underlying cause. Previous cases have followed injury in the region of the soft palate (Braudo, 1956; Fairburn, 1957), severe throat infection (Litchfield, 1938), thrombosis of a patent ductus arteriosus (Gross, 1945; Mymin, 1960), and have been attributed to calcification of the arterial wall (Duffy, Portnoy, Mauro, and Wehrle, 1957), but in the majority no definite pathology could be found. In the middle-aged and elderly the common cause of internal carotid artery occlusion is atheroma, and these cases usually present with a history of intermittent disturbance of cerebral function. The child reported here thus presented with a history similar to that seen in adults and unlike that in the previously reported children, who usually presented with hemiplegia of sudden onset which persisted for days until either death or slow and usually incomplete recovery occurred. Atheroma is very rare in children, particularly in the absence of hypercholesterolaemia.

Surgical intervention in this case seems to have altered for the better what appeared to be a progressive deterioration. However, there is some permanent damage to cerebral function and there would still seem to be reduced flow in his right internal carotid artery. His long-term prognosis must remain uncertain.

The authors would like to thank Dr. D. C. Fison, Medical Superintendent, Brisbane Children's Hospital, Professor T. J. Rendle-Short, and Dr. John M. Sutherland under whose care this child was at the Brisbane Children's Hospital for permission to publish this case.

### References

Brandt. S. (1962). Causes and pathogenic mechanisms of acute hemiplegia in childhood. In *Acute Hemiplegia in Childhood*, ed. M. Bax and R. Mitchell, p. 7. Heinemann, London.

Braudo, M. (1956). Thrombosis of internal carotid artery in childhood after injuries in region of soft palate. *Brit. med. J.*, **1**, 665.

Duffy, P. E., Portnoy, B., Mauro, J., and Wehrle, P. F. (1957). Acute infantile hemiplegia secondary to spontaneous carotid thrombosis. *Neurology (Minneap.)*, **7**, 664.

Fairburn, B. (1957). Thrombosis of internal carotid artery after soft-palate injury. *Brit. med. J.*, **2**, 750.

Faris, A. A., Guth, C., Youmans, R. A., and Poser, C. M. (1964). Internal carotid artery occlusion in children. *Amer. J. Dis. Child.*, **107**, 188.

Gross, R. E. (1945). Arterial embolism and thrombosis in infancy. *ibid.*, **70**, 61.

Litchfield, H. R. (1938). Carotid artery thrombosis complicating retropharyngeal abscess. *Arch. Pediat.*, **55**, 36.

Mymin, D. (1960). Carotid thrombosis in childhood. *Arch. Dis. Childh.*, **35**, 515.

Till, K., and Hoare, R. D. (1962). Cerebral angiography in investigation of acute hemiplegia in childhood. In *Acute Hemiplegia in Childhood*, ed. M. Bax and R. Mitchell, p. 69. Heinemann, London.

Wisoff, H. S., and Rothballer, A. B. (1961). Cerebral arterial thrombosis in children. *Arch. Neurol. (Chic.)*, **4**, 258.

# BRITISH ASSOCIATION OF PAEDIATRIC SURGEONS

The 11th Annual Meeting of The British Association of Paediatric Surgeons took place in Rotterdam from August 31 to September 4, 1964, under the patronage of Her Majesty Queen Juliana of the Netherlands.

The sudden death of J. J. Mason Brown, O.B.E., P.R.C.S. (Ed.), left the Association without a President, and Dr. D. Vervat, of Rotterdam, acted as Chairman of the Meeting.

Over 230 surgeons from 40 countries attended the Meeting, which was inaugurated by a reception given by Her Majesty Queen Juliana to the officers of the Association and the chairmen of the various sections of the Meeting. The Congress was opened by His Excellency Sir Peter Garran, K.C.M.G., Ambassador to the Netherlands, and the Meeting was opened by Miss Isabella Forshall giving the 4th Liverpool Lecture on 'Necrotizing Entero-colitis in Infants'. During the next three days 47 papers were given; some of them are reported in this Surgical Issue of the Archives and the others appear in abstract form below. There were three guest lectures: Sir Russell Brock, M.S., P.R.C.S. (England), lectured on the development of heart surgery in children; Professor A. G. Brom (Leyden) on the treatment of transposition of the great vessels, and Professor M. E. Müller (St. Gall) on hip surgery in children.

On Tuesday, September 1, the members of the Association were received in the Town Hall by the Burgomaster of Rotterdam, and on Wednesday, September 2, they were guests at a scientific session and social programme arranged by Philips Electrical Works at Eindhoven. The official part of the meeting closed with the Annual Dinner at the Rotterdam Hilton Hotel on the evening of Thursday, September 3.

Mr. Wallace Dennison, F.R.C.S., has been elected President of the Association for 1965/66.

The 12th Annual Meeting of the Association will take place in Edinburgh from July 27 to 30, 1965. It will be a combined meeting with the Surgical Section of the American Academy of Pediatrics (President—Dr. L. K. Pickett).

The following are abstracts of papers read at the meeting.

K. Devens (Munich, Germany). 'Atresia of the deferent duct (vas deferens).' Three boys with atresia of the spermatic duct are described. The macroscopic findings were similar in all three: atresia of the vas deferens with separation of testis and epididymis. This separation was present in all three, as was a patent processus vaginalis. There were no malformations of the kidneys. The first two boys also had an undescended testicle, as well as an incomplete descent of the deferent duct, whereas in the third boy the deferent duct had completed its descent leading to an atresia in the proximal part of the vas.

We have found 20 reported cases where there was a lack of fusion between the testis and epididymis. There were reports of about 45 cases of atresia of the spermatic duct, and in 7 of these an undescended testicle was described.

Herbert B. Eckstein (Carshalton, Surrey). 'Urethral Valves: A Review of 104 Cases.' A review of the clinical features, initial definitive treatment, and follow-up of 104 consecutive cases of obstructive valves of the posterior urethra admitted between 1951 and 1963 under the care of Mr. D. Innes Williams, at The Hospital for Sick Children, Great Ormond Street. Primary endoscopic section was possible in 35% of children under the age of 3 months and 67% of children over 3 months: 5 patients had a retropubic resection and 14 died before definitive treatment could be instituted.

Urinary control is normal in 30 patients; 25 are too young or too recent to be assessed; 4 have permanent skin diversion. Of 27 children that died, 21 did so because of renal failure.

J. H. Fisher, Frank G. DeLuca, and Orvar Swenson (Boston, Mass., U.S.A.). 'Rectal Biopsy in Hirschsprung's Disease.' The technique for rectal biopsy as an aid in the diagnosis of Hirschsprung's disease is described. The results during a 13-year period are reviewed. The procedure is a safe and reliable test.

The most frequent indication is to rule out Hirschsprung's disease in those patients suspected of having chronic constipation. The biopsy is performed in infants having symptoms suggestive of Hirschsprung's disease regardless of the findings by barium enema. The biopsy is also valuable in patients with short aganglionic lesions and in those with previous colostomies or inadequate resections.

V. Kafka, M. Krolupper, and L. Paleček (Prague, Czechoslovakia). 'Rhabdomyosarcoma of the Bladder in Childhood.' A report is given of a boy of 2 years who survived for more than 11 years after combined surgical and radiological therapy for rhabdomyosarcoma of the bladder.

The diagnostic and therapeutic principles recommended by the authors are described.

A. H. Loutfi, I. Mehrez, and I. Kamel (Cairo, U.A.R.). 'Masses in the Spermatic Cord in Children.' Three different varieties of spermatic cord solitary masses are presented: a fibrosarcoma, a bilharzial mass, and a tuberculous mass. In all, the testis and epididymis have been unaffected.

The rarity of tumours of the cord compared with testicular tumours is emphasized. The bilharzial mass of the cord occurs because bilharzia is endemic in Egypt. It does not regress with anti-bilharzial treatment and surgery may be indicated. Histology of bilharzia is classically demonstrated. The tuberculous mass of the cord is unassociated with tuberculous epididymitis.

António Gentil Martin (Lisbon, Portugal). 'The Challenge of Xeroderma Pigmentosum.' Xeroderma pigmentosum is a rare disease due to congenital abnormality of the ectodermal elements of the body, which react in a hypersensitive way to any form of radiant energy. This report is based on 4 patients suffering from this condition. The first 3 patients had localized squamous cell carcinomata which were excised and the resulting defect repaired. The fourth patient had disseminated facial cancer. A one stage monoblock total excision of the facial skin and total facial skin replacement were carried out with good final result.

J. C. H. M. van der Meulen and J. C. Raadsveld (Rotterdam, Netherlands). 'Hypospadias.' The morphology of hypospadias was discussed with special reference to the urethral delta and the oblique raphe associated with this condition. Treatment consisted in a Y-V rotation procedure.

A. Oberniedermayr (Munich, Germany). 'Adrenal Surgery.' A survey of adrenal surgery for Cushing's syndrome, the adreno-genital syndrome, and phaeochromocytoma.

The diagnosis, pre- and post-operative treatment are outlined in 11 cases.

J. E. S. Scott (Newcastle upon Tyne, England). 'Upper Ureteric Obstruction in Childhood.' A series of children with obstructive lesions of the upper ureter and pelvi-ureteric junction is described. There were 41 affected kidneys in 36 children.

Nephrectomy was performed on 12 children and conservative operations on the remainder with the exception of one baby who was left untreated. The radiological result of conservative surgery was satisfactory in all the cases on which this was carried out.

The incidence of post-operative urinary infection in those subjected to conservative surgery was high, and a method of detecting which kidneys are affected by chronic pyelonephritis is described.

V. A. J. Swain, L. Stimmler, N. E. France, and S. Tucker (London, England). 'Perinatal Ascites with Extravasation of Urine from the Kidneys.' Two infants with ascites at birth and two developing ascites at 3 and 4 weeks respectively are described. All four were males with posterior urethral valves.

Extravasation of urine from the urinary tract into the perirenal or subcapsular tissue was demonstrated radiologically, operatively, or at necropsy. Drainage of the subcapsular space in one case prevented further recurrence of ascites.

Two cases survived after cauterization of the urethral valves.

E. Tsakayannis, Chr. Moutsouris, and T. Valaes (Athens, Greece). 'Divided Liver: Twisted Pediculated Left Half.' An infant born with exomphalos was admitted in profound oligaemic shock at the age of 8 months. At operation the liver was found to be divided completely in two halves and the left lobe was twisted through about 270°. Cardiac arrest, which occurred both before and after the operation, led to the death of the infant.

A. W. Wilkinson (London, England). 'Biochemical Aspects of Neonatal Surgery.' The body composition and daily intakes and outputs of an adult, a boy of 10 years of age, a baby of 1 year, and a newborn infant are compared. The differences in the proportions of the intakes which are retained or excreted at different ages are described, and their significance in relation to metabolism at these various ages is discussed to emphasize the important differences in scale, both of total body content and daily turnover in the design of post-operative treatment in the newborn. The effects of deviation in the newborn from the normal range of intake as exemplified by human breast milk are illustrated.

W. van Zeben (The Hague, Holland). 'Cervical Lymph Node Tuberculosis Caused by Atypical Mycobacteria.' Eleven cases with enlarged cervical lymph nodes due to atypical mycobacteria are described. The clinical course and the bacteriology are discussed. The special tuberculin tests which are diagnostic for these mycobacteria are described.

Eoin Aberdeen and David Waterston (London, England). 'Preductal Coarctation of the Aorta.' The experience of the operation for coarctation of the aorta in over 200 cases in the 11-year period 1953-63 are discussed. More than half these cases were infants.

The results of operation have varied with age. Patients over 1 year have nearly all done well, but the younger the infant the higher the mortality rate: this is mainly the result of additional cardiovascular defects, and is not explained by the age of the patient. The severest cardiac deformities would be expected to present first. Time is a filter that selects the severe cases, and they present in early infancy. Preductal coarctation of the aorta is one of the severe deformities that commonly present in infancy. Survival after surgical correction of this lesion has improved in recent years and the reasons for this are discussed. Some details of management of respiratory insufficiency are given, since this is such an important part of the management of these infants.

G. Bellmann (Dresden, D.D.R.). 'Congenital Diaphragmatic Hernia.' Four cases with congenital diaphragmatic hernia are described. The diagnosis and treatment is discussed. There was one death.

S. J. Cohen (Manchester, Great Britain). 'Diagnostic Aids for the Unusual Types of Oesophageal Atresia and Tracheo-oesophageal Fistulae.' The diagnosis of the unusual varieties of oesophageal atresia and tracheo-oesophageal fistula is discussed. Techniques that assist in the diagnosis are described.

Francis Daniel, Tivadar Adler, and George Köteles (Budapest, Hungary). 'Surgical Complications of Staphylococcal Pneumonia in Infants.' Infants with the diagnosis of staphylococcal pneumonia are examined first by the paediatrician. The course may change very rapidly, and complications necessitating the surgeon's intervention, such as abscess, pneumothorax, pyopneumothorax, pneumocele with or without tension, may be very sudden in onset.

Before starting treatment, bacterial cultures and antibiotic sensitivity tests are carried out.

Forty-three infants with staphylococcal pneumonia and its complications have been treated surgically in hospital, and 4 of them died. In 3 patients puncture, and in 40 patients continuous closed thoracotomy drainage have been performed, with good therapeutic effects in most cases. Surgical intervention has been carried out in 6 patients because of bilateral, and in 34 patients because of unilateral process.

Edward Drescher (Szczecin, Poland). 'Some Remarks on Congenital Atresia of the Oesophagus.' Tracheo-oesophageal fistula can be diagnosed by noticing a blowing murmur over the left side of the hypogastric region. Phonographic records of this murmur have been made.

An uncommon anatomical variety of congenital atresia of the oesophagus, where both the proximal and the distal segments are joined together by longitudinal muscle fibres, is described.

The treatment of secondary narrowing at the site of anastomosis after a successful operation for oesophageal atresia is discussed.

Werner von Ekesparre (Hamburg-Duvenstedt, Germany). 'The Operative Treatment of Diaphragmatic Hernia and Relaxation.' During the past 5 years the author has operated on 19 children with diaphragmatic hernia or relaxation. Twelve had hernias, 4 had a relaxation, and 3 had a para-oesophageal hernia. Two children died after operation: the first who was premature with a diaphragmatic hernia and also extreme hypoplasia of the left lung, ventricular septal defect, etc., died 3 days after operation because of pneumonia due to aspiration. The second child had a diaphragmatic hernia and extreme hypoplasia of the left lung: after operation an ileus occurred due to adhesions on two occasions, making a further operation necessary. 17 children have developed normally after operation. One child had whooping-cough 2 years after operation; radiographs showed the diaphragm unchanged.

In the author's experience special plastic procedures such as a handled flap of the quadratus lumborum muscle, the psoas muscle, or the anterior abdominal wall, or even the use of alloplastic material can be avoided in the newborn and during the first year of life.

These methods should be employed only in the rare instances of extremely large diaphragmatic defects or the total aplasia of one side of the diaphragm.

H. Hartl (Linz, Austria). 'Intrathoracic Duplications of the Gastro-intestinal Tract and their Complications.' Four cases of intrathoracic duplications in the gastro-intestinal tract are reported. Two of these duplications were cystic and corresponded to a duplication of stomach. One of them was supplied by an artery arising from the abdominal aorta and perforating the diaphragm. One 6-week-old infant was lost. Two tubular forms of duplications were reported, one of them being a duplicate stomach; an ulcer of this duplicate stomach perforated into the right lower lobe and the chronic haemorrhage of this ulcer caused expectoration of haematin-acid gastric juice. The infant was operated on at the age of 16 months, weighing 4,400 g.; within a few weeks the infant had regained its normal weight. Another case with a duplication of oesophagus, a pseudo-stomach, and a duplicate duodenum was successfully operated upon.

The rarity of these malformations, the puzzling symptoms, and possible aetiological explanations are discussed.

Vladislav Rapant, Zdenek Sery, and Vladimir Vojtek (Olomouc, Czechoslovakia). 'Indications and Results of Pulmonary Resections in Children.' An analysis of 260 resections of the lung performed on 251 children under the age of 16 is presented. The mortality rate was 3%, and there were 31 major and 31 minor complications. The highest rate of complications was encountered in the group of 17 resections performed for chronic lung abscess. Most complications occurred during or after pneumonectomies. A definite relation was found between the type of the primary disease, the extent and difficulty of the resection, and the number of severe complications.

During the follow-up period of 204 patients who could be examined or questioned 3 died, the cause of death being decompensated cor pulmonale. In all 3 patients extensive resections had been performed. The late results of pulmonary resections in the four groups of patients described above were satisfactory, especially in those where lobectomy or segmentectomy was performed.

Stefania Reszke, Zdzislaw Rondio, and Stanislaw Kubicz (Warsaw, Poland). 'Suppurative Lesions of the Pulmonary Tissue in Children due to the Presence of Foreign Body in the Bronchus.' In severe pneumonia or pleurisy in a previously healthy child, or in any prolonged suppurative disease of the lung and pleura resistant to conservative treatment, the presence of a foreign body in the bronchus ought to be suspected.

Prolonged suppuration of the lung due to the presence of a foreign body, especially of vegetable origin, leads to an irreversible destruction of the bronchial wall and lung tissue.

Resection of the affected pulmonary tissue allows full recovery.

The sojourn of the foreign bodies in the bronchial tree in our series was prolonged (3 to 20 months). Much earlier recovery could have been obtained if the presence of the foreign body had been suspected earlier.

I. SZÖTS and J. GULYAS (Budapest, Hungary). 'Bronchial Adenoma in Childhood.' Bronchial adenoma is a semi-malignant disease. Its treatment has undergone changes in recent years. At first, the tumour, believed to be benign, was excised via bronchoscopy. In our first case we found that two excisions still failed to produce the desired result, and lobectomy had to be performed.

We no longer believe bronchoscopic excision of the tumour to be sufficient and adequate. The method of choice is resection of the bronchus, at least 10 mm. above the tumour, and the removal of the usually secondarily affected parenchyma. When the parenchyma belonging to the bronchus is intact, reconstruction of the wall may be undertaken in some cases.

Owing to the possibility of late recurrence, evaluation of the results of treatment requires at least 10 years.

KRYSTYNA WYSOCKA (Warsaw, Poland). 'Some Remarks Concerning the Surgical Palliative Treatment of Tetralogy of Fallot in Children.' A Blalock-Taussig type of anastomosis is the best palliative surgical procedure in children with tetralogy of Fallot and can be performed even in the youngest patients.

Mobilization of the aortic arch and carotid artery may be very helpful when the subclavian artery is too short.

Glenn's anastomosis is indicated in cases with total atresia of tricuspid valve.

Moderate hypothermia decreases the risk of operation in patients who are critically ill.

Omentopexy of lung hilus is recommended in cases with total or partial aplasia of pulmonary artery.

G. BRANDESKY (Vienna, Austria). 'On Treatment and Prognosis of Severe Head Injuries in Children.' Children have a much better chance of survival after a severe cranio-cerebral injury than adults. The younger the child the better the chance of complete recovery. Permanent disability occurs only seldom in childhood.

DENIS BROWNE (London, Great Britain). 'Orthopaedics of the Foetus.' The foetus *in utero* is exposed to certain forces of a mechanical (including hydraulic) nature, and these forces can act upon it in a way that can be deduced. The assumption is made that the developing body reacts to forces in much the same way before birth as afterwards. These hypothetical effects may be divided into: (1) differences between the newborn baby and the slightly older child; (2) increased mechanical pressure; (3) malposition; (4) increased hydraulic pressure; and (5) membranous perforation.

ANDREW P. LAIRD (Glasgow, Scotland). 'Operative Treatment for Failed Cases of Talipes Equinovarus.' A detailed description is given of the author's operative methods for failed cases of talipes equinovarus.

O. E. RAISCH (Stuttgart, Germany). 'Treatment of Fractures of the Head of the Radius in Childhood.' Fractures of the head of the radius showing slight luxation require no special treatment: immobilization in plaster bandage can be expected to lead to bony union without functional impairment.

In the case of more pronounced luxation an attempt can be made at atraumatic reposition under fluoroscopic control. If this fails, open reposition must be carried out; the operative technique is described. The results have been good.

In childhood, removal of the head of the radius is ill advised in view of the risk of disturbing the growth of the radius.

In the treatment of obsolete fractures of the head of the radius, which have healed with deformity and impairment of function in the elbow-joint, osteotomy with wire fixation is a promising procedure.

NORMAN SHAW (London, England). 'The Primary Treatment of Congenital Talipes Equinovarus.' In the past 10 years three principal methods have been used for the treatment of talipes equinovarus at The Hospital for Sick Children. None has proved entirely satisfactory.

The three techniques of primary correction used have been (i) serial or kite plasters; (ii) Denis Browne splints; and (iii) Robert Jones' strapping and stretching. Over 100 cases have been reviewed.

The author recommends gentle passive stretching and Robert Jones strapping in the corrected position; this has the merit of simplicity.

# BOOK REVIEWS

**Audiological Evaluation of the Pediatric Patient.** By MAURICE H. MILLER and IRA A. POLISAR. (Pp. xi + 117; 8 figures. $5.75.) Springfield, Illinois: Charles C. Thomas. 1964.

This book is written about the diagnosis of the young deaf child, and from the start much stress is placed on the need for *early* referral of children with speech and hearing problems to centres with adequate diagnostic facilities. Information about the necessary equipment and staff is gathered together in a valuable appendix. The authors emphasize the necessity for the contribution of many different specialties in the work of these centres and consider that the centres should be under medical direction. Both these points coincide with what is increasingly the common practice in this country. It is of course implicit in the title of the book that the deaf child is regarded as a patient, an attitude for which Kerr Love pleaded in this country in the early part of the century. Attention is drawn to the desirability of house staff serving in the centres so that they may receive training in the care of acoustically handicapped patients.

Excellent descriptions are given of various methods of audiometry in children but the book is marred by one all-important defect. A brief mention is made of how some workers have tested the hearing of infants, but no definite advice is given that would enable the reader to carry out these tests so as to arrive at an evaluation of the hearing of an infant referred to him for diagnosis. The authors comment disparagingly that tests in infants must rely on gross responses to uncalibrated sound and apparently think little of such tests because they do not give an accurate description of the hearing in terms of frequencies and intensities. They consider that these two factors must be known in order to reach final conclusions on the status of a child's hearing and that this information is necessary before adequate treatment and rehabilitative procedures can be recommended and initiated. This attitude makes it out of the question to diagnose deafness really early, i.e. during the first year of life. Yet it is at this age that treatment must start if the young deaf child is to have the chance to learn at the same age and in a similar way to the normally hearing infant. Failure to use the vital early years is borne out in the case histories given, for while one child is first seen just under 2 years of age and two others at about 2½, the others are much older and in no case does a diagnosis appear to have been made under 3 years.

There are 23 pages describing the conditioning of the child to carry out a pure tone audiogram, yet the pure tone audiogram will not indicate the use a child will make of his hearing in the acquisition of speech. The authors stress the importance of evaluating the child as a whole, but nevertheless exact and scientific tests of hearing are considered more important than clinical observations and deductions. A further 15 pages describe psychogalvanic skin resistance testing and electroencephalographic audiometry. A full and clear account is given and anyone wishing to know why these tests are not of greater value will find the information here.

It is to be hoped that in a subsequent edition the authors will give equally clear accounts of the clinical methods that are of value in testing the hearing of young infants. Their book will then be an excellent diagnostic manual for workers with deaf children. Until then it is feared that the book may dissuade others from attempting the diagnosis of deafness at the vital time, i.e. in infancy, and may perpetuate the ill results of late diagnosis which the authors themselves deplore.

**The Paediatric Prescriber**. 2nd ed. By PINCUS CATZEL. (Pp. xx + 261. 20s.) Oxford: Blackwell Scientific Publications. 1963.

The purpose of Catzel's 'Paediatric Prescriber' is to provide the practitioner in pocket form with a guide to drugs and dosage for infants and children, and in this respect the new second edition proves most useful.

It contains a wealth of information. The section on neonatal prescribing (Chapter 2) will prove an invaluable guide to many in their first clinical encounter with this age-group.

The author's percentage method, based on surface area (Chapter 1) will prove valuable to many in calculating dosages. His plea for standardizing measures deserves support. The value of this little book is beyond dispute, though had the author selectively omitted some of the less popular preparations, some alternative names, and perhaps the section on milk and milk products, the publishers might have been able to use a print that would have been easier to read. This comment in no way detracts from the reviewer's commendation of this edition, and the suggestion that every newly appointed resident to a paediatric post should invest at once in a copy of this prescriber.

**Diet and Bodily Constitution. Ciba Foundation Study Group No. 17.** In honour of Professor J. F. Brock. Edited by G. E. W. WOLSTENHOLME and MAEVE O'CONNOR. (Pp. 120; 31 figures. 15s.) London: Churchill. 1964.

This symposium, with Professor R. A. McCance in the chair, was arranged in honour of Professor J. F. Brock. Six papers were given each followed by discussion and finally there was a group discussion with Professor Brock in the chair.

Bodily constitution implies human constitution, though much of the information offered has been obtained from animal experiment.

In the first communication Dr. Widdowson establishes that malnutrition means a deficiency of some essential part of the diet for an appreciable length of time and points out that a diet of very low protein-calorie ratio produces a loss of appetite in the animals concerned and hence a reduced intake of calories below the requirement level. She emphasizes that the earlier in development the period of malnutrition the more likely is it to have a permanent effect on ultimate growth. This period may be early in postnatal life but in man it is probably *in utero*. This may affect brain as well as skeletal growth and influence subsequent intellectual development.

Next follows an account by Tanner of the relationship of different bodily tissues during growth and in the adult; work largely carried out at the Harpenden Growth Study; and Scrimshaw discusses the interrelation of nutrition and stress. Stress may precipitate acute malnutrition and conversely individuals with severe deficiency of almost any nutrient are usually more susceptible to infection and trauma, findings that have real significance both in technically under-developed areas and in developed countries.

Passmore discusses some problems of the body stores of carbohydrate and suggests that excess carbohydrate is not immediately converted to fat but probably is stored in the form of glycogen, mostly in the muscles.

The respective roles of the psychological and physiological influences that determine feeding in man are debated by Russell, with particular reference to obesity and anorexia nervosa. He describes several physiological studies in these conditions and then considers the psychological influences, concluding with a somewhat qualified statement that psychogenic mechanisms play an important part in causing feeding disorders.

This is a well-balanced and thoughtful symposium with much provocative discussion. There is an excellent bibliography after each paper and in addition references are given in the context of the discussion. A stimulating book for all who are concerned with growth and development and nutritional disorders.

**Growth Disorders in Childhood and Adolescents.** By SOLOMON A. KAPLAN. (Pp. xv + 202: 56 figures. $8.50.) Springfield, Illinois: Charles C. Thomas. 1964.

This monograph has been written by the Head of the Division of Endocrinology in the Children's Hospital of Los Angeles. Paediatricians interested in the subject of growth will find it a useful text, though it contains less about the biology of growth than does Tanner's *Growth at Adolescence* (1962) and less about disorders of growth than Wilkins' classic work on *The Diagnosis and Treatment of Endocrine Disorders* (1957). It includes, however, references to more recent papers on the subject than are found in the last editions of these works. No book can be up to the minute and the advice given in this book has to be reconsidered in the light of papers published since it was compiled.

For example, the last sentence in the book, summing up a discussion of the use of oestrogen in stopping the growth of tall girls, concludes, 'at present there does not seem to be any real proof that administration of oestrogens will arrest growth in such individuals, and their use cannot be recommended.' This statement takes no account of the paper by Whitelaw, Foster, and Graham (*J. clin. Endocrinol.*, 1963, **23**, 1125) which provides the evidence that if oestrogen therapy is started at an early age, if possible not later than 10 years, growth will indeed be arrested.

There is a useful chapter on growth hormone, its assay and its effects, though here again work is proceeding so rapidly that important papers are not mentioned. In the pages on the treatment of growth retardation the author advises that methyl testosterone should be used in those children in whom treatment is indicated. He gives insufficient warning of the need to watch the effect of anabolic steroids on skeletal maturation and of the need to interrupt the treatment for long periods since there is a delay of many months before the effect of all anabolic steroids on bone development can be assessed. In such common matters the author appears to rely too heavily on the work of others rather than on his own experience. There is no reference to the classic work of Edwards Park in the pages on bone growth.

This book is good enough to demand a critical review, and those who consult it will find it an accurate text. The author has collected together much useful information on many aspects of growth disorders. It certainly should find a place on the shelves of the hospital library. The book contains about 300 selected references from the literature of the past 30 years. Too few are collected from other than United States papers. Even the reference to the growth of Uganda children is from an American source.

**Klinische Diagnostik für den Kinderarzt. Heute gebräuchliche Funktionsprüfungen und Laboruntersuchungen.** By PETER HEINZ KOECHER, under the Editorship of and in collaboration with HANS-GEORG HANSEN, with contributions by G. KLEIN and A. M. EHRING. (Pp. 347; 26 figures + 40 tables, paper cover—DM.75.80; cloth cover—DM.80.) Stuttgart: Ferdinand Enke. 1964.

This manual is an enlarged and extensively revised second edition of the Supplement to the *Archiv für Kinderheilkunde* which appeared nine years ago.

Edited by E. Rominger it was written and compiled by four paediatricians with the intention of helping the clinician in hospital and his colleagues in practice with the correct interpretation of organ function tests and the results of essential laboratory investigations. Stress has, therefore, been laid on the range of normal values and discussion of the factors influencing them, in addition to the exposition of pathological findings.

The content is divided into four chapters: metabolic investigations; organ function tests; coagulation tests and investigations of the corpuscular elements of the blood; and growth and development. The last chapter contains a weight chart for premature infants (according to Holt), somatograms, tables for head and chest circumferences, ossification tables for the assessment of bone age and a brief review of dwarfism.

The first three chapters contain a great deal of useful information which is set out clearly in a pleasantly readable style. The sentences are short, the meaning precise without being epigrammatic. A number of tests are given with details of method and others where the technique is not mentioned but with an adequate evaluation of results. Although it was probably not intended to produce a comprehensive volume certain omissions are regrettable. The xylose absorption test, for instance, is not mentioned, nor are means of assessing disturbances of tryptophane metabolism. Although tryptophane occurs in a table of disturbances of amino acid metabolism, it is not to be found in the index.

The haemoglobinopathies have been ignored, except for haemoglobin F and its occurrence in thalassaemia, and are also omitted from the index. Assessment of labyrinthine, visual, and auditory sensations are rather unexpectedly included among the organ function tests. The function of the kidneys and endrocrine organs are fully dealt with, but the chapter on growth and development is the weakest part of the book and has little more to offer than any standard textbook of paediatrics. The inadequacy of the index is sometimes infuriating and will need a thorough overhaul in the next edition, which this book certainly deserves.

**Pathologie und Klinik in Einzeldarstellungen.** Band XIII: **Normale und Anomale Menschliche Hämoglobine.** By Hans Rudolf Marti. Edited by R. Hegglin, F. Leuthardt, R. Schoen, H. Schwiegk, and H. U. Zollinger. (Pp. viii + 197; 74 figures + 11 tables. DM.48.) Berlin, Göttingen, and Heidelberg: Springer-Verlag. 1963.

This monograph gives a complete account of our knowledge of human haemoglobin, its molecular structure, its function, and its alterations, be they primary changes in the globin moiety or secondary changes in the haem. The author is a clinician and a well-known research worker in this discipline. Thus he deals also with enzymes of the red cell, and their influences on haemoglobin stability, all of them necessary for the normal life span of the erythrocyte, and with laboratory methods. A special section is devoted to thalassaemia, its pathogenesis and its clinical and laboratory diagnosis. Interwoven are personal observations, and one reads with interest that Dr. Marti has encountered much thalassaemia in Switzerland, and has identified amongst his patients at the Medical Polyclinic of Basel University haemoglobins Bart's, H, I, S, Zürich, E, C, and M. The chapters on laboratory methods form one of the best collections published so far of simple yet reliable instructions on how to deal with virtually every diagnostic problem. The detailed list of references, all with full titles, completes the usefulness of this monograph as a textbook, a work of reference, and a bench book for the laboratory.

**Control of Glycogen Metabolism: Ciba Foundation General Symposium.** Consulting Editor: W. J. Whelan. Editor for the Ciba Foundation: Margaret P. Cameron. (Pp. xiv + 434; 72 figures + tables. 60s.) London: Churchill. 1964.

This latest symposium in the series promoted by the Ciba Foundation is concerned with the metabolism of glycogen, a topic as important as any previous one. It is of especial interest to paediatricians since the glycogen storage diseases are fully discussed. All clinicians must nowadays be in part biochemists, and this applies particularly to paediatricians who see the hereditary metabolic diseases in their earliest phase and who should therefore be particularly aware of them. They have a great advantage over the clinician who is concerned only with adult patients and who may at best see these disorders in an advanced state, with secondary complications obscuring the initial onset. Indeed, many children with hereditary metabolic disease may never reach adult life, and the paediatrician can contribute more than any other clinician to our knowledge in this field.

The subject matter of this volume is divided into three sections. The first, occupying about half the text, deals with the basic processes of glycogen metabolism and is a description, fascinating in its complexity, of the properties and characterization of the enzymes concerned in the synthesis and degradation of glycogen. All the papers are lucidly written and, though hard going biochemically, are not so involved as to be beyond the comprehension of the modern paediatrician. It is not obvious why Dahlqvist's paper on the intestinal absorption of disaccharides is in this section, or indeed in the symposium at all, since its link with glycogen is tenuous, but we should be grateful for its inclusion because of its importance in paediatrics. The second section deals with the regulation of glycogen metabolism in liver and muscle, particularly via phosphorylase, and the effect of insulin.

The last part, comprising about one-quarter of the volume, deals with the glycogen storage diseases. The past few years have seen great progress in the biochemical understanding of these conditions, and this has enabled us to classify them on biochemical rather than on clinical grounds, surely a more rational basis for classification since, as one author observes, similar clinical manifestations may arise from differing metabolic disturbances, and, on the other hand, similar enzyme defects may give rise to considerable variability in clinical expression.

After an introductory paper on the clinical manifestation of glycogen storage disease, there are separate communications on Types I, II, and V, and another on Types III, IV, and VI. Though not strictly a glycogen storage disease, glycogen synthetase deficiency is also described. All these papers are of an extremely high standard, which is not surprising since the authors are the foremost in their respective fields. The discussion following each paper is a model of what such discussions should be (but only infrequently are): illuminating, sharp, and clear, and giving an indication of the path ahead. This volume can be unreservedly recommended.

**Disorders of Voluntary Muscle.** Edited by John N. Walton. (Pp. x + 628; 143 figures + tables. 100s.) London: J. & A. Churchill. 1964.

In his preface, Dr. John Walton writes: 'In designing the present volume, therefore, it has been my aim and that of the other twenty-four contributors, each an acknowledged expert in the field, to give an up-to-date and comprehensive yet precise view of disorders of muscle from several stand-points. The book is aimed primarily at the clinician, whether he be a general physician, paediatrician or neurologist, or post-graduate student studying for a higher examination or any doctor wishing to expand his knowledge of this group of disorders.' It must be said at once that the Editor has achieved exactly what he set out to do. The book is comprehensive in the sense that the anatomy, physiology, pathology, and diseases affecting muscle are all discussed by experts who have succeeded to a remarkable extent in covering recent advances in knowledge and in giving copious references. This reviewer found the chapters on the pathology of muscular disorders particularly rewarding. Pearse's 'Histochemical Aspects of Muscle Diseases' and Pennington's 'Biochemical Aspects of Muscle Disease' for example, are remarkable reviews that repay detailed study. The chapters on electrodiagnosis are also excellent for they not only discuss methods of electrodiagnosis but also indicate when and how electrodiagnosis can be helpful in the clinical setting. In comparison, some of the chapters on clinical problems in muscle disease in the third part of the book seem to have rather little to say and that on 'Myopathies in Animals' hardly describes the clinical problems that are likely to be encountered frequently by those for whom the book was written. The chapter on polyneuropathies by Earl is rather sketchy; that on neuromuscular disorders of infancy by Tizzard inevitably contains little new; that by Kloepfer on genetic aspects of neuromuscular disease could have been expanded with advantage, for the large amount of information given in its 16 pages makes for rather heavy reading.

In general, however, there can be few criticisms of this excellent book which is beautifully printed and illustrated. It will be found useful by anybody interested in muscular disorders.

**Tumoren im Kindesalter. Postgraduate Courses in Pediatrics.** Vol. 13. Edited by E. Rossi. (Pp. 107; 24 figures + 15 tables. S.Fr./DM.19.) Basel and New York: S. Karger. 1964.

This Swiss paperback contains 5 essays on childhood neoplasms, 2 in French and 3 in German. It will be useful to the paediatrician and the general pathologist but is too elementary for the paediatric pathologist and the paediatric surgeon.

In the first chapter the late Dr. Bodian gives a clear account of the classification, incidence, treatment, and survival rates of 1,162 neoplasms (excluding leukaemias) seen at Great Ormond Street. It is interesting to note that the percentage of deaths from neoplasia during childhood rose from 10% in 1949 to 20·3% in 1961.

Schweisguth's account to some extent overlaps that of Bodian, though the approach is somewhat more clinical. There are some strange contradictions: in London, Wilms tumour not infrequently calcifies, yet practically never does so in Villejuif. Actinomycin D is useless at Great Ormond Street, but an excellent adjuvant in Berne and Boston. In London, no children with osteosarcoma survive, but 5 to 19% do so in Berne.

There follows an outline of the role of surgery, either alone or in combination with other methods of attack. Most of the quoted results relate to American work.

Wagner and Kaser deal with the effect of chemotherapy on all types of childhood malignancies. This is the best section in the book. The team approach (surgeon, radiotherapist, chemotherapist, and histologist) is rightly stressed. Though it is encouraging that in 60% of cases chemotherapy is beneficial, the list of side-effects makes grim reading.

The last chapter deals very briefly with the excretion of catecholamines in neuroblastoma and phaeochromocytoma.

Three criticisms: there is too much overlap and the editor should try some radical surgery; only two of the five chapters have a bibliography; a 'recent-advances-type' of book is presumably meant for reference, yet this 35s. paperback showed signs of falling apart even after one reading.

## Donald Paterson Prize Essay

A prize essay competition will be held, open to medical practitioners registered in the United Kingdom for not more than ten years. The value of the prize will be twenty-five pounds.

The subject of the essay shall be related to paediatrics but will be chosen individually by candidates. The essay shall consist substantially of unpublished work.

Entry forms and further information may be obtained from the Secretary, British Paediatric Association, Institute of Child Health, Great Ormond Street, London W.C.1. The closing date for applications will be June 30, 1965.

*Arch. Dis. Childh.*, 1965, **40**, 235.



# THE USE OF FIBRINOLYTIC ACTIVATORS IN MENINGITIS AND SIMILAR CONDITIONS

BY

R. L. NEWMAN and G. T. STEWART

*From the Department of Pathology, Queen Mary's Hospital for Children, Carshalton, Surrey*

(RECEIVED FOR PUBLICATION AUGUST 24, 1964)

The deposition of fibrin in the ventricles and subarachnoid cisternae of the brain, which occurs in bacterial meningitis, seldom causes complication in patients who receive adequate chemotherapy, provided the causal organism is quickly eliminated and no anatomical abnormality is present. Fibrin deposition still occurs, however, in certain circumstances, e.g. in children with congenital abnormalities of the central nervous system and after neurosurgical procedures with or without infection. In these cases, infections are often due to staphylococci or Gram-negative bacilli, particularly *Proteus* and *Ps. pyocyanea*, which are relatively resistant to antibiotics. When infection persists, the protein content of the cerebrospinal fluid (CSF) increases to very high levels. Deposition of fibrin from the CSF can then occur leading to loculation, hydrocephalus, and additional difficulties in surgical treatment. It is of interest, therefore, to investigate the possibility of using fibrinolytic agents in preventing the deposition of fibrin in such cases and in the lysis of fibrin already deposited.

The lysis of intravascular thrombi can now be achieved in certain cases by activation of the physiological plasma fibrinolytic system. It has been shown that thrombi contain a high concentration of plasminogen (Blombäck and Blombäck, 1956) and that activator in the surrounding medium diffuses readily into established clots (Alkjaersig, Fletcher, and Sherry, 1959). It is generally agreed that the lysis of intravascular thrombi is, therefore, best achieved by administration of activators of plasminogen such as streptokinase and urokinase, thereby producing a high level of plasmin within the clot itself, without a hyperplasminaemic state in the plasma (Sherry, Lindemeyer, Fletcher, and Alkjaersig, 1959). These considerations would presumably apply also to established fibrin deposits in the subarachnoid and ventricular spaces, but in aiming at the prevention of fibrin formation it would be advantageous to produce a high level of plasmin in the CSF.

Cathie (1949) reported the use of a streptokinase preparation in tuberculous meningitis. The preparations in use at that time, however, were relatively crude and contained many impurities so that serious reactions were often provoked. Fletcher (1954) using a streptokinase-streptodornase preparation concluded that this might be used to induce an effective level of fibrinolytic activity in certain cases, but found some reactions to larger doses and suggested that inhibitors might also be present.

The first necessity when considering treatment of this kind is to demonstrate the components of the fibrinolytic system in the CSF, that is, to ascertain that plasminogen is present and amenable to activation and that inhibitors if present can be neutralized. To investigate these fundamentals, specimens of CSF from cases of meningitis and from post-meningitis cases were examined, together with as many normal specimens as possible, by the techniques described below.

### Preliminary Laboratory Studies

Generally speaking, existing methods for assay of components of the fibrinolytic system are unsuitable for use with CSF, being too insensitive or too time consuming for this purpose. New methods or modifications of existing ones have therefore been devised.

**Plasminogen.** A new method for plasminogen assay was used which has a high degree of sensitivity and is suitable for detection and measurement of plasminogen at low levels (Newman, 1964a). This is a fibrinolytic assay using a standardized bovine fibrin clot. Streptokinase is added to the clot mixture and the lysis time is predictable with known quantities of plasminogen. Plasminogen is supplied by the CSF being tested, and the lysis time depends on the amount of plasminogen present. Lysis times are read visually or by means of a photoelectric instrument (Newman, 1964b). A standard curve can be drawn relating these co-ordinates, which correlates

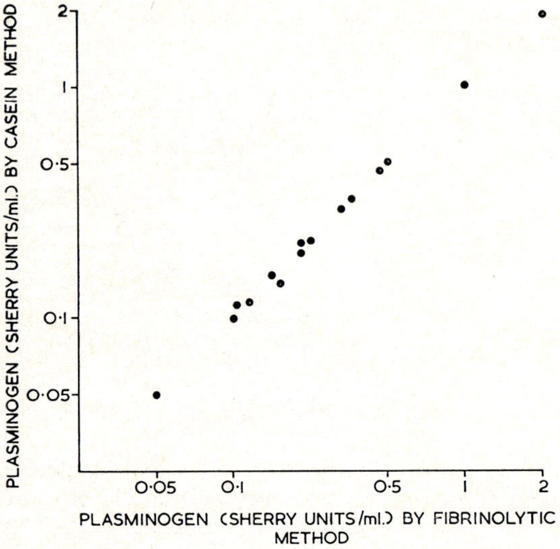


FIG. 1.—Comparison of fibrinolytic and caseinolytic methods of plasminogen assay.

closely with values obtained by caseinolytic assay (Fig. 1).

**Activator.** A modification of the above method proved suitable for detection of activator in small amounts in CSF. This consists of the omission of streptokinase from the clot mixture and enrichment of the clot with added human plasminogen. Lysis time then depends on the amount of activator present, as in the method described below for detection of antibodies.

**Antibodies.** A method was also devised for detection and measurement of anti-streptokinase (Newman, 1965). In this, streptokinase is added to a plasminogen-enriched bovine fibrin clot. Anti-streptokinase is demonstrated quantitatively by alteration of the lysis time caused by addition of CSF to the system.

Seventy-five specimens were examined for plasminogen level and for the presence of activator. Antibody tests were conducted with a few normal specimens and specimens from patients under treatment with activator.

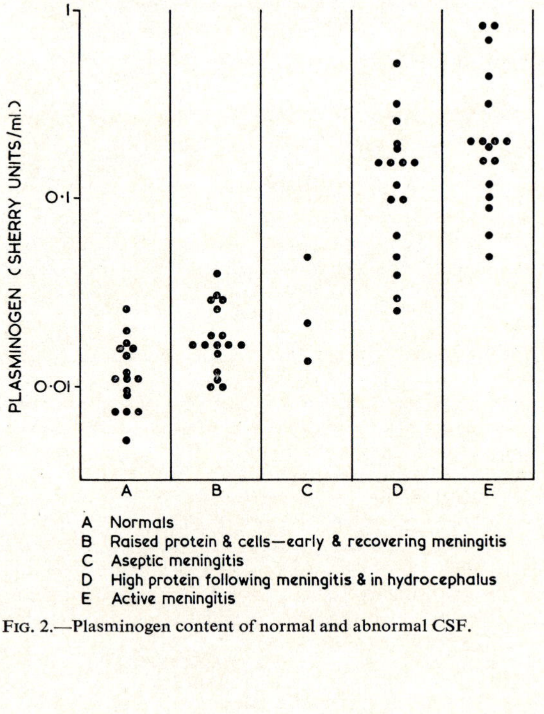


FIG. 2.—Plasminogen content of normal and abnormal CSF.

## Results

**Plasminogen.** All specimens of CSF examined, normal and abnormal, contained plasminogen in varying amount. In normal specimens trace amounts only were found, never exceeding 0·026 Sherry units per ml., which is about 1/100 of the normal plasma level. In nearly all the pathological specimens examined higher levels of plasminogen

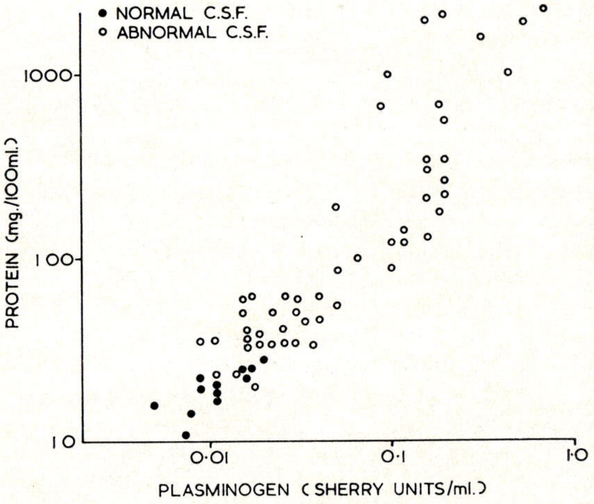


FIG. 3.—Relation between plasminogen and protein in CSF.

were found (Fig. 2). The highest levels occurred in the acute stage of pyogenic meningitis, during the first few days of the disease when organisms were cultured from the CSF and the protein was increased. In very early cases of meningitis (within the first 24 hours of the disease), when the protein was only slightly increased but the cell count raised, smaller increases were found, as also in a few cases of aseptic meningitis or encephalitis with raised lymphocyte counts in the CSF and increased protein. High levels were also found in cases of chronic hydrocephalus where the protein level was raised.

There was fairly close correlation between plasminogen and protein levels in the CSF (Fig. 3).

Paper electrophoresis at *p*H 8·6 of specimens with high protein levels showed patterns similar to the plasma proteins but with relatively less $\alpha_1$- and $\gamma$-globulin and relatively more $\beta$-globulin. Fibrinogen was inconstantly present. After dilution of plasma so that the protein concentration was commensurate with that in the CSF, and electrophoresis as above, comparable zones of lysis appeared around the $\beta$-globulin bands of both fluids when the strips were left overnight on bovine fibrin plates containing streptokinase (Fig. 4). This confirmed the presence of the estimated amount of plasminogen in the $\beta$-globulin band in the CSF. In cases of meningitis where serial CSF specimens were obtained early in the illness, plasminogen rose rapidly to high levels, sometimes within the first 48 hours. The rate of rise in plasminogen was faster than the rate of rise in protein, which sometimes continued to rise thereafter with no further increase in plasminogen.

**Activator.** Of 72 specimens examined, normal and abnormal, no activator was detectable in any of them by the method used.

**Inhibitors.** Not all specimens were examined for inhibitors as the method was developed recently. In those tested no anti-streptokinase was detected.

It is apparent from these results that plasminogen is present in quantity in the CSF in inflammatory and post-inflammatory states, no intrinsic activator is present, and inhibitors are not detectable. The plasminogen is capable of activation *in vitro* by streptokinase and urokinase, and fibrin clots incorporating such CSF in small quantities are lysed by addition of activator. It seems likely, therefore, that intrathecal or intraventricular administration of activators might produce a fibrinolytic state in the CSF.

**Clinical Studies**

The laboratory results described above provide the basis of an exploratory clinical trial in selected patients in whom abnormal deposition of fibrin appeared to be a factor in preventing recovery from meningitis and ventriculitis.

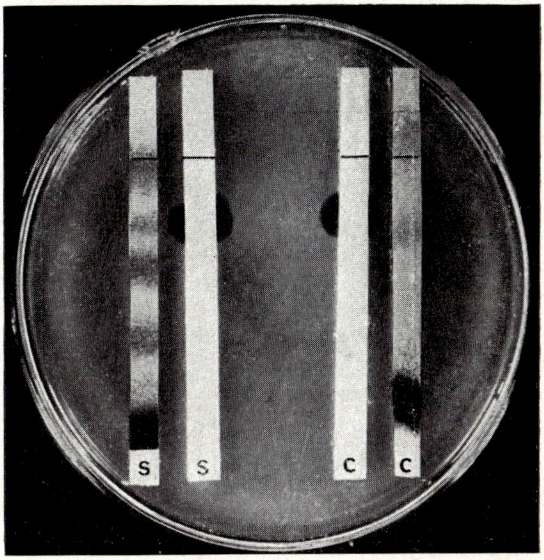


FIG. 4.—Fibrin plate showing comparably the plasminogen content in CSF and diluted serum.

**Selection of Cases.** Seventeen patients were selected for fibrinolytic treatment; of these 16 were babies and one was a child of 5 years (Table 1). Of the 16 babies, 12 were cases of meningitis arising before, or immediately after, repair of a meningomyelocele. In 7 of these the infecting organism was *Ps. pyocyanea* and in 4 it was *Proteus*. In the remaining one the organism was a Gram-negative bacillus which could not be cultured; 2 cases developed subarachnoid blocks during the course of acute coccal meningitis (1 *Staph. aureus*, 1 *Meningococcus*) being treated with antibiotics. Two were cases of ventriculitis and meningitis associated with colonization of Spitz-Holter valves, inserted for relief of congenital hydrocephalus. The older child had a large acrocephalic brain hernia, previously repaired, and developed meningitis due to *Ps. pyocyanea* following a further attempt at surgical repair.

Seven cases were given streptokinase (Kabi) and 10 were given urokinase (Leo). The drug was not selected with any attempt in mind to compare the effects of the two. In most cases it was administered together with the appropriate antibiotic by the intraventricular route,

TABLE 1

| Organism | *Proteus* | *Ps. pyocyanea* | Unident. | Colif. | Staph. | Meningo. | Total |
|---|---|---|---|---|---|---|---|
| Meningocele infected before, during, or after surgical repair | 4 | 6 | 1 | 1 | — | — | 12 |
| Subarachnoid block | — | — | — | — | 1 | 1 | 2 |
| Acrocephalic hernia | — | 1 | — | — | — | — | 1 |
| Infected Spitz-Holter valve | 1 | — | — | — | 1 | — | 2 |
| Total | 5 | 7 | 1 | 1 | 2 | 1 | 17 |

| Case No. | Organism | Activator and Total Dose (units) | Duration of Treatment (days) | No. of Injections | Start of* Treatment | CSF Protein (mg./10( |
|---|---|---|---|---|---|---|
| Group I: Meningocele and Meningitis | | | | | | |
| 1 | *Ps. pyocyanea* | UK 270,000 | 12 | 6† | 7 wk. | Steady fall; 550- |
| 2 | *Ps. pyocyanea* | UK 340,000 | 48 | 20 | 1 day | Steady fall; 1,200- |
| 3 | Unidentified Gram-negative bacillus | UK 150,000 | 15 | 6† | 4 wk. | Steady fall; 2,800-2, |
| 4 | *Ps. pyocyanea* | UK 75,000 | 3 | 3† | 1 day | Holding with rise la |
| 5 | *Ps. pyocyanea* | SK 62,500 | 4 | 4† | 2 days | Irregular; 1,100-1, |
| 6 | *Proteus* | SK 50,000 | 2 | 2 | 1 day | Steady rise; 900-2, |
| 7 | *Ps. pyocyanea* | UK 100,000 | 14 | 7 | 1 day | Steady rise; 840-1, |
| 8 | *Proteus* | SK 100,000 | 5 | 4 | 2 days | Steady fall; 960- |
| 9 | *Proteus* | SK 37,500 | 6 | 3 | 8 days | Steady fall; 800- |
| 10 | *Ps. pyocyanea* | UK 75,000 | 6 | 6 | 3 days | Rise and then during treatme 340-1,100-250 |
| 11 | *Proteus* | SK 75,000 | 5 | 3 | 1 mth. | Irregular; 2,160-2, |
| 12 | Coliform | SK 225,000 | 15 | 9 | 6 wk. | Steady rise; 2,800-4, |
| Group II: Meningitis with Subarachnoid Block | | | | | | |
| 13 | *Staph. aureus* | UK 75,000 | 5 | 3 | 3 days | Holding with su quent rise after tr ment 350-950 |
| 14 | *Meningococcus* | UK 33,000 | 4 | 3 | 5 days | Irregular; over-all 450-100 |
| Group III: Infection of Spitz-Holter Valve | | | | | | |
| 15 | *Proteus* | SK 100,000 | 6 | 3 | 4 days | Rise unaffected treatment; 760-1, |
| 16 | *Staph. albus* | UK 221,000 | 22 | 13† | 17 days | Early rise followed fall during tr ment; 200-500- |
| Acrocephalic Brain Hernia with Meningitis | | | | | | |
| 17 | *Ps. pyocyanea* | UK 225,000 | 14 | 8 | 3 days | Slow rise 300-375 |

* Interval between onset of meningitis and beginning of fibrinolytic treatment. UK = Urokinase; SK = streptokinase. † EEG during i

alternate doses into alternate lateral ventricles, usually daily or on alternate days and for varying periods (Table 2). In one of the cases of subarachnoid block the drug was given by lumbar puncture. Injections consisted of the appropriate dose of activator dissolved in 1 ml. of sterile water and in cases where this was combined with an antibiotic the total volume of injection was usually 2 to 2·5 ml. which was given after withdrawal of a sample of CSF for examination. This enabled laboratory tests to be made of the state of the CSF before each injection, which was normally 24 or 48 hours after the previous one. In every case a sample of CSF was examined before treatment started, to determine dosage and to obtain a base-line. In two cases treated early in the series protamine sulphate was added to the mixture to prolong the effect of the activator. This, however, appeared to make little difference to the clinical or biochemical results and was later omitted.

Each patient was observed carefully to ascertain whether administration of activator in this way had any toxic or other side-effects. CSF specimens were examined for evidence of meningeal irritation such as rise in protein, pleocytosis, eosinophilia, etc. In 4 cases, EEG recordings were taken before, during, and after the injections and in most other cases within 24 hours of the injections. Duration of treatment varied considerably, from 2 to 20 injections over 2 to 48 days. This depended largely on clinical progress and the results of the laboratory tests. Total dose of urokinase ranged from 33,000 to 340,000 Ploug units and of streptokinase from 37,500 to 225,000 Kabi units. Treatment with activators was sometimes delayed for varying periods in the early cases but, as a result of experience gained, the later cases were given treatment as early as possible, normally with the first antibiotic dose. In some cases activator was given later in the course of the disease after the CSF was sterilized to see if the CSF protein could be lowered.

All specimens obtained during the course of treatment were examined for protein and cells and were cultured routinely. Plasminogen and activator levels were also estimated on all specimens except those contaminated with blood which made the tests difficult to interpret. Inhibitor levels were also estimated in the later cases being treated with streptokinase.

| Results | | Necropsy |
|---|---|---|
| Early | Late | |
| ied of acute hydrocephalus during treatment | | Ventricular walls clear; choroid plexus buried in fibrin (collagen + +) |
| SF sterilized; early hydrocephalus arrested temporarily | Good progress; S-H valve; well after 2 yr. | |
| ead diameter increased steadily | Died of acute hydrocephalus | Choroid buried in pyogenic membrane |
| SF sterilized; intracranial pressure fell; head diam. remained static | Died in another hospital; no hydrocephalus | No necropsy |
| ied during treatment of acute hydrocephalus | | No necropsy |
| SF sterilized; hydrocephalus arrested | Discharged with arrested hydrocephalus | |
| SF sterilized but protein continued to rise | Died of acute hydrocephalus | Choroid buried in fibrin; ventriculitis |
| SF sterilized | Died of acute hydrocephalus | No fibrin in ventricles; aqueduct closed |
| ydrocephalus arrested temporarily | Good progress after S-H valve; well 6 mth. later | |
| ecurrence of meningitis with resistant organism | Died of bronchopneumonia | No necropsy |
| SF sterilized; hydrocephalus established 4 wk., no improvement | Died of hydrocephalus | Choroid buried in fibrin (collagen + +) |
| creasing hydrocephalus arrested; head diam. decreased 16-15½ in. | Valve inserted; discharged well | |
| ock relieved after 2nd dose | Poor progress due to brain damage; died from bronchopneumonia | Abscesses in both hemispheres; pus in lateral ventricles; aqueduct blocked by old inflammation |
| ock relieved after 1st dose | Good recovery; well 5/12 later | |
| fection not cleared | Valve replaced; hydrocephalus controlled; well 6 mth. later; infection cleared spontaneously, later | |
| ongenital hydrocephalus; no change | Hydrocephalus controlled by valve; died of bronchopneumonia | |
| o change | Died from *Staph. aureus* septicaemia | Choroid buried in fibrin |

## Results

### 1. Laboratory.

Plasminogen. All the cases treated showed high levels of plasminogen in the CSF before treatment. None showed any activator and, in the specimens so tested, no inhibitor was detected.

In every case the administration of the first dose of activator resulted in a fall in plasminogen level. The rate of fall was difficult to determine as specimens could not normally be obtained less than 18 hours after the first dose, but in every case the plasminogen level fell to zero or to very low values within 24 hours. In one case with an exteriorized Spitz-Holter valve where specimens could be obtained at frequent intervals, plasminogen fell to almost zero within 2 hours of administration of activator. In another such case serial specimens were obtained after a single dose and estimations of streptokinase and plasminogen were carried out. In this case there was some delay in the fall in plasminogen and the greatest fall occurred between 4 and 8 hours after the dose (Fig. 5). In the early cases when smaller doses were given, plasminogen fell to low levels after a dose but the fall was not so great as in later cases with

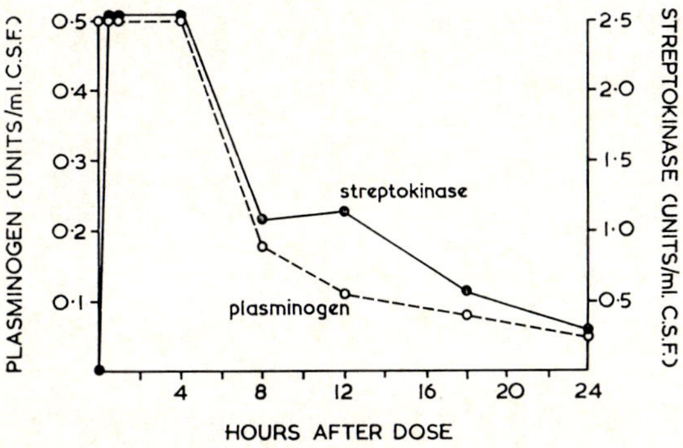


Fig. 5.—Changes in streptokinase and plasminogen levels in CSF after a single intraventricular dose of 25,000 units of streptokinase.

higher dosage. In cases that received frequent doses the plasminogen levels remained low as long as treatment continued. At the end of a short course of treatment, plasminogen rose again, usually to its pre-treatment level, though in most cases levels remained low for at least 48 hours after the last dose and began to rise thereafter. In one case where treatment was discontinued and then started again, a rise in plasminogen occurred during the interval with a fall when treatment was restarted (Fig. 6).

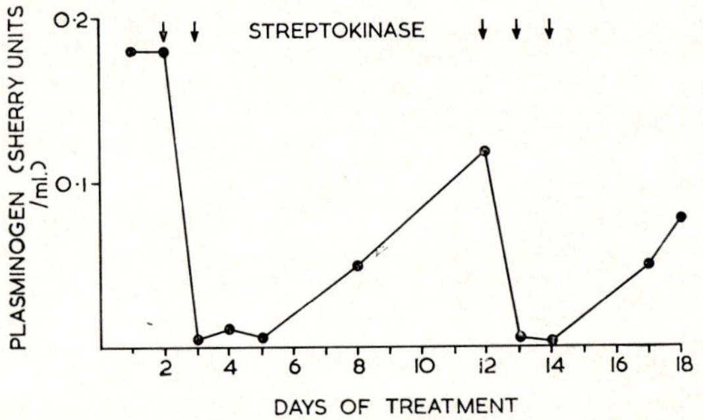


FIG. 6.—Plasminogen levels in cerebrospinal fluid of a patient treated with two courses of intraventricular streptokinase (25,000 units/dose).

*Activator* was demonstrated in a few of the specimens examined during treatment but could not be found in any specimen taken 24 hours after a single dose and was only detected 24 hours after the previous dose when several daily doses had already been given. The amounts found in these circumstances were of the order of 0·5 to 1% of the daily dose and appeared only in cases receiving large amounts (25,000 units daily or more).

*Protein* levels changed in a variable manner during treatment. In all cases protein was increased when treatment began, in a few to a very high level (2 to 3 g./100 ml.). No great increase was seen that could be attributed to the injections of activator. In some cases there was a steady fall throughout and following treatment (Cases 1, 2, 3, 8, 9, 10, 14, 16), in some the established rise continued (Cases 6, 7, 12, 15, 17), while in two others the results were irregular (Cases 5 and 11). In a few cases there was a halt in the rise while treatment was in progress followed by a resumption of the rise when treatment stopped (Cases 4 and 13).

TOXICITY. In none of the cases treated was there any evidence of ill effect from the injections. The CSF cell count showed no adverse change and as a rule decreased as treatment continued. The EEG recordings taken continuously during and after the injections showed no abnormality attributable to the drugs except in a few cases a transient asymmetry. Clinical observation of the patients during injections revealed no sign of irritation of the CNS or of any distress attributable to the drugs.

2. **Clinical.** These results are shown in Table 2.

GROUP I: MENINGOCELE AND MENINGITIS (12 cases). Of the 12 babies with meningitis associated with a meningocele, 6 showed clinical improvement and 6 did not. Clinical improvement or a good result of treatment was judged by arrest of increasing head diameter, and in 5 of the 6 cases this occurred during treatment. In 2 cases the improvement was only temporary and hydrocephalus supervened later. In one case (Case 8) improvement was assumed on the basis of post-mortem findings. Though the patient died of hydrocephalus there was no fibrin deposition in the subarachnoid space and hydrocephalus appeared to be due to the developmental abnormality. In view of the findings at necropsy in cases of this kind not so treated, the absence of fibrin after a severe meningitis was taken to indicate some measure of success. Of the 12 cases 6 were treated with urokinase and 6 with streptokinase. Of the 6 urokinase cases 2 were improved clinically, while of the 6 streptokinase cases 4 were improved. Commencement of treatment was early in 4 of the 6 cases with a good result, but duration of treatment or dosage appeared to be unrelated to the result. Cases 1 and 5 died during treatment. Of the 10 cases that survived, only 4 were alive 6 months after treatment: 5 died of acute hydrocephalus and one of unknown cause at another hospital. *Necropsies* were carried out in 5 cases. In 4 of these the choroid plexus was buried in a dense fibrinous mass, collagenized in most cases. In all 5 there was hydrocephalus with Arnold-Chiari malformation: 3 showed fibrin deposition in the subarachnoid space. In Case 8 there was a non-patent aqueduct. No evidence was seen in any of the cases at necropsy of damage due to the ventricular taps, apart from small areas of old subarachnoid haemorrhage in 2 cases.

GROUP II: MENINGITIS WITH SUBARACHNOID BLOCK (2 cases). Two cases of subarachnoid block during the course of actue meningitis were treated. In both the immediate result was excellent, with disappearance of the block after the first and second injections respectively. Case 13 made poor progress due to brain damage from the meningitis and died later from bronchopneumonia. Abscesses were found in the cerebral hemispheres and the aqueduct was blocked by old inflammatory exudate. Case 14 made a good recovery and is well 5 months later:

some bleeding occurred into the CSF after administration of urokinase intrathecally, but no excess of plasmin was demonstrated in the CSF or plasma, and the bleeding was considered to be traumatic, due to the repeated lumbar punctures.

GROUP III: INFECTION OF SPITZ-HOLTER VALVE (2 cases). Two cases with infection of Spitz-Holter valves and ventriculitis were treated. In both, established hydrocephalus was already controlled by the atrio-ventricular shunt, but from past experience it was thought likely that bacterial colonization was accompanied by deposition of fibrin within the valve. In neither case was the infection cleared by combined intraventricular chemotherapeutic and fibrinolytic treatment, and both had the valves removed and changed. Case 15 later recovered and is well 1 year later. In Case 16, the new valve again became infected and the patient later died from bronchopneumonia.

Case 17, the 6-year-old child with the brain hernia, showed no improvement with treatment. Hydrocephalus persisted and she later died from untreated septicaemia due to *Staphylococcus aureus*. At necropsy the characteristic changes in the choroid plexuses were seen as in the other cases.

## Discussion

In all the cases treated except Cases 13 and 14, congenital abnormalities were present predisposing to hydrocephalus. When meningitis occurs in such cases, necropsy reveals fibrin deposits, variable in extent, in the basal subarachnoid spaces and ventricles; the choroid plexus is often covered by a tough fibrinous deposit and in long-standing cases the lining of the ventricles is usually granular and may show fibrinous deposits as well. It seems likely, though difficult to prove, that deposition of fibrin in these sites might well contribute to the onset of hydrocephalus. In this event, fibrinolytic therapy might be expected to give improvement and, in 8 of the 17 cases treated, some measure of success has been achieved. In some this has been only temporary and surgical treatment has been necessary at a later date. It is difficult in the cases with congenital abnormalities to assess results categorically as the prognosis with or without infection is poor.

With regard to the effects of treatment on protein content in the CSF, plasmin is known to have proteolytic effects on substrates other than fibrin and fibrinogen, and it is possible that the fall in protein level seen in some of our cases might have been due to this effect. Again the results were variable, but the fall was greatest in those cases that received treatment for longer periods.

Reactions to intraventricular or intrathecal injections of streptokinase or urokinase were not seen in any of our cases. The highly purified preparations available at present appear to be free from such effects and are tolerated in large doses in intravascular thrombolytic therapy. Occasional batches, however, have been shown to be pyrogenic (McNicol, Douglas, and Bayley, 1962), and the results of such a reaction within the CNS might well be disastrous.

Antibodies were not detected in any of the cases where this test was made. In some, the treatment was given for too short a time for antibody formation to occur. In two cases treated for longer periods with streptokinase no antibody appeared and no reaction was noted to the later doses. Tillett and Sherry (1949) found that patients given intrapleural streptokinase developed specific anti-streptokinase in both pleural fluid and blood. We have examined the blood antistreptokinase titre in only one of our cases (Case 12), and no rise in titre was found after the course of streptokinase lasting 15 days. It is possible that with lower dosage and rapid local utilization of the streptokinase antibody formation might not be a problem in this type of treatment as it is recognized to be in intravascular therapy, though Tillett and Sherry also found that streptokinase given into the pleural cavity disappeared within a few hours of injection.

The series of cases described here is too small to permit comparison between streptokinase and urokinase; both activators are well tolerated and interact rapidly with plasminogen. Being of human origin, urokinase might be regarded as the more acceptable substance physiologically; some of our preparations showed traces of thromboplastic activity but this was probably unimportant in the presence of degenerative cerebral tissue.

## Summary

The cerebrospinal fluid in health contains only traces of plasminogen but a rapid rise occurs with the onset of meningitis, whether bacterial or viral. This is most marked during the first few days but persists thereafter as long as the protein content remains high. Plasminogen in this form can be activated by streptokinase and urokinase to yield plasmin. With proper dosage of activator, utilization of plasminogen in the CSF is virtually complete.

Given intraventricularly or intrathecally, purified preparations of these activators are well tolerated and appear to induce a fibrinolytic state in the CSF. By this means early deposition of fibrin was probably prevented or cleared in 8 cases of meningitis and ventriculitis out of 17 treated.

Antibodies and inhibitors to these activators were

not detected in the CSF even after repeated administration. Other factors influencing the response to treatment are discussed.

We are grateful to our colleagues, Dr. H. M. T. Coles, Mr. H. B. Eckstein, Mr. D. M. Forrest, and Mr. H. H. Nixon for the opportunity to treat patients under their care, and for their co-operation; we also acknowledge the help of Dr. L. Crome and Dr. M. Erdohazi for necropsies and of junior medical staff and nursing staff, in particular Sister M. Perry; we are grateful to Leo Laboratories Ltd. for supplies of urokinase and to Messrs. Kabi for streptokinase.

### References

Alkjaersig, N., Fletcher, A. P., and Sherry, S. (1959). The mechanism of clot dissolution by plasmin. *J. clin. Invest.*, **38**, 1086.

Blombäck, B., and Blombäck, M. (1956). Purification of human and bovine fibrinogen. *Ark. Kemi.*, **10**, 415.

Cathie, I. A. B. (1949). Bacterial fibrinolysin, its possible therapeutic application in tuberculous meningitis. *J. clin. Path.*, **2**, 73.

Fletcher, A. P. (1954). The preparation of partially purified plasmin, and an account of its intrathecal use in patients. *J. clin. Invest.*, **33**, 1242.

McNicol, G. P., Douglas, A. S., and Bayley, C. (1962). Experience with streptokinase infusions. *Lancet*, **2**, 1297.

Newman, R. L. (1964a). A method for detecting and estimating plasminogen in cerebrospinal fluid. *J. clin. Path.*, **17**, 313.

—— (1964b). An instrument for recording the lysis time of fibrin clots. *ibid.*, **17**, 194.

—— (1965). Method for the detection and measurement of antibodies to streptokinase in the cerebrospinal fluid. *ibid.*, **18**, 256.

Sherry, S., Lindemeyer, R. I., Fletcher, A. P., and Alkjaersig, N. (1959). Studies on enhanced fibrinolytic activity in man. *J. clin. Invest.*, **38**, 810.

Tillett, W. S., and Sherry, S. (1949). The effect in patients of streptococcal fibrinolysin (streptokinase) and streptococcal desoxyribonuclease on fibrinous, purulent, and sanguinous pleural exudations. *ibid.*, **28**, 173.

*Arch. Dis. Childh.*, 1965, **40**, 243.

# A STUDY OF THE IMMUNOGLOBULINS IN PREMATURE INFANTS

BY

J. C. HAWORTH, MARJORIE NORRIS, and LOUISE DILLING

*From the Winnipeg Children's and General Hospitals and the Department of Paediatrics, University of Manitoba, Canada*

(RECEIVED FOR PUBLICATION SEPTEMBER 4, 1964)

The immunoglobulins are a family of proteins which may be identified in the plasma or serum by immunochemical methods. There are three main components (Franklin, 1962):

(1) $\gamma$-globulin ($\gamma_2$) which has a sedimentation constant of 7S and contains about 90% of the acquired antibodies. It has been shown that the concentration of $\gamma$-globulin in the plasma of newborn infants is equal to or higher than that of their mothers because of selective transfer across the placenta. After birth the concentration decreases to reach a low-level trough between 3 and 6 months of age, which may be about one-third of the initial level. This decrease is due to the combined effect of the normal rate of katabolism of the protein and the deficient synthesis of $\gamma$-globulin during the first weeks of life. The concentration then rises again to reach adult levels between the first and second year of life (Knapp and Routh, 1949; Orlandini, Sass-Kortsak, and Ebbs, 1955; Oberman, Gregory, Burke, Ross, and Rice, 1956).

(2) $\gamma_{1A}$-globulin, which is also called $\beta_{2A}$ because it migrates with the $\beta$-globulins on electrophoresis, also has a sedimentation constant of approximately 7S. It does not cross the placenta and has been shown by a number of workers to be absent from the plasma of newborn infants. Synthesis begins about the fourth week of life and the concentration rises slowly but probably does not reach adult levels until puberty (Hitzig, 1957, 1961; Scheidegger and Martin du Pan, 1957; West, Hong, and Holland, 1962). Not much is known about the antibody content of this fraction, but there is recent evidence that some of the skin sensitizing antibodies in allergic individuals may belong to the $\beta_{2A}$-globulins (Heremans and Vaerman, 1962; Rockey and Kunkel, 1962) as well as *Brucella abortus* and diphtheria antibodies (Heremans, Vaerman, and Vaerman, 1963). Colostrum has been found to contain $\beta_{2A}$ antibodies against a number of viruses and bacteria (Hodes, Berger, Ainbender, Hevizy, Zepp, and Kochwa, 1964).

(3) $\gamma_1$-macroglobulin or $\beta_{2M}$ has a sedimentation constant of 19S. This fraction is also not capable of crossing the placenta but synthesis may occur at a slow rate in the foetus. After birth the rate of synthesis increases rapidly and it has been reported that adult levels may be reached at 9 months of age (Hitzig, 1957, 1961; Scheidegger and Martin du Pan, 1957; Franklin and Kunkel, 1958; West *et al.*, 1962). $\beta_{2M}$-globulin contains Gram-negative agglutinins including typhoid O antibody as well as the rheumatoid factor. It has been shown that newborn infants inoculated with vaccines to Gram-negative organisms form antibodies as early as the seventh day of life which are 19S-macroglobulins. After a number of weeks the antibody is found to have changed to a 7S-globulin. In adults, initial antibody formation is also primarily of the 19S variety, but a change to 7S occurs within a few days (Fink, Miller, Dorward, and LoSpalluto, 1962; LoSpalluto, Miller, Dorward, and Fink, 1962; Smith and Eitzman, 1964). Thus the 19S-macroglobulin fraction has been regarded as a more immature and perhaps even vestigial method of producing antibody. This recent work has also indicated that the newborn infant is by no means immunologically incompetent as was once thought, but is in fact perfectly well able to produce a humoral immune response by means of 19S production.

We describe here a study that was made of the immunoglobulins in a group of 19 premature infants who were carefully observed from birth to 1 year of age, and some well into their second year of life. The intention was to record changes in the concentration of the three immunoglobulins in the plasma, and to find whether there was any correlation between these changes in concentration and episodes of naturally occurring infection and routine immunization procedures.

## Material and Methods

The subjects were 19 premature infants (11 males, 8 females) who were born at the Women's Pavilion of the Winnipeg General Hospital. Their birth weights ranged from 850 to 2,438 g. and their estimated gestational ages ranged from 24 to 40 weeks. They were only selected in so far as they were born on the public service, that they were not private patients, and that it would be possible to follow them adequately in the premature baby clinic. They all received artificial milk feedings.

Blood was taken by heel prick as soon after birth as practicable and thereafter at approximately monthly intervals until the infants were 1 year of age. In a few instances it was possible to follow the babies into the second year of life, and blood was also obtained from some of the mothers. The blood was collected into heparinized capillary tubes and, after separation, the plasma was stored at $-20°$ C. until the analyses could be performed. Our pooled adult standard serum was stored under similar conditions and the immunoglobulin content showed no deterioration. We have no reason to believe that any deterioration took place in the samples obtained from the subjects. In a few instances clotted blood was obtained and the serum analysed.

A qualitative analysis of each sample was undertaken by a modification of the micro-immunoelectrophoretic technique of Scheidegger (1955) and the slides were photographed for easier analysis and for permanent record. The three immunoglobulins, $\gamma_2$, $\beta_{2A}$, and $\beta_{2M}$, were analysed quantitatively by the use of 'Immuno plates' (Hyland Laboratories, California, U.S.A.). These are clear plastic slides coated with agar gel which contains standardized specific antihuman $\gamma$-globulin, $\beta_{2A}$-globulin, or $\beta_{2M}$-globulin. Each slide contains 6 wells, into 3 of which were measured pooled control serum. For assay of the $\beta_{2A}$- and $\beta_{2M}$-globulins the control serum was used undiluted and diluted 1 : 2 and 1 : 4. For $\gamma_2$-globulin dilutions of 2 : 5, 1 : 4, and 1 : 10 were used. Into the other 3 wells different unknown plasma samples were measured. After incubation (4 hours at 37° C. in the case of the $\gamma$-globulin 'Immuno plates' and 16 hours at room temperature in the case of the $\beta_{2A}$ and $\beta_{2M}$ plates), the diameter of the zone of precipitate around each well was measured by means of a low power magnification viewer. Measurement was made by two observers and after practice it was found that the readings always agreed within 0·1 mm. Using semi-logarithmic paper the zone size of the pooled standard serum dilutions was plotted on the horizontal arithmetic scale and the globulin concentration on the vertical logarithmic scale. The concentration of the globulins in the unknown plasma samples could then be read from the graph. Samples containing globulins in concentrations too high to be plotted on the graph were diluted. Since only small amounts of each plasma sample were usually available it was necessary to perform the dilutions in the 'Immuno plate' wells, and this introduced some error. Fig. 1 shows typical examples of $\beta_{2A}$- and $\beta_{2M}$-globulin plates.

Each plasma or serum sample tested was compared with pooled adult serum collected from about 100 subjects. Through the courtesy of Dr. Kingdon Lou who recently supplied us with a reference serum with known globulin content established by means of purified antigens, we have been able to perform a quantitative assay of the immunoglobulins in our standard serum. The $\gamma_2$-globulin content was 1,100 mg./100 ml., $\beta_{2A}$ globulin 295 mg./100 ml., and $\beta_{2M}$-globulin 127 mg./100 ml. These concentrations agree fairly well with those reported in the literature for normal adults (Fahey and Lawrence, 1963; Chodirker and Tomasi, 1963). We felt it advisable to express the concentration of the immunoglobulins obtained from the premature infants as a percentage of our normal adult serum rather than in mg./100 ml.

The reproducibility of the quantitation of the immunoglobulins by means of 'Immuno plates' was assessed. In 22 duplicate samples the standard deviation (SD) of the $\gamma$-globulin estimations was $\pm$ 8·8% of normal adult serum, for $\beta_{2A}$ in 25 duplicate samples the SD was $\pm$ 4·7% of normal serum, and for $\beta_{2M}$ at concentrations of 100% or less of the adult serum the SD of 12 duplicate samples

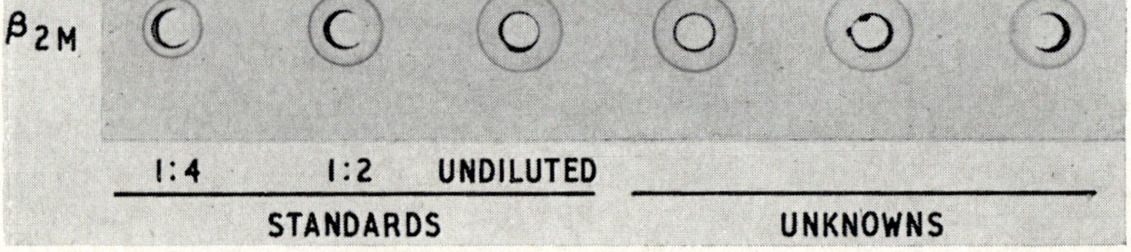


FIG. 1.—Typical examples of $\beta_{2A}$- and $\beta_{2M}$-globulin 'Immuno plates'. In each plate the first 3 wells have been filled with pooled adult serum in dilutions of 1 : 4, 1 : 2, and undiluted, and the next 3 wells with 3 different unknown plasma samples.

was $\pm$ 5·9%. When the concentration of $\beta_{2M}$ was greater than 100% of the normal serum, dilution of the unknown plasma or serum was necessary and the reproducibility was reduced. In 8 duplicate samples the SD was $\pm$ 28·4% of adult normal serum.

A record was kept of all infections that occurred in infants and also of their immunizations.

## Results

Fig. 2 is a scattergram of the concentrations of the $\gamma_2$-globulin in the infants in relation to their age. The range of values at any given age was very wide, but it may be seen that the mean concentration during the first four weeks was a little greater than the adult value. The mean level then decreased rapidly, as expected, to reach 25% of the adult value between 12 and 16 weeks. A slow rise then occurred to approximately 100% again at 1 year of age.

In Fig. 3 the concentrations of $\beta_{2A}$-globulin have been plotted against age. At birth in most cases this fraction was not detectable (mean 2·8% of normal adult serum). A steady but slow rise then occurred in the mean level and at 1 year of age the level was 28%. In only one infant was a level of $\beta_{2A}$ greater than 100% recorded (119% at 16 months in Case 8, see Fig. 7).

In Fig. 4 the $\beta_{2M}$ concentrations are shown. Again there was a wide range of values. The levels at birth were low (mean 25%) but thereafter a rapid increase occurred to reach a mean level of 100% at 20 to 24 weeks of age. Several very high levels were recorded after 20 weeks of age, 15 of 200% or greater and 3 greater than 300%.

Figs. 5-9 illustrate the findings in 5 individual cases. Fig. 5 shows a graph of the immunoglobulin concentrations in Case 9, a male baby of 34 weeks' gestation, birth weight 2,058 g. At 4 days of age he had absent $\beta_{2A}$-globulin, 16% $\beta_{2M}$-globulin, and 64% $\gamma_2$-globulin. By 7 weeks the $\gamma$-globulin line of precipitation was very faint and the $\beta_{2M}$ fraction had increased slightly on quantitative assay though no line could be seen on the immunoelectrophoretic slide. At 25 weeks the gamma globulin level was 56% and the $\beta_{2M}$-globulin had reached 100%. This baby had no infection and thrived normally until 40 weeks of age when he developed bronchitis and 4 weeks later pharyngitis. At this time (44 weeks of age) the $\beta_{2M}$-globulin was 248%, the $\gamma$-globulin 48%, and the $\beta_{2A}$-globulin 25·5%. $\beta_{2A}$-globulin could not be identified by the qualitative technique in any sample.

Case 2 (a male, birth weight 1,134 g., gestation 28 weeks) also had severe hypo-$\gamma$-globulinaemia at 12 to 16 weeks of age (Fig. 6). Unfortunately the sixth-day plasma sample was not suitable for quantitative $\gamma_2$-globulin estimation. This infant was

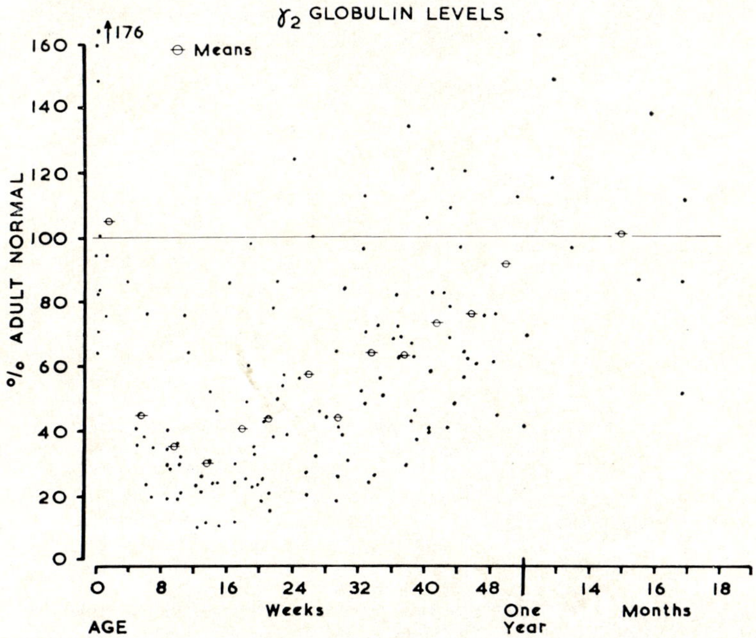


FIG. 2.—Scattergram of the $\gamma_2$-globulin levels in the 19 premature infants expressed as a percentage of the concentration in pooled normal adult serum and plotted against age of the infants. The mean levels (⊖) have been calculated for each four-week period. Values obtained from infants over 1 year of age have been combined as a single mean value.

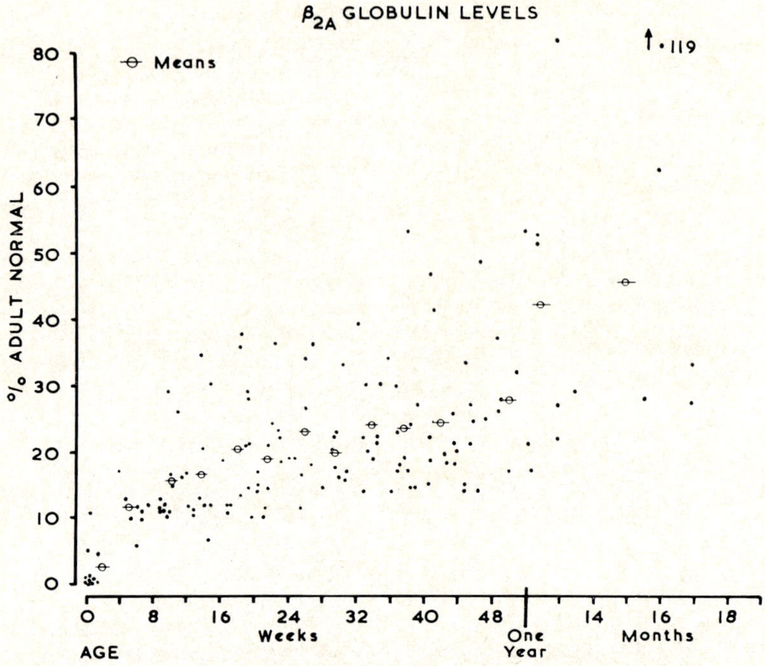


FIG. 3.—Scattergram of $\beta_{2A}$-globulin levels. Legend otherwise as in Fig. 2.

ill with pneumonia at 7 weeks of age and again at 20 weeks of age. The immunoelectrophoretogram of the plasma at 12 weeks of age showed only a trace of $\gamma_2$-globulin (10%) and the $\beta_{2M}$-globulin concentration was 62% of adult normal. By 29 weeks the $\gamma_2$-globulin fraction was clearly visible and the level had risen to 18%. At 30 weeks he was exposed to measles and received 1 ml. of $\gamma$-globulin by intra-

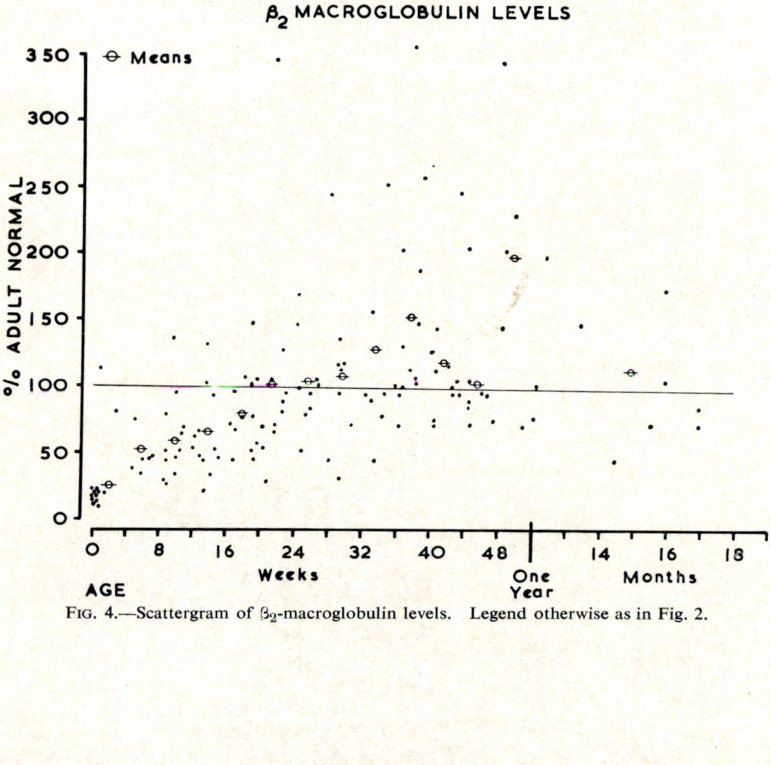


FIG. 4.—Scattergram of $\beta_2$-macroglobulin levels. Legend otherwise as in Fig. 2.

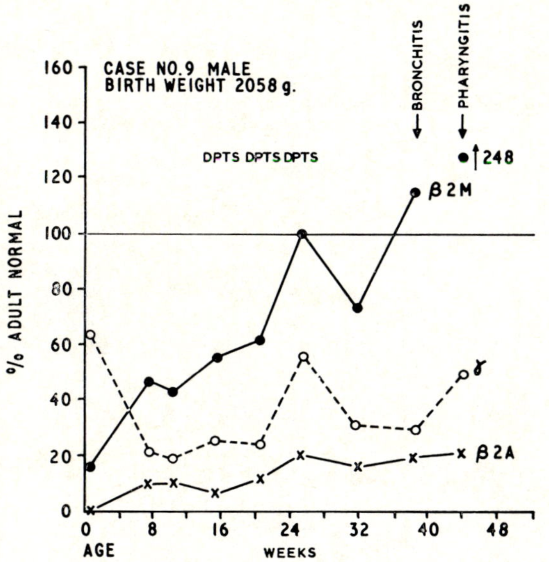


FIG. 5.—The values of the immunoglobulins in Case 9 expressed as a percentage of the concentration in pooled normal adult serum and plotted against age of the child. Episodes of infection are indicated by the arrows. Immunizing injections against diphtheria, pertussis, tetanus, and poliomyelitis (Salk) are indicated by the abbreviations DPTS at the appropriate ages.

muscular injection. Between 27 and 44 weeks he was in and out of hospital with a number of infections and a persistent respiratory infection raised the possibility of cystic fibrosis. However, the sweat chlorides were normal. Two further injections of $\gamma$-globulin were given because of the persistently low plasma $\gamma_2$-globulin level. It should be noted, however, that the $\beta_{2M}$-globulin rose to 100% of normal at 37 weeks. The $\gamma_2$-globulin finally reached normal values at about 1 year of age at which time the $\beta_{2M}$ fraction had decreased again. After the age of 1 year this infant had little infection and thrived normally.

Fig. 7 shows the immunoglobulin levels in another infant (a male, birth weight 2,041 g., gestation 32 weeks) who also had a number of infections during the early weeks and months of life but, unlike Case 2, this infant did not show hypo-$\gamma$-globulinaemia. In fact the $\gamma_2$-globulin level did not decrease in the usual manner from the birth level of 75% of adult normal. The $\beta_{2M}$-globulin level rose fairly rapidly to 69% at 11 weeks of age. This infant at 48 weeks showed one of the highest $\beta_{2M}$-globulin levels we recorded (340%) and was the only case in which the $\beta_{2A}$-globulin reached normal concentrations (119% at 16 months of age).

The infant represented in Fig. 8 (female, birth weight 1,219 g., 29 weeks' gestation) was a tiny baby whose $\gamma$-globulin level decreased rapidly from 148% at birth to 30% at 17 weeks. The $\beta_{2M}$-globulin level rose rapidly to 93% at 17 weeks and to 343% at 22 weeks. This infant remained completely well in spite of the hypo-$\gamma$-globulinaemia and there were no infections until 33 weeks of age.

Case 1 (a female, birth weight 1,673 g., gestation

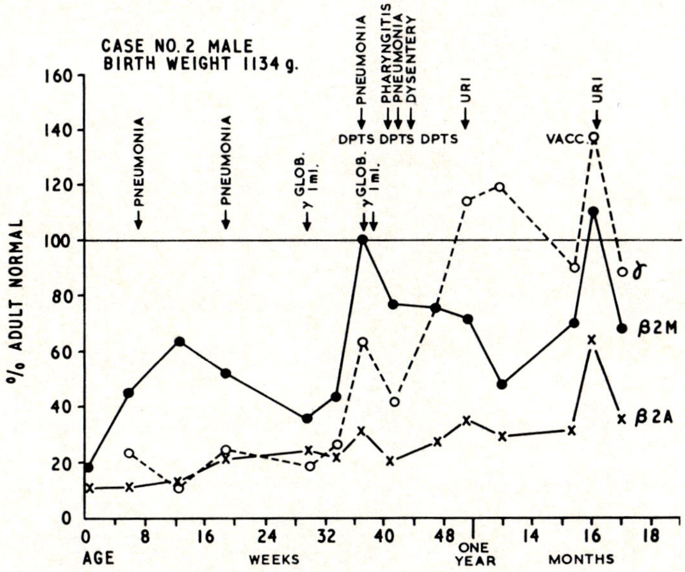


FIG. 6.—Immunoglobulins in Case 2. URI = upper respiratory infection. VACC = vaccination. Legend otherwise as in Fig. 5. This infant also received 3 injections of commercial $\gamma$-globulin as indicated (see text).

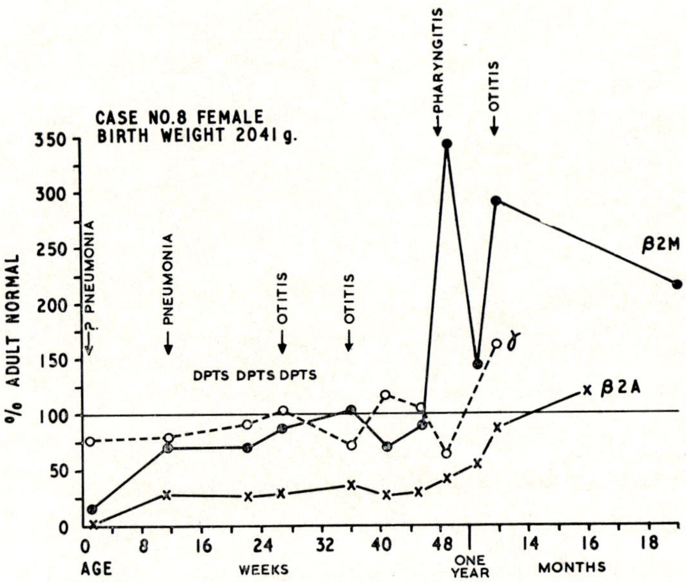


FIG. 7.—Immunoglobulins in Case 8. Legend otherwise as in Fig. 5.

34 weeks) (Fig. 9) was followed until nearly 2 years of age. The $\beta_{2M}$-globulin level rose rapidly to 240% at 28 weeks despite only one minor infection. The $\beta_{2A}$-globulin level in this infant was still only 44% of normal the last time she was seen at $21\frac{1}{2}$ months of age.

The number of infants studied was too small for any statistical analysis of immunoglobulin level in relation to birth weight or gestational age.

It was also not possible to show any statistically significant correlation between the number and severity of infection and the concentrations of any of the three immunoglobulins. In a number of cases a high peak of the $\beta_{2M}$-globulin occurred in association with an infection (e.g. Cases 9 and 8, Figures 5 and 7), but in an equal number of cases there was no such association (e.g. Case 7, Fig. 8). Similarly with the $\gamma_2$-globulin levels there was no correlation between the depth of the 'trough' and the incidence of infection.

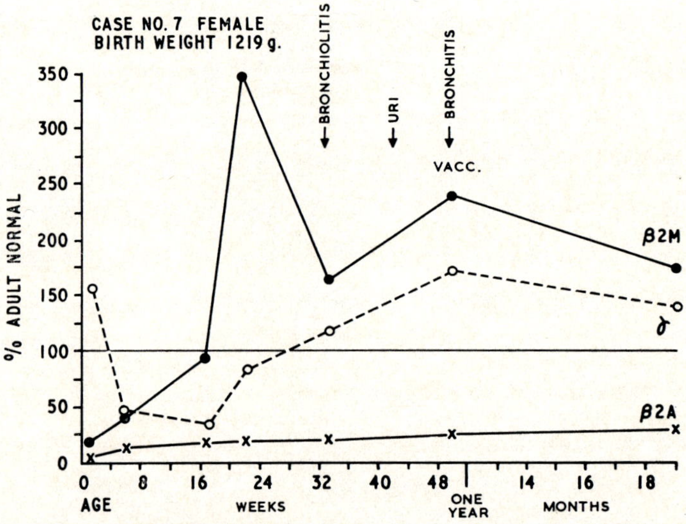


FIG. 8.—Immunoglobulins in Case 7. Legend otherwise as in Figs. 5 and 6.

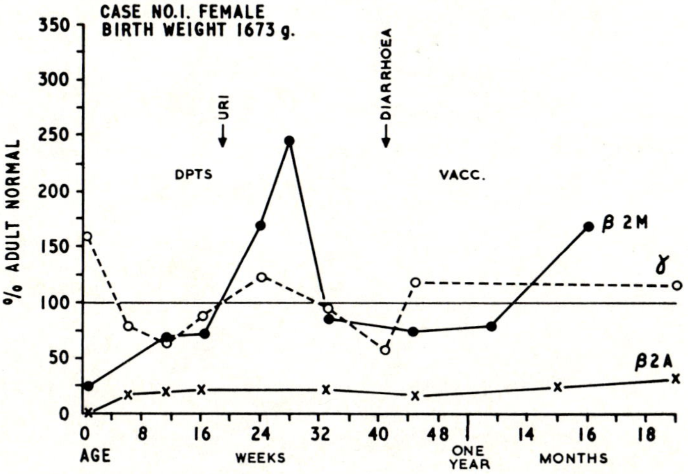


FIG. 9.—Immunoglobulins in Case 1. Legend otherwise as in Figs. 5 and 6.

We were also unable to show any change in immunoglobulin concentration following immunization against diphtheria, pertussis, tetanus, poliomyelitis, and small-pox.

## Discussion

In general the results we obtained in this group of 19 premature infants are in agreement with the results in other studies of immunoglobulin concentrations in young infants (Hitzig, 1957, 1961; Scheidegger and Martin du Pan, 1957; Franklin and Kunkel, 1958; West *et al.*, 1962). Our attempt to follow the changes of immunoglobulin concentration in a group of premature infants during the first year or so of life has, we feel, been of some value even if only to demonstrate the great variability in the values obtained. The changes in the $\beta_{2M}$-globulin concentration were of considerable interest. All infants showed some $\beta_{2M}$-globulin in their plasma by the quantitative assay during the first few days of life, though no line of precipitation could be identified on the immunoelectrophoretogram at levels below about 40% of adult normal. Our finding of low levels of $\beta_{2M}$ at birth, or within a few days of birth, supports the work of others that this protein can be synthesized by the foetus *in utero*, since $\beta_{2M}$-globulin does not cross the placenta. Synthesis after birth evidently continues at a very rapid rate because adult normal values were reached by 20 to 24 weeks of age. This rapid synthesis is occurring at a time when the $\gamma_2$-globulin level is decreasing because of katabolism and little or no synthesis. This supports the recent concept that the premature infant is by no means immunologically incompetent but is able to produce antibody by means of the $\beta_2$-macroglobulin mechanism before $\gamma_2$-globulin synthesis begins (Fink *et al.*, 1962; Smith and Eitzman, 1964).

It appears that the $\beta_{2A}$-globulin synthesis does not occur to any degree in the foetus, but synthesis evidently begins during the first few weeks after birth and increases very slowly during the first year of life. By 1 year the mean concentration in the infants was only 28% of the average normal level. These findings were similar to those of West *et al.* (1962).

We were not able to demonstrate a statistically significant correlation between the concentration of the immunoglobulins in the plasma of the premature infants and the incidence of infection. Such an association might have been missed for several reasons. The follow-up of a few of the infants was not always as good as we would have wished. Some cases attended rather irregularly and we were dependent upon the mother's history about minor infections that had occurred in the interval between two visits if she did not consider the baby ill enough to bring to the hospital at the time of the infection. In addition the total number of infants was too small for much statistical analysis.

Case 2 (Fig. 6) was a very immature baby who had a lot of infection during the first 11 months of life. He had profound and prolonged hypo-$\gamma$-globulinaemia. At 12 weeks of age the $\gamma_2$-globulin concentration was only 10% of the mean adult level which would correspond to 110 mg./100 ml. In addition the $\beta_{2M}$-globulin level remained lower than the average and did not reach the adult mean until 37 weeks. This baby appears to be similar to Cases 11 and 12 of West *et al.* (1962) with transient hypo-$\gamma$-

globulinaemia or a 'slow starter'. Four other infants might also have been considered 'slow starters' with $\gamma_2$-globulin levels of less than 20% (220 mg./100 ml.) of the adult mean and in 3 of them the $\beta_{2M}$-globulin also remained low. One of these infants had no infections at all and the other two had minor infections such as skin pustules and conjunctivitis.

Clearly there is much more to be learned about immunity in the premature infant. We did not measure antibody production in this series of infants, and this will remain a fruitful field for further investigation.

Besides the immunoglobulins, a number of other protein fractions appeared to be diminished or absent on the immunoelectrophoretic slides of the plasma of these infants during the first few weeks of life. These other fractions were not analysed in the present study but it is hoped to do this at a later date.

## Summary

A study was made of the immunoglobulins in a group of 19 premature infants. Blood was collected from the infants during the first few days of life and thereafter at approximately monthly intervals until 12 months of age. In a few cases it was possible to follow the infant in the second year of life.

Each plasma or serum sample was analysed qualitatively by a modification of the micro-immunoelectrophoretic technique of Scheidegger (1955) and the three main immunoglobulins, $\beta_2$-macroglobulin ($\beta_{2M}$), $\beta_{2A}$-globulin, and 7S-$\gamma$-globulin were assayed quantitatively.

The $\beta_{2A}$-globulin was usually found to be absent at birth, confirming the observations of other workers. Thereafter the levels rose very slowly and at 1 year the mean concentration was only 28% of the average adult normal. The mean $\beta_{2M}$ concentration at birth was 25% of the adult value and during the first few months of life rose very rapidly to reach normal adult values between 20 and 24 weeks of age. The levels of $\gamma_2$-globulin approximated the level found in normal adult serum at birth, presumably because of placental transfer from the mother. The levels then declined rapidly to a mean of 25% of normal between 12 and 16 weeks of age, after which a rise occurred to reach the adult average value at 12 months of age.

There was no statistically significant correlation between the incidence of infection in these 19 infants and the level of any of the three immunoglobulins.

We acknowledge the help of Drs. W. L. Parker and H. Taylor in many aspects of this investigation and thank both of them for reviewing the manuscript.

This work was supported by a grant from Parke, Davis and Co. Ltd. and from the Department of National Health and Welfare of Canada.

### References

Chodirker, W. B., and Tomasi, T. B., Jr. (1963). Gamma-globulins: Quantitative relationship in human serum and nonvascular fluids. *Science*, **142**, 1080.

Fahey, J. L., and Lawrence, M. E. (1963). Quantitative determination of 6·6 S $\gamma$-globulins, $\beta_{2A}$- globulins and $\gamma_1$-macroglobulins in human serum. *J. Immunol.*, **91**, 597.

Fink, C. W., Miller, W. E., Jr., Dorward, B., and LoSpalluto, J. (1962). The formation of macroglobulin antibodies. II. Studies on neonatal infants and older children. *J. clin. Invest.*, **41**, 1422.

Franklin, E. C. (1962). The structure, function and significance of the immune globulins. *Vox Sang. (Basel)*, **7**, 1.

——, and Kunkel, H. G. (1958). Comparative levels of high molecular weight (19S) gamma globulin in maternal and umbilical cord sera. *J. Lab. clin. Med.*, **52**, 724.

Heremans, J. F., and Vaerman, J.-P. (1962). $\beta_{2A}$-globulin as a possible carrier of allergic reaginic activity. *Nature (Lond.)*, **193**, 1091.

——, ——, and Vaerman, C. (1963). Studies on the immune globulins of human serum. II. A study of the distribution of anti-brucella and anti-diphtheria antibody activities among $\gamma_{ss}$-, $\gamma_{1M}$- and $\gamma_{1A}$-globulin fractions. *J. Immunol.*, **91**, 11.

Hitzig, W. H. (1957). Die physiologische Entwicklung der 'Immunglobuline' (Gamma- und Beta$_2$-Globuline). *Helv. paediat. Acta*, **12**, 596.

—— (1961). Das Bluteiweissbild beim gesunden Säugling: spezifische Proteinbestimmungen mit besonderer Berücksichtigung immunochemischer Methoden. *ibid.*, **16**, 46.

Hodes, S. L., Berger, R., Ainbender, E., Hevizy, M. M., Zepp, H. D., and Kochwa, S. (1964). Proof that colostrum polioantibody is different from serum antibody. American Pediatric Society, Seattle.

Knapp, E. L., and Routh, J. I. (1949). Electrophoretic studies of plasma proteins in normal children. *Pediatrics*, **4**, 508.

LoSpalluto, J., Miller, W., Jr., Dorward, B., and Fink, C. W. (1962). The formation of macroglobulin antibodies. I. Studies on adult humans. *J. clin. Invest.*, **41**, 1415.

Oberman, J. W., Gregory, K. O., Burke, F. G., Ross, S., and Rice, E. C. (1956). Electrophoretic analysis of serum proteins in infants and children. I. Normal values from birth to adolescence. *New Engl. J. Med.*, **255**, 743.

Orlandini, T. O., Sass-Kortsak, A., and Ebbs, J. H. (1955). Serum gamma globulin levels in normal infants. *Pediatrics*, **16**, 575.

Rockey, J. H., and Kunkel, H. G. (1962). Unusual sedimentation and sulfhydryl sensitivity of certain isohemagglutinins and skin-sensitizing antibody. *Proc. Soc. exp. Biol. (N.Y.)*, **110**, 101.

Scheidegger, J.-J. (1955). Une micro-méthode de l'immuno-électrophorèse. *Int. Arch. Allergy*, **7**, 103.

——, and Martin du Pan, R. (1957). Étude immunoélectrophorétique des protéines sériques du nouveau-né et du nourisson. *Étud. néo-natal.*, **6**, 135.

Smith, R. T., and Eitzman, D. V. (1964). The development of the immune response. Characterization of the response of the human infant and adult to immunization with salmonella vaccines. *Pediatrics*, **33**, 163.

West, C. D., Hong, R., and Holland, N. H. (1962). Immunoglobulin levels from the newborn period to adulthood and in immunoglobulin deficiency states. *J. clin. Invest.*, **41**, 2054.

*Arch. Dis. Childh.*, 1965, **40**, 251.

# 3β: 21-DIHYDROXYPREGN-5-ENE-20-ONE IN URINE OF NORMAL NEWBORN INFANTS AND IN THIRD DAY URINE OF CHILD WITH DEFICIENCY OF 3β-HYDROXYSTEROID-DEHYDROGENASE*

BY

D. M. CATHRO, KATHLEEN BIRCHALL, F. L. MITCHELL, and CONSTANCE C. FORSYTH

*From the Department of Child Health, University of St. Andrews and the Clinical Investigation Unit, Maryfield Hospital, Dundee*

(RECEIVED FOR PUBLICATION OCTOBER 1, 1964)

The unusual patterns of excretion of steroids of adrenal or placental origin occurring in the urine of normal newborn infants have been the subject of previous reports (Birchall, Cathro, Forsyth, and Mitchell, 1961; Cathro, Birchall, Mitchell, and Forsyth, 1963) and have been interpreted as providing evidence that the metabolism of adrenal steroids in early infancy is unique. The presence of atypical urinary neutral steroids is characteristic of the first week of life and one of these has been provisionally identified as the $\Delta^5$-compound 3β: 21-dihydroxy-pregn-5-ene-20-one (Cathro *et al.*, 1963).

Further study of the isolated material (Birchall and Mitchell, to be published) has supported the original provisional identification of the compound as 3β: 21-dihydroxypregn-5-ene-20-one (21-hydroxypregnenolone), and the occurrence of this steroid in the urine of newborn infants is of considerable theoretical importance, since it suggests that in early infancy adrenal steroids may be synthesized by pathways that are unimportant in the adult.

Although 21-hydroxypregnenolone has not been found to be one of the dominant reducing steroids in the urine of newborn infants, it has been shown to be consistently present and to be easily measurable during the first week of life (Cathro *et al.*, 1963). This is in marked contrast to what is found with adult males, in whom urinary excretion of 21-hydroxypregnenolone as the 3 : 21-disulphate occurs in such small quantities that the average value obtained following corticotrophin stimulation is only 70 μg./litre (Pasqualini, 1962; Pasqualini and Jayle, 1962). This low excretion of the steroid by adults is not unexpected, since 21-hydroxypregnenolone is not an intermediary compound in the accepted major pathways for corticosteroid biosynthesis outlined in bold print in Fig. 1.

Examination of the patterns of excretion of neutral steroids in the urine of mothers has shown that a steroid with the properties of 21-hydroxypregnenolone, though usually measurable, has not been prominent in pregnancy urine (Cathro *et al.*, 1963), and this is in agreement with the results of Pasqualini and Jayle (1962), though the average maternal excretion value established in this laboratory at 150 μg./24 hr., corrected for losses incurred during estimation, is somewhat above the level calculable from the data of the Paris workers. The slight difference is possibly due to the fact that the urine specimens analysed in this laboratory were collected during the 24 hours following delivery and may have reflected a temporary increase in adrenal activity.

This output of 21-hydroxypregnenolone by mothers is, nevertheless, small, and it has been the purpose of the present study to examine the excretion levels of this compound in a number of newborn infants, both normal controls and infants undergoing some form of physical stress during the first week of life, in an attempt to elucidate the clinical significance of the excretion of this $\Delta^5$-steroid in infancy urine. 21-hydroxypregnenolone and other neutral steroids have also been measured in the third day urine of a cryptorchid male infant with the type of salt-losing adrenogenital syndrome shown by Bongiovanni (1961) to be due to deficiency of the enzyme 3β-hydroxysteroid-dehydrogenase (3β-ol-dehydrogenase), and the results have contributed valuable circumstantial evidence towards the substantiation of a hypothesis which can explain the appreciable

* Communications on this subject have been presented at the Second and Third meetings of the Paediatric Endocrinology Club at Groningen, Holland, in May 1963, and at Hamburg, West Germany, in April 1964.

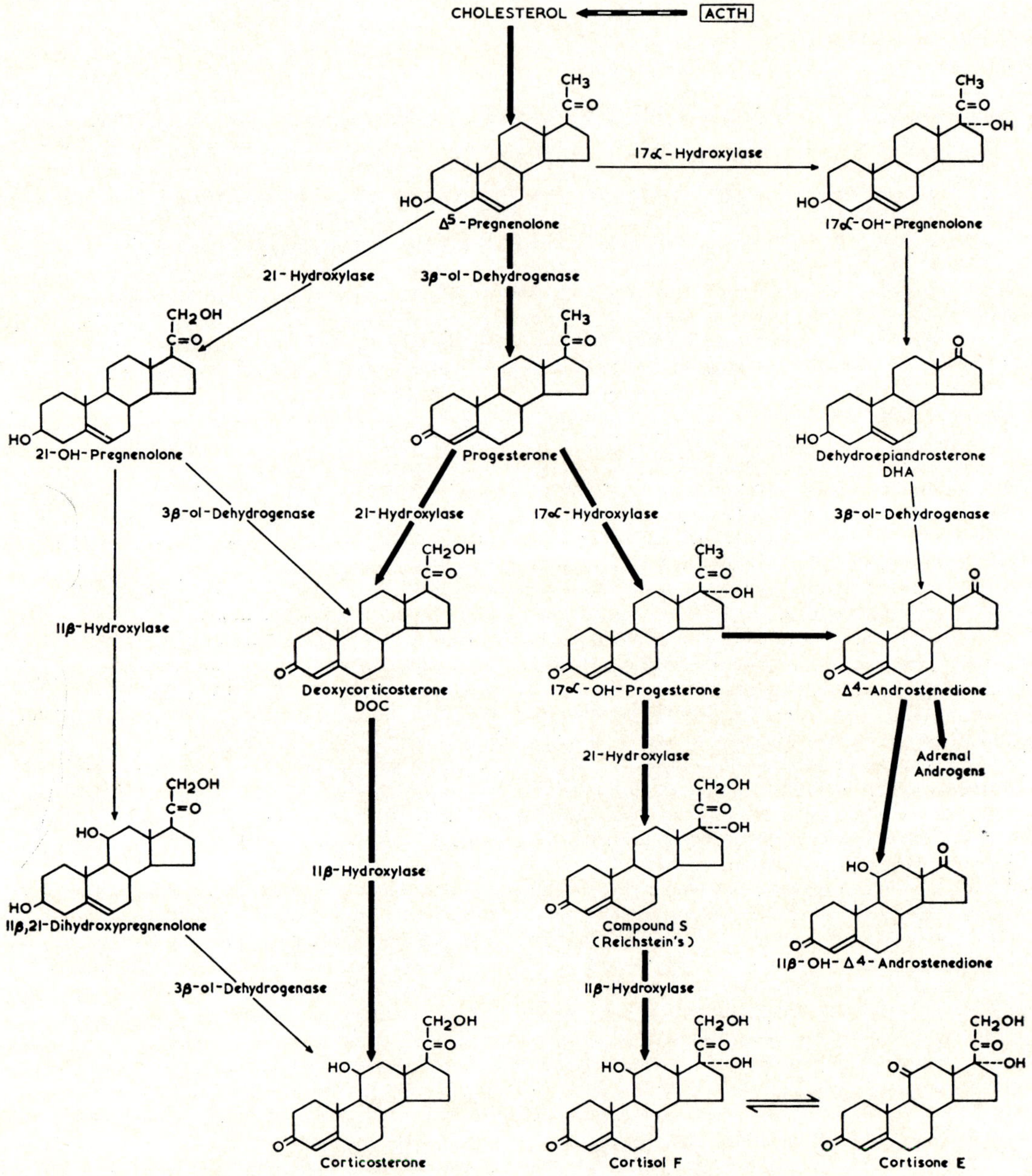


FIG. 1.—Biosynthesis of steroids in the adrenal glands.

excretion of $\Delta^5$-steroids by endocrinologically normal newborn infants.

## Materials and Method

Assays have been carried out only on 24-hour urine specimens considered to be complete, obtained from full-term and from premature male infants on days 1, 2, 3, and 6. One normal infant, born at term, has been studied at intervals up to the age of 3 weeks.

Urine has also been collected on days 1, 2, 3, and 6 from infants born to women with diabetes mellitus and from infants born to women with pre-diabetes. Mothers have been classified as 'diabetic' if they have required treatment with insulin or drugs following the puerperal period and as 'pre-diabetic' if drugs or insulin have been unnecessary following the birth of the baby as a result of improved carbohydrate tolerance.

We are indebted to Dr. W. Hamilton for the provision for analysis of a sample of urine obtained on the 3rd day of life from a patient diagnosed as a case of 3β-ol-dehydrogenase deficiency, and for permission to publish clinical and biochemical data pertaining to this patient. This infant, at birth, somewhat resembled a virilized female, being cryptorchid with scroto-labial folds, but the nuclear sex was male. The urethra opened at the tip of a small, hooded phallus. Urinary pregnanetriol excretion was not abnormal during the first three days of life nor were the plasma electrolytes at this stage. Total 17-oxosteroids were 4·3 mg./24 hr. on day 7 (Medical Research Council Committee on Clinical Endocrinology, 1951) in association with values of 5·2 mg./24 hr. for 17-hydroxycorticosteroids (Appleby, Gibson, Norymberski, and Stubbs, 1955) and 2·1 mg./24 hr. for 21-deoxyketols (Appleby and Norymberski, 1955). By the 9th day there were clinical and biochemical indications of incipient adrenal failure and satisfactory control was achieved by administration of salt, cortisone, and deoxycorticosterone acetate, both steroids being required in very high dosage. The history of salt-losing tendencies and other frank signs of hypoadrenalism in a male child with incomplete masculine development is similar to those recorded in published cases of 3β-ol-dehydrogenase deficiency in male infants (Bongiovanni and Eberlein, 1961; Bongiovanni, 1962; Bongiovanni and Clark, 1962; Bongiovanni and Root, 1963).

In all cases, following preliminary purification of the urinary extracts, the free steroids and those released by a two-stage enzyme hydrolysis have been chromatographed and subjected to staining techniques that have permitted their direct measurement on paper chromatograms (Birchall, Cathro, Forsyth, and Mitchell, 1963). Corrections for losses of steroid during the estimations have been applied on the basis of the recovery values for 4-$^{14}$C steroids added to the urine samples at the outset. Quantitation of 21-hydroxypregnenolone has been based on comparison of the colour developed by this steroid from urinary extracts with the colour developed by standard deoxycorticosterone following staining with blue tetrazolium. This practice has been unavoidable because of the difficulty in obtaining pure 21-hydroxypregnenolone from commercial sources. However, it is not likely to have given rise to significant error since the chromogenicity of pure 21-hydroxypregnenolone has been shown, on average, to be 86% of that of an equivalent quantity of deoxycorticosterone when both compounds have been stained with blue tetrazolium on paper under the same conditions. Similar values, ranging from 80-85% (average 82·8%) for the chromogenicity of 21-hydroxypregnenolone relative to deoxycorticosterone, have been obtained when the two steroids have been assayed in solution using a micro-modification of the reaction of Chen, Wheeler, and Tewell (1953). The values for 21-hydroxypregnenolone represented in the diagrams are therefore marginally low.

## Results

Measurement of 21-hydroxypregnenolone in 18 complete 24-hour urine specimens obtained on days 1, 2, or 3 from 10 normal infants born at term has given a range of values from 11·6 to 146 μg./24 hr. with an average value of 46·1 μg. The average output from 5 normal infants on day 6 has been found to be above this at 63·3 μg./24 hr. (range 14·4 to 129·5 μg.).

The output of 21-hydroxypregnenolone has also been studied in premature infants—prematurity having been arbitrarily defined on the basis of a birth weight of 2·5 kg. or less. Measurement of 21-hydroxypregnenolone in 12 complete 24-hour urine samples obtained on days 1, 2, or 3 from 6 premature infants in good clinical condition has given an average excretion value of 21·5 μg./24 hr. (range 4·3 to 57·6 μg.) for these days, while the 6th day levels from 5 of these infants have given an average value of 36·2 μg./24 hr. (range 3·0 to 69·8 μg.).

Infants who have endured undue stress during the neonatal period have also been studied. Most of these infants suffered moderate or severe asphyxia at the time of birth, while 3 were submitted to exchange transfusion on account of Rhesus incompatibility. The results show a wide scatter, and the average output of 21-hydroxypregnenolone at 59·3 μg./24 hr. (range 11·1 to 131·5 μg.) in 13 urine samples obtained during the first 3 days of life from 7 full-term infants in the stressed category cannot, therefore, be considered significantly higher than that of the normal infants.

Calculation of the daily steroid excretion of individual infants on a basis of body weight has allowed comparison of results from infants of widely differing birth weights, and the results are presented in Figs. 2 and 3. The values for days 1, 2, and 3 have been averaged in each case, and the symbol indicative of the output on day 6 has been joined to the symbol registering the average steroid output of the same infant during the first three days.

By the 6th day, the levels of 21-hydroxypregnenolone seem more often to have remained unchanged or to have risen than to have fallen, but all 3 trends have been observed. Of the two highest day 6 values measured in full-term infants (Fig. 2), one was obtained from a child who was severely asphyxiated at birth following a prolonged labour and a forceps delivery, and whose feeding and general vigour were not quite optimum even by the sixth day; the other high value was given by an infant who had an exchange transfusion at 4 hours.

The results from infants of low birth weight (Fig. 3) show that though there is a wide scatter, there has been a tendency for stressed infants to excrete more 21-hydroxypregnenolone during the first days of life

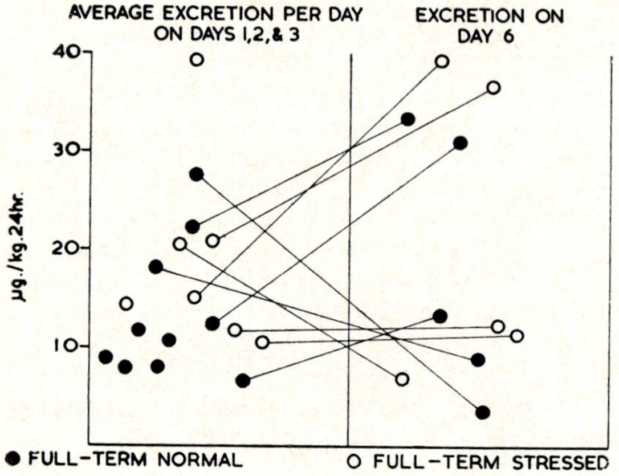


FIG. 2.—Urinary excretion of 21-OH-pregnenolone by full-term infants.

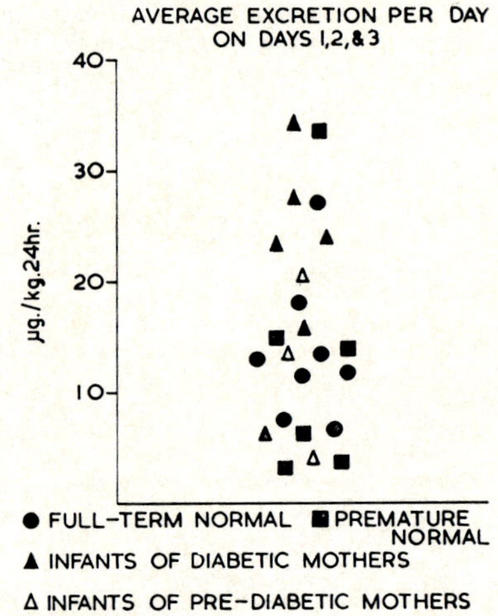


FIG. 4.—Urinary excretion of 21-OH-pregnenolone by infants of diabetic and pre-diabetic mothers, compared with normal term and premature infants.

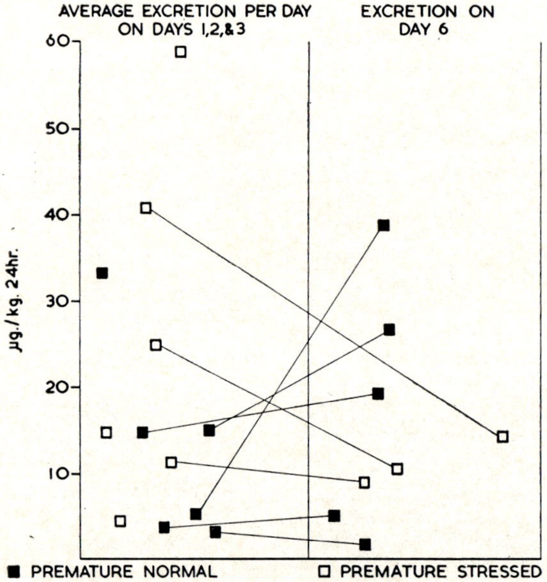


FIG. 3.—Urinary excretion of 21-OH-pregnenolone by premature infants.

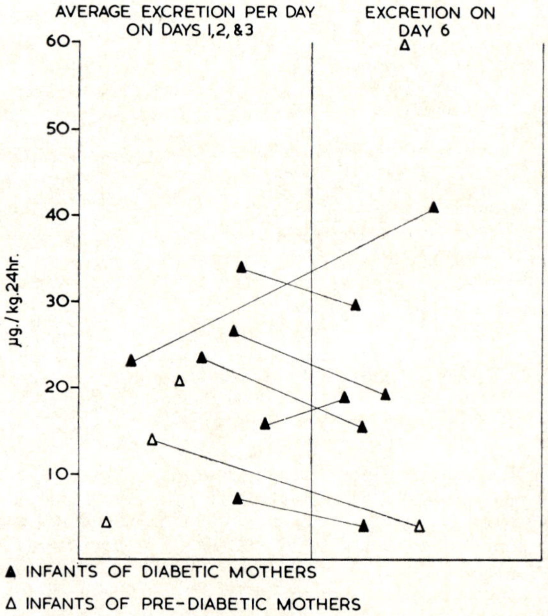


FIG. 5.—Urinary excretion of 21-OH-pregnenolone by infants of diabetic and pre-diabetic mothers.

than infants whose clinical condition has been entirely satisfactory.

The relatively high excretion of 21-hydroxypregnenolone by infants born to diabetic mothers is shown in Fig. 4. The prematurity of these infants (average gestational age between 36 and 37 weeks) may in part have contributed to the high values, but the suggestion of increased adrenal activity in this group cannot be ignored. It is noteworthy that in the urine of two diabetic mothers and in that of one pre-diabetic mother, the excretion of 21-hydroxypregnenolone was no higher than that in the urine of normal mothers. The output of 21-hydroxypregnenolone on day 6 in the infants of diabetic and pre-diabetic mothers is compared with the average output of this steroid during the first three days of life in Fig. 5.

The Table compares the excretion of neutral

TABLE

EXCRETION OF INDIVIDUAL STEROIDS ON DAY 3 BY NORMAL INFANTS AND BY AN INFANT WITH DEFICIENCY OF 3β-OL-DEHYDROGENASE (μg./kg. 24 hr.)

| Clinical Category | 21-OH-pregnenolone | DHA* | U | BT Reducing Steroids THF to F |
|---|---|---|---|---|
| 3β-ol-dehydrogenase deficiency | 132 | 30·3 | 133 | 885 |
| Full-term normal infants | 11·8 av. (5) † range 8·7-15·1 | 2 (7) range 0-4 | 6·5 (7) range 1-10·2 | 131 (11) range 46-322 |
| Full-term stressed infants | 16·2 av. (4) range 11-24 | 2·6 (9) range 1-6·7 | 11·9 (7) range 7·3-17·9 | 295 (9) range 103-879 |
| Full-term infants normal and stressed | 13·7 (9) range 8·7-24 | 2·3 (16) range 0-6·7 | 9 (15) range 1-17·9 | 205 (20) range 46-879 |
| Premature infants normal and stressed | 25·9 (6) range 2-74 | 3·8 (6) range 1·4-7·7 | 10 (15) range 4·9-21 | 246 (10) range 57-549 |
| Infants of diabetic mothers | 26·4 (6) range 4·7-54·6 | 3·3 (8) range 0·5-9·5 | 9·5 (7) range 1·8-19·2 | 360 (7) range 188-866 |
| Infants of pre-diabetic mothers | 7·3 (2) range 1·8-12·8 | 1·95 (3) range 0·5-2·8 | 4·14 (2) range 1·8-6·6 | 102 (3) range 92-112 |

*DHA = dehydroepiandrosterone.
† The numbers of urine specimens analysed are given in parentheses.
U = a Zimmermann-reacting compound with the $R_F$ value of 0·19 in the system LB 21/80.
BT = blue tetrazolium.
THF = tetrahydrocortisol—3α: 11β: 17α: 21-tetrahydroxy-5β-pregnan-20-one, $R_F$ value 0·067 in the system T/75.
F = cortisol —11β: 17α: 21-trihydroxypregn-4-ene-3: 20-dione, $R_F$ value 0·156 in the system T/75.

steroids in the 3rd day urine of normal infants and that of the male child diagnosed as a case of 3β-ol-dehydrogenase deficiency. In addition to values for 21-hydroxypregnenolone and for dehydroepiandrosterone (DHA)—known $\Delta^5$-steroids—values are included for an unknown Zimmermann-reacting compound (U), prominent in first-week urine, with a mobility similar to that of 11β-hydroxyandrost-4-ene-3: 17-dione in the Bush system LB 21/80. Values are also included for the complex of blue tetrazolium-reducing steroids with mobilities ranging from that of tetrahydrocortisol (0·067) to that of cortisol (0·156) in the Bush system T/75.

## Discussion

The biosynthetic pathways by which the major secretory products of the adrenal cortex are formed from cholesterol are now well known (Pincus, 1962). Cholesterol is initially degraded by side-chain scission to pregnenolone, most of which is then converted to progesterone, the corticosteroids, and the androgens (Fig. 1). Two possible pathways for adrenal androgen biosynthesis have been known for some years: one via pregnenolone, progesterone, 17α-hydroxyprogesterone, and androst-4-ene-3: 17-dione: the other via pregnenolone, 17α-hydroxypregnenolone, DHA, and androstenedione, by-passing 17α-hydroxyprogesterone (Neher and Wettstein, 1960; Dorfman, 1962; Pincus, 1962). However, it is only recently that the possibility of corticosteroid biosynthesis by means of secondary pathways from pregnenolone directly to 17α-hydroxypregnenolone or to 21-hydroxypregnenolone, by-passing progesterone, has been described (Berliner, Cazes, and Nabors, 1962; Berliner, Cazes, Nabors, and Dougherty, 1962; Mulrow, Cohn, Kuljian, and Ganong, 1962). The secondary pathway leading to corticosterone formation via 21-hydroxypregnenolone is illustrated in Fig. 1, which shows that in this alternative route for corticosteroid formation, the enzyme system 3β-ol-dehydrogenase takes part at a late stage, whereas in the major route, this enzyme acts prior to the sequence of 17α-, 21-, and 11β-hydroxylations.

The conclusions of Berliner and his colleagues were based on experiments with bovine adrenals, but the discovery of 21-hydroxypregnenolone in small quantities in human urine by the Paris workers (Pasqualini, 1962; Pasqualini and Jayle, 1962) signifies that this subsidiary pathway in which 21-hydroxylase acts directly upon pregnenolone also exists in man. It appears, however, to be of such slight importance in adult life that the occurrence of 21-hydroxylated steroids with the 3β-hydroxy formation in human urine had not been described until as recently as 1961, when Bongiovanni drew attention to the existence of an unidentified, highly polar, non-ketonic steroid, yielding formaldehyde on periodate oxidation, in the urine of an infant with congenital adrenal hyperplasia due to deficiency of 3β-ol-dehydrogenase.

The present study has shown that though 21-hydroxypregnenolone is not a major excretory product in the urine of normal newborn infants, it is nevertheless present in significant amounts. The higher average output of the compound on the 6th day than during the first 3 days of life in infants born at term, and the persistence of the compound in the urine of the one normal infant studied up to the age of 3 weeks, suggests that this steroid is synthesized by infants and that it is not entirely a vestigial product of some foetal or placental system for the biosynthesis or katabolism of steroids which has served its purpose by the time of birth. Two possible explanations exist for the excretion of this steroid in the urine of newborn infants. The first is that there may be increased utilization by the newborn infant of the biosynthetic pathway to corticosterone via 21-hydroxypregnenolone, with resultant overspill of some of the intermediary steroid into the urine. This hypothesis is in agreement with the relatively higher output of corticosterone and its metabolites than of cortisol and its metabolites demonstrable in infancy urine (Birchall *et al.*, 1961; Cathro *et al.*, 1963; Exley and Norymberski, 1963). Supportive evidence for increased use of the pathway via 21-hydroxypregnenolone during disproportionate corticosterone secretion by the adrenal gland has been given in the present study by analysis of pregnancy urine. Although the 21-hydroxypregnenolone output is insignificant in the urine of non-pregnant women, it is small, but easily measurable, during late pregnancy, and Norymberski (1961) has demonstrated that corticosterone secretion is likely to be increased out of proportion to the usual ratio with cortisol at this time when the urinary excretion of 17-deoxycorticosteroids (Exley, Ingall, Norymberski, and Woods, 1961) is rather high.

In pregnancy, both the foetal and the maternal circulations are supplied with large amounts of progesterone synthesized in the placenta (Woolever, Goldfien, and Page, 1961) and, by analogy with the kinetics of other enzyme systems that have been studied, excessive production of progesterone by another organ may inhibit the pregnenolone $\rightarrow$ progesterone stage in the adrenal glands of both foetus and mother, and result in an increased use of the secondary pathways via 21-hydroxypregnenolone or 17α-hydroxypregnenolone.

(If the pathway of cortisol synthesis via 17α-hydroxypregnenolone is of some importance in the non-pregnant woman (Mulrow *et al.*, 1962), increased use of it during pregnancy could give rise to an appreciable excretion of pregnenolone derivatives hydroxylated at C-17 and, possibly, elsewhere in the molecule. If pregnenolones hydroxylated at C-17 are more prominent than pregnenolones hydroxylated at C-21 in pregnancy urine, an explanation is suggested for the hitherto unexplained rise in the excretion of 21-deoxyketols during pregnancy (Appleby and Norymberski, 1957; Schüller, 1957). Likewise, increased excretion of any of the possible $\Delta^5$-pregnenes which may arise by direct hydroxylation of pregnenolone could account for the known rise in urinary Pettenkofer chromogens during pregnancy (Natoli, Nicolosi, and Magliocca, 1957). The possibility of a foetal contribution to the $\Delta^5$-steroids excreted by pregnant women must, however, be considered.)

In the case of the infant, following delivery, some rate-limiting factor in the pregnenolone $\rightarrow$ progesterone conversion could provide a second explanation for formation of 21-hydroxypregnenolone and the formation of the very considerable amounts of 16α-hydroxypregnenolone excreted in the urine of normal newborn infants (Reynolds, 1963b, 1964). A specific factor that would explain the presence of 3β-hydroxylated $\Delta^5$-pregnenes in infancy urine would be a slight or relative deficiency of the enzyme 3β-ol-dehydrogenase in the adrenal glands of the foetus, and the normal newborn infant, and this concept is supported by the results from incubation studies on foetal adrenal glands using pregnenolone as the substrate (Longchampt and Axelrod, 1963). Reynolds (1963a, b) believes that his results from the analysis of infancy urine also support this hypothesis. Enzyme studies on foetal adrenal glands have given evidence for the sequential appearance of the enzymes for 17α-hydroxylation, 21-hydroxylation, and 11β-hydroxylation of steroids at a stage when 3β-hydroxysteroid dehydrogenase activity has appeared to be lacking (Villee, 1963) and the large amount of progesterone synthesized by the placenta has again been under consideration as a possible inhibitory factor to the development of the latter system, or systems, in the foetus, since the possibility of different 3β-hydroxysteroid dehydrogenases for specific substrates has been raised (Weliky and Engel, 1963; Baillie and Griffiths, 1964).

Experiments carried out by Bloch and Benirschke (1962) who incubated slices of foetal zone and slices representative of both zones of foetal adrenal glands with acetate have suggested that 3β-ol-dehydrogenase activity is limited in both zones of adrenal tissue, at least before mid-gestation. Relatively slow development of the 3β-ol-dehydrogenase enzyme system has also been demonstrated in another foetal endocrine gland—the testis—by Acevedo, Axelrod, Ishikawa, and Takaki (1963) who have found that when tritiated 3β-hydroxypregn-5-ene-20-one has been used as the substrate in their incubations, relative deficiency of 3β-ol-dehydrogenase has been the major rate-limiting factor for the biosynthesis of androstenedione and, therefore, of testosterone.

The discovery of severe and persistent deficiency of this enzyme 3β-ol-dehydrogenase as a cause of a rare variant of the adrenogenital syndrome (Bongiovanni, 1961; Bongiovanni and Clark, 1962) has aroused considerable interest amongst paediatricians and has drawn attention to the advisability of studying the excretory pattern of 3β-hydroxy-$\Delta^5$-steroids in all patients in whom a diagnosis of any one of the variant forms of congenital adrenal hyperplasia is suspected (Jacobsohn, 1962). The availability of third-day urine from a child with this syndrome has provided the opportunity for comparison of the excretion of $\Delta^5$-steroids in the syndrome with the excretion levels of these steroids in normal infants and has provided further circumstantial evidence for the validity of the hypothesis of a relative deficiency of 3β-ol-dehydrogenase in all normal newborn infants. Diagnosis of this disorder by means of biochemical findings alone on the third day of life is not easy, and merely qualitative assays seem to be of little value, since the urinary steroid patterns from this child with 3β-ol-dehydrogenase deficiency have been found to resemble the complicated patterns of the normal newborn infant so closely that clinical evidence has been an equally valuable guide to the diagnosis. On theoretical grounds, all infants with the syndrome should produce excessive quantities of 21-hydroxypregnenolone, a steroid which, by virtue of its blue tetrazolium-reducing properties, is easily measurable on paper chromatograms.

The 21-hydroxypregnenolone excretion in the patient described in this report has been considered to be diagnostic as early as day 3. The Table shows that when the results have been expressed in μg./kg. body weight/24 hr. the patient has shown an excretion of 132 μg. against a normal value of 13·7 μg. (range 8·7-24 μg.)

In all published cases of the syndrome of 3β-ol-dehydrogenase deficiency, DHA excretion has been extremely high and diagnostic. Bongiovanni (1961) gave an excretion value of 3·1 mg./24 hr. in an affected infant at the age of 2 weeks but did not report the DHA excretion in a case in which the diagnosis was made at 7 days. Further information on the excretion of DHA during the early days of life in infants with this syndrome would be advantageous to the endocrinologist faced with making a decision on the optimum time for establishing the diagnosis of the disease by means of urinary steroid analysis, since, if a slight or relative deficiency of the enzyme is postulated in the healthy normal infant, some explanation must exist for the minimal excretion of DHA in the urine of endocrinologically normal infants during the first week of life (Birchall *et al.*, 1961; Cathro *et al.*, 1963). It is noteworthy that DHA has been reported to occur in large amounts in meconium (Francis, Shen, and Kinsella, 1960) and to attain higher levels in cord blood than in maternal blood (Migeon, Keller, and Holmstrom, 1955; Colás, Heinrichs, and Tatum, 1964), so that the small amounts found in the urine in the first week of life in the normal child can only be explained by a major excretion of DHA in the form of hydroxylated metabolites such as 16α-hydroxy-DHA (Reynolds, 1964). In this context it is also relevant to quote that Colás *et al.* (1964) have recently shown that 16α-hydroxy-DHA attains levels in foetal blood much higher than those of DHA itself. It has, therefore, been of importance to know whether such hydroxylation or other polyhydroxylation mechanisms in a child with severe enzyme deficiency of 3β-ol-dehydrogenase can mask the excessive DHA production and excretion and, therefore, the diagnosis, during the first days of life. Analysis of urine obtained from the infant reported suggests that hydroxylation of DHA and many of the other peculiarities of steroid metabolism characteristic of normal newborn infants also apply to infants with the syndrome. Nevertheless, estimation of individual compounds, in particular, DHA, 21-hydroxypregnenolone, and other $\Delta^5$-steroids can be used to establish the diagnosis with certainty even on the third day of life, if careful comparison on a quantitative basis is made with the results from normal controls.

The DHA excretion at 3 days in the patient studied was 101 μg./24 hr. in contrast to the milligramme amounts found by Bongiovanni (1961) at 2 weeks in another patient. The day 3 excretion value for DHA in 20 full-term normal infants has been found to average 7·9 μg./24 hr. (range 0 to 21·3 μg.), and thus though DHA excretion in the patient was much less than that reported in other patients with the disorder, it was still five times greater than the highest value in the normal range.

The high excretion of the compound designated U in the Table in the infant with 3β-ol-dehydrogenase deficiency is of interest, since it contributes circumstantial evidence towards this normal constituent of first-week urine having a $\Delta^5$-structure. Information on this compound which is of medium polarity and which gives a greyish-purple Zimmermann colour has already been published (Cathro *et al.*, 1963). It has an ultraviolet absorption maximum at 232 mμ, gives a positive Pettenkofer reaction, and is likely to be a $\Delta^5$-steroid with a hydroxyl group at carbon atom 3.

It has been shown that the pattern of the more polar blue tetrazolium-reducing steroids excreted by newborn infants is extremely complicated (Cathro *et al.*, 1963) and that tetrahydrocortisol and tetrahydrocortisone—the most abundant corticosteroids in the urine of adults—are not the dominant reducing steroids during the first three days of life. In chromatograms of infancy urine, obtained during days 1 to 3, compounds with the mobilities of tetrahydrocortisol and tetrahydrocortisone are less prominent than another reducing compound which is slightly more polar than tetrahydrocortisone.

Another unknown reducing steroid prominent only in the first few days of life has a mobility between that of tetrahydrocortisone and that of cortisol (Cathro *et al.*, 1963). There is evidence, however, for the existence of tetrahydrocortisone in the urine of newborn infants, the proportion of this compound steadily increasing with advancing age (Bertrand, Loras, Gilly, and Cautenet, 1963; Kenny, Malvaux, and Migeon, 1963; Cathro *et al.*, 1963; Cathro, 1964). The values given in the Table represent the total blue tetrazolium-reducing compounds of this order of polarity, namely, those with $R_F$ values ranging from 0·06 to 0·2 in the Bush system T/75 under strictly controlled conditions (Birchall *et al.*, 1963; Cathro, Cameron and Birchall, 1965). Possible $\Delta^5$-constituents of this group of compounds, on theoretical grounds, are 3β: 7α: 16α-trihydroxyandrost-5-ene-17-one, 3β: 16α-dihydroxandrost-5-ene-7: 17-one, 3β: 17α: 21-trihydroxypregn-5-ene-20-one and 3β: 16α: 21: trihydroxypregn-5-ene-20-one, the first of which Bongiovanni (1961) has postulated may be present in the urine of infants with congenital adrenal hyperplasia due to deficiency of 3 β-ol-dehydrogenase. The values listed in the Table are, therefore, likely to be largely indicative of $\Delta^5$-steroid excretion.

Thus, though superficial examination of the corticoid fraction of the urine from the infant with 3β-ol-dehydrogenase deficiency revealed no obvious abnormality, and the complicated patterns of the more polar blue tetrazolium-reducing steroids did not differ significantly from those expected on the third day of life, the Table shows that quantitation of reducing steroid in the tetrahydrocortisol to cortisol area indicates that more was present than was found in control infants whose delivery had been normal and whose course up to day 3 had been uneventful. The marked increase in excretion of these compounds by an infant with severe 3β-ol-dehydrogenase deficiency provides further circumstantial evidence for a high proportion of the unusual blue tetrazolium reducing steroids of this order of polarity found in the urine of normal newborn infants being $\Delta^5$-compounds, resulting from a relative or mild deficiency of 3β-ol dehydrogenase which is physiological in the neonatal period of life.

During analysis of the urine from the affected infant for corticosteroids giving sodium fluorescence, excessive amounts of interfering material were obtained on the chromatograms. The physiologically active $\Delta^4$-corticosteroids, cortisol, cortisone, and corticosterone, or at least steroids with their properties, were present in amounts in the upper part of the wide normal range. These steroids probably represented a maternal or a placental contribution. It is at least possible, on theoretical grounds, that some of these corticosteroids could have been synthesized in the adrenal glands of the affected infant directly from progesterone produced in the placenta. It is noteworthy that signs of incipient adrenal failure were not evident until the ninth day.

Though this study has shown that it is possible to make an accurate diagnosis of the rare condition of permanent 3β-ol-dehydrogenase deficiency by means of elaborate biochemical techniques as early as the third day of life, clinical and theoretical evidence both suggest that the detailed urinary analysis should be deferred until the sixth or seventh day, by which time the urinary steroid patterns become less complicated. During these first few days it is essential to keep a close watch on the clinical condition of the infant and on the plasma electrolytes, since supportive measures may be required soon thereafter to prevent the onset of frank adrenal failure.

## Summary

The occurrence of the steroid 3β: 21-dihydroxypregn-5-ene-20-one in the urine of normal newborn infants is interpreted as signifying that the newborn infant makes use of a pathway for the biosynthesis of corticosteroids involving 21-hydroxypregnenolone which is of little importance in the adult. It is suggested that the significant excretion of $\Delta^5$-steroids by normal newborn infants reflects a relative deficiency of the enzyme 3β-hydroxysteroid dehydrogenase in the adrenal glands at this stage of life.

Although normal newborn infants have a high output of steroids retaining the $\Delta^5$-structure, quantitative comparison of the individual neutral steroids excreted by normal infants and by an infant with permanent deficiency of 3β-hydroxysteroid dehydrogenase has made it possible to diagnose this endocrine abnormality with certainty as early as the third day of life, because of the much greater quantities of $\Delta^5$-steroids excreted by this infant.

This research programme has been supported by a grant from the Scottish Hospital Endowments Research Trust. We have to thank Professor J. L. Henderson for his support and encouragement. We are indebted to Dr. W. Hamilton of the Department of Child Health, University of Glasgow, for provision of a urine specimen from an infant suffering from 3β-ol-dehydrogenase deficiency. We wish to thank Mrs. J. Cameron, Miss M. Philp, and Mr. I. Roberts for technical assistance. Helpful advice has been given by Dr. J. R. Pasqualini.

### References

Acevedo, H. F., Axelrod, L. R., Ishikawa, E., and Takaki, F. (1963). Studies in fetal metabolism. II. Metabolism of progesterone-4-$C^{14}$ and pregnenolone-7α-$H^3$ in human fetal testes. *J. clin. Endocr.*, **23**, 885.

Appleby, J. I., Gibson, G., Norymberski, J. K., and Stubbs, R. D. (1955). Indirect analysis of corticosteroids. I. The determination of 17-hydroxycorticosteroids. *Biochem. J.*, **60**, 453.

——, and Norymberski, J. K. (1955). Indirect analysis of corticosteroids. 2. The determination and identification of urinary 17-hydroxy-20-oxosteroids unsubstituted at $C_{(21)}$. *ibid.*, **60**, 460.

——, —— (1957). The urinary excretion of 17-hydroxycorticosteroids in human pregnancy. *J. Endocr.*, **15**, 310.

Baillie, A. H., and Griffiths, K. (1964). 3β-hydroxysteroid dehydrogenase activity in the mouse Leydig cell. *ibid.*, **29**, 9.

Berliner, D. L., Cazes, D. M., and Nabors, C. J., Jr. (1962). Adrenal 3β-hydroxysteroid dehydrogenase activity on $C_{17}$-hydroxylated $\triangle^5$-pregnenes, $C_{21}$-hydroxylated $\triangle^5$-pregnenes, or both. *J. biol. Chem.*, **237**, 2478.

——, ——, ——, and Dougherty, T. F. (1962). Conversion of $\triangle^5$-pregnene-3β, 21-diol-20-one to DOC and $\triangle^5$-pregnene-3β, 17α, 21-triol-20-one to 'S' of Reichstein by the adrenal gland. *Fed. Proc.*, **21**, 184.

Bertrand, J., Loras, B., Gilly, R., and Cautenet, B. (1963). Contribution á l'étude de la sécrétion et du métabolisme du cortisol chez le nouveau-né et le nourrisson de moins de trois mois. *Path. et Biol.*, **11**, 997.

Birchall, K., Cathro, D. M., Forsyth, C. C., and Mitchell, F. L. (1961). Separation and estimation of adrenal steroids in the urine of newborn infants. *Lancet*, **1**, 26.

——, ——, ——, —— (1963). A method for the separation and estimation of neutral steroids in the urine of newborn infants. *J. Endocr.*, **27**, 31.

Bloch, E., and Benirschke, K. (1962). Steroidogenic capacity of foetal adrenals *in vitro*. In *The Human Adrenal Cortex*, ed. A. R. Currie, T. Symington, and J. K. Grant, p. 589. Livingstone, Edinburgh.

Bongiovanni, A. M. (1961). Unusual steroid pattern in congenital adrenal hyperplasia: deficiency of 3β-hydroxy dehydrogenase. *J. clin. Endocr.*, **21**, 860.

—— (1962). The adrenogenital syndrome with deficiency of 3β-hydroxysteroid dehydrogenase. *J. clin. Invest.*, **41**, 2086.

——, and Clark, A. (1962). Urinary $\triangle^5$-pregnene-3β, 17α, 20α, 21-tetrol in 3β-ol-dehydrogenase deficiency. *ibid.*, **41**, 1346.

——, and Eberlein, W. R. (1961). Defects in steroidal metabolism of subjects with adrenogenital syndrome. *Metabolism*, **10**, 917.

——, and Root, A. W. (1963). The adrenogenital syndrome (continued). *New Engl. J. Med.*, **268**, 1342.

Cathro, D. M. (1964). A Study of Adrenocortical Function in Newborn Infants. Thesis submitted for the degree of M.D., University of Edinburgh.

——, Birchall, K., Mitchell, F. L., and Forsyth, C. C. (1963). The excretion of neutral steroids in the urine of newborn infants. *J. Endocr.*, **27**, 53.

——, Cameron, J., and Birchall, K. (1965). The application of paper chromatography to the study of steroid structure. *J. Chromatog.*, **17**, 362.

Chen, C., Wheeler, J., and Tewell, H. E., Jr. (1953). Methods of estimation of adrenal cortical steroids with tetrazolium salts. *J. Lab. clin. Med.*, **42**, 749.

Colás, A., Heinrichs, W. L., and Tatum, H. J. (1964). Pettenkofer chromogens in the maternal and fetal circulations: detection of 3β, 16α-dihydroxy-androst-5-en-17-one in umbilical cord blood. *Steroids*, **3**, 417.

Dorfman, R. I. (1962). Androgen biosynthesis in adrenal tumours. In *The Human Adrenal Cortex*, eds. A. R. Currie, T. Symington, and J. K. Grant, p. 93. Livingstone, Edinburgh.

Exley, D., Ingall, S. C., Norymberski, J. K., and Woods, G. F. (1961). Indirect analysis of corticosteroids. 5. The determination of 17-deoxycorticosteroids. *Biochem. J.*, **81**, 428.

——, and Norymberski, J. K. (1963). The urinary excretion of 17-deoxycorticosteroids. In *Abstracts of papers presented at the International Symposium on Steroids, Rome, 1963*, p. 40. Arti Grafiche Capaccetti, Rome.

Francis, F. E., Shen, N. C., and Kinsella, R. A., Jr. (1960). Enteric excretion of metabolites of steroid hormones in the human. II. Isolation of $\triangle^5$-androsten-3β-ol-17-one from meconium. *J. biol. Chem.*, **235**, 1957.

Jacobsohn, G. M. (1962). Isolation of 5-pregnenediol from the urine of a patient with congenital adrenocortical hyperplasia. *J. clin. Endocr.*, **22**, 859.

Kenny, F. M., Malvaux, P., and Migeon, C. J. (1963). Cortisol production rate in newborn babies, older infants, and children. *Pediatrics*, **31**, 360.

Longchampt, J., and Axelrod, L. R. (1963). Contribution to steroids biosynthesis in human adrenal. In *Abstracts of papers presented at the International Symposium on Steroids, Rome, 1963*, p. 18. Arti Grafiche Capaccetti, Rome.

Medical Research Council Committee on Clinical Endocrinology (1951). Proposed standard method of 17-ketosteroid determination. *Lancet*, **2**, 585.

Migeon, C. J., Keller, A. R., and Holmstrom, E. G. (1955). Dehydroepiandrosterone, androsterone and 17-hydroxycorticosteroid levels in maternal and cord plasma in cases of vaginal delivery. *Bull. Johns Hopk. Hosp.*, **97**, 415.

Mulrow, P. J., Cohn, G. L., Kuljian, A. A., and Ganong, W. F. (1962). Incorporation of 17-hydroxy-pregnenolone-$H^3$ into cortisol by the human adrenal in vitro and by the dog adrenal in vivo. *J. clin. Invest.*, **41**, 1388.

Natoli, A., Nicolosi, G., and Magliocca, R. (1957). In tema di rapporti tra corticosurrene e gravidanza: l'eliminazione urinaria degli steroidi chetonici Zimmermann—e Pettenkofer—reagenti in donne gravide nei vari mesi di gestazione. *Quad. Clin. ostet. ginec.*, **12**, 31.

Neher, R., and Wettstein, A. (1960). Occurrence of $\triangle^5$-3β-hydroxysteroids in adrenal and testicular tissue. *Acta endocr.* (*Kbh.*), **35**, 1.

Norymberski, J. K. (1961). Methods of group corticosteroid estimation in urine—II. In *The Adrenal Cortex*, ed. G. K. McGowan and M. Sandler, p. 88. Pitman, London.

Pasqualini, J. R. (1962). *Contribution à l'Étude Biochimique des Corticostéroïdes*. R. Foulon, Paris.

——, and Jayle, M. F. (1962). Identification of 3β, 21-dihydroxy-5-pregnene-20-one disulfate in human urine. *J. clin. Invest.*, **41**, 981.

Pincus, G. (1962). The metabolism and mode of action of the adrenocortical hormones: Introductory review. In *The Human Adrenal Cortex*, ed. A. R. Currie, T. Symington, and J. K. Grant, p. 85. Livingstone, Edinburgh.

Reynolds, J. W. (1963a). Salt-losing congenital adrenal hyperplasia with a mixed enzymatic defect. *J. Pediat.*, **63**, 718.

—— (1963b). Isolation of 16 OH pregnenolone from urine of newborn infants. *Proc. Soc. exp. Biol.* (*N.Y.*), **113**, 980.

—— (1964). The isolation of 16-ketoandrostenediol (3β, 17β-dihydroxyandrost-5-en-16-one) from the urine of a newborn infant. *Steroids*, **3**, 77.

Schüller, E. (1957). Corticosteroid-Ausscheidung in der normälen Gravidität. *Acta endocr.* (*Kbh.*), **25**, 345.

Villee, C. A. (1963). The development of enzyme systems. *Acta paediat.* (*Uppsala*), **52**, 205.

Weliky, I., and Engel, L. L. (1963). Metabolism of progesterone-4-$C^{14}$ and pregnenolone-7α-$H^3$ by human adrenal tissue. Formation of 16α-hydroxyprogesterone-$C^{14}$, corticosterone-$C^{14}$, and cortisol-$C^{14}$-$H^3$. *J. biol. Chem.*, **238**, 1302.

Woolever, C. A., Goldfien, A., and Page, E. W. (1961). Studies of the isolated perfused human placenta. II. Progesterone content of perfusates. *Amer. J. Obstet. Gynec.*, **81**, 1137.


## Appendix

The following terms for trivial names have been used in the illustrations and in the text.

| | |
|---|---|
| Androstenedione | Androst-4-ene-3: 17-dione |
| Corticosterone | 11β: 21-Dihydroxypregn-4-ene-3: 20-dione |
| Cortisol (F) | 11β: 17α: 21-Trihydroxypregn-4-ene-3: 20-dione |
| Cortisone | 17α: 21-Dihydroxypregn-4-ene-3: 11: 20-trione |
| Dehydroepiandrosterone (DHA) | 3β-Hydroxyandrost-5-ene-17-one |
| Deoxycorticosterone | 21-Hydroxypregn-4-ene-3: 20-dione |
| 16α-Hydroxydehydroepiandrosterone | 3β: 16α-Dihydroxyandrost-5-ene-17-one |

| | |
|---|---|
| 16α-Hydroxypregnenolone | 3β: 16α-Dihydroxypregn-5-ene-20-one |
| 17α-Hydroxypregnenolone | 3β: 17α-Dihydroxypregn-5-ene-20-one |
| 21-Hydroxypregnenolone | 3β: 21-Dihydroxypregn-5-ene-20-one |
| 17α-Hydroxyprogesterone | 17α-Hydroxypregn-4-ene-3: 20-dione |
| Pregnanetriol | 3α: 17α: 20α-Trihydroxy-5β-pregnane |
| Pregnenolone | 3β-Hydroxypregn-5-ene-20-one |
| Progesterone | Pregn-4-ene-3: 20-dione |
| Testosterone | 17β-Hydroxyandrost-4-ene-3-one |
| Tetrahydrocortisol (THF) | 3α: 11β: 17α: 21-Tetrahydroxy-5β-pregnan-20-one |
| Tetrahydrocortisone | 3α: 17α: 21-Trihydroxy-5β-pregnan-11: 20-dione. |

*Arch. Dis. Childh.*, 1965, **40**, 261.

# ALDOSTERONE AND 17-HYDROXYCORTICOSTEROID EXCRETION FOLLOWING RAMSTEDT'S OPERATION

BY

WILLIAM HAMILTON

*From the University Department of Child Health and the Royal Hospital for Sick Children, Glasgow*

(RECEIVED FOR PUBLICATION NOVEMBER 5, 1964)

The management of infants with pyloric stenosis has local variations. In this department a régime of simplicity has been adopted in which the patient is disturbed as little as possible. The diagnosis is made on palpation of a pyloric 'tumour' during a test feed, and only rarely is diagnostic assistance sought from a barium meal.

A gastric lavage is done not less than four hours before operation. Pyloromyotomy is performed under general or local anaesthesia according to the surgeon's preference and the child is returned to the medical ward. Feeding is recommenced 4 hours after operation with 8 ml. half-cream National Dried Milk alternating hourly with half-strength physiological saline in unrestricted quantities. The volume of milk is gradually increased and also the interval between feeds until on the third post-operative day 45 ml. milk is being given 4-hourly. Water at this stage is given instead of saline. On subsequent days the volume of each milk feed is increased by 15 ml. until an appropriate full feed is reached. The child is discharged on the 5th post-operative day and returns on the 12th day for removal of sutures. Breast-fed infants are given expressed breast milk and allowed home usually on the 2nd post-operative day to continue breast-feeding. The sutures are also removed on the 12th post-operative day.

Biochemical studies are not done routinely and parenteral fluid and electrolyte replacements are undertaken only in the infrequent cases in which dehydration is severe.

During the past 4 years 58 cases, on average, have been treated annually in this unit with one death (a mortality rate of less than 0·5%).

The present study was designed to assess the adrenocortical response to the acute stress of pyloromyotomy as measured by the urinary 17-hydroxycorticosteroid excretion, and to determine the level of free aldosterone excretion in infants.

## Material and Methods

The series comprises 27 male infants with pyloric stenosis admitted to the Royal Hospital for Sick Children, Glasgow. Each child had, on admission, a length of ½ in. (1·27 cm.) wide Paul's tubing secured over the penis with 'Sleek'. The free end was knotted and the urine which collected was transferred at intervals to suitable containers. Five consecutive 24-hour urine collections were made using chloroform as preservative. Urinary 17-hydroxycorticosteroids (17-OHCS) were estimated by Few's (1961) method. Recovery rates were consistently over 80% using cortisol as a model compound. Aldosterone was measured by soda-fluorescence using Brooks' (1960) technique. Recovery rates ranged from 38 to 77%. The fluorimetric readings for standard aldosterone diacetate were linear in the range 0·5 to 2·0 $\mu$g.

## Results and Discussion

**17-Hydroxycorticosteroids.** In non-stressful conditions the pituitary and adrenal cortex act together to maintain optimal plasma cortisol levels. This mechanism is altered during major surgical procedures. Under such stress the pituitary gland continues to secrete ACTH despite a rise in plasma cortisol. An increased urinary excretion of 17-OHCS follows (Tyler, Schmidt, Eik-Nes, Brown, and Samuels, 1954).

In Table 1 the daily urinary 17-OHCS excretion in 12 male infants following pyloromyotomy is shown. Depending on the time of admission of the individual case, pyloromyotomy might have been performed at any time within 24 hours of admission. Any increase in adrenocortical secretion due to the operation in such cases might, therefore, increase the output of urinary 17-OHCS within the first 24 hours. Except for Cases 1 and 3, those with a first day excretion greater than 1 mg. 17-OHCS had the operation within 24 hours of admission. Cases 1 to 8 excreted more than 5 mg. 17-OHCS/24 hours on at least one day in the post-operative period. In Cases

TABLE 1

URINARY 17-HYDROXYCORTICOSTEROID IN CASES OF PYLORIC STENOSIS TREATED BY RAMSTEDT OPERATION

| Case | Age (wk.) | Duration of Vomiting | Birth Weight (kg.) | Admission Weight (kg.) | Anaesthetic | Urinary 17-hydroxycorticosteroids (mg./24 hr.) | | | | | Maximum Daily Excretion (mg./kg. day) |
|---|---|---|---|---|---|---|---|---|---|---|---|
| | | | | | | 1 | 2 | 3 | 4 | 5 | |
| 1 | 9 | 6 wk. | 3·2 | 4·0 | General | 1·8 | 7·1 | 4·8 | 4·3 | 1·9 | 1·77 |
| 2 | 4 | 4 wk. | 3·2 | 3·34 | General | *1·5 | 6·4 | 4·2 | 4·4 | 1·2 | 1·91 |
| 3 | 4 | 2 wk. | 2·86 | 3·2 | General | 1·9 | 7·4 | 7·1 | 4·3 | 2·1 | 2·3 |
| 4 | 8 | 6 wk. | 2·72 | 3·12 | General | *1·2 | 6·1 | 3·5 | 2·3 | 1·3 | 1·95 |
| 5 | 8 | 3 wk. | 3·5 | 5·0 | General | 0·7 | 5·5 | 0·6 | 1·2 | 0·8 | 1·1 |
| 6 | 4 | 2 wk. | 3·2 | 3·2 | General | 0·4 | 6·5 | 1·3 | 1·3 | — | 2·03 |
| 7 | 4 | 7 dy. | 2·44 | 2·64 | Local | *3·4 | 5·8 | 2·6 | 4·0 | 2·6 | 2·19 |
| 8 | 4 | 8 dy. | 3·4 | 3·56 | General | 0·8 | 5·6 | 2·0 | 1·6 | 1·6 | 1·57 |
| 9 | 3 | 10 dy. | 2·58 | 2·15 | General | *1·6 | 0·7 | 1·3 | 2·8 | 3·4 | 1·58 |
| 10 | 2 | 6 dy. | 3·3 | 3·02 | Local | 0·5 | 1·8 | 1·9 | 3·6 | 2·4 | 1·19 |
| 11 | 7 | 7 dy. | 3·85 | 3·45 | General | *1·2 | 3·1 | 3·7 | 2·2 | 2·0 | 1·07 |
| 12 | 5 | 10 dy. | 3·68 | 3·42 | General | 0·3 | 3·6 | 2·1 | 2·3 | — | 1·05 |

A dash (—) indicates incomplete urine collection.
* Operation within 24 hours of admission.

9 to 12 urinary 17-OHCS were less than 5 mg./24 hours. The degree of adrenal response to operation in Cases 1 to 8 as measured by urinary 17-OHCS parallels that expected from a standard corticotrophin stimulation test in the same age-group (author's findings to be published).

It will further be noted from Table 1 that a greater response was seen in those infants who were above their birth weight and in whom vomiting had been less severe though persistent and often over a longer period. The nature of block estimations for urinary steroid metabolites imposes restrictions on the further interpretation of results, but it will be seen that all the cases studied had a maximum excretion of 1-2 mg. 17-OHCS/kg. on at least one day immediately following pyloromyotomy.

**Aldosterone.** The estimation of aldosterone by the method used involves three chromatographic systems. Small losses occur inevitably at various stages and it is necessary to measure the final percentage recovery. This is done by adding 10 mμc (millimicrocurie) 7-$H^3$-aldosterone to the urine before extraction and measuring the specific activity of an aliquot of the diacetate fraction. Another aliquot of this fraction, containing approximately the same amount of aldosterone as the standards to be used, is applied to the final chromatogram. Since the amount of aldosterone likely to be encountered was not known, the optimum aliquot applied to the final chromatograph was found by trial and error. In the early experiments, using 24-hour urine volumes, insignificantly different galvanometer readings for blank and fluorescence were obtained, even when using three-quarters of the aldosterone extract and with satisfactory recovery rates. Subsequently, the urine from each patient was bulked for 5 consecutive 24-hour periods and the daily excretion of free aldosterone taken as one-fifth of the total. Thus in only 7 of the 15 cases studied were reliable results obtained (Table 2). With recovery rates ranging from 43 to 75%, the daily urinary excretion of free aldosterone ranged from 0·6 to 3 μg.

In Table 3 the calculated excretion of free aldosterone for the first 24-hour period in Cases 1-7 is shown.

TABLE 2

URINARY EXCRETION OF FREE ALDOSTERONE IN CASES OF PYLORIC STENOSIS TREATED BY RAMSTEDT OPERATION

| Case No. | Age (wk.) | Urinary Aldosterone (μg.) | | |
|---|---|---|---|---|
| | | 5-day Total | Per Day | Per Day Corrected* |
| 1-7 | | Aldosterone not detected in single 24-hour collections | | |
| 8 | 11 | 11·5 | 2·3 | 3·0 |
| 9 | 6 | 3·0 | 0·6 | 1·0 |
| 10 | 5 | 2·0 | 0·4 | 0·6 |
| 11 | 5 | 2·5 | 0·5 | 1·0 |
| 12 | 3 | 3·0 | 0·6 | 0·8 |
| 13 | 10 | 2·5 | 0·5 | 1·1 |
| 14 | 10 | Nil | — | — |
| 15 | 7 | 7·5 | 1·5 | 2·7 |

* Corrected according to individual recovery rates, which were from 43 to 75%.

TABLE 3

DAILY EXCRETION OF FREE ALDOSTERONE CALCULATED FROM RECOVERY RATES AND FLUORIMETER SENSITIVITY: TOTAL SINGLE 24-HOUR URINE SPECIMENS WERE EXTRACTED

| Case No. | % Recovery | Aliquot of Extract Applied | Calculated Daily Aldosterone Excreted (μg.) |
|---|---|---|---|
| 1 | 54 | 0·25 | 0·7 |
| 2 | 46 | 0·25 | 0·8 |
| 3 | 60 | 0·25 | 0·6 |
| 4 | 60 | 0·5 | 0·3 |
| 5 | 58 | 0·5 | 0·3 |
| 6 | 38 | 0·75 | 0·35 |
| 7 | 62 | 0·75 | 0·2 |

The average paper blank reading in each experiment was equivalent to 0·3 μg. aldosterone. Under test conditions a ratio of 1 to 4 for blank to aldosterone diacetate standard readings was consistently achieved by a minimum of 0·5 μg. amounts. While readings could be obtained for 0·1 μg. aldosterone diacetate a 'noise to signal' ratio of at least 1 to 4 was accepted as a better working rule. It will be seen from Tables 2 and 3 that the calculated daily excretion of free aldosterone and that actually found from bulked 5-day collections of urine are in agreement, and in each case the daily urinary excretion is 3 μg. or less.

The fractions of aldosterone appearing in the urine are free aldosterone, a Δ4-3-oxoconjugate split by acid hydrolysis to yield free aldosterone, and a metabolite, tetrahydroaldosterone conjugated with glucuronic acid. Only the first two fractions are estimated by the method used, and together these fractions represent 5-15% of the total daily secretion of aldosterone by the adrenal cortex (Ross, 1959; Jones, Lloyd-Jones, Riondel, Tait, Tait, Bulbrook, and Greenwood, 1959). Thus daily secretion rates for aldosterone from 5-60 μg. might be expected in infants up to 3 months of age.

Data on the aldosterone secretion rate for infants in this age-group are scant, but Degenhart, Visser, Wilmink, and Croughs (1965), using the double isotope dilution technique of Kliman and Peterson (1960), found the aldosterone secretion rate to be 60 μg./24 hours and 13·5 μg./24 hours in two infants, aged 2 months and 4 months respectively. After 4 to 6 days of salt deprivation the secretion rates were 100 μg./24 hours and 225 μg./24 hours, respectively. In the present series all the urine collections for aldosterone estimation were made after the operation and during the period when an increased salt intake was encouraged. Indeed all cases received during the 3 days after operation more salt than would have been contained in standard milk feeds appropriate for the infants' ages. This might have depressed aldosterone production. It is clear that only small amounts of free aldosterone appear in the urine in this age-group and thus more helpful information will be obtained from the estimation or urinary tetrahydroaldosterone or from measurement of the aldosterone secretion rate.

**Summary**

The daily urinary 17-hydroxycorticosteroid (17-OHCS) excretion was followed during the 5 days following pyloromyotomy in 12 infants with pyloric stenosis treated surgically, and attempts were made to estimate the daily excretion of free aldosterone in 15.

Higher urinary levels of 17-OHCS, of 5 mg. and more per day, were observed in infants who had a more favourable clinical assessment. In these vomiting had been less severe though of longer duration.

Insufficient free aldosterone appears in the urine to permit estimation on a single 24-hour specimen. Using total 5-day urine collections, a free aldosterone excretion of 0·6 to 3 μg. per day was found. It is suggested that measurement of daily aldosterone secretion rates or of urinary tetrahydroaldosterone would yield more helpful information.

I wish to thank Professor J. H. Hutchison for his encouragement in the preparation of this paper and for permission to publish these results from his patients. Thanks are also due to Professor Ivor H. Mills for his helpful criticism of this work, The sodium fluorimeter was made by Mr. D. Rowan, Regional Physics Department of the Western Regional Hospital Board. Part of the expense of these investigations was defrayed by the Rankin Funds of the University of Glasgow.

REFERENCES

Brooks, R. V. (1960). A method for the determination of aldosterone. *Mem. Soc. Endocr.*, **8**, 9.

Degenhart, H. J., Visser, H. K. A., Wilmink, R., and Croughs, W. (1965). Aldosterone and hydrocortisone secretion rates in infants and children with congenital adrenal hyperplasia indicating different degrees of 21-hydroxylation defects in salt-losers and non-salt-losers. Proc. Third Meeting of the European Pediatric Endocrinology Club held at Hamburg, 1964. *Acta endocr.* (*Kbh.*), Suppl. In the press.

Few, J. D. (1961). A method for the analysis of urinary 17-hydroxy-corticosteroids. *J. Endocr.*, **22**, 31.

Jones, K. M., Lloyd-Jones, R., Riondel, A., Tait, J. F., Tait, S. A. S., Bulbrook, R. D., and Greenwood, F. C. (1959). Aldosterone secretion and metabolism in normal men and women and in pregnancy. *Acta endocr.* (*Kbh.*), **30**, 321.

Kliman, B., and Peterson, R. E. (1960). Double isotope derivative assay of aldosterone in biological extracts. *J. biol. Chem.*, **235**, 1639.

Ross, E. J. (1959). *Aldosterone in Clinical and Experimental Medicine*, p. 24. Blackwell, Oxford.

Tyler, F. H., Schmidt, C. D., Eik-Nes, K., Brown, H., and Samuels, L. T. (1954). The role of the liver and the adrenal in producing elevated plasma 17-hydroxycorticosteroid levels in surgery. *J. clin. Invest.*, **33**, 1517.

*Arch. Dis. Childh.*, 1965, **40**, 264.

# THE PLACENTAL TRANSFUSION SYNDROME IN MONOZYGOUS TWINS*

BY

G. CORNEY and W. AHERNE

*From the Departments of Paediatrics and Pathology, United Oxford Hospitals*

(RECEIVED FOR PUBLICATION JULY 6, 1964)

The description in Genesis of the birth of Esau and Jacob records that 'the first came out red'; this may well have been the first description of the birth of a plethoric twin.

It was realized towards the end of the last century that there could be a difference in the haemoglobin values in uniovular twins (Westphalen, 1897, quoted by Price, 1950); a little earlier Schatz (1882 and 1884-1910, quoted by Newman, 1923) had demonstrated communications between the two halves of a monochorionic placenta, but 50 years passed before the syndrome in which one twin is born anaemic, the other polycythaemic, was attributed to such vascular anastomoses (Herlitz, 1941).

A number of cases of the 'placental transfusion syndrome' have now been described, and in this paper the published reports will be reviewed; one further case is described, being of particular interest as the anaemic baby had purpura and thrombocytopenia at birth, and has since been found to have several abnormalities.

## Case History

The mother, a Rhesus positive multigravida aged 39 years, was quite well in the early months of her pregnancy; when seen in the antenatal clinic at the 34th week a diagnosis of twins was made, and, as ankle oedema was present, she was admitted to the Churchill Hospital for rest. Her condition improved sufficiently to allow discharge home two weeks later; she was readmitted two weeks before term in labour.

Five hours after the onset of labour the first twin was delivered as a breech; he was pale and limp, but gasped at once, and regular respirations were established within three minutes. Petechiae were noted at birth and quickly became more marked. The second baby was delivered spontaneously ten minutes later and cried well immediately; he was very red in contrast to the pallor of his twin (Fig. 1).

On examination, Twin I, birth weight 4 lb. (1·8 kg.), was a pale quiet baby (Hb 39%; 5·8 g./100 ml.); petechiae and ecchymoses were present mainly on the face, but also, though to a lesser extent, on the trunk. The liver and spleen were easily palpable, and a systolic murmur could be heard over the whole praecordium, which was maximal in the third and fourth intercostal spaces at the sternal border. The clinical picture was very similar to that seen in a baby with severe anaemia due to haemolytic disease of the newborn. Twin II, birth weight 5 lb. 1 oz.

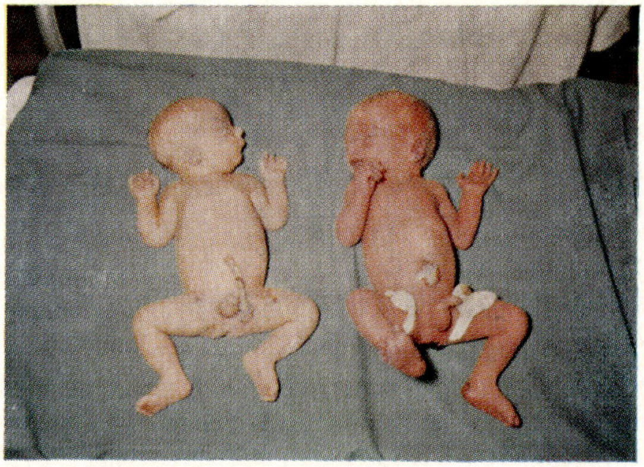

FIG. 1.—Appearance of the twins at birth. Twin I is on the left and Twin II on the right.

(2·3 kg.), was in excellent condition, with a striking plethoric appearance (Hb 170%; 25·2 g./100 ml.); the liver and spleen were easily palpable.

Apart from the extreme difference in the haemoglobin values, the main features in the investigations were the thrombocytopenia and marked normoblastaemia seen in the blood film of Twin I; a further unusual feature of this film was the almost complete absence of lymphocytes which were plentiful in his twin. A full account of the investigations is given in Table 1 and Table 2.

**The Placenta.** The placenta was monochorionic with two amniotic sacs. The two portions were strikingly dissimilar (Fig. 2), that belonging to Twin I being large,

* A paper read at a meeting of the Royal Society of Medicine, Section of Paediatrics, in Oxford, June 1964.

TABLE 1

BLOOD AND URINE FINDINGS IN TWINS AND MOTHER

| | Twin I | Twin II | Mother |
|---|---|---|---|
| Hb .. .. .. .. .. .. .. | 39% (5·8 g./100 ml.) | 170% (25·2 g./100 ml.) | 90% (13·3 g./100 ml.) |
| Platelets .. .. .. .. .. .. | 41,000/c.mm. | Large clusters | 173,000/c.mm. |
| Film—normoblasts .. .. .. .. | 75,000/c.mm. | Very scanty | Nil |
| lymphocytes .. .. .. .. | Scanty | Normal | Normal |
| Direct Coombs test .. .. .. .. | Negative | Negative | — |
| Immune antibodies .. .. .. .. .. | — | — | α-haemolysin, not active against babies' cells |
| Wassermann and Kahn reaction .. .. | Negative | Negative | Negative |
| Toxoplasmosis—Dye .. .. .. .. .. | Positive 1/16 | — | — |
| C/F .. .. .. .. .. | Negative 1/4 | — | — |
| (repeat at age 5 weeks)—Dye .. .. .. | Negative 1/4 | | |
| C/F .. .. .. | Negative 1/4 | | |
| Blood culture .. .. .. .. .. .. | Negative | Negative | Negative |
| Urine inclusion bodies .. .. .. .. .. | Nil | Nil | — |

TABLE 2

BLOOD GROUP OF THE TWINS AND THEIR PARENTS

| | ABO | MNS | $P_1$ | Rh | $Lu^a$ | K | $Le^a$ | $Le^b$ | $Fy^a$ | $Fy^b$ | $Jk^a$ | $Jk^b$ | $Xg^a$ |
|---|---|---|---|---|---|---|---|---|---|---|---|---|---|
| Twin II .. .. | $A_1$ | MNSs | $+^w$ | $R_1 R_2$ | — | — | + | — | — | + | + | + | + |
| Twin I .. .. | $A_1$ | MNSs | $+^w$ | $R_1 R_2$ | — | — | + | — | — | + | + | + | + |
| Father .. .. | $A_1$ | NsNs | + | $R_1 R_1$ | — | — | — | | + | + | + | + | + |
| Mother .. .. | O | MMS | — | $R_2r$ | — | — | + | — | + | + | + | + | + |

pale, and thick, and weighing 678 g.; and that belonging to his twin being small and deeply congested, weighing only 254 g. The two portions were sharply demarcated except at the centre where there appeared to be one or more shared cotyledons. The superficial vessels of the large pale portion were of fine calibre and contained little blood (Fig. 3); the cord, which was marginally inserted, was rather thin (diameter about 0·75 cm.). The vessels of the other half, by contrast, were grossly engorged and tortuous; the cord on this side was thicker (diameter 1·0 cm.) and the insertion was velamentous. Several small anastomoses were visible crossing in the subamniotic tissues from one vascular territory to another. These connected veins to veins. No arteriovenous or other anastomoses were found amongst the superficial vessels.

MICROSCOPICAL FEATURES. The monochorionic structure of the placenta was confirmed. The chorionic villi of the large pale portion were bulky, with prominent trophoblast, frequent Hofbauer cells, and marginated capillaries containing a high proportion of nucleated red cell precursors (Fig. 4). The resemblance to a placenta in severe haemolytic disease was close. The volume of the villous tissue was estimated as 356 ml.; the volume of the intervillous space as 239 ml.; and the total villous surface area as 9·8 sq. m. (These quantitative estimates were made by techniques that will be described by Aherne and Dunnill (in the press.) The small portion of the placenta was histologically normal and mature, but the capillaries were intensely congested; the visible blood was noticeably free from nucleated red cell precursors

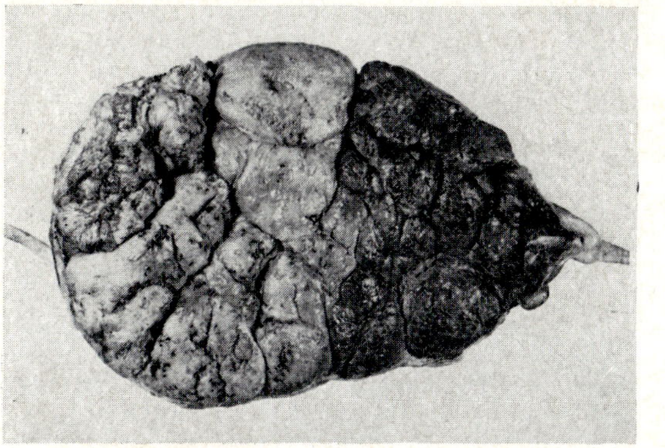

FIG. 2.—Maternal surface of placenta, showing the sharp demarcation into unequal contrasting portions.

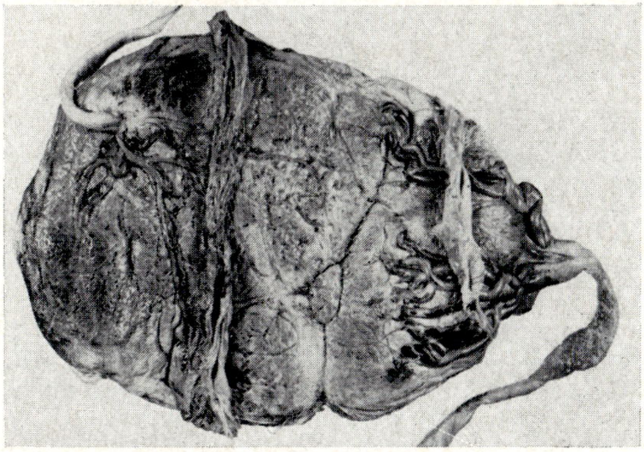

FIG. 3.—Foetal surface of placenta, with amnions peeled back. Note very small size of surface anastomoses between the two vascular systems.

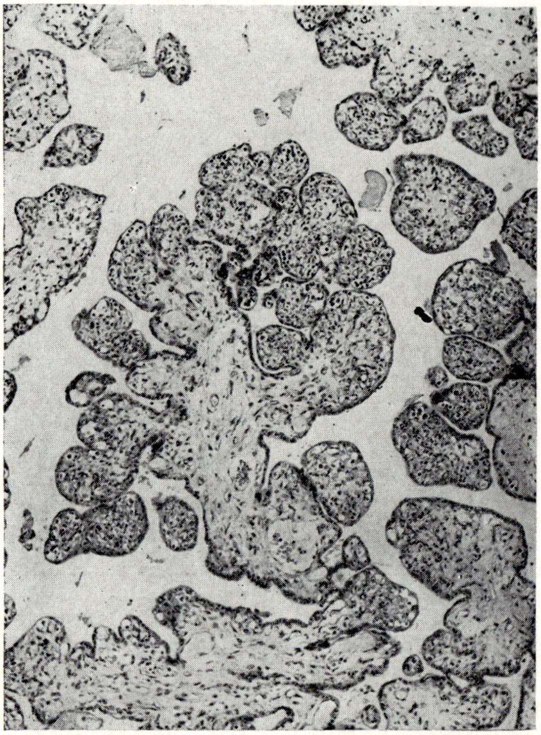

FIG. 4.—Typical villi and villous stem from the larger, pale portion of the placenta. Note the bulbous villi, with marginated capillaries full of nucleated red-cell precursors. (H. and E. × 90.)

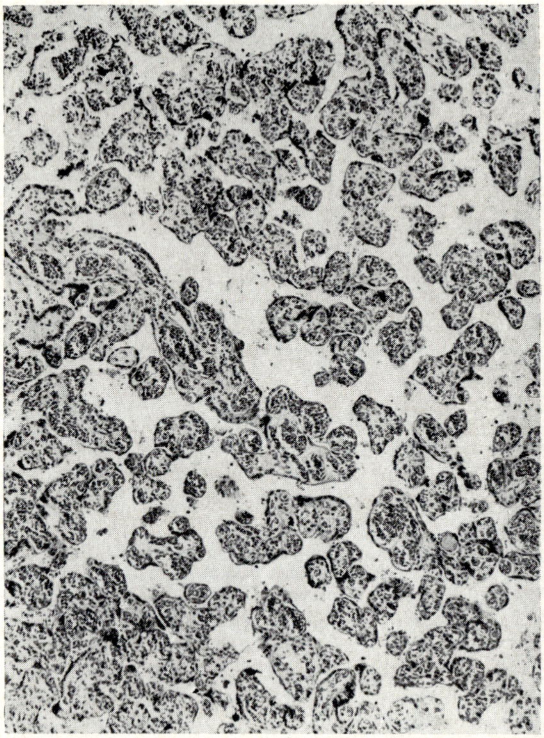

FIG. 5.—Typical villi from smaller portion of placenta. Though the capillaries are deeply engorged the general morphology is normal. (H. and E. × 90.)

(Fig. 5). The volume of the villous tissue in this portion was estimated as 113 ml.; the volume of the intervillous space as 73 ml.; and the total villous surface area as 4·9 sq. m.

These estimates of surface area (Twin I: 9·8 sq. m.; Twin II: 4·9 sq. m.) may be compared with the following estimates of mean villous surface area in five normal placentas at 38-40 weeks' gestation: 12·6, 11·6, 10·6, 10·5, and 9·1 sq. m. (Aherne and Dunnill).

**Treatment and Progress.** Twin I initially developed signs of respiratory distress; in view of the severe anaemia and the possibility of haemolytic disease (which was considered at that early stage), it was decided to perform an exchange transfusion. On completion of this, his condition was slightly improved, and the systolic murmur previously noted was no longer audible. The following day, as the haemoglobin was still only 51% (7·5 g./100 ml.), a simple transfusion of blood (60 ml.) was given. The platelet count remained low.

During the first four days his condition was poor; there were recurrent cyanotic attacks with occasional twitching and jerky movements; crepitations were present in both lungs and on several occasions fresh blood was aspirated from the pharynx and stomach. Digoxin was given, together with a course of tetracycline; sedation with phenobarbitone was used as necessary. Slight jaundice developed, the maximum bilirubin being 5 mg./100 ml. From the fifth day of life, however, there was a steady improvement. The petechiae faded, but the size of the liver and spleen remained essentially unchanged. The systolic murmur previously heard was again heard at this stage, but this gradually became less marked. By the third week of life the platelet count had risen to 215,000/c.mm. and remained at a normal level. Digoxin was discontinued from the fourth week without ill effect. By the sixth week, however, the haemoglobin had fallen to the low level seen at birth—37% (5·5 g./100 ml.), and a third transfusion was, therefore, given.

On discharge from the premature nursery at age 2 months his general condition was very good; a soft systolic murmur could still be heard, the liver and spleen weie still easily palpable. Oral iron, which had been given from the age of 1 month, was continued on discharge.

Twin II was in excellent condition at birth, and remained so, apart from very slight jaundice (maximum bilirubin 4 mg./100 ml.); no treatment was given to this baby. On discharge at the age of 3 weeks the liver and spleen were palpable, but clinical examination was otherwise normal.

**Further Progress.** When seen for review at the age of 4 months, each twin could lift his head from the pillow and both would follow a moving light; the mother felt, however, that Twin II was brighter and more responsive than his brother; he certainly pulled to sitting in a more satisfactory manner and maintained a better posture in this position. Twin I's haemoglobin was again low despite treatment with oral iron.

Shortly after this review Twin I was noticed (by his mother) to have abnormal eye movements, and at the age of 5 months was found to have bilateral lamellar cataracts. It was also apparent that his hearing was less good than that of his twin, and Mr. Gavin Livingstone found that there was impairment of hearing in both ears which was more marked on the left side. Discission operations were performed on the left eye at the age of 11 months by Dr. Sarwar at the Oxford Eye Hospital, the appearance of the fundus was normal; a similar operation is planned for the other eye.

Both twins were seen for review at age 1 year when it was apparent there was a marked difference in development. Twin I weighed 19 lb. 15 oz. (9 kg.), made no attempt to sit, and head lag was still present when he was pulled to the sitting position; he would sit with support, but not well. He was able to follow a moving light, and was obviously able to see the movement of his hands. There was no evidence of congenital heart disease. The teeth were stained yellow, probably due to the tetracycline which had been given in the first week of life. His development was that of a 3-to-4-month-old baby.

Haemoglobin, white cell and platelet counts, urine (including amino acid chromatography), and electrocardiogram were all within normal limits. A radiograph of hand and wrist for bone-age showed identical development with that of his twin.

In marked contrast, Twin II, weight 22 lb. 11 oz. (10·3 kg.), was in all respects a normal little boy who laughed and chuckled, crawled, pulled to standing, and used his hands and fingers quite well. There was no evidence of cataract, and vision and hearing seemed normal for his age. Investigations, performed as for his twin, were all normal.

## Discussion

At present it is assumed that a monochorionic placenta indicates monozygous twinning (Benirschke, 1961); these twins, however, showed many differences, as has been detailed, and it was decided that the fullest study should be made to determine the zygosity.

The twins were of the same sex; 10 blood group systems were studied and found to be identical; and the total finger ridge counts were similar. It was calculated that according to the table of Maynard Smith, and Penrose (1954) the total chance of monozygosity was 99·6%.

To complete the investigation it was decided to exchange skin grafts; this was discussed with the parents, who were fully agreeable, and when the twins were 1 year old, Mr. T. J. S. Patterson transferred 1 $cm.^2$ Wolfe Grafts (full thickness of skin) from the inner side of the upper arm; both homografts and autografts were exchanged. It is not thought that this procedure has been performed previously when there has been complete knowledge of placentation.

The grafts were inspected at weekly intervals; the initial appearances were those of normal human Wolfe grafts; when seen on the 29th day after grafting, however, there was a difference in the appearance of the homografts. The homograft and autograft on Twin I's arm showed the normal appearances of human grafts at this stage, i.e. a thin layer of desquamated epithelium which could easily be peeled off leaving pink skin beneath. The homograft in Twin II's case showed a thick dark crust; this also stripped off easily leaving a pink but rather irregular surface. All grafts maintained their square shape, and there had been no contracture. Subsequent appearances showed little change.

When human skin grafts are rejected there is evidence of contracture (Rogers, 1957), this was not seen in this case, and it is thought that these grafts had taken and confirmed that the twins were uniovular. The difference in the appearance of the grafts cannot be explained.

It would have been interesting to have exchanged second homografts, for if these had been accepted it would have been decisive evidence of compatibility. 'Such compatibility might be due either to the twins being identical, or, alternatively, if they were non-identical, to their having become tolerant as a result of interchange of blood during intra-uterine life' (M. F. A. Woodruff, 1964, personal communication).

Extensive blood group studies have been made and there is no evidence of chimaerism. It was not thought justifiable, however, to perform a further grafting procedure. From all the evidence it was concluded that these were monozygous twins.

The clinical state of the first twin, and the microscopical changes in his placenta, would have been compatible with haemolytic disease of the newborn, cytomegalic inclusion body disease, toxoplasmosis, and perhaps syphilis. All these conditions were excluded. It seemed reasonable to suppose that the changes observed were due to transfusion of blood from the first to the second twin through placental anastomoses.

Anastomoses between the vascular territories of the monochorionic twin placenta were suspected as long ago as the late seventeenth century. The first demonstration of their anatomy was given by

Schatz (1882, 1884-1910) who showed that there were two main types, superficial and deep. The superficial anastomoses, he found, joined artery to artery or vein to vein (both types can be present in the same placenta) on the foetal surface; the deep connexions were constantly arteriovenous. Schatz drew the important conclusion that the superficial anastomoses compensated for the haemodynamic imbalance set up by the deep ones. Both Schatz, and more recently Benirschke (1961), stress that superficial anastomoses are present in the great majority of monochorionic twin placentas, and that it is the absence (or inadequacy) of these communications that may harm the foetus. Anastomoses as found by Benirschke in 60 monochorionic placentas are given in Table 3.

TABLE 3*

VASCULAR ANASTOMOSES IN 60 MONOCHORIONIC PLACENTAS (BENIRSCHKE, 1961)

| Anastomosis | Sets of Twins | |
|---|---|---|
| | Total | Survivors |
| Artery to artery only .. .. .. .. .. | 17 | 12 |
| Artery to artery plus artery to vein .. .. | 17 | 14 |
| Artery to artery plus vein to vein .. .. | 2 | 2 |
| Vein to vein only .. .. .. .. | 3 | 2 |
| Artery to vein only .. .. .. .. | 7 | 3 |
| Artery to vein plus vein to artery .. .. | 2 | 1 |
| Artery to vein plus vein to vein .. .. | 3 | 1 |
| No anastomoses seen .. .. .. .. | 9 | 6 |

* Reproduced by permission of the Editor, *New York State Journal of Medicine*.

It is agreed that transfusion of blood from one foetus to the other may occur; the time at which this happens and the duration of such a transfusion are in dispute. Bergstedt (1957) and Littlewood (1963) believed that in their cases this happened during delivery. Seip (1956) also held this view, though he differed from Bergstedt in supposing that the dynamics of labour tended to make the second twin plethoric and not the first. In fact, a review of the reported cases shows that the first twin is as likely to be plethoric as the second. Herlitz (1941), following Schatz, thought that there must be a 'slow ooze' from one foetus to the other throughout the pregnancy. The finding of normoblastaemia and reticulocytosis together with enlargement of the liver and spleen would seem to favour this view. It is difficult to explain why the nucleated red cell precursors should be present in only one-half of the placenta, unless (as has been described in the similar syndrome in animals described below) the transfusion had at some point ceased.

Further support for the 'slow ooze' theory comes from quantitative analysis of the placenta in the present case. Normally there is a direct and fairly close correlation between foetal weight and placental villous surface area (Aherne and Dunnili). By analogy with normal infants of comparable maturity, the first twin, attached to a villous surface measuring 9·8 sq. m., might have been expected to weigh at least 6 lb. 10 oz. (3 kg.). In fact this baby weighed only 4 lb. (1·8 kg.). On the other hand the second twin possessing a villous surface of only 4·9 sq. m., grew to a vigorous 5 lb. 1 oz. (2·3 kg.) instead of the expected weight of 3 lb. 5 oz. (1·5 kg.) or less. These exceptions to the general rule may be explained by supposing that a prolonged 'slow ooze' from one placenta to the other impoverished the first twin and supplemented the second placenta. This may well have dated from the time of vasculogenesis, as has been previously suggested (Price, 1950).

It must, however, be pointed out that the anaemic baby is not always the smaller twin, as in the cases quoted by Kerr (1959), Valaes and Doxiadis (1960), Littlewood (1963), and Falkner, Datta Banik, and Westland (1962).

Foeto-foetal transfusion may have grave effects, as when acardia is found in one twin, circulation being maintained by his partner. Milder effects are commoner. Benirschke (1958) and Naeye (1963) noted cardiovascular and renal hypertrophy with associated hydramnios in the plethoric twin and converse changes in the anaemic baby. Most attention has been given to the haematological changes already noted and to their clinical concomitants such as hepatosplenomegaly. But thrombocytopenia has not been described previously; Herlitz (1941) in fact reported thrombocythaemia.

Thrombocytopenia has been seen in rubella embryopathy (Berge, Brunnhage, and Nilsson, 1963) and in association with malformations of the limbs (Zetterström and Strindberg, 1958). Platelet formation starts in these early weeks (Fruhling, Rogers, and Jobard, 1949) when the embryo is particularly vulnerable. The association of cataract and impairment of hearing in the anaemic infant is also reminiscent of rubella embryopathy. Since the common causes of these anomalies were excluded, it is tempting to ascribe their occurrence in one of apparently uniovular twins to the abnormal haemodynamics of the milieu in which that twin developed. It must, however, be conceded that the eyes of the anaemic baby were not examined in the neonatal period, and his mother is convinced that he could see in the early weeks. The presence of cataract in the early months, which was *not* present at birth, has been reported (Ryan, 1956) in a baby who was very anaemic (for reasons undetermined) after delivery and required transfusions.

The placental transfusion syndrome has many features in common with the syndrome of 'parabiotic intoxication' (Finerty, 1952) seen in a high percentage of cases when mice or rats are joined by the skin for experimental purposes. If the animals are genetically dissimilar, then the full syndrome with anaemia in the hybrid and polycythaemia in the pure animal is seen; the liver and spleen may enlarge in both and blood pressure changes have been recorded. It has been demonstrated that the anaemia is not due to haemolysis or other mechanisms, and that there is a marked shift of blood from one animal to the other (Tokuda and MacGillivray, 1962.) If the animals are similar genetically, then there is a shift of blood from one to the other, but no other features of 'intoxication'; this has been termed the *primary* phase (Eichwald, Lustgraaf, Fuson, and Weismann, 1961), in the full syndrome, the *secondary* phase is thought to be due to immunological mechanisms not possible in animals with an identical genetic background. This would be very like 'runt disease' (Billingham, 1959); in affected babies, however, changes as seen in runt disease have not been found (Naeye, 1963).

The analogy in the case of human monozygous twins would, therefore, seem to be with the primary phase, i.e. a shift of blood due to pressure gradients; a complete analogy is not possible as the animal studies were of necessity performed on mature animals. In the case of the human foetus, if the transfusion does take place in the early weeks, then this will be before the foetus is immunologically competent.

Present theories for the survival of grafts in monozygous twins are based on the presence of placental anastomoses; there have, however, been no previous reports of grafting in twins known to be affected by the placental transfusion syndrome (K. Benirschke, 1964, personal communication). It is of interest that the appearances of the grafts were unusual, though the significance of this is not certain, and it would be difficult to suggest a mechanism for this. It would be instructive to observe the results of grafts in other twins so affected.

The differing progress made by the present pair of twins in the first year of life is striking. Becker and Glass (1963) reported that the polycythaemic twin made better progress up to the age of 4 months, but at 2 years the status of both infants was similar and normal for age. Herlitz (1941) found that the first set of twins he reported still differed in size at 6 years, but were otherwise normal.

The anaemic baby may seem more in need of treatment, but an analysis of deaths shows that the plethoric twin is just as much at risk, being prone to kernikterus, cyanotic attacks, convulsions possibly due to cerebral thrombosis (Chaptal, Jean, Izarn, Campo, and Menard, 1958), and cardiac failure (Minkowski, 1962).

Neligan and Russell (1954) have suggested that transfusion is indicated if the haemoglobin level falls below 13·3 g./100 ml. in the first 24 hours of life, and stress that the exsanguinated baby may appear deceptively well. Care should be taken not to precipitate cardiac failure, and it was for this reason that we, like others, favoured exchange transfusion initially. Valaes and Doxiadis (1960) used blood from the plethoric baby to restore the haemoglobin level of his twin.

As in haemolytic disease, there appears to be an increased risk of anaemia in the first months of life, even if transfusion has been given initially. It may be that this tendency is only found in infants who have suffered prolonged loss of blood during gestation. In these cases, as in our own case, a further transfusion may be needed, and it seems advisable to give iron therapy for several months.

The plethoric baby may require venesection, followed by an intravenous infusion of saline, glucose-saline, or plasma.


## Summary

Monozygous twins were found to have a gross difference in haemoglobin values at birth, the anaemic baby showing thrombocytopenia; this baby has since been found to be retarded in development, and has cataracts and impaired hearing. Placental vascular anastomoses have been demonstrated, and it is suggested that twin-to-twin transfusion took place from the very early months of the pregnancy.

Skin grafts were performed for the first time in twins affected by this syndrome; these confirmed the fact that the twins were uniovular, but the appearances were somewhat unusual.

Previous case reports are reviewed; comparison is made to a similar syndrome in experimental animals.


We are grateful to Dr. Victoria Smallpeice for permission to publish this report, to Mr. T. J. S. Patterson, Department of Plastic Surgery, United Oxford Hospitals for performing the skin grafts and for his interest in this case, and to Dr. I. B. Shine, Medical Research Council, Population Genetics Research Unit for the genetic studies and help in the preparation of the paper. Blood group studies were performed by Dr. Ruth Sanger at the Lister Institute, London. We would also like to thank Dr. P. A. Davies, Lecturer in Paediatrics, University of Oxford, for her guidance and advice.


### References

Aherne, W., and Dunnill, M. S. In preparation.

Becker, A. H., and Glass, H. (1963). Twin-to-twin transfusion syndrome. *Amer. J. Dis. Child.*, **106**, 624.

Benirschke, K. (1958). In *Gestation. Transactions of the Fifth Conference*, ed. C. A. Villee. Josiah Macy Jr. Foundation, New York.

—— (1961). Twin placenta in perinatal mortality. *N.Y. St. J. Med.*, **61**, 1499.

Berge, T., Brunnhage, F., and Nilsson, L. R. (1963). Congenital hypoplastic thrombocytopenia in rubella embryopathy. *Acta paediat.* (*Uppsala*), **52**, 349.

Bergstedt, J. (1957). Monozygotic twins, one with high erythrocyte values and jaundice, the other with anaemia neonatorum and no jaundice. *ibid.*, **46**, 201.

Billingham, R. E. (1959). Reactions of grafts against their hosts. *Science*, **130**, 947.

Chaptal, J., Jean, R., Izarn, P., Campo, Mme C., and Menard, P. (1958). La polyglobulie pathologique neo-natale: a propos de cinq observations. *Pédiatrie*, **13**, 515.

Eichwald, E. J., Lustgraaf, E. C., Fuson, R. B., and Weismann, I. (1961). Parabiotic anemia-polycythemia. *Proc. Soc. exp. Biol.* (*N.Y.*), **106**, 441.

Falkner, F., Datta Banik, N. D., and Westland, D. R. (1962). Intrauterine blood transfer between uniovular twins. *Biol. Neonat.* (*Basel*), **4**, 52.

Fruhling, L., Rogers, S., and Jobard, P. (1949). L'hématologie normale (tissus et organes hematopoïétiques, sang circulant) de l'embryon, du foetus et du nouveau-né humains. *Sang*, **20**, 313.

Finerty, J. C. (1952). Parabiosis in physiological studies. *Physiol. Rev.*, **32**, 277.

Herlitz, G. (1941). Zur Kenntnis der anämischen and polyzytämischen Zustande bei Neugborenen sowie des Icterus gravis neonatorum. *Acta paediat.* (*Uppsala*), **29**, 211.

Kerr, M. M. (1959). Anaemia and polycythaemia in uniovular twins. *Brit. med. J.*, **1**, 902.

Littlewood, J. M. (1963). Polycythaemia and anaemia in newborn monozygotic twin girls. *ibid.*, **1**, 857.

Maynard Smith, S., and Penrose, L. S. (1954). Monozygotic and dizygotic twin diagnosis. *Ann. hum. Genet.*, **19**, 273.

Minkowski, A. (1962). Le retentissement cardiaque de la polycythémie néo-natale (jumeaux) et post-natale (enfants uniques). *Biol. Neonat.* (*Basel*), **4**, 61.

Naeye, R. L. (1963). Human intrauterine parabiotic syndrome and its complications. *New Engl. J. Med.*, **268**, 804.

Neligan, G. A., and Russell, J. K. (1954). Blood loss from the foetal circulation: a hazard of lower segment Caesarean section in cases of placenta praevia. *J. Obstet. Gynaec. Brit. Emp.*, **61**, 206.

Newman, H. H. (1923). *The Physiology of Twinning.* University of Chicago Press, Chicago.

Price, B. (1950). Primary biases in twin studies. *Amer. J. hum. Genet.*, **2**, 293.

Rogers, B. O. (1957). The genetics of skin homo-transplantation in the human. *Ann. N.Y. Acad. Sci.*, **64**, 741.

Ryan, H. (1956). Postnatal cataracts in a premature infant. *Amer. J. Ophthal.*, **41**, 310.

Schatz, F. (1882). Eine besondere Art von einseigtiger Polyhydramnie mit anderseitiger Oligohydramnie bei eineiigen Zwillingen. *Arch. Gynäk.*, **19**, 329.

—— (1884-1910). Die Gefässverbindungen der Placentakreisläufe eineiiger Zwillinge, ihre Entwickelung und ihre Folgen. *ibid.*, **24**, 337; **27**, 1; **29**, 419; **30**, 169, 335; **53**, 144; **55**, 485; **58**, 1; **60**, 81, 201; **92**, 13.

Seip, M. (1956). A comparison of hemoglobin and erythrocyte values in the first-born and the second-born twin, and in first, second, and third triplet during the neonatal period. *Acta paediat.* (*Uppsala*), **45**, 58.

Tokuda, S., and MacGillivray, M. H. (1962). Parabiotic intoxication, II. The distribution and survival of $Cr^{51}$-labeled red blood cells. *Plast. reconstr. Surg.*, **29**, 462.

Valaes, T., and Doxiadis, S. A. (1960). Intrauterine blood transfer between uniovular twins. *Arch. Dis. Childh.*, **35**, 503.

Westphalen, F. (1897). Ueber der mikrochemischen Nachweis von Eisen im fötalen Organismus nebst Beschreibung eines Falles von Schatz'scher Zwillingsschwangerschaft. *Arch. Gynäk.*, **53**, 31.

Zetterström, R., and Strindberg, B. (1958). Sporadic congenital spherocytosis associated with congenital hypoplastic thrombocytopenia and malformations. *Acta paediat.* (*Uppsala*), **47**, 14.

*Arch. Dis. Childh.*, 1965, **40**, 271.

# FAVISM IN ENGLAND—TWO MORE CASES

BY

J. M. HOLT and R. A. SLADDEN

*From the Nuffield Department of Clinical Medicine, The Radcliffe Infirmary, Oxford, and the Department of Pathology, Northampton General Hospital, Northampton*

(RECEIVED FOR PUBLICATION JULY 27, 1964)

*Vicia faba* (L), the broad bean, contains a potentially toxic substance, the exact nature of which is unknown, capable of producing a haemolytic crisis in a susceptible person. The crisis may be induced by eating the beans raw or, less commonly, cooked, and in some cases by inhalation of the bean pollen. The erythrocytes of susceptible individuals are deficient in the enzyme glucose-6-phosphate dehydrogenase (G6PD). The defect is transmitted as a sex-linked dominant trait, and shows a variable degree of penetrance (Hargreaves, 1963). Favism cannot, however, be induced in all those people who are deficient in erythrocyte G6PD, which suggests that there is a second abnormality in patients with this disease, which has yet to be defined.

Favism has been known for many centuries along the Mediterranean littoral, and it may have been one reason why Pythagoras forbade his followers to eat beans and he himself was slain rather than set foot in a bean field (Arie, 1959).

The condition was first described in Britain only 11 years ago in two Cypriots (Diggle, 1953), and since then only five other cases have been reported in this country. These included a Cypriot child (Gower and Frommer, 1960), an English child of Mediterranean ancestry (Discombe and Mestitz, 1956), an English child (McCarthy, 1955), and two English women (Brodribb and Worssam, 1961; Davies, 1962).

In spite of the ubiquity of the broad bean and the recent increase in immigration from the Mediterranean area, this potentially lethal, yet largely preventable, condition remains little known and rarely described in this country. It may well become more common, and this report of two further cases, one of which might have proved fatal, will serve as a reminder of its existence.

## Case Reports

**Case 1.** J.W., a 14-year-old schoolboy, had been well until early in June 1963, when he began to complain of tiredness and he was noticed to be listless and apathetic. On the evening of July 31 he was extremely tired and the following morning he fainted. Later that day he complained of noises in the ears and he vomited at frequent intervals. He became very drowsy. On the morning of August 2 he was admitted to the Radcliffe Infirmary, Oxford, desperately ill, jaundiced, weak, and barely able to respond to question or command. Examination showed a regular pulse of 132, blood pressure of 105/55 mm. Hg, and temperature of 102° F. (38·9° C.). There was a soft apical systolic murmur and the plantar responses were extensor.

The urine was dark red, and spectrophotometry confirmed the diagnosis of haemoglobinuria.

LABORATORY INVESTIGATIONS. Haemoglobin 4·3 g./100 ml. White cells, 18,100/c.mm.; reticulocytes 29%. Blood film: fragmentation of the red cells; 4 normoblasts/100 leucocytes. Heinz bodies: considerable numbers present. Serum bilirubin 7·0 mg./100 ml. Blood urea 61 mg./100 ml.

Acute haemolytic anaemia was diagnosed and, following the transfusion of whole blood, the boy's condition promptly improved.

About three weeks previously the boy had fallen into the river Thames, but there was no evidence to support a diagnosis of Weil's disease. No malarial parasites were found in thick blood films. On the other hand, the erythrocyte G6PD level (method of Prankerd, 1962) was found to be 0·4 units (normal range 2·1-4·2 units), suggesting that the haemolytic anaemia was related to G6PD deficiency.

On further inquiry, the boy's mother, who was dark skinned and claimed German nationality, admitted that she was of Greek ancestry. The boy was fair complexioned, taking after his English father. It was then found that a neighbour had given the family a large quantity of broad beans which they had been eating daily for a week. A diagnosis of favism was therefore made, and following the initial blood transfusion the boy's recovery was complete and uneventful.

The boy's mother and sister were the only members of the family who were available for investigation. Their erythrocyte G6PD levels were 2·1 and 2·6 units respectively, showing that the mother's level was at the lower limit of the normal range. Broad beans had never made the mother feel ill, though she did not particularly like them.

**Case 2.** P.B., an Italian boy 10 years of age, came to this country from Southern Italy in 1961 with his parents and sister. During the evening of August 11, 1963, he complained to his parents of epigastric pain. He soon became very unwell and lethargic, and developed a headache.

The following morning he was seen by his doctor who found slight conjuctival icterus and who was told by the parents that the boy's urine was dark. No urine was available at this time for examination. The liver edge was palpable and the boy was pyrexial. The doctor suspected infective hepatitis or, possibly, Weil's disease. He attended the boy again the following morning and sent him into Northampton Infectious Diseases Hospital the same day (August 13).

When the boy was examined in hospital he appeared sallow but not jaundiced. The following day various investigations were made.

LABORATORY INVESTIGATIONS. Haemoglobin 6·7 g./100 ml. White cells 4,500/c.mm.; reticulocytes 12%. Serum bilirubin 1·0 mg./100 ml. Liver function tests: normal. Blood film: marked polychromasia; a few normoblasts were present; no spherocytosis seen. Heinz bodies not found.

There was no history of blood loss, and the blood film suggested that a haemolytic episode had taken place. In view of the boy's nationality and the season of the year, a diagnosis of favism was suspected and the boy was transferred to the Northampton General Hospital.

No abnormal pigments, bile salts, or urobilinogen were found in the urine, but the boy later said that his urine had been 'red' at the onset of the illness. The diagnosis was confirmed by the finding of a level of 63 units of erythrocyte G6PD (method of Zinkham, 1959; normal range 150-217 units).

The father was then asked about the eating of broad beans. He said that the boy had often eaten cooked beans without ill effect, but that on the day his illness began he had eaten, for the first time, a lot of raw broad beans. When he later complained of abdominal pain, the parents were inclined to attribute this to indigestion following overindulgence. There was no knowledge of any intolerance to beans in other members of the family, but it was not possible to persuade them to attend for G6PD estimations*.

The boy's condition rapidly improved without any active treatment and he was sent home on the sixth day after admission, when his haemoglobin level was 9·9 g./100 ml.

## Discussion

These two cases illustrate the varying degrees o severity with which favism can manifest itself. The first case might well have proved fatal, and in a large series of cases a mortality rate of 8% in children has been reported (Luisada, 1941). In the second case even the jaundice was transient, and the only real evidence of haemolysis was in the blood film.

The disease tends to be self-limiting once exposure to beans has been stopped, with selective survival of younger erythrocytes in which G6PD levels are relatively high (Beutler, 1960).

G6PD levels usually tend to be lower in affected (hemizygous) males, than in heterozygous females. In the male, the levels are dependent upon the degree of expression of the gene for G6PD deficiency. Beutler and Baluda (1964) have suggested that, in heterozygous females, coexisting populations of normal and enzyme-deficient red cells result from inactivation of the locus for G6PD deficiency in one of the two X chromosomes. The severity of the illness presumably depends not only upon the G6PD level, but also upon the amount of the bean toxin ingested or inhaled and the unknown sensitivity factor. This factor must account for the fact that while the erythrocytes of all individuals who have had favism can be shown to be G6PD deficient, not all those with G6PD deficiency develop a haemolytic anaemia when exposed to the broad bean (Hargreaves, 1963). The relatively less harmful effect on any one subject of cooked beans, as opposed to raw beans, is emphasized by the second case.

Once the condition has been diagnosed, subsequent attacks of favism are preventable in the family concerned. Individuals who are deficient in G6PD are also liable to develop a haemolytic anaemia following the administration of a wide range of drugs or from contact with some industrial chemicals. Comprehensive lists of such substances are given by Beutler (1960) and Vuopio (1963), and include 8-aminoquinoline drugs (primaquine), sulphonamides (including sulphones), vitamin K analogues, salicylates (including aspirin and para-amino salicylic acid), probenecid, and nitrofurantoin. Naphthalene, TNT, and methylene blue show increased toxicity in G6PD-deficient subjects.

## Summary

Two more cases of favism in England are reported, one in an English boy whose mother was of Greek ancestry, the other in an Italian immigrant boy.

* Since this paper was written, an opportunity arose to estimate the G6PD levels in the erythrocytes of other members of the family in Case 2. The results were as follows.

Father: 2·6 units  Mother: 0·78 units
Sister: 2·5 units  P.B. (propositus): 0 units
(Method of Prankerd (1962), normal range 2·1-4·2 units.)

These figures were obtained in the course of a study which was being made by Dr. C. B. Kerr, of the Oxford Population Genetics Unit, to whom we are indebted.

The original blood sample from the propositus examined immediately after the attack of favism contained detectable amounts of G6PD. A probable explanation for this finding is that the blood then contained numerous young erythrocytes, in which small amounts of G6PD may be present, even in G6PD deficient subjects.

The first boy was severely affected by cooked beans; the second had previously eaten cooked beans without ill effect, but was affected by raw beans.

In both cases a deficiency of erythrocyte glucose-6-phosphate dehydrogenase was demonstrated; reference is made to the numerous chemical compounds of an oxidant nature that are capable of causing haemolysis in subjects whose erythrocytes are deficient in this enzyme.

We would like to thank Professor L. J. Witts and Dr. I. H. Gosset, under whose care these two patients were admitted to hospital in Oxford and Northampton, for permission to publish the case reports.*

In Case 1, the estimation of erythrocyte G6PD was suggested by Dr. A. A. Sharp.

REFERENCES

Arie, T. H. D. (1959). Pythagoras and beans. *Oxf. med. Sch. Gaz.*, **11**, 75.

Beutler, E. (1960). Drug induced hemolytic anemia (Primaquine sensitivity). In *The Metabolic Basis of Inherited Disease*, ed. J. B. Stanbury, J. B. Wyngaarden, and D. S. Fredrickson, pp. 1031-1067. McGraw Hill, New York.

——, and Baluda, M. C. (1964). The separation of glucose-6-phosphate-dehydrogenase-deficient erythrocytes from the blood of heterozygotes for glucose-6-phosphate-dehydrogenase deficiency. *Lancet*, **1**, 189.

Brodribb, H. S., and Worssam, A. R. H. (1961). Favism in an Englishwoman. *Brit. med. J.*, **1**, 1367.

Davies, P. (1962). Favism: a family study. *Quart. J. Med.*, **31**, 157.

Diggle, J. H. (1953). Favism in London. *Arch. Dis. Childh.*, **28**, 369.

Discombe, G., and Mestitz, W. (1956). Favism in an English-born child. *Brit. med. J.*, **1**, 1023.

Gower, N. D., and Frommer, E. (1960). Favism in a Cypriot child. *Lancet*, **1**, 628.

Hargreaves, T. (1963). Inherited enzyme defects: a review. *J. clin. Path.*, **16**, 293.

Luisada, A. (1941). Favism: a singular disease chiefly affecting the red blood cells. *Medicine* (*Baltimore*), **20**, 229.

McCarthy, O. R. (1955). A case of favism. *Lancet*, 1, 748.

Prankerd, T. A. J. (1962). *The Determination of Glucose-6-Phosphate Dehydrogenase in Red Cells.* Association of Clinical Pathologists, Broadsheet No. 42 (N.S.).

Vuopio, P. (1963). Red cell enzymes in anemia. *Scand. J. clin. Lab. Invest.*, **15**, Suppl. 72, 24.

Zinkham, W. (1959). An in-vitro abnormality of glutathione metabolism in erythrocytes from normal newborns: mechanism and clinical significance. *Pediatrics*, **23**, 18.

* Dr. Gosset has recently died.

*Arch. Dis. Childh.*, 1965, **40**, 274.

# GONADAL DYSGENESIS WITH UNUSUAL ABNORMALITIES

BY

K. HUGH-JONES, SHEILA J. WALLACE, JANET M. THORNBER, and N. B. ATKIN
*From Mount Vernon Hospital, Northwood, Middlesex*

(RECEIVED FOR PUBLICATION NOVEMBER 19, 1964)

Gonadal dysgenesis is the generic term for a group of conditions characterized by the absence of germ cells, and the presence of female internal and external genital organs. It can occur on its own—ovarian agenesis (Wilkins and Fleischmann, 1944), or in association with short stature—ovarian dwarfism (Varney, Kenyon, and Koch, 1942), or with multiple congenital abnormalities—Turner's syndrome (Turner, 1938). It is an example of the last type that is being reported here. The whole subject has recently been comprehensively reviewed by both Hauser (1963) and Lindsten (1963).

## Case Report

Janet is now 15 years old. Her mother was 33 and her father 31 when she was born. She has a normal sister of 12, and another sib, a girl, died within half hour of birth after a difficult delivery. A paternal great aunt has diabetes.

Turner's syndrome was diagnosed at the age of 7, when she had a plastic operation performed elsewhere to improve the appearance of her webbed neck. She was referred to this hospital because a hearing defect had been discovered by the School Medical Officer. Glycosuria was then discovered during routine examination and further questioning revealed some thirst and loss of weight during the previous year. Her lack of development had not been commented upon by her parents, partly because of natural reserve and partly because she had had two menstrual periods, 4 and 8 months earlier. Otherwise she had enjoyed good health and was of normal intelligence.

**Physical Findings.** She is a short underdeveloped girl, weight 92 lb. (42 kg.), and height 55½ in. (141 cm.); upper segment 29 in. (73½ cm.) and lower segment 26½ in. (67½ cm.) (Fig. 1). Her hair is low on her neck, which is still webbed despite plastic surgery. She has slight epicanthic folds, a receding chin, and pigmented naevi on her face. The ears appear normal but a marked high tone deafness has been demonstrated by audiometry. She has bilateral astigmatism, but no colour blindness by Ishihara's chart tests. There is an increase in the carrying angle at her elbows, and her finger-nails are slightly concave longitudinally with very deep peri-ongular folds. The nipples are hypoplastic with no breast development. There is no axillary and only scanty pubic hair. The external genitalia are normal in appearance. The thyroid is not palpable. In the cardiovascular system the heart is not enlarged, there is a soft apical systolic murmur, the femoral pulses are easily felt and synchronous with the radial, and the blood pressure in the arms is 110/85 and in the legs 140/100 mm.Hg. The remainder of the examination is normal.

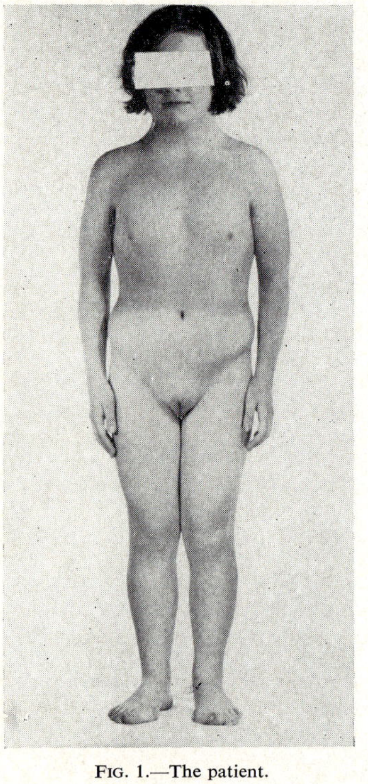

FIG. 1.—The patient.

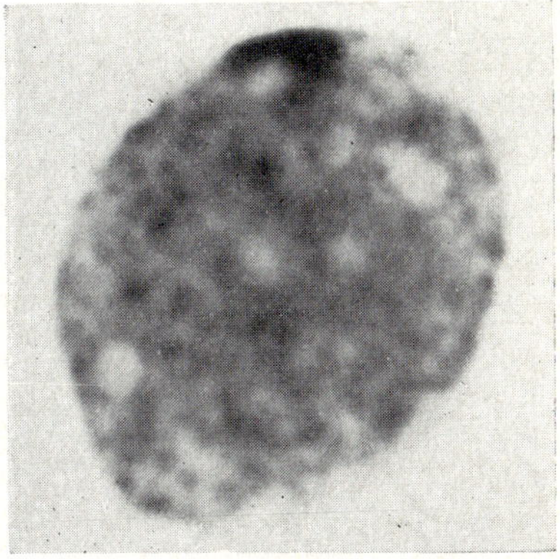

FIG. 2 (a).

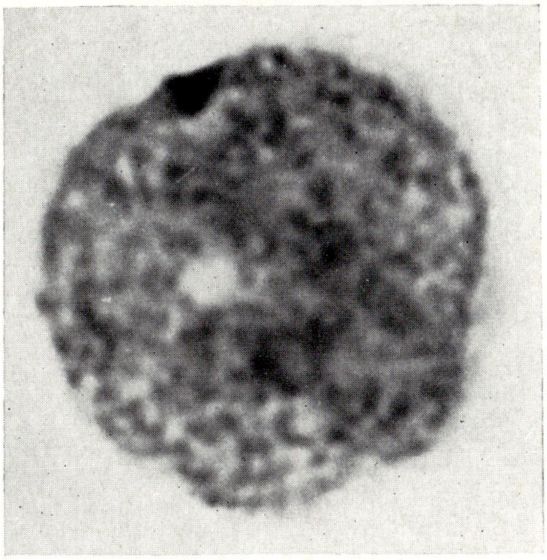

FIG. 2 (b).

FIG. 2.—(a) Buccal epithelial cell, showing large sex chromatin body (Orcein. × 1925.) Compare with (b) from a normal female.

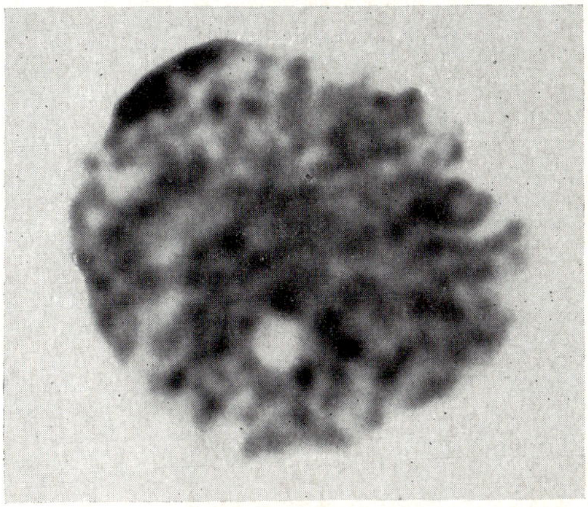

FIG. 3.

FIGS. 3 and 4.—Buccal epithelial cell, showing bipartite form of sex chromatin. (Orcein. × 1925.)

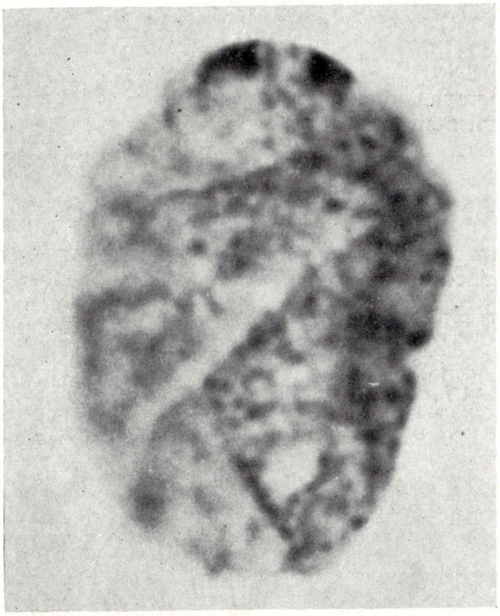

FIG. 4.

**Investigations.** Hb 93%; white blood cells 4,500. Normal differential. Wassermann and Kahn reaction negative. Urine: no protein, deposit normal, culture sterile, 2% sugar. Random blood sugar 273 mg./100 ml. Serum electrolytes, blood urea, normal; protein bound iodine, 7·2µg./100 ml. Glucose tolerance test after 30 g. of glucose is shown below.

| Minutes | 0 | 10 | 20 | 30 | 40 | 50 | 60 | 75 | 90 |
|---|---|---|---|---|---|---|---|---|---|
| Blood sugar mg./100 ml. | 223 | 242 | 303 | 378 | 399 | 395 | 375 | 375 | 392 |

Insulin glucose test: 30 g. glucose + 5U insulin/m². body surface, is shown opposite.

| Minutes | 0 | 10 | 20 | 30 | 40 | 50 | 60 | 75 | 90 |
|---|---|---|---|---|---|---|---|---|---|
| Blood sugar mg./100 ml. | 250 | 218 | 205 | 250 | 258 | 224 | 264 | 245 | 262 |

Urinary 17 ketosteroids 3·9 mg./24 hr. (normal 6-15), 17-OH corticosteroids 10·6 mg./24 hr. (normal 6-20). Urinary gonadotrophins 3·2 HMG 20A units/24 hr. (normal for this age 0·5-3·1). Plasma growth hormone 6·9 mµg./ml. (well within normal range for age). Radiograph of wrist showed bone age of 13 years at chronological age 15. Chest radiograph showed clear lung fields and heart of normal size and shape. Skull

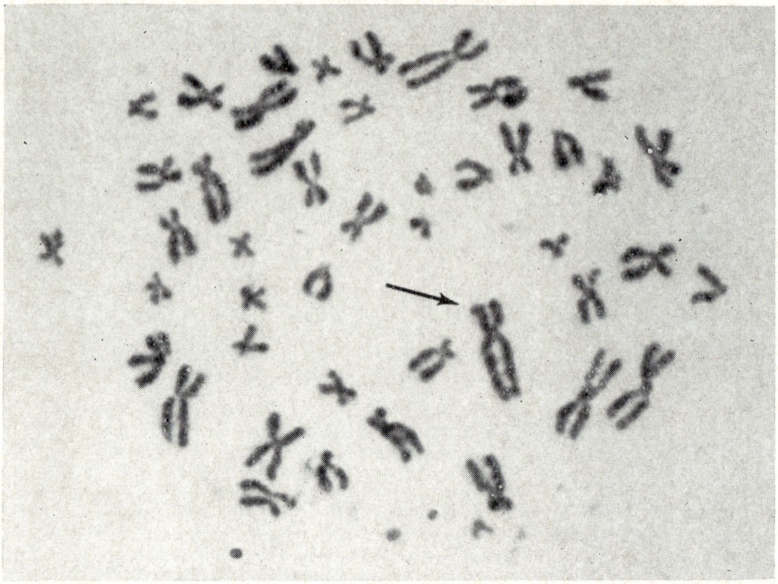

FIG. 5.—A 46-chromosome metaphase showing the large abnormal chromosome (arrowed).

radiograph normal. The intravenous pyelogram showed normal excretion and anatomy of kidneys, ureters, and bladder.

**Chromosome Studies.** Sex chromatin was seen in 50 out of 200 cells (25%) in buccal smears. The sex chromatin bodies were clearly abnormal (Figs. 2-4) and contained more chromatin material than usual; frequently the chromatin was aggregated into two unequal masses which were usually contiguous but sometimes a micron or so apart (Fig. 4). Chromosome counts from two separate leucocyte cultures are summarized in the Table. Analysis of cells with 45 chromosomes revealed an apparently 2A-XO constitution. In all cells with 46 chromosomes, a large abnormal chromosome was present, apparently replacing an X chromosome (there were only 15 chromo-

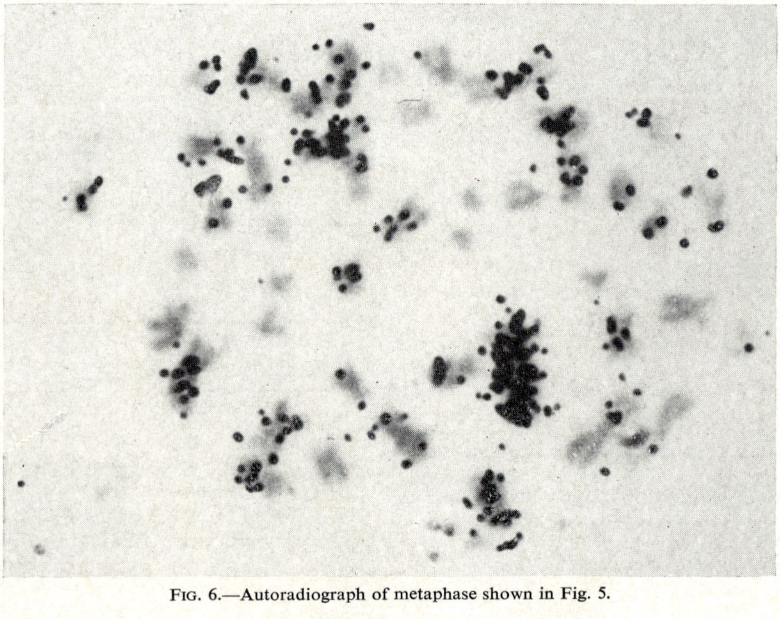

FIG. 6.—Autoradiograph of metaphase shown in Fig. 5.

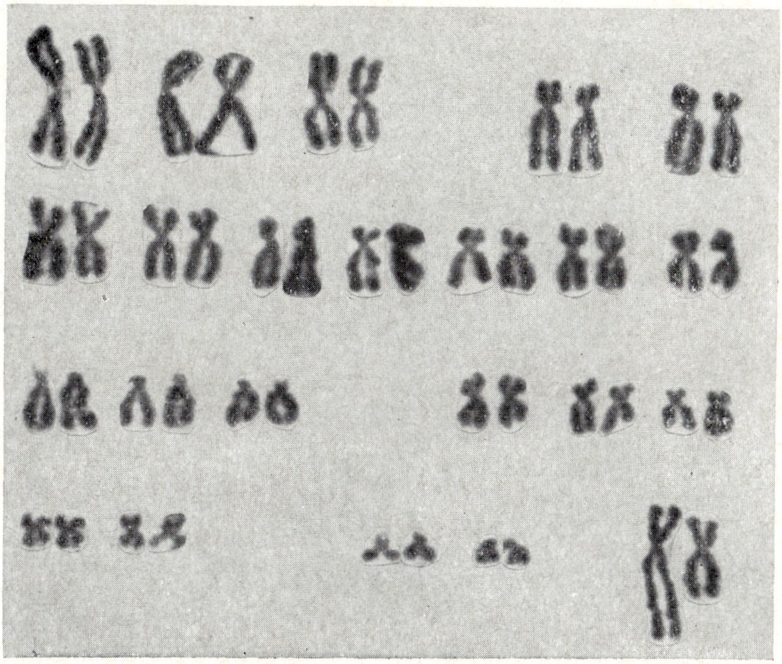

FIG. 7.—Karyotype of a 46-chromosome metaphase. The abnormal chromosome and the presumed normal X are at the right of the bottom row.

TABLE 1

CHROMOSOME COUNTS OF 230 CELLS FROM TWO LEUCOCYTE CULTURES

| | Number of Chromosomes | | | | | Total |
|---|---|---|---|---|---|---|
| | 44 | 44 | 45 | 46 | 46 | |
| No. of cells | 4 | 17 | 164 | 44 | 1 | 230 |

somes in the X-6-12 group). It was as long as, or slightly longer than, the No. 1 chromosomes, and its long arm was about $2\frac{1}{2}$ times its short arm (Figs. 5 and 7). Studies with tritiated thymidine revealed that it was uniformly late-labelling (Fig. 6).

The drumsticks of polymorphs in patients with abnormalities of the X chromosome have recently been studied by Fraccaro, Lindsten, Mittwoch, and Zonta (1964), who found a relation between the size of the drumsticks and that of the abnormal X chromosome. We failed to find any drumsticks among 700 polymorphs in the present case, but on a further blood smear, which was kindly examined by Dr. Ursula Mittwoch, one large drumstick was found among 400 polymorphs (Fig. 8).

The chromosomes of the parents and sister were investigated in peripheral leucocyte cultures. No abnormalities were found; a late-labelling chromosome in a culture from the mother treated with $^3$H thymidine had the morphological characteristics of a normal X chromosome.

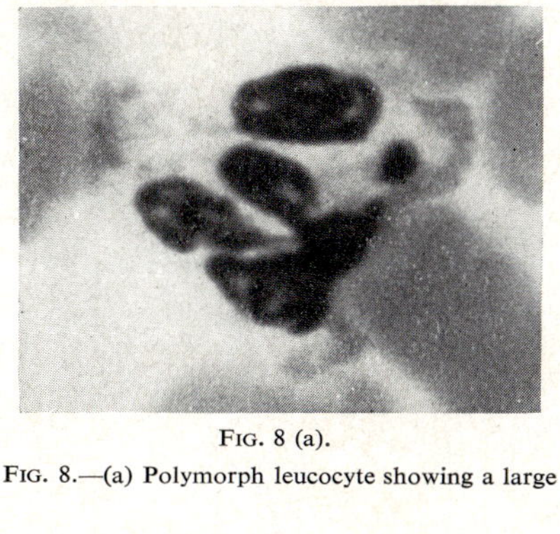

FIG. 8 (a).

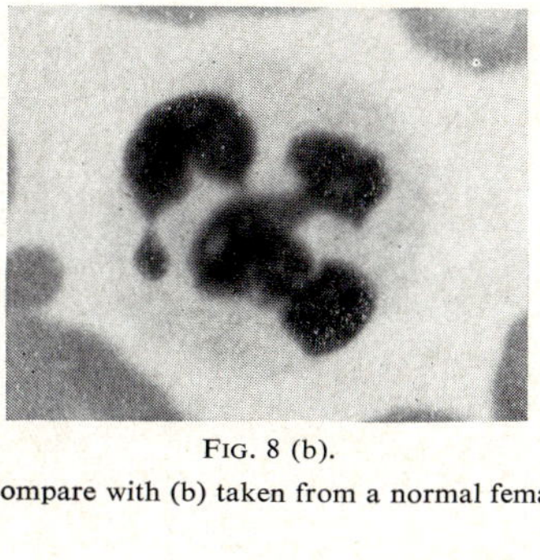

FIG. 8 (b).

FIG. 8.—(a) Polymorph leucocyte showing a large drumstick. (× 2200.) Compare with (b) taken from a normal female.

## Discussion

The unusual clinical features of this case of gonadal dysgenesis were first that Janet was referred because of her deafness and, secondly, during routine medical examination, glycosuria was discovered. Deafness of sufficient severity to be the presenting factor is rare. Hauser (1963), in his review of about 1,000 cases of gonadal dysgenesis, had 5 examples of clinical deafness, but as Lindsten points out in his monograph, slight hearing loss when tested for by audiometry is relatively common. Of 41 cases tested, 28 had a hearing loss of at least 20 decibels and broader than one octave. Of these, 20 were pure perceptive hearing losses, the commonest curve being with a central dip. 3 cases had a high tone deafness similar to this case.

Frank diabetes has not been frequently observed in gonadal dysgenesis, but Lichtwitz, Grivaux, and Delaville (1948) reported that hyperglycaemic glucose tolerance curves were not uncommon. Forbes and Engel (1963) found 6 cases of diabetes amongst 41 examples of gonadal dysgenesis. They suggested that the reason that this had not been noticed before was that the average age of reported examples of gonadal dysgenesis was 21 years, whereas the average age of their own was 51, which is within a few years of the mean age of onset of diabetes. But they may have somewhat overstated their case. In 2 instances the diagnosis of gonadal dysgenesis appeared to have been made just on the absence of secondary sexual characteristics. In their third case a normal chromosomal constitution was found and their fifth case was not examined for this. It was interesting that in the 3 remaining cases in which they examined the chromosomes they discovered an abnormal X chromosome (a presumptive isochromosome for the long arm): on 2 occasions this was the only abnormality in a normal chromosome count of 46, and on the third it was associated with a mosaicism with the usual XO constitution as seen in the present case. In our case the diabetes was noted at the age of 15, was sensitive to insulin, and was initially controlled by a low carbohydrate diet. However, because of subsequent weight loss, the treatment has been changed to chlorpropamide 125 mg. daily. This controlled the glycosuria.

The low incidence of sex chromatin suggested a mosaicism. This is relatively common in gonadal dysgenesis (Polani, 1962). The large abnormal chromosome seen in the cells with 46 chromosomes clearly contains more chromosomal material than a single X chromosome, yet from the position of its centromere it is not an isochromosome. In view of its late-labelling properties, and because of the large size of the sex chromatin body, it is presumably this chromosome that forms the Barr body in interphase. It might be assumed to consist entirely of 'hot' chromosome material; however, Ohno and Cattanach's (1962) studies on an X autosome translocation in the mouse have shown that an X chromosome composed partly of X chromosome and partly of autosomal material can manifest positive heteropycnosis along its entire length. It is possible, therefore, that the abnormal chromosome is the result of a structural rearrangement either between two X's or between an X and an autosome. If the former is the case, it could represent a duplication or duplication-deficiency chromosome, such as might arise through crossing-over within a pericentric inversion in a parent who was heterozygous for this inversion (P. E. Polani, personal communication). The fact that the mother's late-labelling X appears structurally normal, though not lending direct support to this hypothesis, does not of course rule it out. It appears that, as in other patients with gonadal dysgenesis having a cell-line with two X chromosomes, one abnormal and the other normal, it is the abnormal chromosome that is late-labelling and forms a Barr body in interphase.

## Summary

A case of gonadal dysgenesis with typical body configuration is described. The girl also had a high-tone deafness and hyperglycaemia. Chromosome studies revealed a mosaicism of cells with 45 chromosomes of 2A-XO constitution, and cells with 46 chromosomes in which an unusually large submetacentric late-labelling chromosome replaced one of the X chromosomes.

We would like to thank Professor P. E. Polani for his helpful advice and Miss Christine Hawes for assistance in preparing the autoradiographs.

The urinary gonadotrophins were estimated under the guidance of Dr. Barbara Clayton by a method devised by W. H. E. Fitschen in the Department of Chemical Pathology, Hospital for Sick Children, Great Ormond Street, London.

The plasma growth hormone was estimated by W. M. Hunter by the method described by Hunter and Greenwood (1962) (*Biochem. J.*, **85**, 39P).

### References

Forbes, A. P., and Engel, E. (1963). The high incidence of diabetes mellitus in 41 patients with gonadal dysgenesis, and their close relatives. *Metabolism*, **12**, 428.

Fraccaro, M., Lindsten, J., Mittwoch, U., and Zonta, L. (1964). Size of drumsticks in patients with abnormalities of the X-chromosome. *Lancet*, **2**, 43.

Hauser, G. A. (1963). Gonadal dysgenesis. In *Intersexuality*, ed. Claus Overzier, p. 298. Academic Press, New York.

Lichtwitz, A., Grivaux, M., and Delaville, M. (1948). Deux cas de nanisme avec insuffisance ovarienne totale et hypersécretion d'hormone gonadotrope. (Syndrome de Turner.) *Sem. Hôp. Paris*, **24**, 2823.

Lindsten, J. (1963). *The Nature and Origin of X Chromosome Aberrations in Turner's Syndrome.* Almqvist and Wiksell, Stockholm.

Ohno, S., and Cattanach, B. M. (1962). Cytological study of an X-autosome translocation in *Mus musculus*. *Cytogenetics*, **1**, 129.

Polani, P. E. (1962). Sex chromosome anomalies in man. In *Chromosomes in Medicine*, ed. J. L. Hamerton, p. 73. Wm. Heinemann (Medical Books), London.

Turner, H. H. (1938). A syndrome of infantilism, congenital webbed neck, and cubitus valgus. *Endocrinology*, **23**, 566.

Varney, R. F., Kenyon, A. T., and Koch, F. C. (1942). An association of short stature, retarded sexual development and high urinary gonadotropin titers in women. *J. clin. Endocr.*, **2**, 137.

Wilkins, L., and Fleischmann, W. (1944). Ovarian agenesis. *ibid.*, **4**, 357.

## Addendum

While this girl has been under observation she has recently been started on stilboestrol 0·5 mg./day for one month, then 1·0 mg./day for one month. After 9 weeks she began a heavy period. Examination under anaesthetic during a dilatation and curettage revealed normal female anatomy. Curettings were normal and showed the same nuclear chromatin pattern, i.e. a low incidence of Barr bodies, which were larger than normal. Stilboestrol has since been stopped and there is no further bleeding. Recently she has had to go on to insulin for treatment of her diabetes.

*Arch. Dis. Childh.*, 1965, **40**, 280.

# NEONATAL JAUNDICE ASSOCIATED WITH FAMILIAL G6PD DEFICIENCY IN ISRAEL

BY

S. FREIER, K. MAYER, C. LEVENE, and A. ABRAHAMOV

*From the Children's Department, the General Jewish Hospital 'Shaare Zedek', Jerusalem, and the Children's Department and Blood Bank, Hadassah University Hospital, Jerusalem*

(RECEIVED FOR PUBLICATION JULY 30, 1964)

It is now well established that hyperbilirubinaemia and even kernikterus may occur in the newborn in association with glucose 6 phosphate dehydrogenase (G6PD) deficiency, in the absence of any of the other causes of neonatal jaundice (Panizon, 1960a, b; Doxiadis, Fessas, and Valaes, 1960; Doxiadis, Fessas, Valaes, and Mastrokalos, 1961; Fessas, Doxiadis, and Valaes, 1962; Smith and Vella, 1960; Weatherall, 1960; Flatz, Szingam, Premyothin, Penbharkkul, Ketusingh, and Chulajata, 1963).

In Israel, in spite of the high incidence of G6PD deficiency in some communities, a retrospective survey of 42,000 births undertaken by Szeinberg, Oliver, Schmidt, Adam, and Sheba (1963), revealed only one case of severe neonatal jaundice that could possibly be ascribed to the enzyme deficiency. We wish to report here 8 cases of severe neonatal jaundice which occurred in G6PD-deficient infants in a Jerusalem hospital (Shaare Zedek), and to submit evidence suggesting that an antiseptic dye applied to the umbilicus was the precipitating haemolytic agent.

## Material and Methods

Each newborn was examined daily, and in every case of moderate or severe jaundice the serum bilirubin was determined. If the result was over 18 mg./100 ml. a detailed history was taken of the mother including her country of origin, past and family history of anaemia, jaundice, or favism, and details of drugs taken in the perinatal period. Whenever Rh iso-immunization could be excluded, the blood of the infant and of the parents was examined for G6PD deficiency by the semi-quantitative method of Motulsky and Campbell as described by Doxiadis *et al.* (1961).

The test is based on the time taken to decolorize a solution of 'brilliant-cresyl-blue' (National Aniline Division) mixed with the blood to be examined. If decolorization occurred after 60 minutes enzyme deficiency was considered to be present, values between one and two hours suggesting heterozygosity.

For blood group studies clotted venous blood was used. The blood groups of the mothers and the babies were determined for the following red cell antigens: ABO, Rh (including C, c, $D^u$, E, e) MN, Kell, and Duffy. The direct Coombs test was performed on the blood of the infants. The serum of the mothers was screened against a panel of group O red cells for the presence of antibodies belonging to the following blood group systems: MNS, P, Lutheran, Rh, Kell, Duffy, Kidd, and Lewis. The red cell antigen typing of the panel cells was performed for us by Dr. A. G. Mourant of the Lister Institute, London. The screening techniques were performed using the panel cells suspended in saline, and also using the same cells treated with ficin. The saline tubes were incubated both at room temperature and at 37° C. and were followed by the indirect Coombs test. The ficinized cells were incubated at 37° C. Titres for complete and incomplete anti-A and/or anti-B were performed where indicated by the ABO groups of the mothers and babies. A dextran medium was used for the detection of the incomplete anti-A and anti-B (Mollison, 1961). The techniques used were the standard methods described by Race and Sanger (1954).

## Description of Cases

The criterion of severe neonatal jaundice in this report is a total serum bilirubin level of 18 mg./100 ml. or above on one or more occasion. Exchange transfusion was performed in all but one of the cases here described. During the period July 1962 until February 1963 (incl.) there were 10 cases of severe neonatal jaundice: in 2 of these there was evidence of Rh incompatibility; G6PD deficiency was present in the other 8. The details are presented in Table 1. Most of the parents were Jewish immigrants from Kurdistan among whom the incidence, in males, of G6PD deficiency is 58·2%—the highest of any Jewish community in Israel (Sheba, Szeinberg, Ramot, Adam, and Ashkenazi, 1962). Kurdish infants constitute less than one-fifth of the infants born in this hospital. The sudden increase in the proportion of Kurdish infants requiring exchange transfusion during the period in question is shown in the Figure. ABO

TABLE 1

CLINICAL AND LABORATORY FINDINGS IN EIGHT JAUNDICED INFANTS WITH G6PD DEFICIENCY

| Case No. | 1 | 2 | 3 | 4 | 5 | 6 | 7 | 8 |
|---|---|---|---|---|---|---|---|---|
| Birth date | 30.6.62 | 5.7.62 | 16.7.62 | 23.12.62 | 10.1.63 | 5.8.62 | 30.10.62 | 4.2.63 |
| Sex | F | M | M | F | M | F | M | F |
| Birth weight (g.) | 2,850 | 3,460 | 2,950 | 2,420 | 3,550 | 2,210 | 3,410 | 1,970 |
| Mother's origin | Kurdistan | Kurdistan | Kurdistan | Syria | Kurdistan | Kurdistan | Kurdistan | Kurdistan |
| Father's origin | Kurdistan | Kurdistan | Kurdistan | Morocco | Morocco | Kurdistan | Kurdistan | Kurdistan |
| *Enzyme Tests** | | | | | | | | |
| Mother | – | – | – | – | ± | ± | ? | – |
| Father | – | + | – | + | – | – | ? | – |
| Infant | – | – | – | ± | – | – | – | – |
| *ABO Groups* | | | | | | | | |
| Mother | A | A | O | O | O | O | O | O |
| Father | A | A | O | O | A | A | B | AB |
| Infant | A | A | O | O | A | A | B | B |
| A, B antibody | | | | | Anti A | Anti A | ? | Anti B |
| Titre complete | | | | | 1 : 64 | 1 : 32 | | 1 : 256 |
| Incomplete | | | | | 1 : 64 | 1 : 256 | ? | 1 : 1024 |
| Onset of jaundice (hr.) | 24 | 96 | 96 | 24 | 48 | 10 | 72 | 24 |
| Highest bilirubin direct/indirect | 0/34 | 0/29 | 0/18 | 0/22 | 0/26 | 0/19 | 0/25 | 0/25 |
| Exchange transfusions | 2 | 1 | – | 1 | 1 | 1 | 1 | 2 |
| Haemoglobin on discharge (g./100 ml.) | 12·1 | 12·7 | ? | 8·6 | 10 | 11·8 | ? | 11·2 |
| Condition on discharge | ? Neurological signs | Good | Good | Good | Good | Good | Good | Good |

* Key for enzyme tests: + normal, – deficient, ± intermediate, ? not tested.

TABLE 2

MODE OF DELIVERY, POSTNATAL COMPLICATIONS, AND ANTIBIOTIC TREATMENT OF INFANTS

| Case No. | 1 | 2 | 3 | 4 | 5 | 6 | 7 | 8 |
|---|---|---|---|---|---|---|---|---|
| Complications of delivery | BBA* | Breech | N | N | N | Asphyxia | N | N |
| Hypothermia | + | – | – | + | – | – | – | – |
| Diarrhoea | + | – | + | + | – | + | – | – |
| Septicaemia | + | – | – | – | – | – | – | – |
| Conjunctivitis | – | + | – | – | – | – | – | – |
| Penicillin | + | – | – | + | – | + | – | – |
| Erythromycin | + | – | – | + | – | – | – | – |
| Neomycin | + | – | – | – | – | – | – | – |
| Tetracycline | – | – | – | + | – | – | – | – |

* Born before arrival in hospital. N = None.

TABLE 3

DRUGS ADMINISTERED TO MOTHERS

| Drugs | Case No. | | | | | | | |
|---|---|---|---|---|---|---|---|---|
| | 1 | 2 | 3 | 4 | 5 | 6 | 7 | 8 |
| Tetracycline and dicoumarol | – | – | – | – | + | – | – | – |
| Pitocin | – | – | – | + | – | – | – | – |
| Magnesium sulphate | – | + | – | – | – | – | – | – |
| Vitamins | + | – | – | + | + | + | + | – |
| Chloramphenicol | + | – | – | + | – | + | – | – |
| Sulphonamides, opium, chlorpromazine | – | – | – | – | – | – | – | + |

incompatibility was present in Cases 6 and 8 as shown by the titres of complete and incomplete anti A and anti B antibody respectively. In Case 7, ABO incompatibility could not be excluded as insufficient blood was available. The direct Coombs test was negative in the 8 cases, and no incompatibility in the CDE, Kell, Duffy, and MN systems could be found. Irregular blood group antibodies in the mother's serum were not detected. Details of the delivery and of drugs administered are given in Tables 2 and 3. With the exception of mild analgesics, of whose administration no record is kept, no drug was given uniformly to all the mothers. The vitamins administered to the mothers consisted of a multiple preparation without vitamin K. Although Case 1 also had signs of systemic infection, these were not considered to be responsible for his jaundice since jaundice was marked within 24 hours, whereas signs of infection appeared only on the fifth day.

Triple dye was used in this hospital as prophylactic treatment against umbilical sepsis. This dye is applied

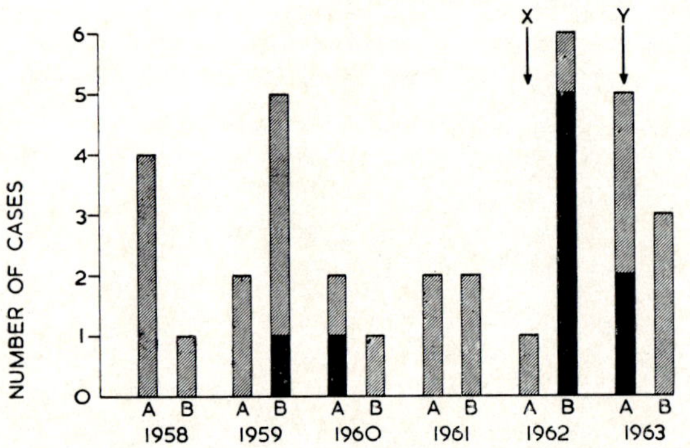


FIG. 1.—Incidence of exchange transfusions. The solid black area indicates exchange transfusions to Kurdish Jewish infants; the hatched area indicates total number of transfusions. X = triple dye begun in April 1962; Y = triple dye discontinued in April 1963. A, first six months of year; B, second six months of year.

while the infant is still in the delivery room and thereafter daily in the nursery. The three premature infants received vitamin K in a dose of 1 mg., intramuscularly. Antibiotics were administered as shown in Tables 2 and 3. A history of severe neonatal jaundice in previous infants was obtained in only one family.

## Discussion

In previous years between two to five exchange transfusions were performed yearly. A sudden increase in the need for exchange transfusion, such as here described, suggested the possibility of a laboratory error in the estimation of bilirubin. Such an error would not explain why the proportion of Kurdish infants requiring exchange transfusion should rise suddenly. Neither the total number of births nor the ethnic composition of the hospital population had changed in recent years. As the Kurdish community in Israel is unique in its particularly high incidence of G6PD deficiency, suspicion was immediately cast on this fact as being related to the jaundice. We could demonstrate this enzyme deficiency in all infants requiring exchange transfusion in the nine months under review, apart from two in whom Rh incompatibility was the obvious cause. Prematurity and ABO incompatibility were present in some cases but there was an associated G6PD deficiency. No exchange transfusions were required for the first two reasons alone during the period under review.

Hyperbilirubinaemia in newborn infants may be due to increased cell destruction or to inhibition of the conjugating capacity of the liver. That increased haemolysis had occurred in our cases can be assumed by the early onset of jaundice in some cases and the low haemoglobin values on discharge. The sudden appearance of a comparatively large number of cases of jaundice of this type, which heretofore was almost non-existent in Israel (Szeinberg *et al.*, 1963), led to a search for changes in treatment which might have given rise to haemolysis in enzyme-deficient infants.

As jaundice appeared within 24 hours in five infants, a hypothetical haemolytic agent in the breast milk could not have been the precipitating factor. None of the mothers ate beans at the time of delivery and the cases were not confined to the season in which favism occurs. It was suggested to us by Professor E. Goldschmidt that a likely cause was the antiseptic dye used in treating the umbilicus. The reason for implicating this substance is as follows: as jaundice due to enzyme deficiency was confined to our hospital, the provoking agent must be confined to that hospital. The other hospitals in this town use either 'brilliant green' alone or no dye at all, whereas in our hospital a 'triple dye' was used to prevent umbilical sepsis, as recommended in the control of staphylococcal infections in newborn nurseries (American Academy of Pediatrics, 1958). The B.P.C. preparation of 'triple dye' consists of a mixture of brilliant green, crystal violet, and proflavine hemisulphate, but instead of the last, the closely related ethacridine lactate ('Rivanol') was used. By April 1963 the evidence against this dye was strong enough to warrant using brilliant green alone, which was the practice in a neighbouring hospital where G6PD deficiency jaundice was not occurring in newborn infants. In the nine months following the discontinuation of its use, only one Kurdish infant had severe neonatal jaundice.

In order to test the potential haemolytic properties of our 'triple dye', it was incubated with enzyme-deficient red cells. There was no abnormal decrease of reduced glutathione and we, therefore, failed to confirm such a haemolytic effect *in vitro* (E. Heimann-Hollaender and S. Freier, 1963, unpublished observations). This, however, does not exclude the possibility that one of the breakdown products of these dyes present in the patient's plasma may be responsible for haemolysis. The amount of substance that can be absorbed through the umbilicus is obviously very small, but cases of G6PD-deficient jaundice are on record where the offending substance was probably a comparably small amount of naphthalene present in clothes impregnated with this substance (Zinkham and Childs, 1958; Dawson, Thayer, and Desforges, 1958; Jim and Chu, 1963). The evidence is, therefore, strongly in favour of an external factor being the cause of G6PD-deficient neonatal jaundice in Israel.

The rarity of severe neonatal jaundice due to G6PD deficiency in African infants in America and in infants of Oriental Jews in Israel as opposed to the high incidence of such jaundice in Greece, Italy, and Singapore, has given rise to the suspicion that some, as yet unrecognized, toxic substance is responsible for increased haemolysis in those countries. Our findings support such a theory. On the other hand Fessas *et al.* (1962) have adduced evidence for a familial tendency for enzyme-deficient neonatal jaundice. They suggest that a second genetic factor inherited independently of G6PD deficiency may exist in these families. As deficiencies of other enzymes, namely acid phosphomonoesterase and catalase, are known to occur in the erythrocytes of some G6PD deficient subjects (Tarlov and Kellermeyer, 1961; Oski, Shahidi, and Diamond, 1963) this possibility must be seriously considered. The relative importance of hereditary as opposed to environmental factors in enzyme-deficient jaundice in newborn infants, therefore, awaits further evaluation.

## Summary

Eight infants with severe neonatal jaundice associated with deficiency of G6PD were observed in a Jerusalem hospital. Incompatibility of the ABO groups of mother and infant possibly contributed to the jaundice in three cases. In spite of the high incidence of G6PD deficiency among Kurdish Jews in Israel, neonatal jaundice of this type is known to be uncommon in this country. An antiseptic preparation applied to the umbilicus was considered to be the most likely cause of the haemolysis in our cases.

We wish to thank most sincerely Professor E. Goldschmidt for her help at all stages of this work, and Miss Lia Cividalli for carrying out the Motulsky test.

### References

American Academy of Pediatrics (1958). *Suggestions for Control of Staphylococcal Infections in Newborn Nurseries.* Evanston, Illinois.

Dawson, J. P., Thayer, W. W., and Desforges, J. F. (1958). Acute hemolytic anemia in the newborn infant due to naphthalene poisoning. *Blood*, **13**, 1113.

Doxiadis, S. A., Fessas, Ph., and Valaes, T. (1960). Erythrocyte enzyme deficiency in unexplained kernicterus. *Lancet*, **2**, 44.

——, ——, ——, and Mastrokalos, N. (1961). Glucose-6-phosphate dehydrogenase deficiency. A new aetiological factor of severe neonatal jaundice. *ibid.*, **1**, 297.

Fessas, Ph., Doxiadis, S. A., and Valaes, T. (1962). Neonatal jaundice in glucose-6-phosphate-dehydrogenase deficient infants. *Brit. med. J.*, **2**, 1359.

Flatz, G., Szingam, S., Premyothin, C., Penbharkkul, S., Ketusingh, R., and Chulajata, R. (1963). Glucose-6-phosphate dehydrogenase deficiency and neonatal jaundice. *Arch. Dis. Childh.*, **38**, 566.

Jim, R. T. S., and Chu, F. K. (1963). Hyperbilirubinemia due to glucose-6-phosphate dehydrogenase deficiency in a newborn Chinese infant. *Pediatrics*, **31**, 1046.

Mollison, P. L. (1961). *Blood Transfusion in Clinical Medicine*, 3rd ed. Blackwell Scientific Publications, Oxford.

Oski, F. A., Shahidi, N. P., and Diamond, L. K. (1963). Erythrocyte acid phosphomenoesterase and glucose-6-phosphate dehydrogenase deficiency in Caucasians. *Science*, **139**, 409.

Panizon, F. (1960a). Erythrocyte enzyme deficiency in unexplained kernicterus. *Lancet*, **2**, 1093.

—— (1960b). L'ictère grave du nouveau-né à une déficience en glucose-6-phosphate déhydrogenase. *Biol. Neonat.* (*Basel*), **2**, 167.

Race, R. R., and Sanger, R. (1954). *Blood Groups in Man*, 2nd ed. Blackwell Scientific Publications, Oxford.

Sheba, C., Szeinberg, A., Ramot, B., Adam, A., and Ashkenazi, I. (1962). Epidemiologic surveys of deleterious genes in different population groups in Israel. *Amer. J. publ. Hlth*, **52**, 1101.

Smith, G. D., and Vella, F. (1960). Erythrocyte enzyme deficiency in unexplained kernicterus. *Lancet*, **1**, 1133.

Szeinberg, A., Oliver, M., Schmidt, R., Adam, A., and Sheba, C. (1963). Glucose-6-phosphate dehydrogenase deficiency and haemolytic disease of the newborn in Israel. *Arch. Dis. Childh.*, **38**, 23.

Tarlov, A. R., and Kellermeyer, R. W. (1961). The hemolytic effect of primaquine. XI. Decreased catalase activity in primaquine-sensitive erythrocytes. *J. Lab. clin. Med.*, **58**, 204.

Weatherall, D. J. (1960). Enzyme deficiency in haemolytic disease of newborn. *Lancet*, **2**, 835.

Zinkham, W. H., and Childs, B. (1958). A defect of glutathione metabolism in erythrocytes from patients with a naphthalene-induced hemolytic anemia. *Pediatrics*, **22**, 461.

*Arch. Dis. Childh.*, 1965, **40**, 284.

# A RELIABLE RAPID SCREENING TEST FOR SULPHATIDE LIPIDOSIS

BY

BRIAN D. LAKE

*From the Department of Morbid Anatomy, The Hospital for Sick Children, Great Ormond Street, London W.C.1*

(RECEIVED FOR PUBLICATION AUGUST 17, 1964)

The tests devised by Austin (1957) for the detection and isolation of metachromatic material from urine as a screening test for sulphatide lipidosis (metachromatic leucodystrophy) have been shown not to be entirely reliable because of the high incidence of false positives (Helfant, Börgeson, and Hellström, 1962). Even biochemical estimation showing raised amounts of urinary sulphatide cannot be taken as a reliable guide, since increased sulphatide excretion is also found in demyelinating diseases and in normal infants of less than 1 year (Hagberg and Svennerholm, 1960).

We have been using a simpler method than that of Austin for the screening of mentally retarded children, and have found that in 10 cases of sulphatide lipidosis all gave a positive result on urine sediment examination. There have been no false positives in 128 cases examined. The diagnosis was confirmed by rectal and peripheral nerve biopsies (Bodian and Lake, 1963) or by brain biopsy. Two cases in the series have come to necropsy, and together with five other available necropsy cases, the renal deposition of sulphatide was readily demonstrated in frozen sections by the same staining procedure.

## Method

The urine, which must be fresh and preferably not an early morning specimen, is centrifuged at 2,000-3,000 r.p.m. for 10 minutes. The supernatant is decanted, and 6 smears from the sediment are made on glass slides and then fixed in formalin vapour at 60°C. for one hour. The slides are washed in water and stained at room temperature for 10 minutes in a 1% aqueous solution of cresyl fast violet (E. Gurr, or Hopkins and Williams), the *p*H of which has been adjusted to 3·5-3·6 with acetic acid. The smears are washed in water and mounted in glycerin jelly.

## Results

A positive result is indicated by the presence of brown metachromatic staining material in the cytoplasm of renal epithelial cells (see Table). In all cases of sulphatide lipidosis examined in this series, there has been intracellular brown metachromatic material present. Only intracellular material is to be regarded as positive. Extracellular brown material is often seen and may be related to release of sulphatide in other types of demyelinating process, but it is so often seen that some other explanation is more likely.

TABLE

| No. of Urines Examined | No. Negative | No. Positive | No. Subsequently Shown to Have Sulphatide Lipidosis | No. of False Positives |
|---|---|---|---|---|
| 128 | 118 | 10 | 10 | 0 |

## Discussion

There are two explanations to account for the presence of sulphatide in the urine in sulphatide lipidosis. The first is that it is an excretion phenomenon related to removal of sulphatide from sites of demyelination. The second is that sulphatide lipidosis is a generalized enzymopathy and that wherever sulphatide is metabolized, i.e. in the kidney, accumulation takes place with subsequent excretion. The bulk of evidence supports the latter theory since excess sulphatide is observed in a variety of sites not related to myelinated nerves, i.e. gall-bladder, liver, pancreas, lamina propria of the colon, and the kidney. All myelinated nerves are also affected. Certain organs will become affected at an earlier stage by virtue of a normally high sulphatide metabolism, and as the kidney is always grossly involved it may be possible to provide an early preclinical diagnosis by examination of the urinary sediment. This test may appear positive before a diagnosis is possible by the conventional procedure of biopsy of peripheral nerve or rectum. Sulphatide lipidosis is a hereditary disorder and an early diagnosis is of the utmost importance so that the requisite advice may be given to the parents.


## Summary

A simple reliable method for the diagnosis of sulphatide lipidosis is described. Used in conjunction with other urine tests, i.e. phenistix and amino acid chromatography, it is a reliable guide on which to base subsequent investigations of mentally retarded children.


This work was supported by a grant from the Joint Research Board of the Institute for Child Health, Great Ormond Street, W.C.1.

### References


Austin, J. H. (1957). Metachromatic form of diffuse cerebral sclerosis. *Neurology* (*Minneap.*), 7, 415, 716.

Bodian, M., and Lake, B. D. (1963). The rectal approach to neuropathology. *Brit. J. Surg.*, **50**, 702.

Hagberg, B., and Svennerholm, L. (1960). Metachromatic leucodystrophy—a generalized lipidosis. Detection of sulfatides in urine, blood plasma and CSF. *Acta paediat.* (*Uppsala*), **49**, 690.

Helfant, M. H., Börgeson, M., and Hellström, B. (1962). The value of urinary sediment examination as a screening method in suspected cases of metachromatic leucodystrophy. *ibid.*, **51**, 49.

*Arch. Dis. Childh.*, 1965, **40**, 286.

# NEONATAL FITS ASSOCIATED WITH HYPOMAGNESAEMIA

BY

J. A. DAVIS, D. R. HARVEY, and J. S. YU*

*From the Nuffield Neonatal Research Unit, Institute of Child Health, Hammersmith Hospital, London W.12*

(RECEIVED FOR PUBLICATION SEPTEMBER 21, 1964)

Kruse, Orent, and McCollum (1932) were the first to show conclusively that experimental magnesium deficiency in rats causes clinical symptoms. The magnesium deficiency syndrome in man has been reviewed by MacIntyre (1963). The cardinal feature of severe magnesium deficiency is fits; other symptoms and signs are muscular weakness, vertigo, mental changes, gross tremor, and alteration in the electroencephalographic pattern.

There are few reports of symptomatic magnesium deficiency in the paediatric literature and few data about normal serum magnesium levels (Gittleman, Pincus, Schmerzler, and Saito, 1956). The case reported here is, we believe, the first in which there are adequate data to support a diagnosis of hypomagnesaemic fits in the neonatal period.

### Case Report

**Clinical History.** Infant Nigel B. was born on April 12, 1964 at 38 weeks' gestation and weighing 2,520 g. at birth.

His mother was 23 years and this was her first pregnancy. Coeliac disease was diagnosed when she was 7 years old and she was treated with a starch-free diet in 1949. She had a dramatic gain in weight and returned to a normal diet in 1951; since then she has had intermittent steatorrhoeic diarrhoea but is often constipated. At the 29th week of pregnancy she developed a megaloblastic anaemia (haemoglobin 9·0 g./100 ml.; serum folic acid 1·0 mμg./ml., and serum B12 240 μμg./ml.) which was treated with folic acid and iron. Her haemoglobin rose to 13·0 g./100 ml. in mid-April.

She was fully investigated two weeks after delivery. Physical examination was normal except that she was small, being only 155 cm. in height. A jejunal biopsy showed a flat mucosa, and barium follow-through demonstrated dilatation of the duodenum and jejunum with thickened primary folds. Serum calcium levels were 3·9-4·3 mEq, magnesium 1·3-1·4 mEq, and phosphate 1·6-1·7 mEq/l., and the phosphate excretion index was + 0·088 (normal). Folic acid absorption was low, 7% of a 50 μg. dose excreted in a 24-hour collection of urine. She is now on a gluten-free diet.

* Present address: Institute of Child Health, Royal Alexandra Hospital for Children, Sydney, N.S.W., Australia.

She was delivered by forceps, because of delay in the second stage of labour.

The baby was in good condition at birth and remained well until he was 8 days old. He was breast fed for five days but on the sixth day complementary feeds of evaporated cows' milk were introduced. From the 8th day he was fed entirely on evaporated cows' milk.

On the 8th day (April 19, 1964) generalized clonic convulsions began, this first episode of fits lasting 8 minutes. Physical examination showed no neck stiffness, fever, or tetany, but there were imposable tonic neck reflexes. The head circumference was 33·5 cm. There was severe oral thrush.

**Investigations.** Haemoglobin 15·1 g./100 ml. White cell count 17,000/c.mm.; neutrophils, 7,650; lymphocytes, 7,480; eosinophils, 1,530; monocytes, 340; and platelets, 20,000/c.mm.

*Cerebrospinal fluid* (obtained by cisternal puncture) was clear. There were 20 white cells/c.mm.; it was sterile on culture; glucose 55 mg./100 ml.; protein 85 mg./100 ml. *Blood sugar* was 22·5 mg./100 ml.; *serum calcium*, 2·6 mEq/l.; and *serum magnesium* 0·9 mEq/l.

**Progress.** Because of the equivocal cell count in the CSF, the baby was given a two-week course of the antibiotics (chloramphenicol, polymyxin, and cloxacillin). He was also given nystatin for the oral thrush. These were begun on the eighth day of life.

The fits continued throughout the next two days increasing in intensity and frequency, and they could not be adequately controlled by paraldehyde and chloral. On the tenth day, the baby had spasms of the limbs, as shown by episodic slow extension of his leg and dorsiflexion of his foot. Trousseau's sign was negative but Chvostek's sign was positive.

We have compressed the biochemical data into a chart (see Fig.). On the morning of the 11th day the baby was convulsing continuously and an EEG was taken while various substances, which might stop the convulsions, were injected intravenously. Pyridoxine 50 mg., 10 ml. 10% glucose, and 2 mEq calcium as 10% calcium gluconate, were given at 10-minute intervals; there was no change in the clinical state nor in the EEG, though after the calcium injection the serum calcium had returned to normal levels. After half an hour's delay, 2·5 mEq of

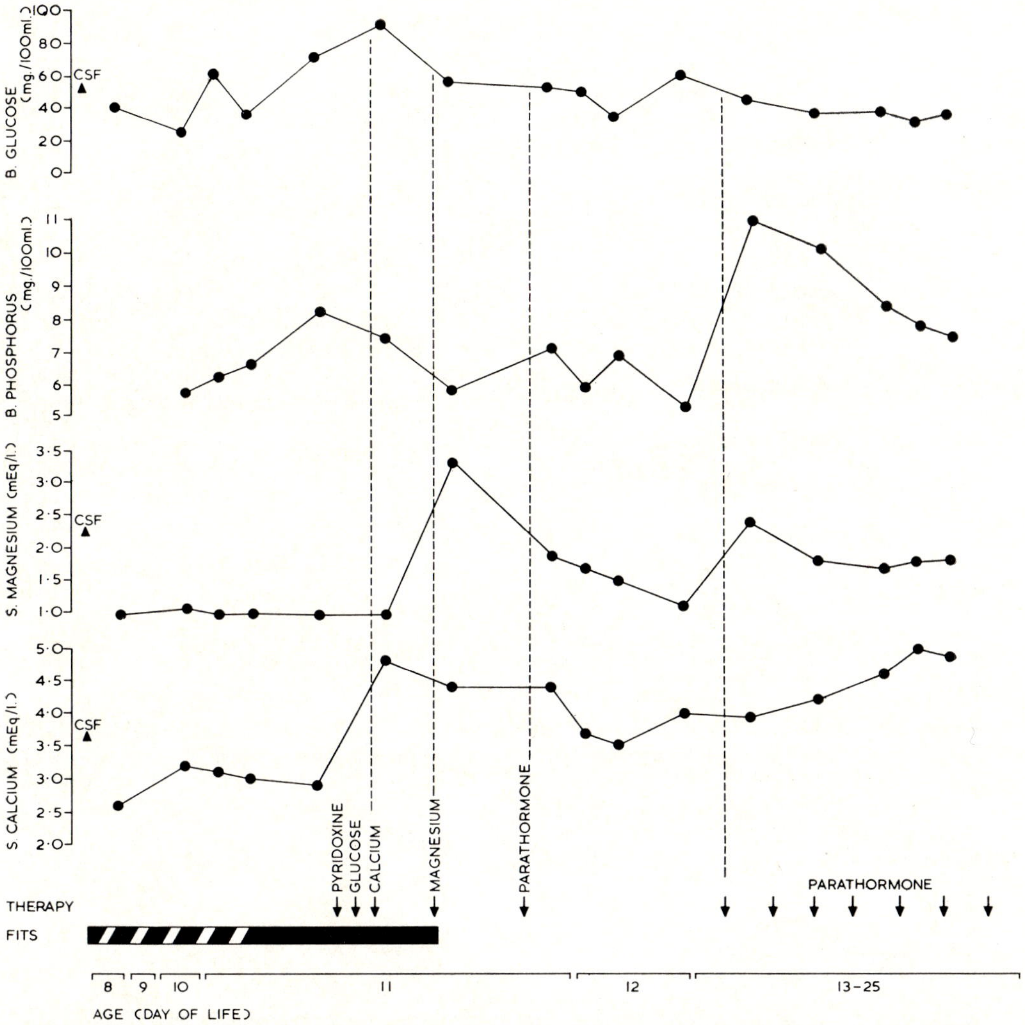


FIG.—Showing biochemical data. The pied strip indicates intermittent fits and the rest indicates continuous fits.

magnesium were given intravenously and produced a dramatic response. The clonic convulsions ceased in 30 seconds and Chvostek's sign, which was *strongly* positive just after the injection, rapidly became negative. There was no immediate change in the EEG, but 2 days later it was nearly normal, and after 6 days it was entirely normal.

There were occasional bilateral myoclonic jerks involving the proximal limb muscles during the 24 hours following the magnesium injection, but no further convulsions.

Three clearances of calcium, magnesium, and phosphorus were estimated before and after treatment and these are shown in the Table. The second study, made after 15 USP units of parathyroid extract had been given, showed a marked reduction of calcium and magnesium excretion. On April 24 (at 13 days of age) the serum magnesium level had again fallen to 1·1 mEq/l. Since the evidence suggested a functional hypoparathyroidism, a course of parathyroid extract given by intramuscular injection was begun.

On the 13th day he had 7 USP units of parathyroid

TABLE

RESULTS OF THE CLEARANCE STUDIES (ml./hr.)

| Clearance | Before Parathormone | After Single Dose of 15 USP Units of Parathormone | When Stabilized on Parathormone |
|---|---|---|---|
| Phosphate (ml.) | 5·6 | 7·8 | 14·7 |
| Calcium (ml.) | 1·6 | 0·3 | 1·7 |
| Magnesium (ml.) | 5·5 | 0·4 | 1·8 |

extract, on the next day 7 and 5 units, and thereafter 1 unit twice daily. His serum calcium and magnesium levels having returned to normal, treatment was stopped after 14 days of therapy. He was discharged on the 27th day and has since remained well, with no evidence of neurological damage.

**Special Investigations.** (1) CLEARANCE STUDIES. Serum calcium and magnesium were determined by a flame spectrophotometric method (Alcock, MacIntyre, and Radde, 1960), phosphate by the Fisk and Subarrow method, using phosphomolybdic acid, and glucose by glucose-oxidase (Marks, 1959). Serum cortisol levels were determined fluorimetrically.

The clearance studies were all done during the same 12-hour period to minimize errors due to diurnal variation. The baby was given the same volume and strength of processed evaporated cows' milk.

Clearance figures have been used as one index of calcium, magnesium, and phosphate homeostasis: the lack of normal values for the neonatal period precludes the use of more complex expressions. Three serum levels were taken during each clearance study, and from these a mean clearance was derived. The results are shown in the Table.

At the time of the third clearance study the baby was clinically well, and the serum calcium and magnesium levels were 4·6 and 1·8 mEq/l. respectively.

During the period when the infant was convulsing continuously, the plasma cortisol levels were 19-37 μg./100 ml. Thirty minutes after the convulsions had stopped, the cortisol had fallen to 8 μg./100 ml., and it remained within this range for the rest of the study period.

(2) ELECTROENCEPHALOGRAMS. Nine electrodes were used, the connexion being bipolar (scalp to scalp). Electrocardiogram and respiratory rate were recorded simultaneously.

(a) *At the age of 8 days and 10 hours.* The baby appeared clinically in the second stage of sleep for long periods, as judged by regular respiration (45/min.) and absence of eye movements, but the EEG did not show the episodic activity usually associated with this stage of sleep. Instead, it showed runs of unusually rhythmic activity usually at 4 to 7 c/s. (40 μV amplitude) appearing independently from either side of the head. On a few occasions there were short runs of slow activity 1·5 c/s.) and once clear spike and wave activity at this frequency from both anterior leads. During the recording there were numerous episodes of single twitches of a limb or a digit, but there were no corresponding changes in the EEG. On the other hand, there were rather frequent instances of sharp waves on one or other side showing phase reversal about the midline. Very occasionally there was a bilaterally synchronous single sharp wave.

(b) *At the age of 8 days and 15 hours.* He was given 0·3 ml. paraldehyde 3½ hours before recording. Background activity was the same as in the previous record. One fit was observed. Clinically this consisted of an odd cry followed by twitching of the left leg preceding twitching of all limbs. During the fit there were only brief periods of apnoea. The EEG changes lasted about 50 seconds. At first there were alternate low amplitude spikes and high amplitude slow waves at 1·5 c/s. from the right hemisphere only, but after a few seconds the left hemisphere was also involved. Almost continuous spike and wave activity continued, but the rate varied from 1 to 5 c/s., the faster activity replacing the slow spike and wave in runs of a few seconds only. The spike and wave complex showed phase reversal about the midline on both sides. After the fit the record was flat for about half a minute.

(c) *At the age of 10 days.* Background activity was similar to that seen in previous records, but there were numerous instances of single monophasic sharp waves showing phase reversal about the midline on one or other side. Occasionally these sharp waves occurred in runs of a second or two, and occasionally there was a bilateral burst of irregular sharp and slow waves of about the same duration. During the recording there were no major fits, but frequent jerks of different parts of the body—single or repeated jerks lasting several seconds. However, there did not appear to be any association between these apparent focal fits and the sharp wave discharges on the EEG.

Following intravenous injections of 50 mg. pyridoxine, 10 ml. 10% glucose, and 2 mEq calcium as 10% calcium gluconate, there was no change in the clinical state nor in the EEG record.

Immediately after intravenous injection of magnesium chloride (2·5 mEq) the almost continuous jerking ceased. There was no immediate change in the EEG, and sharp waves from one or other hemisphere continued to appear. Gradually, however, the record became episodic, with bursts of higher amplitude activity of varying frequencies against a rather flat background about every 10 seconds. These bursts differed from normal episodic sleep activity only in that they contained moderate to high amplitude sharp waves on one or other or both sides.

(d) *At the age of 12 days.* The recording was made during varying stages of sleep. The earlier part of the record showed less rhythmic activity in the $\theta$ frequency range, was of higher amplitude, and contained more delta waves than previously seen. There were only a few sharp waves. The next section was very similar in background activity to the earliest records, and no sharp waves were seen. In the last section there was a return to the higher amplitude arrhythmic appearance with episodic sleep bursts containing sharp elements as in the last recording.

(e) *At the age of 16 days.* When the baby was awake the record was of low amplitude and arrhythmic containing elements at all frequencies. There were a few low amplitude sharp waves not showing phase reversal and of doubtful significance. During sleep rather indistinct episodic activity was seen.

(f) *At the age of 97 days.* An EEG recording was normal.

## Discussion

Serum calcium and magnesium levels in infants of birth weight 1,500-2,500 g. vary considerably during the first 48 hours, falling to a minimum level at 18-24 hours before rising again. At 48 hours serum calcium is 4·4 ± 0·3 SD mEq/l. (W. W. Payne, 1964, personal communication). Hypocalcaemia by adult standards is frequently seen in normal asymptomatic newborn infants.

Levels of serum calcium and magnesium in the neonatal period depend on the type of feed given. Breast-fed infants tend to have slightly higher calcium and magnesium levels at 5 days, while babies having processed cows' milk with added vitamin D have significantly lower calcium and magnesium levels at 5 days than on the first day of life (Gittleman, Pincus, and Schmerzler, 1964). Tufts and Greenberg (1938) showed that nursing rats with deficient magnesium diets have lower than normal quantities of magnesium in their milk and that their suckling young, even though their birth weight and initial serum magnesium may be normal, develop the magnesium deficiency syndrome at 2 to 3 weeks of age.

By the standards of this laboratory, the levels of both calcium and magnesium were low throughout the entire symptomatic period. The causes of these deficiencies may have been both pre- and postnatally determined. The blood glucose level remained within the normal range for a newborn infant of this weight.

At the time of the intravenous test doses of pyridoxine, glucose, calcium, and magnesium, the baby had been convulsing continuously for 4 hours and looked very ill. The tests were performed under continuous EEG control.

The one indisputable clinical fit that occurred during recording was accompanied by striking electroencephalographic abnormalities, showing sharp and slow wave complexes from the contralateral hemicranium, when the fit was lateralized, and then from leads on both sides. The interseizure records were not strikingly abnormal: the single focal sharp waves differed from those seen in recordings from normal newborn babies only in being more numerous and they did not coincide with single limb jerks. They did, however, disappear gradually following restoration of normal serum magnesium levels, and the other noticeable change was the appearance, for the first time following this treatment, of normal episodic sleep activity which had not accompanied the second stage of sleep in previous recordings (Harris and Tizard, 1960).

After the successive injections of pyridoxine, glucose, and calcium there was no improvement clinically or on the EEG tracing. Thirty minutes later 2·5 mEq of magnesium were given, and within 30 seconds the convulsing ceased, not to recur, though the EEG changes persisted for 24 hours.

Whether the magnesium alone would have stopped the fits we cannot say, since it seems probable that calcium and magnesium are interrelated in their actions on the nervous system. Though it cannot be excluded, the dose of magnesium given was not thought to be sufficient to cause pharmacological CNS depression, and paraldehyde had had no effect.

In looking for a cause for the baby's hypomagnesaemia, it may be relevant that his mother had coeliac disease and suffers from intermittent diarrhoea on a normal diet. Booth, Babouris, Hanna, and MacIntyre (1963) described 42 cases of malabsorption of whom 15 had subnormal serum magnesium levels. After the dramatic response to magnesium in this baby, investigation of the mother showed a pathologically flattened jejunal biopsy with a low serum calcium 3·9-4·3 mEq/l. and a serum magnesium of 1·3-1·5 mEq/l. which is at the lower limits of the normal adult range (MacIntyre, 1963); a skeletal survey showed mild cortical thinning.

One can speculate that the mother's homeostatic mechanisms for magnesium conservation were under stress during her pregnancy, and that there was a compensatory increase in parathyroid activity. It also seems likely that her milk would be deficient in magnesium (Tufts and Greenberg, 1938). The lack of clinical evidence to support a diagnosis of hyperparathyroidism may be the result of an associated vitamin D deficiency which also occurs in malabsorption.

Impaired activity of the parathyroid glands has been suggested as a cause of the observed fall in serum calcium and magnesium in the first 48 hours of life in normal newborn infants (Smith, 1959). A high maternal parathormone level might depress the activity of the foetal parathyroid still further, and so delay the acquisition of normal function in the newborn infant.

In the absence of compensating parathyroid activity, the substitution of breast milk in the baby's diet by processed cows' milk, containing vitamin D, and an increased phosphate load, would tend to lower subsequent calcium and magnesium levels.

The clearance studies after a test dose of parathormone (15 USP units) suggest that the baby's own parathyroid gland had been unable to respond to low blood levels of calcium and magnesium by reducing urinary loss of these elements. When the plasma levels of magnesium and calcium were depressed to 0·9 and 2·6 mEq/l., respectively, the infant was still excreting large quantities of magnesium and calcium in his urine. This is grossly abnormal. Parathyroid extract then caused a dramatic fall in the urinary excretion of calcium and magnesium. MacIntyre, Boss, and Troughton

(1963) showed a similar response to pure parathormone in parathyroidectomized rats with magnesium deficiency, but were not able to demonstrate this response in normal rats.

The phosphate excretion did not increase significantly with parathyroid extract, a phenomenon recognized in newborn infants on the first day of life (Connelly, Crawford, and Watson, 1962).

After parathyroid extract had been administered for 6 days, in a dosage of 1 USP unit per day, the serum magnesium had risen to 1·8 mEq/l. At this serum level the urinary clearance of magnesium was 1·8 ml. per hour, which is still less than the excretion at the time when the serum magnesium was only 0·9 mEq/l. and before any parathyroid extract had been given.

These clearance studies, which closely parallel experimental findings in parathyroidectomized rats, strongly support the existence of a functional hypoparathyroidism during the initial illness of this infant.

## Summary

The case of a newborn infant with persistent convulsions associated with low serum calcium and magnesium levels is described. Magnesium deficiency in the mother, as a result of coeliac disease, together with a diet of cows' milk containing vitamin D, are suggested as factors in the baby's hypomagnesaemia and hypocalcaemia.

Evidence is presented suggesting that the baby was deficient in parathormone and that a low serum magnesium level was a cardinal factor in the aetiology of the convulsions.

It is a pleasure to thank Professor J. P. M. Tizard for his EEG reports, Dr. I. MacIntyre for the calcium and magnesium estimations, and Dr. W. W. Payne for his advice and guidance.

Laboratory facilities were provided by the Sir William Coxen Trust.

### References

Alcock, N., MacIntyre, I., and Radde, I. (1960). The determination of magnesium in biological fluids and tissues by flame spectrophotometry. *J. clin. Path.*, **13**, 506.

Booth, C. C., Babouris, N., Hanna, S., and MacIntyre, I. (1963). Incidence of hypomagnesaemia in intestinal malabsorption. *Brit. med. J.*, **2**, 141.

Connelly, J. P., Crawford, J. D., and Watson, J. (1962). Studies of neonatal hyperphosphatemia. *Pediatrics*, **30**, 425.

Gittleman, I. F., Pincus, J. B., and Schmerzler, E. (1964). Interrelationship of calcium and magnesium in the mature neonate. *Amer. J. Dis. Child.*, **107**, 119.

——, ——, ——, and Saito, M. (1956). Hypocalcemia occurring on the first day of life in mature and premature infants. *Pediatrics*, **18**, 721.

Harris, R., and Tizard, J. P. M. (1960). The electroencephalogram in neonatal convulsions. *J. Pediat.*, **57**, 501.

Kruse, H. D., Orent, E. R., and McCollum, E. V. (1932). Studies on magnesium deficiency in animals. Symptomatology resulting from magnesium deprivation. *J. biol. Chem.*, **96**, 519.

MacIntyre, I. (1963). Magnesium metabolism. *Sci. Basis Med. Ann. Rev.*, 216.

——, Boss, S., and Troughton, V. A. (1963). Parathyroid hormone and magnesium homeostasis. *Nature (Lond.)*, **198**, 1058.

Marks, V. (1959). An improved glucose-oxidase method for determining blood, c.s.f. and urine glucose levels. *Clin. chim. Acta*, **4**, 395.

Smith, C. A. (1959). *Physiology of the Newborn Infant*, 3rd ed., p. 300. Blackwell, Oxford.

Tufts, E. V., and Greenberg, D. M. (1938). The biochemistry of magnesium deficiency. I. Chemical changes resulting from magnesium deprivation. *J. biol. Chem.*, **122**, 693.

*Arch. Dis. Childh.*, 1965, **40**, 291.

# THE OSMOTIC CONCENTRATING ABILITY IN HEALTHY INFANTS AND CHILDREN

BY

E. POLÁČEK, J. VOCEL, L. NEUGEBAUEROVÁ, M. ŠEBKOVÁ, and E. VĚCHETOVÁ

with the technical co-operation of M. Křišťan and B. Trousilová

*From the Institute for Research in Child Development, Pediatric Faculty, Prague, First and Second University, Children's Departments, Prague, Infant Home, Prague-Krč, Children's Home, Kunratice, Czechoslovakia*

(RECEIVED FOR PUBLICATION OCTOBER 16, 1964)

The concentrating ability of the kidney changes with age: after birth it increases (Smith, 1959), and in old age it falls (Lindeman, van Buren, and Raisz, 1960). The maximum osmolality during the newborn period is much lower than in adults (Heller, 1944; Smith, Yudkin, Young, Minkowski, and Cushman, 1949; Barnett and Vesterdal, 1953; Hansen and Smith, 1953; McCance and Widdowson, 1954; Calgagno and Rubin, 1960; Fisher, Pyle, Porter, Beard, and Panos, 1963). This smaller concentrating ability rapidly increases after birth, as shown by the significantly higher maximum osmolality of the urine in mature and some premature children in the second to fourth week of life (Pratt and Snyderman, 1953; Edelmann, Barnett, and Troupkou, 1960), and may reach 1,473 mOsm./l. at the age of 35 days (Pratt, Bienvenu, and Whyte, 1948), and 1,570 mOsm./l. at 73 days (Drescher, Barnett, and Troupkou, 1962). The osmolality of the urine of premature infants in the first month of life can be low (Calgagno, Rubin, and Weintraub, 1954), particularly in premature infants with a birth weight below 2,250 g. in comparison with that of mature infants of the same age (Vocel, Poláček, Neugebaurová, and Šebková, 1963). Results in a number of series of children investigated with various tests showed a tendency for maximum osmolality to increase after the second month of life (Winberg, 1959; Poláček and Polanská, 1962; Martínek, Janovský, and Stanincová, 1962) and even after the first year of life (Winberg, 1959; Poláček, 1962). The comparison of these data is difficult because the methods used to achieve increasing concentration of urine were diverse. For this reason it seemed desirable to investigate subjects from the early postnatal period up to adult life, using a single method. Since premature infants with a low birth weight react to fluid restriction with lower concentration of urine, and sometimes even by haemoconcentration and raised non-protein nitrogen (Vocel *et al.*, 1963; Fisher *et al.*, 1963), only those premature infants with a birth weight over 2,250 g. were included in the series.

### Material and Methods

The following 212 children were included in the investigation: 32 newborn infants from the First University Obstetric Department, 13 premature infants with a birth weight above 2,250 g. in the First University Children's Department in Prague, 79 toddlers from the Children's Home in Kunratice, and 57 pre-school and school children in the Educational Department of the First University Children's Department in Prague. Children affected with serious disease and convalescents after acute illness were excluded. The concentration test was carried out by giving the children dried milk dissolved in half the usual amount of water with sugar added, for 24 hours, in amounts corresponding to their usual calorie intake. The preparation of full-cream milk was used for older children and a half-cream milk in younger infants. The urine was collected at intervals of about three hours and stored in the refrigerator. The temperature of infants and young children was taken frequently. If it rose above 37·5° C. the experiment was stopped, but the result of this abbreviated test was also taken into the series. Osmolality was determined cryoscopically by a thermistor connected up to a Wheastone bridge. The accuracy of the method was repeatedly checked by determining the depression of the freezing point on the same sample by the Beckmann thermometer. The difference between two measurements did not exceed 1%. Maximum osmolality was taken as the highest osmotic value attained in the urine samples. Unusually high osmolality was determined at least three times and the probability of the results confirmed by determining specific gravity and concentrations of Na, K, Cl, and urea.

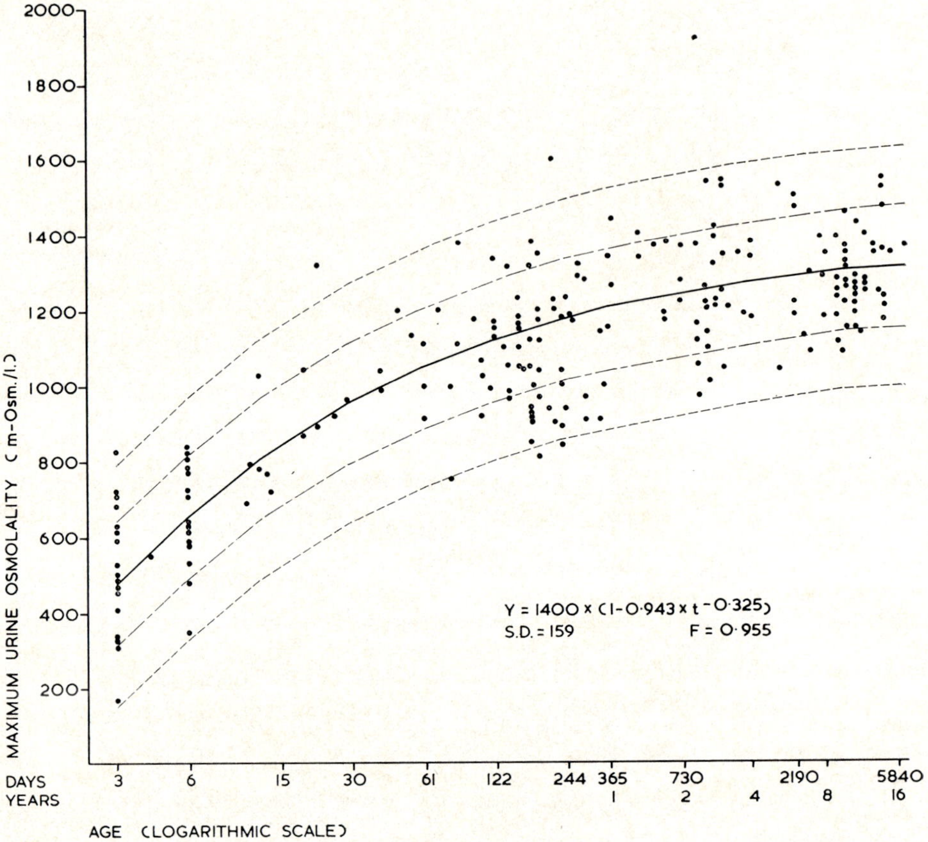


FIG. 1.—Relation of maximum urine osmolality to age in healthy infants and children. Maximum urine osmolality of urine samples in course of 24-hour concentration test by means of double concentrated milk. Logarithmic scale for age.

TABLE 1

AVERAGE AND MAXIMUM URINE OSMOLALITY OF PREMATURE AND FULL-TERM INFANTS DURING FIRST WEEK OF LIFE

| Reference | Description of Infants | Diet | Urine Osmolality (mOsm./l.) on Different Days | | | | | |
|---|---|---|---|---|---|---|---|---|
| | | | 1 | 2 | 3 | 4 | 5 | 6 |
| Heller (1944) | 23 full-term | Normal fluid intake | 350–450 | 280–530 | 120–440 | 80–700 | 50–360 | 120–150 |
| McCance and Widdowson (1954) | 18 full-term | 25 ml. water for first 48 hr. | 375<br>± 91·5 | 465<br>± 51 | — | — | — | — |
| Smith *et al.* (1949) | 10 prematures (1,530-2,260 g.) | Fluid withheld 52·5- 112 hr. | — | — | Maximum urine osmolality: 400–624 | | | — |
| Hansen and Smith (1953) | 3 full-term<br>6 prematures | Fluid withheld for first 72 hr. | 200*–530* | 350*–600* | 400*–680 | — | — | — |
| Calgagno and Rubin (1960) | 4 full-term | Cows' milk | — | Average urine osmolality: 318 (184–449) | | | | — |
| | 12 full-term | Low osmolar milk | — | Average urine osmolality: 157 (77–492) | | | | — |
| | 14 full-term | Modified evaporated milk + carbohydrate formula | — | Average urine osmolality: 204 (114–454) | | | — | — |
| | 9 full-term | Colostrum | — | Average urine osmolality: 273 (70–408) | | | | — |
| | 2 full-term | Transitional milk | — | — | — | — | — | 77 and 164 |
| Barnett and Vesterdal (1953) | 4 prematures<br>5-8 days | 4 hr. after last feeding | — | — | — | — | 5th to 8th day<br>610 | (432–778) |
| Fisher *et al.* (1963) | 60 full-term | 5% glucose first 24 hr., then evaporated milk with 1½ parts water | 291<br>(120–460) | 309<br>(140–460) | 240<br>(70–587) | 187<br>(58–480) | — | — |
| | 15 prematures | Fluid withheld 72 hr., then 5% glucose for 24 hr., then breast milk | 230<br>± 56<br>Serum Na<br>145 mEq/l. | 293<br>± 40<br>— | 441<br>± 69<br>Serum Na<br>150 mEq/l. | —<br>— | 149<br>± 24<br>— | 94<br>± 51<br>Serum Na<br>142 mEq/l. |

* Results given only in figures. Values estimated.

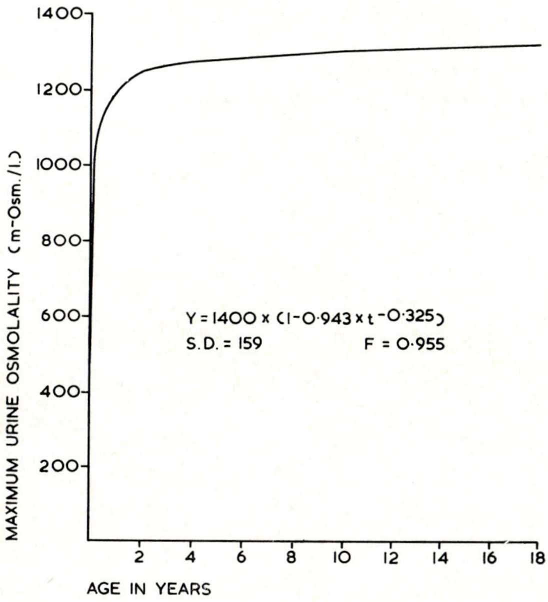


FIG. 2.—Regression line of maximum urine osmolality. Normal scale for age.

## Results

The general results are given in Fig. 1 in which the age is expressed logarithmically, and it shows that the maximum osmolality of the urine tends to increase with age. However, the regression line does not run linearly ($F = 1 \cdot 4$; $F (0 \cdot 05, 200, 500) = 1 \cdot 2$), but exponentially ($F = 0 \cdot 955$). The unconverted course of the regression line is given in Fig. 2, which shows that the average maximum osmolality of the urine increases rapidly in the first few months of life and that subsequently the rate of increase progressively slows down.

## Discussion

All authors give much lower values for the osmolality of the urine in the first week of life than at a later age. In Table 1 are set out the results of a number of investigations on the concentrating ability of premature and full-term infants during the first week of life.

In our series the average maximum osmolality of the urine was 515 mOsm./l. (S.D. 172, $n = 17$) on the 3rd day, which is in good accord with findings of Hansen and Smith (1953) who found values of 400-680 mOsm./l. in 3-day-old infants without fluid intake.

In our series the average maximum osmolality on the 6th day was 663 mOsm./l. (S.D. 133, $n = 16$), which is significantly higher than on the third day ($p < 0 \cdot 01$) and corresponds approximately to values found by Barnett and Vesterdal (1953) in premature infants aged 5-8 days (432-778 mOsm./l.), but much higher than those quoted by Heller (1944) (on the 6th day 120-150 mOsm./l.) and by Fisher *et al.* (1963) (on the 6th day 94 mOsm./l. $\pm$ 51). These considerable differences in the results can be explained by the fact that in the last two groups the infants were given a small osmotic load with adequate fluid intake. Great diversity in the osmolality of the urine has been recorded from the end of the first week to the end of the first year. For this reason comparison should be restricted to investigations in which an increased osmotic load or a restriction of fluid intake has been employed or a combination of both. In Table 2 are set out the results of investigations in infants aged over 1 week up to 3 months.

We found that at the age of 10-30 days maximum osmolality of the urine amounted to an average value of 896 mOsm./l. (S.D. 179, $n = 12$). This value is significantly higher than the average maximum osmolality in this series at 6 days ($p < 0 \cdot 001$). This corresponds to the osmolality of the urine reached by infants of Edelmann *et al.* (1960) fed on 8-9 g. protein/kg.

The maximum osmolality noted in our infants aged 1-2 months reached an average of 1,054 mOsm./l. and is in agreement with the average osmolality in the infants of Pratt *et al.* (1948) after the first 24 hours of water restriction.

The osmolar concentrating ability of infants aged over 2 months was investigated by Winberg (1959). He first gave an intramuscular injection of pitressin tannate in oil (0·5 pressure units per 6 kg. body weight) and then deprived the infants of all fluid for 16 hours by leaving out one or two feeds. The regression line in Winberg's series rose up to 1 to 1½ years. In children older than 3 years, Winberg recorded an average maximum osmolality of the urine of 1,069 mOsm./l. (S.D. 127, $n = 16$). Increase in urine osmolality with age in infants on a decreased fluid intake was noted by Martínek *et al.* (1962, Table 2).

In our series the regression line rises throughout the entire first year of life. In the children aged 10-12 months maximum urine osmolality reached an average of 1,118 (S.D. 154, $n = 7$) and was significantly higher than in infants aged 2-5 weeks ($p < 0 \cdot 02$). The increase in the regression line persists, though more slowly after the first year of life. At 14-18 years the average osmolality of the urine reaches 1,362 (S.D. 109, $n = 9$), which is significantly higher than at the end of the first year ($p < 0 \cdot 01$).

It is very probable that some children in our series

TABLE 2

MAXIMUM URINE OSMOLALITY OF INFANTS AGED 1 WEEK TO 3 MONTHS: RESULTS OF INVESTIGATIONS BY VARIOUS METHODS OF CONCENTRATION

| Reference | Description and Age of Infants | Description of Diet | Maximum Urine Osmolality mOsm./l. | Results After Age of 3 mth. |
|---|---|---|---|---|
| Calgagno *et al.* (1954) | 5 prematures 5-25 dy. | 12-18 hr. without fluid | 617 (588-648) | |
| Pratt and Snydermann (1953) | 6 prematures 11-23 dy. | Evaporated milk with small amounts of water for 3 dy. | 637-985 | |
| Edelmann *et al.* (1960) | Prematures 7-39 dy. | Various diets for 3-7 dy. | | |
| | No. 4 | 8-9 g. protein/kg. + restricted water | 857-993 | |
| | No. 5 | 8-9 g. protein/kg. + normal water intake | 707-1,139 | |
| | No. 4 | 4 g. protein/kg. + restricted water | 615-864 | |
| | No. 1 | Loaded with urea | 825 | |
| | No. 1 | Loaded with 250 mg. NaCl/kg. | 616 | |
| Vocel *et al.* (1963) | 28 prematures 26 full-term 10-90 dy. | Dried milk + ½ water content up to 24 hr. | Full-term and prematures over 2,250 g. in 16 hr. above 700 Prematures 1,400-2,250 g.: 36% under 700 in 24 hr. | |
| Drescher *et al.* (1962) | 6 full-term 2 wk.-2 mth. | Various protein and urea loads with restricted water for 3 dy. | 905*-1,570* Highest value in infant 73 dy. old | |
| Pratt *et al.* (1948) | 5 infants 30-65 dy. | 130 cals/kg./day: Evaporated milk with carbohydrate without added water | After 24 hr.: 914-1,177 after 5-6 dy.: 973-1,473 | |
| Martínek *et al.* (1962) | Infants | Dried breast-milk with ⅓ water content for 24 hr. | | |
| | 16-19 dy. | | 694 | |
| | 6 wk. | | 919 | |
| | 2½-3 mth. | | 1,012 | 4½ mth. 1,082 mOsm./l. |
| Winberg (1959) | 10 infants from 1 mth. up | Fluid withheld 16 hr. + pitressin tannate in oil | 500*-960* | 31 children 3-36 mth.: 580*-1,320* 16 children above 3 yr.: 1,069 (S.D.127·5) |

* Results given only in figures. Values estimated.

did not reach their maximum concentrating ability in the course of 24 hours. Others perhaps did not need to reach this limiting concentration. The results of Pratt *et al.* (1948), Drescher *et al.* (1962), and Sargent and Johnson (1954, 1956) furnish evidence that some children and young men can attain higher concentrations of the urine by more prolonged water restriction combined with adequate osmotic loading. Our experience (Poláček and Polanská, 1962) shows, however, that some healthy infants do not tolerate this prolonged water restriction without greatly increased temperature and other disturbances. The method described in this paper permitted the investigation of children in the same manner from the neonatal period up to puberty while sufficiently high values of urine osmolality were obtained.

## Summary

A concentrating test was carried out in 212 children aged from 3 days to 18 years by giving them dried milk made up with half amount of water for 24 hours with addition of sugar and limited to the usual intake of calories. Urine was collected at three-hour intervals, and maximum osmolality of the urine was taken as the highest value found in the separate urine samples. This maximum urine osmolality increases with age from birth to puberty. The average maximum urine osmolality values increase rapidly in the first months of life and then the increase is slower. There are significant differences between the average values of maximum urine osmolality on the 3rd day (515 mOsm./l.), the 6th day (663 mOsm./l.), the first month excluding the first week (896 mOsm./l.), the end of the first year (1,118 mOsm./l. at 10-12 months), and at puberty (1,362 mOsm./l. at 14-18 years). The regression line has an exponential character ($Y = 1{,}400 \times (1 - 0{\cdot}943 \times t^{-0{\cdot}325})$).

### REFERENCES

Barnett, H. L., and Vesterdal, J. (1953). The physiologic and clinical significance of immaturity of kidney function in young infants. *J. Pediat.*, **42**, 99.

Calgagno, P. L., and Rubin, M. I. (1960). Water requirements for renal excretion in full-term newborn infants and premature infants fed a variety of formulas. *ibid.*, **56**, 717.

——, ——, and Weintraub, D. H. (1954). Studies on the renal concentrating and diluting mechanisms in the premature infant. *J. clin. Invest.*, **33**, 91.

Drescher, A. N., Barnett, H. L., and Troupkou, V. (1962). Water balance in infants during water deprivation. *Amer. J. Dis. Child.*, **104**, 366.

Edelmann, C. M., Jr., Barnett, H. L., and Troupkou, V. (1960). Renal concentrating mechanisms in newborn infants. *J. clin. Invest.*, **39**, 1062.

Fisher, D. A., Pyle, H. R., Jr., Porter, J. C., Beard, A. G., and Panos, T. C. (1963). Control of water balance in the newborn. *Amer. J. Dis. Child.*, **106**, 137.

Hansen, J. D. L., and Smith, C. A. (1953). Effects of withholding fluid in the immediate postnatal period. *Pediatrics*, **12**, 99.

Heller, H. (1944). The renal function of newborn infants. *J. Physiol. (Lond.)*, **102**, 429.

Lindeman, R. D., van Buren, H. C., and Raisz, L. G. (1960). Osmolar renal concentrating ability in healthy young men and hospitalized patients without renal disease. *New Engl. J. Med.*, **262**, 1306.

Martínek, J., Janovský, M., and Stanincová, V. (1962). Regulace hospodaření vodou a elektrolyty za dehydratace u kojenců. *Čs. Fysiol.*, **11**, 459.

McCance, R. A., and Widdowson, E. M. (1954). Normal renal function in the first two days of life. *Arch. Dis. Childh.*, **29**, 488.

Poláček, E. (1962). Vývoj koncentrační schopnosti ledvin. 100 let. St. zdrav. nakl. Praha. p. 257.

——, and Polanská, M. (1962). Koncentrační pokus u kojenců. *Čs. Pediat.*, **17**, 1.

Pratt, E. L., Bienvenu, B., and Whyte, M. M. (1948). Concentration of urine solutes by young infants. *Pediatrics*, **1**, 181.

——, and Snyderman, S. E. (1953). Renal water requirement of infants fed evaporated milk with and without added carbohydrate. *ibid.*, **11**, 65.

Sargent, F., II, and Johnson, R. E. (1954). Solute load and the renal osmotic parameters of chronically dehydrated men. *J. clin. Invest.*, **33**, 962.

——, and —— (1956). The effects of diet on renal function in healthy men. *Amer. J. clin. Nutr.*, **4**, 466.

Smith, C. A. (1959). *The Physiology of the Newborn Infant*, 3rd ed., p. 331. Blackwell, Oxford.

——, Yudkin, S., Young, W., Minkowski, A., and Cushman, M. (1949). Adjustment of electrolytes and water following premature birth. *Pediatrics*, **3**, 34.

Vocel, J., Poláček, E., Neugebaurová, L., and Šebková, J. (1963). Koncentrační test u nedonošenců a mladých kojenců. *Čs. Pediat.*, **18**, 774.

Winberg, J. (1959). Determination of renal concentration capacity in infants and children without renal disease. *Acta paediat. (Uppsala)*, **48**, 318.

*Arch. Dis. Childh.*, 1965, **40**, 296.

# INTELLECTUAL IMPAIRMENT IN MUSCULAR DYSTROPHY

BY

VICTOR DUBOWITZ
*From the Department of Child Health, University of Sheffield*

(RECEIVED FOR PUBLICATION AUGUST 7, 1964)

The association of intellectual retardation with childhood muscular dystrophy was noted many years ago. Duchenne (1872) thought that 5 of his 13 cases were retarded. Gowers (1879), on the other hand, found evidence of mental retardation in only 2 of his 24 patients, and he thought that it was not a feature of the muscle disease but that there was probably a higher incidence of muscular dystrophy in mentally retarded children. In Erb's (1891) review of 83 cases of muscular dystrophy there are 25 whose case histories conform to the Duchenne-type: mental retardation was recorded in 5 of these, the intelligence was said to be normal in 7, and there was no comment about the others.

In recent years there has been some controversy about the presence of intellectual impairment in muscular dystrophy. Walton and Nattrass (1954) studied 48 cases of Duchenne-type muscular dystrophy and concluded that, in spite of clinical impressions, no patient was mentally defective and only four were slightly backward. They thought that this clinical impression of backwardness could be attributed to loss of education, or to the reaction of these patients to their physical disability. Truitt (1955) also concluded that the mental ability of a series of patients with pseudohypertrophic muscular dystrophy was 'within the limits of normal expectation for the socio-economic group', that it was commensurate with the intelligence of their sibs, and that it did not decrease with advanced age or progression of the disease.

On the basis of the verbal part of the Wechsler Intelligence Scale for children, Morrow and Cohen (1954), in a study of 29 cases, found a mean IQ of 94. Although this was below average, they concluded, on the basis of other psychological data, that the lowered intellectual functioning resulted from the social and educational consequences of the disease and was not a primary consequence of the muscular dystrophy. They also found that in schooling about one-half of the patients were in grades one or more years behind other children of the same age and that 15 out of 23 children over 8 years of age showed reading retardation, while about 50% were retarded in number skills.

Del Carlo Giannini and Marcheschi (1959) studied 18 cases of muscular dystrophy, including 7 of the Duchenne-type: 5 of the latter group had a marked reduction in IQ.

More recently Allen and Rodgin (1960) found a mean IQ of 82 in a series of 30 boys with muscular dystrophy, ranging in age from 2 to 23 years. Various standard tests were used and the IQ ranged from 14-117. There were 15 boys with an IQ over 95. There was no correlation between the degree of intellectual impairment and the severity of the physical disability. While they also found evidence for depression of intellectual function related to emotional problems associated with the physical handicaps, they did not think this in itself could explain the intellectual impairment.

Worden and Vignos (1962) made a detailed study of the intelligence in 38 cases of progressive muscular dystrophy. All but one were over the age of 7. The mean IQ was 83, with a range of 46-134. Only 3 were above 110, while 26 were below 90. There was also evidence of special difficulties with reading and mathematics, and the mean educational quotients in these two fields were 83 and 87 respectively. They found no correlation between the IQ and the disability grading of the disease and no evidence of a progressive mental deterioration with advance of the disease. In a comparative study of 27 unaffected sibs of these patients they obtained a mean IQ of 110 and in a series of 16 cases of 'amyotonia congenita' with equivalent or more severe physical handicap, the mean IQ was 118.

## Material and Methods

This investigation of the intellectual development in progressive muscular dystrophy falls into three parts.

TABLE

PSYCHOMETRIC ASSESSMENT OF 27 CASES OF MUSCULAR DYSTROPHY CORRELATED WITH CLINICAL DATA

| Case No. | Chronological Age (yr.) | Mental Age (yr.) | IQ | Clinical* Rating | Motor Milestones (age in months) | | |
|---|---|---|---|---|---|---|---|
| | | | | | Sat Unsupported | Stood Unsupported | Walked Unaided |
| 16 | 16 + | 17 9/12 | 118 | A | 9 | 12 | 12 |
| 4 | 15 2/12 | 15 7/12 | 103 | A | 4 | 10 | 15 |
| 36 | 12 6/12 | 12 7/12 | 101 | B | 9 | 16 | 24 |
| 31 | 12 4/12 | 12 2/12 | 99 | A | 5 | 10 | 18 |
| 43 | 12 2/12 | 11 2/12 | 92 | A | 8 | 13 | 16 |
| 37 | 16 1/12 | 12 2/12 | 81 | A | 9 | 20 | 24 |
| 12 | 11 6/12 | 8 10/12 | 77 | A | 9 | 11 | 12 |
| 20 | 12 7/12 | 9 6/12 | 76 | C | 9 | 12 | 24 |
| 27 | 9 5/12 | 6 10/12 | 73 | C | 7 | 15 | 17 |
| 48 | 16 + | 10 8/12 | 71 | C | 7 | 12 | 18 |
| 45 | 15 10/12 | 10 | 67 | C | 12 | 18 | 24 |
| 55 | 14 6/12 | 9 2/12 | 65 | A | 8 | 14 | 16 |
| 1 | 14 1/12 | 8 10/12 | 64 | B | 12 | 18 | 18 |
| 28 | 8 | 5 1/12 | 64 | C | 8 | 18 | 24 |
| 22 | 9 9/12 | 5 10/12 | 60 | C | 9 | 20 | 48 |
| 42 | 9 9/12 | 5 10/12 | 59 | C | 12 | 18 | 20 |
| 33 | 11 8/12 | 6 10/12 | 59 | C | 6 | 12 | 18 |
| 35 | 13 2/12 | 7 6/12 | 57 | C | 12 | 18 | 30 |
| 23 | 15 6/12 | 8 4/12 | 56 | C | ? | ? | 24 |
| 15 | 10 8/12 | 6 2/12 | 55 | C | 8 | 11 | 12 |
| 41 | 11 3/12 | 6 | 53 | C | 12 | 24 | 27 |
| 53 | 16 + | 8 | 53 | C | 12 | ? | 18 |
| 40 | 14 7/12 | 7 2/12 | 51 | C | 15 | 24 | 30 |
| 14 | 12 8/12 | 6 6/12 | 51 | C | 9 | 11 | 12 |
| 25 | 12 11/12 | 6 2/12 | 48 | C | ? | ? | 24 |
| 32 | 15 7/12 | 7 | 47 | C | 8 | 15 | 24 |
| 26 | 12 11/12 | 5 5/12 | 42 | C | 9 | 24 | 24 |

* A, normal intelligence; B, probably retarded; C, retarded.

**Part I:** A clinical assessment of intelligence in the course of a comprehensive study of 65 patients with Duchenne-type muscular dystrophy (Dubowitz, 1960). This was based on the clinical history of milestones, which was obtained from the parents, and on the clinical impression of intelligence assessed in a fairly empirical way on the basis of simple reading, writing, arithmetical, and general knowledge tests appropriate to the age. On this basis the children were divided into three groups: A, normal intelligence; B, possibly retarded; and C, definitely retarded.

**Part II:** A psychometric assessment of 27 long-term in-patients by the Terman-Merrill revision of the Stanford-Binet test (form L). All these children had attended the hospital school for at least 6 months.

**Part III:** Three patients, who were diagnosed early, have been studied prospectively. Various tests of intellectual as well as motor and manipulative abilities were performed at frequent intervals. Comparative studies in unaffected sibs were also done along similar lines. These three patients will be described in detail.

## Results

**Part I.** Of the 65 patients in this study, 63 were male and 2 were female. Their ages ranged from 3-19 years.

MILESTONES. An arbitrary upper limit of normal for sitting without support, standing unsupported, and walking unaided, was taken as 9 months, 14 months, and 18 months, respectively. A delay in walking plus one of the other motor milestones was considered a delay, and a delay in walking alone or in both sitting and standing a doubtful delay.

On this basis the motor milestones were normal in 27 cases, there was a delay in 28 cases, and a doubtful delay in 9. In one instance no information was available.

Of the 34 children who were not walking by 18 months, 29 did not walk till the age of 2 years or over.

CLINICAL ASSESSMENT. 30 children (46%) were considered to be of average or above average intelligence (category A), 21 (32%) retarded (category C), and 14 (22%) possibly retarded (category B).

Of the 30 children in category A, 18 had normal motor milestones, 9 had delayed milestones, and 3 possibly delayed milestones. Of the 21 cases in category C, 5 had normal milestones, 11 were delayed, and 4 doubtfully delayed. In the intermediate category B, 4 had normal milestones, 8 were delayed, and 2 doubtfully delayed.

**Part II.** The results of the psychometric testing of the 27 children are given in the Table. Ten patients had an IQ above 70 (37%); 14 (52%) had an IQ score of between 50 and 70 and 3 (11%) below 50. The clinical rating correlated fairly well with the IQ assessment in the majority of these cases. With regard to the motor milestones, of the 10 patients with an IQ over 70, 7 were walking at the age of 18 months, while of the 17 with an IQ of under 70 only 5 were able to walk by that age. Using the same criteria as in Part I above, the motor milestones were considered to be normal in 7 of the 10 patients with an IQ above 70, delayed in 2, and doubtfully delayed in 1. In the group with an IQ less than 70, 4 had normal milestones, 10 had delay, and 3 doubtful delay.

**Part III.** On the basis of the detailed developmental history and the repeated assessment of various intellectual, manipulative, and other abilities, it was concluded that all three children had intellectual impairment out of proportion to their physical handicap. Detailed case histories are included in the appendix.

The degree of intellectual impairment in Case 3 was less marked than in the other two cases.

Serial examination in Case 1 suggested a deterioration in intellectual function, in that certain previously acquired skills were subsequently lost. Moreover in other intellectual spheres this child was fairly static and not advancing at a normal rate. This would imply a fall in IQ with increasing age. In Case 2, the history suggested that some of the child's previous skills, such as counting, had deteriorated.

## Discussion

There are numerous difficulties in trying to assess intelligence in children with severe physical handicap. Many of the standard tests for older children are weighted for general knowledge and experience which may be limited because of physical disabilities. In infancy many of the tests depend on manipulation and co-ordination which can be affected by muscular weakness.

It is deceptive to assess intelligence on clinical impression, because the physically handicapped child may become introverted and apathetic and thus give the impression of a lower intelligence than he in fact has.

In spite of the criticism that may be levelled at each approach, there has been a fairly uniform pattern of results and a number of interesting correlations have become apparent. In most children, the clinical assessment correlated fairly well with the psychometric testing. In both less than half were in the normal range.

There was a significant correlation between delayed motor milestones and intellectual retardation In the children judged to have a normal intelligence by psychometric testing 70% had normal milestones, while in those judged to be subnormal under 25% had normal milestones. Similarly in the clinical assessment there was a significantly higher proportion of children with normal milestones in category A (normal intelligence) than in category B or C.

A positive family history was much less frequent in the cases of normal intelligence than in the retarded ones. Of 10 patients with IQ above 70 on psychometric testing, only 2 had a positive family history (Table, Cases 27 and 48). Of the 17 with IQ below 70, 10 had a positive history. In category A (normal intelligence) on clinical assessment, the family history was positive in 4 (all definite sex-linked recessive), negative in 24, and the 2 affected sisters had consanguineous parents, indicating an autosomal recessive inheritance. In category C, 10 had a positive family history and 11 a negative one, while in category B the figures were 8 and 6 respectively.

Why are some children with typical Duchenne-type muscular dystrophy of grammar school intelligence, while others, with equal muscular involvement, are ineducable? The higher incidence of negative family histories in the more intelligent group suggests that a larger proportion of these may have an autosomal recessive rather than a sex-linked recessive inheritance with a different disease pattern.

An alternative explanation is that separate genes are responsible for the muscular dystrophy and the intellectual impairment. Perhaps under these circumstances one would expect to find intellectual impairment without muscular dystrophy in some sibs, but this was not the case.

The possibility of intellectual impairment being a sequel of the physical handicap is not borne out by the detailed studies of the three early cases. The severe intellectual impairment in all three was out of proportion to the physical disability. In 2 of them, younger sibs had already overtaken them in intellectual development.

In this context, it is also of interest that the intelligence was normal in 12 patients with a slowly progressive form of infantile muscular atrophy where the onset was usually earlier and physical disability more severe than muscular dystrophy (Dubowitz, 1964).

The most likely explanation for the intellectual impairment in progressive muscular dystrophy is a biochemical abnormality affecting the metabolism of brain as well as muscle. The apparent absence of progression of the intellectual impairment may be due to maximal involvement in early life, when the brain is most vulnerable, and an imperceptible deterioration thereafter. In those with normal intelligence, the initial onset may be less acute and severe, thus also explaining the higher incidence of normal motor milestones in this group.

## Conclusions

Severe intellectual impairment is a commonly associated feature of progressive muscular dystrophy of the Duchenne-type. It may already be present before the onset of the severe physical disability. It is probably an integral part of the disease process, and any theory of the aetiology of the disease should take this into account. It may, therefore, not be entirely accurate to look upon muscular dystrophy as a disease confined to voluntary muscle.

It is difficult to explain why some children should have a normal intelligence, in contrast to others who are severely retarded, in spite of similar severity of muscular involvement. A possible explanation in some of these cases is a different gene inherited by an autosomal recessive rather than a sex-linked recessive mechanism, or that separate genes are responsible for the intellectual impairment and the muscular involvement. A more likely explanation is a single biochemical lesion affecting brain and muscle, but with less acute onset in those with normal intelligence. Alternatively, a product of the muscle destruction may affect the developing brain.

I wish to thank Professor R. S. Illingworth for his help and advice, Dr. David Lawson for the facilities he afforded me at Queen Mary's Hospital for Children, Carshalton, and Miss E. J. Shearn for the psychometric tests.

This work has been supported by grants from the Muscular Dystrophy Group of Great Britain and the Sheffield University Research Fund.

### References

Allen, J. E., and Rodgin, D. W. (1960). Mental retardation in association with progressive muscular dystrophy. *Amer. J. Dis. Child.*, **100**, 208.

Del Carlo Giannini, G., and Marcheschi, M. (1959). Sui disturbi psichici nella distrofia muscolare primitiva. *Sist. nerv.*, **11**, 461.

Dubowitz, V. (1960). Progressive Muscular Dystrophy in Childhood. M.D. Thesis, University of Cape Town.

—— (1964). Infantile muscular atrophy. A progressive study with particular reference to a slowly progressive variety. *Brain*, **87**, 707.

Duchenne, G. B. (1872). *De l'Electrisation Localisée et de Son Application à la Pathologie et à la Thérapeutique*, 3rd ed. Bailliere, Paris.

Erb, W. (1891). Dystrophia muscularis progressiva. Klinische und pathologisch-anatomische studien. *Dtsch. Z. Nervenheilk.*, **1**, 13, 173.

Gowers, W. R. (1879). *Pseudo-hypertrophic Muscular Paralysis. A Clinical Lecture.* Churchill, London.

Morrow, R. S., and Cohen, J. (1954). The psycho-social factors in muscular dystrophy. *J. Child. Psychiat.* (*N.Y.*), **3**, 70.

Truitt, C. J. (1955). Personal and social adjustments of children with muscular dystrophy. *Amer. J. phys. Med.*, **34**, 124.

Walton, J. N., and Nattrass, F. J. (1954). On the classification, natural history and treatment of the myopathies. *Brain*, **77**, 169.

Worden, D. K., and Vignos, P. J., Jr. (1962). Intellectual function in childhood progressive muscular dystrophy. *Pediatrics*, **29**, 968.

## Appendix

**Case 1.** This boy, born October 18, 1960, was referred on June 14, 1963, at the age of 2¾, because his father thought that 'he had no sense'.

He did not sit unsupported till 10 months. He stood with support at about 16 months and on his own at 18 months. He walked without support at about 20 months. At 2¾ he was still not very stable on his feet and fell frequently. He had slight difficulty in getting up from the floor. He was not able to run, skip, or jump and had difficulty in stepping on to a pavement or climbing steps. He had no difficulty with chewing or swallowing. He did not learn to drink from a cup until the age of 2. He was able to feed himself with a spoon but still messed a lot. He had no bowel or bladder control.

He was very late in speaking and had only recently acquired the single words—'daddy, mummy, van, and baby'. He made no attempt to put words together.

He did not imitate any activities of his parents or sibs. He was not able to dress or undress himself. He did not obey commands or bring objects he was asked for. His mother thought he needed more coaxing and was less interested in things than before, but there was no obvious regression in intellectual activity. However, he did seem fairly static and improvement in intellectual function was barely perceptible.

Clinical Examination. He walked with a slight waddle, supported a hand on the knee when getting up from the prone, and could be diagnosed as an early muscular dystrophy on clinical grounds.

He had a mature two-finger grasp for small objects. He was able to match two cubes and make a tower of 3 cubes. He made no attempt to make a train or bridge with cubes. He was unable to place the blocks in a simple formboard, but piled them on top of each other. He did not copy a line, but only scribbled with a pencil. His grasp of the pencil was immature. He turned a few pages of a book at a time, and was unable to turn them singly. He did not point to pictures.

On the basis of the history and clinical assessment his intellectual development was considered to be less than that of an 18-month-old child in all spheres.

The diagnosis of muscular dystrophy was confirmed by the raised serum enzymes levels (SGOT 220 units, SGPT 292 units, aldolase 154 units, and creatine kinase 570 $\mu$M/ml./hr.); and the typical histological features on muscle biopsy.

Family History. The mother has a brother suffering from muscular dystrophy, and an affected son by a previous husband.

Sibs. His 15-month-old male sib cruised at 10 months and was just about walking without support. His speech was much more advanced; he had a vocabulary of at least 10 words and was putting words together. He was able to feed himself with a cup and spoon from the age of 11 months.

On detailed assessment his intelligence was judged to be normal for his age and in many respects in advance of his affected brother.

An older male sib, aged 4½, walked at 10½ months. His intelligence was normal on assessment.

FOLLOW-UP OF PATIENT. One month later there was no change in his speech, or general intellectual and manipulative abilities, though he did manage to build a tower of 8 cubes.

In November 1963, aged 3 years, he was saying more words, but not putting two words together. He was able to take off his shoes. He placed a circle in the simple formboards, and could adapt. He was only able to build a tower of 3 bricks.

In December 1963, there were no new achievements.

In January 1964, he was saying more single words, but not putting words together yet. He placed the circle in the simple formboard and could adapt. He made a tower of two bricks only. He refused to page a book. He could not copy pencil strokes, and did not identify pictures. He had not yet acquired sphincter control.

In April 1964, aged 3½, he had not shown any improvement in intelligence. Mother said he was not able to say as many words as before and had not acquired any new ones. He did not help with dressing or undressing. He only obeyed an occasional command. He was not yet using a potty. Often when asked to do something he stared as if he did not understand. He tended to be introverted, would not play with other children, and was content to sit and play with his cars. He was able to make a tower of 4 cubes only and they were poorly aligned. He would not place the circle in the simple formboard. He was unable to copy a straight line or circle, and the only command he obeyed was 'open the door'.

There was very little change in his motor disability, but there appeared to be a deterioration in his intellectual capacity.

**Case 2.** This boy, born on March 22, 1957, was first seen in November 1962, aged 5 years and 8 months. He had never been an active child. He sat without support at 11 months, stood up at 18 months, shuffled on his bottom at 20 months and walked at 26 months. He had a waddling gait and had difficulty with running and climbing stairs.

He did not say single words until 18 months and started to put words together at about 2½ years. He seemed to have no power of concentration and his mind seemed to wander.

He had recently started school and was not making any progress. He could not write or draw and only scribbled. At one time he was counting up to 10, but when examined he could only count to 2 and then repeat it.

EXAMINATION. In November 1962 he showed the typical clinical features of muscular dystrophy. He was able to obey single commands but not multiple ones. He could not copy any geometric forms. In repeating sentences he only said the last one or two words. He did not know his age. He made a tower of 6 cubes and nearly managed to make a bridge with three cubes. He completed the Goddard formboard test in 90, 70, and 60 seconds, respectively, on three successive occasions. With the Goodenough 'draw a man' test, he did not score at all.

His intelligence was judged to be below the 3-year level in all spheres.

The diagnosis of muscular dystrophy was confirmed by abnormally high levels of serum enzymes, namely, SGPT 580, SGOT 318, aldolase 208 units, and creatine kinase 800 $\mu$M/ml./hr.

FAMILY HISTORY. The mother's twin sister has an affected child (Case 3 below), and three affected cousins (Cases 26, 27, and 28) have been assessed previously.

SIB. A younger sib, aged 19 months, sat unsupported at 8 months, stood on his own at 10 months, crawled at 9 months, and walked at 14 months. He was saying single words from 8 months, and at 19 months was putting 2 or 3 words together. He was able to make a tower of 4 cubes, and placed the circle and square in the simple formboard. His intelligence was regarded as normal.

FOLLOW-UP OF PATIENT. Three months later there was little change. By July 1963 there had been some improvement in his speech and he was saying more words. He was able to copy a square and a cross, but not a circle. He made a tower of 9 cubes without difficulty.

After three trials he was able to repeat 3 digits. He was still only able to remember one command. He was unable to say any nursery rhymes and he only repeated the first and last words of sentences given to him. On three attempts the best time for the Goddard formboard was 46 seconds. He made no score on the Goodenough 'draw a man' test.

In October 1963 his performance was about the same. In February 1964, aged 6 years and 11 months, there was some further improvement in his speech, and he was making full sentences. At school he was in a class of average age 5½ to 6 years, and was not showing much progress. He was unable to do sums or to write. He was still unable to count beyond 2. He repeated 2 digits correctly on 3 successive attempts, but was unable to repeat 3 digits on 3 trials. He was unable to name coins. He still left out parts of sentences he was asked to repeat. He could point to parts of his anatomy and knew left from right. His best time with the Goddard formboard was 55 seconds.

He made a tower of 10 cubes without difficulty, a bridge spontaneously, and a gate after being shown. He was readily distracted from what he was doing. With the Goodenough 'draw a man' test he scored at the 4-year level.

There had been some decline in his motor power, but he was still able to walk well and to get up after falling. He had great difficulty in climbing steps. His intellectual development was still below the 4-year level.

In contrast his sib, at 3 years, was able to make a tower of 10 cubes, to repeat 2 digits in each of the three trials, and 3 digits in 1 out of 3 trials. He was speaking in full sentences and his speech was more advanced than his older brother.

**Case 3.** This is a cousin of Case 2, born on April 23, 1961. He was first seen in November 1962, aged 19 months. He had smiled at 6 weeks and cooed at the same age. He made no attempt to roll from prone to supine or vice versa. He sat unsupported at 9 months. He shuffled on his bottom from the age of 13 months. At 19 months he could stand with support, but not unaided, and was not cruising. He started casting at 1 year but did not wave bye-bye till 16 months. He said single words with meaning from about 18 months, but was was not putting words together.

Examination. He stood well with support and walked with two hands held. He had a mature grasp and instant finger thumb apposition. He was uncooperative with any further tests.

In January 1963, aged 21 months, he was cruising with the furniture. He was putting words together. He built a tower of 2 cubes but was unable to place the blocks in a simple formboard. He seemed more alert and interested than previously.

At 22 months he was able to pull up into a standing posture, and started walking at the age of 2. He went upstairs on all fours and down on his bottom.

At 2 years and 10 months, he was putting 3 or 4 words into sentences. He pointed to objects in a book, but could not repeat nursery rhymes. He was able to feed himself with a spoon. He had bladder control by day. He used a pot when given one, but did not ask for it.

He made a tower of 5 cubes and aligned them into a train. He placed the circle in the simple formboard, but had difficulty in adapting. He was unable to copy a line or a circle, but only scribbled. He could point to parts of his face and he named objects in a book.

Clinically there were signs of early muscular dystrophy. The diagnosis was confirmed by a raised serum creatine kinase level of 680 $\mu$M/ml./hr. and the pathological changes on muscle biopsy.

His general intellectual performance was considered to be less than the 2-year level.

His sister aged 5 years was of normal intelligence in all respects.

*Arch. Dis. Childh.*, 1965, **40**, 302.

# CEREBELLO-THALAMO-SPINAL DEGENERATION IN INFANCY: AN UNUSUAL VARIANT OF WERDNIG-HOFFMANN DISEASE

BY

R. M. NORMAN and J. M. KAY*

*From the Burden Neuropathological Laboratory, Frenchay Hospital, Bristol, and the Department of Pathology, University of Bristol*

(RECEIVED FOR PUBLICATION SEPTEMBER 22, 1964)

The stereotyped clinical picture of hypotonic muscular weakness presented by the majority of children suffering from Werdnig-Hoffmann disease gives little indication of the wealth of neuropathological findings which examination of the brain may sometimes reveal. In such cases the lesions found in the spinal white matter, the cerebellum, or the basal ganglia remain clinically silent because they are masked by the widespread degeneration of the anterior horn cells.

The patient to be described in this paper was an exception to this rule, for spasticity rather than hypotonia was the salient feature, and the diagnosis of Werdnig-Hoffmann disease was not suggested during life. Yet neuropathological changes characteristic of this disease were present, and the atypical clinical picture must be attributed to the unusual distribution of the lesions.

### Case Report

K.M., a girl, was the third child of healthy parents who were not blood relatives.

The first child, a boy, came under observation at the age of 11 months because of his failure to sit up or take interest in his surroundings. Examination showed a convergent strabismus, a generalized increase in muscle tone, which was more pronounced in the lower limbs, brisk reflexes, and a head circumference of 18·75 in. (48 cm.). Pneumoencephalography was performed when the child was 18 months: this showed a mild degree of symmetrical hydrocephalus probably compensatory to cerebral hypoplasia or atrophy. He was admitted to a home for mentally retarded children where he died at the age of 28 months. At necropsy the head circumference was 19 in. (48 cm.), the cerebral white matter was thin, the ventricles were dilated, and the subarachnoid space increased in width. No microscopical examination was made.

The second child is a normal healthy girl.

K.M. was born after an uneventful full-term pregnancy and a normal delivery. She was admitted to hospital for investigation at the age of 11 months because of failure to reach her milestones, difficulty in feeding, and failure to gain weight. On examination it was found that she was unable to sit up and could not roll from the prone to the supine position. The head circumference measured 17·25 in. (44 cm.), the weight was 16·75 lb. (7·6 kg.) and length 27 in. (69 cm.). Muscle tone was generally increased but more so in the lower limbs. The thumbs were maintained abducted across the palms. The cranial nerves were normal. The tendon reflexes were uniformly brisk. An extensor plantar response was elicited on the left side. Examination of the urine for phenylketones, amino acids, reducing substances, and metachromatic fat granules yielded negative results. Serological tests for syphilis and toxoplasmosis were negative. Radiological examination of the skull showed no abnormality. An electroencephalogram taken on this admission was normal. The child's condition remained virtually the same until the age of 22 months when she was admitted for further investigation. At this time her head circumference was 18 in. (46 cm.), her weight was 16 lb. (7·3 kg.) and length 27 in. (69 cm.). She could not sit up, but lay in bed with her legs semi-flexed at the knee and hip joints. An electroencephalogram recorded extremely low potential, slow components from the right hemisphere and virtually nothing from the left side of the head, which was interpreted as indicating an atrophic or dystrophic condition of the brain. Shortly after admission she developed a high temperature for which no cause could be found; penicillin was administered and the temperature subsided. Twelve days later, however, she suddenly collapsed and died.

**Necropsy.** A full necropsy revealed no abnormalities outside the nervous system. Microscopically the lungs, heart, spleen, liver, pancreas, and psoas major muscle showed no significant pathological changes. A cause for the child's sudden death could not be found.

### Neuropathology

MACROSCOPIC. The fixed brain weighed 880 g., of

* Present address: Department of Pathology, University of Birmingham.

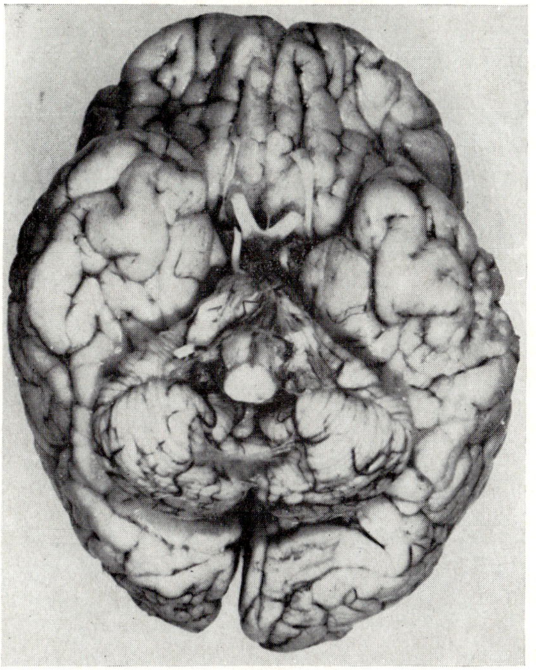

FIG. 1.—Base of brain showing small size of cerebellum and widely separated lateral lobes.

which the cerebellum and brain-stem accounted for 49 g. (normal 120 g.). The convolutional pattern, cranial nerves, and basal vessels were normal. On coronal section the ventricles were slightly enlarged and the thalami appeared small. There was no hypoplasia of the corpus callosum. The cerebellum was small, and there was an undue separation of the lateral lobes which allowed the tonsils and inferior vermis to be easily seen (Fig. 1).

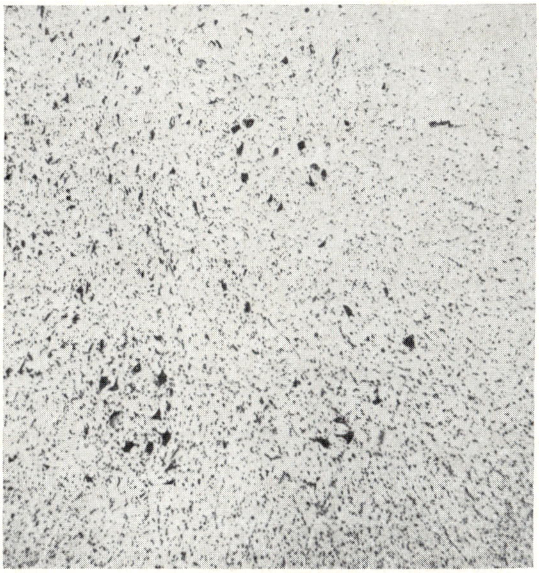

FIG. 2.—C7. Anterior horn showing poverty of nerve cells in the antero-lateral area. The antero-median cell group is well preserved. (Carbol azure. × 45.)

MICROSCOPIC. Representative parts of the cerebral hemispheres, cerebellum, brain-stem, and spinal cord were stained by standard methods in celloidin and frozen sections. The cerebellum, brain-stem, and segments of the cervical and lumbar cord were studied in spaced serial sections.

*Spinal Cord.* In the cervical region the anterior horn cells were reduced in number, the amount of neuronal loss varying considerably in the individual cell groups at different levels (Fig. 2). In most sections there were one to five degenerating nerve cells of ovoid or round shape which had lost their Nissl bodies and stained a pale, uniform blue, the nucleus retaining its neucleolus and membrane, and being usually displaced to the margin of the cell (Fig. 3a). Sometimes a remnant of the Nissl substance was present at the periphery of the cyton (Fig. 3b). Microglial nuclei were often abnormally numerous but there were no figures of neuronophagia. In the thoracic cord the loss of nerve cells was less conspicuous. Clarke's column was preserved in the thoracic segments which were sampled, one chromatolytic cell being seen. At the level of L1, however, there was almost complete loss of nerve cells and several greatly inflated chromatolytic cells (Fig. 3c). The myelin picture showed the normal configuration of the nucleus with spaces devoid of nerve cells ('empty cell beds'). The lumbar enlargement seemed at first sight normal in its neuronal population, but here and there, at different levels, the same distinctive chromatolytic change was found in isolated cells (Fig. 3d).

In sections stained for *myelin* the cervical cord showed a marked pallor in the lateral columns and a slight pallor at some levels in the columns of Goll (Fig. 4a). In the thoracic segments the myelin stained poorly in the whole cord except in the posterior columns, and in the lumbar region the pallor was confined to the pyramidal tracts. *Fibrous gliosis* was increased throughout the cord, the ventral part of the anterior horns being specially affected (Fig. 4b). In the white matter the gliosis was usually but not invariably accentuated in the areas of myelin pallor. In the cervical region the columns of Goll were distinguished by the denser gliosis present in them. There were no sudanophil products of myelin breakdown, and the axis cylinders in transverse and longitudinal sections showed no significant differences from those in a normally myelinated cord coming from a 2-year-old epileptic child. The *nerve roots* appeared normal except in the cervical region where the anterior roots were often extremely small and contained less densely packed myelinated fibres than the posterior roots (Fig. 4a).

*Brain-stem.* Both superior vestibular nuclei showed a loss of nerve cells and contained several swollen, chromatolytic cells analogous to those in the spinal cord (Fig. 5a). The hypoglossal nucleus on one side also showed a patch of neuronal loss with one degenerating nerve cell. There

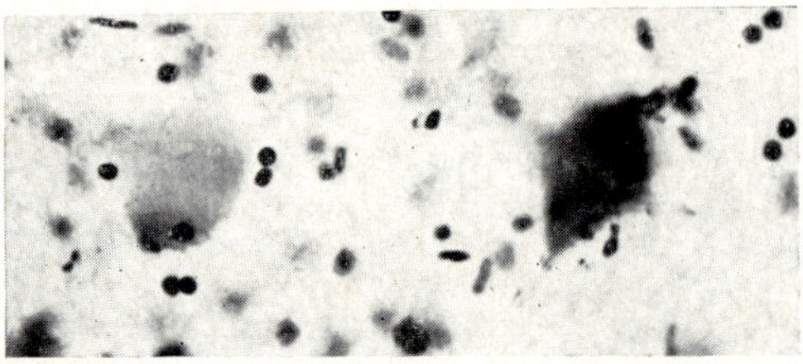

(a)

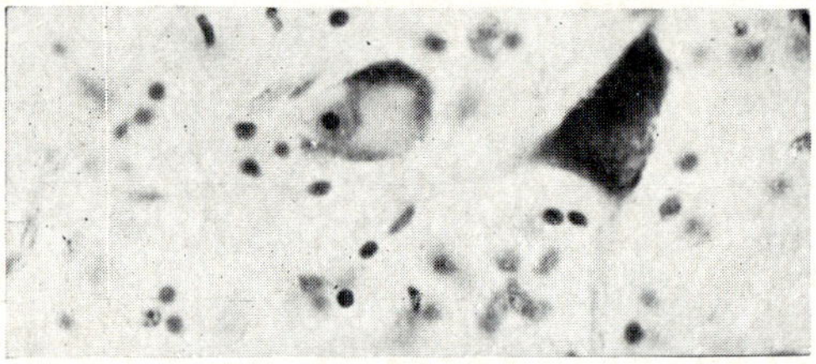

(b)

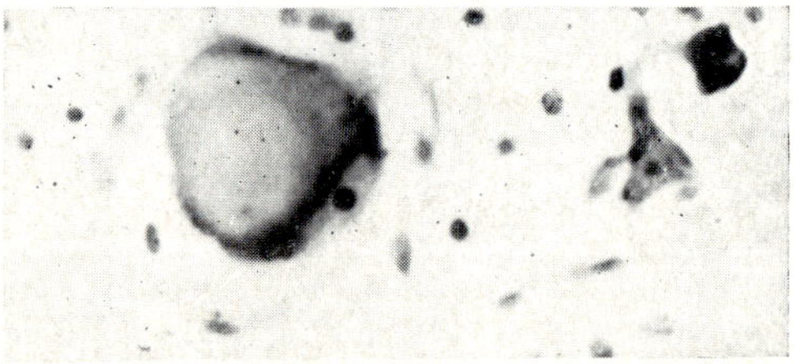

(c)

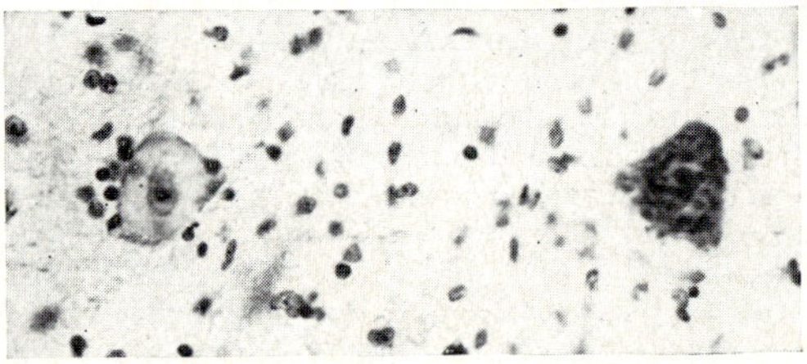

(d)

FIG. 3.—Chromatolytic anterior horn cells. (a) and (b) from the cervical region; (c) from Clarke's column at L1 level (all × 400) and (d) from the lumbar region (× 282.)

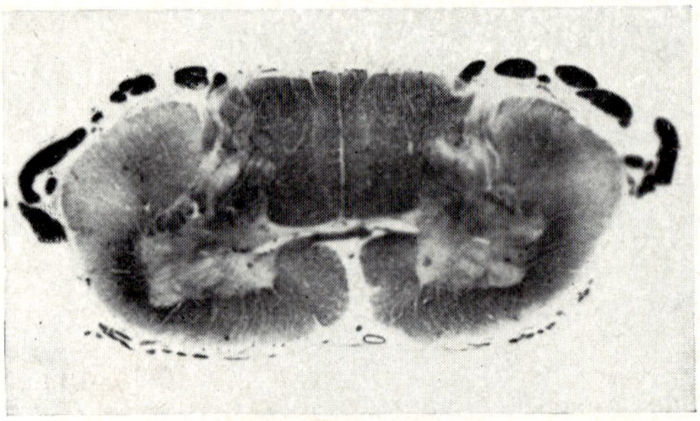

(a)

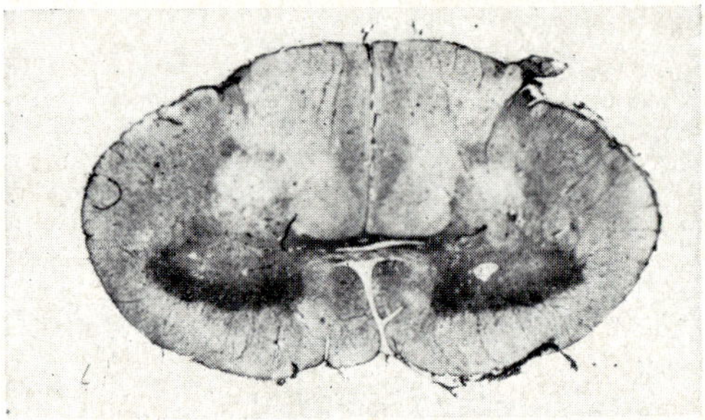

(b)

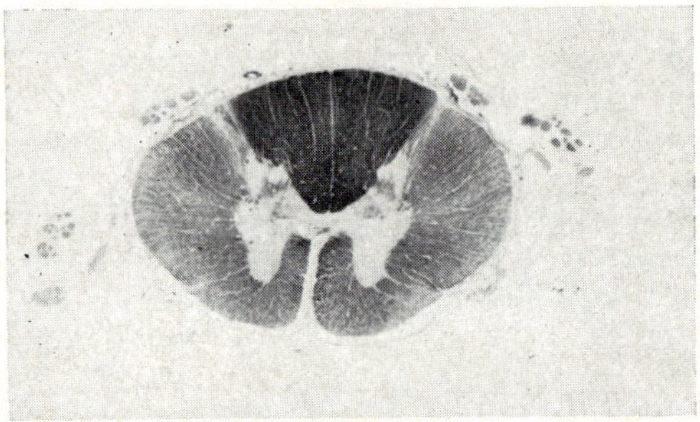

(c)

FIG. 4.—(a) Cervical cord showing pallor predominantly in the lateral columns, and atrophy of the anterior roots. (Heidenhain. × 5·4.) (b) Cervical cord showing gliosis in the anterior horns, lateral columns and tracts of Goll. (Holzer. × 4·8.) (c) Thoracic cord showing normal myelination only in the posterior columns. (Heidenhain. × 7·3.)

was a marked increase in fibrous neuroglia throughout the brain-stem, both in the nuclei and fibre tracts, but the myelination was unaffected. The medullary pyramids and pes pontis were of normal size.

*Basal Ganglia.* Severe pathological changes were found in the thalami where large parts of the lateral nuclei were almost devoid of nerve cells and showed marked fibrous gliosis (Fig. 6). The fibres of passage were normally myelinated. The principal anterior nuclei also showed widespread degeneration while the accessory anterior nucleus of each side had retained most of its cells (Fig. 7). Patchy nerve cell loss and gliosis were present in the medial nuclei and in the pulvinars. In the partially degenerated areas there were several slightly swollen neurones that had completely lost their Nissl substances and stained a uniform pale blue (Fig. 5b). These chromatolytic cells were sharply distinguishable from the healthy nerve cells which greatly outnumbered them There was little microglial activity except for a few clusters suggestive of neuronophagia. One binucleate nerve cell was seen. A few chromatolytic cells were found in the external geniculate body. The corpus striatum, subthalamic nucleus, and globus pallidus of

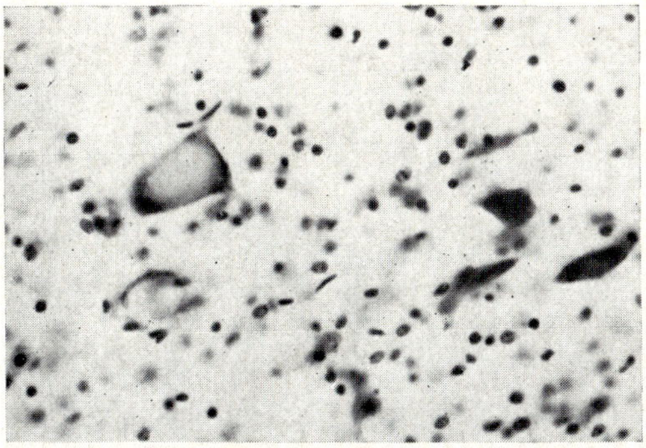

(a)

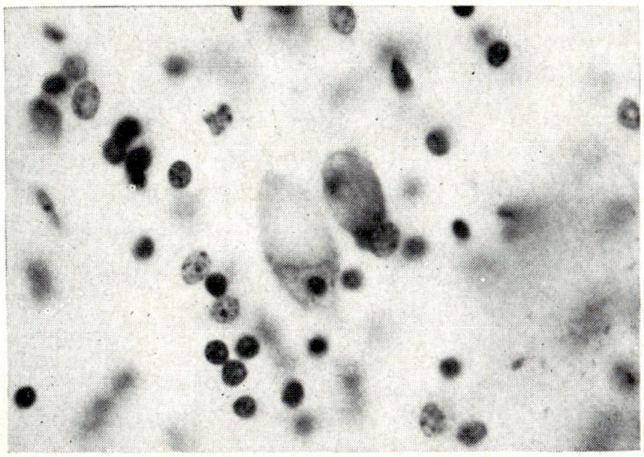

(b)

FIG. 5.—(a) Chromatolytic nerve cell in the superior vestibular nucleus. (Carbol azure. × 263.) (b) Chromatolytic cell in the pulvinar of the thalamus. (Carbol azure. × 518.)

each side were normal except for a mild fibrous gliosis in the latter nucleus, which was unaccompanied by myelin loss.

*Cerebellum.* The granular layer of the cortex of the lateral lobes and vermis showed a diffuse reduction in cellular density. Very few healthy Purkinje cells were seen, the great majority presenting the appearance of simple atrophy with marked shrinkage of the nucleus and cell body, the latter often showing vacuolation (Fig. 8a). There were only minor losses of Purkinje cells, and usually the apparent gaps in this layer contained barely visible remnants of atrophic neurones. Silver impregnation showed that the dendrites of the remaining cells and the tangential and basket fibres were present, but the latter were often feebly represented. There was a marked fibrous gliosis in the whole of the central white matter and the folial cores, and a moderate proliferation of the Bergmann fibrils throughout the molecular layer. A slight pallor of myelin staining was seen in the posterior part of the left lateral lobe and also in the hila of both dentate nuclei where gliosis was particularly intense (Fig. 9). The nerve cells of the dentate nuclei showed considerable shrinkage but no numerical reduction. Several chromatolytic cells and a few figures of neuronophagia were seen in the nucleus emboliformis.

*Other Parts of the Brain.* The cerebral cortex, including the hippocampal formations, were normal in every respect. A slight fibrous gliosis without detectable

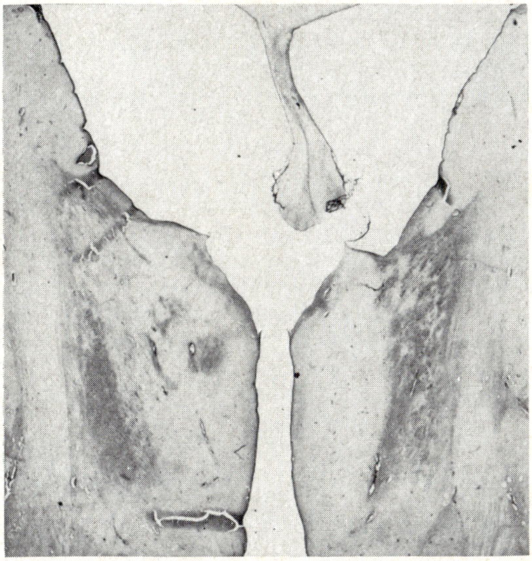

FIG. 6.—Thalami showing dense fibrous gliosis in the lateral nuclei. (Holzer. × 3·7.)

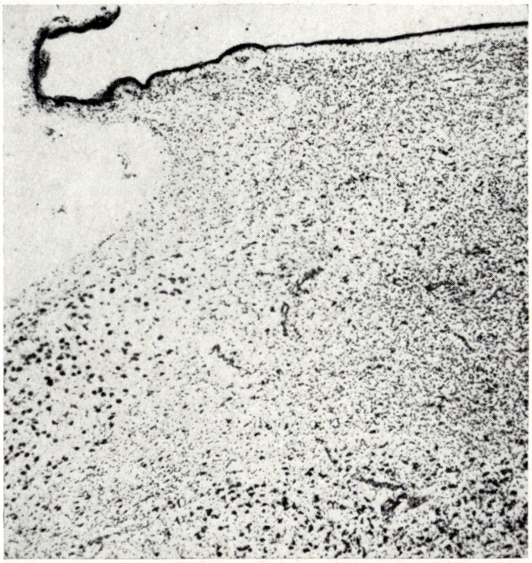

FIG. 7.—Thalamus showing almost complete loss of nerve cells and greatly increased glial nuclei in the principal anterior nucleus. Cells are seen in the accessory anterior nucleus (left). (Carbol azure. × 3·3.)

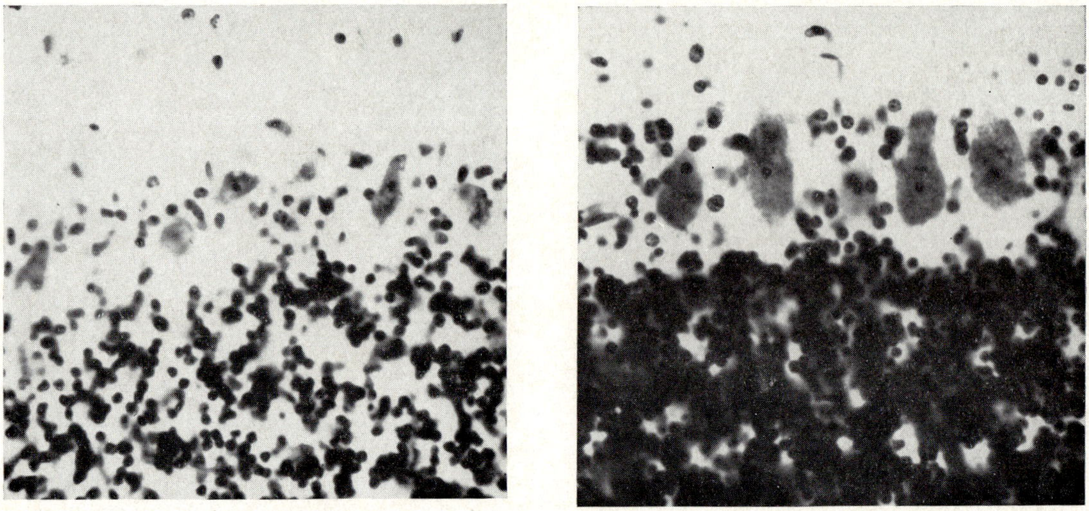
(a) (b)

FIG. 8.—(a) Cerebellar cortex showing rarefied granular layer and atrophy of Purkinje cells (b) Normal cerebellar cortex in child of 2 years. (Carbol azure. × 382.)

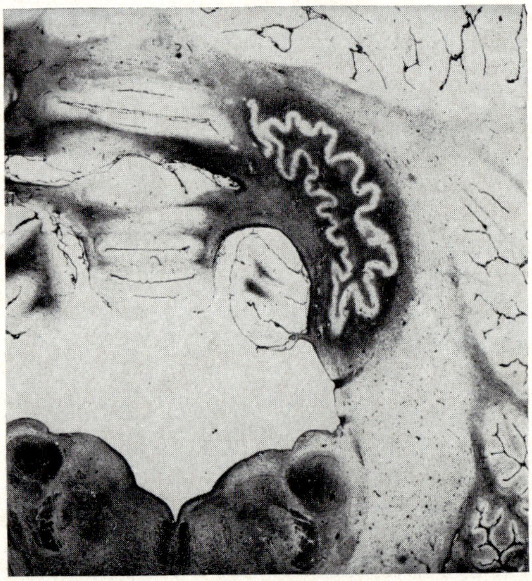
FIG. 9.—Fibrous gliosis in the dentate nucleus and brain-stem. (Holzer. × 3·5.)

defect of myelin was present throughout the centrum ovale, gyral cores, optic nerves, and tracts. The choroid plexuses, ependyma, leptomeninges, and blood vessels were normal.

## Discussion

The diagnosis of Werdnig-Hoffmann disease in this case rests on the neuropathological findings, since persistent spasticity of the legs and a positive Babinski response have never been described in this condition. Nevertheless, the classical features of the disease were seen in the loss of anterior horn cells, the atrophy of the anterior roots, and the presence of swollen, chromatolytic nerve cells, not only in the spinal cord, but in some of the brain-stem nuclei and the thalamus. It has been realized since the time of Conel's papers (Conel, 1938, 1940) that the latter change is more characteristic of the disease than small size or dark staining of nerve cells, the significance of which is difficult to assess in the immature nervous system. This form of neuronal degeneration has often been likened to the central chromatolysis that occurs after axonal lesions and it has been aptly named *gonflement bulleuse* by Thieffry, Arthuis, and Bargeton (1955). One cannot say that this form of neuronal degeneration *per se* is pathognomonic of Werdnig-Hoffmann disease, but when the distribution of the lesions is taken into account, we know of no other heredo-degeneration occurring in this age-group with which the condition might be confused. Except in Werdnig-Hoffmann disease we have only once seen acute anterior horn cell changes of approximately the same type, namely, in a child of 2 years with precocious Friedreich's ataxia (as described by André-van Leeuwen, 1949), and in this case there were the distinguishing features of degeneration of the posterior columns and of the visual pathways.

An atypical feature of the present case, and one that seems to be partly responsible for the clinical condition, was the predominant involvement of the cervical in contrast with the lumbar region of the cord. There is some evidence that this disease may start in certain segments and even become localized in them for a considerable time. Thus De Lange (1937) found intact lumbar segments in an infant who died on the 20th day of life, and Thieffry *et al.* (1955) noted that muscular weakness was confined to the lower limbs in 2 of the 40 patients they studied. The relative integrity of the lumbar cord in our patient, combined with the lesions present in the lateral columns, may be held responsible for the spasticity observed during life. These changes in the white matter, though unusually extensive, were similar in type to those often described in other cases of Werdnig-Hoffmann disease, i.e. pallor of myelin staining, not sharply confined to individual tracts and varying somewhat in intensity, in distribution, and in the associated gliosis, according to the level examined. Radermecker (1951), in particular, has drawn attention to these lesions which he believes are degenerative in character, but in view of the changes described in our case it seems more likely that defective myelination had occurred.

The exceptionally severe atrophy of the thalami and cerebellum in this brain invites comparison with the suprasegmental lesions found in the case recently reported in this journal by Norman (1961). In this instance, the cerebellum weighed only 21 g. and showed a combination of malformation (retarded convolutional development) and atrophy, which was regarded as an early manifestation of Werdnig-Hoffmann disease. This interpretation did not go unchallenged, for after the publication of the paper more than one correspondent suggested that birth injury was a more plausible explanation for the lesions, particularly in view of the clinical history. This opinion failed to take into account the acute neuronal changes in the spinal cord and basal ganglia which were typical of Werdnig-Hoffmann disease, but at that time the possibility of a double pathology could not be entirely ruled out. The present case removes any lingering doubt as to the propriety of attributing such severe suprasegmental lesions to a degenerative disease. There was no clinical suggestion of birth trauma, and the cerebellar cortical changes were those of a diffuse degenerative process of slow tempo which had introduced an element of hypoplasia into the post-natal growth of the organ. The exceptionally severe loss of nerve cells in the thalami may have accounted for the abnormalities shown in the second electroencephalogram.

In conclusion it may be pointed out that the brother of this patient had died at about the same age and had also shown spasticity and mental retardation. At necropsy the dilated lateral ventricles with no associated enlargement of the head had suggested an atrophic process, but since the brain was not examined histologically no further comparison is possible. However, it seems likely that both children suffered from the same genetic condition. The final diagnosis depends upon the propriety of including such atypical cases within the category of Werdnig-Hoffmann disease. For reasons already given, we believe that our patient did, in fact, suffer from an unusual variant of this disease. The neuropathological findings add no new dimension to its definition: they merely confirm the wide range of variation that may exist in the distribution and severity of the degenerative process.

**Summary**

A girl aged 23 months at death had failed to achieve normal motor development and was regarded clinically as a case of spastic cerebral palsy of unknown origin. Another sib had died at 28 months with similar clinical features. Neuropathological examination in the first case showed acute changes in the anterior horn cells, brain-stem nuclei, and thalamus, which were histologically typical of Werdnig-Hoffmann disease. The spinal cord changes were atypical in so far as the cervical segments were much more affected than the lumbar as regards loss of anterior horn cells. In myelin preparations, the spinal cord showed marked pallor of the antero-lateral areas, which was interpreted as the consequence of defective myelination rather than true tract degenerations. Supra-segmental lesions were particularly impressive in this brain. The cerebellum was small and showed mild diffuse atrophy of the granular layer, marked shrinkage of the Purkinje cells, gliosis of all the cortical layers and of the central white matter, especially in the hila of the dentate nuclei. The thalami showed an extensive loss of nerve cells, with corresponding gliosis, particularly in the lateral nuclei.

It is suggested that this thalamic lesion was responsible for the abnormal EEG recorded in the later stages of this child's illness.

These findings have been compared with those in a previously reported case of Werdnig-Hoffmann disease, which also showed unusually severe supra-segmental lesions.

We wish to thank Professor A. V. Neale and Professor T. F. Hewer for their kindness in making their records available to us.

References

André-van Leeuwen, M. (1949). Sur deux cas familiaux de maladie de Friedreich avec atrophie optique précoce globale et grave (observation de dix années). *Rev. neurol.*, **81**, 941.

Conel, J. L. (1938). Distribution of affected nerve cells in a case of amyotonia congenita *Arch. Neurol. Psychiat.* (*Chic.*), **40**, 337.

—— (1940). Distribution of affected nerve cells in amyotonia congenita (second case). *Arch. Path.*, **30**, 153.

De Lange, Cornelia (1937). Studien über angeborene Lahmungen bzw. angeborene Hypotonie. *Acta paediat.* (*Uppsala*), **20**, Suppl. 3.

Norman, R. M. (1961). Cerebellar hypoplasia in Werdnig-Hoffmann disease. *Arch. Dis. Childh.*, **36**, 96.

Radermecker, J. (1951). L'amyotrophie spinale de l'enfance (Werdnig-Hoffmann) comme hérédo-dégénérescence. *Rev. neurol.*, **84**, 14.

Thieffry, S., Arthuis, M., and Bargeton, E. (1955). Quarante cas de maladie Werdnig-Hoffmann avec onze examens anatomiques. *ibid.*, **93**, 621.

*Arch. Dis. Childh.*, 1965, **40**, 309.

# METHODS OF ROUTINE HAEMOGLOBINOMETRY IN CHILDHOOD: EVALUATION OF COPPER SULPHATE DENSITOMETRY

BY

HANAN COSTEFF*

*From the Beer-Sheva District Health Office, Israel Ministry of Health, Israel*

(RECEIVED FOR PUBLICATION OCTOBER 26, 1964)

A routine haemoglobin determination is generally recommended as part of the health supervision of infants and children. This is easily done in hospital settings or private practice, but is far more difficult in mass child health supervision among deprived populations. Standard haemoglobinometry methods such as photoelectric colorimetry are poorly adapted to such a purpose because of their expense and their need for trained personnel. The ideal routine haemoglobin examination in settings such as child health surveys in slums or undeveloped regions would permit a provisional diagnosis of anaemia on the spot by relatively untrained personnel, using simple cheap equipment. It would accurately distinguish between anaemia and normality but need not be precise beyond that point.

The determination of whole blood specific gravity in copper sulphate solutions has been described (van Slyke, Phillips, Dole, Hamilton, Archibald, and Plazin, 1950; Phillips, van Slyke, Hamilton, Dole, Emerson, and Archibald, 1950) as having most of the features required for mass screening for anaemia, and has been used for screening blood-bank donors (Heim and Ammon, 1952). It has not yet been standardized or evaluated in children.

This paper reports the standardization and evaluation of the whole blood specific gravity determination as a screening test for anaemia in infancy and early childhood.

## Material and Methods

Copper sulphate solutions were prepared by a modification (Simmons and Gentzkow, 1955) of the method of Phillips and van Slyke (Phillips *et al.*, 1950). Copper sulphate crystals of 'chemically pure' grade were used. Specific gravity of solutions was checked by pycnometry and Westphal balance. Concentration of solutions was measured frequently by iodometric titration of copper content with 0·1 N sodium thiosulphate solution. Determination of whole blood and plasma specific gravity followed the method of Phillips and van Slyke (Phillips *et al.*, 1950). Haemoglobin was measured by photoelectric colorimetry of cyanmethaemoglobin in a 1 : 201 dilution of blood in Drabkin's solution. The standard solution of cyanmethaemoglobin was matched throughout the study against cyanmethaemoglobin solutions of known iron content. In the study of venous bloods, 1 ml. amounts were drawn in 1 mg. of double oxalate, and haemoglobinometry was performed on 0·1 ml. aliquots.

Venous blood in anticoagulant was drawn from 60 infants aged 5-7 months attending child health conferences in the Beer-Sheva area. Haemoglobin, specific gravity of whole blood, and specific gravity of plasma were measured.

The same examinations were performed on the venous blood of 34 children aged 11-14 months in the same setting.

502 consecutive children aged 6 months to 6 years were examined in the same child health conferences. Physical examination was performed, a clinical suspicion of anaemia or its absence was recorded, and a lateral skin puncture was performed on the middle finger with a hypodermic needle. Free blood flow was established in most cases, but minimal squeezing was sometimes necessary. Blood was collected in a 20 c.mm. pipette which was emptied into 4 ml. Drabkin's solution for cyanmethaemoglobin colorimetry, and in a microhaematocrit tube from which it was dropped into a copper sulphate solution of specific gravity 1·0458. Specific gravity of blood was read as greater than, equal to, or less than, 1·0458.

Capillary blood in three 20 c.mm. pipettes was collected from 27 children aged 4 months to 5 years, in the same setting and by the same technique. Physical examination was performed first and a clinical prediction of the haemoglobin value was recorded. The bloods underwent one haemoglobin determination by the acid haematin method of Sahli and two separate haemoglobin determinations by photoelectric colorimetry of cyanmethaemoglobin. The first of the two colorimetric determinations was arbitrarily accepted as the 'true' value in calculations of standard error.

* Present address: Yale University Child Study Center, New Haven, Connecticut, U.S.A.

TABLE 1

CORRELATION BETWEEN HAEMOGLOBIN CONCENTRATION AND SPECIFIC GRAVITY OF VENOUS BLOOD

| | Group 1 (5-7 mth.) | Group 2 (11-14 mth.) |
|---|---|---|
| Number of samples | 60 | 34 |
| Haemoglobin (g./100 ml.)* | 11·75 ± 2 (0·99) | 11·14 ± 2 (1·27) |
| S.G.* of whole blood | 1·0472 ± 2 (0·0020) | 1·0480 ± 2 (0·0023) |
| S.G.* of plasma | 1·0249 ± 2 (0·0011) | 1·0267 ± 2 (0·0014) |
| r | + 0·83 | + 0·92 |
| Regression equation | Hb − 11·75 = 420 (S.G. − 1·0472) | Hb − 11·14 = 520 (S.G. − 1·0480) |
| Standard error of haemoglobin estimate from specific gravity of whole blood (g./100 ml.) | 0·59 | 0·46 |

* Recorded as mean ± 2 (S.D.).

TABLE 2

CORRELATION BETWEEN ANAEMIA AND SPECIFIC GRAVITY SCREENING TEST

| Age (mth.) | Hb < 10·0* S.G. ≦ 1·0458 | Hb ≧ 10·0 S.G. > 1·0458 | Hb < 10·0 S.G. > 1·0458 | Hb ≧ 10·0 S.G. ≦ 1·0458 | Total |
|---|---|---|---|---|---|
| 6-12 | 20 | 74 | 3 | 17 | 114 |
| 12-60 | 42 | 326 | 4 | 16 | 388 |
| Total | 62 | 400 | 7 | 33 | 502 |

Hb in g./100 ml.

## Results

The correlation between haemoglobin concentration and specific gravity of venous blood was high in both groups of infants, as shown in Table 1 and in Figs. 1 and 2. The specific gravity of whole blood could be used with small error as an estimate of haemoglobin both in the 5-7-month-old infants and in those of 11-14 months, though the estimates were not identical for the two groups because of a difference in plasma specific gravity.

The effectiveness of a one-drop screening test of whole blood specific gravity as an examination for anaemia (haemoglobin less than 10 g./100 ml.) in 502 children aged 6-72 months is shown in Fig. 3 and in Table 2. Of 69 cases of anaemia, including all but one with haemoglobin values under 9·5 g./100 ml., 62 had specific gravities equal to or less than 1·0458. All the 62 bloods with specific gravities of less than 1·0458 had haemoglobin values of 10·8 g./100 ml. or less, and 53 of them were anaemic. Of the 33

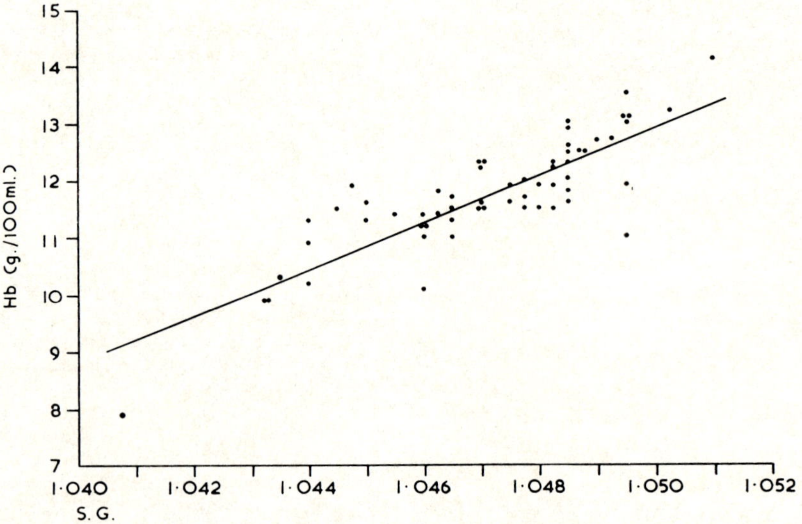


FIG. 1.—Relation between specific gravity and haemoglobin concentration of venous blood in 60 infants aged 5-7 months.

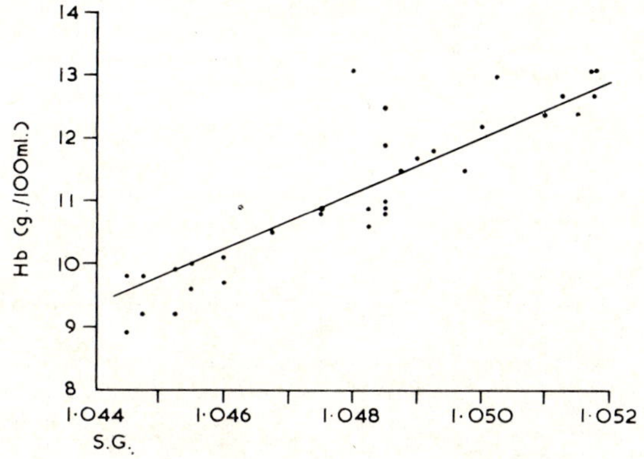


FIG. 2.—Relation between specific gravity and haemoglobin concentration of venous blood in 34 infants aged 11-14 months.

bloods with specific gravities equal to the test solution of 1·0458, 9 were anaemic. Of the 95 bloods with specific gravities equal to or less than 1·0458, 62 were anaemic. By comparison, physical examination alone gave a presumptive diagnosis of anaemia in 15 of the 433 children with a normal haemoglobin and in only 18 of the 69 anaemic children. Table 2 shows that the specific gravity is a somewhat more

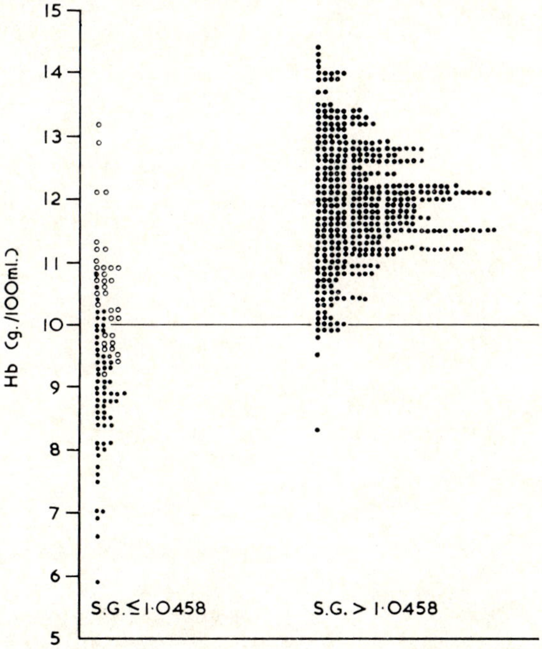


FIG. 3.—Distribution of haemoglobin concentration of capillary blood in 502 children aged 6-60 months. Circles at left represent bloods with S.G. ≦ 1·0458. Solid dots at left represent bloods with S.G. < 1·048.

accurate test for anaemia in children over the age of 12 months than in infants. The over-all number of false positive and false negative results indicates a standard error of about 0·71 g./100 ml.

This standard error of estimate may be compared with the standard error of estimate derived for the clinical guess, the Sahli method, and the cyanmethaemoglobin method in a group of 27 children. Table 3 demonstrates that photoelectric colorimetry of cyanmethaemoglobin was somewhat more accurate than the specific gravity determination, the Sahli examination less accurate, and the clinical guess so inaccurate as to be almost valueless.

TABLE 3

RELATIVE ACCURACY OF CAPILLARY HAEMOGLOBIN DETERMINATIONS FROM THE SAME FINGER PUNCTURE

| Type of Examination | No. of Examinations | S.E.* (g./100 ml.) | Cases of Verified Anaemia† Detected |
|---|---|---|---|
| Clinical estimate . . | 27 | 1·60 | 3 |
| Sahli method . . . . | 27 | 0·88 | 6 |
| Second photoelectric colorimetry . . . . | 26 | 0·46 | 6 |

* S.E. = Standard error from 'true value' measured by first photoelectric colorimetry.

† Verified anaemia indicates a haemoglobin of under 10·0 g./100 ml. on the first photoelectric colorimetry. There were 7 such cases.

The different haemoglobin examinations were timed. The one-drop screening examination required a total of 45-60 seconds to perform, including finger-prick. The Sahli examination required about 5 minutes. The various steps of photoelectric colorimetry (pipeting Drabkin's solution, finger-stick, withdrawal, expression, and mixing of blood, reading of solution and standard, and rinsing of tube) required a total of 3-4 minutes per examination.

Stored copper sulphate solutions were repeatedly examined by weighing and thiosulphate titration. The solutions remained stable except for the effect of evaporation. When bottles with mouths of 1·0-1·5 cm. diameter remained unstoppered on laboratory benches during a hot dry summer (laboratory temperatures 24°-29° C., relative humidity 30-50%) the rate of evaporation ranged from 100 mg. to 350 mg. per 24 hours. Evaporation was 15-19 mg. per day in loosely stoppered bottles and negligible over a period of months in bottles tightly closed with rubber stoppers.

## Discussion

The results indicate that copper sulphate densitometry is a simple, rapid, and accurate screening test for anaemia. One solution of specific gravity

1·0458 can be used by semi-skilled personnel to screen for anaemia in the entire 6-month to 6-year age-group at a rate of better than one examination a minute and with less error than the Sahli method in good hands. The total cost is that of one micro-haematocrit tube per examination plus 2 to 4 hours of a laboratory technician's time whenever new solution has to be prepared. Since the solution can be prepared in batches of several litres or more, and since each litre suffices for 1,000 examinations, this adds little to the expense. Specific gravity of stock solutions can be checked at preparation and thereafter as needed either by Westphal balance or by iodometric titration with 0·1 N sodium thiosulphate solution. 5 ml. copper sulphate solution of specific gravity 1·0458 will be neutralized by 14·38 ml. of the thiosulphate solution.

The standard errors found in the various haemoglobin estimates are compatible with those previously reported. Macfarlane, King, Wootton, and Gilchrist (1948) found an even greater error in the Sahli method than that reported here. The error of photoelectric colorimetry of cyanmethaemoglobin in this study was similar to that reported by King, Bartholomew, Geiser, Ventura, Wootton, Macfarlane, Donaldson, and Sisson (1951) but somewhat greater than that reported earlier by the same workers (King, Gilchrist, Wootton, Donaldson, Sisson, Macfarlane, Jope, O'Brien, Peterson, and Strangeways, 1948) and by Macfarlane *et al.* (1948). Since their studies were performed on pooled venous blood rather than capillary samples, their smaller errors are not surprising.

The variance of haemoglobin estimate by copper sulphate densitometry is similar to that reported by van Slyke *et al.* (1950) in a small group of adults, but the regression equation is different, probably because of lower plasma protein concentration in childhood.

For practical purposes evaporation was not a problem in stoppered bottles even in a warm dry climate. Changes of less than 0·0002 in specific gravity of copper sulphate solutions are negligible in calculating haemoglobin, and it would take a total evaporation of 0·44% (440 mg. of the contents of a 100 ml. bottle) to produce this change. Even in unfavourable climates this could be avoided by keeping the stock solution in tightly stoppered bottles and by replenishing the solution in examination bottles every two weeks.

## Summary and Conclusions

The van Slyke 'falling drop' specific gravity measurement of whole blood was correlated with haemoglobin concentration in 94 venous bloods and 502 capillary bloods of children aged 5 months to 6 years. This method was evaluated as an estimate of haemoglobin and as a screening test for anaemia in comparison with acid haematin haemoglobinometry, photoelectric colorimetry of cyanmethaemoglobin, and physical examination. It was found less accurate than photoelectric colorimetry but more accurate than the other methods. In addition the van Slyke method was found to be rapid, cheap, and easy to teach to semi-skilled personnel. It may be recommended as a routine in mass child health supervision.

The Department of Environmental Medicine of the Beer-Sheva Institute for Arid Zone Research provided the facilities for this study. I am grateful to its director Dr. K. Furman, to Anita Levy and Chava Mendel of his staff, and to Louis Fisher of the University of London for their help.

### References

Heim, W., and Ammon, G. (1952). Mitteilung uber die Anwendung eines Hb-Schnelltestes zu Spenderuntersuchungen. *Dtsch. med. Wschr.*, **77**, 51.

King, E. J., Bartholomew, R. J., Geiser, M., Ventura, S., Wootton, I. D. P., Macfarlane, R. G., Donaldson, R., and Sisson, R. B. (1951). Determination of haemoglobin; VIII. Accuracy of methods applied to abnormal bloods. *Lancet*, **1**, 1044.

——, Gilchrist, M., Wootton, I. D. P., Donaldson, R., Sisson, R. B., Macfarlane, R. G., Jope, H. M., O'Brien, J. R. P., Peterson, J. M., and Strangeways, D. H. (1948). Determination of haemoglobin; V. Precision of colorimetric methods. *ibid.*, **2**, 563.

Macfarlane, R. G., King, E. J., Wootton, I. D. P., and Gilchrist, M. (1948). Determination of haemoglobin; III. Reliability of clinical and other methods. *ibid.*, **1**, 282.

Phillips, R. A., van Slyke, D. D., Hamilton, P. B., Dole, V. P., Emerson, K., Jr., and Archibald, R. M. (1950). Measurement of specific gravities of whole blood and plasma by standard copper sulfate solutions. *J. Biol. Chem.*, **183**, 305.

Simmons, J. S., and Gentzkow, C. J. (1955). *Medical and Public Health Laboratory Methods*, p. 358. Lea and Febiger, Philadelphia.

van Slyke, D. D., Phillips, R. A., Dole, V. P., Hamilton, P. B., Archibald, R. M., and Plazin, J. (1950). Calculation of hemoglobin from blood specific gravities. *J. biol. Chem.*, **183**, 349.

*Arch. Dis. Childh.*, 1965, **40**, 313.

# URINARY WHITE CELL EXCRETION IN CHILDHOOD

BY

I. B. HOUSTON

*From the Department of Child Health, St. Mary's Hospital, Manchester* 13

(RECEIVED FOR PUBLICATION OCTOBER 8, 1964)

In recent years more attention has been paid to the diagnosis of pyelonephritis, and this has made accurate estimation of pyuria more necessary. Houghton and Pears (1957), Hutt, Chalmers, MacDonald, and de Wardener (1961), and Little (1962) have all reported their experience in measuring the rate of urinary white cell excretion. Their figures are very largely derived from adults; the present report is designed to provide a comparable set of values during infancy and childhood. Such figures have a direct relevance to the diagnosis of chronic pyelonephritis, other renal diseases, and also to the interpretation of the 'prednisolone provocative test' (Little and de Wardener, 1962; Katz, Velasquez, and Bourdo, 1962) when this is performed on a child.

## Material and Methods

Carefully timed specimens of urine were collected by a clean voiding technique from 141 children (85 male, 56 female) of varying ages. The problems inherent in collecting timed specimens of urine from small infants necessitate their presence in hospital, and in consequence the urine specimens were collected from children already in hospital convalescing from a variety of illnesses. Any child who was febrile, who had had any disease remotely likely to influence the cellular composition of the urine, or who was receiving steroid, antibiotic, or salicylate therapy was excluded from the study.

For continent children able to micturate on request there is no problem about collecting a timed specimen of urine, though with some it is preferable to allow them to micturate spontaneously, carefully noting the times. In consequence, though most specimens were collected over an interval of two hours, there was a variation of 23 to 267 minutes.

Incontinent infants and toddlers present greater difficulties; these were surmounted by using a special machine which gave immediate audible warning of the fact that an infant had micturated. The time of passing the first specimen was noted and the specimen was discarded. The next time micturition occurred the specimen was collected, unless the time interval between specimens was less than an hour, in which case more specimens were collected and pooled together for examination, the total time being carefully noted. The duration of these specimens varied from 60 to 290 minutes.

The white cell excretion rate of each urine specimen was determined by the method of Houghton and Pears (1957). A few minor modifications in technique were made: 10 ml. urine were centrifuged at 2,000 r.p.m. for 10 minutes and the sediment resuspended in 0·5 ml. fluid (instead of 1 ml.) thus concentrating the urine 20 times. This was found generally to produce a more convenient concentration of white cells for counting in a Fuchs-Rosenthal chamber. An attempt was made to count only leucocytes and, to facilitate this, 2 drops of 0·1% Nile-blue stain were allowed to dry on the cover slip before use.

The height, weight, and age of each child were noted and their body surface area calculated from nomograms.

## Results

In Figs. 1-4 the urinary white cell excretion rates are plotted against the age, height, weight, and surface area of individual patients. There is clearly a relation between white cell excretion and the individual's size, best shown in respect of height and surface area. Six of the values are so different, however, that it must be assumed that these patients had pathologically raised excretion rates. Careful reappraisal of these cases has not revealed a cause; one was awaiting tonsillectomy, the others suffered respectively from asthma, Fallot's tetralogy, idiopathic thrombocytopenic purpura, temporal lobe epilepsy, and muscular dystrophy.

In 20 patients, further estimates of the white cell excretion rate were made at intervals varying between 3 days and 6 months. 13 patients had two, 5 patients three, 1 four, and 1 five specimens of urine collected. The results are shown in Table 1. In 15 patients the initial result was within the normal range and so were all except one of the subsequent values, though they sometimes varied considerably from the original one. Of the 6 patients with unusually high values, 5 had repeat estimates performed: 2 remained abnormal and the others became normal.

In 5 children consecutive urine specimens were collected over a complete 24-hour period (Table 2).

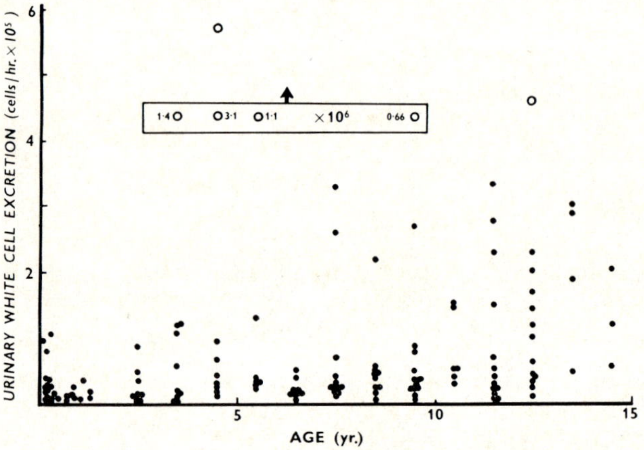


FIG. 1.—Relationship of white cell excretion to age. In the first two years of life, age is plotted to the nearest month. The rings represent fortuitously abnormal results.

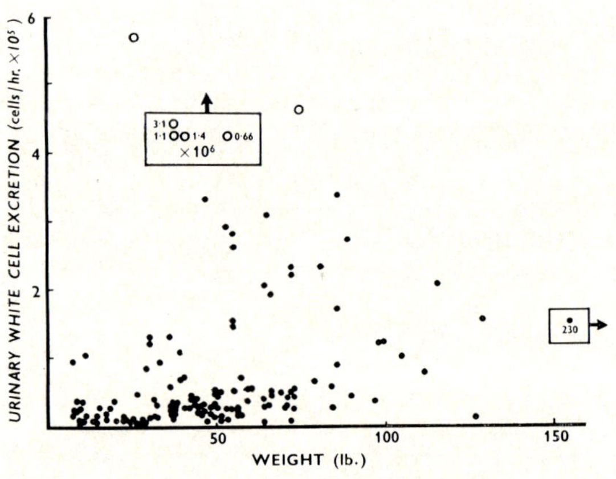


FIG. 2.—Relationship of white cell excretion to weight.

There was sometimes a five- or sixfold difference between minimal and maximal excretion rates in any one day, but there was sufficient consistency in the results to define whether the figures fell, over-all, into a normal or abnormal pattern. Some of this variation could be due to the failure of some children to empty their bladders completely when micturating; collection by catheter would obviate this possibility but cannot be justified in view of the known risks of the procedure.

## Discussion

Hodson, Drewe, Karn, and King (1962) have shown that, in childhood, the length and cross-sectional area of the kidneys are closely related to the child's height and weight, especially the height. The present study suggests that urinary white cell excretion is also a function of body size and,

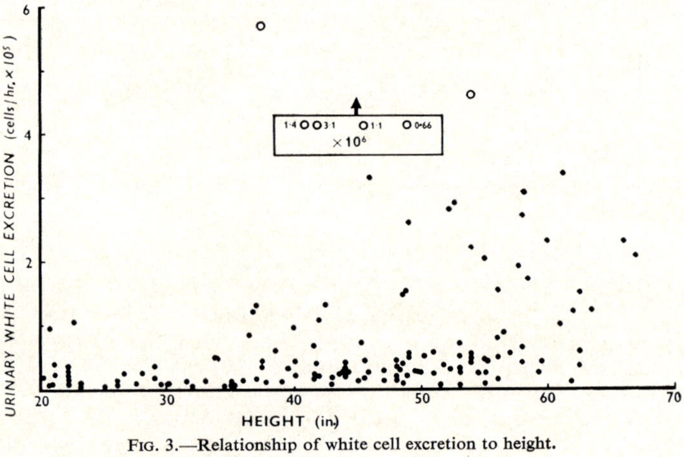


FIG. 3.—Relationship of white cell excretion to height.

TABLE 1

URINARY WHITE CELL EXCRETION RATES FROM INDIVIDUAL PATIENTS WITH VARYING INTERVALS BETWEEN SPECIMENS

| Patient | Urinary White Cell Excretion (cells/hr.) | | | | |
|---|---|---|---|---|---|
| | 1 | 2 | 3 | 4 | 5 |
| A.M. | 39,000 | 22,000 | 17,000 | 16,000 | 15,000 |
| P.R. | 17,000 | 34,000 | | | |
| D.Br. | 190,000 | 32,000 | 75,000 | | |
| M.B. | 2,000 | 7,000 | 8,000 | | |
| A.D. | 11,000 | 23,000 | 14,000 | | |
| T.P. | 24,000 | 31,000 | | | |
| R.M. | 42,000 | 17,000 | 69,000 | | |
| B.N. | 230,000 | 45,000 | | | |
| W.St.L. | 53,000 | 95,000 | 172,000 | 120,000 | |
| P.C. | 18,000 | 12,000 | | | |
| M.J. | 26,000 | 61,000 | | | |
| A.J. | 55,000 | 41,000 | | | |
| K.L. | 260,000 | 99,000 | | | |
| D.Bo. | 104,000 | 19,000 | | | |
| S.E. | 330,000 | 1,100,000 | | | |
| R.F. | 460,000 | 290,000 | | | |
| P.N. | 570,000 | 96,000 | 35,000 | | |
| J.F. | 660,000 | 2,000,000 | | | |
| D.McC. | 1,400,000 | 79,000 | | | |
| W.H. | 3,100,000 | 170,000 | | | |

TABLE 2

URINARY WHITE CELL EXCRETION RATES, CONSECUTIVE SPECIMENS OVER A 24-HOUR PERIOD*

| Time of Day | White Cell Excretion Rate (cells/hr.) | | | | |
|---|---|---|---|---|---|
| | P.C. | M.J. | M.F. | P.N. | M.G. |
| | | 8,000 | | 35,000 | |
| A.M. | 12,000 | 61,000 | | 16,000 | 27,000 |
| | 5,000 | 41,000 | 1,500,000 | 14,000 | 50,000 |
| | | 29,000 | 260,000 | | 80,000 |
| | 33,000 | 16,000 | 200,000 | 7,000 | 29,000 |
| P.M. | | | 510,000 | | 21,000 |
| | 10,000 | 7,000 | 1,040,000 | | |
| | 21,000 | | 660,000 | 6,000 | 21,000 |
| A.M. | | 18,000 | 700,000 | | |
| | 9,000 | | 320,000 | | |

* In 4 of the 5 patients, the highest rate was recorded between 6 a.m. and midday.

presumably, of renal size. The majority of adults have urinary white cell excretion rates of less than 200,000 cells/hr., and though a few exceed this value it rarely reaches more than 400,000 cells/hr. (Houghton and Pears, 1957; Hutt *et al.*, 1961; Little, 1962). Even the lower of these figures would be quite abnormal for a small child or infant and a separate set of standards must be applied to results obtained from children. Infants up to 36 in. (91 cm.) or 0·55 sq. m. in height or surface area respectively rarely exceed an excretion rate of 50,000 white cells/hr.; with increasing size the acceptable upper limit gradually increases to 100,000 white cells/hr. for a child of 45 in. (114 cm.) or 0·8 sq. m. and eventually reaches an approximately adult level with a height of about 52 in. (132 cm.) or a surface area of 1·0 sq. m. (approximately 8 to 10 years of age). The only comparable report on this subject is that of Gekle (1964) who, from 50 children (2 to 14 years old) obtained figures to suggest that 40,000 white cells/hr. was the normal upper limit of white cell excretion. His results are compatible with the hypothesis that body (or renal) size is a factor in determining white cell excretion; the discrepancy in results in later childhood between that report and the present one may be attributable to the difference in numbers of specimens examined or possibly to the fact that catheterization was the method by which specimens were obtained by Gekle.

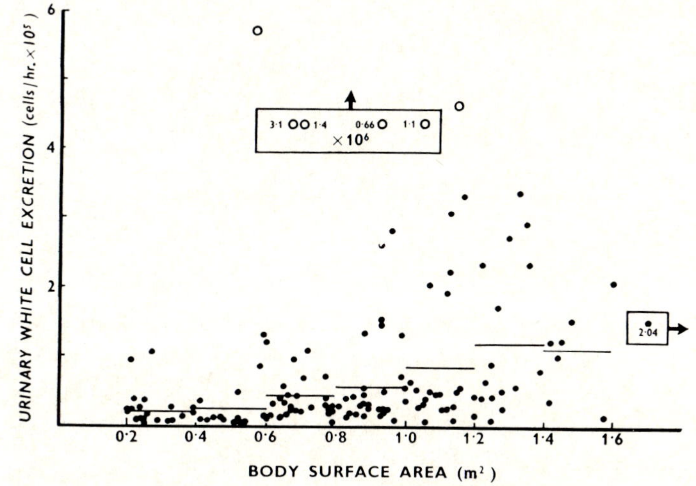


FIG. 4.—Relationship of white cell excretion to surface area. The mean values for patients in 0·2 sq. m. groups is shown by the horizontal lines. They are respectively (from the left) 20,000, 24,000, 45,000, 58,000, 87,000, 120,000, and 112,000/hour.

There is a disappointingly wide variation in excretion rates in the same child on different days and even at different times of the same day, which makes changes of excretion rate induced by prednisolone or bacterial pyrogen difficult to evaluate. It is desirable not to rely too heavily on the results of a single observation in assessing renal status, though a repeat measurement will usually yield a result sufficiently like the first to say with some certainty that it is, or is not, normal.

As will be seen, the measurement of white cell excretion in the urine has drawbacks, but if the correct set of standards for the child's size are applied, this sensitive technique can supply very valuable information.

## Summary

A set of standards is described relating urinary white cell excretion rates to the size of the child. Though the variation in excretion rates in the same child at different times is sometimes appreciable, the results can usually be quite easily interpreted and can be of great assistance in assessing cases of 'subclinical' renal disease.

I should like to thank Dr. H. B. Marsden for his helpful advice and for permitting me to use the facilities of his laboratory. My appreciation is also due to Professor Wilfrid Gaisford for his support and assistance and to the Department of Medical Illustration, Manchester Royal Infirmary, for the figures.

### References

Gekle, D. (1964). Untersuchungen über die physiologische Leukocyturie im Kindesalter und die Beeinflussung der Leukocytenausscheidung durch Prednisolon bei chronischer Pyelonephritis. *Ann. paediat.* (*Basel*), **203**, 113.

Hodson, C. J., Drewe, J. A., Karn, M. N., and King, A. (1962). Renal size in normal children; a radiographic study during life. *Arch. Dis. Childh.*, **37**, 616.

Houghton, B. J., and Pears, M. A. (1957). Cell excretion in normal urine. *Brit. med. J.*, **1**, 622.

Hutt, M. S. R., Chalmers, J. A., MacDonald, J. S., and de Wardener, H. E. (1961). Pyelonephritis. *Lancet*, **1**, 351.

Katz, Y. J., Velasquez, A., and Bourdo, S. R. (1962). The prednisolone provocative test for pyelonephritis. *ibid.*, **1**, 1144.

Little, P. J. (1962). Urinary white-cell excretion. *ibid.*, **1**, 1149.

——, and de Wardener, H. E. (1962). The use of prednisolone phosphate in the diagnosis of pyelonephritis in man. *ibid.*, **1**, 1145.

*Arch. Dis. Childh.*, 1965, **40**, 317.

# HISTOLOGICAL OBSERVATIONS ON GLYCOGEN RESERVES OF THE FOETUS AND NEWBORN INFANT

BY

JEAN M. SCOTT

*From the Royal Maternity Hospital, Glasgow*

(RECEIVED FOR PUBLICATION OCTOBER 15, 1964)

Every observer must be impressed by the ability of the foetal heart to continue beating under conditions of extreme oxygen lack. It has been known for many years that the foetus is specially endowed in this respect, but only recently has animal experimental work shown that survival may well be determined by the level of the foetal glycogen reserves, especially those of the myocardium (Shelley, 1961; Mott, 1961). Histological studies in this department over the past four years have shown that in stillbirths these levels vary considerably, but in newborn infants they are invariably low (Scott, 1961). Recently, however, our paediatric colleagues started to treat respiratory distress syndrome (RDS) of the newborn by means of intravenous alkalies and laevulose (Hutchison, Kerr, Douglas, Inall, and Crosbie, 1964). Striking differences in the glycogen reserves, even in babies coming to necropsy, were immediately noted, and these formed an interesting comparison with our earlier findings.

### Materials and Methods

Post-mortem material was used. The bodies were refrigerated immediately after death and the majority of necropsies were carried out within 24 hours. Control cases were drawn from the original untreated series of 72 babies (Scott, 1961) and compared with 35 RDS babies, given bicarbonate and laevulose. Sections of liver and heart were examined as before for glycogen and fat, using a lead tetra-acetate Schiff method (LTAS) after picric alcohol fixation for the former and Sudan IV for the latter. The slides were graded on a +, ++, +++ basis, and the assessment made without reference to the clinical history or the therapy given.

### Results

Though this paper is mainly concerned with the newborn infant, a few of the more important changes noted in stillbirths should be briefly mentioned here, as factors operative in intrauterine life undoubtedly influence the neonatal period, and some of these were not fully dealt with in the original paper. Nine stillbirths examined at that time showed variable amounts of glycogen in the myocardium. Seven, including two that were premature, had no stainable glycogen in their livers. The baby with the greatest amount of glycogen in its liver died from intracranial haemorrhage due to bilateral tentorial tears: death was sudden and unexpected and only a few cells in the periportal region of the liver lobule showed any sign of glycogen depletion; they failed to stain with LTAS, and in H. and E. sections glycogenic vacuolation was absent and the cytoplasm became shrunken and eosinophilic. Other similar cases have since been examined and it has been confirmed that in mature babies, where stress is of short duration, only the periportal region is affected, but, as foetal distress increases, depletion spreads throughout the whole lobule. Thus glycogen reserves may vary considerably in mature babies, but where the infant is premature the levels are invariably low.

Apart from cases of placental insufficiency, foetal blood loss, and Rhesus incompatibility, fatty change is uncommon in the myocardium of stillbirths (Scott, 1961), and this is also true of the liver. Only traces of fat were found in 2 of the 9 livers examined. One was a delayed labour with cord round the neck, the other an *abruptio placentae* and both were mature.

In the neonatal group, the 21 control cases and the 35 treated babies were compared and the amounts of glycogen found in the livers and hearts of both groups are shown in Table 1. In untreated control cases no stainable glycogen was found in the liver, but in those receiving laevulose, 57% had one plus or more. Cardiac glycogen stores were also enhanced. Only 33% of controls were positive and these merely one plus, but with treatment 76% became positive and 17% were actually ++ or more.

Fatty change in each group is shown in Table 2. At first the results seemed disappointing. More

TABLE 1

GLYCOGEN CONTENT OF LIVER AND HEART IN BABIES TREATED WITH LAEVULOSE

| Organ | Group | No. | Glycogen Grading (% incidence) | | | |
|---|---|---|---|---|---|---|
| | | | 0 | + | ++ | +++ |
| Liver | Treated | 35 | 43 (15) | 23 (8) | 23 (8) | 11 (4) |
| | Control | 21 | 100 (21) | | | |
| Heart | Treated | 29 | 24 (7) | 59 (17) | 14 (4) | 3 (1) |
| | Control | 21 | 67 (14) | 33 (7) | | |

Figures in brackets represent the number in each group.

TABLE 2

FATTY CHANGE IN LIVER AND HEART IN BABIES TREATED WITH LAEVULOSE

| Organ | Group | No. | Fat Grading (% incidence) | | | |
|---|---|---|---|---|---|---|
| | | | 0 | + | ++ | +++ |
| Liver | Treated | 32 | 10 (3) | 31 (10) | 40 (13) | 19 (6) |
| | Control | 21 | 33·3 (7) | 33·3 (7) | 33·3 (7) | |
| Heart | Treated | 25 | 56 (14) | 4 (1) | 36 (9) | 4 (1) |
| | Control | 21 | 19 (4) | 28·5 (6) | 28·5 (6) | 24 (5) |

Figures in brackets represent the number in each group.

fatty change was evident in the livers of treated cases. Only 10% were negative compared with 33% of controls, and 59% showed ++ or more. Less fatty change, however, was seen in the myocardium of the treated babies; 44% were positive compared with 81% of controls. This problem will be discussed later, but two important points should be mentioned here; first, the treated babies lived longer on the average (Fig. 1) and, secondly, 46% of them had terminal intraventricular haemorrhages.

Since administration of laevulose could obviously replenish glycogen stores, the next step was to see

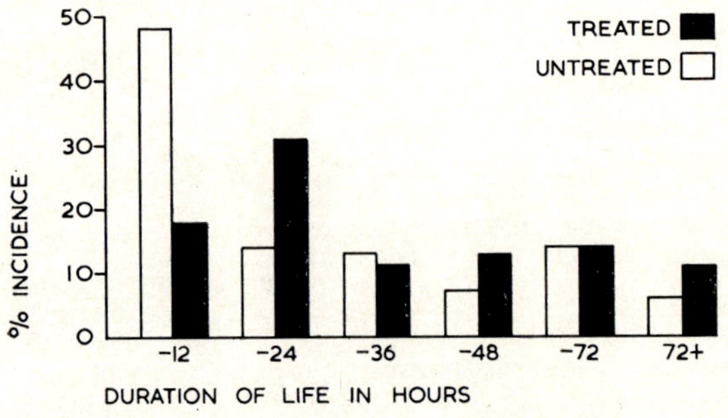


FIG. 1.—Duration of life in control and treated series.

whether there was any relation between the amount given and the glycogen assessed histologically. The quantity of laevulose each baby received varied very much from case to case depending on the severity of the respiratory and metabolic acidosis and the necessity to give bicarbonate. As biochemical correction was achieved, however, maintenance therapy with 20% laevulose as well as bicarbonate could be given, the proportions depending on the Astrup readings (Hutchison *et al.*, 1964). A total fluid intake of 60 ml./kg. in 24 hours was allowed. Thus it was possible, though highly unlikely, that all this could be given as laevulose, and for comparative purposes this amount of laevulose was taken as the ideal maximum on which all others were based, the values being expressed as percentages of it. The range was wide (7 to 85%) but when the percentages were compared with the liver glycogen grading, it was found that if the very immature babies (less than 1,000 g.) and those mature babies over 2,500 g. were excluded, some correlation was evident. The individual results of 27 babies whose weights fell into this range are shown in Fig. 2 and apart from one case, which has been ringed, it can be seen that as the percentage of laevulose rose, so the glycogen grading in the liver also increased. Considerable overlap is evident between the various groups, as one

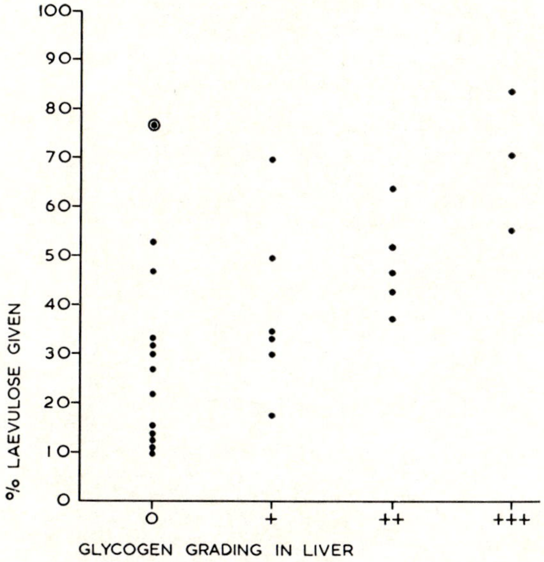


FIG. 2.—Glycogen grading in liver in relation to amount of laevulose given in 27 babies of 1·0-2·5 kg.

might expect, where gradings based on a relatively crude histological assessment are used. The exception (ringed in Fig. 2) was a baby who, in spite of having 78% of the possible laevulose dose, had no stainable glycogen in its liver: it weighed only 1,030 g. and like 3 other babies under 1,000 g. it seemed to be incapable of laying down glycogen adequately, even when laevulose was available. Only one baby under 1,000 g. had any stainable glycogen in its liver and then only one plus, despite the fact that it had been given 83% of the possible laevulose dose. Three mature babies with weights over 2,500 g. died of respiratory distress syndrome and were included in the treated series. The percentages of laevulose given were 22, 24, and 43 and the liver glycogen gradings +++, +, and +++, respectively. The numbers are small, but the lack of correlation is obvious.

Glycogen gradings in the myocardium were also analysed and related as before to the amount of laevulose administered during life, but for reasons that will be discussed later no correlation was found. It was also impossible to correlate glycogen storage with true blood glucose and fructose levels. In their clinical analysis Hutchison *et al.* (1964) showed that in 27 babies examined blood glucose levels were also raised after laevulose therapy but wide variations occurred. Of this group, 13 eventually came to necropsy, but the numbers were too small to form any opinion.

Deposition of glycogen itself within the various organs was interesting. Fig. 3 shows a liver with +++ glycogen grading. All the parenchymal cells contain glycogen, but in addition material giving a positive reaction is seen lying in portal veins. Presumably this represents carbohydrate that has been precipitated in processing. Livers with less glycogen tended to concentrate what they had round portal tracts (Fig. 4), but this was not always true. Sometimes glycogen could be seen round central veins as well as portal tracts, leaving the mid-zone free. On the other hand, it might be concentrated in one or other of these two sites in different lobules of the same liver (Fig. 5).

In the heart, heaviest concentrations were seen beneath the endocardium and round smaller vessels in the myocardium. Only rarely, with +++ grading, did the glycogen extend out to the pericardial surface.

## Discussion

Histological assessment of glycogen from tissues obtained at necropsy has its limitations, but in the present circumstances the effects of therapy were so striking that grading was remarkably easy. This was partly due to the fact that most of the babies requiring treatment were premature and had RDS. Their initial glycogen reserves were therefore minimal. Certainly this was the case in the untreated control series (Scott, 1961), and similar findings have since been reported by Shelley (1964), using a more accurate chemical method.

This being so, the effects of therapy would naturally be more obvious, provided of course that the baby could utilize the laevulose presented to it. The findings show that the majority were capable of doing so. 57% had one plus or more glycogen in their livers, and this figure would probably have been higher had it been possible to give more laevulose in certain cases. Reference to Fig. 2 will show that 7 babies, or one-fifth of the series, had less than 25% of the possible laevulose dose.

In those given adequate amounts only the extremely premature babies around 1,000 g. seemed to be incapable of laying down glycogen. There were three such cases in the present series and it is possible that like very young unhatched chicks studied by Gill (1938) and early foetal guinea-pigs (Nemeth, Insull, and Flexner, 1954), their enzyme systems were incomplete, especially those concerned with glycogen synthesis. Certainly if these extremely premature babies are excluded, the rest of the premature babies lay down glycogen in their livers in amounts roughly proportional to the quantity of laevulose administered.

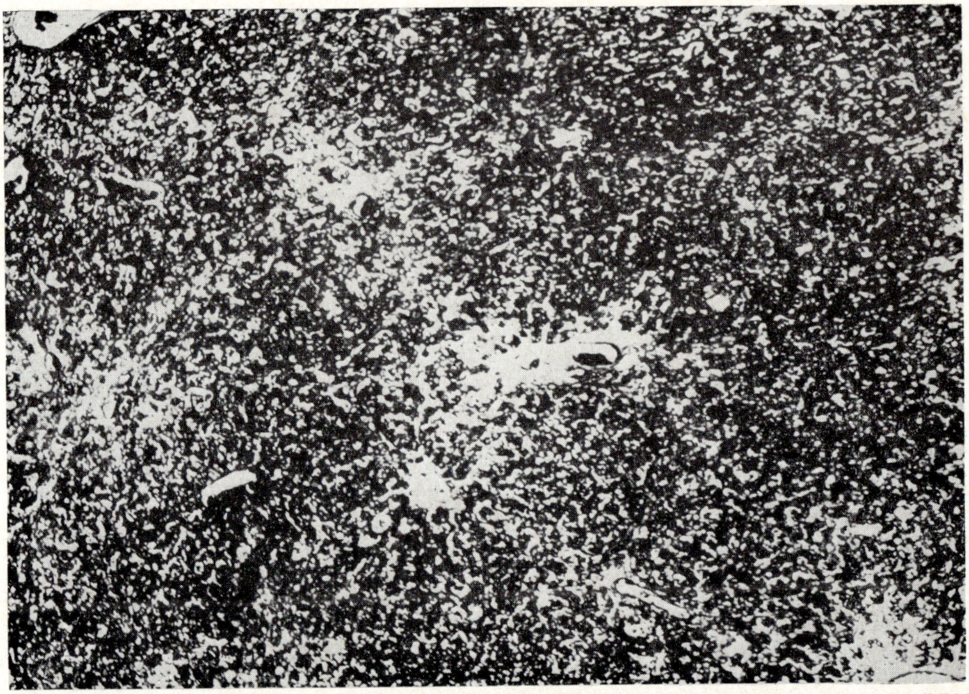

FIG. 3.—Liver, treated series, graded + + + for glycogen. Note positive material in portal tracts and central veins. (LTAS × 55.)

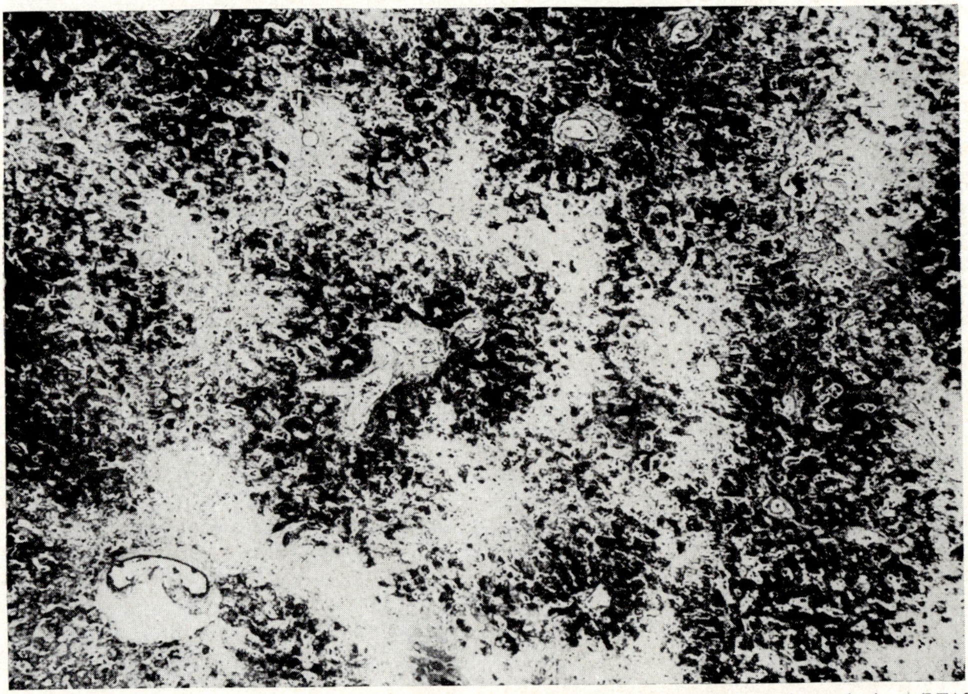

FIG. 4.—Liver, treated series, graded + + for glycogen. Most of the material is round portal tracts less round central veins. (LTAS × 55.)

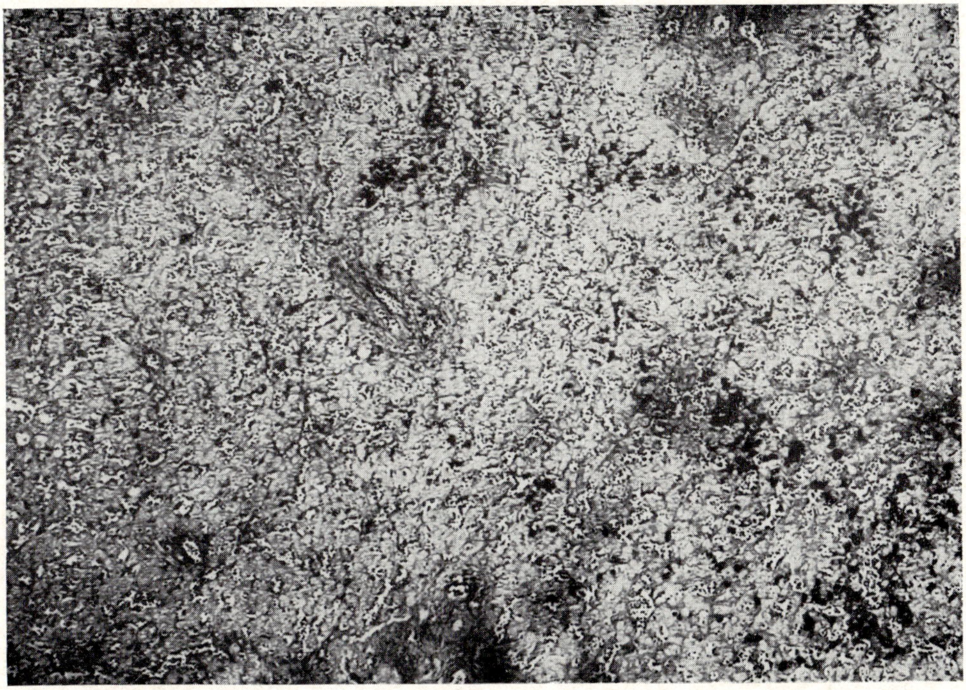

FIG. 5.—Liver, treated series, graded + for glycogen, which is irregularly distributed throughout the lobules. (LTAS × 55.)

Whether the same is true of mature babies is by no means certain. The number of cases studied here is too small to come to any definite conclusion, but even with larger numbers, it is doubtful if the findings would be comparable. In mature babies there is such a wide range in liver glycogen at birth (Shelley, 1964, and personal observations) that any effect of therapy in the immediate neonatal period could easily be obscured.

Myocardial glycogen showed even less correlation with treatment given. Though twice as many positive cases were found in the treated group, there was no evidence of any quantitative relationship even in premature babies. However, the presence of intraventricular haemorrhage here (46%) may well have altered the picture, for it has been shown that glycogen depletion is usually less marked, when this complication arises (Scott, 1961).

Fatty change in the myocardium was also less frequent in the treated group, only 44% compared with 81% in controls, but again this cannot be wholly attributed to treatment since intraventricular haemorrhage might also influence the picture (Scott, 1961).

Treatment certainly seemed to have no influence on fatty change in the liver. 90% of treated babies being positive for this compared with only 33% of controls. This was a disappointment, for it had been hoped that increase of hepatic glycogen would reduce fatty change. However, one has to remember that in a survey such as this only those babies coming to necropsy are seen, and the picture may be entirely different in survivors. Moreover the treated babies lived considerably longer than their control opposite numbers, 50% of whom died within 12 hours. One would, therefore, not expect to see much fatty change in the latter group. Indeed it only begins to appear with long and continued distress.

Apart from quantitative assessment of the glycogen, its distribution in histological sections was also interesting. In the heart it was found at 'points of entry' beneath the endocardium and around small vessels in the myocardium. In the liver, appearances were sometimes more difficult to explain. The administration of laevulose was often interrupted, when demands for bicarbonate increased, and the baby would then have to draw on its own glycogen reserves. If the depletion pattern followed that seen in stillbirths, then those cells around portal tracts would be the first to lose glycogen, followed later by cells in the mid-zone, until a stage would be reached when only small amounts might be found round central veins. Further administration of laevulose, at this point, would immediately replenish the stores of those cells nearest the periphery and possibly some in the mid-zone. Thus, if one takes into account the various stages in the above process, a ready explanation can be found for any of the irregular distribution patterns found in post-mortem material.

## Summary

A histological assessment of glycogen storage and fatty change has been made on the livers and hearts of 35 babies treated with bicarbonate and laevulose via umbilical vein catheter for respiratory distress syndrome, and the findings have been compared with an earlier control series.

Apart from the very immature baby who seems to have reduced ability to lay down glycogen, storage increases roughly in proportion to the amount of laevulose administered. Myocardial glycogen also increases, though not proportionately as in the liver, and the reasons for this are discussed.

Fatty change was more common in the livers of treated babies but this could be due to the fact that they lived longer. On the other hand the myocardium showed less fatty change.

I should like to thank Dr. A. D. T. Govan for his advice and encouragement, and I am also grateful to Mr. David Johnston for technical assistance, to Mr. J. Sommerville for blood glucose estimations, and to Mr. Andrew Fraser and Mr. T. Pearston for photographic illustrations. Professor Hutchison very kindly gave me access to his clinical records.

### References

Gill, P. M. (1938). The effect of adrenaline on embryonic chick glycogen *in vitro* as compared with its effect *in vivo*. *Biochem. J.*, **32**, 1792.

Hutchison, J. H., Kerr, M. M., Douglas, T. A., Inall, J. A., and Crosbie, J. C. (1964). A therapeutic approach in 100 cases of the respiratory distress syndrome of the newborn infant. *Pediatrics*, **33**, 956.

Mott, J. C. (1961). The ability of young mammals to withstand total oxygen lack. *Brit. med. Bull.*, **17**, 144.

Nemeth, A. M., Insull, W., Jr., and Flexner, L. B. (1954). Glycogenesis in the liver of the fetal guinea pig. *J. biol. Chem.*, **208**, 765.

Scott, J. M. (1961). Fatty change in the myocardium of the newborn. *Brit. med. J.*, **2**, 1746.

Shelley, H. J. (1961). Glycogen reserves and their changes at birth and in anoxia. *Brit. med. Bull.*, **17**, 137.

—— (1964). Carbohydrate reserves in the newborn infant. *Brit. med. J.*, **1**, 273.

*Arch. Dis. Childh.*, 1965, **40**, 323.

# VENOUS PRESSURE MEASUREMENT IN EXCHANGE TRANSFUSION

BY

DENNIS COTTOM and MAUREEN YOUNG
*From St. Thomas' Hospital, London*

(RECEIVED FOR PUBLICATION AUGUST 5, 1964)

Exchange transfusion in small infants carries a mortality of 4-7·5% (Van Praagh, 1961; Boggs and Westphal, 1960). Many factors such as hypocalcaemia, circulatory overloading, hyperkalaemia, acidosis, citrate toxicity may be responsible, and the mode of death, whatever the aetiology, is usually thought to be acute cardiac failure (O'Neill and Gordon, 1959; Robinson and Barrie, 1963), and commonly the infant shows signs of cardiac failure at necropsy. When cardiac failure occurs the venous pressure, as measured through the exchange catheter, rises; however, central venous pressure will only be recorded if the catheter tip passes through the ductus venosus and into the inferior vena cava.

Recently three observers (Rudolph, Drorbaugh, Auld, Rudolph, Nadas, Smith, and Hubbell, 1961; Burnard and James, 1963; Jegier, Blankenship, and Lind, 1963) have shown that the mean venous pressure in the normal newborn infant, whether it be measured in the right atrium or the inferior vena cava, is approximately 0 cm. $H_2O$ and similar to the central venous pressure in the adult; these pressures were measured with electrical manometers from catheters introduced through the umbilical vein and related to the sternal angle. Both Rudolph *et al.* and Jegier *et al.* noted that it was not always possible to pass a catheter through the ductus venosus and therefore, before any interpretation of venous pressure is made, it must be known with certainty that the catheter is in the inferior vena cava. The site of the catheter can be readily determined by watching for the pressure drop of 5-10 cm. $H_2O$ as the tip is advanced from between 8 to 12 cm. from the umbilicus; the respiratory pressure swings are also considerably larger in the thoracic inferior vena cava than in the portal sinus (Fig. 1).

The data reported below confirm the findings just described and give some indication of the expectancy of passing an umbilical vein catheter through the ductus venosus during the first two days of life.

## Methods and Material

The observations were made on 32 infants, 1 hour to 31 hours old, and ranging from 2·3-5·8 kg. in weight. They were part of a study of hypoglycaemia of the newborn in which glucose was given parenterally and blood samples taken from the umbilical vessels; at the time the venous pressure was measured the infants were considered to be normal from the circulatory standpoint. Parental permission was always obtained from one or both parents when normal babies were investigated.

The venous pressure was measured with a New Electronic Products (N.E.P.) inductance manometer; the recordings were made with the N.E.P. recorder through pencil-type mirror galvonometers with an ultraviolet light source and print-out recording paper. The manometer was approximately level with the heart. The catheter was filled with heparin saline (0·25 ml. 5,000 i.u./ml. heparin in 100 ml. saline). The frequency response of the catheter manometer system was 30 cycles/second.

The observations were made in the premature baby nursery using sterile technique; the room temperature was 76° F. (24° C.). The infants were clothed and lay comfortably in the supine position on a mattress on a

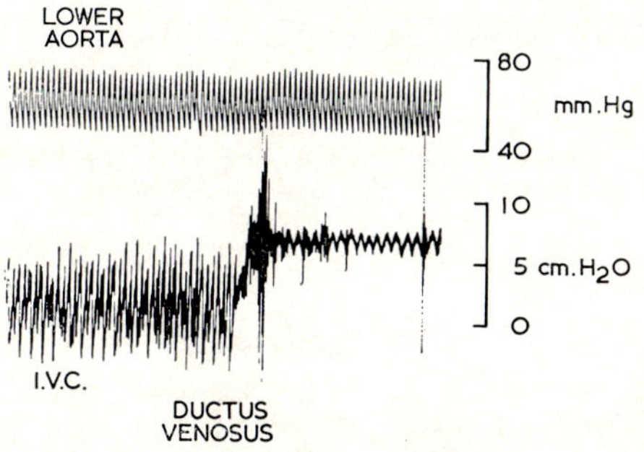


FIG. 1.—The lower pressure tracing shows, from left to right, (a) the relatively large respiratory pressure swings around the mean of zero recorded from the inferior vena cava above the ductus venosus; (b) a disturbance as the catheter is drawn through the ductus venosus; and (c) the small respiratory pressure swings around the mean of 7 cm. $H_2O$ in the umbilical vein below the ductus venosus. The upper pressure trace is from the lower aorta.

small instrument table to which they were lightly bandaged. A No. 6 (F.G.) 'Portex' catheter with 2 side holes, attached by a short length of saline-filled polythene tubing to the manometer, was introduced into the umbilical vein. It entered easily for the first 8 cm. until the ductus venosus was reached. In two-thirds of the infants the catheter tip passed through a slight resistance when a pressure drop and more marked respiratory fluctuations were observed. In the remaining one-third this was not possible, and no pressure drop was observed; occasionally a little blood flowed back around the catheter when its tip coiled in the sinus below the ductus venosus.

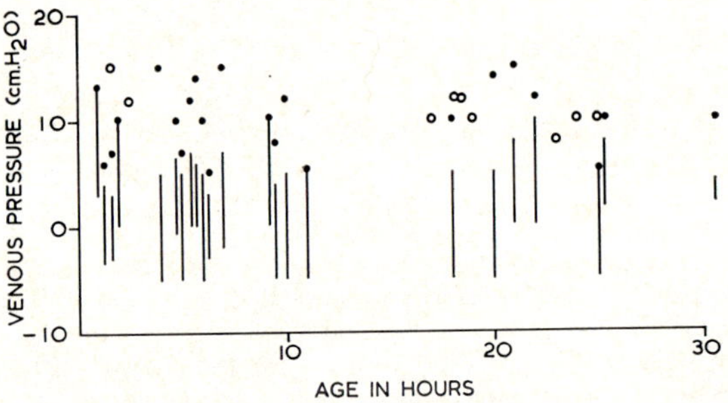


FIG. 2.—To demonstrate the different relationships between the mean pressure in the umbilical vein below the ductus venosus, and in the inferior vena cava above the ductus venosus, in 31 infants. In 9 of these it was impossible to pass the catheter beyond the ductus venosus. Pressure in IVC, vertical lines; in portal sinus ●; and in portal sinus when ductus impassable ○.

## Results

The venous pressure measured in the portal sinus below the ductus venosus ranged from + 5 to 15 cm. $H_2O$, with an average of 9·9 (SD ± 3·2) cm. $H_2O$; respiratory swings of only 2-4 cm. $H_2O$ were observed. In the inferior vena cava the mean pressure ranged from + 5 to − 0·5 cm. $H_2O$ with an average of + 1·4 (SD ± 2·0) cm. $H_2O$; the respiratory fluctuations were large and ranged from 5 to 13 cm. $H_2O$, as observed by Boggs and Westphal (1960). It was possible to pass the catheter through the ductus venosus in 22 out of 31 infants and a record of the pressure drop is shown in Fig. 1. The 9 failures to reach the inferior vena cava with the catheter advanced 10-12 cm. from the umbilicus occurred most frequently in infants over 18 hours of age (Fig. 2).

## Discussion

It was not possible to introduce a catheter beyond the ductus venosus in 30% of cases, a figure similar to that found by Rudolph *et al.* (1961) during the first 2 days of life. A recent necropsy study by Lind (unpublished observations) has demonstrated that this may be due to absence of the ductus venosus, a particularly small lumen, or an abnormal anatomical arrangement. Peltonen and Hirvonen (1963) have demonstrated by angiography that the ductus venosus may be open *in vivo* 12 days after birth.

The high venous pressure figures acceptable as normal in infants (Mollison and Cutbush, 1949; Bonham Carter, Bound, and Smellie, 1956) and during exchange transfusion (Boggs and Westphal, 1960; Walker and Neligan, 1955; Wright, 1961; Farquhar and Smith, 1958) suggest that the measurements have been made with the catheter tip in the portal sinus. Farquhar and Smith (1958) preferred this site for exchange transfusion since they had encountered cyanosis in the lower limbs, which they thought was due to spasm of the inferior vena cava if the catheter was advanced more than 7 to 8 cm. from the umbilicus. The disadvantages of having the catheter in the portal sinus below the ductus venosus are twofold. First, it is possible that the perfusion of the slightly acid stored blood directly into the liver may be a factor in the development of portal vein thrombosis reported by Tizard (1962) and Oski, Allen, and Diamond (1963); in a recent study of the aetiology of portal vein thrombosis Thompson and Sherlock (1964) found no relationship to exchange transfusion. Secondly, it is difficult to interpret the venous pressures measured because the relation between central venous pressure and pressures measured in the portal sinus has not been fully explored. Our findings suggest that there is no constant relation between central venous pressure and pressure in the portal sinus, but the readings have not been compared over a wide range of pressures in the same infant.

It is usually assumed that the venous pressure will rise in the infant with inadequate cardiac function as it does in the adult, and may be a warning of early cardiac failure. For this reason the blood volume is frequently reduced during an exchange transfusion. The extrapolation from adult to infant may not, however, be justified. Moss and Duffie (1962) did not observe a raised right atrial pressure in infants of up to 2 years of age with other clinical signs of congestive cardiac failure. Both Burnard and James (1963) and Jegier *et al.* (1963) observed only a small rise in venous pressure lasting 6 hours in infants who had a blood transfusion from the placenta, equal to about 50% of their blood volume at birth. Further, Burnard and James (1963) found particularly low venous filling pressures in asphyxiated infants with enlarged hearts. The absence of an expected rise in venous pressure in the newborn might be due to the distribution of high venous filling pressures between both auricles, while the foramen ovale is patent, and to relative inactivity of reflex venous control at this age (Sharpey-Schafer, 1963). The latter is suggested because both baroreceptor and chemoreceptor reflex regulating mechanism appear to be relatively unreactive in the newborn period (Young and Cottom, unpublished observations). It is also possible that the venous pressure measurements during cardiac failure in infants are incorrect, for tachypnoea is also commonly present and the mean intrathoracic pressure is therefore likely to be low. Measurements of intraoesophageal pressure simultaneously with the inferior venal caval pressures will be needed to obtain the true venous filling pressure.

## Summary

Catheterization of the inferior vena cava through the umbilical vein and ductus venosus was possible in 60% of 31 infants, 1-31 hours old.

In confirmation of other workers, the mean central venous pressure at heart level was similar to that found in the adult, but the respiratory swings were frequently as large as 13 cm. $H_2O$; the mean pressure below the ductus venosus in the portal sinus was + 7 to + 10 cm. $H_2O$.

No relation was observed between the pressures measured in the inferior vena cava and the portal sinus. The latter should not be used as a substitute for central venous pressure in assessing the 'deficit' with which the baby should be left at the end of exchange transfusion.

We are most grateful for the interest and co-operation of the nurses in charge of the Premature Baby Unit, Nurse Theodosius, Nurse Bywaters, and Nurse Miller-Jones.

This investigation was supported by the Endowment Funds of St. Thomas' Hospital, to whom we offer our thanks.

Dr. M. Young also wishes to acknowledge a grant from the National Spastics Society for the support of Miss Audrey Butler who gave invaluable technical assistance.

### References

Boggs, T. R., Jr., and Westphal, M. C., Jr. (1960). Mortality of exchange transfusion. *Pediatrics*, **26**, 745.

Bonham Carter, R. E., Bound, J. P., and Smellie, J. M. (1956). Mean venous pressures in the first hours of life. *Lancet*, **2**, 1320.

Burnard, E. D., and James, L. S. (1963). Atrial pressures and cardiac size in the newborn infant. *J. Pediat.*, **62**, 815.

Farquhar, J. W., and Smith, H. (1958). Clinical and biochemical changes during exchange transfusion. *Arch. Dis. Childh.*, **33**, 142.

Jegier, W., Blankenship, W., and Lind, J. (1963). Venous pressure in the first hour of life and its relationship to placental transfusion. *Acta paediat.* (*Uppsala*), **52**, 485.

Mollison, P. L., and Cutbush, M. (1949). Haemolytic disease of the newborn: Criteria of severity. *Brit. med. J.*, **1**, 123.

Moss, A. J., and Duffie, E. R. (1962). Congestive heart failure in infancy: significance of the venous pressure. *J. Pediat.*, **60**, 346.

O'Neill, E. M., and Gordon, R. R. (1959). Extended exchange transfusion in pre-hydropic infants. *Arch. Dis. Childh.*, **34**, 174.

Oski, F. A., Allen, D. M., and Diamond, L. K. (1963). Portal hypertension—a complication of umbilical vein catheterization. *Pediatrics*, **31**, 297.

Peltonen, T., and Hirvonen, L. (1963). The ductus venosus. *Acta paediat.* (*Uppsala*), **52**, 202.

Robinson, A., and Barrie, H. (1963). The electrocardiogram during exchange transfusion. *Arch. Dis. Childh.*, **38**, 334.

Rudolph, A. M., Drorbaugh, J. E., Auld, P. A. M., Rudolph, A. J., Nadas, A. S., Smith, C. A., and Hubbell, J. P. (1961). Studies on the circulation in the neonatal period. *Pediatrics*, **27**, 551.

Sharpey-Schafer, E. P. (1963). Venous tone: effects of reflex changes, humoral agents and exercise. *Brit. med. Bull.*, **19**, 145.

Thompson, E. N., and Sherlock, S. (1964). The etiology of portal vein thrombosis with particular reference to the rôle of infection and exchange transfusion. *Quart. J. Med.*, **33**, 465.

Tizard, J. P. M. (1962). Portal hypertension following exchange transfusion through the umbilical vein. *Proc. roy. Soc. Med.*, **55**, 772.

Van Praagh, R. (1961). Causes of death in infants with hemolytic disease of the newborn (erythroblastosis fetalis). *Pediatrics*, **28**, 223.

Walker, W., and Neligan, G. A. (1955). Exchange transfusion in haemolytic disease of the newborn. *Brit. med. J.*, **1**, 681.

Wright, T. (1961). A new technique in exchange transfusion. *Arch. Dis. Childh.*, **36**, 400.

*Arch. Dis. Childh.*, 1965, **40**, 326.

# AN UNUSUAL CASE OF SUBCUTANEOUS FAT NECROSIS IN A NEWLY BORN INFANT

BY

W. S. CRAIG

*From the Department of Paediatrics and Child Health, University of Leeds*

(RECEIVED FOR PUBLICATION SEPTEMBER 29, 1964)

Sclerema, scleroderma, and scleroedema are terms used to describe various conditions in the newly born with swelling and induration of areas of skin and the underlying subcutaneous tissues. Confusion, described by Macgregor (1960) as 'chaotic', has arisen from a loose use of the terms. McIntosh, Waugh, and Ross (1938) explain the historical origins of the confusion and mention the tendency for the term 'sclerema neonatorum' to be replaced by 'subcutaneous fat necrosis'. Credit for first describing this condition is usually accorded to Cruse (1875, 1879), but McIntosh and his co-workers consider that Usenbenzius (1722) was responsible for the first description.

In the newly born baby described below, bilateral axillary swellings were unexpectedly shown by biopsy examination to be the sites of fat necrosis.

## Case Report

**Obstetrical History.** The infant was a male and the fourth child of a mother aged 38 years. There was no history of miscarriages, and the three older children are alive and well. The mother suffered from severe toxaemia, and labour was induced by artificial rupture of the membranes at the 39th week. There was no history of maternal diabetes mellitus or of familial fat necrosis. Presentation was by the vertex. Irregularity of the foetal heart was noted before the onset of labour. Pethidine was administered three hours before delivery which was spontaneous.

**The Baby at Birth.** Weight 9 lb. 4 oz. (4,195 g.): length 24 in. (61 cm.).

The infant was asphyxiated. Respirations commenced four minutes after delivery and were persistently irregular, shallow, and accompanied by intercostal inspiratory indrawing for 36 hours. Traumatic cyanosis of the face and generalized hypotonicity were features, and the baby was semicomatose for 24 hours. Resuscitative measures included extraction of mucus, oxygen by mask, and the intramuscular administration of nalorphine (0·4 mg.). A large quantity of foul-smelling blood-stained mucus was aspirated from the stomach.

**Subsequent Clinical Course.** The infant was nursed in an incubator from the time of birth. Initial difficulty was experienced in controlling body temperature which rose to 100° F. (37·8° C.) on the third day and thereafter fluctuated between 100° F. (37·8° C.) and 99° F. (37·2° C.) for over two weeks. During the first 36 hours the cry was shrill though weak. On the second and third days of life large amounts of red urine were passed, containing massive quantities of urates and uric acid crystals but no red blood cells. The liver was enlarged and the spleen palpable but of normal size and consistence. Occasional regurgitation began on the third day and later acquired the character of moderately forceful vomiting which occurred irregularly once or twice daily for a fortnight. The general condition remained precarious until the fourth day, by which time the infant had lost 12 oz. (340 g.) in weight. Thereafter the weight trend was reversed and progressed uninterruptedly, the baby being discharged home at the age of 5 weeks.

**The Axillary Swellings** (Fig. 1). On the 13th day of life painless swellings in both axillae were noted for the first time. At first the swellings lacked precise definition and were of uncertain consistence. There was no crepitus to suggest surgical emphysema. On pressure the swellings disappeared into the depths of the axillae, and within 72 hours had grown sufficiently in size to be obvious to the naked eye. With continued increase in size they protruded from the axillae when the baby cried, but had neither the consistence nor definition of glands. Extremely mobile and without attachment to either the skin or underlying hard structures, the swellings felt fleshy on palpation, though the fleshy mass had embedded in it a curious ribbon-like meshwork of firmer consistence. There was no suggestion of matting, induration, or nodularity. Some five days after they were first noticed the swellings became more clearly defined and their mobility lessened. It was estimated that the mass in each axilla was 0·5 in. (1·2 cm.) in depth and had a maximum surface breadth of 1·5 in. (3·5 cm.). At no time was there any discoloration of the skin over the affected areas. A portion of the swollen tissues in the left axilla was taken on the 29th day of life for biopsy examination.

At the age of 2 months the axillary swellings were less obvious and by the age of 12 weeks had diminished greatly

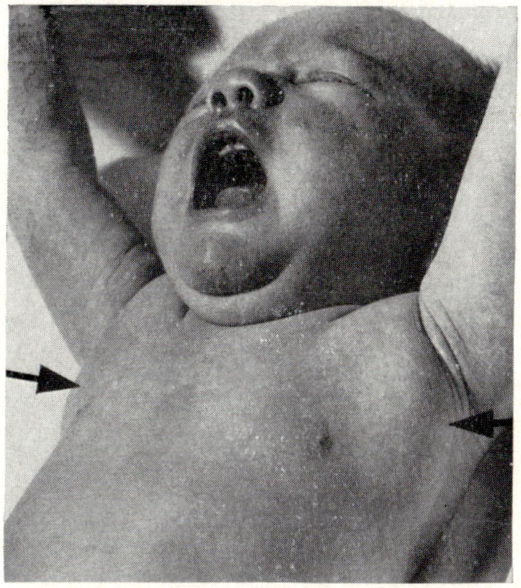

FIG. 1.—Swellings in the axillae on the 18th day of life.

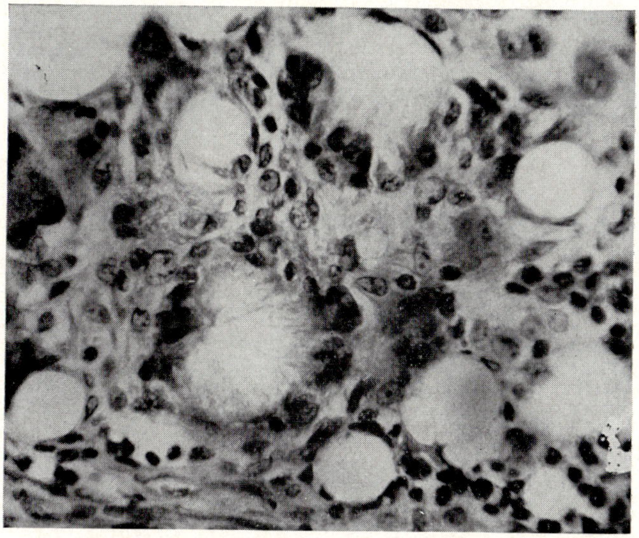

FIG. 2.—Multinucleate giant cells, containing sheaves of spaces representing crystals, in the granulation tissue. (H. and E. × 390.)

in size. Spontaneous disappearance was complete by the 4th month of life. Healing at the site of the biopsy scar was normal. There had been no recurrence of swellings when the child was re-examined at 2 years and again at 5 years of age.

**Miscellaneous Investigations.** *Chest radiographs* showed soft tissue swellings in the axillae but no evidence of calcium deposits. Lung fields were clear and there was no enlargement of mediastinal lymph nodes or of the thymus. *Blood* (at 15 days of age): WBC 10,000; polymorphs 22%, lymphocytes 75%, monocytes 2%, myelocytes 1%. No abnormal leucocytes or erythroblasts. Culture, sterile. *Blood urea* (at 15 days of age), *serum* calcium (at 18 days and 2 months), and serum potassium and sodium (at 18 days) all normal. Wassermann reaction negative; Mantoux test negative (1/1,000) (at 2 months).

**Micro-pathology** (Dr. T. W. Sutherland). 'Lobulated adipose tissue, comprising most of the specimen, showed areas of necrosis sometimes associated with a pronounced but patchy granulomatous reaction.

'In some areas sheets of necrotic adipose-tissue cells were associated with little or no granulomatous reaction. Here the altered cells showed faintly eosinophilic, blurred cell-outlines, nuclear karyolysis, and calcification.

'In other parts a granulomatous reaction was associated with accumulations of foamy, sometimes multinucleate macrophages, as well as infiltrations of eosinophil polymorphs and lymphoid cells. Prominent giant cells were associated with fan-like arrangements of slender spaces—representing spicular crystals (Fig. 2).

'There was no evidence of recent haemorrhage, and no evidence of haemosiderin deposition, so that old haemorrhage was unlikely. Vessels appeared normal. A little normal-looking lymphoid tissue was also present.'

## Discussion

Biopsy examination established the diagnosis which was not suspected clinically. Possibilities were considered with dermatological and surgical colleagues, and diagnoses tentatively suggested, only to be discarded, included surgical emphysema, lymphangioma, reticulosis, and neurofibromatosis. The fact that fat necrosis was not seriously considered is explained by the absence of attachment of the skin to the underlying lesions (Fox, 1933; Papadia and Fransvea, 1958; Hering and Undeutsch, 1956), and of discoloration of the skin in the neighbourhood of the lesions (Papadia and Fransvea, 1958; Hering and Undeutsch, 1956). The sites of the lesions differed from those most commonly involved (Papadia and Fransvea, 1958; Hering and Undeutsch, 1956; Wesener, 1957; Fox, 1933). There was no local tenderness or plaque-like induration (Papadia and Fransvea, 1958; Fox, 1933; Wesener, 1957).

By way of contrast the case resembled others previously recorded in the onset of abnormal signs within three weeks of life (Papadia and Fransvea, 1958; Fox, 1933; Hering and Undeutsch, 1956; McIntosh *et al.*, 1938), followed by disappearance within a few months (Papadia and Fransvea, 1958; Hering and Undeutsch, 1956; Wesener, 1957); birth at or after term with an average or above average birth weight (Papadia and Fransvea, 1958; Fox,

1933); normal haematological and biochemical findings (Papadia and Fransvea, 1958; Hering and Undeutsch, 1956); and a tendency for the necrotic lesions to be distributed symmetrically (Fox, 1933).

## Summary

An unusual case of subcutaneous fat necrosis appearing on the 13th day of life and disappearing spontaneously by the age of 4 months is described.

I am indebted to Dr. T. W. Sutherland for the pathological reports; to Mr. G. R. Pendrill, Librarian, Royal College of Physicians, Edinburgh for help with foreign literature; and to Dr. W. Goldie, Professor J. T. Ingram, and Mr. J. M. P. Clark, F.R.C.S., for their interest.

### References

Cruse, P. (1875). Ein Fall von Sclerodermie (sogenannt sclerodermia adultorum) bei einem Säugling. *St. Petersb. med. Ztschr.*, **5**, 306. (Quoted by Hering and Undeutsch, 1956.)

—— (1879). Ueber sclerodermie bei neugeborenen sauglingen. *Jb. Kinderheilk.*, **13**, 35.

Fox, H. (1933). Subcutaneous fat necrosis of the new-born. *Arch. Derm. Syph. (Chic.)*, **27**, 237.

Hering, H., and Undeutsch, W. (1956). Zur Klinik und Pathogenase der adiponecrosis subcutanea neonatorum. *Derm. Wschr.*, **134**, 917.

Macgregor, A. R. (1960). *Pathology of Infancy and Childhood*, p. 579. E. & S. Livingstone, Edinburgh and London.

McIntosh, J. F., Waugh, T. R., and Ross, S. G. (1938). Sclerema neonatorum (subcutaneous fat necrosis). *Amer. J. Dis. Child.*, **55**, 112.

Papadia, J., and Fransvea, P. (1958). Adiponecrosi del sottocutaneo del neonato. *Minerva pediat.*, **10**, 238.

Usenbenzius, J. A. (1722). Partus octimestris vivus, frigidus et rigidus. *Acad. nat. curios. ephem.*, **9**, 62.

Wesener, G. (1957). Zur Klinik und Therapie der Adiponecrosis subcutanea neonatorum. *Arch. klin. exp. Derm.* **206**, 531.

*Arch. Dis. Childh.*, 1965, **40**, 329.

# CHOLEDOCHAL CYST: A CASE REPORT AND DISCUSSION OF AETIOLOGY

BY

R. H. BURNELL and G. B. MARKEY
*From the Department of Child Health, University of Adelaide, Adelaide Children's Hospital, North Adelaide, South Australia*

(RECEIVED FOR PUBLICATION OCTOBER 20, 1964)

Choledochal cyst is an uncommon condition, though more than 400 cases have been described, the first by Vater in 1723 (Aird, 1957). In recent years, as the nature of the disease has become more widely recognized, the frequency of reports has increased considerably. Parallel with this, and with each succeeding review, the number of theories of aetiology has multiplied.

As Gross (1953) states, 'With such a multiplicity of explanations it it entirely possible that we are dealing with a heterogeneous group of lesions which may be produced in several ways, for while many of the theories are plausible, no one explanation fulfils the condition found in all cases.'

A recent case in this hospital, diagnosed pre-operatively as suffering from choledochal cyst, and coincidentally possessing a congenital hydroureter and hydronephrosis, has suggested another cause. Indeed, a review of some of the published reports suggests that this hypothesis may be a plausible explanation for quite a large number of cases.

## Case Report

The patient, a male aged 1 year and 4 months, was admitted to the Adelaide Children's Hospital on January 6, 1964. He was the first and only child of Australian parents, the product of a forceps-assisted birth. His birth weight was 4 kg. and he had progressed normally, with no significant illness, until two days before admission.

At this time he developed intermittent abdominal pain, vomiting, and constipation. Examination on admission showed a well-nourished, well-hydrated baby. No significant cause for his illness could be found. Abdominal findings were entirely negative. Microscopic examination of the urine, and the blood picture, were normal.

Intermittent abdominal colic and vomiting continued without detectable cause until January 9, when jaundice was first noticed. Serum bilirubin at this time was 2·4 mg./100 ml.

Barium meal performed on January 9, showed marked displacement of the duodenum anteriorly and medially, with no evidence of obstruction.

At intravenous cholangiogram on January 10, the liver excreted dye in fair concentration, outlining dilated hepatic ducts, and, apparently, a small choledochal cyst in the region of the common bile-duct. The gall-bladder appeared normal. A coincidental finding was gross left hydronephrosis and hydroureter apparently due to uretero-vesical obstruction. The right kidney and ureter appeared normal.

It was thought that, of the two lesions found, the renal tract obstruction was the more urgent. Cystoscopy on January 13 confirmed that the obstruction was at the lower end of the left ureter, the right ureteric orifice and bladder being normal. After this examination, he developed a high fever, apparently due to urinary tract infection. The only suitable antibiotic for the responsible organism, a *B. proteus*, was chloramphenicol, of which a full course was given with satisfactory response.

On January 21 a simple transvesical left ureteric meatotomy was performed, accepting the risk of later ureteric reflux. Recovery from this operation was uneventful.

However, the patient continued miserable, with intermittent abdominal pain and occasional fever. This was at first thought to be due to persisting urinary infection, though repeated examination of the urine showed a progressive return to normal. In view of the possibility of ascending cholangitis being a cause of the continuing fever, it was decided to proceed with the definitive operation on the biliary system.

The second operation was performed on February 7, through a horizontal rectus-cutting incision. There was a moderate excess of bile-stained peritoneal fluid. The region of the common bile-duct and porta hepatis was walled off by omental adhesions, producing a cyst-like cavity containing dark green bile. The gall-bladder appeared normal, though somewhat thick-walled.

The adhesions were broken down (Fig.), revealing two ragged perforations in the anterior wall of the common bile-duct, at and just distal to its junction with the cystic duct. The perforations were of approximately equal size and measured 3-4 mm. in diameter. The more proximal perforation seemed to involve the distal part of the cystic duct. The remainder of the common bile-duct seemed only slightly dilated, but the anterior duct wall surrounding the perforations and extending both proximally and

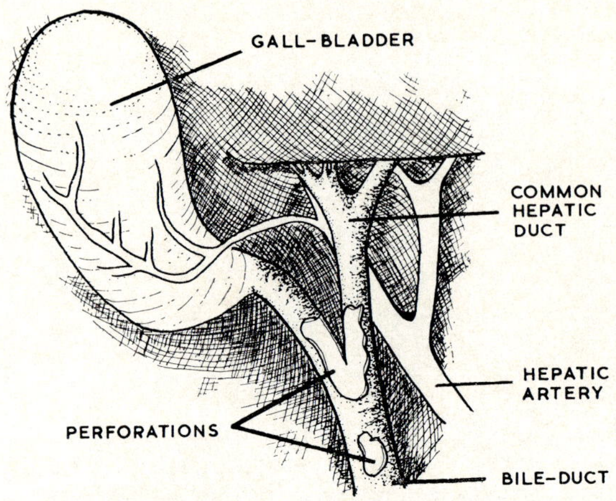


FIG.—Diagrammatic representation of conditions found at operation.

distally about 1 cm. appeared almost necrotic, rather suggestive of an infarct.

Exploration of the bile-ducts and choledochogram failed to prove patency into the duodenum, due to obstruction of unknown nature just proximal to the sphincter. The perforations were joined by excising part of the anterior wall of the common bile-duct between them, and choledocho-jejunostomy was performed on the Roux-Y principle. No other disease could be found so the wound was closed with drainage to the operation site.

Post-operative recovery was quite uneventful, and he was discharged home on February 20, progressing well. When last seen on May 4, he continued well, and was gaining weight satisfactorily. Serum bilirubin at this time was 0·8 mg./100 ml.

## Discussion

Spontaneous perforation of the bile-ducts, like choledochal cyst, is rare. Johnston (1961) in a review of neonatal cases found only 12. However, it seemed likely, as suggested by Aird (1957) and others, that many cases of spontaneous bile peritonitis are due to small perforations in the bile-duct system which either seal off before discovery, or are missed at operation.

A possible relation between spontaneous perforation of the bile-ducts and choledochal cyst has been suggested previously by Johnston (1961) and Caulfield (1936), and the present case, as well as those reported, provide some evidence in support of this.

Both conditions are commoner in females. Aird (1957) states that choledochal cyst is four times more common in females, and this ratio is supported by most other writers. An analysis of cases collected by McLaughlin (1946) shows that perforation of the bile-ducts and idiopathic bile peritonitis in the absence of other gross biliary tract disease is also four times more common in females. In the series of McWilliams (1912), including many cases with stones, there are twice as many females as males.

Allied to this evidence, both diseases are associated with the younger age-groups. Thus Alonso-Lej, Rever, and Pessagno (1959) found that 82% of cases of choledochal cyst were diagnosed before the age of 30 years. Johnston (1961) states that spontaneous perforation of the bile-ducts is found almost exclusively in newborn infants. Though this is not strictly true, and exact figures of age incidence of idiopathic bile peritonitis are not quoted or are not available, an analysis of the cases of McLaughlin (1946), Cope (1925), McWilliams (1912), and Johnston (1961), shows a similar age incidence. A significant fact related to age incidence is that choledochal cyst is singularly uncommon in newborn infants, surely unusual for a purely congenital malformation of this nature. Thus Alonso-Lej *et al.* (1959) could find only 5 cases diagnosed before the age of 3 months, from a total of 92. In the same series 18% were found before the age of 1 year.

As Aird (1957) and McLaughlin (1946) state, sterile bile produces only mild peritonitis in humans, though its ability to stimulate fibrosis with prolonged action is well known. Because of this it is suggested that leakage of bile, in the absence of other gros pathology of the biliary tree, is, in many cases, effectively contained by the normal defences of the peritoneal cavity. Such an event would produce an illness not unlike acute cholecystitis or even acute hepatitis, and would be expected to settle without operative treatment. The histories of many reported cases of choledochal cyst do start with such an incident, and give a history extending over weeks or months, but not often years. This suggests an acquired condition, and certainly not one present since birth. Even though the basic defect may be congenital, such as the 'protodilatational state' as postulated by Alonso-Lej *et al.* (1959), it seems likely that the cyst is a secondary manifestation.

Although the evidence is incomplete, it seems certain that a high percentage of choledochal cysts have no, or little, epithelial lining, and a fibrous wall containing no smooth muscle (Gross, 1933, 1953; Alonso-Lej *et al.*, 1959; Gilliland, Holloway, and Lange, 1950; Wrightson, 1953; Shallow, Eger, and Wagner, 1943; Tsardakas, and Robnett, 1956). This finding is usually explained by the occurrence of infection, but it can equally well be explained by the present theory which would be untenable if there was always a complete epithelium. In fact, many cases give a relatively short history, and produce very little clinical evidence of infection severe enough to produce ulceration within the cyst. Certainly epithelial loss is not a usual feature of cholangitis.

A significant percentage of cases of choledochal cyst show some intrinsic obstruction to the distal bile-duct, usually incomplete. This could also be related to bile leakage or perforation of the duct, though, as Aird (1957) states, obstruction of the common bile-duct rarely leads to such an event. The present case, however, does fit into this category, but as is so often the case, the presence of a normal gall-bladder suggests that obstruction is only a minor factor in aetiology.

Thus the present hypothesis is that many, but not all, choledochal cysts are formed following spontaneous perforation of the bile-duct. The subsequent leakage of bile is then contained by the usual defences within the peritoneal cavity, probably mainly by omental adhesions around the affected area. Cases operated on at this stage are classified as spontaneous perforation of the bile-duct or bile peritonitis. However, once the bile leakage is contained, symptoms subside and the true nature of the condition is hidden. This is particularly the case in infants, where symptoms are few, and signs of peritonitis often masked or missed. Progressive thickening of the wall surrounding the extravasation eventually produces the 'cyst' found at later operation. If operation is delayed long enough it may even be possible to find some patches of epithelium spreading from the adjacent duct.

The cyst retains its connexion with the bile-duct system via the original perforation, preventing complete absorption of the contained bile, or conversion to a true abscess.

Collapse of the cyst is prevented by two main factors. One is the narrowness of the connexion between the cyst and the bile-duct. The other is that the wall of the cyst will not contract, both because of the absence of muscle in its wall, and also because of the positive pressure within the biliary system, maintained by the gall-bladder which is usually normal in this condition.

Removal of this positive pressure is the basis of the usual method of operative treatment. As Gross (1953) states, 'There has been ample opportunity to demonstrate the potentiality of the cyst to shrink to small dimensions when adequate drainage has been established.' This is not the behaviour of a congenital cyst.

The present case provided a convincing example of the course of events. Although intravenous cholangiography before operation had shown the picture of choledochal cyst, at operation it was recognized that the condition was spontaneous perforation of the bile-duct. The 'cyst' was well on the way to completion by the time of operation, and it is suggested that a further delay of two or three weeks would have produced a classical picture of choledochal cyst.

## Summary

A case of spontaneous perforation of the common bile-duct in an infant is presented.

Coincidental left hydronephrosis and hydroureter is described.

A causal relation between local bile peritonitis and choledochal cyst is suggested and discussed.

Our thanks are due to Professor G. M. Maxwell and Mr. G. G. Wyllie, under whose care the patient was admitted; and to Dr. W. McCoy for the radiological investigations.

### References

Aird, I. (1957). *A Companion in Surgical Studies*, 2nd ed., p. 1012. Livingstone, Edinburgh.

Alonso-Lej, F., and Rever, W. B., Jr., and Pessagno, D. J. (1959). Congenital choledochal cyst, with a report of 2, and an analysis of 94, cases. *Int. Abstr. Surg.*, **108**, 1.

Caulfield, E. (1936). Bile peritonitis in infancy. *Amer. J. Dis. Child.*, **52**, 1348.

Cope, Z. (1925). Extravasation of bile. *Brit. J. Surg.*, **13**, 120.

Gilliland, M. B., Holloway, C. E., and Lange, J. H. (1950). Congenital choledochus cyst. *J. Pediat.*, 37, 387.

Gross, R. E. (1933). Idiopathic dilatation of the common bile duct in children. *ibid.*, 3, 730.

—— (1953). *The Surgery of Infancy and Childhood.* Saunders, Philadelphia.

Johnston, J. H. (1961). Spontaneous perforation of the common bile duct in infancy. *Brit. J. Surg.*, **48**, 532.

McLaughlin, E. F. (1946). Choledochus cyst. *Ann. Surg.*, **123**, 1047.

McWilliams, C. A. (1912). Acute, spontaneous perforation of the biliary system into the free peritoneal cavity. *ibid.*, **55**, 235.

Shallow, T. A., Eger, S. A., and Wagner, F. B. (1943). Congenital cystic dilatation of the common bile duct. *ibid.*, **117**, 355.

Tsardakas, E., and Robnett, A. H. (1956). Congenital cystic dilation of the common bile duct. *Arch. Surg.*, **72**, 311.

Wrightson, P. (1953). Congenital cystic dilatation of the common bile duct: a case occurring in infancy. *Aust. N.Z. J. Surg.*, **23**, 110.

*Arch. Dis. Childh.*, 1965, **40**, 332.

# PAEDIATRIC PATHOLOGY CLUB

## Proceedings of the Tenth Annual Meeting

The Tenth Annual Meeting was held in Manchester on October 16, 1964, at the Clinical Sciences Building and Royal Infirmary, and on October 17 at the Children's Hospital, Pendlebury. Drs. Jennison, Langley, Marsden, and White acted as chairmen. Dr. A. D. Bain was elected President for 1965 and the members of the Committee of Paediatric Pathology were all re-elected. A proposal to change the name of the Club to the 'Paediatric Pathology Society' was carried. 38 members signed the attendance book.

### Scientific Communications

The following papers were read at Manchester.

H. B. MARSDEN (Manchester). 'Addison's Disease and Cerebral Sclerosis.' Addison's disease due to cytotoxic atrophy was described in a 7-year-old boy with sudanophilic cerebral sclerosis. The accumulating reports suggest that the association is due to more than chance. The aetiology was discussed and it was considered that the most important feature was that all the recorded cases were young males, suggesting genetic or endocrine influences affecting the integrity of myelin. (To be published in full.)

J. L. EMERY (Sheffield). 'Nuclear Abnormality and Cytomegaly in the Islets of Langerhans of Newborns.' While examining the islets of Langerhans of stillborns and neonatal deaths, we noticed that the islets occasionally contained larger cells with big hyperchromatic irregular nuclei. These cells appear very like those seen in the involuting foetal cortex of the adrenal. It has been shown that there is a physiological partial involution of the islets of Langerhans following birth (Emery and Bury, 1964).* It is now suggested that the abnormal nuclei seen are due to endo-reduplication associated with this involution.

J. HUBER (Groningen). 'Hereditary 18-oxidation Defect in the Biosynthesis of Aldosterone.' A girl of 7 months with a salt-losing syndrome died with hyperpyrexia and dehydration probably caused by an intercurrent virus infection. During life aldosterone was absent even after ACTH stimulation. The child had been maintained on a salt-rich diet and DOCA therapy.

The adrenals were of normal weight, the outer layer of the cortex showed tubular atrophy and locally an adenomatous aspect, with total lack of lipid matter. The juxta-glomerular apparatus and the axial areas of the glomeruli showed hypertrophy and accumulation of PAS-positive material.

Upon post-mortem analysis of the adrenals no aldosterone was found, while precursors were present. The salt-losing syndrome was in all probability due to an isolated enzyme defect of 18-oxidation, the last step in the synthesis of aldosterone. The pedigree of the family, traced back for six generations, revealed 16 consanguineous marriages and 2 more salt-losers in the patient's generation with similar features, pointing to an inborn error of metabolism due to a recessive autosomal gene with clinical expression in the homozygous state.

G. R. OSBORNE (Derby). 'Congenital Diabetes.' K.O. died on September 16, 1963, at the age of 14 days. Two previous babies were full-term and weighed just over 7 lb. (4,535 g.). This baby was also full-term but weighed only 2 lb. 10 oz. (1,190 g.). Delivery was normal and the condition at birth was good, though the baby was described as scraggy. When 4 days old he had an attack during the night, becoming pale and grey with shallow respirations and startled movements; he improved after 1 hour. Clinical diagnosis of hypoglycaemia was made and 20% glucose was given. His condition was then good until 11 days old when it was noted that weight was static and that he was still very scraggy, and had neither gained nor lost weight. When 14 days old the blood sugar was found to be 585 mg./100 ml. He was given 2 units of soluble insulin before each feed, later the same day the blood sugar had risen to 1,090 mg./100 ml. and the soluble insulin was increased to 3 units. The following day he vomited after feeds, had an apnoeic attack, and died. Blood sugar at time of death was 1,450 mg./100 ml.

At necropsy the brain, heart, and lungs appeared normal. The abdomen was grossly distended, mostly the result of acute dilatation of the stomach which was filled with milk curds. Milk curds formed discrete hard masses throughout the majority of the small bowel. The liver was only about one-third normal size. Remaining abdominal organs appeared normal. Microscopically the liver cells had rather scanty eosinophilic cytoplasm, the intralobular bile canaliculae contained inspissated bile. The pancreas showed unusually large numbers of islets of Langerhans.

* *Reference:* Emery, J. L., and Bury, H. P. R. (1964). *Biol. Neonat.* (*Basel*), **6**, 16-25.

M. SANDLER and C. R. J. RUTHVEN (London). 'Catecholamine Metabolites in Neuroblastoma.' Children with tumours belonging to the dopamine-secreting neuroblastoma-ganglioneuroma group rarely present with any severe degree of hypertension, in contrast to subjects with phaeochromocytoma, though both tumours elaborate large amounts of noradrenaline.

In the present study, by measurement of urinary 0-methylated metabolites (normetadrenaline plus metadrenaline) and deaminated metabolites (4-hydroxy-3-methoxymandelic acid and 4-hydroxy-3-methoxyphenylglycol), data were obtained suggesting that the tumours fall into distinct biochemical groups: the ratio of 0-methylated to deaminated metabolites was always greater than 0·2 in phaeochromocytoma and less than 0·1 in neuroblastoma and in normals. In accordance with the findings of other workers in the experimental animal, this finding indicates the following: that whereas in phaeochromocytoma free catecholamine is released directly into the blood stream to be inactivated primarily by catechol 0-methyl-transferase (COMT), further metabolism and inactivation of the amines is likely to occur by both COMT and monoamine oxidase in the tumour tissue itself in neuroblastoma.

B. IVEMARK and B. ROBERTSON (Stockholm). 'Pulmonary Microangiography in Congenital Malformations of the Heart.' In the normal full-term neonatal lung the bronchial arteries can be filled by injection of contrast medium into the pulmonary artery. The communication seemed to be localized at capillary level, around peripheral intralobular bronchi. The bronchial arteries always followed the course of the bronchi in the normal lung.

In 8 cases, aged 1 day to 7 weeks, with transposition of the great arteries, an abnormal pattern of the bronchial arteries was found. In all cases the bronchial arteries were wider and more tortuous than normal and gave off abnormal branches which left the bronchial wall to ramify in the adjacent pulmonary parenchyma. Many alveolar groups displayed a double arterial vascularization, and there seemed to be widespread capillary anastomoses between branches of the pulmonary and bronchial arteries. In addition, some vessels with the structure and course of bronchial arteries were found to be branches of the pulmonary artery, originating near the hilum. Particularly wide and tortuous bronchial arteries and a marked capillary filling were present in the case that survived for seven weeks.

In transposition, the abnormalities are apparently already present at birth. Whether the arterial abnormalities in transposition are the result of an intrauterine adaptation to the malformation of the great trunks or a collateral malformation, cannot as yet be established. Their functional significance cannot be ascertained from this study, but the findings suggest an intrapulmonary shunt between the two arterial systems. A study of the pulmonary vasculature in other types of cardiovascular malformations is in progress.

F. A. LANGLEY (Manchester). 'Thymic Hyperplasia and the Choice of a Suitable Biometric Framework.' During late foetal life the weight of the thymus increases proportionately with the body weight. In large babies born after term this relation does not hold. After birth the thymus grows little, if at all, in relation to the body weight for the first six to nine months of life. Parallel with this there is a diminution in the number of PAS positive cells in the organ. Based on these studies a case of thymic hyperplasia is assessed. It occurred in an infant who had been given vole bacillus BCG at 9 days and died at 7 months with acute meningitis. There was generalized lymphoid hyperplasia, some glands showing tuberculous lesions and an increase in the PAS positive cells in the thymus.

Using maturity, based on the mother's menstrual history, as the independent variable, it can be shown that there is a linear relation between the logarithm of the thymus weight and the maturity of stillborn infants and infants dying under 24 hours. On this basis it can be shown that there is no hyperplasia of the thymus in anencephalic foetuses.

M. ELVES (Manchester). 'Recent Studies on the Thymus.' Recent studies have shown that the small lymphocyte is a relatively long-lived cell which is produced at a slow rate. A smaller proportion of the small lymphocytes of the peripheral blood are, however, short lived with a life-span of about two weeks; these cells are produced at a more rapid rate. The high lymphocyte output from the thoracic duct into the blood stream is due to the recirculation of the long-lived lymphocytes via the lymph nodes.

Removal of the thymus causes a marked fall in the thoracic duct output in young rodents. After neonatal thymectomy the weight of the lymph nodes decreases, and the number of small lymphocytes in the peripheral blood falls to about 60% of the normal value. There is a marked lymphocytic aplasia in such animals. These facts clearly suggest that the thymus is an important source of small lymphocytes.

Using tritiated thymidine it has been shown that a majority of the thymic small lymphocytes are of the short-lived variety, in contrast to those of the thoracic duct and the lymph glands. There is evidence that the thymus also produces many of the long-lived cells of the body.

The small lymphocytes are formed in the thymic cortex, probably by the maturation of reticulum cells. From the cortex they pass into the medulla where they become actively amoeboid and eventually enter the blood by crossing the walls of the venules via the perivascular channels.

Neonatal thymectomy results in a severe impairment of the immunological capacity of the animal. This is associated with a failure of development of lymphoid germinal centres. The small lymphocyte has also been shown to play an important role in immunological responses. It may, therefore, be postulated that the thymus is the chief producer of the lymphocytes of the body, and as the long-lived cells are immunologically competent, the thymus is important for the immune response.

A. H. Cameron (Birmingham). 'Malformations of the Thymus and Cardiovascular System.' In the past six years, necropsy disclosed no evidence of thymic tissue in 4 infants. In 4 other infants the thymus was extremely small and anomalous in position, being either entirely cervical or entirely within the thorax. In all, there were major anomalies of the cardiovascular system including defects of the ventricular septum, common truncus, Fallot's tetralogy, atresia and coarctation of the aortic arch, right aortic arch, and anomalous subclavian arteries.

Two further infants with hypoplasia and anomalous location of the thymus had almost identical associated malformations, the most striking being an enormous pulmonary artery of almost saccular proportions. In both, the pulmonary valve was represented by a hypoplastic fringe without stenosis and there was a small VSD. The ductus arteriosus was absent and the innominate artery lay behind the innominate vein. There was anomalous lobation of the lungs with emphysematous enlargement of the right lower lobe due to compression of the bronchus.

None of the 10 cases showed asplenia which is also associated with cardiovascular anomalies, and none showed positive evidence of immunological incompetence. Nor was there any indication of hypoparathyroidism. The development of the thymus and the arterial trunks in relation to the branchial arches was briefly discussed.

H. Fox (Manchester). 'The Villous Cytotrophoblast as an Index of Placental Ischaemia.' Langhan's cells can be demonstrated in many of the terminal villi of the mature placenta. Using a PAS stain the negatively staining cytoplasm of these cells contrasts well with the weakly positive cytoplasm of the syncytial trophoblast. With a PAS stain the trophoblastic basement membrane is also stained and confusion with stromal cells is hence avoided. In the normal mature placenta usually less than 20% of the terminal villi contain Langhans' cells, but there is a tendency for proliferation of these cells in the placentae of elderly mothers, in the placentae of 'grand multipara', and in placentas delivered at or after the 42nd week of gestation. There is a marked tendency to proliferation of villous Langhans' cells in toxaemia of pregnancy and the degree of proliferation is related both to the severity of the toxaemic process and to the length of time for which symptoms have been present. In the placentae of anoxic stillbirths there is a marked proliferation of villous Langhans' cells.

A high villous Langhans' cell count in the placenta is related to a high incidence of foetal distress during labour and with a high incidence of neonatal asphyxia. It is suggested that proliferation of villous Langhans' cells is an indication of placental ischaemia and that a villous Langhans' cell count may enable a quantitative assessment of the degree of such ischaemia.

P. K. Kalpaktsoglou (Athens). 'Crown-rump Length in Vital Statistics of the Newborn.' The purpose of this study was to determine in the living newborn child which of the measurements, weight, gestation age, or length, gives the least variability when related to the other two. Greek babies born between February and July 1964 were observed at the University Maternity Hospital 'Alexandra', in Athens. There were 1,590 babies, all apparently normal, of which 841 were boys and 749 girls.

The material was first classified according to sex and then the data were analysed in three ways. First, each criteria was charted arithmetically against the other two, then, using the same method, we studied the difference of the mean values of body weight and crown-rump length between boys and girls. Finally, we charted the logarithms of the mean values of each criteria against the other two.

There appeared to be a greater uniformity of growth pattern when the crown-rump length was used than with weight or gestation age. By using the crown-rump length, the difference between the sexes was least, which suggests that using this criteria, girls and boys can most safely be studied together.

J. O'H. Tobin and L. L. R. White (Manchester). 'Virus Isolation from Manchester Children with Acute Respiratory Disease.' From November 1961 to March 1964, 878 viruses were isolated by the direct inoculation of rhesus monkey kidney and HeLa cultures with throat swabs from children admitted to Booth Hall and other hospitals in South-east Lancashire. Swabs were taken in the admission room or at the bedside and, after incubation for up to four days locally, were sent to the Public Health Laboratory, Manchester, for further examination.

In children without respiratory disease virus was found in 7%, mainly herpes virus from cases of stomatitis, and enteroviruses and adenoviruses from cases of Bornholm disease, pyrexia, meningitis, or mediastinitis.

About one-third of the cases of respiratory disease yielded virus. The commonest was respiratory syncytial virus (439 strains), mainly from infants with lower respiratory infections. This virus caused epidemics during each of the three winters of the study. Parainfluenza viruses (111 strains) were less frequent; though present throughout the period, an increased incidence was associated with a rise in the number of cases of croup. The commonest manifestation of this virus, however, was upper respiratory tract infections with or without coryza. Adenoviruses (83 strains) produced tonsillitis more frequently than the other viruses, while the enteroviruses (64 strains) were the commonest cause of respiratory disease during the summer.

The respiratory syncytial virus was found before death four times and after death once in infants who died with respiratory disease. The morbid anatomical findings included changes described by Adams in 1941* as 'Primary Virus Pneumonitis with Cytoplasmic Inclusion Bodies'. One case showed extensive pneumonia with hyaline membrane formation, and in another the lung changes resembled those commonly encountered in 'cot deaths'.

J. R. S. More and Banti Devi (Manchester). 'A Case of Bilateral Pulmonary Agenesis and the First of Total Tracheo-pulmonary Agenesis.' In addition to absence of

* *Reference:* Adams, J. M. (1941). *J. Amer. med. Ass.*, **116**, 925.

the lower portion of the larynx, the trachea, and the lungs, there were a number of cardiac abnormalities, including a common atrio-ventricular canal, a common truncus arteriosus, and total absence of the pulmonary trunk and arteries. Additional malformations included absence of the spleen, gastric hypoplasia, and a hemi-vertebra. The embryology of the defects was discussed with particular reference to their time of onset and the important findings compared with those of the previously published cases.

P. E. CONEN and B. ERKMAN (Toronto). 'Chromosome Studies in Paediatric Intersex Problems.' A review of these studies during the past 4 years at The Hospital for Sick Children was illustrated by typical and atypical cases. Two infants with chromatin-positive Klinefelter's syndrome (47/XXY) had a bifid scrotum and penile hypospadias. Phenotypic females with some features of Turner's syndrome showed a spectrum of X chromosome abnormalities. These included 45/XO, 45/XO-46/XX, and 45/XO-46/X isochromosome long arm X mosaics and 46/X-isochromosome long arm X and a case with a deletion of part of the X chromosome. One of these patients has been menstruating regularly. An infant with an XO chromosome pattern was found to have normal ovaries. A boy with Turner's syndrome had 45/XO-46/XY mosaicism in blood with only the XO cell line in skin, muscle, and testes tissue cultures. Double chromatin masses in buccal smears and a 47/XXX super-female chromosome pattern in blood cultures from a girl with Turner's syndrome suggested the presence of an additional undetected 45/XO cell line. One other super-female girl (47/XXX) was detected during investigation of patients with multiple anomalies.

A 14-year-old true hermaphrodite with 46/XX pattern and an infant true hermaphrodite with a mosaic 46/XX-46/X deletion short arm X were described. Several variants of male pseudo-hermaphroditism were also presented.

J. H. EDWARDS (Birmingham). 'Classification of Malformations.'* Since the classification of malformations is mainly based on structure rather than mechanism, the method of classification must be based on the presence or absence of a multiplicity of signs, and this involves procedural difficulties in analysis.

Some problems of classification were discussed and a classification designed to conform to the limitations of conventional punch-cards was presented.

K. M. LAURENCE (Cardiff). 'Progressive Familial Infantile Cerebral Cortical Degeneration.' This condition arose in 2 sisters of a sibship of 4, who suffered from progressive spasticity and retardation and repeated sweating attacks. Pregnancy, delivery, the neonatal period, and development in the first three months were normal. One died of bronchopneumonia at 10 months, the other of diarrhoea and vomiting at 8 months. In both the main post-mortem findings were confined to the central nervous system. The brains were almost identical and weighed 188 g. and 230 g. They showed gross atrophy of the whole of the cerebral hemispheres which resembled large walnut kernels with severe external and internal hydrocephalus. Microscopically the cortical neurones had disappeared, with some neurophagocytosis still evident. There was microglial proliferation, compound granular corpuscle formation, myelin loss, and gliosis. The basal nuclei were almost normal and the cerebellum and brain-stem appeared to be completely spared.

The condition bears a resemblance to Alper's disease but affected the whole of the cerebral hemispheres without softening or severe changes in the basal nuclei and cerebellum. It is open to question whether this is yet another form of Alper's disease or is a separate entity. In any case, it is likely to be a hereditary condition due to a recessive gene.

A. E. CLAIREAUX (London). 'Congenital Renal Anomalies in the Newborn.' Between 1947 and 1963, 2,287 necropsies were performed at Queen Charlotte's Maternity Hospital and these yielded 50 severe congenital malformations of the kidney, an incidence of 2·2%. There were 17 examples of bilateral cystic dysplasia (34%), 10 of bilateral hydronephrosis (20%), and 7 of bilateral renal agenesis (14%). In 35 of the 50 cases (70%) other severe malformations such as anencephalus, hydrocephalus, or congenital heart disease were present. The striking facial appearances commonly associated with bilateral renal agenesis were also observed in over half the cases of cystic dysplasia and in one-fifth of the cases of bilateral hydronephrosis. Of the 50 infants, 31 were stillborn and only 5 survived longer than 48 hours. In 8 of the 50 infants severe pulmonary hypoplasia was noted. The high incidence of associated malformations appears to indicate that surviving children with severe unilateral renal disease may also be suffering from other congenital anomalies.

B. OCKENDEN (London). 'Absent Abdominal Muscles and Associated Genito-urinary Abnormalities.' 16 cases of the rare but well-recognized syndrome of absent abdominal muscles, megaureters, and undescended testes have been seen at The Hospital for Sick Children: of these 9 have died. Necropsies were carried out on 6, all under 7 months of age: 5 had a variable degree of renal cystic dysplasia; they all had complete or almost complete absence of the anterior abdominal wall muscles, and intra-abdominal testes attached to the lateral aspects of dilated, tortuous, thin-walled ureters; 4 had one or more ureteric stenoses but all had patent ureteric orifices; only 2 showed dilatation of the renal pelves. In all cases the bladders were large, pear shaped and very thick walled without gross trabeculation; 3 had abnormal trigones with a central pouch in the interureteric bar. The bladder apex was elongated and attached to the anterior abdominal wall near the umbilicus. In 3 cases the urachus was patent, and in these there was urethral obstruction due to atresia of the penile and/or membran-

* *Reference:* Edwards, J. H., Leck, I., and Record, R. G. (1964). A classification of malformations. *Acta genet.* (*Basel*), **14**, 76.

ous urethra. The prostatic urethra was funnel shaped in 1 and dilated in the other 5 cases. Other associated congenital anomalies were partial universal mesentery in 5, bilateral talipes equinovarus in 4 and left talipes equinavarus with agenesis of the right leg in one.

The clinical features were compared with the post-mortem findings to show that once the abnormal abdominal musculature is recognized one can fairly accurately predict the underlying genito-urinary abnormalities.

Chromosome studies have been performed in one living boy and the karyotype was normal.

(To be published in full elsewhere.)

J. L. S. SMITH and J. K. STEWART (Manchester). 'Spontaneous Regression of Retinoblastoma.' Since 1900 there have been 160 proven cases of retinoblastoma in the Manchester Hospital Region, in addition to approximately 50 children who had one or both eyes removed with a purely clinical diagnosis of retinoblastoma. Of these, 75% were cured. By examining the eyes of the survivors or relatives it was possible to find 7 cases of spontaneous regression of the tumour.

The end result of spontaneous regression was either a shrunken eye with a characteristic histological picture, or a sighted eye which showed chorio-retinal atrophy, raised grey masses, and good preservation of the retinal vessels.

Since multifocal and bilateral tumours regressed, a general factor must be implicated. Regression seemed more common in boys than girls and could occur in infancy. In affected families one sib might die of the disease while in another the tumour might regress.

A. M. MACDONALD (Glasgow). 'A Case of Apparent Adrenal Hypoplasia in the Neonate.' Reference was first made to a previous paper (Boyd and MacDonald, 1960)* describing adrenal cortical hypoplasia in sibs. The third member of this family has since died of this lesion, the adrenal glands being identical with those seen in the other sibs.

A case was then presented of a male infant with the clinical features similar to those in the family with adrenal hypoplasia. The diagnosis was based on the urinary steroid analysis and the clinical features of failing to regain birth weight by the 10th day, vomiting, and a high serum potassium. There was no response to ACTH stimulation. Only on the last day of life, aged 15 days, were coliform organisms grown from the urine and the probability of a renal lesion recognized. The blood urea was 400 mg./100 ml.

At necropsy both adrenals were normal in size and in their histology, but both kidneys showed gross hypoplasia with superadded pyelonephritis. This infers that urinary steroid analysis provides insufficient evidence for the diagnosis of adrenal hypoplasia, as low levels of urinary corticosteroids may be due to gross renal hypoplasia or dysfunction, with failure of steroid excretion. A method of estimating plasma corticosteroids must be developed.

S. F. CAHALANE (Dublin). 'Pinealoma with Aldosterone-like Activity.' Hyperaldosteronism with recovery in a woman who had a hyperplastic pineal gland removed has been recently described.

This patient was admitted when 2½ years old for investigation of abdominal pain and vomiting and she was treated for *Esch. coli* urinary infection and severe anaemia. A low serum potassium (2·2 to 2·5 mEq/litre) and a high urinary output of potassium (up to 25 mEq per day) with consistently dilute and generally alkaline urine were features throughout her hospital stay. A second admission was necessary for return of symptoms, and eventually a renal calculus was removed. Muscle weakness, lethargy, vomiting, and pyuria continued, and the hypokalaemia and urinary findings persisted until she died.

At necropsy a 2 cm. rounded firm grey mass occupied the site of the pineal and the liver was enlarged and yellow. Histologically, the tumour was composed mainly of rather plump cells arranged in an alveolar pattern with copious interstitial acellular stroma. There were some clumps of small round cells and no calcification. The picture recapitulated the developmental stage of the normal gland in a child of some 18 months. The liver sections showed diffuse toxic changes with cell necrosis, fatty metamorphosis, and portal lymphocytic infiltration. The renal tubules exhibited well-marked cytoplasmic vacuolization. The adrenal glands were normal.

K. and J. BOROWICZ (Warsaw). 'The Mouse Placenta in Experimental Toxoplasmosis.' Gravid mice were infected with *Toxoplasma gondii* by intraperitoneal injection. Nodular lesions of the liver developed in 49 of the 56 mice and most contained toxoplasms. Lesions in the spleen were not so intense. The mucosa of the uterus showed no evidence of infection, but there were lesions in the tunica serosa, uterine muscle, and broad ligament.

Histological examinations were carried out on 346 placentas from 56 mice. The placentas from 15 mice showed toxoplasma in a free extracellular form, with no inflammatory or degenerative changes in the trophoblast. In 22 mice there were aggregates of degenerate leucocytes, among which there were 'toxoplasma-like bodies'. In 19 mice there was no evidence of toxoplasma infection of the placenta. The foetuses from 38 infected mice showed no evidence of toxoplasma infection on histological examination. However, toxoplasms were identified biologically in the liver and brain of the foetuses from 18 mice, and in 10 the toxoplasms were identified by both biological and histological examination. In 8 cases with positive biological tests there was no histological evidence of toxoplasms in the placenta.

It was concluded that the placenta did not appear to be a suitable substrate for multiplication of toxoplasms and that lesions in the placenta were not essential for passage of infection from mother to foetus.

In man, congenital toxoplasmosis appears to be related to parasitaemia in the mother during the primary infection or during exacerbation of a chronic infection.

* *Reference:* Boyd, J. F., and MacDonald, A. M. (1960). *Arch. Dis. Childh.*, 35, 561.

# BOOK REVIEWS

**Neurological and Encephalographic Correlative Studies in Infancy.** Edited by PETER KELLAWAY and INGEMAR PETERSÉN. (Pp. x + 364; illustrated. $14·75) New York: Grune and Stratton. 1964.

This volume is made up of the collected papers and discussions of a Symposium sponsored by the World Federation of Neurology in 1963. It must have been a most stimulating meeting for the participants, because not only were their numbers kept small (28) but the content of the papers and the discussions showed several interesting trends. The studies of the changes in structure and in function of the brain have recently gained impetus from various causes, more especially since the techniques of the neurophysiologists have been turned loose on human and animal problems not strictly within the narrow province of the 'pure' neurophysiologist. Perhaps this is best exemplified by the chapter by Dominick Purpura on the 'Relationship of seizure susceptibility to morphologic and physiologic properties of normal and abnormal miniature cortex'. This worker's approach to the problem of seizures is broad and catholic so that he can write with equal intimacy of the details of synaptic contacts in electron micrographs, patterns of dendrite branching in golgi preparations of neurones, and the significance of electrical activity in cortex and hippocampus. This correlative approach to brain development forms the central chapter of the symposium, and approximates as far as is possible to the ideal approach, for each single technical study inevitably leaves the reader with a sense of incompleteness. Grafstein's chapter on the 'Post natal development of the Corpus Callosum in the Cat' shows how the use of electrical methods can demonstrate lack of homogeneity in the myelination of fibres in the corpus callosum, and thereby emphasize problems of morphology and cell relationships that cannot be high-lighted by any other method. The use of the 'spreading depression' phenomenon for studying the development of neuroglial function (Bures, Fifkora, and Mares), and correlation of such findings with assessment of cytoplasmic volume and electrolyte content of neuroglia (Schade) in both normal and anoxic brains, is an exciting approach to elements hitherto only capable of being studied under the microscope, or by crude and indirect chemical methods.

A good part of the book is taken up with electro-encephalographic observations on young animals and humans, particularly in relation to seizure activity. The parameters of normality in this field are less clear than one would wish because of the limitations of the technique. Their analysis is important and must go on for practical clinical reasons, but the final interpretations will be dependent on the critical results of the experimentalist working on well-defined experimental systems.

This book is recommended to anyone interested in brain function whether they have personal experience of the techniques or not. It will certainly be of interest to those handling brain-damaged and epileptic children, and it is hoped that in it even the neuropathologist might find instruction.

**Pediatric Neurology.** Edited by THOMAS W. FARMER. (Pp. xiv + 690; illustrated. $18.50; 137s.) London and New York: Haeber Medical Division, Harper and Row. 1964.

Any work on paediatric neurology invites comparison with Frank Ford's monumental and highly personal volume on the same subject—a book that transcends its title to furnish an outstanding text of general neurology as well as of paediatric nervous disease.

Dr. Farmer's book is different but entirely admirable. The work of 13 authors, it is nevertheless much shorter than Ford and lacks the revealing clinical vignettes that make the larger volume so readable. The present work is, however, clearly written, elegantly produced, and superbly illustrated. The editor's preface suggests that it is intended for medical students, hospital residents, and practitioners, but it must be doubted whether many British medical students will read and fewer still purchase any volume on paediatric neurology. Nor is the present work sophisticated enough for the professed neurologist. Its use seems to be mainly for the clinical paediatrician, for whom it certainly provides an attractive up-to-date and well-documented guide to a field that is sadly neglected, especially in Britain. Many of the contents of *Pediatric Neurology* are of course covered by any of the standard neurological texts, but the authors, most of whom hail from the University of North Carolina School of Medicine at Chapel Hill, are both experienced and articulate, and the work abounds in evidence of the close clinical observation which characterizes the best paediatric practice.

If only as a valuable epitome of recent literature and for its treatment of the newer biochemical approaches to neurology this book should be in the library of every children's hospital and department. It will not replace Ford but it is a useful supplement and a not inconsiderable competitor.

**Nelson Textbook of Pediatrics.** 8th Edition. (Pp. xx + 1636; 471 figures + 144 tables. 126s.) Philadelphia and London: W. B. Saunders. 1964.

Years of ownership of successive editions of 'Griffith-Mitchell' and later 'Nelson' (usually of two copies, one at home and one at hospital), and the countless times your reviewer has turned to the book to look up facts, has gradually engendered in him a profound admiration for its qualities. These qualities are the comprehensive cover of the subject, so that it is rare not to find what one needs in the index; the balanced presentation of difficult, obscure, or controversial subjects; the intelligent choice of relatively few but key references; the remarkably uniform and effective literary style, terse without being staccato; and the 'up-to-dateness' made possible by a new edition every five years or so. The editor's ability to impose these qualities on all 85 contributors is indeed marvellous.

The new (8th) edition will certainly maintain the richly deserved success of its predecessors.

**Practical Paediatric Problems.** By JAMES A. HUTCHISON. (Pp. xii + 514; 87 figures + 5 tables. 50s.) London: Lloyd-Luke. 1964.

On setting out to write a textbook, the author's first rule should be to keep clearly in mind who his readers are going to be, and whom he is aiming to instruct. It is almost impossible to write effectively for more than one class of reader at once, but Professor Hutchison has aimed at doing so. He states that his intention was to produce a book intermediate in size between the usual undergraduate text and the large work of reference, yet covering the problems of the paediatrician and the family doctor. In the event he has written a textbook, parts of which are sufficiently detailed to be of use to the paediatrician (e.g. the clearly explained biochemistry of the metabolic disorders) but most of which is likely to be more valuable for the paediatric house officer or postgraduate student with some previous knowledge of paediatrics. Surely it is not a family doctor's book, for the author has purposely omitted so much that would be of importance for him? There is no section on the common infectious fevers, skin diseases or ear and eye disorders, and the word 'worms' does not appear in the index. No account of the normal child and how to assess deviation from normal development is included.

With these reservations, the book is carefully planned and well written. The word 'Practical' in the title is justified by the attention to detail in describing methods of diagnosis and treatment, including dosage of drugs. This is usually given on a bodyweight basis, though occasionally the dose recommended aims to ignore the age and size of the child, e.g. morphine gr. 1/6 (10 mg.) as part of the treatment of left ventricular failure in acute nephritis.

The metabolic and endocrine disorders are described with a clarity that is unusual in general textbooks of paediatrics. Enough biochemistry is included to explain the errors involved without drowning the reader in a sea of complex formulae. The advice on infant feeding is brief and reflects the author's individual views on the subject, which are easy to follow. The chapter on emotional disorders is the least valuable and perhaps reflects an outdated approach in dealing mainly with such things as thumb-sucking, nail-biting, and masturbation, which most paediatricians regard as relatively unimportant matters compared with the rest.

The illustrations are all well chosen and clear.

There is little doubt that Professor Hutchison has produced a book that will establish itself firmly amongst the several other British paediatric textbooks, but one cannot help regretting that he did not undertake the much needed full work of reference.

**Praxis der Antibiotikatherapie im Kindesalter ihre Anwendung.** Edited by WALTER MARGET and MALTE KIENITZ. (Pp. xi + 296; 37 figures + 39 tables. DM. 25) Stuttgart: Georg Thieme. 1964.

As the present fashion, this book is based on a symposium on modern trends and practice of chemotherapy in childhood. Organized by the editors, who are senior members of the medical staffs in the paediatric departments of the Universities of Tübingen and Münster, it was held at Reutlingen in South West Germany. In addition to contributions by 22 participants the book also includes relevant observations made during discussion. Skilful editing has by these means stressed controversial aspects and allowed differences of opinion to become evident where dogmatic statements might have incurred lively criticism.

No doubt dictated partly by the individual experience of the contributors and their special fields of interest, the topics in this treatise range somewhat haphazardly over more general subjects in the nature of the 'basis of antibiotic treatment'—antibiotics, steroids, $\gamma$-globulins; synergism and antagonism in infectious diseases; and 'The effect of chemotherapy on micro-organisms' to the more detailed exposition of the treatment of infections caused by specific organisms such as streptococcal diseases, tuberculosis, pertussis, listeriosis, toxoplasmosis, leptospiroses, and mycoses. Some contributors approached the main theme from a different angle by discussing the infections of particular organ systems. Thus the therapy of respiratory disorders, throat, nose, and ear infections, and diseases of the urinary and alimentary tracts are dealt with according to the organ system involved. Other authors preferred to expound their views on selected disease entities of varying aetiology such as purulent meningitis, osteomyelitis, septicaemia, and bacterial endocarditis. We were astonished to find that in the management of meningococcal meningitis Friederiscik recommends penicillin as the only drug to be given in maximal doses, i.e. 1 mega unit per kg. body weight per day to infants and 500,000 units/kg. body weight per day to older children and disregards completely the sulphonamides, a view that is not generally shared in this country. However, his results seemed to be very gratifying for, of 117 patients, only one died. Surprising also seemed the claim of a cure in one-third of all the patients with Waterhouse-Friderichsen syndrome.

Werner of Berlin regards tetracycline as the drug of choice in pertussis. Antibiotics are given to young infants and toddlers with the aim of preventing complications. J. Sutherland's article on chemotherapy in the newborn contains an interesting approach to the problem of dosage based on studies of streptomycin clearance. Very useful are the chapters on the side-effects of the antibiotics and a concise but relatively comprehensive survey of the individual antibiotics regarding antibacterial activity, administration, absorption, and excretion.

The list of references at the end of each chapter is well chosen and up to date.

The print is pleasing and the diagrams clear but the captions occasionally too brief, with the exception of Fig. 2 covering pages 90 and 91 relating the number of rheumatic fever relapses to continued penicillin prophylaxis, which has none.

This is a timely and very helpful manual of antibiotic treatment. To the younger paediatrician and to the family doctor it offers a well of sound information that will readily guide him through the maze of modern antibiotics.

**Klinik und Therapy der Vergiftungen.** 4th ed. By Sven Moeschlin. (Pp. xxii + 750; 99 figures. DM. 66) Stuttgart: Georg Thieme. 1964.

Four editions within 12 years is probably the best index of the value and popularity of any medical textbook. But if it deals with such a relatively limited subject as the symptomatology and treatment of poisonings it is indeed a sign of widespread recognition. In addition to the fourth German edition, translations of this manual have appeared in Italian, Polish, Spanish, and now also in English.

The special sections are preceded by a general discussion on incidence, distribution and principles of treatment of poisonings with a useful chapter on the most important antidotes which should be available in every hospital. The detailed account of poisonings due to inorganic and organic substances is followed by the toxicology of important drugs such as sedatives, antipyretics, hypnotics, tranquillizers, anticonvulsants, vitamins, hormones, antibiotics etc. Particular attention has been paid to some substances that have become ubiquitous in our modern society, such as insecticides and plastics. Included in the book also is a chapter on poison gases prepared during World War II and other chemicals for mass extermination. The author acknowledges there his indebtedness to a number of informants who preferred to remain anonymous.

Very helpful are the instructions on treatment of the common complications of poisonings, particularly of shock and disturbances of water and electrolyte metabolism.

A tabulation of guiding symptoms at the end of the book should facilitate greatly a correct diagnosis, which may be extremely difficult in the absence of any history or in the unconscious patient, where the nature of the poison is unknown.

Since the author is a physician in charge of a large medical unit his experience is based mainly on observation of the industrial and suicidal poisonings while the paediatrician is faced mainly with accidental poisoning. However, the author has not neglected the aspects of poisoning in childhood, and the paediatrician will find relevant, though somewhat summary, up-to-date information. Interestingly, calomel disease is not regarded as identical with acrodynia but only as a part of the syndrome. A strong plea is made to remove calomel from the national pharmocopœias.

Printing, paper, reproduction of photographs, and diagrams are of excellent quality and a credit to the publishers.

This book is an essential requisition for all concerned with the treatment of poisonings.

**Iron Metabolism, An International Symposium Sponsored by CIBA.** Aix-en-Provence, 1st-5th July, 1963. Chairmen J.-C. Dreyfus and G. Schapira. Edited by F. Gross with the assistance of S. R. Naegeli and H. D. Philps. (Pp. xi + 629; 234 figures + tables. DM. 45.) Berlin, Göttingen, Heidelberg: Springer-Verlag. 1964.

In July 1963, CIBA of Basle sponsored an international symposium at Aix-en-Provence on the subject of iron metabolism. Fifty-eight workers whose interest in this field is well known were invited to attend. The papers given and the discussion arising from these papers are now published in this volume. The book is divided into sections dealing with biochemistry, physiology, iron deficiency and overload, and finally therapeutics. Each section contains approximately 6 chapters followed by relevant discussion. The book is not intended as, and does not fulfil the requirements of, a textbook. Some of the contributions include a review of the literature, but in most cases the main part of the contribution is a review of the author's own work. The book therefore presents a very good cross-section of the research, both basic and applied, in iron metabolism.

The book is well illustrated; most of the illustrations have been taken from lantern slides, and in certain cases these do not fit neatly into the published text. However, this aesthetic loss is more than compensated for by the speed with which the editor has produced the book.

Naturally the standard of contribution and the style of composition vary from one chapter to another. One variation, however, that can be critized on editorial grounds is the quotation of references. In some chapters these are designated by numbers only, in others by the leading author, and in others still by both author and number. However, invariably at the end of each chapter the references are given in a continuous form, using abbreviations for journals which are not always those internationally accepted. The index appears perfectly adequate.

This book will provide little help to anyone whose main interest is the therapuetic aspects of iron. However, it will prove invaluable to those who wish to improve their knowledge of iron metabolism. The wide coverage of the subject and the extensive list of references quoted in each chapter make it a good starting point for further reading.

**Our Blind Children, Growing and Learning with Them.** 2nd ed. By Berthold Lowenfeld. (Pp. xiv + 240; illustrated. $7·00) Springfield, Illinois: Charles C. Thomas. 1964.

Having met the writer of this book on various occasions, and knowing of his international repute in the field of the education of blind children, one is privileged to have a preview of this second edition of Dr. Lowenfeld's book.

Throughout the whole of this work Dr. Lowenfeld has the sound educational approach to the blind child, in showing that though blind he is first and foremost a baby or a child. His analysis of early parental thoughts on the blind baby within the family will greatly assist such parents and his insistence on normalcy does not affect the awareness nor the unawareness that often accompany blindness both collectively and individually. His advice and guidance to parents of blind children are succinct and equally sound for all those who have to work with young blind children.

Dr. Lowenfeld has a wide knowledge of the problems of blindness and does not seek to hide them. He does, however, give advice and observations which help to modify these problems, and place them in their proper perspective. He avoids despair as he also avoids over-optimism, and his guidance will be of great value to parents and families who have a blind child.

In his references to the business of growing up, his understanding of children and of blind children is always evident. His suggestions on the need for tactual demonstration replacing lack of sight, and for a blind child's need for maximum opportunities for manipulation, adaptation, and touch discrimination, will be fully agreed and accepted by all who have experience in working with blind children. But with all the positive assertions that Dr. Lowenfeld so rightly illustrates in his book, he does not minimize the isolation and frustration that can loom so large in the life of the blind child or indeed, of any blind person: but he helps to lessen the isolation and frustration by his own deep psychology and experience of blind persons. At no time is this book dogmatic or dictatorial, though the author is always sure in his observations and advice. He wisely avoids too many definite conclusions, and constantly reminds his readers that the blind child is first and foremost an individual, so there can be no general classification of the effects of the blindness.

This book will be a direct help to many parents of blind children; it will be equally helpful to those who work with blind children in residential accommodation, public school classes, itinerant services, or in any other form of collective or individual work for children who are blind and need special educational facilities.

In recent years two methods have loomed large in the education of blind children—segregation and integration. In putting forward the pros and cons of present systems Dr. Lowenfeld has wisely steered a middle course in quoting 'that each blind child should be educated according to his individual needs, and that not for a long, long time—if ever—will any of the three types of education listed above eliminate the other two'. Time and again in his writings Dr. Lowenfeld returns to what may be called the time requirement of blindness. This is of vital importance in the education of blind children, and is something that must be faced by educationalists in evaluating educational programmes. In giving his own views on the experience and information necessary to all blind children, the author never overlooks the need of the blind child to have opportunity, time and guidance in learning, to encourage the child's development to his fullest potential.

This book confirms what many experienced teachers of blind children have felt and learned through their work with pre-school and school age blind children. Perhaps Dr. Lowenfeld was a little ambitious in his writing on the question of colour and light, with their meanings to the totally blind child. To the child who has enjoyed sight these things have positive meaning even when such meaning eventually comes only through memory because of total blindness. In the case of the child who is totally blind from birth, the interpretation and understanding of light and colour, particularly light, are hardly explained with cetainty. I doubt if Dr. Lowenfeld himself is satisfied with these two pages of his book. In fact he passes the question back to others to a considerable degree by writing 'you yourselves will find some way in which you can explain them to your child.'

*Our Blind Children, Growing and Learning with Them*, is a valuable contribution to the literature on blindness and blind persons. It will certainly serve an important purpose in assisting many parents of blind children throughout the world; and will be of great value to all teachers of blind children and particularly in those areas of the world where such education and provisions are in their infancy.

**Research in Deafness in Children.** Edited by L. Fisch. (Pp. xiv + 103; illustrated. 15s.) Oxford: Blackwell Scientific Publications. 1964.

Deafness in children is an important and topical subject and there has been a need for a guide on the subject for paediatricians and other doctors working with children. This little book goes far to supply this need and to that extent is very welcome. Furthermore, the length of the book is quite adequate without being too long to read in an evening, and the price is reasonable.

It is not in fact greatly concerned with research, apart from one section in which some suggestions are thrown out as to the more important aspects of deafness requiring exploration. A more serious criticism is that the title fails to disclose that most of this book is an almost verbatim account of a conference held in the Spring of 1963. Consequently, a great deal of it, especially in the first half, is subject to the comment recently made about another book, that to put it in print between hard covers was rather like preserving one's fingernail parings in a matchbox, and about as useful.

This is certainly not true of the very professional and useful commentaries and contributions by the editor. Perhaps it is not too much to hope that he might be the author or at least the editor, with a few selected contributors, of a future book on deafness, and that that one will have the virtues of brevity and simplicity that this one possesses, but without the dead wood.

In the meantime, in spite of this criticism, most of us will find much of value in it and much to learn from the proceedings of this Oxford conference, with its variety of eminent participants. By the way, how quiet the teachers of the deaf seem to have been.

**The Child Who Does Not Talk.** Report of an International Study Group, St. Mary's College, Durham, 1963, on the Development and the Disorders of Hearing, Language and Speech in Children. (Clinics in Developmental Medicine No. 13). Edited by CATHERINE RENFREW and KEVIN MURPHY. (Pp. 220; illustrated, 30s.; $5.) The Spastics Society Medical Education and Information Unit in Association with William Heineman Medical Books Ltd., London.

Once again the Spastics Society puts us in their debt by publishing this book, the 13th in the notable series of Clinics in Developmental Medicine (but it is a pity that the apt term Little Club Clinics has been dropped). This is a report of an international study group at Durham in the Autumn of 1963, which brought together audiologists, neurologists, phoneticians, psychologists, paediatricians, psychiatrists, surgeons, linguists, speech therapists, and remedial teachers.

Papers are grouped under these titles: Normal Development and Background to Communication; Diagnosis; General Principles of Treatment; The Child with Mental Defect; The Non-communicating Child; Cerebral Palsy; Stammering. The subject matter is necessarily one where little solid fact of an anatomical or numerical kind is applicable, and perhaps because of this the papers make less immediate impact on the reader than they evidently did when delivered in their context at the opening of a discussion. One infers that the main achievement of the conference was to bring into sharper focus those aspects of the subject requiring particular study, and to underline the necessity for a team approach (exemplified by this study group) to the usually complex problems of the speechless child.

Like the others in this series, the format is notably agreeable.

**Cerebral Palsy. The Pioneer Years of Occupational Therapy in Scotland.** By A. KATHARINE LEVIN. (Pp. xi + 120; 97 figures + 3 tables. 30s.) Edinburgh and London: E. and S. Livingstone. 1964.

This book is an historical account of the development of the occupational training unit at Westerlea with a description of its present make-up. Of the 120 pages, the first 57 are text and the remaining pages are photographs of varying interest.

The text makes interesting and informative reading and one must realize that much of the work was pioneer work involving trial and error, and this account tells how ideas arose and were developed. Some 17 pages are thus devoted to the history of the development of the unit.

Occupational therapy has been divided into 3 main sections: (1) activities of daily living; (2) remedial games; and (3) remedial craftwork. It is gratifying to see that the first of these developed into the most important aspect of the work, i.e. feeding, dressing, toileting, etc.

While not everyone will agree with the particular philosophy or physiological ideas behind some of the work, it can still be said that many beneficial activities were devised even if for a reason or by reasoning not acceptable to all.

An account is given of an out-patient unit operating on the same lines and there is a further account of the development of a sheltered workshop in the form of a laundry, which enable a number of spastics to be self supporting and at the same time provide a useful service to the community. The work has been very much along the lines of developing skills in connexion with daily living, and it is on much firmer ground in this respect than when directed to remedial activities. No attempt has been made to analyse individual cases or groups of cases nor to give figures or results statistically. For those concerned with setting up such a unit this book will provide much useful information, and indeed it is a pity that greater detail of methods and apparatus is not always given, though the main interest of the photographs is when they provide this information.

**Humangenetik. Ein kurzes Handbuch in fünf Bänden.** Band II. Edited by P. E. BECKER. (Pp. xv + 663; 425 figures. DM. 198.) Stuttgart: Georg Thieme. 1964.

This is the first volume to appear and is second in a series of five volumes in German on Human Genetics, and deals with the skeleton. The Editor of the series is Professor Becker of Göttingen, well known for his contribution to the clinical and genetic classification of muscular dystrophy.

Paediatricians and orthopaedic surgeons will find the volume a most valuable source of references, especially references from continental literature. Certain of the individual chapters are well written, for example, that by Lenz on anomalies of growth and body build, in which is discussed most of the syndromes associated with dwarfism; that of Schulze on the anomalies of the teeth and jaws; and that of Degenhardt on the anomalies of the skull and back-bone. Other sections, such as that on generalized diseases of the skeleton and the limb bones, are complete, but do not attempt to integrate what is known of the genetics, probably because the authors are experienced clinicians rather than geneticists.

All those interested in genetics will look forward to the appearance of the other four volumes.

**Tuberculosis in Twins.** By BARBARA SIMONDS. (Pp. 81; 31 tables + appendixes. 10s. 6d.) London: Pitman. 1964.

From 1950 to 1957 Dr. Barbara Simonds conducted an inquiry on behalf of the Prophit Committee of the Royal College of Physicians into 'the genetic variation of resistance to tuberculosis by a study of twins on the lines of research carried out in New York by Dr. F. J. Kallman and Dr. D. Reisner'. Those workers, after a study in their own city, had concluded that the chance of developing tuberculosis increases in strict proportion to the degree of blood relationships to a tuberculous index case. The inquiry was, therefore, into the hereditary component of resistance to tuberculosis.

The report is short but is presented with great clarity and economy of language and space in six chapters in 45 pages; the remaining 35 pages contain necessary statistical appendixes.

The first and second chapters survey previous similar investigations and describe the methodology of this study and the diagnosis of zygosity: the method of sampling the twins was seen to be crucial and was therefore carefully planned. Eventually a group of 150 dizygotic and 55 monozygotic pairs was obtained. In the third chapter the diagnosis and outcome of tuberculosis and the contact history are considered. The fourth and fifth chapters contain the results in two parts; in the first part the mono- and dizygotic twin samples are shown to be comparable with regard to sex and age and the nature and fate of the tuberculous disease. The only difference revealed was a relative increase in size of the 20-30 age-group of monozygotic female co-twins.

When both twins of a pair developed the disease the twins were defined as concordant, and when only one twin was affected the pair was said to be discordant. Study of concordance showed that a significantly greater proportion of the co-twins of monozygotic index cases ($\chi^2 = 7\cdot986$; $p < 0\cdot01$) and that the number of concordant pairs were significantly greater in female monozygotic twin pairs than in female dizygotic or concordant dizygotic twin pairs with a female index. This finding was not present in male concordant monozygotic twin pairs. Concordant twins were much more likely to have a tuberculous parent than discordant twins.

There were differences between the findings in this study and that of Kallmann and Reisner. Simonds' study suggests that the higher concordance rate from tuberculosis in monozygotic twin pairs is due to increased exposure to index cases with a positive sputum and by a larger number of susceptible females in the monozygotic twin pairs. It is suggested that the differences in findings between the studies are due to a more complete method of collecting twins and a greater knowledge of the clinical differences between twin-pairs.

Emphasizing as it does that it is contact with an index case rather than blood relationship that is all important in the development of tuberculosis, this report should help to dispel any lingering thoughts about the hereditary nature of tuberculosis and should be further valuable evidence for the epidemiologists who believe that it is both practical and sensible to attempt to eradicate the disease. It is good to know that it has been published, and there is no doubt that it will often be used as a point of reference when questions of hereditary resistance are discussed.

**Babies and Young Children. Feeding, Management and Care.** 3rd Ed. By RONALD ILLINGWORTH and CYNTHIA ILLINGWORTH. (Pp. vii + 317; 24 figures + 50 sketches. 18s.) London: Churchill. 1964.

In this third edition the authors have completely revised the text. Without lengthening the book many alterations and additions have been made to ensure that it meets the accepted present-day practice. There are chapters on all the aspects of child care from clothing to emotional disturbance. The wisely chosen words of advice aiming to inform as completely as possible without alarming are directed mainly towards parents. However, hospital and nursery nurses, health visitors, and others engaged in child welfare would find the material helpful and interesting. The delightful pen sketches and plates amusingly and often very pertinently illustrate the text.

Though the text is simply written to avoid confusion in the minds of parents, most of it would not conflict with the views of any paediatrician unless he held particularly dogmatic views.

There are chapters on the feeding and clothing of infants and older children, on the avoidance and management of feeding problems, on play, toys, books, sleep and sleep disturbances. There are also useful and comforting remarks about minor ailments and disturbing habits such as thumb sucking and masturbation. The section on 'first aid' gives clearly sensible 'do's and don'ts' on the emergency management of sudden illnesses like croup and convulsions, and accidents such as burns and fractures and inhaled foreign bodies.

Troublesome children are dealt with especially aiming to give an insight into the underlying causes of various behaviour disturbances. Advice is also given on the nursing of the sick child and on keeping him occupied when confined to bed.

There are also hints on holidays and journeys, advice on immunization schedules, and a recommended list of other books on child care.

This is a well-presented 'paper back' with a good index which is easily read and very informative.

## Paediatric Research Society

The 6th meeting of the Paediatric Research Society (Secretary, B. D. Bower) was held in the Department of Child Life and Health, University of Edinburgh, on October 23 and 24, 1964: 25 members and guests were present.

The following papers were read:—

'Some aetiological associations in studies of congenitally determined disabilities.' By Cecil Drillien.

'Lipoma of the cauda equina.' By Victor Dubowitz.

'Adrenocortical function in newborn infants.' By D. Methven Cathro.

'The leucocyte pattern in the neonatal period.' By Elizabeth M. Innes.

'Histamine in human diseases.' By Ross Mitchell.

'Urinary cortisol excretion as a test of adrenal cortical function.' By William Hamilton.

'Paediatrics in India.' By J. W. Farquhar.

On October 23 a visit was made to the unit for dysmelic children at the Princess Margaret Rose Hospital (Dr. Werner Schutt and colleagues).

*Review Article*

*Arch. Dis. Childh.*, 1965, **40**, 343.

# IRON DEFICIENCY AND IRON OVERLOAD

BY

R. SEPHTON SMITH*

*From the Department of Pediatrics, University of Southern California and Children's Hospital of Los Angeles, U.S.A.*†

(RECEIVED FOR PUBLICATION MARCH 29, 1965)

Iron is essential to most, if not all, living organisms, and the higher animals and man have employed it for many purposes essential to life. The readiness with which iron undergoes oxidation and reduction is utilized in many of the enzymes of electron transport, and in a number of other enzymes whose function is not understood. Furthermore, the combination of iron with porphyrin and protein leads to complexes that have the property of binding large amounts of oxygen in a readily reversible fashion. Haemoglobin and myoglobin are complexes of this nature, which serve the function of oxygen transport and storage. About three-quarters of the iron in a normal man (between 4 g. and 5 g.) is incorporated in circulating haemoglobin. Less than 5% is present in myoglobin, various enzymes, or in transport in the plasma. The remainder, about 20% of the total, is present in the tissue stores, much of it as the iron-protein complex ferritin (Drabkin, 1951). Very little iron is excreted, as the iron from broken-down aged red cells is returned to the marrow for re-use in haemoglobin synthesis. The iron content of the body is achieved during periods of growth, and maintained thereafter at a steady level, through control of the amount absorbed. As the amount of iron utilized in haemoglobin synthesis is so much greater than the quantity of new iron absorbed, it is perhaps not surprising that iron deficiency is so common. It is the most frequent cause of anaemia, and the most important deficiency state in countries with good economic means. Iron deficiency is particularly common in early infancy, as the requirements of rapid growth exceed the infant's capacity to absorb enough iron from food. Iron in excess is toxic: acute iron poisoning follows ingestion of large amounts of iron salts, and is one of the most common and serious forms of poisoning seen in young children. The progressive deposition of iron in the tissues from excess intestinal absorption or after repeated transfusions leads eventually to impaired organ function. In children chronic iron overload is increasingly seen, now that the availability of blood transfusion and improved medical care have prolonged the survival in conditions such as thalassaemia, and the hypoplastic and aplastic anaemias. The development of new iron-chelating agents raises the possibility of removing excess iron in these conditions, and offers specific therapy for acute iron poisoning. In this review, the aspects of iron deficiency and iron excess of special interest to the paediatrician will be considered in relation to our basic concepts of iron metabolism.

## Iron Absorption

The classic observations of McCance and Widdowson (1937) that the ability to excrete iron was very severely limited, led to the concept that the absorptive process must be of paramount importance in regulating the body's content of iron. Our knowledge of the mechanism of iron absorption and of the factors that control it is incomplete. Chemical balance studies of iron absorption are notoriously difficult for technical reasons, and most of our knowledge has come from studies using tracer doses of radioactive isotopes. Such studies limit our observations to the absorption of a measured dose of a single labelled substance. Their applicability to the absorption of iron from a whole meal, or a complete diet, is doubtful. The iron in food exists in a number of different chemical forms, each of which may be absorbed by a different process. Some food iron is present in the ionized form (Ascham, Speirs, and Maddox, 1938; Bergeim and Kirsch, 1949), but there will also be varying amounts of tightly-complexed iron, such as haemoglobin,

* Formerly Research Fellow in Haematology, The Hospital for Sick Children, Great Ormond Street, London.

† Postal address: 4614 Sunset Boulevard, Los Angeles, California 90027, U.S.A.



2

TABLE 1
FACTORS INFLUENCING IRON ABSORPTION

| Factor | Effect on Absorption of Inorganic Iron | | Reference |
|---|---|---|---|
| | Increase | Decrease | |
| *Iron stores:* | | | |
| Iron deficiency | + | | Bothwell *et al.* (1958), Callender (1964) |
| Iron overload | | + | Bothwell *et al.* (1958), Pirzio-Biroli *et al.* (1958) |
| *Bone-marrow:* | | | |
| Increased erythropoiesis | + | | Mendel *et al.* (1963), Pirzio-Biroli *et al.* (1958) |
| Erythroid hypoplasia | | + | Mendel *et al.* (1963), Pirzio-Biroli *et al.* (1958) |
| *Peripheral blood:* | | | |
| Anaemia | + | | Mendel *et al.* (1963), Schiffer *et al.* (1965) |
| Hypoxia | + | | Mendel (1961) |
| Hypertransfusion | | + | Mendel (1961) |
| *Pancreas:* | | | |
| Destruction of pancreas | + | | Davis and Badenoch (1962) |
| Pancreatin administration | | + | Callender and Malpas (1963) |
| Reducing agents, ascorbic acid | + | | Brise and Hallberg (1962) |
| Phosphates, phytates | | + | Turnbull *et al.* (1962) |

myoglobin, and ferritin, in meats and liver. Iron can be absorbed at any level when placed in direct contact with the gut mucosa (Valquist, Neander, and Neander, 1945), but absorption is largely confined to the duodenum and upper small bowel when iron salts are given by mouth (Brown and Justus, 1958). The amount of iron absorbed seems to depend on a number of unrelated factors (Table 1).

**Type of Iron.** Ferrous iron is absorbed to a greater extent than the ferric form, when placed in a gut loop (Groen, Van Den Broeck, and Veldman, 1947). When given by mouth, ferric iron is absorbed to a greater extent, though still not as well as the ferrous form (Brise and Hallberg, 1962): the use of a ferrous complexing agent blocks the absorption of both forms (Venkatachalam, Brading, George, and Walsh, 1956), so it appears that ionized iron is reduced before its absorption. Furthermore, the absorption of iron salts can be increased by adding reducing substances such as ascorbic acid (Moore, Bierman, Minnich, and Arrowsmith, 1940; Brise and Hallberg, 1962). Absorption may be reduced by binding substances such as phosphates and phytates (McCance, Edgecomb, and Widdowson, 1943; Turnbull, Cleton, and Finch, 1962). When iron salts are given with food, absorption is reduced (Pirzio-Biroli, Bothwell, and Finch, 1958), and if baked in bread, they are less than half as well absorbed as when given alone (Steinkamp, Dubach, and Moore, 1955). Studies of the absorption of haemoglobin, in which the iron is present as a complex with porphyrin, show that in a dose of 5 mg. this type of iron is about half as well absorbed as ferrous sulphate (Callender, 1964). Moreover, the absorption of this type of iron is not enhanced by ascorbic acid, or blocked by the presence of a meal or phytate (Turnbull *et al.*, 1962). This finding is of great interest and suggests that the mechanism of absorption of haemoglobin iron may differ fundamentally from the absorption of iron salts. It is possible that the iron in porphyrin complexes is absorbed as such, without conversion into free ionized iron. Sanford (1961) demonstrated that less than 12% of the iron in liver or haemoglobin could be split off by peptic or tryptic digestion. On the other hand, patients with iron-deficiency anaemia may absorb as much as 68% of a dose of haemoglobin iron (Callender, 1964).

**Amount of Iron.** The quantity of iron administered to some extent determines the amount absorbed. Studies using graded doses of radioiron have shown that at each increasing dose level, although the proportion of the dose absorbed was reduced, the actual amount of iron absorbed increased (Smith and Pannacciulli, 1958). About 50% (0·05 mg.) of a dose of 0·1 mg. ferrous iron is absorbed by a normal man, compared with 5-10% (5-10 mg.) of a dose of 100 mg. (Bothwell and Finch, 1962, p. 98).

**Effect of Gastric Secretion.** The site of maximal iron absorption has focused attention on the possible role of gastric and duodenal juice in the regulation of iron absorption. It is well known that iron absorption is decreased after partial gastrectomy (Baird, Podmore, and Wilson, 1957; Stevens, Pirzio-Biroli, Harkins, Nyhus, and Finch, 1959), but this may not be the result of achlorhydria. Although Goldberg, Lochhead, and Dagg (1963) found decreased iron absorption in anaemic patients with achlorhydria, Moore and Dubach (1956) were unable to increase it in such patients by the administration of hydrochloric acid. It may be that anatomical continuity of the stomach and intestine, rather than the presence of acid, is necessary for adequate absorption of iron.

**Effect of Pancreatin.** Recent work suggests that pancreatic secretions may have a much more important role in the regulation of iron absorption than was formerly realized. In 1935 Taylor, Stiven, and Reid showed that iron deposition developed rapidly following ligation of the pancreatic duct in cats. More recently, Davis and Badenoch (1962) showed that iron absorption was significantly increased in 6 patients with severe chronic pancreatitis. In one patient, iron absorption was reduced by the administration of pancreatic extract. Further studies have shown that the administration of pancreatic extracts will reduce the absorption of iron in patients with cirrhosis of the liver and haemochromatosis (Biggs and Davis, 1963; Callender and Malpas, 1963). It has also been shown that children with cystic fibrosis, treated by pancreatic extracts, absorb iron poorly and show evidence of iron deficiency (Smith, 1964a). The mechanism of this action of pancreatin is not understood. It is not likely to be due to a direct absorptive effect, as it has been shown that pancreatin can absorb only negligible amounts of iron (Biggs and Davis, 1963). Furthermore the inhibitory effect on iron absorption is found with haemoglobin iron as well as with iron salts (Callender and Malpas, 1963).

**Mucosal Factors.** The transfer of iron from the gut lumen is effected through the mucosal cell as an active metabolic process (Dowdle, Schachter, and Schenker, 1960). It appears that the entry of iron into a mucosal cell stimulates the production of the protein apoferritin which then combines with iron to form ferritin (Gabrio and Salomon, 1950; Granick, 1946). This has led to much speculation as to whether ferritin accumulation inhibits or facilitates iron absorption. In early experiments with dogs, it was found that iron absorption was much depressed when a loading dose had been given several hours previously (Hahn, Bale, Ross, Balfour, and Whipple, 1943), and the concept of the 'mucosal block' was formed in which it was suggested that the mucosal cells, when saturated with ferritin, had the ability to prevent the absorption of further iron. This old concept, however, does not stand examination in the light of modern experience. The massive absorption in acute iron poisoning shows that the block is, at best, incomplete, and more recent experiments have shown that when iron is infused continuously, or in sequential doses, iron absorption in appreciable amounts may continue for 4 to 6 hours (Brown, Dubach, and Moore, 1958; Hallberg and Sölvell, 1960). However, there is good evidence that the mucosal cell does play an active part in the regulation of iron absorption. Recent autoradiographic studies (Conrad and Crosby, 1963) suggest that absorption of iron proceeds in two distinct stages. Following the initial rapid uptake of iron by the mucosal cell, ferritin is formed, after which the iron may enter the blood stream, or remain, if not needed, to be shed into the gut as the mucosal cell desquamates. The role of the mucosal cell in iron absorption is reviewed in detail by Crosby (1963). The regulation of transfer of iron from the mucosal cell into the circulation is not well understood. At least three factors, or combinations of them, seem to be involved: the size of the iron stores, the rate of erythropoiesis, and the haemoglobin level in the blood.

**Size of Iron Stores.** There is good evidence that the size of the iron stores influences the amount of iron absorbed. Absorption is increased in iron-deficiency anaemia, or when the stores are diminished, and iron overload leads to a reduction in iron absorption (Bothwell, Pirzio-Biroli, and Finch, 1958; Callender, 1964; Pirzio-Biroli *et al.*, 1958; Moore, 1955). Similar variations were seen in a study in which iron absorption was measured in normal subjects, in whom the iron stores were varied over a period of three years (Pirzio-Biroli and Finch, 1960). From a normal mean absorption of 6% of a tracer dose of iron added to food, absorption was reduced to 3% when the stores were increased by 1·5 g., and conversely was increased to about 20% after iron depletion. These variations were not dependent on the level of haemoglobin, plasma iron, or transferrin. The results suggest that throughout life iron absorption may be modified in a way to maintain optimal body stores. During periods of growth, or after blood loss, absorption may be augmented until adequate stores have been achieved. At the present time, the mechanism by which the level of body iron stores can influence the absorption of iron is obscure. It is evidently not accomplished through changes in the degree of saturation of the plasma transferrin. which have been found to have no influence on iron absorption (Wheby and Jones, 1963).

**Erythropoiesis and Anaemia.** There is a wealth of evidence that iron absorption varies with alterations in the rate of erythropoiesis: increased erythropoiesis is accompanied by increased iron absorption, and conversely when erythropoiesis is reduced or abolished, iron absorption is diminished. The evidence is well reviewed by Bothwell and Finch (1962, p. 108). This view is supported by the finding that iron overload frequently develops in patients with chronic haemolytic anaemias of various aetiology. Unfortunately, many of the patients and experimental models studied have additionally some degree of anaemia or iron-loading or both, so that it is not always possible to conclude that an alteration in iron absorption noted is solely or mainly the consequence of an alteration in erythropoiesis. Mendel (1961) and Mendel, Weiler, and Mangalik (1963) studied this problem in mice where erythropoiesis had been abolished by splenectomy and administration of radioactive strontium. It was, therefore, possible to study independently the effects of changes in the rate of erythropoiesis and in the haemoglobin level. It was found that iron absorption was enhanced not only by increased erythropoiesis, but also by anaemia or hypoxia not associated with increased erythropoiesis. The increase in iron absorption following erythropoietin administration was also clearly shown to be due to increased erythropoiesis: no effect was seen in animals without erythropoiesis. A recent study of iron absorption in aregenerative anaemia (Schiffer, Price, and Cronkite, 1965) has also clearly demonstrated that anaemia, even in the presence of decreased erythropoiesis, may be associated with increased absorption of iron.

In summary, there is good evidence that the size of the iron stores has an important role in regulating iron absorption in health, and in promoting increased absorption in iron deficiency. The pancreatic secretions may also play an important part in preventing excess absorption of iron. In many haemolytic and refractory anaemias, anaemia and sometimes increased erythropoiesis might be expected to increase iron absorption, and increased iron stores to reduce it. The balance of these opposing forces must vary, though most of the evidence suggests that the inhibiting effect of increased iron stores can be overcome, so that these patients develop a progressive overloading with iron.

### Iron Excretion

Although iron is often referred to as a 'one-way' substance, minute amounts are lost in the urine, faeces, sweat, and exfoliated cells. Many attempts to measure these losses by chemical methods have given erroneously high values, as it is almost impossible to prevent external contamination of the body surface. By the use of radioactive iron, the total loss from all these sources has been estimated to be between 0·5 mg. and 1·0 mg. daily (Dubach, Moore, and Callender, 1955). A second isotopic method has been to label the total body iron, and follow the radioactivity of the red cell mass for several years (Finch, 1959). By this method an average total daily iron loss of 0·6 mg. was calculated for normal men. It seems reasonable to conclude that adult men will lose on average slightly less than 1 mg. daily. The figure will be higher for women during the child-bearing years, due to additional losses from menstruation and pregnancy. No data are available for children, but it may be assumed that boys of all ages and girls in the years preceding the onset of menstruation will not lose more iron than adult men, and will probably in fact lose considerably less, perhaps in proportion to their surface area. Newborn infants appear to be an exception, and may lose up to 3 mg. daily in the stools during the first few days of life (Cavell and Widdowson, 1964). This interesting finding might be explained by failure of the immature newborn liver to conserve some of the iron from red-cell breakdown. It is not yet known at what age these high faecal losses of iron cease.

In iron-deficient subjects, the loss of iron is reduced (Dubach *et al.*, 1955). Patients with iron loading might be expected to excrete more iron than normal men, due to the increased iron content of exfoliated cells and secretions, but this has not yet been proved. However, a daily iron loss of about 4 mg. was estimated for a single patient (Crosby, Conrad, and Wheby, 1963).

### Iron Nutrition in Childhood

When growth has ceased, adults remain in iron balance by absorbing from food sufficient iron to replace normal losses, between 0·5 mg. and 1 mg. daily in adult men. During infancy and childhood, an additional amount will have to be absorbed to meet the requirements of growth, as the child's haemoglobin mass and iron content increase. The amount will be greatest during periods of rapid growth, but over the whole period of childhood, 0·6 mg. of iron daily will be required. The total iron content of a normal diet in Great Britain is about 14 mg. per day (Davidson and Passmore, 1963). The intake of food iron in children receiving a normal diet will vary in proportion to the amount eaten, and in the case of the younger ones, may be substantially less than this. Healthy adult men do not become iron deficient or iron laden, and iron deficiency is not common in growing boys, or in girls in the years preceding the onset of menstruation. We may therefore conclude that enough iron to meet the normal losses and requirements of growth is absorbed from a diet containing quantities of iron up to 14 mg. Growing children might therefore be expected to absorb more iron than adult men, to

TABLE 2

ABSORPTION OF FOOD IRON

| Type of Food | Amount of Iron (mg.) | Mean % Absorbed* | | | | Reference |
|---|---|---|---|---|---|---|
| | | Normal | | Iron-deficient | | |
| | | Adults | Children | Adults | Children | |
| Haemoglobin | 5 | 12 (25) | 22 (8) | 25 (27) | — | Bannerman *et al.* (1964), Callender (1964) |
| Chicken liver | 6·5 | 7·7 (5) | 8 (3) | — | — | Moore and Dubach (1951) |
| Chicken muscle | 9 | 11 (5) | — | 30 (2) | — | Moore and Dubach (1951) |
| Egg | 6 | 1·4 (14) | — | — | — | Chodos *et al.* (1957) |
| | 3·5 | 3·8 (8) | — | 3·8 (5) | — | Moore and Dubach (1951) |
| | 1·2 | — | 8·6 (52) | — | — | Schulz and Smith (1958a) |
| Egg and milk | 1·2 | — | 5·8 (5) | — | 17 (6) | Schulz and Smith (1958a) |
| Milk | 0·3 | 2·8 (6) | — | — | — | Schulz and Smith (1958a) |
| | 0·1 | — | 9·5 (14) | — | 16 (4) | Schulz and Smith (1958a) |
| Vegetables (Swiss chard, beet greens) | 3 | 1·1 (6) | — | — | — | Chodos *et al.* (1957) |
| Fortified cereals | 3 | — | 12·3 (16) | — | — | Schulz and Smith (1958a) |
| Enriched bread | 3 | 5 (28) | — | 55 (3) | — | Steinkamp *et al.* (1955) |

* Number of observations indicated by figures in parentheses.

meet the additional requirements of growth, though their iron intake may be slightly less. Studies of absorption of food iron, particularly in children, are not numerous (Table 2). Schulz and Smith (1958a) found a mean absorption of 10·6% of a dose of 0·1 mg. of iron in 6 oz. of milk, whereas adult men absorbed only 2·8% of a comparable intake. An average of 8% of chicken liver iron was absorbed, and 8·6% of egg iron. It was further demonstrated that children under 3 years of age absorbed egg iron about twice as well as the older ones. In similar studies with adults, Moore and Dubach (1956) found absorption of 3·8% of egg iron. Schulz and Smith also found a mean absorption of 12·3% of iron in enriched cereals. The portions served were 6 g., with 2 oz. of milk, containing a total of 3 mg. of iron. Bannerman, Callender, Hardisty, and Smith (1964) found that children absorbed a dose of 5 mg. of iron as haemoglobin approximately twice as well as adults. The mean values for iron absorption found in this study were 22% for the children, and 12% for the adults. Comparison of the absorption of various kinds of food iron in children shows that haemoglobin iron was absorbed to the greatest extent, even though the amount of iron was larger. Studies of absorption of food iron in adults (Chodos, Ross, Apt, Pollycove, and Halkett, 1957; Moore and Dubach, 1956) have also shown that there is a wide variation in absorption of iron in different kinds of food. These studies suggest that the iron in muscle meats is absorbed about four times as well as egg iron, and about 10 times as well as vegetable iron. Children may, therefore, derive a very substantial proportion of their food iron from meat, rather than from milk, eggs, or vegetables. Enriched cereal products represent a further valuable source of iron when these are given: although iron in this form may be slightly less readily absorbed than meat iron, the amount of iron in the portions normally served is many times greater than the iron in milk or vegetables. We may conclude that children normally absorb between 10 and 20% of the iron in meat, eggs, enriched cereal products, and milk. This corresponds to between 1 and 2·5 mg. of iron, if the diet is normal, and agrees well with the theoretical requirement based on normal losses and the requirements of growth.

Studies of iron absorption in infancy are limited to a small number of observations with $^{59}$Fe-labelled milk. Garby and Sjölin (1959) showed that newborn infants below the age of 1 month absorbed a mean of 72% of radioiron in milk, decreasing to 30% at 3 months of age. In similar studies with premature infants, Gorten, Hepner, and Workman (1963) found a mean absorption of 31·5%, and noted that the highest iron absorption values were obtained in the most rapidly growing infants. It is interesting to consider the question of iron deficiency and anaemia in early infancy in the light of these observations. Although growing infants may absorb iron well, a normal infant may treble his birth weight in the first year of life; the increase will be even greater in premature infants. Little stored iron is present at birth, probably not more than 10 to 25 mg. (McCance and Widdowson, 1951), but the high haemoglobin level in the normal infant at birth provides a source of some iron, the destruction of the excess red cells providing enough for the increase in the infant's size during the first two to four months of life. Studies with radioactive iron (Smith, Caton, Roby, Reid,

Caswell, and Gibson, 1950) have confirmed that little, if any, exogenous absorbed iron is used in haemoglobin formation during this period, and if anaemia develops it is the result of decreased erythropoiesis rather than iron deficiency (Gairdner, Marks, and Roscoe, 1952; Seip, 1955; Garby, Sjölin, and Vuille, 1963). Thereafter, the rate of growth is so rapid that the iron requirement exceeds the amount which can be absorbed from the available diet, even though the iron may be well absorbed. The iron content of infant foods varies widely, and though some infants receiving heavily iron-enriched formulas may ingest 5 to 10 mg. of iron per day in food, those fed on milk alone may receive as little as 0·14 mg. per day (Sturgeon, 1956). By calculation from the birth weight and haemoglobin level, the anticipated increase in haemoglobin mass in a normal infant will require the absorption of about 2 mg. iron daily from the fourth month of life onwards. It is obvious that this cannot be achieved by the use of milk feeding without iron supplements, and iron-deficiency anaemia may be expected to follow. It is also generally conceded that the early institution of mixed feeding will not lead to higher haemoglobin levels in either full-term or premature infants. Brokaw, Sedam, and Cassirer (1942) could demonstrate no difference in haemoglobin levels in normal infants fed solids early, as compared with those kept on milk during the first 12 months of life. This is perhaps not surprising, as the quantity of iron in such foods is relatively small in relation to the infant's requirements.

The deficiency of iron in many infant foods, including normal human breast milk, has led paediatricians to accept, as normal, levels of haemoglobin in infancy, which are considerably lower than those found in older children and adults. Sturgeon (1956) showed that this physiological anaemia of late infancy might be prevented by the parenteral administration of iron. 30 infants within the ages of 8 to 10 months were each given a total of 250 mg. of iron as iron dextran, and after 3 months they were found to have significantly higher haemoglobin levels than the untreated controls. Premature infants, whose iron requirement is even greater due to the initial greater iron deficit coupled with a more rapid rate of growth, almost invariably become anaemic, and this may be prevented by the administration of parenteral iron as iron dextran (Gaisford and Jennison, 1955; Elliott, 1962).

There is now good evidence that the prophylactic administration of oral iron, or the use of iron-enriched cereals in infant feeding, will lead to higher haemoglobin levels and prevent much of the iron-deficiency anaemia seen in otherwise normal infants. Niccum, Jackson, and Stearns (1953) and Sturgeon (1958) showed that supplementation with oral medicinal iron will prevent iron-deficiency anaemia and lead to a higher mean haemoglobin level during infancy. Farquhar (1963), in a double blind controlled study of 44 infants, found higher levels of haemoglobin at 3, 6, 9, and 12 months in the experimental group who were given 5 mg. of iron as ferric pyrophosphate daily from the age of 1 month. A most noteworthy recent contribution in this field has been the work of Moe in Norway (1963). The effect of diets of varying iron content was studied in 255 normal healthy babies, who were divided into four groups, and given varying dietary iron intakes from the age of 3 months onwards. One group received no supplements, the remainder were fed cereals with an iron content of 5 mg./100 g., 12·5 mg./100 g., or 20 mg./100 g. The last group also received 15 mg. medicinal iron daily (0·6 ml. Fer-In-Sol) to ensure a high iron intake. The two groups receiving the highest iron intakes had significantly higher haemoglobin levels at 1 year of age than the group receiving cereals containing 5 mg. iron/100 g., or the unsupplemented diet. Dietary histories were kept, and it was found that the actual iron intakes of the two groups with the highest supplements were over 20 mg., and 8·6-13·5 mg. It was concluded that an iron content of 12·5 mg./100 g. of cereal will assure an adequate iron supply for the normal infant, when cereals are fed regularly twice a day from the age of 3½ months. In an extension of the study (Moe, 1964) in which these infants were followed up to the age of 3 years, it was found that the infants in the two groups which had received cereals with the highest iron content maintained normal haemoglobin levels, and showed a negligible incidence of iron-deficiency anaemia. On the other hand, iron-deficiency developed in nearly one-third of the children receiving diets without iron supplements.

It is evident that the iron content of many infant diets is insufficient to meet the needs of growth. A high incidence of iron-deficiency anaemia can be prevented by supplements of oral iron which can be given conveniently and cheaply by feeding iron-fortified cereals. A daily iron intake of 10-12 mg. by the end of the first year seems to be necessary. It is also possible that the lower levels of haemoglobin found in apparently normal infants fed without iron supplements may indicate some degree of latent iron deficiency. Mackay (1931) demonstrated a decrease in resistance to infections in infants with iron-deficiency anaemia; iron medication was followed by a marked reduction in morbidity. It would be of great importance, in view of current interest in the effects of tissue iron deficiency without anaemia, to know whether the small increase in haemoglobin achieved by feeding iron-enriched cereals was accompanied by any improvement in rate of growth, and any decrease in the instance of infections. It still remains to be shown whether the premature infant requires medicinal iron to avoid the anaemia which is almost invariably seen in late infancy, or whether this could be prevented by the provision of a diet with a sufficiently high iron content. This problem deserves further study, as suitable iron-enriched formulas and cereals could easily be prepared, and it is known that these infants absorb iron salts well.

### Iron Deficiency

**Aetiology.** Iron deficiency occurs when the body's need for iron to meet the requirements of growth or to replace normal or pathological losses of iron is not met by alimentary absorption. This may be due to nutritional insufficiency, intestinal malabsorption of iron, or blood loss, which is the only way in which significant pathological amounts of iron can be lost from the body. More than one of these factors may contribute to the presence of iron deficiency in the individual patient.

*Dietary insufficiency* is probably the commonest cause of iron deficiency in infancy and childhood. It has already been shown that even in countries with a high standard of living, the usual types of infant foods contain an inadequate amount of iron, unless supplements are given; it is therefore not surprising that these infants have an incidence of iron-deficiency anaemia of 15-30%. A much higher incidence of iron deficiency is found in areas inhabited by families of poorer economic means. Davis, Marten, and Sarkany (1960) found evidence of iron deficiency in 22·4% of white children in London, while the incidence in West-Indian immigrants was 53·5%. The incidence of iron deficiency in children under the age of 3 years was stated to be approaching 30% in Cincinnati (Guest and Brown, 1957) and in Oslo (Moe, 1964). Among the poorer inhabitants of North East Scotland, 42% of infants under 2 years had a haemoglobin level more than 10% below the accepted normal (Davidson, Donaldson, Dyar, Lindsay, and McSorley, 1942). Incidences over 50% have been reported in Mauritius and in the Philippines (Stott, 1960; Stransky and Dauis-Lawas, 1948). Sturgeon (1954), using measurements of plasma iron and iron-binding capacity as an index of iron deficiency, found evidence of iron deficiency in approximately half of a group of infants from homes with good economic means. He suggested that a more rapid rate of growth in well-nourished children might account for the high incidence of iron deficiency.

In addition to inadequacy of the dietary supply of iron, a number of other factors modify the iron content of the newborn infant, and thus his subsequent iron requirement during infancy. In prematurity or twinning, the birth weight may be much lower than in normal single full-term births and the combination of the lower initial body iron content with a more rapid rate of growth leads to the development of iron deficiency in a very high proportion of such babies. The manner in which the cord is ligated will also influence the amount of iron present in the infant at birth. By draining the placenta through gravity, or by stripping the umbilical cord, the infant's blood volume may be increased by 20%, with a consequent gain of about 50 mg. of iron by the infant. Simple delay in ligation of the cord has no such effect (Whipple, Sisson, and Lund, 1957). The infant's iron content does not seem to be adversely affected by maternal iron deficiency, unless it is very severe. Strauss (1933) found that anaemia during the first year was much more frequent in infants of mothers with a mean haemoglobin level of 5·3 g./100 ml. at term, and the studies of Sisson and Lund (1957) showed a significant reduction in red cell mass in the infants of anaemic mothers, compared with those born to women without significant anaemia. In contrast to this, Woodruff and Bridgeforth (1953) found no difference in haemoglobin levels up to 1 year of age in infants born to two groups of mothers, with mean haemoglobin levels of 9·9 g./100 ml. and 13·9 g./100 ml. at term. Furthermore Sturgeon (1959) showed that supplementation with oral iron or even the administration of large doses of parenteral iron to mothers during pregnancy did not influence the haemoglobin levels of their infants at 6, 12, or 18 months. It may be concluded that the infant's iron stores cannot be significantly increased, or the subsequent development of anaemia prevented, by the administration of iron to the mother during pregnancy, unless severe iron-deficiency anaemia is present.

*Pathological blood loss* is of considerable importance in the aetiology of iron-deficiency anaemia in infancy and childhood. Bleeding may be due to generalized bleeding disorders, such as haemophilia, familial telangiectasia, and idiopathic thrombocytopenic purpura. Frequent bleeding episodes in these and similar conditions often lead to iron-deficiency anaemia which may be overlooked in the child's management. In the adolescent girl, heavy menstrual losses at the time of the menarche is a frequent cause of iron-deficiency anaemia, particularly as this occurs at a period of rapid growth.

Significant amounts of blood can be lost from the gastro-intestinal tract, without being noticed by the parents or physician. Such losses may be due to generalized bleeding disorders, or to local lesions such as Meckel's diverticulum, angioma, hiatus hernia, and in older children, regional enteritis and ulcerative colitis. On a global level, a major cause of iron-deficiency anaemia through bleeding is hookworm infestation. When iron-deficiency fails to respond to adequate treatment, or recurs rapidly, causes for occult gastro-intestinal bleeding should be sought.

Of particular interest is the very high incidence of occult blood loss in iron deficiency in infancy. Using radioactive iron, Hoag, Wallerstein, and Pollycove (1961) found significant blood loss in all of 13 infants studied. The amount of blood lost varied between 7 ml. and 107 ml. over a period of three to four weeks. Wilson, Heiner, and Lahey (1962) found occult blood in the stools of 41% of the infants studied, and many of these infants also had precipitins to cows' milk in their serum, and evidence of loss of significant quantities of serum proteins into the gastric juice. Whatever the primary cause, it appears that iron-deficiency anaemia may frequently occur in infancy from gastro-intestinal bleeding in the absence of anatomical lesions.

*Malabsorption of iron* is probably the least important cause of iron deficiency. This is not surprising, since the duodenum, which is the site at which iron is best absorbed, is rarely involved in pathological processes. The most important condition associated with the malabsorption of iron is idiopathic steatorrhoea, and coeliac disease in childhood. The block in iron absorption has been clearly demonstrated in studies using radioactive iron, and it can be shown that iron absorption returns to normal after treatment (Badenoch and Callender, 1954, 1960). Iron deficiency and malabsorption of iron have also recently been shown to be present in children with cystic fibrosis, possibly a consequence of prolonged treatment with pancreatin (Smith, 1964a). When iron deficiency cannot be corrected by oral iron in adequate doses, and careful search has failed to reveal any evidence of blood loss, malabsorption of iron may be suspected: this may prove to be part of a more generalized but unrecognized malabsorption syndrome (Whitehead, Carter, and Sharp, 1965). Malabsorption can be documented with certainty by means of radioactive iron absorption tests; a much less time-consuming procedure is the 'iron tolerance test' (Verloop, Meeuwissen, and Blokhuis, 1958). Serial measurements of serum iron are made after a loading test dose of iron. If iron absorption is unimpaired, a single serum iron measurement, 30 minutes or one hour after the test dose, may be sufficient to exclude malabsorption as the cause of the iron deficiency.

**Tissue Iron Deficiency.** It has been well known for many years that many of the tissue changes seen in iron-deficiency anaemia are not found in other types of anaemia of equal severity. These changes include alterations in the epithelium of the mouth and alimentary tract, which may also be seen in patients without significant anaemia, but with evidence of reduced iron stores. The severity of the symptoms in patients with iron-deficiency anaemia is frequently unrelated to the haemoglobin level, and iron treatment may be followed by marked improvement in symptoms, which precedes the eventual haemoglobin rise. Beutler (1964) reviews the evidence that the tissues may be deprived of essential iron in the absence of anaemia. In experimental animals, it was shown that a number of enzymes, particularly aconitase and cytochrome C, become very depleted in the earliest phases of iron deficiency, when haemoglobin levels are only slightly reduced. Although it has not yet been possible to relate any specific enzyme depletion in man with the symptomatology of iron deficiency, it is clear that the old-fashioned concept that enzyme iron is inviolate is not true. Anaemia may not always be the first symptom of iron deficiency, and at the present time the extent of morbidity from tissue deprivation of iron is unknown. Beutler, Larsh, and Gurney (1960) suggest that iron therapy may be of value in patients with chronic fatigue and malaise, normal haemoglobin levels, but reduced marrow iron stores.

These findings are of great interest to the paediatrician. Although we know that iron deficiency is very common in infancy and childhood, and that haemoglobin and serum iron levels are lower in infancy than in later childhood and adult life, we have no information on the extent of tissue iron deprivation in infancy and childhood, nor of its consequences. It would be of great importance to know whether the supplementation of infant foods with iron in sufficient quantities to raise the haemoglobin and serum iron levels will be accompanied by an increase in the rate of growth, or a reduction in morbidity from infections.

**The Diagnosis of Iron Deficiency.** Anaemia is the finding that most frequently alerts the paediatrician to the presence of iron deficiency, and the diagnosis normally rests on the demonstration of the presence of anaemia, and on the proof that iron deficiency is the factor limiting erythropoiesis. In most instances, a correct diagnosis can be made from the haemoglobin level, and examination of a stained peripheral blood smear, in which varying degrees of microcytosis, anisocytosis, poikilocytosis, and hypochromia are seen. In mild or early cases, estimation of the mean corpuscular volume (MCV), mean corpuscular haemoglobin (MCH), and mean corpuscular haemoglobin concentration (MCHC) may be helpful. Of these, the MCHC is the simplest, as it can be calculated from the haemoglobin level and the haematocrit, and a red cell count is not required. Normal values in childhood are approximately 32-36%, and in iron deficiency values below 30% are usually seen (Wintrobe 1961, pp. 105, 745).

There are several additional tests that may be of value in the demonstration of iron deficiency with minimal or insignificant changes in the peripheral blood, and in the differential diagnosis of hypochromic anaemia due to causes other than iron deficiency.

*Plasma iron and iron-binding capacity.* These measurements provide a very good index of the adequacy with which iron is being supplied to the marrow. In iron deficiency, plasma iron levels are low, and transferrin levels, measured by the total iron-binding capacity of the plasma, are raised. The ratio of the plasma iron to the total iron-binding capacity is expressed as the percentage saturation of the iron-binding capacity or transferrin. In iron deficiency, there is usually less than 20% saturation of the plasma transferrin, compared with 30-40% in normal subjects (Beutler, Robson, and Buttenwieser, 1958, Verloop *et al.*, 1958). On the other hand, normal or raised levels of plasma iron, with normal or reduced levels of transferrin, and high levels of transferrin saturation are characteristically found in the hypochromic anaemias due to disorders of haemoglobin synthesis in the presence of an adequate iron supply, such as thalassaemia and the sideroachrestic and pyridoxine-responsive anaemias.

*Marrow haemosiderin.* Assessment of the quantity of haemosiderin in bone-marrow reticuloendothelial cells is the most useful method to determine the adequacy of the body's iron stores. It is generally agreed that the absence of haemosiderin indicates iron depletion, whereas if haemosiderin is present, the anaemia is almost certainly not due to iron deficiency, and iron therapy will be useless or even harmful. Beutler *et al.* (1958) found that assessment of the marrow haemosiderin provided a better indication of the adequacy of the body iron stores than plasma iron or transferrin saturation. It may, therefore, be a useful test when iron deficiency is suspected in spite of normal levels of plasma iron and transferrin. It is also helpful in differentiating between iron deficiency and anaemia due to infection, where increased quantities of marrow haemosiderin may be found in association with reduced saturation of the plasma transferrin. In such patients iron therapy is of no value.

*Marrow sideroblasts and siderocytes.* When the marrow normoblasts and reticulocytes are stained for iron, one or more aggregates of ferritin may be seen as small particles. In iron deficiency, these siderotic granules are absent, and in conditions such as thalassaemia, where hypochromic red cells are the result of a block in haem synthesis, siderotic granules are present in increased numbers. From a practical point of view, enough material for examination can frequently be obtained from the buffy coat of the peripheral blood, particularly in anaemia associated with a hyperplastic bone-marrow (Bothwell and Finch, 1962, p. 331).

Determinations of plasma iron and iron-binding capacity, marrow haemosiderin, and sideroblast and siderocyte iron, may be of help in documenting the presence of iron deficiency when blood counts are within normal limits, or when anaemia is due to infection rather than iron deficiency. They will also lead the clinician to suspect the correct diagnosis when hypochromic anaemia is due to a block in haem synthesis rather than to iron deficiency. The possibility of thalassaemia should always be considered when hypochromic anaemia fails to respond to iron treatment. This disease is seen increasingly in England, and in addition to cases arising in immigrants of Mediterranean origin, examples of homozygous and heterozygous thalassaemia have now been described in subjects of Anglo-Saxon stock (Lloyd and Brown, 1964). When the disease is suspected on clinical grounds, a diagnosis may be made by the demonstration of a marked increase in alkali-resistant haemoglobin.

There are a number of other rare causes of refractory hypochromic anaemia, all of which can be distinguished from iron deficiency on the basis of these tests. Of these the least uncommon are the sideroachrestic anaemias, which include the pyridoxine-responsive anaemias. These anaemias also seem to be due to a block in haemoglobin synthesis in the presence of adequate or excess iron (Bourne, Elves, and Israëls, 1965; MacGibbon and Mollin, 1965). Very rarely, hypochromic anaemia may be due to a defect in iron transport to the developing erythroblasts. A case of congenital absence of plasma transferrin has been described (Heilmeyer, Keller, Vivell, Keiderling, Betke, Wöhler, and Schultze, 1961); in another study, there was evidence of impaired transport of iron to the marrow in the presence of normal transferrin levels (Shahidi, Nathan, and Diamond, 1964).

### The Treatment of Iron-deficiency Anaemia

The basis of iron therapy is to supply optimal amounts of iron to the marrow while avoiding toxic reactions. A wide variety of suitable oral and parenteral preparations are available for this purpose. When the degree of anaemia is life-threatening, transfusion may be needed, usually when iron deficiency is complicated by continuing blood loss which exceeds the regenerative capacity of the marrow. Transfusion is not often required in iron deficiency when active bleeding is not present, as the regenerative capacity of the marrow in infancy and childhood is very great. In these patients oral or parenteral iron is frequently followed by a rapid increase in haemoglobin level.

**Oral Iron Therapy**. In trying to formulate a rational basis for the use of oral iron, it is of interest to consider the maximum amount of iron which the marrow can handle in a state of blood regeneration from the stimulus of anaemia. Experiments using phlebotomy or ferrokinetics, and observations of the rate of response in patients under treatment, suggest that the optimal iron requirement varies between 0·3 mg. and 0·8 mg. per kg. body weight daily (Finch, Haskins, and Finch, 1950; Coleman, Stevens, Dodge, and Finch, 1953; Giblett, Coleman, Pirzio-Biroli, Donohue, Motulsky, and Finch, 1956). Sufficient iron must be given to ensure that at least these quantities are absorbed. Iron salts have been shown to be well absorbed in iron deficiency (Bothwell *et al.*, 1958; Callender, 1964), but allowance must be made for wide individual variations. Thus Callender (1964) found that 19 adults with iron deficiency absorbed between 14 and 94% of a dose of 5 mg. of iron as ferrous sulphate, and Riley (1960) obtained levels of absorption of between 10 and 92% of a dose of 30 mg. of iron as ferrous sulphate in anaemic infants. Schulz and Smith (1958b) found an average of 12-15% absorption of 30 mg. ferrous iron in children. These figures suggest that dosage up to 5 mg./kg. daily may be needed to achieve an optimal erythropoietic response. As absorption of iron salts decreases in proportion to increasing dosage, and is to some extent reduced by the presence of food, it seems logical to divide the dose and administer it between meals.

The number of available oral iron preparations is perplexing. There is no doubt that ferrous salts are better absorbed than ferric salts, and it seems that ferrous sulphate is probably absorbed as well as any other. Studies have shown that the sulphate is absorbed as well as other ferrous salts, such as the succinate, gluconate, fumarate, lactate, citrate, and others (Brise and Hallberg, 1962). As ferrous sulphate is the cheapest, and apparently absorbed as well as any other, it seems to be the drug of choice, provided that it is well tolerated by the patient. Much has been written on iron intolerance, and it appears that the incidence is probably overestimated, and that psychological factors may enter into tolerance to a great extent (Girdwood, 1952; Kerr and Davidson, 1958). Children usually tolerate oral iron preparations well, unless excessive doses are given. In the event of intolerance to the sulphate a wide range of alternative tablets are available. For those unable to swallow tablets, either ferric ammonium citrate mixture BPC, or the least expensive of the proprietary preparations, such as 'Feravol Syrup', 'Fersamel Syrup', and 'Sytron elixir', (*Brit. med. J.*, 1963), should be tried.

A great variety of more complex iron preparations are available, many of which claim advantages without foundation in fact, such as increased availability of iron, decreased toxicity, or the presence of additives which are supposed to assist the patient's response to iron therapy. At the present time, there is very little published evidence to indicate that any iron compound is superior to ferrous sulphate or similar salts. Although ascorbic acid can cause an increase in iron absorption (Brise and Hallberg, 1962), ferrous salts are absorbed so well alone, that the possible advantage of the additional ascorbic acid is probably hardly worth the expense. There are also a number of iron complexes, for which advantages are claimed, which are definitely *less* well absorbed than ferrous salts. These include certain carbohydrate-bound complexes, and iron versenate (Brise and Hallberg, 1962). The use of iron compounds containing other so-called haematinics is to be condemned. Recovery in iron-deficiency anaemia is not assisted by vitamin supplements or minerals (Moore, Minnich, Vilter, and Spies, 1943), and if other specific deficiencies are present it is important to identify them rather than to obscure their presence by multiple therapy.

Oral iron therapy in adequate doses may be expected to show rapid results, with reticulocytosis within three days, and a haemoglobin response up to 0·3 g./100 ml. per day when the initial haematocrit is below 20%. Response is usually less when the initial haematocrit is higher. When the haemoglobin level has been restored to normal, iron therapy should be continued, probably for at least two to three months, in an attempt to replenish the stores.

**Parenteral Iron Therapy.** Although most cases of iron deficiency will respond to oral iron, and can be treated satisfactorily in this way, the availability of parenteral iron therapy is of great value when oral therapy is ineffective or unsuitable for any reason. It is specifically recommended when there is evidence of malabsorption of iron, and the anaemia cannot be corrected by oral therapy, or when the patient is completely unable to tolerate any kind of oral iron. It may also be necessary when there is chronic blood loss, and it proves impossible to correct the anaemia and replenish the stores by oral iron alone. A further indication may be in severely anaemic children, in whom prolonged oral therapy is needed, and the parents cannot be relied upon to follow the instructions.

If parenteral iron therapy is required, there are a number of available preparations: saccharated iron oxide and iron-dextrin are probably less suitable for use in children, as they must be given intravenously, and a number of excellent preparations are available for intramuscular use. Of these, iron-dextran (Imferon) and iron citric acid sorbitol complex (iron-sorbitol, Jectofer) are most frequently used at the present time. Both tend to cause a little aching after injection, but differ somewhat in the way in which they are handled by the body. Studies with $^{59}$Fe-labelled iron-dextran have shown that though the majority of the injected dose is rapidly used in haemoglobin synthesis, significant amounts remain at the site of injection, and are little mobilized for periods up to 100 days (Grimes and Hutt, 1957). The persistence of significant amounts at the site of injection may lead to skin staining, and it has been postulated, on the basis of animal experiments, that iron-dextran may be a local carcinogen (Richmond, 1959; Haddow and Horning, 1960). It must be stressed, however, that these results were obtained with massive doses, and there is no available evidence at the present time that the doses used in man are carcinogenic. There seems to be no good reason why the compound should not be given, if there are clear-cut indications for parenteral iron therapy.

Iron-sorbitol has overcome some of the drawbacks in the use of iron-dextran, and studies with $^{59}$Fe-labelled material (Pringle, Goldberg, Macdonald, and Johnston, 1962; Wetherley-Mein, Buchanan, Glass, and Pearce, 1962) have shown that it is also well utilized in haemoglobin synthesis and is almost completely removed from the injection site in 24 hours. As a result, skin staining is seen less frequently than with iron-dextran, and so far no carcinogenic effect has been found, even using high doses in animals (Fielding, 1962). However, it suffers from the disadvantage that about 30% of the dose is excreted in the urine which turns black on standing (Boyle, Dellipiani, Owen, Seaton, and Tonkin, 1964), due to the formation of iron sulphide. This may be disconcerting to the patient, but more serious is the apparent ability of the iron to exacerbate pyelonephritis as it passes through the kidney (Scott, 1963; Briggs, Kennedy, and Goldberg, 1963). It therefore seems unwise to use this preparation in patients with urinary tract infection. Side-effects such as headache, dizziness, nausea, and vomiting have also been observed, possibly due to the concomitant administration of oral iron preparations (Scott, 1963). It seems advisable to discontinue oral iron therapy before starting treatment with any kind of parenteral iron. It appears that iron-sorbitol and iron-dextran are both suitable for parenteral iron therapy in children. Another suitable compound may be iron polyisomaltosate (Mereu and Tonz, 1962). As a practical choice, many physicians may prefer to use iron-sorbitol, except in the presence of renal infection, until more information is available on the possible though remote risk that iron-dextran may be a local carcinogen.

These preparations all suffer from the disadvantage that repeated injections are needed. An interesting recent development is the administration of the total requirement of iron in a single intravenous dose (Marchasin and Wallerstein, 1964). In Great Britain there are a number of reports of the administration of 25-35 ml. of iron-dextran by slow intravenous infusion in 500-1,000 ml. 5% glucose or normal saline in pregnant women with severe iron-deficiency anaemia (Basu, 1963; Powell, 1963). Although serious reactions to this form of treatment were noted in one study (Clay, Rosenberg, Sampson, and Samuels, 1965), this has not been the experience in a number of other centres, where total-dose-infusions of iron-dextran have been given safely (Goldthorp, Spencer, and Dawson, 1965). Further experience is needed, but if this form of therapy is found to be free from serious side-effects, total-dose-infusion of iron might be a welcome alternative to long courses of intramuscular injections in severely anaemic children.

### Toxic Effects of Excess Iron

It is well known that an excess of iron in the

tissues is toxic. Acute poisoning with iron salts is common in infancy, and if enough is ingested may lead to death within a short period. The toxic effects of chronic iron deposition in the tissues have been recognized for many years in idiopathic haemochromatosis, and more recently in transfusion haemosiderosis. Iron overload is seen more frequently in children, now that improved medical care and blood transfusions have prolonged survival in conditions such as thalassaemia, and the hypoplastic and aplastic anaemias.

**Iron-chelating Agents.** Until recently there was no specific therapy for acute iron poisoning, or chronic iron overload. However, the advent of repeated venesection therapy for haemochromatosis showed that large quantities or iron could be mobilized, even after many years' storage in the tissues. This finding suggested that chelating agents might be used as an alternative method to bind and remove excess iron. Suitable chelating agents might be expected to render harmless unabsorbed iron in the gut and excess circulating iron in the blood and tissues in acute iron poisoning, and mobilize excess stored iron in conditions of chronic iron overload. However, the use of iron-chelating agents raises many problems. Iron, unlike toxic substances such as lead which are present in relatively small amounts, is a physiological substance; the quantities that cause toxicity, and which therefore must be bound and removed to achieve a useful therapeutic effect, are massive. Suitable chelating agents must therefore be non-toxic even when given in very large doses; they must have a high affinity for iron, yet their affinity for essential substances such as calcium and magnesium must be low enough to prevent significant depletion of these substances during therapy. On the other hand, the chelating agent should not interfere with the normal process of iron metabolism by removal of iron from haemoglobin or essential enzymes, or inhibit haemoglobin synthesis by removal of essential iron from the plasma transferrin or developing erythroblasts.

Some iron can be mobilized and removed by the use of ethylenediaminetetra-acetic acid (EDTA) or British-anti-Lewisite (Ohlsson, Kullendorff, and Ljungberg, 1953; Seven, Gottlieb, Israel, Reinhold, and Rubin, 1954). The limited quantities of iron removed, combined with possible side-effects of long-term administration, suggest that these substances are of little value in the treatment of chronic iron overload, although EDTA may be of therapeutic value in acute iron poisoning (Covey, 1964). In recent years three new chelating agents have been developed, which have been shown to be much more effective in the removal of iron from the body. Two of these are synthetic substances: ethylenediamine di-ortho-hydroxyphenyl acetic acid (EDDHA) (Korman, 1960), and trisodium calcium diethylene-triaminepenta-acetate (DTPA) (Fahey, Rath, Princiotto, Brick, and Rubin, 1961). Early experiences with these substances showed that up to 100 mg. of iron could be removed from patients with iron storage by a single infusion of either substance (Cleton, Noyes, Turnbull, and Finch, 1961; Fahey *et al.*, 1961).

A different kind of iron-chelating agent was prepared by removing iron from the highly stable iron-chelate ferrioxamine which was isolated from *Streptomyces pilosus*. The iron-free substance, desferrioxamine, was found to have a very high affinity for iron but not for any other metals or the alkaline earths. One molecule of desferrioxamine combines with a single atom of trivalent iron: 9·3 mg. of iron can theoretically combine with 100 mg. of desferrioxamine (Vischer, 1961). *In vitro* studies showed that desferrioxamine was capable of removing iron from haemosiderin and ferritin, the main iron storage complexes, and administration to iron-laden animals and patients was followed by mobilization and excretion of iron without any interference with erythropoiesis, or depletion of essential substances (Wöhler, 1961). After parenteral administration, it seems that desferrioxamine combines with stored iron, after which it circulates as ferrioxamine until removed by excretion through the kidney. This takes place rapidly during the first 6 hours after administration and is virtually complete in 24 hours (Nielsen, 1963).

Desferrioxamine, DTPA, and EDDHA, all have a much higher affinity for iron than the earlier chelating agents. There have been no further reports on the use of EDDHA, but desferrioxamine has now been successfully used in the treatment of iron poisoning, and both desferrioxamine and DTPA have given promising results in the management of chronic iron storage in adults and children.

**Acute Iron Poisoning.** Iron is one of the most important causes of accidental poisoning in Great Britain. This is probably because iron deficiency is common, and many oral iron preparations are presented as attractively coloured tablets, similar to some of the most popular brands of sweets. The clinical course is often severe, characterized by vomiting, gastro-intestinal bleeding, and peripheral vascular collapse, followed by severe shock, with cyanosis, lethargy, and restlessness. Vigorous supportive therapy may lead to improvement, but subsequent relapse several hours or one to two days later is not uncommon. The mortality rate approaches 50%, and some of the children who recover face the prospect of scarring, leading to stricture of the stomach, and pyloric stenosis (Ross, 1953; Shepherd, 1955; Jacobziner and Raybin, 1962). The lower limit of the toxic dose of iron in children is not known, but severe symptoms were seen in a 2-year-old boy who ingested only eight 0·3 g. ferrous sulphate tablets (Jacobziner and Raybin, 1962), while death from late sequelae occurred in one child who may have ingested as few as six tablets (Ross, 1953). It therefore seems wise to institute appropriate therapy, unless it is known with absolute certainty that not more than two or three tablets have been ingested.

*Immediate treatment.* Attempts should be made to induce vomiting, and to delay any further absorption of iron by reducing its solubility. For this purpose, sodium bicarbonate, eggs, and milk may be helpful. Gastric lavage should be carried out as soon as possible, and the stomach irrigated with sodium bicarbonate solution. For this purpose a wide-bore tube should be used if possible, in order to aspirate any undissolved tablets.

*Supportive measures.* Shock needs urgent therapy, and the serum electrolytes, especially bicarbonate, should be determined. Alterations in acid-base balance should be corrected by intravenous fluids, and oxygen therapy may be needed.

*Specific therapy: chelation of iron.* This has a twofold aim: first, to prevent further absorption by binding any residual iron in the gastro-intestinal tract, and secondly, to chelate the excess iron in the plasma and tissues so that it is converted into a non-toxic form which can be excreted rapidly. Desferrioxamine was suggested for this purpose by Moeschlin and Schnider (1963) on the basis of animal studies. Henderson, Vietti, and Brown (1963) describe the treatment of a 14½-month-old infant who had ingested a large quantity of ferrous gluconate tablets. 5 g. desferrioxamine were given through a naso-gastric tube, together with 800 mg. intravenously: further intravenous doses of 800 mg. were given 12 and 24 hours later. Clinical improvement was marked, and the serum iron, which had initially been 2,500 μg. per 100 ml., fell within 5 hours to a normal level; 25 mg. of iron were excreted in the urine. Desferrioxamine has also been used successfully in the treatment of iron poisoning by Powell and Dugdale (1964) and Whitten, Gibson, Good, and Goodwin (1964). In the latter study, 13 children who had ingested varying amounts of iron were treated, and all survived. However, hypotensive attacks were noted when some of the children were given intravenous desferrioxamine in doses up to 1·5 g. in 15 minutes or less. This type of side-effect has not been seen after intramuscular injection, or when slow intravenous infusion is used.

Although the clinical reports are few so far, it seems that desferrioxamine has a valuable and possibly life-saving role in the management of iron poisoning. Treatment with desferrioxamine should be instituted without delay, using both the oral and parenteral routes. After gastric lavage, 5 g. desferrioxamine should be introduced into the stomach. This can be dissolved in as little as 20 ml. of water, and is enough to bind over 400 mg. iron, or the amount contained in 10-12 ferrous sulphate tablets. The dose of oral desferrioxamine may possibly be increased if there is reason to believe that more than this amount remains in the stomach, but at present it is not known whether any adverse effect results from the administration of larger quantities by mouth. Desferrioxamine should also be given parenterally: rapid intravenous injections should be avoided and the drug administered intramuscularly, or by slow intravenous infusion, or by both methods in combination. It is known that desferrioxamine is rapidly absorbed after intramuscular injections, though the rate may be lower in children with severe peripheral circulatory collapse. Accordingly, 2 g. desferrioxamine should be given intramuscularly without delay, supplemented by intravenous administration of a further amount, which should not exceed 15 mg./kg. hour, or a maximum of 80 mg./kg. in 24 hours. In the event of relapse, additional intramuscular injections of 2 g. desferrioxamine can be given at 12-hourly intervals. It is possible that these dosages will need modification in the light of experience and that it will prove perfectly safe to give much larger amounts of desferrioxamine by the intravenous route. Experience in the use of desferrioxamine in children with chronic iron overload (Smith, 1964b) has shown that much larger amounts can be given to small children without side-effects, provided that they are infused slowly.

The reports of its successful use, and the fact that it is readily available in Great Britain, suggest that desferrioxamine (Desferal) is at the present time the specific chelating agent of choice in the treatment of acute iron poisoning. The drug should be available at general and children's hospitals and poison centres throughout the country, so that there is no delay in its use when indicated. As an alternative, EDTA or DTPA might be used if they are readily available in the absence of desferrioxamine. Other methods of removing iron from the body that have been tried in iron poisoning include peritoneal dialysis (Covey, 1964) and exchange transfusion (Amerman, Brescia, and Aftahi, 1958; Jacobziner and Raybin, 1962). Although some iron is removed by either of these methods, the amounts are much smaller than can be achieved by the use of desferrioxamine, which also has the important advantage that it forms a non-toxic chelate with the iron. It is doubtful whether these measures now have any place in the management of acute iron poisoning.

**Chronic Iron Overload.**

Repeated blood transfusion over many years leads to a progressive deposition of iron in children with thalassaemia, congenital pure red cell aplasia, and some hypoplastic, aplastic, and haemolytic anaemias. Many of these anaemic children also absorb iron through the intestinal tract in increased amounts. Although these children may tolerate the deposition of large quantities of iron for many years without ill effect, impairment of organ function is eventually seen, leading to death from cardiac or hepatic failure.

**Pathogenesis.** The quantity of iron accumulated through blood transfusion is more readily assessed than that absorbed from food. Although it is frequently stated that a bottle of blood contains 250 mg. iron, the haemoglobin level and amount transfused from a single bottle suggest that a more realistic figure is 200 mg. In a study of the amount transfused to 18 children with thalassaemia or pure red cell aplasia, varying between 3 and 15 years of age (Smith, 1964b), it was found that the daily iron gain from transfused red cells varied between 2·2 and 17·0 mg. per day, or 0·73 to 6·2 g. per year. Most of the children over 5 years were shown to be accumulating about 3 to 4 g. or iron per year from transfusions. The massive quantity of iron accumulated is at once apparent: in comparison with a normal adult's iron stores of about 1 g., many of these children, if transfused from early infancy, will accumulate between 50 and 200 g. of iron from blood transfusions, by the time they reach adult life.

An additional quantity of iron will inevitably be absorbed through the intestinal tract from food. Although there are many studies suggesting that iron absorption is reduced in the presence of iron loading, these children always show some degree of anaemia, and many have hyperplastic bone-marrows, both of which factors might be expected to increase iron absorption. Several recent studies suggest that many iron-laden anaemic patients have increased absorption of iron. Robertson, Maxwell, and Elliott (1963) found increased absorption of small doses of ferric chloride in children with thalassaemia, all of whom had been repeatedly transfused and showed evidence of iron overload. Erlandson, Walden Stern, Hilgartner, Wehman, and Smith (1962) measured the absorption of a dose of 5 mg. of iron as ferrous sulphate in 19 anaemic children with thalassaemia or sickle-cell disease. A mean absorption of 45% was found, compared with 14% in the control group. On the other hand, when the absorption of 5 mg. of iron as haemoglobin was studied by Bannerman *et al.* (1964), it was found that most of the thalassaemic children absorbed less iron than the control group. Anaemic patients with hypoplastic bone-marrows may also absorb more iron than normal controls (Schiffer *et al.*, 1965). It has been further demonstrated that the increased iron absorption found in these anaemic patients can be reduced to levels approaching normal when the patient's haemoglobin level is raised by transfusion; this has been demonstrated in anaemic patients with both hypoplastic and hyperplastic bone-marrows (Erlandson *et al.*, 1962; Schiffer *et al.*, 1965). The available evidence suggests that anaemia, whether associated with a hyperplastic or hypoplastic bone-marrow, is frequently associated with increased absorption of inorganic iron, even in the presence of iron loading. Absorption is reduced when the haemoglobin level is raised by transfusion, but even then some absorption of iron persists.

The absorption of haemoglobin iron on the other hand may be reduced in anaemic children with iron loading. It may be concluded that these children will accumulate significant amounts of iron from food over the years, though it is not possible to assess the amount of iron absorbed daily on the basis of these studies. The finding that it is *inorganic* iron that is absorbed most avidly by these children suggests that iron-enriched cereal foods may contribute more to their load than foods containing iron-porphyrin complexes, such as meat or liver. However, it is possible that 1 g. of iron or more might be absorbed from food each year, particularly by the older children, fed a normal diet including the usual iron-enriched foods.

It can be seen that many of these anaemic children accumulate iron from transfusions and alimentary absorption at a rate of 5 g. or more yearly, of which the greater proportion is derived from transfusions. If fewer transfusions are given, the amount absorbed from food will increase. In assessing the net iron gain, allowance must be made for any loss of iron from the body. It is not known how much iron is excreted by these children: a single observation in an adult with transfusion haemosiderosis indicated a daily iron loss of 4 mg. (Crosby *et al.*, 1963). This increased iron loss is probably mainly derived from the increased iron content of desquamated cells and secretions: children might be expected to lose less, in proportion to their size, and on this basis we may conjecture that they lose amounts up to 20 mg./kg. year. If this is so, the rate of iron deposition will be reduced by less than 20% as a result of iron loss.

It is of interest to speculate why some of these children, who develop a load of over 50 g. of iron, mostly from transfusions, show minimal evidence of impaired organ function. In contrast to this, patients with idiopathic haemochromatosis, where the iron load is derived from alimentary absorption, may show evidence of damage to the liver and pancreas, when the total amount of excess iron in the body is less than 20 g. It has been suggested that iron derived from transfused red cells is less toxic to the tissues than iron absorbed from the intestine. It is certainly true that the initial handling is different: in conditions associated with iron storage, iron from transfused red cells is deposited in reticuloendothelial cells and may remain there for long periods, whereas iron absorbed through the intestinal mucosa gains immediate access into the plasma, and a high proportion finds its way into the parenchyma of organs such as the liver. This difference in handling is reflected in the pathological findings. In haemochromatosis, the deposition of iron is mostly parenchymal, and hepatic cirrhosis is present. A similar pattern of iron deposition with cirrhosis may be seen in thalassaemia (Witzleben and Wyatt, 1961; Fink, 1964). Intestinal absorption clearly makes a significant contribution to the deposition of iron in this disease, especially when transfusions are given only infrequently, and cases have been reported where more iron was found at necropsy than could be accounted for by transfusion (Ellis, Schulman, and Smith, 1954).

On the other hand, in patients who have received numerous transfusions, the deposition of iron is predominantly in the reticuloendothelial system, and cirrhosis is less frequently seen. Cappell, Hutchison, and Jowett (1957) showed extensive iron deposition, which was predominantly reticuloendothelial in distribution, but no cirrhosis, in a number of patients who had received multiple transfusions, including 2 patients in whom over 50 g. of iron were found in the liver alone. Oliver (1959) found that cirrhosis was the accompaniment of iron deposition most frequently in patients with disorders associated with a hyperplastic bone-marrow, who might be expected to have parenchymal iron deposition from increased intestinal absorption. However, impaired organ function and cirrhosis were found in a number of patients with aplastic bone-marrows, who had received over 30 g. of iron in transfusions.

It is difficult to escape the conclusion that even though red-cell iron may be deposited initially in the reticuloendothelial system, redistribution of iron with eventual parenchymal damage to vital organs must occur. The time taken by this process may well vary in different patients, and it is possible that marrow hyperplasia with an associated rapid plasma iron turnover may hasten parenchymal damage by speeding the redistribution of reticuloendothelial iron as well as enhancing intestinal absorption. If so, the child with erythroid aplasia should be able to tolerate the greatest iron load before the inevitable redistribution of iron and parenchymal organ damage is seen.

**Therapy.** Until recently, attempts to remove significant amounts of iron from the body have been unsuccessful, and the management of these patients has consisted in restricting the amount transfused to the lowest possible limit, in order to delay the ultimate inevitable onset of organ damage. Pancreatic involvement is not seen as frequently as in idiopathic haemochromatosis, and when diabetes occurs it can be treated with insulin. Cardiac and hepatic failure are more common, and usually lead to death within a few months (Witzleben and Wyatt, 1961; Engle, 1964).

*Removal of stored iron by chelating agents.* There is now a wealth of evidence showing that significant amounts of iron can be removed from patients with iron overload by the use of desferrioxamine or DTPA. Parenteral administration is essential: oral doses of desferrioxamine or DTPA produced no significant level of iron excretion in four heavily iron-laden patients, all of whom showed marked iron excretion when the drugs were given parenterally Bannerman, Callender, and Williams, 1962; Smith, 1964b). The intravenous and intramuscular routes have been used successfully with both drugs.

*Intravenous route.* In the earliest studies with DTPA (Fahey *et al.*, 1961), adults with iron-storage disease were given intravenous infusions of 2·4-4 g., after which up to 100 mg. of iron was excreted in the urine. Robertson *et al.* (1963) used infusions of 60-80 mg. DTPA/kg. body weight in thalassaemic children, which removed up to 33 mg. of iron. In most of the studies with intravenous desferrioxamine, lower doses have been used; in a large number of observations on the treatment of adults with haemochromatosis, and of adults and children with transfusion haemosiderosis, infusions of 0·2-1·2 g. of desferrioxamine were used, with a maximum excretion of 40 mg. of iron (Wöhler, 1961, 1963; Smith, 1962). The effects of intravenous infusions of equal doses of desferrioxamine and DTPA were compared in iron-laden children with thalassaemia or pure red cell aplasia (Smith, 1964b); it was found that infusions of 1 or 2 g. of desferrioxamine or DTPA were followed by comparable levels of iron excretion, with an average of 20-25 mg. of iron excreted per g. of chelating agent administered. However, when doses of 3-6 g. were studied in three of the most heavily iron-laden children, it was found that in two of the three, the excretion of iron following desferrioxamine did not exceed the level achieved on a dose of 2 g., while 100-230 mg. of iron were removed after doses of 4-6 g. DTPA. In this study, the chelating agents were given at the time of blood transfusion, the dose being divided and mixed in the blood or sedimented red cells: though doses up to 180 mg./kg. of desferrioxamine or DTPA were given, the dose rate was never higher than 20 mg./kg. hour. No toxic effects were observed with either drug when given in this way.

*Intramuscular route.* There are a number of studies in which patients have received intramuscular or subcutaneous injections of 0·4-1·2 g. of desferrioxamine daily. In this dose range, the quantity of iron removed is about the same whether the intravenous or intramuscular route is used (Bannerman *et al.*, 1962; Wöhler, 1963; Norman, 1964; Smith, 1964b). When given daily the average amount of iron excreted may be slightly less, but may reach an impressive total amount, over a period of weeks, months, or years. For example, Wöhler (1963) reported that a 4-year-old boy with congenital pure red cell aplasia excreted 12-14 mg. or iron daily during a 7-month period of treatment, which would amount to the removal of 4 g. of iron from the body in a year. Moeschlin and Schnider (1963) treated an 8-year-old boy with thalassaemia with daily desferrioxamine injections for two months, and then with intermittent courses; in a little over 6 months, 675 mg. of iron were removed. Over a period of three months, iron excretion levels averaging 10 mg. a day were found in several heavy iron-laden children with red-cell aplasia or thalassaemia, when treated by daily injections of 0·5 g. desferrioxamine. If continued, this would amount to the removal of about 3·5 g. of iron in one year (Smith, 1964b).

It seems possible that very large amounts of iron can be removed from some patients by prolonged desferrioxamine treatment over many months or possibly years. In the treatment of adults with haemochromatosis, using larger intramuscular doses, quantities of iron up to 18 g. have been removed in little over a year (Heilmeyer and Wöhler, 1963). No toxic effects have yet been noted in patients following prolonged administration of desferrioxamine, and the injections are not painful, even when long courses are given.

DTPA can also be given by intramuscular injection, but has several important disadvantages. The injections are very painful (Robertson *et al.*, 1963) unless mixed with procaine. Although DTPA was given on alternate days to one patient for a period of 17 days without ill effects (Fahey *et al.*, 1961), long-term studies with this drug have not been made. Heilmeyer and Wöhler (1963) state that DTPA is too toxic for long-term use, and the studies of Muller-Eberhard, Erlandson, Ginn, and Smith (1963) showed that administration of DTPA to thalassaemic children was followed by a marked increase in the amount of magnesium in the urine, accompanied by a significant fall in the serum magnesium levels. It appears wise to limit the use of this drug to intermittent infusions.

*Choice of drug and route of administration.* It can be seen from these reports that it is possible to remove significant amounts of iron from the body by the use of either intravenous infusions or intramuscular injections of chelating agents. If treatment is to be effective, we must aim to remove from the body an amount of iron equalling or preferably exceeding the rate of accumulation; this amounts to 5 g. a year or even more in many cases. Available reports suggest that on average not much more than 20 mg. of iron is removed by each g. of chelating agent, irrespective of the route of administration, and this means that 250 g. of chelating agent must be given to remove 5 g. of iron. We must, therefore, select a plan of therapy that enables amounts of this order to be administered without causing toxicity, and with a minimum of discomfort to the child. 3-4 g. of iron a year can probably be removed from many of these children by a daily injection of 0·5 g. of desferrioxamine. This amount can be dissolved in 2 ml. of water with the formation of an isotonic solution, which can be injected painlessly without any local side-effects by the subcutaneous route. It is possible that the rate of iron removal could be increased by using larger doses, or by giving two doses daily instead of one. Wöhler (1963) has reported the use of 1·2 g. desferrioxamine daily in an adult for over a year, and 0·6 g. daily in a 4-year-old boy with red-cell aplasia.

As an alternative or supplement to prolonged courses of injections, intravenous infusion should be considered. A single infusion of desferrioxamine or DTPA may remove as much iron as 20 injections; unfortunately many of these children are the most difficult of subjects for repeated intravenous work, and furthermore slow infusions require hospitalization, at least for the day. Most of these children, however, receive periodic blood transfusions, and this procedure provides a useful opportunity for the administration of a large therapeutic dose of a chelating agent. For this purpose DTPA was found superior, and on some occasions infusions of 4 or 6 g. of DTPA removed over 200 mg. of iron (Smith, 1964b). If iron can be removed regularly at this rate, 1-2 g. of iron can be removed each year by this means, depending on the frequency of transfusion. As transfusions are widely spaced in time, the possibility of magnesium depletion from the large dose of DTPA used seems to be remote. If this scheme of therapy is chosen, it seems wise to begin with to give alternate doses of desferrioxamine or DTPA at successive transfusions, increasing the dose progressively. On the basis of the figures of iron output obtained, a logical choice of drug and dose can be made.

It seems that intravenous and intramuscular therapy can be combined; it was found that desferrioxamine injections could be resumed, with continuing output of iron, only 48 hours after a large infusion of desferrioxamine or DTPA had been given, which had removed over 200 mg. of iron from the body (R. S. Smith, 1965, unpublished observations). One patient, a 14-year-old girl with thalassaemia, and another 14-year-old boy with pure red-cell aplasia, had been trained to dissolve the drug and give themselves their own injections at home.

*Selection of patients for treatment.* It has been found that significant levels of iron excretion following chelating agents are only achieved in patients with evidence of iron deposition. In practice, it seems that useful levels of iron output can usually only be achieved in children who have received repeated transfusions for 4 years or longer (Muller-Eberhard *et al.*, 1963; Smith, 1964b). Infants with thalassaemia who had never been transfused excreted less than 2 mg. of iron after an infusion of 1 g. of desferrioxamine or DTPA. It therefore seems unlikely that iron-loading can be prevented by the prophylactic administration of chelating agents. In selecting patients for treatment, the simplest practical measure is to administer a test dose, either intramuscularly or intravenously, and measure the iron output. This might be given by infusion when the child is receiving a blood transfusion, or as an intramuscular dose. As the iron chelate is mostly excreted in the first few hours after the dose (Nielsen, 1963), collection of urine for 6 hours is adequate. The quantity removed will indicate whether a worth-while output of iron will be achieved on continuous treatment. It may be useful to study the effect of a test dose of desferrioxamine at yearly intervals in children receiving regular blood transfusions, in order to ascertain the point at which useful therapy can be begun.

The collection of urine for 6 hours after an intramuscular injection of desferrioxamine is a simple and safe procedure that can be readily carried out on out-patients. In addition to the selection of patients for treatment with chelating agents, such a test may be of value in determining the presence of increased iron stores in children with refractory or haemolytic anaemia, or in the sons of men with haemochromatosis.

*Results of therapy.* The amount of iron removed can be determined from the iron content of the urine. For this purpose, wet-ashing is not necessary, and simple colorimetric methods can be used (Bannerman *et al.*, 1962; Smith, 1962; CIBA, 1964). The patient and nurses should not be alarmed if the urine becomes red-brown after desferrioxamine, as this is due to the colour of ferrioxamine: the iron-chelate formed with DTPA is colourless. When children are receiving daily injections of desferrioxamine at home, 24-hour daily urine collections may be impracticable: in these patients the rate of iron removal can be estimated from one or more 24-hour collections at intervals, always beginning immediately after an injection.

In measuring iron excretion great care must be taken that all urinals, bedpans, and specimen bottles are iron free. The plastic bags and tubes used to collect urine from infants should be tested: in one study they were found to be free of iron (Smith, 1962).

It is not yet known to what extent these iron-laden children will benefit from the removal of iron. It is well known that many of the signs and symptoms of haemochromatosis improve after venesection: removal of iron by means of chelating agents might be expected to give similar results. During treatments there is often subjective improvement and reduction in pigmentation; improvements in plasma protein levels and liver function tests have also been noted. In one patient with thalassaemia, from whom 14 g. of iron were removed by desferrioxamine therapy, liver biopsies before and after treatment showed that almost all the liver iron had been mobilized (Wöhler, 1963). Not infrequently these children show only minimal alterations in plasma proteins and liver function tests, even when there is massive iron loading, until abrupt deterioration occurs at termination (Witzleben and Wyatt, 1961). It may, therefore, only be possible to assess the therapeutic value of chelating agents in terms of prolonged survival and decreased morbidity resulting from long-term therapy. Serum iron levels may be expected to remain high until a large proportion of the excess stored iron has been removed. It is possible, however, that the removal of even small quantities of iron may be of benefit, even if the total amount of iron in the body is only slightly reduced. It is evident that many of these children can tolerate a very large excess of iron for prolonged periods: the improvements that have followed the removal of relatively small amounts of iron suggest that desferrioxamine may perferentially remove iron from areas where it exerts its most toxic effects.

An important additional benefit has been seen in patients with sideroachrestic anaemia, where removal of iron by desferrioxamine has been accompanied by an increase in the haemoglobin level, and a decrease in red-cell and urine porphyrins. It has been postulated that this is due to removal from the bone-marrow of the excess iron which blocks some of the enzymes involved in haem synthesis (Wöhler, 1963). Steiner, Baldini, and Damashek (1964) also found a decrease in marrow non-haem iron, and an increased activity of haem-synthesizing enzymes in a patient with thalassaemia, treated by desferrioxamine. The possibility may, therefore, exist that increased erythropoiesis and a decrease in transfusion requirements might result in thalassaemia, if enough iron could be removed.

*Control of iron absorption and accumulation.* The rate of iron accumulation would be significantly reduced if alimentary absorption could be prevented. Wöhler (1963) suggested that desferrioxamine should also be given routinely by mouth to block iron absorption in patients with iron overload, but recent studies cast doubts on the usefulness of this measure. Although desferrioxamine will block the absorption of inorganic iron, it does not reduce the absorption of iron incorporated in haemoglobin, or in chicken liver or meat (Bannerman and Malpas, 1965; Hwang and Brown, 1965). Furthermore, although it has been shown that desferrioxamine will block the absorption of a test dose of inorganic iron, studies have not yet been made of its effect on the absorption of the inorganic iron in a meal. It is possible that the effect of desferrioxamine in this situation might be influenced by the bulk of the meal, or by the presence of other substances in food. As the absorption of tightly-complexed organic food iron is not influenced by desferrioxamine, and its effect on the absorption of the inorganic part of food iron is not yet known, it seems unjustified at the present time to administer large doses of this expensive drug by mouth for this purpose.

It is also possible that the absorption of food iron might be reduced by the use of pancreatic extracts. It has been shown that the absorption of both inorganic iron and iron-porphyrin is reduced in the presence of pancreatin (Biggs and Davis, 1963; Callender and Malpas, 1963). It is not yet known whether this effect of pancreatin is due to a single enzyme: if so, the appropriate factor might be given in concentrated form as an alternative to the rather bulky preparations of whole pancreas.

Attention might profitably be directed to ways in which the iron intake might be reduced by restriction of the dietary iron content. Comparison of the available data suggests that thalassaemic children absorb inorganic iron to a much greater extent than porphyrin-iron (Erlandson *et al.*, 1962; Robertson *et al.*, 1963; Bannerman *et al.*, 1964). It therefore seems possible that the inorganic part of food iron may contribute far more to the iron load than the tightly-complexed iron in meat. Much of the inorganic iron in food consists of iron salts added in the fortification of flour and cereals, and it may be of value to explore the possibility of feeding these children with suitable flour and cereal products which have not been enriched with iron. In addition, it is evident that the iron load in these children will increase rapidly when unwary physicians prescribe iron for them. It is of great importance that long-term treatment with iron should only be given when it is certain that the anaemia is due to iron deficiency.

There is also good evidence that the amount of iron absorbed is less when anaemic patients are transfused (Erlandson *et al.*, 1962; Schiffer *et al.*, 1965). This appears to be due to the correction of the anaemia, and also in some patients to the decrease in erythropoiesis which follows transfusion. The practice of restricting transfusion to a minimum may, therefore, contribute to an increase in alimentary iron absorption, although the accumulation of iron from transfused blood will be reduced. In most instances the quantity of iron accumulated through transfusions is greater, but the possibility remains that iron absorbed from the intestine may be more harmful, due to immediate parenchymal deposition. These anaemic children may also grow and develop more rapidly, and have fewer infections, if maintained at a minimum haemoglobin level of 8 g./100 ml. by frequent transfusions (Wolman, 1964). Now that the consequent increased iron deposition can be treated by the use of chelating agents, it seems possible that the advantages of maintaining a high minimum haemoglobin level may outweigh the disadvantages.

In conclusion, it is evident that iron overload can now be treated by the removal of excess iron with chelating agents. To be successful, this needs massive doses, and most probably a schedule involving daily injections. This seems well worth while in patients with marked iron loading, where some subjective and objective improvement, and possibly prolonged survival, may be expected. It has not yet been shown that prophylactic administration of chelating agents is of any value in preventing iron accumulation, though the effect of desferrioxamine on haem synthesis in some refractory anaemias deserves further study, and effective means have still to be found to block the absorption of food iron. Useful as they are, it is to be hoped that the existing chelating agents will eventually be supplemented by others that can be given by mouth.

Part of this work was carried out during tenure of a Research Fellowship supported by the Joint Research Board of the Institute of Child Health, London University, and The Hospital for Sick Children, Great Ormond Street, London.

## References

Amerman, E. E., Brescia, M. A., and Aftahi, F. (1958). Ferrous sulfate poisoning. *J. Pediat.*, **53**, 476.
Ascham, L., Speirs, M., and Maddox, D. (1938). The availability of iron in various foods. *J. Nutr.*, **16**, 425.
Badenoch, J., and Callender, S. T. (1954). Iron metabolism in steatorrhea. The use of radioactive iron in studies of absorption and utilization. *Blood*, **9**, 123.
——, and —— (1960). Effect of corticosteroids and gluten-free diet on absorption of iron in idiopathic steatorrhoea and coeliac disease. *Lancet*, **1**, 192.
Baird, I. McL., Podmore, D. A., and Wilson, G. M. (1957). Changes in iron metabolism following gastrectomy and other surgical operations. *Clin. Sci.*, **16**, 463.
Bannerman, R. M., Callender, S. T., Hardisty, R. M., and Smith, R. S. (1964). Iron absorption in thalassaemia. *Brit. J. Haemat.*, **10**, 490.
——, ——, and Williams, D. L. (1962). Effect of desferrioxamine and D.T.P.A. in iron overload. *Brit. med. J.*, **2**, 1573.
——, and Malpas, J. S. (1965). Studies on desferrioxamine in relation to the absorption of iron. *Brit. J. Haemat.*, **11**, 15.
Basu, S. K. (1963). Rapid administration of iron-dextran in late pregnancy. *Lancet*, **1**, 1430.
Bergeim, O., and Kirsch, E. R. (1949). Reduction of iron in the human stomach. *J. biol. Chem.*, **177**, 591.
Beutler, E. (1964). Tissue effects of iron deficiency. In *Iron Metabolism, an International Symposium*, ed. F. Gross. Springer, Berlin.
——, Larsh, S. E., and Gurney, C. W. (1960). Iron therapy in chronically fatigued, nonanemic women: a double-blind study. *Ann. intern. Med.*, **52**, 378.
——, Robson, M. J., and Buttenwieser, E. (1958). A comparison of the plasma iron, iron-binding capacity, sternal marrow iron and other methods in the chemical evaluation of iron stores. *ibid.*, **48**, 60.
Biggs, J. C., and Davis, A. E. (1963). Relationship of diminished pancreatic secretion to haemochromatosis. *Lancet*, **2**, 814.
Bothwell, T. H., and Finch, C. A. (1962). *Iron Metabolism.* Little, Brown, Boston.
——, Pirzio-Biroli, G., and Finch, C. A. (1958). Iron absorption. I. Factors influencing absorption. *J. Lab. clin. Med.*, **51**, 24.
Bourne, M. S., Elves, M. W., and Israëls, M. C. G. (1965). Familial pyridoxine-responsive anaemia. *Brit. J. Haemat.*, **11**, 1.
Boyle, D., Dellipiani, A. W., Owen, J. A., Seaton, D. A., and Tonkin, R. W. (1964). Black urine after 'jectofer' injections. *Brit. med. J.*, **1**, 285.
Briggs, J. D., Kennedy, A. C., and Goldberg, A. (1963). Urinary white-cell excretion after iron-sorbitol-citric-acid. *ibid.*, **2**, 352.
Brise, H., and Hallberg, L. (1962). Iron absorption studies. A method for comparative studies on iron absorption in man using two radioiron isotopes. II. *Acta med. scand.*, **171**, Suppl. 376, 7.
*Brit. med. J.* (1963). To-day's drugs, Iron. Iron metabolism. **2**, 367.
Brokaw, K. F., Sedam, M. S., and Cassirer, A. M. (1942). The influence of diet on the physiologic anemia of infants. *J. Pediat.*, **21**, 769.
Brown, E. B., Jr., Dubach, R., and Moore, C. V. (1958). Studies in iron transportation and metabolism. XI. Critical analysis of mucosal block by large doses of inorganic iron in human subjects. *J. Lab. clin. Med.*, **52**, 335.
——, and Justus, B. W. (1958). *In vitro* absorption of radioiron by everted pouches of rat intestine. *Amer. J. Physiol.*, **194**, 319.
Callender, S. T. (1964). Digestive absorption of iron. In *Iron Metabolism, an International Symposium*, ed. F. Gross. Springer, Berlin.
——, and Malpas, J. S. (1963). Absorption of iron in cirrhosis of liver. *Brit. med. J.*, **2**, 1516.
Cappell, D. F., Hutchison, H. E., and Jowett, M. (1957). Transfusional siderosis: the effects of excessive iron deposits on the tissues. *J. Path. Bact.*, **74**, 245.
Cavell, P. A., and Widdowson, E. M. (1964). Intakes and excretions of iron, copper, and zinc in the neonatal period. *Arch. Dis. Childh.*, **39**, 496.
Chodos, R. B., Ross, J. F., Apt, L., Pollycove, M., and Halkett, J. A. E. (1957). The absorption of radioiron labeled foods and iron salts in normal and iron-deficient subjects and in idiopathic hemochromatosis. *J. clin. Invest.*, **36**, 314.
CIBA (1964). *Desferal. A Specific Iron Chelating Agent for the Treatment of Chronic Iron Overload, Acute Iron Poisoning and for Diagnosis.* Ciba Laboratories, Horsham.
Clay, B., Rosenberg, B., Sampson, N., and Samuels, S. I. (1965). Reactions to total dose intravenous infusion of iron dextran (imferon). *Brit. med. J.*, **1**, 29.
Cleton, F. J., Noyes, W. D., Turnbull, A., and Finch, C. A. (1961). The use of chelates in the treatment of iron overload. *Clin. Res.*, **9**, 91.
Coleman, D. H., Stevens, A. R., Jr., Dodge, H. T., and Finch, C. A. (1953). Rate of blood regeneration after blood loss. *Arch. intern. Med.*, **92**, 341.
Conrad, M. E., Jr., and Crosby, W. H. (1963). Intestinal mucosal mechanisms controlling iron absorption. *Blood*, **22**, 406.
Covey, T. J. (1964). Ferrous sulfate poisoning. *J. Pediat.*, 64, 218.
Crosby, W. H. (1963). The control of iron balance by the intestinal mucosa. *Blood*, **22**, 441.
——, Conrad, M. E., Jr., and Wheby, M. S. (1963). The rate of iron accumulation in iron storage disease. *ibid.*, 22, 429.
Davidson, L. S. P., Donaldson, G. M. M., Dyar, M. J., Lindsay, S. T., and McSorley, J. G. (1942). Nutritional iron deficiency anaemia in wartime. Part I. The haemoglobin levels of 831 infants and children. *Brit. med. J.*, **2**, 505.
Davidson, S., and Passmore, R. (1963). *Human Nutrition and Dietetics*, 2nd ed. Livingstone, Edinburgh.
Davis, A. E., and Badenoch, J. (1962). Iron absorption in pancreatic disease. *Lancet*, **2**, 6.
Davis, L. R., Marten, R. H., and Sarkany, I. (1960). Iron-deficiency anaemia in European and West Indian infants in London. *Brit. med. J.*, **2**, 1426.
Dowdle, E. B., Schachter, D., and Schenker, H. (1960). Active transport of $Fe^{59}$ by everted segments of rat duodenum. *Amer. J. Physiol.*, **198**, 609.
Drabkin, D. L. (1951). Metabolism of the hemin chromoproteins. *Physiol. Rev.*, **31**, 345.
Dubach, R., Moore, C. V., and Callender, S. T. (1955). Studies in iron transportation and metabolism. IX. The excretion of iron as measured by the isotope technique. *J. Lab. clin. Med.*, **45**, 599.
Elliott, W. D. (1962). The prevention of anaemia of prematurity. *Arch. Dis. Childh.*, **37**, 297.
Ellis, J. T., Schulman, I., and Smith, C. H. (1954). Generalized siderosis with fibrosis of liver and pancreas in Cooley's (Mediterranean) anemia, with observations on the pathogenesis of the siderosis and fibrosis. *Amer. J. Path.*, **30**, 287.
Engle, M. A. (1964). Cardiac involvement in Cooley's anemia. *Ann. N.Y. Acad. Sci.*, **119**, 694.
Erlandson, M. E., Walden, B., Stern, G., Hilgartner, M. W., Wehman, J., and Smith, C. H. (1962). Studies on congenital hemolytic syndromes. IV. Gastrointestinal absorption of iron. *Blood*, **19**, 359.

Fahey, J. L., Rath, C. E., Princiotto, J. V., Brick, I. B., and Rubin, M. (1961). Evaluation of trisodium calcium diethylenetriamine-pentaacetate in iron storage disease. *J. Lab. clin. Med.*, **57**, 436.

Farquhar, J. D. (1963). Iron supplementation during first year of life. *Amer. J. Dis. Child.*, **106**, 201.

Fielding, J. (1962). Sarcoma induction by iron-carbohydrate complexes. *Brit. med. J.*, **1**, 1800.

Finch, C. A. (1959). Body iron exchange in man. *J. clin. Invest.*, **38**, 392.

Finch, S., Haskins, D., and Finch, C. A. (1950). Iron metabolism. Hematopoiesis following phlebotomy. Iron as a limiting factor. *ibid.*, **29**, 1078.

Fink, H. (1964). Transfusion hemochromatosis in Cooley's anemia. *Ann. N.Y. Acad. Sci.*, **119**, 680.

Gabrio, B. W., and Salomon, K. (1950). Distribution of total ferritin in intestine and mesenteric lymph nodes of horses after iron feeding. *Proc. Soc. exp. Biol. (N.Y.)*, **75**, 124.

Gairdner, D., Marks, J., and Roscoe, J. D. (1952). Blood formation in infancy. Part II. Normal erythropoiesis. *Arch. Dis. Childh.*, **27**, 214.

Gaisford, W., and Jennison, R. F. (1955). Intramuscular iron in infancy. *Brit. med. J.*, **2**, 700.

Garby, L., and Sjölin, S. (1959). Absorption of labelled iron in infants less than three months old. *Acta paediat. (Uppsala)*, **48**, Suppl. 117, 24.

——, ——, and Vuille, J. C. (1963). Studies on erythro-kinetics in infancy. III. Disappearance from plasma and red-cell uptake of radio-active iron injected intravenously. *ibid.*, **52**, 537.

Giblett, E. R., Coleman, D. H., Pirzio-Biroli, G., Donohue, D. M., Motulsky, A. G., and Finch, C. A. (1956). Erythrokinetics: quantitative measurements of red cell production and destruction in normal subjects and patients with anemia. *Blood*, **11**, 291.

Girdwood, R. H. (1952). Treatment of anaemia. *Brit. med. J.*, **1**, 599.

Goldberg, A., Lochhead, A. C., and Dagg, J. H. (1963). Histamine-fast achlorhydria and iron absorption. *Lancet*, **1**, 848.

Goldthorp, W. O., Spencer, D., and Dawson, D. W. (1965). Reactions to intravenous iron dextran. *Brit. med. J.*, **1**, 316.

Gorten, M. K., Hepner, R., and Workman, J. B. (1963). Iron metabolism in premature infants. I. Absorption and utilization of iron as measured by isotope studies. *J. Pediat.*, **63**, 1063.

Granick, S. (1946). Protein apoferritin and ferritin in iron feeding and absorption. *Science*, **103**, 107.

Grimes, A. J., and Hutt, M. S. R. (1957). Metabolism of $^{59}$Fe-dextran complex in human subjects. *Brit. med. J.*, **2**, 1074.

Groen, J., Van Den Broek, W. A., and Veldman, H. (1947). Absorption of iron compounds from the small intestine in the rat. *Biochem. biophys. Acta (Amst.)*, **1**, 315.

Guest, G. M., and Brown, E. W. (1957). Erythrocytes and hemoglobin of the blood in infancy and childhood. III. Factors in variability, statistical studies. *A.M.A. Amer. J. Dis. Child.*, **93**, 486.

Haddow, A., and Horning, E. S. (1960). On the carcinogenicity of an iron-dextran complex. *J. nat. Cancer Inst.*, **24**, 109.

Hahn, P. F., Bale, W. F., Ross, J. F., Balfour, W. M., and Whipple, G. H. (1943). Radioactive iron absorption by gastro-intestinal tract. Influence of anemia, anoxia and antecedent feeding. Distribution in growing dogs. *J. exp. Med.*, **78**, 169.

Hallberg, L., and Sölvell, L. (1960). Iron absorption during constant intragastric infusion of iron in man. *Acta med. scand.*, **168**, Suppl. 358, 43.

Heilmeyer, L., Keller, W., Vivell, O., Keiderling, W., Betke, K., Wöhler, F., and Schultze, H. E. (1961). Congenital transferrin deficiency in a seven-year-old girl. *Germ. med. Mth.*, **6**, 385.

——, and Wöhler, F. (1963). The treatment of haemochromatosis with desferrioxamine. *ibid.*, 8, 133.

Henderson, F., Vietti, T. J., and Brown, E. B. (1963). Desferrioxamine in the treatment of acute toxic reaction to ferrous gluconate. *J. Amer. med. Ass.*, **186**, 1139.

Hoag, M. S., Wallerstein, R. O., and Pollycove, M. (1961). Occult blood loss in iron deficiency anemia of infancy. *Pediatrics*, **27**, 199.

Hwang, Y. F., and Brown, E. B. (1965). Effect of desferrioxamine on iron absorption. *Lancet*, **1**, 135.

Jacobziner, H., and Raybin, H. W. (1962). Iron intoxication. *N.Y. St. J. Med.*, **62**, 85.

Kerr, D. N. S., and Davidson, S. (1958). Gastrointestinal intolerance to oral iron preparations. *Lancet*, **2**, 489.

Korman, S. (1960). Iron metabolism in man. *Ann. N.Y. Acad. Sci.*, **88**, 460.

Lloyd, J. K., and Brown, G. A. (1964). Homozygous thalassaemia in an English child. *Arch. Dis. Childh.*, **39**, 625.

MacGibbon, B. H., and Mollin, D. L. (1965). Sideroblastic anaemia in man: observations on seventy cases. *Brit. J. Haemat.*, **11**, 59.

Mackay, H. M. M. (1931). Nutritional anaemia in infancy with special reference to iron deficiency. *Spec. Rep. Ser. med. Res. Coun. (Lond.)*, **157**, 65.

Marchasin, S., and Wallerstein R. O. (1964). The treatment of iron-deficiency anemia with intravenous iron dextran. *Blood*, **23**, 354.

McCance, R. A., Edgecomb, C. N., and Widdowson, E. M. (1943). Phytic acid and iron absorption. *Lancet*, **2**, 126.

——, and Widdowson, E. M. (1937). Absorption and excretion of iron. *ibid.*, **22**, 680.

——, and —— (1951). The metabolism of iron during suckling. *J. Physiol. (Lond.)*, **112**, 450.

Mendel, G. A. (1961). Studies on iron absorption. I. The relationships between the rate of erythropoiesis, hypoxia and iron absorption. *Blood*, **18**, 727.

——, Weiler, R. J., and Mangalik, A. (1963). Studies on iron absorption. II. The absorption of iron in experimental anemias of diverse etiology. *ibid.*, **22**, 450.

Mereu, I., and Tonz, O. (1962). The treatment of iron deficiency anaemia in children with iron polyisomaltosate. *Germ. med. Mth.*, **7**, 82.

Moe, P. J. (1963). Iron requirements in infancy. Longitudinal studies of iron requirements during the first year of life. *Acta paediat. (Uppsala)*, Suppl. 150.

—— (1964). Iron requirements in infancy. II. The influence of iron-fortified cereals given during the first year of life, on the red blood picture of children at 1½-3 years of age. *ibid.*, **53**, 423.

Moeschlin, S., and Schnider, U. (1963). Treatment of primary and secondary hemochromatosis and acute iron poisoning with a new potent iron-eliminating agent (desferrioxamine-B). *New Engl. J. Med.*, **269**, 57.

Moore, C. V. (1955). The importance of nutritional factors in the pathogenesis of iron-deficiency anemia. *Amer. J. clin. Nutr.*, **3**, 3.

——, Bierman, H. Q., Minnich, V., and Arrowsmith, W. R. (1940). Studies in iron absorption with special reference to the relationship of iron metabolism to ascorbic acid. In *Blood, Heart, and Circulation*, ed. F. R. Moulton (Amer. Assoc. Advanc. Sci. Publ. No. 13). Science Press, Lancaster, Pa.

——, and Dubach, R. (1951). Observations on the absorption of iron from foods tagged with radioiron. *Trans. Ass. Amer. Phycns*, **64**, 245.

——, and —— (1956). Metabolism and requirements of iron in the human. *J. Amer. med. Ass.*, **162**, 197.

——, Minnich, V., Vilter, R. W., and Spies, T. D. (1943). Hypochromic anemia in patients with deficiency of the vitamin B complex; response to iron therapy with and without yeast. *ibid.*, **121**, 245.

Muller-Eberhard, U., Erlandson, M. E., Ginn, H. E., and Smith, C. H. (1963). Effect of trisodium calcium diethylenetriaminepentaacetate on bivalent cations in thalassemia major. *Blood*, **22**, 209.

Nielsen, J. B. (1963). Influence of desferrioxamine on the renal excretion of iron. *Acta med. scand.*, **173**, 499.

Niccum, W. L., Jackson, R. L., and Stearns, G. (1953). Use of ferric and ferrous iron in the prevention of hypochromic anemia in infants. *Amer. J. Dis. Child.*, **86**, 553.

Norman, C. S. (1964). The treatment of iron overload with desferrioxamine B. *Irish J. med. Sci.*, 13.

Ohlsson, W. T. L., Kullendorff, G. T., and Ljungberg, L. K. (1953). Transfusion hemosiderosis. Report of a case treated with BAL. *Acta. med. scand.*, **145**, 410.

Oliver, R. A. M. (1959). Siderosis following transfusions of blood. *J. Path. Bact.*, **77**, 171.

Pirzio-Biroli, G., Bothwell, T. H., and Finch, C. A. (1958). Iron absorption. II. The absorption of radioiron administered with a standard meal in man. *J. Lab. clin. Med.*, **51**, 37.

——, and Finch, C. A. (1960). Iron absorption. III. The influence of iron stores on iron absorption in the normal subject. *ibid.*, **55**, 216.

Powell, L. W., and Dugdale, A. E. (1964). Desferrioxamine and iron. *Lancet*, **1**, 934.

Powell, R. (1963). Iron-dextran: total-dose infusion technique. *ibid.*, **2**, 252.

Pringle, A., Goldberg, A., Macdonald, E., and Johnston, S. (1962). $^{59}$Fe iron sorbitol cirtic-acid complex in iron-deficiency anaemia. *ibid.*, **2**, 749.

Richmond, H. G. (1959). Induction of sarcoma in the rat by iron-dextran complex. *Brit. med. J.*, **1**, 947.

Riley, I. D. (1960). Absorption of radioactive iron by anaemic infants. *Arch. Dis. Childh.*, **35**, 355.

Robertson, E. F., Maxwell, G. M., and Elliott, R. B. (1963). Studies in thalassaemia major. *Med. J. Aust.*, **2**, 705.

Ross, F. G. M. (1953). Pyloric stenosis and fibrous stricture of the stomach due to ferrous sulphate poisoning. *Brit. med. J.*, **2**, 1200.

Sanford, R. (1961). The effect of enzymic digestion of foods on the liberation of iron. *Aust. Ann. Med.*, **10**, 288.

Schiffer, L. M., Price, D. C., and Cronkite, E. P. (1965). Iron absorption and anemia. *J. Lab. clin. Med.*, **65**, 316.

Schulz, J., and Smith, N. J. (1958a). A quantitative study of the adsorption of food iron in infants and children. *Amer. J. Dis. Child.*, **95**, 109.

——, and —— (1958b). Quantitative study of the absorption of iron salts in infants and children. *ibid.*, **95**, 120.

Scott, J. M. (1963). Iron-sorbitol-citrate in pregnancy anaemia. *Brit. med. J.*, **2**, 354.

Seip, M. (1955). The reticulocyte level, and the erythrocyte production judged, from reticulocyte studies in newborn infants during the first week of life. *Acta paediat. (Uppsala)*, **44**, 355.

Seven, M. J., Gottlieb, H., Israel, H. L., Reinhold, J. G., and Rubin, M. (1954). N-hydroxyethylethylenediamine triacetic acid, Versenol in the treatment of hemochromatosis. *Amer. J. med. Sci.*, **228**, 646.

Shahidi, N. T., Nathan, D. G., and Diamond, L. K. (1964). Iron deficiency anemia associated with an error of iron metabolism in two siblings. *J. clin. Invest.*, **43**, 510.

Shepherd, J. A. (1955). Ferrous sulphate poisoning with gross stricture of the stomach. *Brit. med. J.*, **2**, 418.

Sisson, T. R. C., and Lund, C. J. (1957). The influence of maternal iron-deficiency on the newborn. *Amer. J. Dis. Child.*, **94**, 525.

Smith, C. A., Caton, W. L., Roby, C. C., Reid, D. E., Caswell, R. S., and Gibson, J. G., II (1950). Transplacental iron; its persistence during infancy as studied isotopically. *ibid.*, **80**, 856.

Smith, M. D., and Pannacciulli, I. M. (1958). Absorption of inorganic iron from graded doses; its significance in relation to iron absorption tests and the 'mucosal block' theory. *Brit. J. Haemat.*, **4**, 428.

Smith, R. S. (1962). Iron excretion in thalassaemia major after administration of chelating agents. *Brit. med. J.*, **2**, 1577.

—— (1964a). Iron absorption in cystic fibrosis. *ibid*, **1**, 608.

—— (1964b). Chelating agents in the diagnosis and treatment of iron overload in thalassemia. *Ann. N.Y. Acad. Sci.*, **119**, 776.

Steiner, M., Baldini, M., and Dameshek, W. (1964). Enzymatic defects of heme synthesis in thalassemia. *ibid.*, **119**, 548.

Steinkamp, R., Dubach, R., and Moore, C. V. (1955). Studies in iron transportation and metabolism. VIII. Absorption of radio-iron from iron-enriched bread. *Arch. intern. Med.*, **95**, 181.

Stevens, A. R., Jr., Pirzio-Biroli, G., Harkins, H. N., Nyhus, L. M., and Finch, C. A. (1959). Iron metabolism in patients after partial gastrectomy. *Ann. Surg.*, **149**, 534.

Stott, G. (1960). Anaemia in Mauritius. *Bull. Wld Hlth Org.*, **23**, 781.

Stransky, E., and Dauis-Lawas, D. F. (1948). On iron deficiency anemia in infancy and childhood in the tropics. *Ann. paediat. (Basel)*, **171**, 139.

Struass, M. B. (1933). Anemia of infancy from maternal iron deficiency in pregnancy. *J. clin. Invest.*, **12**, 345.

Sturgeon, P. (1954). Studies of iron requirements in infants and children. I. Normal values for serum iron, copper and free erythrocyte protoporphyrin. *Pediatrics*, **13**, 107.

—— (1956). Iron metabolism. A review with special consideration of iron requirements during normal infancy. *ibid.*, **18**, 267.

—— (1958). Studies of iron requirements in infants and children. IV. Recommended daily dietary allowances. In *Iron in Clinical Medicine*, ed. R. O. Wallerstein, and S. R. Mettier. University of California Press, Berkeley.

—— (1959). Studies of iron requirements in infants. III. Influence of supplemental iron during normal pregnancy on mother and infant. B. The infant. *Brit. J. Haemat.*, **5**, 45.

Taylor, J., Stiven, D., and Reid, E. W. (1935). Experimental and idiopathic siderosis in cats. *J. Path. Bact.*, **41**, 397.

Turnbull, A., Cleton, F., and Finch, C. A. (1962). Iron absorption. IV. The absorption of hemoglobin iron. *J. clin. Invest.*, **41**, 1897.

Vahlquist, B., Neander, G., and Neander, E. (1945). Studies on the absorption of iron. I. Absorption of iron from the stomach. *Acta paediat. (Uppsala)*, **32**, 768.

Venkatachalam, P. S., Brading, I., George, E. P., and Walsh, R. J. (1956). An experiment in rats to determine whether iron is absorbed only in the ferrous state. *Aust. J. exp. Biol. med. Sci.*, **34**, 389.

Verloop, M. C., Meeuwissen, J. E. Th., and Blokhuis, E. W. M. (1958). Comparison of the 'iron absorption test' with the determination of the iron-binding capacity of serum in the diagnosis of iron deficiency. *Brit. J. Haemat.*, **4**, 70.

Vischer, E. (1961). Chemistry of desferrioxamine B. In *Experience to Date with Desferrioxamine in the Treatment of Diseases Involving a Pathological Deposition of Iron in the Organism.* Report (compiled by Dr. P. Imhof, Ciba, Basle) on a meeting of clinical investigators.

Wetherley-Mein, G., Buchanan, J. C., Glass, U. H., and Pearce, L. C. (1962). Metabolism of $^{59}$Fe-sorbitol complex in man. *Brit. med. J.*, **1**, 1796.

Wheby, M. S., and Jones, L. G. (1963). Role of transferrin in iron absorption. *J. clin. Invest.*, **42**, 1007.

Whipple, G. A., Sisson, T. R. C., and Lund, C. J. (1957). Delayed ligation of the umbilical cord. *Obstet. and Gynec.*, **10**, 603.

Whitehead, R., Carter, R. L., and Sharp, A. A. (1965). Anaemia in occult intestinal malabsorption. *J. clin. Path.*, **18**, 110.

Whitten, C. F., Gibson, G., Good, M., and Goodwin, J. F. (1964). Experiences with desferrioxamine in the treatment of acute iron poisoning. *J. Pediat.*, **65**, 1050.

Wilson, J. F., Heiner, D. C., and Lahey, M. E. (1962). Studies on iron metabolism. I. Evidence of gastrointestinal dysfunction in infants with iron deficiency anemia: a preliminary report. *J. Pediat.*, **60**, 787.

Wintrobe, M. M. (1961). *Clinical Hematology*, 5th ed. Lea and Febiger, Philadelphia.

Witzleben, C. L., and Wyatt, J. P. (1961). The effect of long survival on the pathology of thalassaemia major. *J. Path. Bact.*, **82**, 1.

Wöhler, F. (1961). Clinical and experimental results with desferrioxamine. In *Experience to Date with Desferrioxamine in the Treatment of Diseases Involving a Pathological Deposition of Iron in the Organism.* Report (compiled by Dr. P. Imhof, Ciba, Basle) on a meeting of clinical investigators.

—— (1963). The treatment of haemochromatosis with desferrioxamine. *Acta haemat. (Basel)*, **30**, 65.

Wolman, I. J. (1964). Transfusion therapy in Cooley's anemia: growth and health as related to long-range hemoglobin levels. A progress report. *Ann. N.Y. Acad. Sci.*, **119**, 736.

Woodruff, C. W., and Bridgeforth, E. B. (1953). Relationship between the hemogram of the infant and that of the mother during pregnancy. *Pediatrics*, **12**, 681.

*Arch. Dis. Childh.*, 1965, **40**, 364.

# A DEFICIENCY STATE ARISING IN INFANTS ON SYNTHETIC FOODS

BY

TREVOR P. MANN, K. MARGARET WILSON, and BARBARA E. CLAYTON
*From the Royal Alexandra Hospital for Sick Children, Brighton, and The Hospital for Sick Children and the Institute of Child Health, Great Ormond Street, London*

(RECEIVED FOR PUBLICATION DECEMBER 10, 1964)

Severe extensive skin eruptions coupled with failure to thrive have been observed in infants fed on a synthetic low-phenylalanine diet (Moncrieff and Wilkinson, 1961; Brimblecombe, Blainey, Stoneman, and Wood, 1961; Wilson and Clayton, 1962). An investigation of this problem by Wilson and Clayton (1962) drew attention to the need to consider all nutrients carefully when constructing synthetic diets. The interdependence of various nutritional factors and the rapidity with which deficiencies could develop in infancy were particularly stressed. The publication of this work led one of us (T.P.M.) to realize that he had observed rashes somewhat similar to those described by Wilson and Clayton in galactosaemic infants receiving the low lactose-containing food, Galactomin (Trufood Ltd.). Similar features have subsequently been observed in 3 infants, one receiving a low sodium milk (Edosol, Trufood Ltd.), another low calcium milk (Locasol, Trufood Ltd.), and a third fed low lactose milk (Low lactose milk food, Cow and Gate Ltd.).

These synthetic milks are prepared by precipitating the casein in cows' milk, washing it to free it from other components and then mixing it with carbohydrate, fat, and a mineral mixture using a spray-drying process. During the initial precipitation and washing procedure, many nutrients are washed out too. Vitamins B1, B2, and nicotinamide are added to Edosol and Locasol, but not to Galactomin* or Low lactose milk food. Edosol also contains added vitamins A and D.

The nutritional properties of these four milks have been studied in weanling rats, and in the light of our experiments recommendations can be made for suitable vitamin supplements, their efficacy having been demonstrated in some infants.

* Trufood Ltd. have already taken note of the experimental and clinical findings reported in this paper, and Galactomin now contains added choline, and the label carries detailed advice about vitamin requirements.

### Milk Preparations Studied

Galactomin, Edosol, Locasol, and Low lactose milk food were fed to the infants as the preparations available commercially.

Special batches of Edosol and Locasol, in which lactose was replaced by dextrimaltose, were used for the feeding experiments in rats, since lactose causes diarrhoea in this species (Mitchell, 1927). 0·3 g. sodium as sodium chloride and 0·6 g. calcium as calcium gluconate were added to 100 g. of Edosol and Locasol, respectively, in order to increase the amounts of sodium and calcium to the levels present in breast milk. Galactomin and Low lactose milk food were fed to rats as the preparations available commercially.

The percentages of protein in Galactomin, Edosol, Locasol, and Low lactose milk food were 22·3, 27·8, 21·4, and 27·8, respectively of the dried food.

### Vitamin Preparations

Details of the preparations of vitamins used for treating the infants, and for the feeding experiments in rats are shown in Table 1. For the purpose of this communication the term 'vitamin' includes choline.

### Case Reports

Two galactosaemic infants who developed the deficiency state while receiving Galactomin are described.

**Case 1.** A.R., a female infant, aged 7 days, was admitted in June 1959, to the Royal Alexandra Hospital for Sick Children, Brighton, for further investigation of galactosaemia. On the 4th day of life galactose had been found in the urine while she was receiving breast milk.

A previous child had been similarly affected, the diagnosis being made on the 10th day of life. On Galactomin there had initially been a good response in this other sib, but vomiting then occurred and she ceased to thrive normally. A soya-bean product was tried with no better response, and while still on this preparation and

TABLE 1

COMPONENTS OF PREPARATIONS OF VITAMINS USED IN INFANTS AND EXPERIMENTAL STUDIES

| Preparation | A (i.u.) | D (i.u.) | B1 (mg.) | B2 (mg.) | B6 (mg.) | Nicotinamide (mg.) | C (mg.) | Other Vitamins |
|---|---|---|---|---|---|---|---|---|
| Abidec (Parke Davis & Co. Ltd. 0·3 ml.) .. | 2,500 | 500 | 0·5 | 0·2 | 0·25 | 2·5 | 12·5 | |
| Adexolin (Glaxo Laboratories Ltd.) 0·3 ml. .. | 3,000 | 300 | | | | | | |
| Becosym elixir (Roche Products Ltd.) 1·0 ml. | | | 1·0 | 0·4 | 0·4 | 4·0 | | |
| Betalin complex (Eli Lilly Ltd.) 1·0 ml. .. .. | | | 25·0 | 6·0 | 10·0 | 100·0 | 150·0 | |
| Compound vitamin drops (Paines & Byrne Ltd.) 0·6 ml. .. .. .. | 5,000 | 400 | 1·0 | 0·4 | 0·5 | 5·0 | 50·0 | |
| Ketovite tablets (Paines & Byrne Ltd.) One tablet + Ketovite supplement syrup (Paines & Byrne Ltd.) 5·0 ml. | 2,500 | 400 | 1·0 | 1·0 | 0·33 | 3·3 | 16·0 | Calcium pantothenate 117 mg. α-tocopheryl acetate 5·0 mg. Inositol 50·0 mg. Biotin 0·17 mg. Folic acid 0·25 mg. Choline chloride 150 mg. Vitamin B12 12·5 μg. |
| Parentrovite (Vitamins Ltd.) No. 1 5·0 ml. + No. 2 5·0 ml. | | | 250·0 | 4·0 | 50·0 | 160·0 | 500·0 | |

in hospital she suddenly collapsed and died at the age of 7 weeks. There was no record of skin lesions in this earlier case, and no cause for death was found at necropsy; the liver was large and fatty.

On *examination* the second affected baby weighed 6 lb. 6 oz. (2,891 g.) at the age of 7 days (birth weight 7 lb. 4 oz. (3,288 g.)). There was slight jaundice of 24 hours' standing and the liver was enlarged, but there were no lens opacities or retinal disease.

*Investigations* revealed a generalized aminoaciduria, and an excessive accumulation of galactose-l-phosphate. Liver function tests were normal.

On admission the infant was given 6 × 2½ oz. feeds of Galactomin each 24 hours, increasing to 6 × 5 oz. feeds on discharge, together with Abidec (Parke Davis) 0·3 ml. daily, throughout. She gained weight steadily and the liver became normal in size. The urine was occasionally positive to Benedict's test. She was discharged aged 7 weeks, weighing 9 lb. 10 oz. (4,365 g.) and in good health. She was readmitted at the age of 4 months in October 1959, having made good progress until a month previously when she had developed soreness of the lips followed by angular fissuring. At the time of her readmission she had a worsening cough, was reluctant to finish feeds, and was vomiting.

On *examination* her weight was 10 lb. 5 oz. (4,677 g.). Her lips were sore and fissured with angular cracking and ulceration. Similar fissuring and ulceration were present at the outer canthi of the eyelids. The buttocks and groins were red, raw, and weeping. There were bronchitic signs in the chest.

She was now receiving Galactomin as six 6-oz. feeds in 24 hours, together with Abidec 1 ml. daily. An initial 8-day course of tetracycline was given for her chest infection.

A dermatological opinion was obtained 5 days after readmission. Dr. Colin Jones considered the baby had a seborrhoea with associated cheilosis. He thought a nutritional deficiency likely and advised the administration of vitamin B and topical neomycin with hydrocortisone ointment to eyelids and mouth. In spite of this application, together with Becosym (Roche) (1·5 ml. daily for 48 hours) and then Betalin complex (Lilly) (4 daily injections each of 0·5 ml.), the various skin lesions failed to heal. Two weeks after starting this intensive treatment, a blood-stained purulent discharge was a feature of the various angular lesions. Also at this time weeping sores developed over the ears. At this stage the dose of Abidec was increased from 1 to 2 ml. daily.

A fortnight after her readmission septic lesions appeared in the sacral region, and though she was given chloramphenicol (7 days by the intramuscular route and 7 days by mouth) multiple abscesses requiring incision developed over the buttocks and lower back. *Staphylococcus pyogenes*, type 80, was isolated from the pus and was sensitive to the antibiotic used. There was an associated profound anaemia, the haemoglobin falling from 13·1 g./100 ml. on admission to 4·0 g. three weeks later, notwithstanding a blood transfusion five days previously.

After an initial 14-oz. (396 g.) weight gain during the first week in hospital, the infant failed to thrive. Vomiting, progressive abdominal distension, and nocturnal restlessness became noticeable features as deterioration set in. Her cough returned pre-terminally. The child suddenly collapsed and died 26 days after admission. Necropsy was refused by the parents.

**Case 2.** T.M., a male infant was admitted to the Royal Alexandra Hospital for Sick Children, Brighton, in September 1962 at 15 days of age, weighing 7 lb. 2 oz. (3,232 g.) (birth weight 7 lb. 11 oz. (3,486 g.)). His parents had been married for 10 years and had two adopted children.

On *examination* he was irritable and wasted but not jaundiced, with a unilateral purulent ophthalmia, a paronychia of one finger, and a sticky umbilicus: *Staph. pyogenes* was isolated from all three sites. His liver was large and there were lens opacities in both eyes (Mr. D. St. Clair Roberts). The urine gave a positive reaction with Clinitest but a negative one with Clinistix, and paper chromatography showed that galactose was present. Uridyl transferase was absent from the red cells (Dr. V. Schwarz, Manchester). Liver function tests were normal and there was no aminoaciduria.

He was placed on Galactomin and Abidec, 1 ml. daily, with an immediate good response. His urine became free of sugar, the vomiting stopped, his liver decreased in size, and his weight increased. He was discharged after 12 days, weighing 7 lb. 10 oz. (3,458 g.).

He was readmitted in November 1962 at 2 months of age because of failure to thrive and recent diarrhoea. He had been snuffly and coughing for a few days but was not vomiting. Glucose feeds had been substituted for Galactomin just before readmission.

On *examination* he was emaciated and dehydrated and weighed 8 lb. 3 oz. (3,713 g.). The lenses were normal. There was crusting around the anterior nares. The lips were dry, fissured, and bled easily. He had a napkin erythema extending to his inner thighs. His liver was normal in size. No reducing substances were found in the urine and no pathogens in the stools.

Galactomin was reintroduced the day after admission and continued until five days before death, when Low lactose milk food and Moll's pudding were tried in succession. He was receiving Abidec 1·8 ml. daily at this time. Tube feeding was necessary to maintain an adequate calorie intake.

Ten days after readmission abdominal distension with umbilical protrusion was first observed and this progressed until death a month later. At the same time both lips became more fissured and the skin eruption over the buttocks and thighs spread to the scrotum and penis. The ankles became similarly affected. The skin of the left external ear was noted to be pink and moist.

The cracked lips and extensive skin eruption responded neither to various topical applications (including corticosteroid preparations) nor to 10 mg. nicotinic acid daily (given for the last month of the illness), nor to two intramuscular injections each of 1·0 ml. of Parentrovite (Vitamins Ltd.). A dermatological opinion was obtained a month after admission. Dr. S. P. Hall-Smith thought the plaques over the buttocks and elsewhere could be labelled psoriasis, though he preferred to consider the eruption as a seborrhoeic dermatitis. Shortly after this opinion was obtained, fissures appeared for the first time at the corners of the mouth and the outer canthi of the eyelids. Also both ears became pink and moist, the exudate tending to crust. Two days before death the main skin lesions (shown in Fig. 1a, b) were summarized as follows by Dr. Hall-Smith.

(1) Muco-purulent nasal discharge with crusting of anterior nares.
(2) External ears pink and glazed especially helices, with a tendency to crusting.
(3) Haemorrhagic fissures of the upper and lower lip surfaces and the angles of the mouth.
(4) Eyes: fissuring and scaling at outer canthi.
(5) A widespread and confluent demarcated pink infiltrated plaque covering the left buttock, with a central island of normal skin. Postero-lateral and postero-medial aspects of left thigh, sacrum, perianal region, perineum, scrotum, and penis all similarly affected.
(6) Pink moist intertrigo groins with follicular eruption in the pubic area.
(7) Pink irregular patches on the posterior aspect of the left lower leg with superimposed flaccid blisters.

Restlessness, irritability, reluctance to feed, and vomiting were features noted by the nursing staff during the infant's five-week stay on the ward. Repeated testing failed to detect reducing substances in the urine. He was afebrile until the last three days of his illness when his temperature rose to 100° F. (37·8° C.) and 48 hours later to 102° F. (38·9° C.). During the last week a five-day course of oxytetracycline was administered, followed by oral chloramphenicol 25 mg. 6-hourly pre-terminally, when a heavy growth of *B. pyocyaneus*, sensitive to this second antibiotic, was isolated from the baby's nose, throat, and skin lesions.

Five weeks after readmission to hospital the infant suddenly collapsed and died after passing a fluid stool.

Necropsy (Dr. R. I. K. Elliott): Salient naked eye and histological features were as follows.

*Skin*. There was a crusted eruption in the distribution already described. Microscopically the skin in the affected areas showed some hyperplasia of the epithelial layer with elongation of the papillae combined with oedema and considerable vascular dilatation. Great masses of parakeratotic keratin were piled up above these dilated papillae; the bulk of the crust was obviously increased by exudation of serum. Some spongiosis was present though it was less striking than one would have expected. The lesion was interpreted as an active eczematous reaction with some degree of lichenification.

*Lungs*. There was bilateral *B. pyocyaneus* pneumonia with multiple abscesses. The histology suggested bronchogenic rather than haematogenous spread.

*Liver*. This looked normal to the naked eye. Microscopy showed a heavy inflammatory infiltration, mainly of lymphocytes and polymorphs, in the portal tracts. In some of the latter there was an increase of fibrous tissue.

*Kidneys*. These looked macroscopically normal. Microscopically, the lining cells of the first convoluted tubules showed considerable degenerative changes; many of these cells had disintegrated and formed a sponge-like meshwork inside the tubules.

*Adrenals*. These were normal in size and appearance. Sections showed a broad hyaline zone between the lower cortex and the medullary cells. In this situation the blood vessels were very dilated and there were scattered

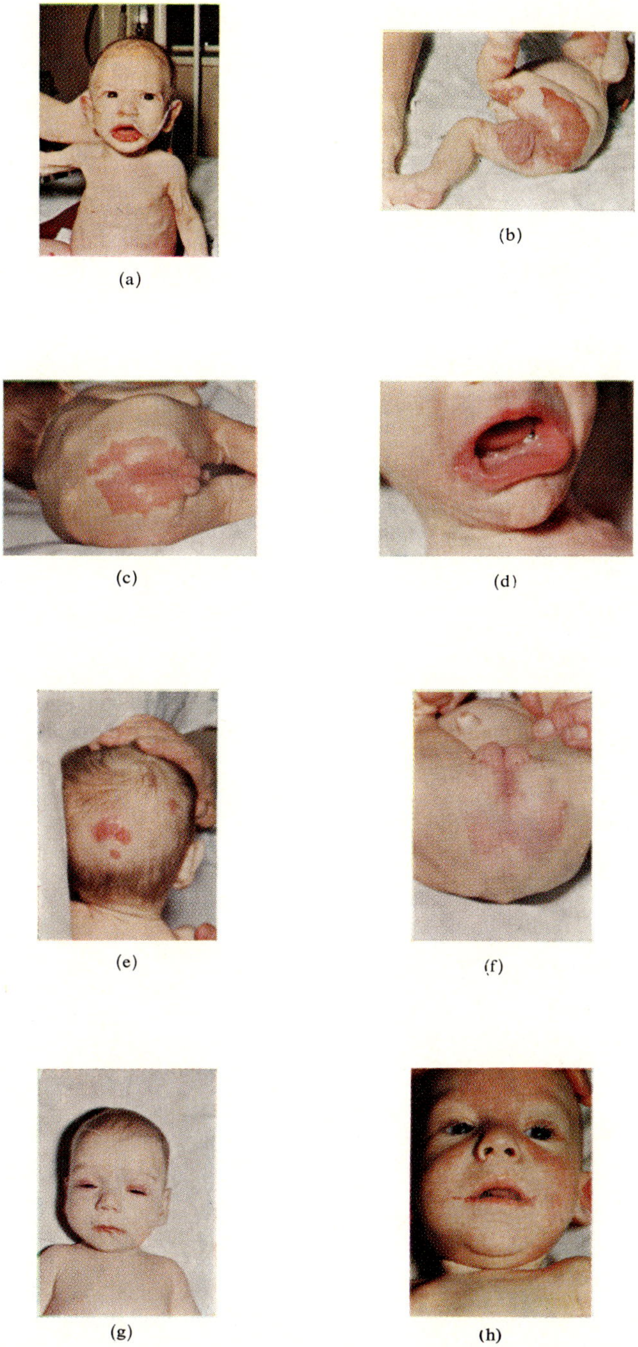


FIG. 1.—(a) (Case 2). Taken a few days before death, showing alert expression, generalized skin pallor, and emaciation. The scabbed external nares, the fissured lips, and the skin lesions at the outer canthi of the eyelids are visible. (b) (Case 2). Well-demarcated pink and glazed buttock eruption suggestive of psoriasis. (c) (Case A). Circumscribed psoriasiform buttock eruption. (d) (Case A). Angular fissuring of the mouth with superimposed whitish film. (e) (Case A). Psoriasiform patches in occipital region. (f) (Case A). The healing buttock eruption one week after the introduction of Ketovite tablets (no topical application), compare Fig. 1 (c). (g) (Case B). Angular fissuring and red eyelids. (h) (Case C). Fissuring of the angles of the mouth and outer canthi of the eyes.

cells containing dark pigment, which were probably not an artefact. In the cortex there was some vascular dilatation and the cells here showed considerable depletion of lipoid.

The recognition of a possible deficiency state in the two galactosaemic infants led to animal experiments with Galactomin which we shall now describe. These studies were later extended to Edosol, Locasol, and Low lactose milk food.

### Animal Experiments

Female Sprague-Dawley rats, obtained from Animal Supplies (London) Ltd., weighed 60 to 90 g. when experiments were begun. Rat cubes containing 20% protein (number 86, from J. C. Withers & Co. Ltd.) were used as a control diet. Tap water was available. Animals were housed in cages with grids so that they could not eat their faeces, and were kept for at least three days before experiments were begun. The number of rats per group and the duration of feeding with the diet are given subsequently for each experiment.

All foods and their vitamin supplements were mixed to a batter-like consistency with water and placed in troughs in the cages. The amount of food eaten each day was measured so that an approximate calorie intake could be determined. For pair feeding, when it was necessary for all groups to consume an equal number of calories, the amount eaten by the group with the poorest appetite was determined each day, and this weight of food was then given to each of the other groups for the next 24 hours.

The rats were weighed to the nearest gram except on Sundays. The percentage changes in body weight during the experiments were calculated. *t* tests for probability of difference were determined for the absolute body weights of groups of rats at the end of each experiment, and the results are given in the Tables when relevant. At the end of each experiment, the rats were killed with ether and dissected. General appearance of fur, tails, and ears was noted, and the abdominal fat pads, uteri, and vaginae were examined.

### Results

In the experiments subsequently described, *all young rats fed on Galactomin, Edosol, Locasol, and Low lactose milk food, without vitamin supplements* had a similar appearance. They failed to thrive and were less lively than controls. Their fur became dull and staring, and in some places, especially round the neck, there were bare patches. Brown discoloration was frequently present on their ears and tails. At necropsy the vaginae were closed, the uteri ill developed, and the abdominal fat pads were absent. The rats were more severely affected by Galactomin (see Fig. 2b) or Low lactose milk food (see Fig. 3a) than by Edosol or Locasol.

When these preparations were supplemented with Ketovite tablets + Ketovite supplement syrup (KT + KS) (see Table 1), the rats thrived, were active, and completely normal in appearance (see Fig. 3b).

**Galactomin.** *Experiment 1: Effect of feeding Galactomin, with and without a complete vitamin supplement, to young rats.* Three groups of rats were fed *ad lib.* with cubes, Galactomin, and Galactomin + KT + KS. Details of the experiment and the results are shown in Table 2 (Groups a, b, c).

Rats in Group b which received Galactomin had the ill appearance already described (see Fig. 2b). They ate less than those in Group c which thrived well, and loss of appetite was probably the result of a deficiency of B vitamins. The difference in body weight between Groups b and c reflected a difference in calorie intake, as well as a deficiency of vitamins. In a further investigation (Groups d, e, and f, Table 2), Groups d and f were pair-fed with Group e so that all the rats received the same calorie intake (see Fig. 4).

The difference in percentage change in body weight between Groups e and f (23% and 48%) was a true reflection of the effect of vitamin content on calorie utilization.

*Experiment 2: Effect of feeding young rats with Galactomin, supplemented with the vitamins given to patient A.R. (Case 1).* Patient A.R. at one period received Galactomin + 1·3 ml. Abidec + 1·7 ml. Becosym elixir daily (i.e. 10,000 i.u. A, 2,000 i.u. D, 3·5 mg. B1, 1·4 mg. B2, 1·6 mg. B6, 50 mg. ascorbic acid, and 16 mg. nicotinamide). Groups of rats were fed on Galactomin with and without various supplements, including a group receiving A.R.'s vitamins.

Details of the experiment and the results are given in Table 3 and the growth curves are plotted in Fig. 5. There were highly significant differences in the body weights attained by the groups except that Groups b and c did not differ from each other. It appeared that one or more of the factors present in KT + KS, but not in Abidec + Becosym + choline, affected appetite, the utilization of calories, and growth.

The vitamins prescribed for A.R., while receiving Galactomin, did not support optimum growth in the young rat.

*Experiment 3: Effect of feeding young rats on A.R.'s diet of Galactomin + Abidec + Becosym, together with choline and various combinations of other vitamins.* Eight groups of rats received Galactomin and various combinations of vitamins. Details of the experiment and the results are shown in Table 4. Adequate amounts of vitamins A, B1, B2, B6, C, D, nicotinamide, and choline were given to all groups.

Rats given supplements which included pantothenic acid achieved considerably greater increases

(a)

(b)

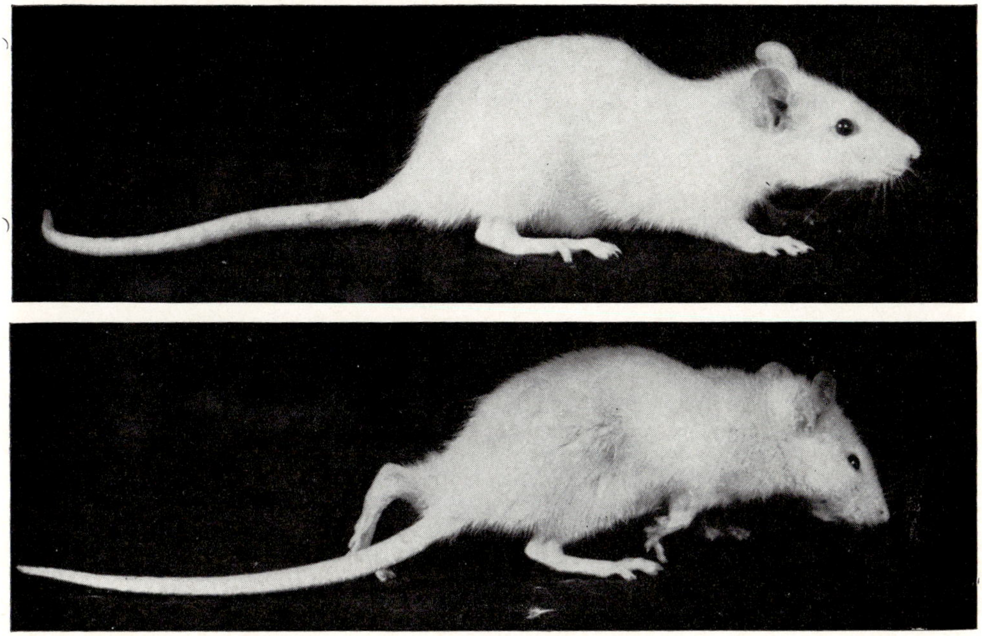

FIG. 2.—Appearances of young rats after 10 days on a diet. (a) Cubes *ad lib.* (Table 2, Group a). (b) Galactomin *ad lib.* (Table 2, Group b).

TABLE 2

EFFECT OF FEEDING GALACTOMIN WITH AND WITHOUT A COMPLETE VITAMIN SUPPLEMENT, TO YOUNG RATS

| Group* | Basic Diet | Supplement to Diet | Approximate Daily Calorie Intake/Rat | % Change in Body Weight During Experiment (Mean ± Standard Error) | *t* test for Probability of Difference Between Groups |
|---|---|---|---|---|---|
| a | Cubes *ad lib.* | None | 60 | 76 ± 1·9 | a compared with b: $p < 0{\cdot}001$<br>a compared with c: $p > 0{\cdot}05$ |
| b | Galactomin *ad lib.* | None | 42 | 17 ± 3·2 | b compared with c: $p < 0{\cdot}001$ |
| c | Galactomin *ad lib.* | KT + KS† | 59 | 70 ± 1·9 | |
| d | Cubes, pair fed with Group e | None | 36‡ | 42 ± 0·6 | d compared with e: $p < 0{\cdot}001$<br>d compared with f: $p > 0{\cdot}05$ |
| e | Galactomin *ad lib.* | None | 43 | 23 ± 1·6 | e compared with f: $p < 0{\cdot}001$ |
| f | Galactomin, pair fed with Group e | KT + KS† | 43 | 48 ± 3·5 | |

The experiment was continued for 10 days.
* 6 rats in each group except b, which had 5. † 100 g. Galactomin + 3 Ketovite tablets + 5 ml. Ketovite supplement syrup.
‡ Owing to a technical difficulty, d received slightly fewer calories than e.

TABLE 3

EFFECT OF FEEDING GALACTOMIN, WITH AND WITHOUT SOME VITAMIN SUPPLEMENT, TO YOUNG RATS

| Group | Supplement to Galactomin | Approximate Daily Calorie Intake/Rat | % Change in Body Weight During Experiment (Mean ± Standard Error) | *t* test for Probability of Difference Between Groups |
|---|---|---|---|---|
| a | None | 34 | −3 ± 3·1 | a compared with b: $p < 0{\cdot}005$<br>a compared with d: $p < 0{\cdot}005$ |
| b | Abidec + Becosym elixir* as given to Case 1 | 40 | 40 ± 10·7 | b compared with c: $p > 0{\cdot}05$<br>b compared with d: $p < 0{\cdot}02 > 0{\cdot}01$ |
| c | Abidec + Becosym elixir + choline chloride† | 41 | 59 ± 9·5 | c compared with d: $p < 0{\cdot}05 > 0{\cdot}01$ |
| d | KT + KS‡ | 60 | 75 ± 12·1 | |

3 rats in each group; experiment terminated after 19 days; feeding was *ad lib.*
Supplements to 100 g. Galactomin:
* 10,000 i.u. A, 2,000 i.u. D, 3·5 mg.B1, 1·4 mg.B2, 1·6 mg.B6, 16 mg. nicotinamide, 50 mg. ascorbic acid.
† As group b + 150 mg. choline chloride. ‡ 3 Ketovite tablets + 5 ml. Ketovite supplement syrup.

(a)

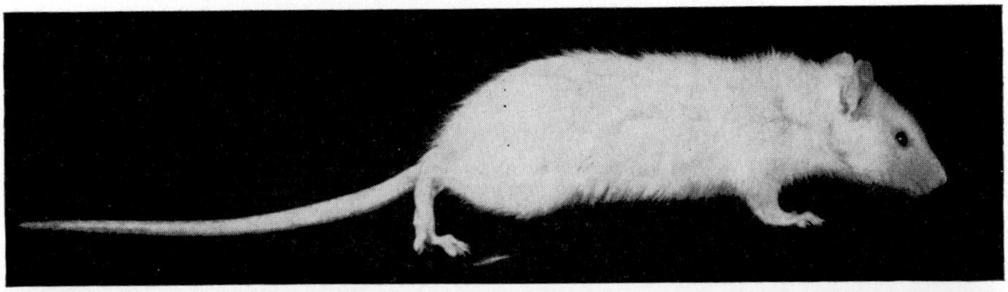

(b)

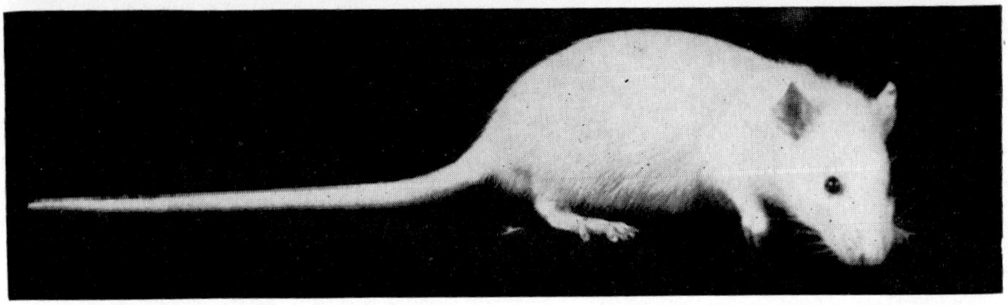

FIG. 3.—Appearance of young rats after 14 days on a diet. (a) Low lactose milk food *ad lib.* (Table 5, Low lactose milk food, Group a). (b) Low lactose milk food *ad lib.* + KT + KS (Table 5, Low lactose milk food, Group b).

in body weight than the others and were of a healthier appearance. There was a significant difference ($p < 0 \cdot 01$) between Group a as compared with Groups e, f, g, and h. Group a did not differ from Groups b and d ($p > 0 \cdot 05$) but was just different from Group c at the $p < 0 \cdot 05$ level; the reason is not apparent but probably depends on the variation encountered with small numbers of animals.

Amongst the groups given pantothenic acid, Group e did not differ from Groups f or g ($p > 0 \cdot 05$) but was different from Group h ($p < 0 \cdot 05$).

No clear-cut trends were evident with α-tocopheryl acetate, B2, folic acid, biotin, and inositol in this experiment.

**Edosol, Locasol, and Low Lactose Milk Food.** Groups of young rats were now fed on Edosol, Locasol, and Low lactose milk food with and without vitamin supplements. Details of the experiments and the effects on body weight are shown in Table 5. Fig. 6 illustrates the growth curves obtained with Locasol.

Young rats fed on these preparations, without vitamin supplements, had poor appetites, failed to thrive, and developed appearances similar to those of the rats fed on Galactomin, except that the changes were less marked with Edosol and Locasol. If a supplement of KT + KS was added, caloric intake, growth, appearance, and liveliness were as satisfactory as with rat cubes. *t* tests for probability of differences between the body weights of groups are given in Table 5 and show highly significant differences between groups receiving the synthetic milk only, and those receiving KT + KS in addition.

Ideally, studies on nutrition should be performed on the human subject, but during infancy this is usually impossible. Soon after the animal studies were completed three infants receiving Edosol, Locasol, and Low lactose milk food came to our notice. The infants had failed to thrive and had developed rashes similar to those of A.R. and T.M. As a result of the conclusions drawn from the animal studies, these infants were given complete vitamin supplements in the form of KT + KS, and the clinical response was in each case dramatic and sustained.

## Case Reports

**Case A.** L.K., a female infant, was first admitted in November 1963 to the Royal Alexandra Hospital for Sick Children, Brighton, at the age of 10 weeks with increasing cough, cyanosis, difficulty with feeding, and failure to thrive.

On *examination* the infant was ill, febrile, dehydrated, and wasted, weighing 7 lb. 2 oz. (3,232 g.) (birth weight 6 lb. 6 oz. (2,891 g.)). There was consolidation of the right lower lobe, and a systolic murmur along the left sternal border was attributed, after radioscopy and electrocardiography, to a left-to-right shunt through a large ventricular septal defect.

The baby received intramuscular penicillin and streptomycin for 7 days, continuous oxygen for 25 days, and 8 daily 75 mg. doses of chlorothiazide. Feeds of Edosol were commenced 3 days after admission (480 cal. in 24 hours) and compound vitamin drops 1 ml. daily.

**TABLE 4**

EFFECT OF FEEDING YOUNG RATS ON DIET OF CASE 1, i.e. GALACTOMIN + ABIDEC + BECOSYM, TOGETHER WITH CHOLINE AND VARIOUS COMBINATIONS OF OTHER VITAMINS

| Group | No. of Rats | Basic Diet | Additional Supplement Added to 100 g. Diet | Approximate Daily Calorie Intake/Rat | % Change in Body Weight During Experiment (Mean ± Standard Error) |
|---|---|---|---|---|---|
| a | 6 | 100 g. Galactomin + 1·2 ml. Abidec + 1·5 ml. Becosym + 150 mg. choline chloride } Case 1's diet | None | 39 | 65 ± 4·9 |
| b | 6 | As Group a | α-tocopheryl acetate 15 mg. | 36 | 68 ± 1·9 |
| c | 5 | As Group a | Folic acid 0·75 mg. B12 10 μg. | 37 | 88 ± 4·8 |
| d | 5 | As Group a | Folic acid 0·75 mg. B12 10 μg. α-tocopheryl acetate 15 mg. | 38 | 69 ± 2·5 |
| e | 6 | As Group a | Calcium pantothenate 3·48 mg. | 42 | 98 ± 3·3 |
| f | 6 | As Group a | Calcium pantothenate 3·48 mg. folic acid 0·75 mg. B12 10 μg. α-tocopheryl acetate 15 mg. | 43 | 102 ± 4·7 |
| g | 6 | As Group a | As for Group f + Biotin 0·51 mg. + inositol 150 mg. | 43 | 96 ± 4·7 |
| h | 6 | Galactomin | KT + KS | 50 | 108 ± 5·5 |

The experiment lasted 16 days; feeding was *ad lib.*

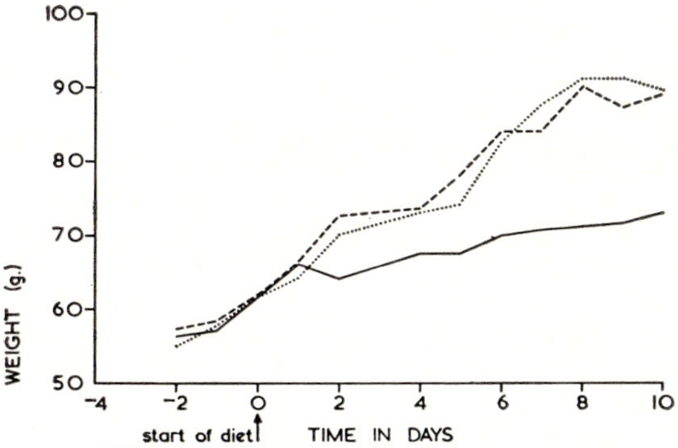


FIG. 4.—Growth curves of groups of weanling rats fed on cubes, Galactomin alone and Galactomin + KT + KS.
-------------- cubes
———— Galactomin alone
................ Galactomin + KT + KS
} pair-fed

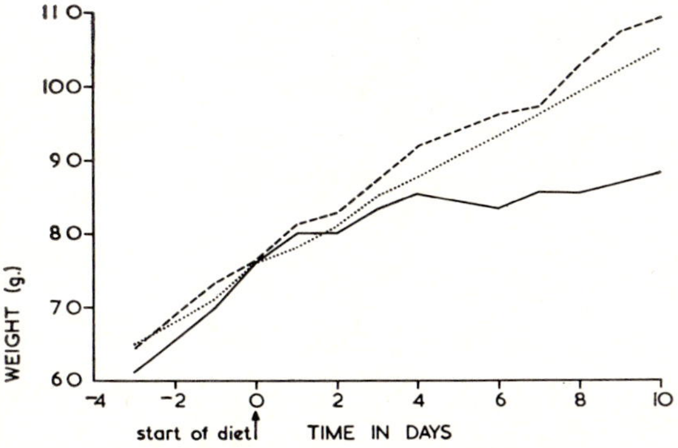


FIG. 6.—Growth curves of groups of weanling rats fed on Locasol; on Locasol + KT + KS: and on cubes.
———— Locasol
............ Locasol + KT + KS
----------- cubes
} pair-fed

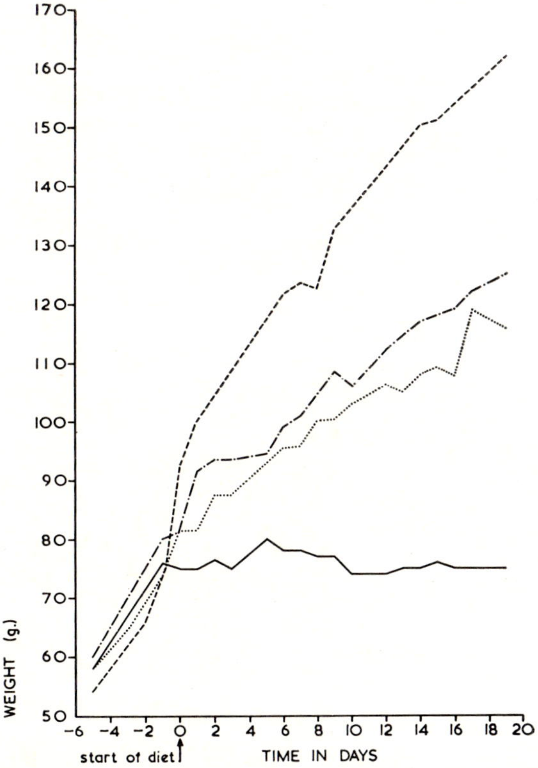


FIG. 5.—Growth curves of groups of weanling rats fed on Galactomin alone; on Galactomin + Abidec + Becosym; on Galactomin + Abidec + Becosym + choline; and on Galactomin + KT + KS. ———— Galactomin alone; ............... Galactomin + Abidec + Becosym; — - — - Galactomin + Abidec + Becosym + choline; ------ Galactomin + KT + KS.

TABLE 5

EFFECT OF FEEDING EDOSOL, LOCASOL, AND LOW LACTOSE MILK FOOD TO YOUNG RATS

| Group | No. of Rats | Basic Diet | Supplement Added to 100 g. Basic Diet | Approx. Daily Calorie Intake/Rat | % Change in Body Weight During Experiment (Mean ± Standard Error) | *t* test for Probability of Difference Between Groups |
|---|---|---|---|---|---|---|
| *Edosol* | | | | | | |
| a | 11 | Edosol *ad lib.* | None | 34 | 21 ± 2·5 | a compared with b: $p < 0·001$ |
| b | 11 | Edosol pair fed with Group a | KT + KS | 34 | 32 ± 2·2 | a compared with c: $p < 0·001$ |
| c | 9 | Edosol *ad lib.* | KT + KS | 44 | 45 ± 3·6 | b compared with c: $p < 0·001$ |
| d | 9 | Cubes *ad lib.* | None | 50 | 44 ± 3·5 | c compared with d: $p > 0·05$ |
| *Locasol* | | | | | | |
| a | 6 | Locasol *ad lib.* | None | 42 | 15 ± 2·3 | a compared with b: $p > 0·001 < 0·005$ |
| b | 6 | Locasol pair fed with Group a | KT + KS | 42 | 44 ± 7·1 | a compared with c: $p > 0·001 < 0·005$ |
| c | 6 | Cubes pair fed with Group a | None | 42 | 38 ± 4·0 | b compared with c: $p > 0·05$ |
| *Low lactose* | | | | | | |
| a | 6 | Low lactose *ad lib.* | None | 38 | 18 ± 5·0 | a compared with b: $p < 0·001$ |
| b | 6 | Low lactose *ad lib.* | KT + KS | 63 | 66 ± 6·6 | a compared with c: $p < 0·001$ |
| c | 5 | Cubes *ad lib.* | None | 48 | 56 ± 2·3 | b compared with c: $p > 0·05$ |

The diet was continued for 10 days.

She was critically ill for the first week with slow improvement subsequently. She was discharged 6 weeks after admission weighing 7 lb. 10 oz. (3,458 g.), on digoxin, Edosol (480 cal./24 hours), and compound vitamin drops 1 ml. daily.

She was readmitted in February 1964, aged 5½ months, i.e. 6 weeks after discharge from hospital, because of failure to thrive, anorexia, vomiting, and cough. Two weeks previously an eruption had appeared over the buttocks and back of the scalp, with no associated pain or irritation. She had periods of irritability and screaming at night possibly due to abdominal pain. Edosol and the drugs were maintained.

On *examination* her temperature was 101° F. (38·3° C.) on admission, but there were no signs of infection. She was alert, responsive, grossly marasmic (weight 8 lb. (3,628 g.)), and irritable when handled. Her lungs were normal and there were no signs of heart failure. Her lips were cracked and bleeding, and there was an eruption on the buttocks and scalp as described below.

She was given an initial 8-day course of demethylchlortetracycline (40 mg./day), and was afebrile within 48 hours of admission.

One week later the striking similarity between this baby and the two galactosaemic ones described earlier led to a diagnosis of a deficiency state associated with Edosol. This synthetic milk (540 cal./24 hr.) was maintained, compound vitamin drops were discontinued, and Ketovite syrup 5 ml. daily was introduced.

Two weeks after admission she was deteriorating and her weight was 8 lb. 1½ oz. (3,670 g.). There were frequent regurgitations and sometimes vomiting after coughing. Her skin lesions were virtually unchanged and, indeed, since being on Ketovite syrup, fissures had appeared at the upper junction of the left ear and scalp. At this point the dermatological picture was summarized by Dr. Hall-Smith as follows.

'Circumscribed psoriasiform lesion with clear-cut edge involving the sacral and coccygeal regions, both buttocks for a distance of one inch on each side and both labia (see Fig. 1c).
Dry linear intertrigo in depths of groin creases. Minimal fissuring at left outer canthus of eye. Fissuring of left retro-auricular ear adjacent to upper pole of left ear.
Angular cheilosis with superimposed whitish film (see Fig. 1d).
Crescentic-shaped psoriasiform patch occiput with two small satellite lesions (see Fig. 1e).'

At this stage, i.e. two weeks after admission, as well as Ketovite syrup (5 ml. daily), compound vitamin drops were reintroduced, 1 ml. daily. In addition, calcium pantothenate 3 mg. and folic acid 0·75 mg. were given daily (i.e. approximate amounts of these nutrients in 3 Ketovite tablets).

48 hours later there was further deterioration with a 3 oz. (85 g.) weight loss and complete refusal to feed. She had implacable screaming and restlessness throughout the night, possibly due to abdominal colic (similar attacks had occurred at home in the fortnight prior to her readmission). One Ketovite tablet daily was then introduced for the first time and the Ketovite syrup was reduced from 5 to 3 ml. daily and compound vitamin drops were discontinued. Edosol (540 cal./24 hr.) was continued by intragastric tube.

48 hours after introducing one Ketovite tablet daily a remarkable change had taken place in the baby's condition. She became contented and peaceful for the first time, and she started to feed hungrily so that the caloric intake was increased from 540 to 660 cal./24 hr. Most dramatic of all was the rapid regression of all the skin lesions without topical applications. A week after starting the Ketovite tablets in addition to Ketovite syrup, all the skin lesions had healed with faint scarring over the buttocks (see Fig. 1f) and scaling over the posterior scalp, and the baby was taking Edosol (780 cal./24 hr.) from the bottle. At this point, she developed styes over both upper eyelids with associated low-grade pyrexia. A

penicillin-resistant staphylococcus was isolated from the pus and methicillin 125 mg. was accordingly given by the intramuscular route 6-hourly for 5 days.

Two weeks after commencing KT + KS the patient looked alert and well, her residual scarring was fading, and her styes were healing. After three weeks she had gained 14 oz. (396 g.) and weighed 9 lb. (4,082 g.), her skin was normal, and she was discharged home. One month later she weighed 10 lb. 5 oz. (4,677 g.) and was changed to a standard dried milk.

**Case B.** K.Y., a male infant aged 2 months was admitted to The Hospital for Sick Children, Great Ormond Street, in October 1963, for the investigation of vomiting and failure to thrive; a diagnosis of early idiopathic hypercalcaemia was made. He was discharged one month later on Locasol, together with 2,500 vitamin A, 150 mg. choline chloride, 12·5 μg. B12, and 3 tablets of Ketovite daily. He thrived and gained 5 oz. (142 g.) weekly until the middle of January 1964, when he weighed 14 lb. 2½ oz. (6,421 g.). At this stage his Ketovite tablets were stopped but the other vitamins were continued. Two weeks later his weight had dropped to 13 lb. 13 oz. (6,264 g.) and the out-patient notes stated that 'he had developed small red spots on his face and then on his legs'. After a further month he was readmitted because his weight had fallen to 12 lb. 1 oz. (5,471 g.), he had begun to vomit, was anorexic, and had a rash.

On *examination* he was a very restless, wasted infant of 12 lb. 1 oz. (5,471 g.), with striking pallor. He had a moderate degree of angular fissuring at the mouth, his eyelids were red (see Fig. 1g), and over the napkin area there was a bright red psoriasiform rash with well-demarcated raised edges.

*Investigations* revealed plasma calcium 6·3 mg./100 ml.; the urinary amino acid pattern showed a raised excretion of glutamine, threonine, serine, and glycine with other amino acids at the upper level of normal; in addition, each 100 ml. of urine contained 500 mg. lactose and 200 mg. sucrose, but less than 5 mg. of galactose, glucose, and fructose.

Two days after admission, the infant was placed on Low lactose milk food, three tablets of Ketovite, and 5 ml. Ketovite supplement syrup daily. Improvement began within 24 hours and five days later the child was feeding well, had gained 12 oz. (340 g.), and the rash was much improved. Three weeks later when he weighed 13 lb. 12 oz. (6,236 g.) he was changed to cows' milk. The lactosuria did not recur and he was discharged well.

**Case C.** G.R., a male infant, was admitted to The Hospital for Sick Children, Great Ormond Street, at the age of 4 months for surgical correction of a large patent ductus arteriosus. Before operation he developed heart failure and pneumonia, and probably a staphylococcal septicaemia. At the age of 6 months he developed lactosuria and was placed on Low lactose milk food, together with 3 drops of halibut liver oil and vitamin C daily. 10 days later his ductus was successfully ligated. 29 days after commencing Low lactose milk food he developed sore buttocks and then fissuring of the angles of the mouth and outer canthi of the eyes (see Fig. 1h). The skin lesions failed to respond to topical treatment. Six days later he was given three tablets of Ketovite and 5 ml. Ketovite supplement syrup daily. There was rapid improvement and after four days the rash had almost gone. The development of the rash was not accompanied by a failure to gain weight in this patient.

## Discussion

The feeding experiments in young rats reported here demonstrated that the synthetic foods studied were unable to support adequate growth and that this could be corrected by the administration of a complete vitamin supplement. Though great caution must always be exercised in applying the results of animal experiments to man, these investigations supported the hypothesis that there was a vitamin deficiency in the human infants. This was subsequently shown to be so, as evidenced by the prompt and dramatic clinical improvement in Cases A, B, and C when adequate vitamins were given.

Admittedly, with the synthetic foods investigated, the appetite of the rats was poor and hence their total calorie intake was lower than that of controls. However, in pair-feeding experiments with Galactomin and Edosol it was shown that there was an actual inability to utilize the calories provided when there was a deficiency of vitamins.

Although the animal feeding experiments using various combinations of vitamins (see Table 4) gave no clear-cut indication of the cause of the deficiency state which developed in the babies described above, the clinical evidence derived from feeding vitamins to Case A suggested that the missing factor or factors might belong to the tocopheryl—inositol—biotin group. However, the interdependence of various nutritional factors made a precise assessment difficult. Furthermore, because of the critical condition of Case A it became necessary to abandon the piecemeal introduction of the components of Ketovite tablets upon which we had embarked. It could, of course, be argued that had we persisted with the calcium pantothenate and folic acid for longer than 48 hours (she was at this stage still receiving vitamins A, B1, B6, B12, C, D, and choline chloride), the unremitting deterioration would have been halted and reversed with the addition of these two vitamins alone. In other words, the suggestion would be that these particular nutrients were not given enough time to take effect. One thing is certain, and that is that a most dramatic change for the better occurred within 48 hours of introducing Ketovite tablets.

There are few data on the minimal requirements of the human infant for individual vitamins, and these,

TABLE 6
TIME OF APPEARANCE OF THE RASH

| | Case | | | | |
|---|---|---|---|---|---|
| | 1 | 2 | A | B | C |
| Age of patient when synthetic food and incomplete vitamin supplement first given .. .. | 7 days | 15 days | 10 weeks | 5 months | 6 months |
| Period on diet before rash appeared .. .. | 10 weeks | 7 weeks | 10 weeks | 2 weeks | 4 weeks |

therefore, have to be decided largely on theoretical grounds, after considering the composition of breast milk. The levels of pantothenate, folate, and thiamine have been measured by Baker, Frank, Pasher, Ziffer, and Sobotka (1960), in the foetus, newborn, and mother. They found that the levels rose in the foetus during gestation, so that the values at birth were 3 to 7 times greater than in the mother. It appears then that high levels of vitamins may be necessary for optimal growth in the early months of life when metabolism is proceeding at a very rapid rate. In this connexion we have indicated in Table 6 the ages at which the synthetic food together with the inadequate vitamin supplements were first given, and also the time taken for the rash to appear thereafter. Although it is impossible to assess the part played by the primary disease under treatment in the time taken for the rash to develop, it is of interest that the most rapid appearance of the eruption was in Cases B and C, the oldest of the series, whose vitamin reserves may have been by this time less plentiful.

The clinical picture found in the babies with this deficiency state is a striking one. Most distinctive are the various skin lesions which, in the florid case, may be itemized as follows.

(1) A well-demarcated pink psoriasiform eruption affecting particularly the buttocks. The rash may extend forwards to involve the perineum and the external genitalia and posteriorly to the natal cleft and sacral region. Similar lesions may occur elsewhere; thus they have been seen over the scalp and the lower limbs. The rash could be moist at first, with blistering on occasions, later becoming dry, scaly, and glazed.

(2) A pink, moist, or dry intertrigo of the groins.

(3) Cracking of the lips often associated with exudation and bleeding.

(4) Fissuring at the angles of the mouth and the outer canthi of the eyelids, again with exudation and sometimes bleeding.

(5) Pink exudative lesions over the external ears especially the helices, with a tendency to crusting. The retro-auricular reflection of skin could be similarly affected, particularly superiorly.

(6) In one fatal case crusting of the external nares was a persistent feature and assumed to be part of the generalized eruption.

Other recurring features noted in the three severe cases were skin pallor, emaciation, anorexia, and fatigue while feeding. Vomiting occurred frequently and was easily induced if milk was pressed on the baby. Coughing could also be troublesome on such occasions and often lead to retching with loss of calories. Irritability and restlessness, particularly at night, were impressive behaviour disturbances, though, contrary to what one might expect from the appearance of the skin lesions, the deeply cracked lips and the sore-looking buttocks did not seem to cause either pain or discomfort. Abdominal distension was a constant development as the child's condition slowly deteriorated. There was a striking tendency for septic lesions to be a late complication. Death in our two fatal cases occurred abruptly and unexpectedly, both babies remaining alert and responsive until near the end. Sudden death was also reported to us in the sib of our first case (Case 1) who had died earlier in another hospital while under treatment for galactosaemia.

The unusual and distinctive lesions affecting the lips and eyes in the present cases are a feature of these nutritionally disturbed infants. While lip fissuring alone has been described in cases of riboflavine deficiency (Spies, Vilter, and Ashe, 1939), it should be emphasized that the patients reported here were not only receiving adequate amounts of this vitamin but failed to respond to additional large supplements.

The Report of the Committee on Nutrition (1963) stressed both the importance of the awareness of composition and nutritional properties of synthetic diets, and the need to give adequate vitamins. The Report also drew attention to the paucity of knowledge concerning the long-term effects of synthetic diets in infancy.

Three recommendations are made as a result of our experience.

(1) The exact composition of synthetic foods, so far as this is known, should be readily available to the clinician.

(2) When the synthetic food is known to be nutritionally incomplete, the label should clearly state this and give definite advice concerning any necessary additions to the diet. It is not sufficient to make the general statement that 'vitamins should be given'.

(3) If an infant is receiving a synthetic food, the clinician should be wary about assuming that the disease under treatment is necessarily the cause of failure to thrive.

## Summary

A deficiency state characterized by disseminated skin lesions of a distinctive kind coupled with failure to thrive is reported in 5 infants who received various synthetic milks: 2 deaths occurred before the nature of the disturbance was appreciated.

The synthetic milks were found not to support adequate growth of young rats but this could be corrected by the administration of a complete vitamin supplement, namely Ketovite syrup together with Ketovite tablets (Paines & Byrne Ltd.). These experiments supported the clinical impression that the two infant deaths were due to a hitherto unrecognized deficiency state. This was subsequently shown to be likely when complete vitamin supplements were given to three other similarly affected infants and led to rapid clinical improvement.

The supplements included choline chloride, calcium pantothenate, inositol, biotin, α-tocopheryl-acetate, and vitamin B12 and folic acid in addition to those provided by conventional vitamin therapy.

We thank Sir Wilfrid Sheldon and Dr. G. H. Newns for permission to investigate their patients. We are grateful for all the help given by Dr. S. P. Hall-Smith, Sister M. Gibson, Sister M. Leavesly, Sister B. Wellar, Mrs. J. Shepherd, and Mrs. C. King. We received invaluable help from Mr. S. T. Higgins and Mr. D. Martin who took the photographs. Financial assistance from The Joint Research Board of the Hospital for Sick Children and the Institute of Child Health was much appreciated. Trufood Ltd. kindly contributed towards the cost of the coloured plates, and it is a great pleasure to acknowledge the close collaboration of Mr. J. V. Hyde of Trufood Ltd., throughout this work.

### References

Baker, H., Frank, O., Pasher, I., Ziffer, H., and Sobotka, H. (1960). Pantothenic acid, thiamine and folic acid levels at parturition. *Proc. Soc. exp. Biol. (N.Y.)*, **103**, 321.

Brimblecombe, F. S. W., Blainey, J. D., Stoneman, M. E. R., and Wood, B. S. B. (1961). Dietary and biochemical control of phenylketonuria. *Brit. med. J.*, **2**, 793.

Mitchell, H. S. (1927). Comparative physiological values of five carbohydrates, based on growth and fecal analysis. *Amer. J. Physiol.*, **79**, 537.

Moncrieff, A., and Wilkinson, R. H. (1961). Further experiences in the treatment of phenylketonuria. *Brit. med. J.*, **1**, 763.

Report of the Committee on Nutrition (1963). Appraisal of nutritional adequacy of infant formulas used as cow milk substitutes. *Pediatrics*, **31**, 329.

Spies, T. D., Vilter, R. W., and Ashe, W. F. (1939). Pellagra, beriberi and riboflavin deficiency in human beings. *J. Amer. med. Ass.*, **113**, 931.

Wilson, K. M., and Clayton, B. E. (1962). Importance of choline during growth, with particular reference to synthetic diets in phenylketonuria. *Arch. Dis. Childh.*, **37**, 565.

*Arch. Dis. Childh.*, 1965, **40**, 376.

# AETIOLOGY OF ATHETOSIS WITH SPECIAL REFERENCE TO NEONATAL ASPHYXIA, IDIOPATHIC ICTERUS, AND ABO-INCOMPATIBILITY*

BY

P. PLUM

*From the University Clinic of Paediatrics, Rigshospital, Copenhagen, Denmark*

(RECEIVED FOR PUBLICATION AUGUST 27, 1964)

In the present paper the aetiology of congenital athetosis has been studied by examining the relative importance of the following factors: (1) neonatal asphyxia without icterus, (2) neonatal icterus of unknown origin, (3) neonatal icterus due to ABO- and Rh-sensitization, and (4) prematurity.

## Material and Methods

The case material comprises all patients with congenital athetosis seen in our clinic from 1949 to 1963 inclusive, a total of 173. The age of the patients at first examination, last examination, and death, is given in Figs. 1 and 2.

It is seen that most of the deaths during childhood occur within the first three years of life: 85 patients, 49%, were seen during their first year of life; of these 85 patients, 41%, died. Of patients first seen after their first year of life, only 7% died. All patients have been examined by the author, in most cases repeatedly.

**Neonatal History.** There were 96 children born in hospital or in a private clinic, and 32 children born at home but admitted to hospital during the neonatal period. Information was obtained from the hospital records for these 128 children. The remaining 45 were born at home and not admitted to hospital during the first weeks of life; in these, information was supplied by the parents and by their physicians. All parents in addition filled in a detailed questionnaire, and later the questionnaire was discussed, usually on several occasions. The reliability of the information given by parents was checked by comparing it with that obtained from hospitals, and was found satisfactory.

**Serological Examinations.** These were carried out in children and their mothers in practically all cases. Most of the serological examinations were carried out at the Blood Bank of the Rigshospital (Head: Erik Freiesleben, M.D.) and some at the Blood Group Department of the State Serum Institute. The following laboratory tests were made. (a) *The child:* ABO and Rh groups, direct

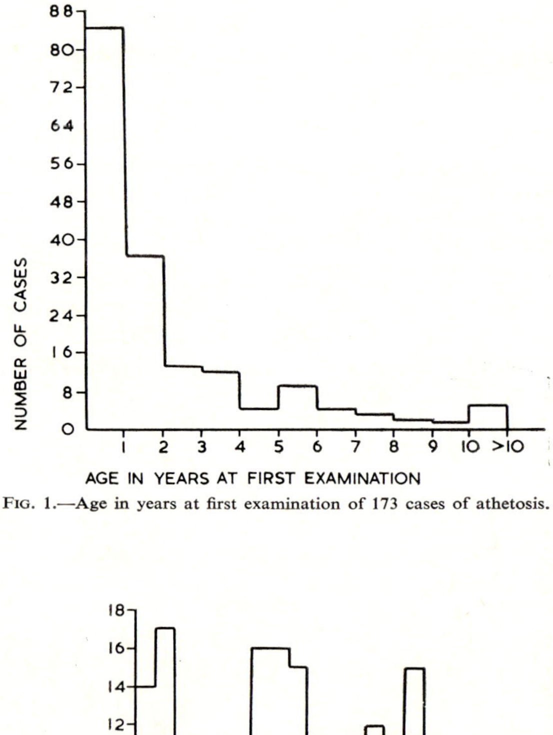


FIG. 1.—Age in years at first examination of 173 cases of athetosis.

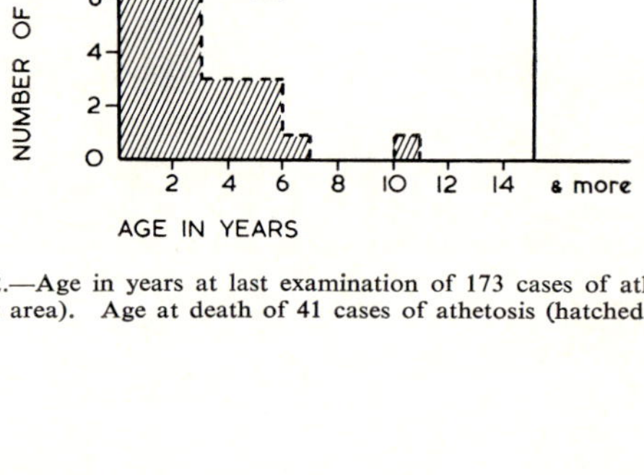


FIG. 2.—Age in years at last examination of 173 cases of athetosis (white area). Age at death of 41 cases of athetosis (hatched area).

* This study was supported by a PHS Research Grant B-2408 from The National Institute of Neurological Diseases and Blindness, Bethesda, U.S.A., and by The Danish Cerebral Palsy Fund.

Coombs test, and a direct Munk-Andersen (1956) conglutination test in the newborn, if the child's red cells were found to be ABO-incompatible with the serum of the mother. (b) *Compatibility test between the child's red cells and the mother's serum:* the test was performed with a saline suspension at 37° C. and followed by an indirect Coombs test. (c) *The mother:* ABO and Rh groups; examination for complete and incomplete antibodies. If ABO incompatibility was found, the mother's serum was examined for specific haemolysins and immune antibodies against the child's ABO antigens.

### Definitions

*Athetosis:* a non-progressive condition, characterized by involuntary movements, lack of co-ordination, paresis, and intermittent hypertonicity. The irregular hyperkinetic movements may appear spontaneously or only under emotional or intentional stress. Only congenital cases have been included.

*Kernikterus.* The following signs have been considered as clinical evidence of kernikterus in the newborn baby: opisthotonus, head bent backwards, increased muscular tone, convulsion-like attacks, attacks of crying, cyanotic attacks, flaccidity, trembling, abnormal eye movements, abnormal jerky or 'fighting' movements of upper extremities, oblique position of head, fever, abnormal respiration, poor feeding, or swallowing.

*Icterus I:* mild neonatal jaundice of a few days' duration; *icterus II:* pronounced neonatal jaundice lasting less than 3 weeks; *icterus III:* pronounced neonatal jaundice lasting for more than 3 weeks.

*Asphyxia I:* mild neonatal asphyxia, lasting in most cases only for a few minutes and in no case for more than 15 minutes; *asphyxia II:* pronounced neonatal asphyxia, lasting for 15-29 minutes; *asphyxia III:* pronounced neonatal asphyxia, lasting for 30 minutes or more.

*Blood-group Immunization.* In cases of Rh incompatibility, the usual criteria were followed. In cases of ABO incompatibility the criteria of the Blood Bank of the Rigshospital were accepted. Antibodies against A or B were described as being of immune character, only if the antibody titre in the indirect Coombs test was three dilutions or more higher than the saline antibody titre. If, for example, the saline titre was 256 and the indirect Coombs titre was 2,048, the antibody was described as immune. If the saline titre was 2,048 and the indirect Coombs titre was 4,096, the antibody was described as not being of immune character. A positive direct Munk-Andersen test on the red cells of the child was considered to be supporting evidence for the presence of immune antibodies.

*Hyperkinesia I:* spontaneous or induced hyperkinetic movements of slight degree; *hyperkinesia II:* of moderate degree; *hyperkinesia III:* of excessive degree.

*Motor handicap I:* does not prevent the patient from carrying out the movements necessary in daily life. *Motor handicap II:* renders it impossible to carry out ordinary movements in a normal manner, and when they are carried out there is considerable exertion. *Motor handicap III:* prevents the patient from carrying out voluntary movements in an efficient manner.

*Speech handicap I:* speech is easily understandable, but not normal for the age; *speech handicap II:* the patient can speak, but is understood with difficulty; *speech handicap III:* the patient has practically no spoken language, perhaps a few words.

### Results

**Neonatal Asphyxia as a Cause of Athetosis.** During 1949 to 1963 inclusive, when the cases of athetosis were observed, changes had taken place with regard to the relative frequency of the possible aetiological factors, namely icterus of unknown origin (idiopathic icterus), icterus due to blood-group immunization, and asphyxia. The case material of athetosis has been presented with respect to these factors in Table 1. The series shows a relative and absolute decrease in frequency of cases with a history of asphyxia without icterus: this tendency may probably be explained by the increasing interest of obstetricians in preventing neonatal asphyxia.

The correlation between degree of icterus, degree of asphyxia, immunization, and prematurity is presented in Table 2, which shows that in all but 5 cases, the children had either neonatal icterus or neonatal asphyxia, or both. In 31, there was neonatal asphyxia without icterus. It can also be seen that asphyxia in these 31 children was most often pronounced and that most of them were full-term infants. In addition, it is clear that the combination of neonatal icterus and neonatal asphyxia is less frequent in cases where the icterus is due to immunization than in cases where it is not due to immunization.

Another explanation for the relative increase in post-icteric cases (Table 1), and the corresponding decrease in post-asphyxial cases, might be that some years ago neonatal icterus was more often overlooked or forgotten. When, however, the group of cases with a history of neonatal asphyxia *without* neonatal icterus is compared with the group of cases *with* a history of neonatal icterus, with or without neonatal asphyxia, such a conclusion is seen to be statistically most unlikely.

In Tables 3 and 4, all cases of athetosis are divided into three groups (A, B, and C) according to the presence or absence of neonatal icterus and neonatal asphyxia. In Table 3 groups A, B, and C are correlated with other factors, such as birth weight, complicated delivery, history of icterus in sibs, and

TABLE 1

179 CASES OF CONGENITAL ATHETOSIS: YEAR OF BIRTH IN RELATION TO NEONATAL ICTERUS, ASPHYXIA, AND BLOOD SENSITIZATION

| Year of Birth | No. of Cases* | Icterus (%) | Icterus and Sensitization (%) | Icterus Without Sensitization (%) | Asphyxia (%) | Asphyxia Without Icterus (%) | Insufficient Information (%) |
|---|---|---|---|---|---|---|---|
| Before 1949 | 32 | 53 | 19 | 34 | 44 | 22 | 22 |
| 1949-53 | 65 | 69 | 31 | 38 | 38 | 17 | 8 |
| 1954-58 | 62 | 82 | 45 | 37 | 32 | 15 | 2 |
| 1959-63 | 20 | 100 | 25 | 75 | 20 | 0 | 0 |

* All cases of athetosis were included, but 6 infants who died with kernikterus in 1963 could not be included in the statistical analysis.

TABLE 2

DISTRIBUTION OF 173 CASES OF ATHETOSIS WITH REGARD TO DEGREE OF NEONATAL ICTERUS, DEGREE OF NEONATAL ASPHYXIA, BLOOD GROUP SENSITIZATION, AND BIRTH WEIGHT

| Degree of Icterus | | | | | | Sensitization | | | Asphyxia | | | | | Birth Weight | |
|---|---|---|---|---|---|---|---|---|---|---|---|---|---|---|---|
| I | II | III | Degree Unknown | — | No Information | + | — | Unknown | I | II | III | — | Unknown | ≦ 2,500 g. | > 2,500 g. |
| 8 | | | | | | 2 | | | 1 | | | | | 0 | 1 |
| | | | | | | | | | | | | 1 | | 0 | 1 |
| | | | | | | | 6 | | 3 | | | | | 1 | 2 |
| | | | | | | | | | | 1 | | | | 0 | 1 |
| | | | | | | | | | | | 1 | | | 1 | 0 |
| | | | | | | | | | | | | 1 | | 1 | 0 |
| | 48 | | | | | 18 | | | 2 | | | | | 1 | 1 |
| | | | | | | | | | | | | 16 | | 3 | 13 |
| | | | | | | | 28 | | 7 | | | | | 3 | 4 |
| | | | | | | | | | | | 2 | | | 1 | 1 |
| | | | | | | | | | | | | 19 | | 10 | 9 |
| | | | | | | | | 2 | | | | 2 | | 1 | 1 |
| | | 77 | | | | 39 | | | 3 | | | | | 0 | 3 |
| | | | | | | | | | | 1 | | | | 0 | 1 |
| | | | | | | | | | | | 1 | | | 0 | 1 |
| | | | | | | | | | | | | 34 | | 10 | 24 |
| | | | | | | | 36 | | 7 | | | | | 6 | 1 |
| | | | | | | | | | | 3 | | | | 0 | 3 |
| | | | | | | | | | | | 2 | | | 2 | 0 |
| | | | | | | | | | | | | 23 | | 13 | 10 |
| | | | | | | | | | | | | | 1 | 0 | 1 |
| | | | | | | | | 2 | | | | 2 | | 2 | 0 |
| | | | 1 | | | | 1 | | 1 | | | | | 1 | 0 |
| | | | | 37 | | 2 | | | | | 1 | | | 0 | 1 |
| | | | | | | | | | | | | | 1 | 0 | 1 |
| | | | | | | | 31 | | 3 | | | | | 0 | 3 |
| | | | | | | | | | | 8 | | | | 2 | 6 |
| | | | | | | | | | | | 15 | | | 2 | 13 |
| | | | | | | | | | | | | 5 | | 0 | 5 |
| | | | | | | | | 4 | | 1 | | | | 0 | 1 |
| | | | | | | | | | | | 3 | | | 0 | 3 |
| | | | | | 2 | | 1 | | | 1 | | | | 1 | 0 |
| | | | | | | | | 1 | | 1 | | | | 1 | 0 |
| Totals: 8 | 48 | 77 | 1 | 37 | 2 | 61 | 103 | 9 | 27 | 16 | 25 | 103 | 2 | 62 | 111 |
| 173 | | | | | | 173 | | | 173 | | | | | 173 | |

TABLE 3

RELATION BETWEEN NEONATAL HISTORY WITH REGARD TO ICTERUS AND ASPHYXIA, AND SOME OTHER FACTORS

| | Neonatal | | No. | Birth Weight ≤ 2,500 g. | Asphyxia | | Complicated Delivery | Immune Anti-bodies Found | History of Icterus in Sibs |
|---|---|---|---|---|---|---|---|---|---|
| | Icterus | Asphyxia | | | I | III | | | |
| A | + | — | 98 | 38·8% | — | — | 38·8% | 52·0% | 34·7% |
| B | + | + | 35 | 45·7% | 68·6% | 17·1% | 51·4% | 22·9% | 11·4% |
| C | — | + | 31 | 12·9% | 9·7% | 61·3% | 61·3% | 3·2% | 9·7% |
| Difference A-B | | | | 6·9 | | | 12·6 | 29·1 | 23·3 |
| p % | | | | >5 | | | >5 | 0·1 | 0·1 |
| Difference B-C | | | | 32·8 | 58·9 | 44·2 | 9·9 | 19·7 | 1·7 |
| p % | | | | 0·2 | <0·1 | <0·1 | >5 | 1·0 | >5 |
| Difference A-C | | | | 25·9 | | | 22·5 | 48·8 | 25·0 |
| p % | | | | <0·1 | | | 2·5 | <0·1 | <0·1 |

presence of immune antibodies. Table 3 shows that Group C, cases with a history of asphyxia but no icterus, differ significantly in several respects from both groups of cases with neonatal icterus.

In Table 4 the three groups A, B, and C are correlated with various neurological defects. Here again group C, post-asphyxial without icterus, differs significantly from the post-icteric groups. The differences are especially significant with regard to degree of motor handicap, impaired hearing, and impairment of upward gaze, in spite of the fact that only a minority of patients were examined for the last-mentioned sign. The post-icteric cases have less motor handicap, less hyperkinesia, less speech defect, and less epilepsy; they have more often normal intelligence and more often a normal electroencephalogram. On the other hand, they have more often strabismus. Reduced hearing and impairment of upward gaze are only found among post-icteric cases.

The difference with respect to hearing loss between the post-icteric and post-asphyxic cases was described in 1957 by the present author, and in 1963 by Churchill and Colfelt, who also emphasized the difference with regard to impairment of upward gaze.

The two groups of cases in the present athetosis series, (A) cases with icterus and without asphyxia, and (C) cases without icterus and with asphyxia (Table 4), were examined for other possible neurological differences. Since a clinical classification into the post-icteric or the post-asphyxial group does not seem to be possible in the individual patient on the basis of his neurological signs, an analysis has been made of all the patients of each group, with regard to five clinical signs: Babinski, ankle clonus, increased knee-jerk, rigidity, and contracture. The frequency with which any one of the signs was absent in the patients of each group, as well as how often two, three, four, or all five signs were absent, have been examined. A significant

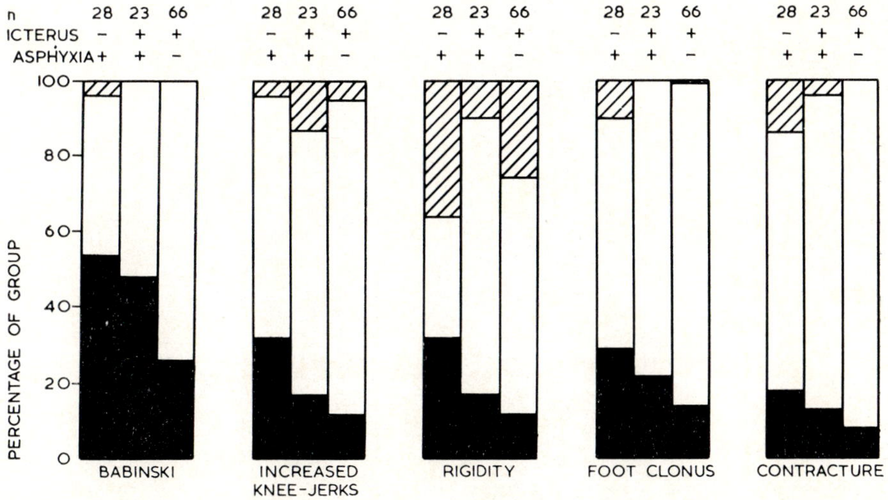


FIG. 3.—Correlation between neonatal history of icterus and asphyxia, and late neurological signs. Black area = positive sign; white area = negative sign; and hatched area = doubtful sign or not examined.

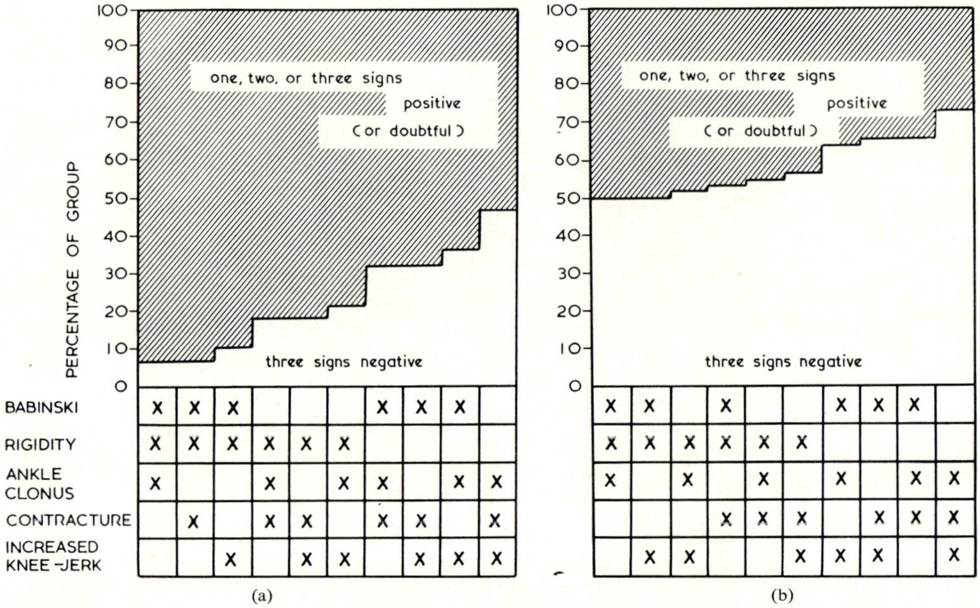


FIG. 4.—Correlation between neonatal history of icterus and asphyxia, and late neurological signs. (a) 31 cases with asphyxia and without icterus. (b) 98 cases with icterus and without asphyxia.

difference between the two groups of patients, the post-icteric and the post-asphyxial cases, was found in all but one of the 31 possible combinations of signs.

Some of the data from this analysis are presented graphically in Figs. 3 and 4.

The over-all result of the neurological analysis of the material is that the post-asphyxial cases of athetosis are more often 'spastic' than the post-icteric cases. On the other hand, no one of the five signs, by its presence or absence, permits a classification of an individual patient in either group, nor does any combination of negative signs permit such a classification.

COMBINED NEONATAL ASPHYXIA AND ICTERUS. Cases with neonatal icterus not due to immunization have neonatal asphyxia in 37·1% and cases with icterus due to immunization have neonatal asphyxia in 13·6% (Table 2). This difference is not likely to be due to chance (p 0·13%). Since the incidence of neonatal asphyxia is higher in both groups than normally, it must be assumed that asphyxia in some way facilitates the damaging effect of hyperbilirubinaemia. It seems difficult, however, to understand why neonatal asphyxia should play a greater aetiological role in cases without than in cases with immunization.

Lucey, Hibbard, Behrman, Esquivel de Gallardo,

RELATION BETWEEN NEONATAL HISTORY, WITH RE

| | Neonatal | | No. | Degree of Motor Handicap | | Degree of Hyperkinesia | | Degree of Speech | |
|---|---|---|---|---|---|---|---|---|---|
| | Icterus | Asphyxia | | I | III | I | III | I | I |
| A | + | − | 66 | 50·0% | 28·8% | 44·0% | 13·6% | 30·3% | 28· |
| B | + | + | 23 | 34·8% | 26·1% | 47·8% | 26·1% | 21·7% | 47· |
| C | − | + | 28 | 10·7% | 64·3% | 21·4% | 53·5% | 7·1% | 46· |
| Difference A-B .. | .. | .. | .. | 15·2 | 2·7 | 3·8 | 12·5 | 8·6 | 19· |
| p % .. | .. | .. | .. | > 5 | > 5 | > 5 | > 5 | > 5 | > 5 |
| Difference B-C .. | .. | .. | .. | 24·1 | 38·2 | 26·4 | 27·4 | 14·6 | 1· |
| p % .. | .. | .. | .. | 3·6 | 0·3 | 4·2 | 3·7 | > 5 | > 5 |
| Difference A-C .. | .. | .. | .. | 39·3 | 35·5 | 22·6 | 39·9 | 23·2 | 17· |
| p % .. | .. | .. | .. | < 0·1 | 0·1 | 2·2 | < 0·1 | 0·2 | > 5 |

*Note:* All patients with athetosis, 4 yea

and Windle (1964) injected indirect-reacting bilirubin into newborn rhesus monkeys. Only when the monkeys were asphyxiated for 10-12 minutes during caesarean section before the bilirubin injections, was it possible to produce clinical and histological signs of kernikterus.

When the cases with neonatal icterus with and without neonatal asphyxia are compared with regard to birth weight, incidence of complications at delivery (Table 3, A and B), and with regard to late clinical signs (Table 4, A and B), no differences are found. The neurological signs, however, show a systematic difference. Fig. 3 shows that each of the five neurological signs is positive more often in cases with both icterus and asphyxia than in cases solely with icterus. Even though none of the observed differences are significant, the constant finding of more positive signs in the post-asphyxial icteric cases seems to indicate that the asphyxia has modified or aggravated the brain pathology.

To conclude, it must be assumed that the presence of neonatal asphyxia in icteric infants affects both the occurrence of the brain injury and the nature of the anatomical lesion.

Degree of Neonatal Asphyxia and Late Symptoms. The question whether a correlation could be demonstrated between degree of asphyxia and late clinical signs was examined. The numbers are small (Table 2), and no conclusions can be drawn.

**Neonatal Icterus of Unknown Origin as a Cause of Athetosis.** The following problems arise. (1) Can physiological or idiopathic icterus, in the same way as icterus due to blood-group immunization, cause cerebral damage resulting in kernikterus and athetosis? (2) If so, what is the relative importance of physiological icterus in causing athetosis? (3) Is there any difference between the sensitized and the non-sensitized cases of athetosis? (4) Must the existence of unknown factors, which determine whether the icteric newborn is brain-damaged or not, be assumed?

(1) In this series, 71 cases of athetosis had a history of neonatal icterus without immunization, and 59 cases had a history of neonatal icterus that was probably due to blood-group immunization. The immediate answer to the first question must, therefore, be in the affirmative. The cases of this series have been grouped in Table 5 according to blood group compatibility or incompatibility of mother and child, and according to presence or absence of immune antibodies.

Reverting to the question of whether cases of athetosis with neonatal icterus not due to immunization are caused by this idiopathic icterus, or whether other aetiological factors should be considered, asphyxia is seen to be present in 26 (37%) of these 71 cases. Thus asphyxia may have played a role in the aetiology of these 26 cases, but it was absent in the majority.

(2) The relative incidence of athetosis with a history of neonatal icterus of unknown origin seems to have been increasing during the past 15 years (Table 1). This is probably due to the fact that newborns with icterus due to immunization have been treated more intensively by exchange transfusion than those without immunization. It would actually seem that during the past few years, more cases of athetosis have been caused by idiopathic icterus than by icterus due to immunization.

(3) Statistical analysis of the data* has shown that in certain respects cases with a history of idiopathic icterus differ from those with icterus due to immuni-

* The author is willing to supply these statistical data on request.

...TERUS AND ASPHYXIA, AND SOME LATE SIGNS

| ...normal ...lligence | Impaired Hearing | Impairment of Upward Gaze | | | Squint | Epilepsy | Abnormal EEG |
|---|---|---|---|---|---|---|---|
| | | – | + | ? | | | |
| ·2% | 51·5% | 13·6% | 22·7% | 63·7% | 34·8% | 4·5% | 19·7% |
| ·8% | 47·8% | 26·1% | 13·0% | 60·9% | 26·1% | 4·4% | 21·7% |
| ·1% | 0 | 28·6% | 0 | 71·4% | 14·3% | 21·4% | 46·4% |
| ·6 | 3·7 | | 9·7 | | 8·7 | 0·1 | 2·0 |
| | > 5 | | > 5 | | > 5 | > 5 | > 5 |
| ·7 | 47·8 | | 13·0 | | 11·8 | 17·0 | 24·7 |
| | < 0·1 | | > 5 | | > 5 | > 5 | 5 |
| ·9 | 51·5 | | 22·7 | | 20·5 | 16·9 | 26·7 |
| ·2 | < 0·1 | | < 0·1 | | 2·0 | 3·8 | 1·2 |

last examination are included.

T

CORRELATION BETWEEN BLOOD GROUPS, IMMUNE ANTIBODIES, AND S

| No. | Blood Groups of Mother and Child with Regard to: A and B | | Rh | | Immune Anti-A or B in Mother's Blood: Examined | | | Immune Anti-Rh in Mother's I: Examined | | |
|---|---|---|---|---|---|---|---|---|---|---|
| | Compatible | Not Compatible | Compatible | Not Compatible | Not Found* | Found | Not Examined | Not Found | Found | N Exan |
| 66 | + | | + | | + | | | + | | |
| 5 | + | | + | | | | + | + | | |
| 9 | + | | + | | | | + | | | + |
| 5 | + | | | + | | | | + | | |
| 14 | | + | + | | + | | | + | | |
| 2 | | + | | + | + | | | + | | |
| 101 | | | | | | | | | | |
| 29 | + | | | + | | | | | + | |
| 27 | | + | + | | | + | | + | | |
| 1 | | + | | + | | + | | | + | |
| 4 | | + | | + | | | + | | + | |
| 61 | | | | | | | | | | |
| 1 | | + | | + | | | + | + | | |
| 2 | | | | | | | + | + | | |
| 8 | | | | | | | + | | | - |
| 11 | | | | | | | | | | |
| Total 173 | | | | | | | | | | |

* Also exami

zation. Cases with idiopathic icterus are more often premature and they are more often asphyxiated neonatally than those with icterus due to immunization. On the other hand, there are fewer neonatal signs of kernikterus, impaired hearing, and sibs with neonatal icterus. There are no significant differences in this series with regard to the degree of icterus, the degree of motor handicap, the incidence of subnormal intelligence, the incidence of epilepsy, and the incidence of neurological signs indicating spasticity.

Fifteen of the non-sensitized children with athetosis died during early childhood. Necropsy was performed in 5 and histological signs characteristic of kernikterus were found in 4 (to be reported by Inge Tygstrup). The death rate was 29·5% in the sensitized and 17·8% in the non-sensitized group; this difference is not significant.

It is general clinical experience that the bilirubin values during the first days of life show an earlier and more rapid rise in sensitized than in non-sensitized icteric newborn. It has not been possible to obtain information on this problem from this series of cases of athetosis, since bilirubin determinations have been made in only 9 sensitized and 9 non-sensitized cases.

(4) Though it seems likely that prematurity and neonatal asphyxia add to the risk of idiopathic neonatal icterus, it is not possible at the moment to explain why an infant is affected or escapes. A search for some other factor of contributory or decisive importance seems indicated. Waters and Porter (1964) have reported that the determination of the reserve albumin-binding capacity of serum adds valuable information. If there is no albumin left for binding the unconjugated bilirubin the risk of kernikterus is great, in spite of a low serum bilirubin.

**ABO Sensitization.** Although there is still some uncertainty associated with demonstrating ABO sensitization in the individual case, it is generally accepted that ABO sensitization is of aetiological importance for neonatal icterus and subsequent brain disease.

To elucidate the question as to whether a relationship could be demonstrated between ABO incompatibility and athetosis the following analyses were made. (a) A comparison between the blood groups of mother and child in the present material and the general population. (b) A comparison of the incidence of various neonatal and late signs within the three groups of cases, ABO-incompatibility, Rh-incompatibility, and post-icteric cases without incompatibility.

(a) Dr. J. Schultz-Larsen, Institute of Human Genetics, University of Copenhagen, has kindly carried out the calculations. The main results were as follows. The total material shows that the number of observed cases of ABO-incompatibility and Rh-incompatibility are significantly greater than in the general population ($\chi^2 = 6{\cdot}4$, $f = 1$, $2\% > p$

NESTIC DATA IN THE ATHETOSIS SERIES (ABSOLUTE NUMBERS; ALL CASES INCLUDED)

| h :ht g. | Neonatal Icterus | | | | Neonatal Asphyxia | | | Icterus in Sibs | Signs of Kernikterus | Reduced Hearing | − Icterus + Asphyxia |
|---|---|---|---|---|---|---|---|---|---|---|---|
| | + | − | Unknown | Icterus III | + | − | Unknown | | | | |
| | 46 | 20 | 0 | 23 | 34 | 32 | 0 | 10 | 19 | 16 | 16 |
| | 5 | 0 | 0 | 2 | 1 | 4 | 0 | 0 | 2 | 2 | 0 |
| | 4 | 4 | 1 | 2 | 8 | 1 | 0 | 0 | 4 | 1 | 4 |
| | 4 | 1 | 0 | 1 | 4 | 1 | 0 | 1 | 2 | 1 | 1 |
| | 10 | 4 | 0 | 7 | 5 | 8 | 1 | 1 | 3 | 2 | 3 |
| | 2 | 0 | 0 | 1 | 0 | 2 | 0 | 0 | 1 | 1 | 0 |
| | 71 | 29 | 1 | 36 | 52 | 48 | 1 | 12 | 31 | 23 | 24 |
| | 29 | 0 | 0 | 21 | 3 | 26 | 0 | 14 | 22 | 15 | 0 |
| | 25 | 2 | 0 | 15 | 5 | 22 | 0 | 13 | 17 | 12 | 1 |
| | 1 | 0 | 0 | 1 | 0 | 1 | 0 | 1 | 0 | 1 | 0 |
| | 4 | 0 | 0 | 2 | 1 | 3 | 0 | 2 | 2 | 2 | 0 |
| | 59 | 2 | 0 | 39 | 9 | 52 | 0 | 30 | 41 | 30 | 1 |
| | 1 | 0 | 0 | 1 | 0 | 1 | 0 | 0 | 1 | 0 | 0 |
| | 1 | 1 | 0 | 1 | 1 | 1 | 0 | 0 | 1 | 1 | 1 |
| | 2 | 5 | 1 | 0 | 6 | 2 | 0 | 0 | 1 | 2 | 5 |
| | 4 | 6 | 1 | 2 | 7 | 4 | 0 | 0 | 3 | 3 | 6 |
| | 134 | 37 | 2 | 77 | 68 | 104 | 1 | 42 | 75 | 56 | 31 |

r immune antibodies.

$> 1\%$, and $\chi^2 = 49 \cdot 6$, $f = 1$, $p < 0 \cdot 1\%$, respectively).

The Rh-compatible part of the material shows that the observed number of cases of ABO-incompatibility is significantly greater than expected ($\chi^2 = 10 \cdot 1$, $f = 1$, $p < 0 \cdot 1\%$).

The ABO-compatible part of the material shows that the observed number of cases of Rh-incompatibility is significantly greater than expected ($\chi^2 = 56 \cdot 7$, $f = 1$, $p < 0 \cdot 1\%$). The Rh-incompatible part of the material shows that the observed number of cases of ABO-incompatibility is not greater than expected. The ABO-incompatible part of the material shows that the observed number of cases of Rh-incompatibility is not greater than expected. The expected frequencies of compatibility and incompatibility between mother and child with respect to ABO were calculated on the basis of the gene frequencies given by Goldschmidt (1961), and with respect to Rh on the basis of the gene frequencies given by Gürtler and Henningsen (1954).

(b) The ABO-incompatible cases lie between the ABO- and Rh-compatible and the Rh-incompatible cases with regard to the incidence of the various signs examined, suggesting that ABO-incompatibility is of importance, but less so than Rh-incompatibility. Cases with immune anti-A or immune anti-B lie between those without immune antibodies and those with Rh-antibodies. The greatest difference between ABO-sensitized and Rh-sensitized children is the greater incidence of prematurity in the former, which likewise includes a greater number of patients with neonatal asphyxia.

If those cases without neonatal icterus are ignored, no differences with regard to late signs were found between sensitized and non-sensitized cases.

**Prematurity.** Prematurity was found in 35% of the total series of athetosis cases, in 40% in the group of athetosis with neonatal icterus, and in 56% in the group of athetosis with idipoathic icterus. With respect to idiopathic icterus, it must be supposed, therefore, that premature infants are either 20 times (i.e. $\frac{94}{6} \times \frac{56}{44}$) as often jaundiced as full-term infants, or that they are 20 times as sensitive to the same level of hyperbilirubinaemia as full-term infants. Since it was found that a certain high bilirubin level was reached only about four times as often by prematures as by full-term infants, it must be concluded either that premature infants are five times as sensitive as full-term infants at a certain degree of hyperbilirubinaemia, or that the critical level of bilirubin is lower for prematures. Trolle (1965) in an examination for the incidence of icterus of unknown origin, found that only duration of pregnancy was of importance. Of children with a birth weight from 2,000 to 2,500 g., those born at term had lower serum bilirubin than those born before term. Trolle suggested that this was probably due to an enzyme deficiency in the liver cells of the premature infants.

On the basis of the present series of athetosis cases, the figures have been examined for any correlation between birth weight and late signs. Only one difference was found, matures were more often of subnormal intelligence than prematures. The difference, however, was of slight significance (p = 3·8%).

### Summary and Conclusions

Based on a series of 173 cases of congenital athetosis, the relative importance of the following aetiological factors was examined: neonatal asphyxia, idiopathic or physiological icterus, ABO- and Rh-sensitization, and prematurity.

Of 173 patients, 31 had a history of neonatal asphyxia without neonatal icterus. This group of post-asphyxial cases differed significantly in several respects from the group of post-icteric cases. The most pronounced differences were found with respect to impaired hearing and impairment of upward gaze, these signs being present only in the post-icteric group. An analysis of the neurological signs showed significant differences between the two groups, the post-asphyxial group showing more cases with signs of spasticity than the post-icteric group.

A history of both neonatal asphyxia and neonatal icterus was less often found in the blood-group sensitized children than in the non-sensitized. The group with both asphyxia and icterus showed a greater incidence of neurological signs indicating spasticity than the post-icteric group, but a smaller incidence of such signs than the post-asphyxial group.

Neonatal asphyxia must be supposed to facilitate the pathological process leading to kernikterus.

More cases developed athetosis from idiopathic icterus than from icterus due to immunization. The group with idiopathic icterus differed significantly from that with icterus due to sensitization in the following respects: birth weight, incidence of neonatal asphyxia, incidence of kernikteric signs, incidence of impaired hearing, and incidence of cases with icterus among sibs. There were no significant differences between the two groups with regard to degree of icterus, degree of motor handicap, incidence of subnormal intelligence, incidence of epilepsy, and incidence of neurological signs indicating spasticity.

Of the 71 non-sensitized infants with athetosis, 15 died during early childhood. Necropsy showed histological signs characteristic of kernikterus in 4 out of 5 (Dr. Inge Tygstrup).

The question of ABO-sensitization is still associated with difficulties of definition. The incidence of ABO- and Rh-incompatibility between mother and child has, therefore, been examined in the athetosis series and compared with the corresponding incidence in the general population. The results indicate that ABO-immunization is of aetiological importance in neonatal icterus.

With regard to the incidence of certain neonatal factors, the group of cases with ABO immune antibodies was found to lie between the group without immune antibodies and the group with Rh-antibodies.

The incidence of prematurity was greater in post-icteric than in post-asphyxia cases, and greater in non-sensitized than in sensitized cases. The susceptibility of premature infants to kernikterus is about 5 times greater than that of full-term infants.

#### References

Churchill, J. A., and Colfelt, R. H. (1963). Etiologic factors in athetotic cerebral palsy. *Arch. Neurol. (Chic.)*, **9**, 400.

Goldschmidt, E. (1961). Variations in the ABO blood group distribution in Denmark. *Acta genet. (Basel)*, **11**, 85.

Gürtler, H., and Henningsen, K. (1954). Rh-chromosome frequencies in the Danish population. *Acta. path. microbiol. scand.*, **34**, 493.

Lucey, J. F., Hibbard, E., Behrman, R. E., Esquivel de Gallardo, F. O., and Windle, W. F. (1964). Kernicterus in asphyxiated newborn rhesus monkeys. *Exp. Neurol.*, **9**, 43.

Munk-Andersen, G. (1956). A dextran serum medium for the demonstration of incomplete anti-A and anti-B. *Acta path. microbiol. scand.*, **38**, 259.

Plum, P. (1957). Etiology of congenital athetosis. *Ann. Paediat. Fenn.*, **3**, 589.

Trolle, D. (1965). *Danish med. Bull.* In the press.

Waters, W. J., and Porter, E. (1964). Indications for exchange transfusion based upon the role of albumin in the treatment of hemolytic disease of the newborn. *Pediatrics*, **33**, 749.

*Arch. Dis. Childh.*, 1965, **40**, 385.

# CORRECTION OF ACIDOSIS IN THE RESUSCITATION OF THE COLLAPSED CHILD

BY

M. E. DODSON and A. L. STEAD

*From the Department of Anaesthesia, Alder Hey Children's Hospital, Liverpool*

(RECEIVED FOR PUBLICATION NOVEMBER 17, 1964)

We present the case histories of 4 severely ill children in whom the decisive factor in survival was thought to have been the correction of their metabolic acidosis with sodium bicarbonate. In 3 of the cases respiratory failure was probably mainly responsible for the child's collapse.

## Methods

The biochemical estimations were made on capillary blood samples using a Vibron *p*H meter with a Robinson-Mattock electrode. It is appreciated that the figures given are only a measurement of the metabolic state of the blood at the site from which it was drawn. From other experiments the authors know that the figures are sufficiently accurate, however, to form a basis for clinical treatment, as 3 of these 4 cases confirm.

**Case 1.** S.H., age 3 years, weight 15 kg., had injured his hip five days previously, and was admitted in a semi-conscious state. A diagnosis of septic arthritis of the hip and septicaemia was made. Within an hour, and despite 200 ml. plasma, his pulse and blood pressure became unrecordable. He was cyanosed and in severe peripheral circulatory failure. A further 200 ml. plasma and 400 ml. blood with intravenous hydrocortisone, Methedrine, and oxytetracycline were given. Oxygen was administered continuously. His condition, however, continued to deteriorate, and his pupils became widely dilated and unreactive.

With difficulty, enough capillary blood was obtained to estimate his base deficit, which was found to be 20 mEq/l. 60 mEq sodium bicarbonate were given rapidly intravenously and his peripheral circulation improved slightly. Repeated estimations showed a decreasing base deficit which was steadily corrected by a further 60 mEq bicarbonate given over the following 3 hours (Table 1); 5½ hours after admission, his pupils were of normal size and reacting to light, he responded to painful stimuli, and his systolic blood pressure was 90 mm. Hg.

His convalescence was prolonged but he slowly recovered complete cerebral function. This case is reported more fully elsewhere (Ellis and Dodson, 1964).

**Case 2.** J.E., age 3 weeks, weight 1·8 kg., a premature baby, was admitted with urinary retention due to urethral valves. His blood urea was 260 mg./100 ml. Under anaesthesia the urethral valves were resected.

Next morning, he collapsed and became cyanosed with laboured respirations and impalpable pulse. It was thought that he had regurgitated and inhaled vomit. He improved slightly after intubation and inflation with oxygen, but there was no obvious respiratory cause for his collapse. His metabolic state was therefore assessed, and the *p*H was found to be 6·69. This was so low that the base deficit could not be estimated from the Siggaard Andersen and Engel nomogram. His alkali reserve was 8 mEq/l. and he was given 4·5 mEq bicarbonate intravenously. One hour later, the *p*H was 6·70.

Within 6½ hours of his first *p*H measurement, he had received 22 mEq bicarbonate; the *p*H was then 7·07 and base deficit 20·5 mEq/l. The further bicarbonate required to correct this is shown in Table 2.

It is interesting that his temperature was 87° F. (30·5° C.) when he was extremely acidotic, and the reduction in metabolism which this produced, may have contributed to his survival (Clowes, Neville, Sabga, and Shibota, 1958).

Twelve hours after his initial collapse, when his condition had been considered hopeless, he was lively and a good colour. Next day, the *p*H was 7·3 and his metabolic state was normal. Should he require further surgery, his acid-base state will be observed closely.

**Case 3.** A.M., aged 1 day, weight 2·3 kg., was cyanosed from birth and was operated on for a supposed diaphragmatic hernia when 12 hours old.

At operation, no hernia was found, but there were numerous cysts of the lower lobe of the left lung, a condition that can produce a similar radiological picture. The left upper lobe was collapsed and could not be inflated. The cystic lobe was resected and an intrapleural drain was inserted. The child's immediate post-operative condition was satisfactory.

Next day she was semi-conscious and cyanosed, with irregular grunting respirations at a rate of 90, indicating severe respiratory insufficiency. Her pulse was 170, and she was in peripheral circulatory failure. At this time, 18 hours after operation, the *p*H was 7·17, $P_{CO_2}$ 40 mm.

TABLE 1

CASE 1: CORRECTION OF ACIDOSIS BY INTRAVENOUS SODIUM BICARBONATE

| Date and Time | | $pH$ | $P_{CO_2}$ (mm.Hg) | Standard Bicarbonate (mEq/l.) | Base Deficit (mEq/l.) | Bicarbonate Given (mEq) |
|---|---|---|---|---|---|---|
| 27.6.63 | 3.45 p.m. | | | 11·6 | 20 | 60 |
| | 4.40 p.m. | 7·30 | 30 | 16·0 | 10 | 30 |
| | 6.0 p.m. | 7·40 | 26 | 19·0 | 6 | 55 |
| | 11.30 p.m. | 7·45 | 23·5 | 20·5 | 3 | 0 |
| 28.6.63 | 9.30 a.m. | 7·45 | 21 | 20·5 | 0 | 0 |

TABLE 2

CASE 2: CORRECTION OF ACIDOSIS BY INTRAVENOUS SODIUM BICARBONATE

| Date and Time | | $pH$ | $P_{CO_2}$ (mm.Hg) | Standard Bicarbonate (mEq/l.) | Base Deficit (mEq/l.) | Bicarbonate Given (mEq) |
|---|---|---|---|---|---|---|
| 3.10.63 | 2.45 p.m. | 6·69 | | | | 4·5 |
| | 4.0 p.m. | 6·70 | | | | 18 |
| | 9.15 p.m. | 7·07 | 34 | 10·5 | 20·5 | 9 |
| 4.10.63 | 9.30 a.m. | 7·3 | 45 | 20 | 4 | 0 |

TABLE 3

CASE 3: CORRECTION OF ACIDOSIS BY INTRAVENOUS SODIUM BICARBONATE

| Date and Time | | $pH$ | $P_{CO_2}$ (mm.Hg) | Standard Bicarbonate (mEq/l.) | Base Deficit (mEq/l.) | Bicarbonate Given (mEq) |
|---|---|---|---|---|---|---|
| 12.12.63 | 12.30 p.m. | 7·17 | 40 | 14 | 15 | 4·5 |
| | 3.0 p.m. | 7·32 | 33 | 17·5 | 7 | 4·5 |
| | 7.30 p.m. | 7·32 | 34 | 15 | 13 | 9 |
| | 11.0 p.m. | 7·36 | 45 | 23 | 0 | 0 |

Hg, and the base deficit 15 mEq/l. Sodium bicarbonate was given intravenously to correct this partially, and $2\frac{1}{2}$ hours later, the base deficit had decreased to 7 mEq/l. Following this, her clinical condition deteriorated again, and this corresponded with an increase in the acidosis (Table 3), requiring further bicarbonate therapy. She thereafter made an uninterrupted recovery.

**Case 4.** K.F., aged 8 weeks, weight 4 kg. This case illustrates that it can be reasonable to give sodium bicarbonate in the absence of measured $p$H changes.

On the morning of admission, this baby became ill at home, and was described by the mother as 'listless and breathing badly'. In the ambulance on the way to hospital he deteriorated further, becoming cyanosed, and by the time he reached the ward at midday he was gasping occasionally and had an irregular bradycardia. External cardiac massage was applied until the child could be intubated and inflated with oxygen. His heart rate and respiration then improved, but he remained cyanosed and began to have continuous convulsions. His temperature was 103° F. (39·5° C.) and he was very dehydrated.

Intravenous fluids were started and in view of the gravity of his clinical state, his base deficit was assumed to be at least 5-10 mEq/l. 150 ml. plasma and 6 mEq bicarbonate were given over the next $1\frac{1}{2}$ hours and by this time his colour was much better. He had peripheral pulses and though his limbs were stiff, he only twitched occasionally. He was breathing well, but was nursed in moist oxygen with the endotracheal tube in place for a further hour. The tube was then removed and he started to take feeds eagerly.

Over the next 24 hours, cyanosis disappeared, and two weeks after admission he was ready for discharge. During this time his prepuce sloughed, an indication of the severity of the initial peripheral circulatory failure. The aetiology of this child's fulminating illness remains obscure.

## Discussion

Many varied disease processes may produce a state of metabolic acidosis, poor tissue perfusion being the common factor in these conditions. Tissue perfusion is dependent upon capillary blood flow, which in itself depends on such factors as arterial pressure, vasoconstriction and blood viscosity.

Many conditions influence these factors. Among them are hypoxia, hypercarbia; severe infections and toxaemias; the occlusion of major arteries; cardiac failure; hypovolaemia and hypotension.

The reduced tissue perfusion results in lowered oxygen supply to the tissues and accumulation of metabolites, including lactic and pyruvic acids.

These cause a fall in tissue and later in blood *p*H. This fall in *p*H, especially if it is accompanied by decreased arterial oxygen tension, is followed by depression of cardiac and vasomotor function. If the acidosis is allowed to persist, a stage will be reached where, though the metabolic disturbance is corrected, death still occurs (Thrower, Darby, and Aldinger, 1961).

Several conditions contributed to the production of the acidosis in the four patients quoted.

Case 1 was hypotensive and hypovolaemic. The hypotension that occurs in severe infections and septic shock is due mainly to vascular changes. Following loss of vasomotor control, redistribution of blood takes place, with reduced venous return and cardiac output (Gilbert, 1960). In addition to these vascular changes, this child had also lost fluid from his circulation into the affected leg.

Cases 2 and 4 were dehydrated, and renal function was depressed in Case 2. Both children had almost stopped breathing when first seen, and cardiac arrest appeared to be imminent in Case 4. Hypoxia, hypercarbia, and low cardiac output were, therefore, contributory factors. Clowes, Sabga, Konitaxis, Tomin, Hughes, and Simeone (1961) have demonstrated the high mortality, experimentally and clinically, of a combination of hypoxia and hypercapnia, and also showed that hypoxia alone produces more severe metabolic and circulatory changes than hypercapnia alone. Case 3, who was cyanosed from birth, was hypoxic and probably also hypercapnic before operation. At operation, oxygenation was improved and $CO_2$ removed by ventilation with a 50 : 50 nitrous oxide-oxygen mixture. This temporarily improved the metabolic and respiratory acidosis, but after operation, the hypoxia recurred and with it a metabolic acidosis.

**Treatment of Acidosis.** The correction of the acidosis should be started as early as possible. Enzymes are active only within a narrow range of *p*H and are inhibited and ultimately destroyed at *p*H's beyond these limits (Carter and Thompson, 1959).

Using the formula $0 \cdot 3 \times$ body weight (kg.) $\times$ base deficit (Astrup, Jørgensen, Andersen, and Engel, 1960), the bicarbonate (mEq) required was calculated. The strength of the sodium bicarbonate was $2 \cdot 5\%$. This is a hypertonic solution containing approximately 300 mEq/l. No venous damage from this solution has been seen, but 5% $NaHCO_3$ has caused erythema when injected into small veins. The usefulness of hypertonic solutions in states of metabolic acidosis has recently been emphasized by Brooks, Williams, Manley, and Whiteman (1963). An article in the *Lancet* (1963) suggests that these solutions may act by preventing the passage of sodium ions and water into damaged cells. Sodium bicarbonate is the logical choice as it is the most important buffer of the plasma.

Two other buffers may be considered.

(a) *Tris-hydroxy-amino-methane.* This hydrogen ion acceptor is effective in restoring *p*H but may have other undesirable effects (Kaplan and Fox, 1961). It could be of use in cases where the administration of large quantities of sodium with bicarbonate is undesirable, e.g. Case 2, where kidney function was depressed.

(b) *Sodium lactate.* This widely used substance was originally introduced as an alternative to bicarbonate in solutions given by the intraperitoneal and subcutaneous routes, as the *p*H of bicarbonate solutions was too high for this purpose (*Amer. J. Med.*, 1962). Now that the intravenous route is so readily available, it is illogical to use sodium lactate in cases of severe metabolic acidosis. Oxygen required to convert the lactate to bicarbonate is not likely to be readily available, and the delay in effective treatment while this oxidation is taking place will be hazardous.

## Summary and Conclusions

Four cases are described of very ill children who received sodium bicarbonate to correct their metabolic acidosis.

The factors that may lead to the production of a metabolic acidosis are discussed and its treatment is outlined.

Metabolic acidosis frequently presents primarily as a respiratory problem, as it did in 3 of the cases. It should always be considered as a possible factor when the patient does not respond to other resuscitative measures. The failure of many cases of 'irreversible' shock to respond to treatment may be due to failure to correct an acidotic state.

While a *p*H meter is essential equipment in any modern hospital, it is practicable, if the clinical state indicates prolonged reduced tissue perfusion, to use an assumed base deficit of 5-10 mEq/l. as a basis for treatment.

Our thanks are due to Mr. G. Shatwell, Mr. H. Johnston, Dr. R. Smithells, and Miss I. Forshall, for permission to publish these cases and to the staff of the respiratory unit for the biochemical estimations.

### References

*Amer. J. Med.* (1962). Lactate versus bicarbonate: a reconsideration of the therapy of metabolic acidosis. (Editorial). **32**, 831.

Astrup, P., Jørgensen, K., Andersen, O. S., and Engel, K. (1960). The acid-base metabolism; a new approach. *Lancet*, **1**, 1035.

Brooks, D. K., Williams, W. G., Manley, R. W., and Whiteman, P. (1963). Respiratory changes in haemorrhagic shock. *Anaesthesia*, **18**, 363.
Carter, C. W., and Thompson, R. H. S. (1959). *Biochemistry in Relation to Medicine*, 3rd ed. Longmans, London.
Clowes, G. H. A., Jr., Neville, W. E., Sabga, G., and Shibota, Y. (1958). The relationship of oxygen consumption, perfusion rate, and temperature to the acidosis associated with cardiopulmonary circulatory bypass. *Surgery*, **44**, 220.
——, Sabga, G. A., Konitaxis, A., Tomin, R., Hughes, M., and Simeone, F. A. (1961). Effect of acidosis on cardiovascular function in surgical patients. *Ann. Surg.*, **154**, 524.
Ellis, W., and Dodson, M. E. (1964). Severe septic shock treated successfully with sodium bicarbonate. *J. Bone Jt Surg.* **46-B**, 746.
Gilbert, R. P. (1960). Mechanisms of the hemodynamic effects of endotoxin. *Physiol. Rev.*, **40**, 245.
Kaplan, S., and Fox, R. P. (1961). Amine buffers in the management of respiratory and mixed acidosis. In Transactions of the American Pediatric Society. *Amer. J. Dis. Child.*, **102**, 695.
*Lancet* (1963). Hypertonic sodium for 'irreversible' oligaemic shock. **1**, 539.
Thrower, W. B., Darby, T. D., and Aldinger, E. E. (1961). Acid-base derangements and myocardial contractility. *Arch. Surg.*, **82**, 56.

*Arch. Dis. Childh.*, 1965, **40**, 389.

# REVERSIBLE MYOCARDITIS DUE TO CHRONIC LEAD POISONING IN CHILDHOOD

BY

RONALD FREEMAN*

*From the Royal Alexandra Hospital for Children, Sydney, Australia*

(RECEIVED FOR PUBLICATION NOVEMBER 26, 1964)

Chronic lead poisoning in childhood, though a relatively uncommon disease, remains a problem in some parts of the world. Between 1948 and 1962, 49 children were treated at the Royal Alexandra Hospital for Children, because of chronic lead poisoning. 48 of the children obtained the lead by ingestion of flaking paint over periods of many months. Encephalopathy was diagnosed in 34 children and 9 of these died. Of the whole group, 21 children have been followed-up adequately and only 8 are known to be well and free of residual effects of the lead poisoning.

Myocardial disease seems to be a rare manifestation of chronic lead poisoning. In children chronic lead poisoning most often presents with a gastro-intestinal illness and pallor which may be followed by an acute encephalopathy at any time (Chisolm and Harrison, 1957; Cohen and Ahrens, 1959; Byers, 1959). In Queensland nephropathy has been found commonly to be a late manifestation of the disease (Nye, 1933; Henderson and Inglis, 1957).

There have been few reports of myocarditis due to lead. Hirschfeld (1926) described 4 young men with 'Angina Pectoris Saturnina', the term introduced by Andral (1843) who thought that the lead caused spasm of the coronary vessels. Haubrich (1947) was the first to claim that lead could involve the myocardium directly. He described a 26-year-old woman with lead poisoning who developed what was thought to be an aneurysm of the left atrium due to the lead; 12 years later, however, thoracotomy revealed a malignant thymoma and there was no sign of an aneurysm (Fritze and di Biasi, 1962). Read and Williams (1952) described a man with chronic occupational lead poisoning who complained of chest pain and was found to have an abnormal electrocardiogram. Following treatment of the lead poisoning he lost his chest pain and the electrocardiogram returned to normal. In reviewing the published reports since 1916, Read and Williams could not find a well-substantiated case of myocarditis directly due to lead. Myerson and Eisenhauer (1963) reported atrio-ventricular conduction defects in 2 adults with chronic lead poisoning. The electrocardiograms returned to normal after treatment of the lead poisoning.

Recently chronic myocarditis was found at necropsy in 5 children dying from lead encephalopathy (Kline, 1960), but myocarditis due to lead poisoning, with recovery, has not hitherto been described in childhood.

It is the purpose of this report to record an account of the illness in a girl aged 3 years with chronic lead poisoning associated with myocarditis. When this child presented with lead encephalopathy she was found to have signs of heart failure which was finally attributed to myocarditis directly caused by the lead. Recovery after treatment with sodium calciumedetate (calcium disodium ethylenediaminetetra-acetic acid; Ca $Na_2$ EDTA) was apparently complete.

## Case Report

P.P., a girl, aged 3 years, was admitted to the Royal Alexandra Hospital for Children on February 6, 1961. She was born in Malta and emigrated with her family to Australia when she was 18 months old. Her early development had been normal and she walked at the age of 12 months and had a fairly good vocabulary on arrival in Australia. She continued to progress well up to the time of the present illness. Her symptoms began 6 weeks before admission to hospital and consisted of anorexia, pallor, vomiting, constipation, irritability, weight loss, and unsteadiness in walking. The vomiting initially occurred 2 to 3 times daily but increased in frequency up to 5 to 6 times each day, becoming projectile and occasionally bile-stained. The other symptoms also became more marked as the illness progressed. Her parents and 2 sibs aged 7½ years and 3 weeks were in good health and there were no significant illnesses in the family.

**Physical Examination on Admission.** She was obviously underweight, pale, and extremely irritable, so that

* Present address: School of Paediatrics, Prince of Wales Hospital, Randwick, New South Wales, Australia.

detailed examination was at first impossible. Following heavy sedation a more complete examination was performed. She weighed 21 lb. 1 oz. (9·6 kg.) and her height was 32 in. (80 cm.), both below the 10th percentile for age. There was clinical evidence of congestive cardiac failure; the relevant findings were heart rate of 150 a minute, jugular venous pressure 5 cm. above the sternal angle, a gallop rhythm, and the liver palpable 3 cm. below the costal margin. There was no oedema. Her blood pressure was 95/50 mm. Hg and the femoral pulses were normal. The apex beat could not be localized. A grade 2 pansystolic murmur heard all over the praecordium was maximal in the 4th and 5th left intercostal spaces.

Neurological assessment was difficult but was considered normal apart from possible slight weakness of her legs. The optic fundi were normal. Her head circumference was 18·5 in. (46 cm.). She was afebrile and the remainder of the physical examination revealed no abnormality.

**Investigations.** The haemoglobin concentration was 7·6 g./100 ml., the haematocrit 28%, the red cell count 4,850,000/c.mm., reticulocytes 250,000/c.mm. (5%), total leucocyte count 10,000/c.mm. (neutrophils 63%, lymphocytes 30%, eosinophils 7%). Marked coarse basophilic stippling and a moderate number of nucleated red cells were seen on the blood smear, together with some anisocytosis, polychromasia, poikilocytosis, and hypochromia. Platelets were numerous on the blood smear. Sickle-cell and Heinz body preparations were negative. Haemoglobin electrophoresis, using Tris buffer showed slight increase of the $A_2$ fraction; this was also found in the father and thought to be consistent with a thalassaemia trait.

The urine contained traces of sugar and albumin and was normal on microscopy; the specific gravity of early morning specimens exceeded 1,023 on several occasions. The cerebrospinal fluid contained 40 mononuclear cells per c.mm. and 100 mg. protein/100 ml. Radiographs showed scattered flecks of radio-opaque material in the large bowel, lines of increased density at the metaphyses of the long bones, a normal skull, enlargement of the cardiac silhouette, and some increase in the lung markings (Fig. 1). The electrocardiogram showed flattening of the T wave in leads I, II, AVF, V5, and V6 (Fig. 2).

The blood urea was 27 mg./100 ml. Other investigations, including serum electrolytes, serum proteins, and electroencephalography, were normal. No pathogens were isolated from the throat and the tuberculin skin test was negative. The anti-streptolysin-0 titre was 80 Todd units/ml. (normal up to 200).

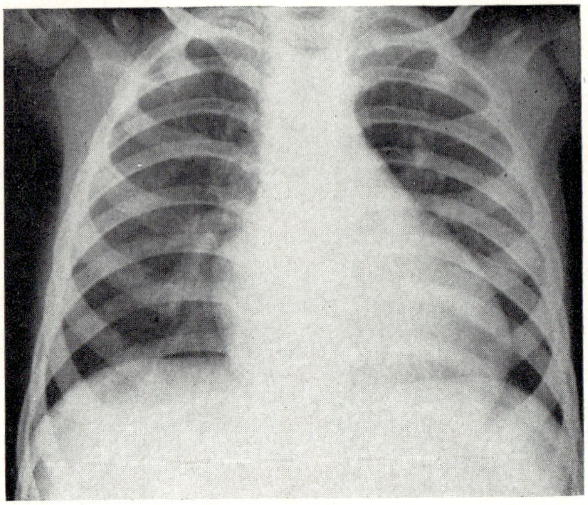

FIG. 1.—Chest radiograph showing enlargement of the heart and increase in lung markings.

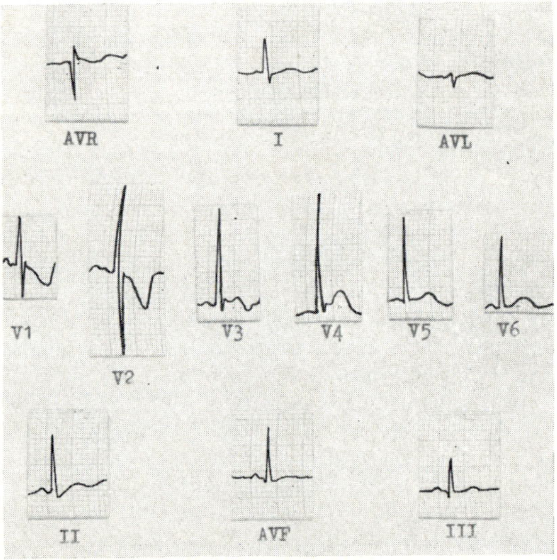


FIG. 2.—Electrocardiogram on February 10, 1961 (shortly after admission to hospital) showing flattened T waves in leads I, II, AVF, V5, and V6.

**Clinical Progress.** A presumptive diagnosis of lead intoxication with encephalopathy was made, but the nature of the cardiac lesion was uncertain. Further questioning of the parents revealed that they were living in a house more than 100 years old. The house was in a poor state of repair, paint peeling off the walls both inside and outside. The child had been frequently observed picking the paint off the walls and eating it. A visit to the house substantiated the parents' description and paint scrapings from the walls were examined by the N.S.W. Government Analyst; all were found to contain lead. Further investigations disclosed marked coproporphyrinuria and the diagnosis of lead poisoning was confirmed by chemical examination of the lead content in the urine; 2 mg. of lead was excreted/litre of urine 24 hours (normal up to 0·05 mg.).

Removal of the radio-opaque material from the bowel by catharsis and enemata was confirmed radiologically. Sodium calciumedetate, 60 mg./kg. 24 hours, was given in two divided doses by intravenous infusion and the fluid intake was limited to 1,200 ml. daily. She was closely observed for deterioration in her cardiac state, but there

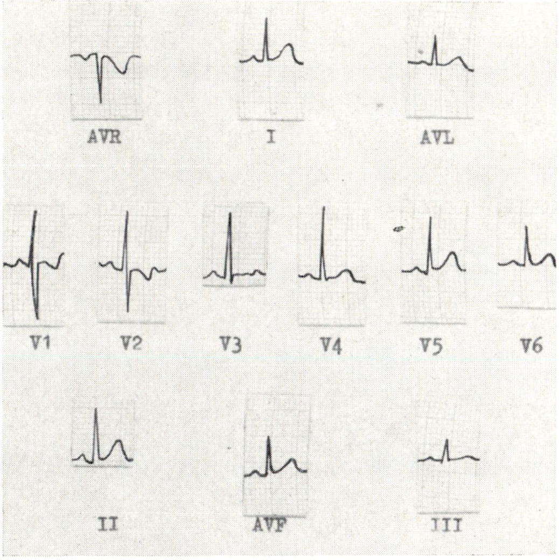


FIG. 3.—Electrocardiogram on March 15, 1961. The T wave voltage is now normal.

was rapid improvement, and after 4 days of sodium calciumedetate therapy signs of congestive cardiac failure had disappeared: the tachycardia had subsided, the jugular venous pressure was not raised, the gallop rhythm had disappeared, and the liver was only just palpable. The praecordial systolic murmur was softer. The electrocardiogram was essentially unchanged, but the chest radiograph showed some decrease in cardiac size and normal lung markings. Her appetite improved, the vomiting ceased, and she was less irritable and withdrawn. 10 days after the course of sodium calciumedetate the copropophyrinuria had disappeared and the urinary lead excretion had fallen to 0·1 mg./litre 24 hours.

By March 3, 1961, the patient looked well, the praecordial systolic murmur was no longer heard, the voltage of the T waves on the electrocardiogram was normal (Fig. 3), and the heart was normal in size, clinically and radiologically. The cytology and protein content of the cerebrospinal fluid had returned to normal.

Despite further clinical improvement the output of lead in the urine remained high and the anaemia persisted. At the end of March 1961 she was given a further course of sodium calciumedetate and a transfusion of 200 ml. of packed red cells. Her subsequent progress was excellent; she gained weight and appeared to be a happy normal child. She remained in hospital until the end of May 1961 due to delay in renovating the home; the old paint was removed and replaced by lead-free paint. At the time of discharge from hospital she weighed 28 lb. 8 oz. (13 kg.) and was very well with no signs of cardiac disease. The haemoglobin concentration was 12·5 g./100 ml. and the blood film was normal with no basophilic stippling of the red cells. The urine was free of sugar, albumin, and coproporphyrins, and several estimations of the lead output in the urine were within the normal range.

She was seen at intervals at the out-patient department and on her last visit in January 1962 she was well, weighing 34 lb. 1 oz. (15·5 kg.), and no abnormality could be found on physical examination. Apart from the metaphysial changes in the long bones, all investigations, including blood count, electrocardiogram, chest radiograph, and blood and urine lead levels, were normal. The parents declined further follow-up visits to the hospital as they considered her to be well; a recent home visit confirmed this impression.

## Discussion

A history of eating lead-containing paint, together with gastro-intestinal symptoms, hyperirritability, and weakness of the legs constitute a fairly typical presentation of chronic lead poisoning in childhood. The presence of radio-opaque material in the abdomen, dense lines at the metaphyses of the long bones, anaemia with basophilic stippling of the red cells, and marked coproporphyrinuria support this diagnosis in the patient described. The changes in the cerebrospinal fluid were characteristic of lead encephalopathy (Chisolm and Harrison, 1957) and the greatly increased rate of excretion of lead in the urine provided proof of lead intoxication (Byers, 1959).

The presence of cardiac failure of obscure origin, a pansystolic murmur, and T-wave changes in the electrocardiogram suggested a generalized disease of the myocardium (Brigden, 1957; Goodwin, Gordon, Hollman, and Bishop, 1961). There were no clinical or laboratory findings to suggest that the heart failure might have been due to acute glomerular nephritis or to acute rheumatic fever; a haemolytic streptococcus was not isolated and the anti-streptolysin-0 titre was not raised. There was no evidence of lead nephropathy. The complete disappearance of signs of a cardiac disorder excluded the possibility of congenital heart disease. Severe anaemia, as seen in thalassaemia major, may precipitate cardiac failure, but the anaemia was not severe enough to have been the primary cause of cardiac failure in this patient.

One must admit that it is very difficult, if not impossible, to make a certain diagnosis of lead-induced myocarditis in the living subject, as the possibility of a coincident viral myocarditis cannot be absolutely ruled out. Nevertheless, the diagnosis of lead myocarditis seems to be justified in this child. The concurrence of signs of myocardial insufficiency with those of lead encephalopathy, the rapid disappearance of signs of heart disease during treatment of the lead poisoning with sodium calciumedetate, and evidence from other sources (to be reviewed) leave no doubt as to the toxic effect of lead on the myocardium.

In their monograph on lead poisoning, Aub, Fairhall, Minot, and Reznikoff (1925) state:

'The heart as might be expected from clinical observation shows nothing remarkable as a result of lead intoxication. . . .'
'Most observers believe that the heart undergoes no real change, certainly none due to the direct action of lead.'

Several reports in recent years are in conflict with this statement. Kline (1960) reviewed the necropsy findings in 5 children aged 1 to 2 years, who died from lead encephalopathy. Numerous sections of the heart were examined and chronic myocarditis was found in all 5 children; the changes consisted of cloudy swelling of the myocardial fibres, interstitial fibrosis with a serous exudate, and relatively few inflammatory cells. The myocarditis was considered to be the cause of death of 2 of the children and contributory in the remainder. A review of the clinical findings revealed that all the children had some features of heart failure before death, but these were thought to be due to the encephalopathy. Kline suggested that the serous inflammation, possibly due to intramyocardial vascular changes, was a precursor to fibrosis; he further suggested that vascular changes might be initiated by hypersensitivity, but no vascular changes were demonstrable histologically.

The work of Kośmider and Sroczyński (1961) provides further evidence of the myocardial toxicity of lead. They induced lead intoxication in 10 rabbits by weekly injections of lead acetate and observed the animals for a period of 83 to 180 days. Progressive lead intoxication was confirmed by increasing anaemia, basophilic stippling of the red cells, and rising levels of blood and urine lead. All the rabbits developed abnormal electrocardiographic patterns, of which T wave changes and abnormal QRS complexes were the most common. The electrocardiographic changes were associated with histological changes of the cardiac muscle in the 6 rabbits subsequently subjected to pathological examination. The findings included loss of definition of the muscle structure, degenerative changes of the muscle fibres, and focal fibrosis; inflammatory exudate, however, was seen only in 1 case. They considered that the lead might have a direct effect on the myocardium itself or act indirectly by disturbing the coronary circulation. Species difference and the method of poisoning the rabbits make these changes questionable in relation to man; however, the histological changes do resemble the findings of Kline (1960).

Kośmider and Petelenz (1962) who examined 38 adults over 46 years of age with chronic lead poisoning found organic electrocardiographic changes in 66%, which was 4 times more common than in a control group. Flattening of the T waves and depression of the S-T segment were the most frequent changes, but other findings included short P-R interval, low voltage QRS complexes, and conduction defects. The lead compounds were thought to act by blocking enzymes concerned in cardiac metabolism, leading to subsequent damage. The patient studied by Read and Williams (1952) was a 39-year-old negro male suffering from lead poisoning. He complained of mid-sternal pain, and his electrocardiogram revealed marked depression of the conducting system with inverted T waves in left praecordial leads. 6 days after treatment for lead poisoning his electrocardiogram was essentially normal and he was asymptomatic. Depression of the conduction tissue with toxic changes in the myocardium as the result of lead poisoning was postulated as an explanation of the cardiac findings.

Myerson and Eisenhauer (1963) reported 2 adults with chronic lead poisoning who developed atrioventricular conduction defects; first degree heart block was found in one, and ectopic atrial pacemakers, at times associated with first degree heart block, in the other. The electrocardiogram returned to normal in both patients after treatment with sodium calciumedetate. Increased vagal tone due to the lead was thought to be the mechanism of these conduction defects.

In Queensland, where lead poisoning in children was prevalent in the early part of the century, chronic nephritis in young adults is a common sequel of childhood plumbism (Nye, 1933; Henderson and Inglis, 1957). Hypertension due to lead nephropathy represents an indirect mechanism by which lead might impair the myocardium, and this was the probable cause of the cardiac changes found at necropsy in the 53-year-old man with 'Saturnine Myocardiopathy', reported by Sessa and Guarino (1957).

The mechanism by which lead may impair the heart directly is purely speculative. Lead may be a direct irritant to the myocardium, it may inhibit enzyme systems concerned with cardiac metabolism or it may selectively disturb the coronary circulation. There are very few necropsy reports in which the lead content of the heart has been analysed. Minot and Aub (1924) found 0·3 mg. of lead in the heart of an infant who died of lead encephalopathy; the total soft tissue lead exceeded 31 mg. It is of interest that relatively small amounts of lead have been found at necropsy in the brains of patients dying from lead encephalopathy; the liver and kidney in most cases were found to contain far higher concentrations (Minot and Aub, 1924; Chisolm and Harrison, 1956; Popoff, Weinberg, and Feigin, 1963). Perhaps certain tissues, such as the brain, are particularly susceptible to traces of lead which might disturb the metabolic functions of the organ or result in vascular damage (Popoff *et al.*, 1963). One might postulate that lead causes a similar disturbance of the myocardium, resulting in a serous exudate which subsequently stimulates new growth of connective tissue. There is no evidence that lead impairs the coronary circulation in man, and the absence of vascular changes in the hearts examined by Kline (1960) tends to discount a vascular mechanism. Possibly a metabolic disturbance of the myocardium might result from the direct action of lead, for lead ions have been shown to impair certain enzymes involved in porphyrin metabolism (Watson, Decker, and Lichtman, 1958; Lichtman and Feldman, 1963).

### Summary and Conclusions

The case history of a 3-year-old girl with myocarditis occurring in the presence of chronic lead poisoning and encephalopathy is described. The diagnosis of lead poisoning was made on a history of eating lead-containing paint, and confirmed by laboratory investigations and the response to sodium calciumedetate. Myocarditis was diagnosed by the presence of cardiac failure in association with T wave changes in the electrocardiogram.

The rapid reversal of the clinical and electrocardiographic signs of myocarditis during treatment of the lead poisoning with sodium calciumedetate implies that the lead was responsible for the cardiac changes.

Myocardial impairment in chronic plumbism may result from direct cardio-toxicity of lead, or indirectly from hypertensive changes due to lead nephropathy. The absence of hypertension and of signs of nephropathy exclude the latter mechanism, and infer that the myocarditis was due to the direct action of lead on the heart.

The mechanism by which lead directly affects the myocardium is unknown. There is no evidence of a selective vascular disturbance. Possibly the lead inhibits enzyme systems in the myocardium; this metabolic disturbance might cause an interstitial serous exudate which subsequently stimulates new growth of connective tissue. The complete return to normal of the cardiac status in the child described implies a reversible impairment of myocardial function. Perhaps effective removal of the lead by sodium calciumedetate enabled the exudative reaction to resolve before fibrosis ensued.

The rarity of myocarditis in chronic lead poisoning is unexplained, but it appears to occur in the more seriously poisoned child in whom the features of encephalopathy may overshadow or be thought responsible for the cardiac signs.

The inference to be drawn from this report is that careful assessment and observation with electrocardiographic studies for possible myocardial damage should be part of the management of a patient with chronic lead poisoning. Supportive measures, though not necessary in this child, may be life-saving in children with lead encephalopathy, because undiagnosed myocarditis could be responsible for the death of such a child.

Careful histological examination and chemical estimation of lead content of the heart in patients dying from chronic plumbism may prove of interest. The awareness of myocarditis as a complication of chronic lead poisoning may reveal that cardiac involvement is not as rare as it seems to be.

I thank Dr. S. E. L. Stening, Senior Paediatrician, Royal Alexandra Hospital for Children, for permission to publish this case. I am grateful to Professor John Beveridge and Dr. Graeme Morgan for their helpful criticism in preparing this report.

References

Andral, G. (1843). *Medizinische Klinik*, Uebersetzt von H. E. Flies, 4th ed., bd. II, teil 2. [Quoted by Read, J. L., and Williams, J. P. (1952). *Amer. Heart J.*, **44**, 797.]
Aub, J. C., Fairhall, L. T., Minot, A. S., and Reznikoff, P. (1925). Lead poisoning. *Medicine (Baltimore)*, **4**, 1.
Brigden, W. (1957). Uncommon myocardial diseases; the non-coronary cardiomyopathies. *Lancet*, **2**, 1179.
Byers, R. K. (1959). Lead poisoning: Review of the literature and report on 45 cases. *Pediatrics*, **23**, 585.
Chisolm, J. J., Jr., and Harrison, H. E. (1956). The exposure of children to lead. *ibid.*, **18**, 943.
——, —— (1957). The treatment of acute lead encephalopathy in children. *ibid.*, **19**, 2.
Cohen, G. J., and Ahrens, W. E. (1959). Chronic lead poisoning: review of 7 years' experience at the children's hospital, District of Columbia. *J. Pediat.*, **54**, 271.
Fritze, E., and di Biasi, W. (1962). Herzaneurysma nach Bleivergiftung. *Arch. Gewerbepath. Gewerbehyg.*, **19**, 340.
Goodwin, J. F., Gordon, H., Hollman, A., and Bishop, M. B. (1961). Clinical aspects of cardiomyopathy. *Brit. med. J.*, **1**, 69.
Haubrich, R. (1947). Mitteilung eines Falles von Herzwandaneurysma nach akuter Bleivergiftung. *Klin. Wschr.*, **24-25**, 754.
Henderson, D. A., and Inglis, J. A. (1957). The lead content of bone in chronic Bright's disease. *Aust. Ann. Med.*, **6**, 145.
Hirschfeld, E. (1926). Angina Pectoris Saturnina. *Z. klin. Med.*, **104**, 698.
Kline, T. S. (1960). Myocardial changes in lead poisoning. *Amer. J. Dis. Child.*, **99**, 48.
Kośmider, S., and Petelenz, T. (1962). Zmiany elektrokardiograficzne u starszych osob z przewlekym zawodowym zatruciem ołowiem. *Pol. Arch. Med. wewnet.*, **32**, 437.
——, and Sroczyński, J. (1961). Zmiany elektrokardiograficzne w przewlekłej doświadczalnej ołowicy u królików. *Postępy Hig. Med. dósw.*, **15**, 353.
Lichtman, H. C., and Feldman, F. (1963). *In vitro* pyrrole and porphyrine synthesis in lead poisoning and iron deficiency. *J. clin. Invest.*, **42**, 830.
Minot, A. S., and Aub, J. C. (1924). Lead studies, V. C. The distribution of lead in the human organism. *J. industr. Hyg.*, **6**, 149.
Myerson, R. M., and Eisenhauer, J. H. (1963). Atrioventricular conduction defects in lead poisoning. *Amer. J. Cardiol.*, **11**, 409.
Nye, L. J. J. (1933). *Chronic Nephritis and Lead Poisoning.* Angus and Robertson, Sydney.
Popoff, N., Weinberg, S., and Feigin, I. (1963). Pathologic observations in lead encephalopathy; with special reference to the vascular changes. *Neurology (Minneap.)*, **13**, 101.
Read, J. L., and Williams, J. P. (1952). Lead myocarditis; Report of a case. *Amer. Heart J.*, **44**, 797.
Sessa, T., and Guarino, A. (1957). Su di un caso di miocardiopatia saturnina: considerazioni diagnostiche e medico-legali. *Folia med. (Napoli)*, **40**, 273.
Watson, R. J., Decker, E., and Lichtman, H. C. (1958). Hematologic studies of children with lead poisoning. *Pediatrics*, **21**, 40.

*Arch. Dis. Childh.*, 1965, **40**, 394.

# SOME CLINICAL NOTES AND ELECTROENCEPHALOGRAPHIC FINDINGS IN CEREBRAL PALSY

BY

GRACE E. WOODS*

*From the Cerebral Palsy Assessment Clinic, Children's Hospital, Bristol*

(RECEIVED FOR PUBLICATION NOVEMBER 13, 1964)

During the past 10 years, electroencephalographic recordings have been taken on children with cerebral palsy, who were attending a special clinic at the Royal Hospital for Sick Children, Bristol. In this paper an attempt has been made to evaluate these records and, in particular, to assess their importance to the clinician.

The published findings on the electroencephalogram (EEG) in cerebral palsy are not extensive possibly because of the difficulty in obtaining records from these severely handicapped children. An early survey was made by Perlstein, Gibbs, and Gibbs (1946). Aird and Cohen (1950) found that 85% of spastics and 60% of athetoids gave abnormal records, but that there was focal pathology in only 32% of athetoids. They suggest that if the EEG shows no evidence of epileptiform disturbance, the chance of a fit occurring is only 1 in 8. They found no correlation between an abnormal EEG and the intelligence quotient.

Pampiglione (1958) reviewing the literature says that there is considerable agreement on four points: (a) asymmetry between the records from the two hemispheres is commoner in hemiplegia, (b) EEG abnormalities are recognizable in most cerebral palsy patients who have seizures, (c) one-third of the cases show normal records, and this is commoner with athetoids than with spastics, (d) there is a smaller proportion of abnormal EEGs among patients whose condition is ascribed to prematurity or anoxia than in those who have a known cerebral injury or infection.

Denhoff and Robinault (1960) found that 24% of a group of 95 cerebral-palsied children had normal records. Lundervold (1960) compared air-encephalographic and electroencephalographic findings and showed that the combined results had some prognostic significance.

Melin (1962) stressed the importance of serial EEG examinations and stated that 80 to 85% of cerebral-palsied children with a history of convulsive disorders showed an abnormal EEG. He particularly mentioned the cases where the EEG findings predicted a future convulsive disorder, and recommended close supervision of the patient and possibly prophylactic anticonvulsant therapy.

Jabbour and Lundervold (1963) obtained EEG records on 43 hemiplegic children. They found that epilepsy occurred in equal proportions among those with normal or near normal records, and those with severely abnormal records. But the follow-up showed better control of the epilepsy in children with more nearly normal records. His records appear to have been taken in very young children.

Lesny (1963) investigated cerebellar disorders in childhood and stated that a 'synchronous bi-occipito-temporal slow wave activity inhibited by eye-opening' was a fairly common finding. Ounsted (1963) made EEG studies of 20 children with cerebellar disease and found 7 with normal records, and varying abnormalities in the remainder.

## Present Findings

In reporting the present series of EEG findings, the patients are analysed in rather arbitrary groups according to the major movement handicap of the child. Records were obtained on the majority of patients with cerebral palsy who were being supervised and treated in the clinic. Usually an EEG record was obtained once in early childhood at about the age of 3 years, and again during school life. In patients with epilepsy more frequent records were taken.

**Athetosis.** In this group of cases 62 records were obtained from 35 patients under the age of 16 years. All showed athetosis. In a few patients there was

* Present address: St. Ebba's Hospital, Epsom, Surrey.

TABLE 1

ANALYSIS OF EEG RECORDS IN INDIVIDUAL CASES OF ATHETOSIS

| Name | EEG | Aetiology | Birth Weight (g.) | IQ | Severity | Remarks | No. of Records |
|---|---|---|---|---|---|---|---|
| A.B. | N | Asph. | 3,175 | 120 + | Mod. | | 1 |
| R.H. | N | Asph. | 1,814 | Average | Mild | | 1 |
| M.B. | N | Asph. | 3,628 | Average | Mild | | 1 |
| C.E. | N | ? | 3,061 | Average | Mild | | 3 |
| B.A. | N | ? | 1,360 | ESN | Mod. | | 1 |
| J.C. | N | Rh. jaund. | 2,635 | Average | Mild | Deaf | 1 |
| J.B. | N | ? | 3,571 | ESN | Mild | | 1 |
| J.W. | Abn. → N | Jaund. | 1,870 | Average | Mild | | 2 |
| D.K. | N | Rh. jaund. | 2,267 | Average | Mod. | Deaf: *P. mal.* | 3 |
| J.H. | N | Jaund. | 2,267 | Average | Severe | Deaf | 1 |
| A.H. | N | R. jaund. | 2,267 | Average | Mod. | Deaf | 1 |
| M.P. | ES | Jaund. | 1,587 | Average | Mod. | Deaf | 1 |
| R.P. | LV | Jaund. | 2,578 | Average | Mod. | Deaf | 2 |
| V.T. | LV | Jaund. | 2,437 | Average | Severe | Deaf | 2 |
| F.G. | LV | Jaund. | 1,360 | ESN | Severe | Deaf | 1 |
| D.H. | LV | Rh. jaund. | 2,041 | Average | Mod. | Deaf | 2 |
| R.R. | ES | Jaund. | 3,175 | Average | Mild | Deaf | 3 |
| A.P. | LV | Rh. jaund. | 3,770 | Ineduc. | Severe | Deaf | 1 |
| J.B. | S | Asph. | 1,671 | ? ESN | Severe | Epileptic | 1 |
| R.F. | ES | ? | 3,402 | Ineduc. | Mod. | | 1 |
| M.R. | LV | Asph. | 1,927 | Average | Mild | | 2 |
| P.L. | Abn. | Asph. | 1,615 | Ineduc. | Mod. | Epileptic | 1 |
| A.B. | LV | Jaund. | 2,125 | ESN | Severe | | 1 |
| S.H. | N → LV | ? | 3,117 | Average | Severe | Deteriorating | 3 |
| C.T. | Abn. → N | Asph. | 3,798 | Univ. 140 + | Mild | | 1 |
| T.S. | LV | Asph. | 2,607 | Ineduc. | Severe | Epileptic | 1 |
| T.C. | N → S | ? | 1,814 | 120 + | Mod. | Deaf | 2 |
| S.T. | LV | Jaund. | 1,814 | Average | Severe | Deaf | 2 |
| M.L. | Abn. + S → LV | Asph. | 2,493 | ESN | Severe | | 4 |
| S.M. | Abn. + S | Asph. | 2,834 | Average | Severe | | 1 |
| G.H. | S → N | Asph. | 2,948 | Average | Severe | | 7 |
| F.B. | Abn. | Asph. + jaund. | 2,976 | Average | Mod. | Deaf | 1 |
| J.S. | N | ? | 1,785 | Average | Mod. | Deaf | 2 |
| D.H. | S | Asph. | 2,891 | Average | Severe | | 3 |
| M.C. | ES | Asph. + jaund. | 2,749 | ESN | Severe | | 1 |

N = normal; Abn. = abnormal; LV = low voltage; ES = electric silent; S = spikes; Asph. = neonatal asphyxia; Jaund. = neonatal jaundice; ESN = educationally subnormal.

super-added spasticity. The patients were designated mild, moderate, or severe on a functional basis. The mild patients (9 in number) had fitted into normal school in spite of incoordinated hand movements. The moderate ones (12 in number), though attending a special school, were thought likely to be fit for some gainful employment in later years and were able to attend to their bodily needs. The severe ones (14 in number) needed help with feeding and other necessary functions, and had little control over hand movements.

The aetiology was fairly clearly divided between 14 patients where it followed neonatal asphyxia, and 14 that followed neonatal jaundice. In the 7 with no history of either condition, 3 had been very immature. In all, 18 were premature. 15 patients showed mild to severe high frequency hearing loss. Three had infrequent *grand mal* fits and one had *petit mal* attacks. The EEG findings are analysed in Table 1.

Of particular interest in athetosis are the number of cases, 14 in all, that repeatedly gave low voltage or electrically silent records. This was reported altogether in 21 records, and suggests that this is a likely EEG finding in patients where the damage is presumed to be in the basal ganglia. Of these 14 patients, 7 were deaf, 8 had been premature, and 8 were severely affected. All 14 were very handicapped physically. This finding does not appear to have been emphasized in published reports, possibly because of the difficulty in obtaining records in severe cases of athetosis (Fig. 1).

Of the 11 children with normal records, 5 were mildly affected and 5 moderately affected, 8 were of good average intelligence, and 1 at least was of Grammar School ability. Of the 4 children where a change occurred to a later normal record, 2 were severely affected. Both showed right-sided spikes in earlier records, though neither were epileptic. One record that changed to normal was taken from a mildly affected boy who is now at University. As these children grew older there was a normal development of alpha rhythm which was physically responsive.

Some children showed runs of theta rhythm, frequently of low potential, which might suggest an involvement of deeper structure.

Of the 4 clinical epileptics, one showed a normal record, one a mildly abnormal one, one was a silent record, and only one showed spikes suggesting an epileptic disturbance. These findings only illustrate trends, and some EEG findings were surprising, as is true in all cases of brain pathology. Of the normal

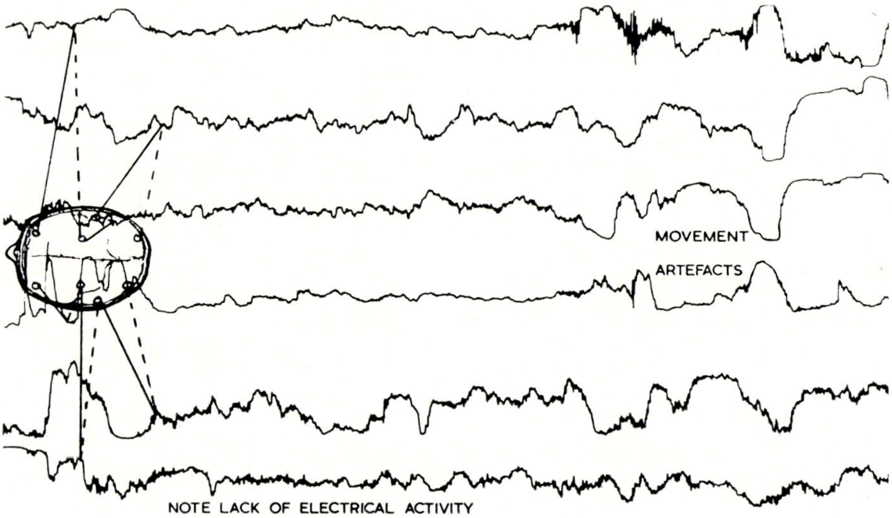


FIG. 1.—Recording of an athetoid patient aged $6\frac{1}{2}$ years, showing low potential in all regions. The swings in the recording are due to movement artefacts.

records, 3 were found in severely physically affected patients, but in all patients with low voltage records the child was very handicapped physically. All the children had been given a prolonged educational trial and only 4 were considered ineducable, and these 4 had very abnormal records.

**Hemiplegia.** There were 200 records taken of 100 children. These were representative of the various types of hemiplegic children and include cases of severe mental subnormality and some of above average intelligence. There were 61 right and 39 left hemiplegias. In 72 patients the condition appeared to date from birth, and may have been due to cerebral trauma in the perinatal period. In 28 there was a clear history of postnatal cerebral trauma, infection, or ill-defined illness as the cause of the hemiplegia. As there is a high incidence of epilepsy in hemiplegia, the EEG records are of clinical importance. Of these children 41% (27 right and 14 left) were epileptic, having had either a solitary or occasional fit, or more frequent attacks. There were 12 (42·8%) epileptic patients in the acquired group of 28 hemiplegias, and 29 (40·3%) in the remaining 72, showing no difference in the incidence of epilepsy between the acquired and congenital cases.

Of the 100 patients, 14 showed persistently normal records. In 10 of these, the children were of good average or above average intelligence. In one boy there was a history of three fits at intervals, but three normal EEG records were obtained. In another boy with a recurring normal record there was an air-encephalographic finding of severe cerebral atrophy on the suspected side. The boy had an IQ of 80 and no history of fits up to the age of 17 years. Presumably one normal hemisphere was responsible for a normal EEG. In a few cases a normal record in early childhood was followed by a record during school-life showing mild abnormality. These mild changes appeared to be associated with increasing age and had no clinical significance or prognosis. It is wondered if the high incidence of normal records in Lundervold's series (1960) might not be related to the young age of her cases.

In 5 patients the records became more abnormal and were associated with clinical and educational deterioration. In 2 boys, the hemiplegic condition had been caused by a cerebral-vascular incident associated with Fallot's tetralogy. In one girl, the condition had followed tuberculous meningitis, and the deterioration of the EEG record coincided with x-ray evidence of intracerebral calcification. In another girl the deterioration in the EEG was reported at the same time as an increased incidence of epilepsy and a school report of unexpectedly poor performance, and a drop in IQ from 117 to 87. An air-encephalogram showed cerebral atrophy of the expected side. In a fifth case the girl had a progressive condition.

Three children produced a normal record after one reported as abnormal. It showed normal maturation of alpha rhythm. This was associated with complete control of fits in 2 patients.

The records were not a completely reliable indication of the side of the lesion. In some cases the abnormalities in the EEG were diffuse, and there

TABLE 2
RELATION BETWEEN INTELLIGENCE AND ONSET OF FITS

| Intelligence Rating | Normal | Educationally Sub-normal | Inedu-cable | Total |
|---|---|---|---|---|
| No epilepsy .. .. | 63 | 8 | 6 | 77 |
| Epilepsy before 3 years .. | 12 | 11 | 17 | 40 |
| Epilepsy after 3 years .. | 14 | 5 | 2 | 21 |
| Total .. .. | 89 | 24 | 25 | 138 (3 too young) |

TABLE 3
ANALYSIS OF EEG RECORDS IN HEMIPLEGIA

| EEG Findings | Right Hemiplegia | Left Hemiplegia |
|---|---|---|
| Normal .. .. .. .. .. .. | 9 | 5 |
| Abnormal → normal .. .. .. | 4 | 1 |
| Normal → abnormal .. .. .. | 6 | 3 |
| Left-sided spikes .. .. .. .. | 7 | 1 |
| Right-sided spikes .. .. .. .. | 3 | 11 |
| Wave and spike .. .. .. .. | 2 | 3 |
| Diffuse spikes .. .. .. .. | 6 | 0 |
| Low voltage .. .. .. .. .. | 10 | 2 |
| Abnormal record .. .. .. .. | 8 | 10 |
| Asymmetry only (affected hemisphere—quiescent or electrically silent) .. | 8 | 3 |
| | 63 | 39 |

were no focal abnormalities. In 6 the EEG recorded a focal abnormality on the ipsilateral side of the movement handicap: 5 of these were epileptic and 5 of low intelligence; and it is possible that the damage in one hemisphere was responsible for the hemiplegia and in the other for the epilepsy. In two patients the air-encephalogram finding supported this view. In 12, asymmetry between the two hemispheres, taking the form of a low voltage record from the affected hemisphere, was recorded. In some the whole hemisphere was involved and in others the low potential records were focal. In 6 patients the affected hemisphere was silent. These 6 were associated with epilepsy, not easily controlled, and in 5 with severe mental subnormality. A generalized low potential record was obtained in a few patients (Fig. 2a, b) being similar to findings in other types of cerebral palsy.

The EEG records were not a definite indication as to whether clinical epilepsy was occurring. In 40 out of 41 patients with epilepsy, the records were abnormal, and in 29 spikes were recorded. The other records were not specifically epileptic but showed abnormalities such as asymmetry; low potential records, runs of focal delta and theta rhythm, and prolonged following response to photic stimulation. There is a correlation between an abnormal EEG and epilepsy. There is an additional correlation between epilepsy and lowered intelligence, as shown in Table 2, taken from a slightly larger group of 138 cases (Woods, 1963), suggesting that all three factors are evidence of more pronounced brain damage. In 5 patients a wave and spike discharge was recorded but in only one boy was there evidence of *petit mal* attacks.

In 15 patients, spikes were reported and epilepsy predicted where there was a clear negative history of epilepsy. In 9 children, epilepsy occurred later. The fact that the epileptic record was known to the clinician led to rapid institution of anti-convulsant treatment. Six never developed epilepsy and five have been followed to adult life. This raises the question as to whether, following an epileptic record, mild anti-epileptic therapy should be instituted as a routine. This has been carried out in 2 patients with marked improvement in the EEG and no occurrence of fits. In this series there were no patients showing aggressive disturbances associated with a temporal lobe focus (Table 3).

**Spastic Diplegia.** In this series of 50 patients who are variously called spastic paraplegics, spastic diplegics, spastic quadriplegics, and bilateral hemiplegics, there are a mixed group of patients with varying aetiology, severity of handicap, and intelligence range. However, some of them fall into fairly clear-cut aetiological and clinical groups.

DIPLEGIA OF PREMATURITY. One group are patients with symmetrical or near symmetrical spasticity, with lower limbs more affected than upper limbs, the condition following a very premature birth. These can be divided into two grades: (1) where from a functional angle the disability only occurs in the legs and the child has normal control of hands and arms, though neurologically there may be minimal evidence of increased tone and reflexes; and (2) where the upper limbs are functionally affected and the clinical condition of the child is worse. This group of spastic cases has the best prognosis for training and education and forms the bulk of the cases of severe spasticity, able to attend a special school for cerebral palsy.

In the first grade (1) there were 24 patients, and 34 electroencephalographic records were obtained: 13 had normal records and 2 were doubtful. All 13 were of good intelligence (one had an IQ of 140). Three showed evidence of visuo-perceptual difficulties which have been described in these children. One boy, who weighed 2 lb. (908 g.) at birth, showed these learning difficulties to a marked extent and had four normal records over a period of four years.

Of the remaining 9 patients who had abnormal

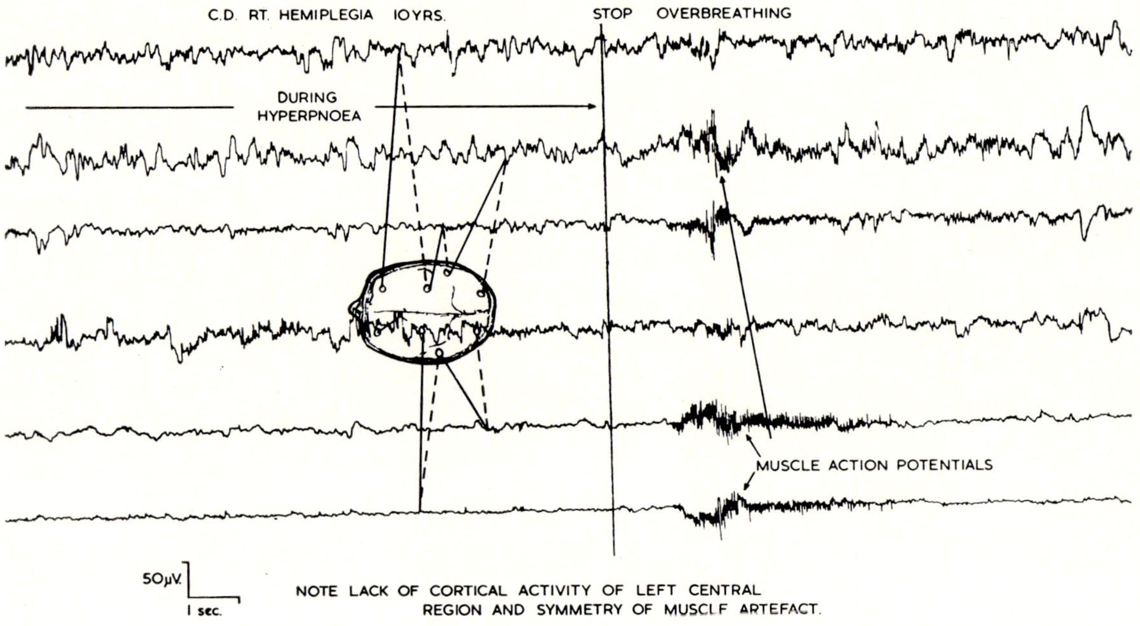


(a)

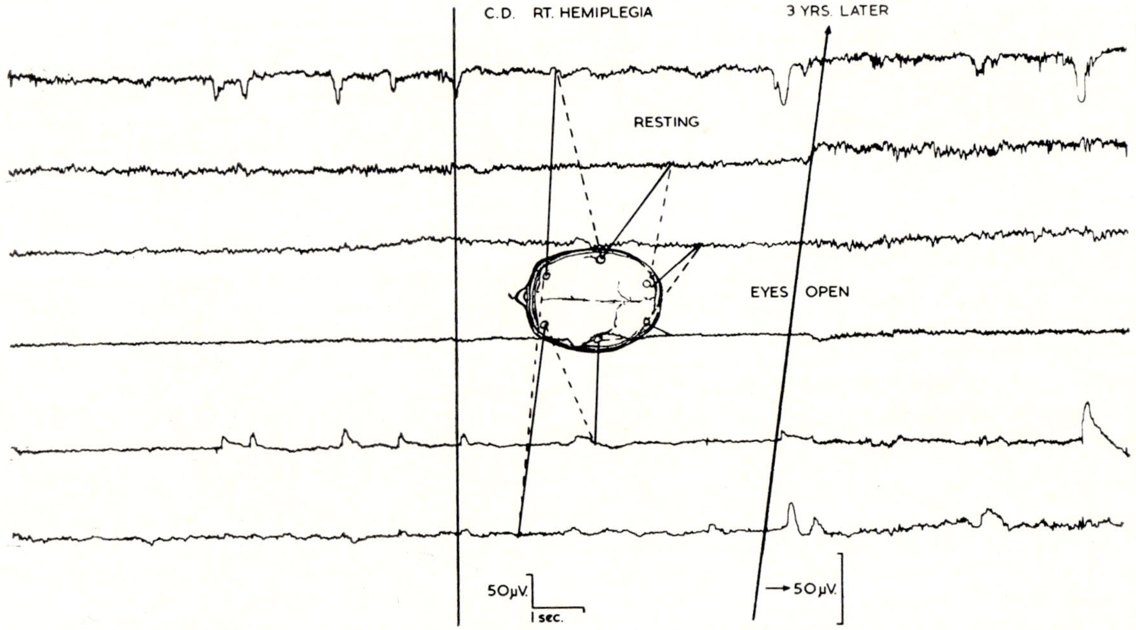


(b)

FIG. 2.—Two recordings of an epileptic girl with right hemiplegia. IQ 100, (a) Aged 10 years, during and after overbreathing, showing the silent area in the left central region. (b) Aged 13 years. During resting the silent area is still apparent.

TABLE 4

ANALYSIS OF EEG RECORDS IN SPASTIC DIPLEGIA

| Aetiology | No. of Patients | No. of Records | No. of Patients With Normal Records | Low Voltage | Mildly Abnormal | Spikes | Epileptic | No. Ineducable |
|---|---|---|---|---|---|---|---|---|
| Prematurity: | | | | | | | | |
| Mild | 24 | 34 | 13 | 0 | 2 | 5 | 2 | 2 |
| Severe | 13 | 20 | 1 | 4 | 2 | 7 | 5 | 12 |
| Abnormal birth | 14 | 31 | 0 | | 4 | 10 | 6 | 8 |
| Genetic | 5 | 7 | 5 | | | | | 2 |
| No apparent aetiology | 3 | 5 | 2 | | 9 | | | |
| Postnatal | 1 | 2 | 1 | | | | | 1 |
| | 60 | 99 | 22 | 4 | 17 | 22 | 13 | 25 |

records, 5 were of low intelligence, 2 coming within the ineducable range. Two with abnormal records had epilepsy, and one a severe behaviour disorder, necessitating institutional care, which may have been partially environmental. There were no low potential records.

In grade (2) 20 records were obtained from 13 patients. One was epileptic and ineducable.

The EEG findings were variable. One gave a normal record and this was a girl of above average intelligence who showed interesting visuo-perceptual difficulties. Four gave low potential or electrically quiet records. There were 7 children showing focal spikes and 5 of these had had one or more epileptic fits. The possibility of epilepsy occurring at any time is a serious factor in the prognosis of these children. In one boy who is educationally and physically making good progress, there is deterioration in the EEG records with a spike and wave focus reported for the first time in the left temporal region at 7 years. The significance of this has not yet been determined. The underlying pathology in this interesting group of symmetrical spasticity following a premature birth, with near normal intelligence, has not yet been determined. Abnormality in the EEG record does appear to be correlated with severity of handicap or the likelihood of epilepsy.

DIPLEGIA FOLLOWING SUSPECTED BIRTH TRAUMA. A further 14 cases followed an abnormal birth, either slight prematurity, breech delivery, twin birth, or pre-eclampsia. In nearly every one there was mild to severe neonatal illness suggesting cerebral trauma. Four of them could be considered bilateral hemiplegias in that one side was more involved than the other and at least one arm was the most severely affected limb. The other 8 were diplegics and clinically similar to the premature group, though 2 were hydrocephalic.

All records were abnormal—4 mildly abnormal and 10 very abnormal and showing spikes. Of these 10, 5 were epileptic. Three showed low potential records. One microcephalic, ineducable epileptic girl gave repeated low voltage records. One showed a temporal lobe focus.

Seven of this group were severely mentally subnormal and one mildly subnormal. Yet two children with very abnormal EEG records attended Grammar Schools, and a gross error of judgement was made in one of them by giving a poor prognosis on the basis of an EEG finding.

DIPLEGIA FOLLOWING OTHER CAUSES. There remain 9 patients with varying aetiology: 5 were genetically determined and gave normal records; there were other affected sibs; only the lower limbs were involved.

One boy who had bilateral hemiplegia following a cerebral infection at the age of 1 month, gave two normal records after an interval of five years, suggesting that the cortex was little affected; his intelligence and insight were above normal and he was a stable, mature boy.

There were 3 patients in whom the clinical condition appeared identical with the previous group and yet the birth was full term and the evidence for genetic or perinatal causation was unconvincing. Two gave normal EEG records, one boy having an IQ of 117. One showed marked deterioration in the EEG records with occurrence of spikes and coinciding evidence of some physical and mental deterioration (Table 4).

**Ataxias.** A further group of cerebral-palsied children are classified as ataxics. They had a defect of balance and co-ordination, but it was not possible to be certain that the lesion was cerebellar in origin. Some showed considerable hypotonia, but a few were hypertonic and could be classified as ataxic diplegics. Two had nystagmus and several showed incoordinated eye movements. Four were epileptic and three ineducable. Of 19 children in this group

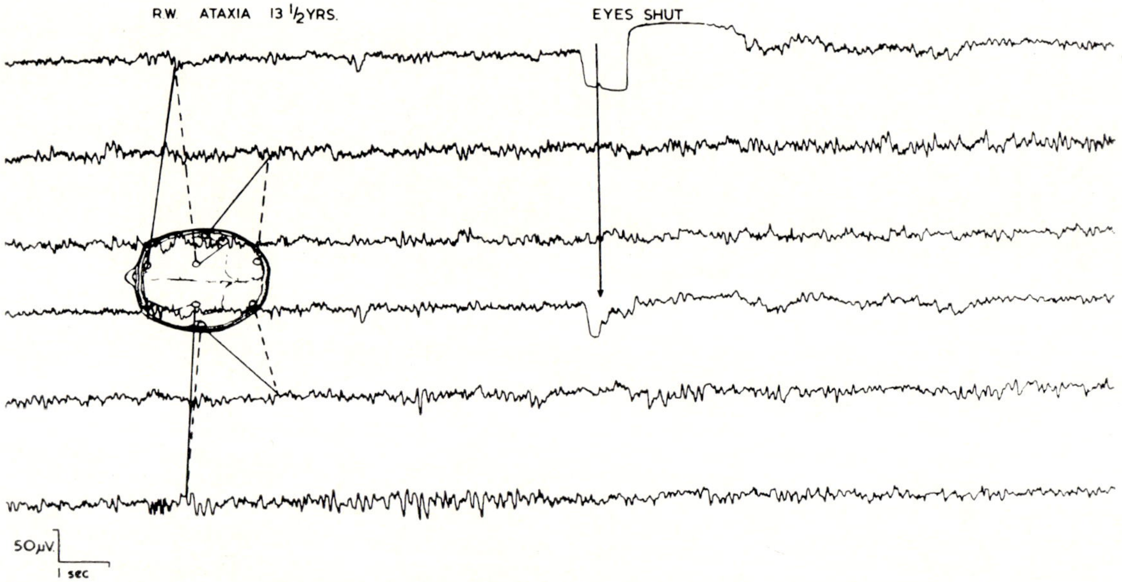


FIG. 3.—Recording of an ataxic patient aged 13½ years, showing diffuse theta activity and some delta mainly from the left central regions, unchanged when the eyes were closed.

from whom 36 EEG records were obtained, the aetiology was varied. Two followed measles encephalitis, were ineducable, and gave very abnormal records; 4 were premature and 6 followed a period of neonatal disorder suggesting cerebral trauma; 2 had arrested hydrocephalus. In 5 no apparent cause for the condition was found and all may have been developmental in origin, though one hypotonic child appeared to be deteriorating and had been called psychotic.

As in the group described by Ounsted, the EEG findings varied, but all but four of the records were abnormal. One measles encephalitic child and one presumed post-encephalitic child gave low potential records. Four showed spikes and two of these were epileptic. Eight showed the slow waves in the occipital or occipito-temporal regions, reported by Lesny. Photic stimulation caused no alteration in the slow waves in some patients, and in one patient, eye opening suppressed the waves. These records from 8 patients appeared to be of a different nature from other records in cerebral palsy and may represent a distinct group of cases with dysplasia of the cerebellum. Lesny's cases were confirmed by an air-encephalography which was not performed in this series (Fig. 3).

**Minimal Movement Defect.** A number of patients were referred to the clinic with minimal movement defect. There was often evidence of other neurological deficit. Many had been referred through school medical officers, as a child's total handicap became obvious when seen with a group of normal children. The movement defects were such conditions as a mild generalized spasticity, athetosis, monoplegia, or general incoordination. There was often an abnormal reflex pattern such as increased arm and leg jerks and extensor plantar responses. The majority had an additional handicap. Of 24 patients, 13 were of below average intelligence, 4 were epileptic, and 5 had a speech defect, a dysarthria or dysphasia. In a number of patients there was a clear history of perinatal or postnatal illness. In some cases there remained a doubt whether the total defect was organic in origin or emotionally or environmentally determined. An EEG record was additional evidence of underlying brain pathology. Forty records were obtained.

In 4 patients the EEG was normal. All had minimal spasticity and attended school. One had an aphasic element.

The remaining 20 children showed varying degrees of abnormality. Two had electrically quiet records: both had been premature babies and the movement defect suggested minimal athetosis. Five showed immature records for the child's age. There were 13 records that were more abnormal, showing focal or diffuse delta and theta rhythm and, in one case, alphoid rhythm. Seven records revealed spikes and in four of these the children were epileptic.

These very abnormal records emphasized the fact

that this rather indefinite group of patients contained children with considerable brain disease.

## Discussion

From these findings it cannot be suggested that the EEG records give a firm indication of the severity of the physical handicap, the occurrence of epilepsy, or the level of intelligence. But after a full clinical appraisal of the child the EEG has some confirmatory and prognostic value.

A normal record appeared to be related to a mild degree of physical handicap. It occurred in 7 out of 9 cases of mild athetosis, and in only 1 out of 14 with severe athetosis. Similarly, a normal record was obtained in 18 out of 19 diplegics with involvement of legs only, and in 4 out of 28 where all 4 limbs were involved. Normal records were obtained in the genetically determined cases.

Normal records were obtained in only two children who suffered from epilepsy. One was a young hemiplegic boy and the other an athetoid girl, where the mother's history of *petit mal* attacks may have been misleading. In all types of movement defect the EEG records did not give an indication of the occurrence of epilepsy, but the more abnormal the record the more likely was the incidence of epilepsy. Fits were occurring in patients who, though giving abnormal records, did not show typical spike or wave and spike discharges; and vice versa, epilepsy up to 10 years did not occur in children who gave a record strongly suggestive of epilepsy. The value of these records was the indication they gave that epilepsy might occur and that the patient should be carefully watched and followed up.

The EEG records appeared to be a poorer indication of intelligence rating than of degree of physical handicap or occurrence of epilepsy. An abnormal record frequently did not indicate poor intelligence and vice versa.

The records did not tend to change to any significant degree over the years, which suggests the static nature of the lesions. In 1 athetoid, 5 hemiplegics, and 1 quadriplegic, there were deteriorating records, and in all but the last patient there was accompanying clinical evidence of deterioration.

Of particular interest is the incidence of low voltage and electrically silent records. This finding occurred in all groups but particularly in cases of severe athetosis.

On several occasions a request was made for an EEG due to a severe behaviour disorder in the child. Many of these children show aggressive behaviour and temper tantrums during periods of stress. This has been particularly noted when a younger sib has commenced to walk and overtaken the handicapped patient. In some cases the disturbance has been so severe as to suggest epilepsy, but in no case has there been a change in the EEG recording.

## Summary

The results are recorded of 382 electroencephalograms in 206 cerebral-palsied children. The findings have been classified under headings which indicate the movement handicap, athetosis, hemiplegia, diplegia, ataxia, and minimal movement defect.

My thanks are due to Mrs. V. Aldridge who carried out the majority of the EEG recordings. I am also grateful to Professor A. V. Neale under whose direction the work has been carried out, and for the facilities for EEG recording at the Bristol Children's Hospital, which made the task of testing these handicapped children so much easier.

### References

Aird, R. B., and Cohen, P. (1950). Electroencephalography in cerebral palsy. *J. Pediat.*, **37**, 448.

Denhoff, E., and Robinault, I. P. (1960). *Cerebral Palsy and Related Disorders.* McGraw, New York.

Jabbour, J. T., and Lundervold, A. (1963). Hemiplegia: a clinical and electroencephalographic study in childhood. *Develop. Med. Child Neurol.*, **5**, 24.

Lesny, I. (1963). E.E.G. in cerebellar disease. *Little Club Clin. dev. Med.*, **8**, 91.

Lundervold, A. (1960). E.E.G. in cerebral palsy. *Cerebr. Palsy Bull.*, **2**, 82.

Melin, K. A. (1962). E.E.G. and epilepsy in cerebral palsy. *Develop. Med. Child Neurol.*, **4**, 180.

Ounsted, C. (1963). E.E.G. anomalies associated with benign congenital cerebellar dysplasia in childhood. *Little Club Clin. dev. Med.*, **8**, 93.

Pampiglione, G. (1958). Electroencephalography in cerebral palsy. *Cerebr. Palsy Bull.*, **1**(3), 16.

Perlstein, M. A., Gibbs, E. L., and Gibbs, F. A. (1946). The electroencephalogram in infantile cerebral palsy. *Res. Ass. nerv. ment. Dis. Publ.*, **26**, 377.

Woods, G. E. (1963). Some observations on 141 cases of infantile hemiplegia. *Cerebr. Palsy Rev.*, **24**, 11.

*Arch. Dis. Childh.*, 1965, **40**, 402.

# THE ELECTROCARDIOGRAM IN RESPIRATORY DISTRESS SYNDROME*

## THE PRAECORDIAL P WAVE AS AN AID TO ASSESSMENT

BY

G. J. SUTIN, RUTH HORNER, H. DE V. HEESE, and A. F. MALAN†

*From the Department of Child Health, University of Cape Town, South Africa*

(RECEIVED FOR PUBLICATION NOVEMBER 30, 1964)

Although the respiratory distress syndrome (RDS) has been the subject of extensive study and review, the clinical and prognostic evaluation, and the therapy, still present considerable difficulties. This report concerns a progressive change in the electrocardiogram, which was found to be of value in assessing severity and prognosis. Attention was drawn to these variations in pattern in a recent brief communication to the *Lancet* (Sutin and Heese, 1964).

### Material and Methods

Electrocardiographic tracings were routinely obtained on infants as soon as possible after admission into a special unit for the intensive investigation and treatment of RDS. This unit is in Groote Schuur Hospital, associated with the University of Cape Town, and staffed by members of the Department of Child Health. All the tracings were recorded on a Sanborn direct-writing Visocardiette, conventionally standardized, and run at paper speed of 25 mm. per second. Attempts were made to obtain the 6 standard limb leads and the praecordial leads V1 to V6 in every instance.

This is a retrospective study on these initial tracings, and concerns the 34 graphs in which the behaviour of the P wave and the QRS deflection in V1 and V2 could be clearly interpreted.

All these tracings were taken within the first 48 hours of life. Of these infants, 27 belonged to the White, 6 to the Coloured, and 1 to the Bantu racial group.

During analysis of the tracings, special emphasis was placed on the pattern of the P wave in the right praecordial leads. This wave was considered to be notched when there was a second peak irrespective of the width or depth of the intermediate phase. Attention was also paid to the Index of Macruz (Macruz, Perloff, and Case, 1958), namely, the ratio of the width of the P wave to the corresponding P-R segment. Constant correlation of a specific electrocardiographic pattern with single factors such as blood *p*H, potassium, and total plasma carbon dioxide, could not be obtained. Attention was then directed at seeing whether any pattern could be related to the over-all clinical condition at the time, and/or the possible outcome.

### Results

Our findings in leads V1 and V2 are shown in the Table. When R was clearly greater than S in the right praecordial leads (Group 1), clear-cut right ventricular dominance was generally present. When R was either equal to, or less than, S in V1 or V2 or both (Group 2), R was usually dominant in V6, indicating a more balanced ventricular pattern or left ventricular preponderance. The P wave is shown as being either peaked, biphasic, notched, or inverted. The average and the range of weights of infants with a specific pattern in V1 and V2 are also shown, as well as the number of survivors and deaths among these particular infants.

From the Table it can be seen that there were 2 deaths in Group 1. One was associated with notching of the P wave in both praecordial leads, and the other with notching in V1 and inversion in V2. In Group 2 there were 11 deaths, i.e. a 50% mortality rate. Of these deaths, 10 occurred in infants showing notching present in V2, and 7 of these had notching present in V1 as well. There were no survivors in Group 2 when notching was present in both praecordial leads.

From the weights it can be seen that the smaller infants tended to fall within Group 2. Two of the smallest infants weighing 2 lb. 12 oz. (1,247 g.) and 2 lb. 15 oz. (1,332 g.) survived. In both these, the P wave was either peaked or biphasic in the right praecordial leads.

Fig. 1 illustrates some of the patterns described.

---

* Paper presented at 6th Congress of the South African Paediatric Association, October 1964.

† Senior Bursar, Council for Scientific and Industrial Research.

TABLE

ELECTROCARDIOGRAPHIC FINDINGS (LEADS V1 AND V2) IN 34 CASES

| P Wave | | Weight (g.) | | Survivors | Deceased |
|---|---|---|---|---|---|
| V1 | V2 | Mean | Range | | |
| *Group I: R > S in V1 and V2* (12 *cases*) | | | | | |
| Peaked or biphasic | Peaked or biphasic | 1,956 | 1,247-3,117 | 4 | 0 |
| Peaked or biphasic | Notched | 2,607 | 2,323-2,834 | 2 | 0 |
| Normal | Notched | 2,295 | 1,814-2,721 | 3 | 1 |
| Normal or inverted | Inverted | 2,210 | 2,041-2,352 | 1 | 1 |
| *Group II: R < S or R = S in V1 and/or V2* (22 *cases*) | | | | | |
| Peaked or biphasic | Peaked or biphasic | 2,182 | 1,332-3,061 | 3 | 1 |
| Peaked or biphasic | Notched | 2,069 | 1,587-2,891 | 8 | 2 |
| Normal | Notched | 1,558 | 1,275-2,295 | 0 | 7 |
| Inverted | Notched | 1,473 | — | 0 | 1 |

## Discussion

Previous studies (Usher, 1959, 1961; Keith, Rose, Braudo, and Rowe, 1961) have shown that left ventricular preponderance tends to occur in the more severe forms of the RDS. This is borne out in our series of predominantly White infants. This electrocardiographic finding may be of lesser significance in our Coloured and Bantu, as an interracial difference in normal full-term newborn infants has recently been shown (Sutin and Schrire, 1964). This interracial factor is being considered in establishing normal standards for premature infants. Right ventricular dominance, noted in those less severely involved, is less suggestive of abnormality in the early neonatal period.

Usher (1959) also drew attention to the 'broadening and flattening' of the P wave, and the absence of the P wave sometimes encountered in this syndrome. He related changes to serum potassium levels. In this study the character of the P wave is reported in greater detail and, as already stated, no constant correlation with serum potassium levels was found. A definite sequence did exist, indicating a progressively more serious prognosis when the P wave was interpreted with due regard to the associated QRS deflection.

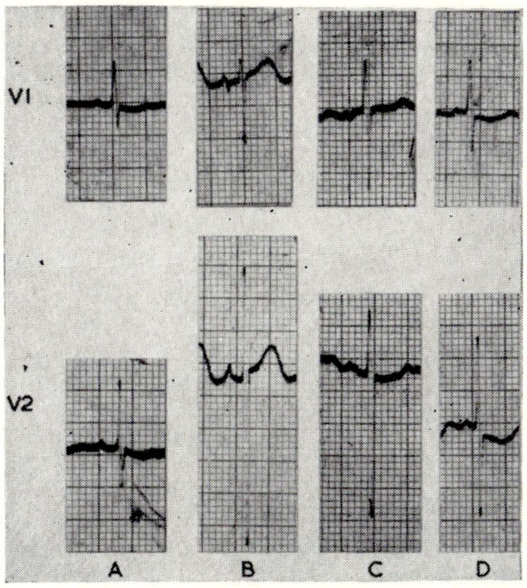


FIG. 1.—Examples of the P wave patterns encountered. (a) Peaked P in V1 and V2. (b) Biphasic P in V1, peaked P in V2. (c) Biphasic P in V1, notched P in V2. (d) Notched P in V1 and V2 (note short P-R segment).

The P wave pattern was found to be variable when the R to S ratio was greater than 1 in V1 and V2. This variability is a well-recognized phenomenon in the normal full-term infant, and has recently been documented by DePasquale and Burch (1963). Walsh (1963) stated that the P wave in the premature infant differed from that in the full-term in voltage rather than contour except that the P waves in the former tended to be more peaked. Essentially, therefore, the P and QRS patterns encountered in Group 1, i.e. those infants usually mildly involved, might well be variations of the normal.

In those infants in Group 2, who were clinically more severely involved, the P wave behaved in a definite manner. When the P wave was peaked or biphasic in V1 and V2, the prognosis proved to be good. The outlook progressively worsened with the appearance of notching, and there was no survivor in Group 2 when notching was present in both the praecordial leads. From our current experience it appears that progression is from notching, through notching associated with an Index of Macruz greater than 1·6, to complete absence of the P wave which is a terminal event.

The value of interpretation of the electrocardiogram relative to the clinical condition at the time is illustrated in Figs. 2 and 3. The successive tracings in Fig. 2 are from a White infant in whom some dispute existed as to the severity of the clinical status on admission. From the initial graph a serious prognosis could be anticipated. The P wave was inverted in V1 and clearly notched in V2, with R less than S in V2 and a dominant R in V6. Within hours

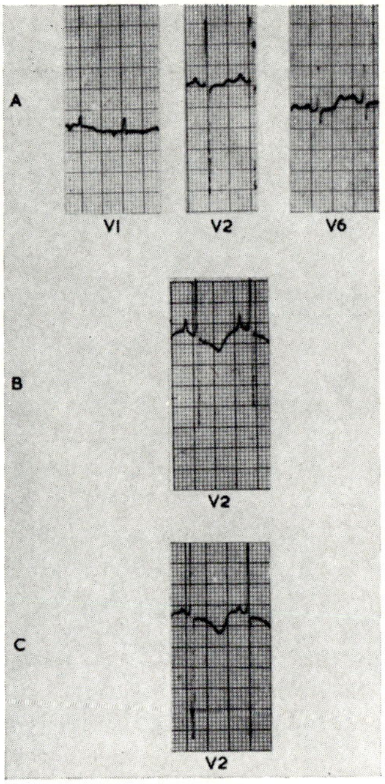


FIG. 2.—Tracings from an infant with severe RDS who succumbed. For discussion see text.

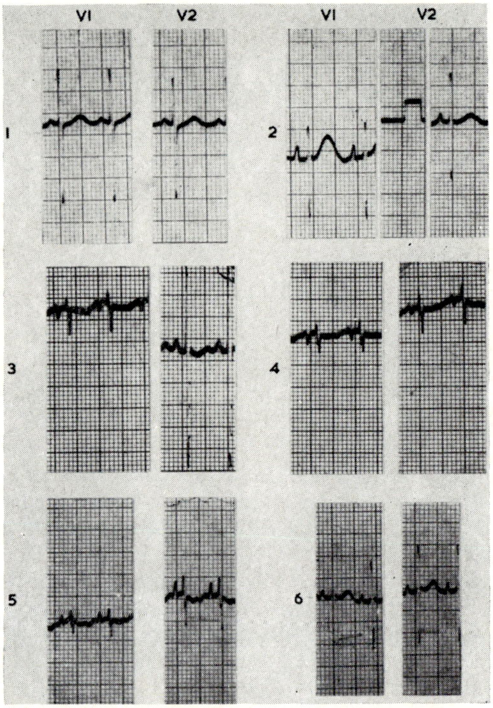


FIG. 3.—Tracings from an infant with severe RDS who survived. For discussion see text.

this infant was on intermittent positive-pressure assisted respiration, with considerable improvement in circulatory status. This was associated with marked peaking of the P wave as shown on the second tracing. Subsequent deterioration was heralded by the reappearance of notching in V2, and the infant died soon after this third electrocardiogram.

The tracings in Fig. 3 are from an infant who survived a very stormy clinical course. Initially, with S clearly dominant over R in V1 and V2, the P wave was peaked. This peaking was more obvious in the next tracing. With deterioration, the P wave became inverted in V1, and subsequently biphasic in V2 (tracings 3 and 4). When recovery began, peaking again occurred while R was still clearly less than S in V1 and V2 (tracing No. 5). With progressive recovery, the P wave remained peaked, while R and S tended to equalize (tracing No. 6). It must be noted that notching was never manifest, and this infant never required mechanical respiratory assistance.

In our present state of knowledge the explanation of the patterns encountered can only be speculative. Nadas (1963) states that accentuation of the negative component of a biphasic P wave in V1 and V2 may be compatible with left atrial hypertrophy. Left atrial hypertrophy is further indicated by a P wave of prolonged duration and two notches of at least 0·05 second apart. Macruz *et al.* (1958) consider left atrial enlargement to be present when their index exceeds 1·6 in lead II regardless of age. Katz (1946) mentions the variations in P wave contour that may occur with respiration and also states that the 'mitral' P wave need not necessarily be notched in the chest leads, but can be biphasic. It is felt that, even if our tracings in the more severely involved do not fulfil the accepted criteria for left atrial hypertrophy, they indicate at least left atrial dominance. This dominance in the presence of left ventricular dominance may indicate a further stage in left-sided overload, and a much more serious disturbance of the haemodynamic status than reflected by the QRS alone. The combined pattern might be a reflection of the size of the left-to-right shunt shown to be present by Rudolph, Drorbaugh, Auld, Rudolph, Nadas, Smith, and Hubbell (1961) in those more severely involved. This shunt would in turn be inversely related to the pulmonary vascular resistance and changes in the latter might well be the primary factor. Left atrial dominance *per se* could indicate that functional closure of the foramen ovale has occurred.

## Summary and Conclusions

The praecordial P and QRS patterns in V1 and V2 in the electrocardiographic tracings on admission on 34 infants with the respiratory distress syndrome are presented. In this retrospective study emphasis is placed on the characteristics of the P wave.

Interpretation of the P wave contour with due regard to the concomitant QRS deflection reveals changes of pattern associated with progressive worsening in prognosis. The evolution is from a variable P wave associated with an R to S ratio greater than 1 in both V1 and V2, through a peaked or biphasic P wave, subsequently becoming notched and finally absent, with an R less than or equal to S in V1 or V2 or both. These changes are sufficiently constant to warrant the routine use of the electrocardiogram as an additional parameter in assessment of severity and prognosis. The possible mechanism by which these patterns could be produced is discussed.

Thanks are due to Dr. J. G. Burger, Medical Superintendent of Groote Schuur Hospital, for permission to publish; the Nursing Staff for willing and vigilant assistance; the Cardiac Clinic for technical assistance; the Department of Chemical Pathology, the Staff Research Fund (Teaching Hospitals Board) and the Dr. C. L. Herman Bequest Award for financial assistance; paediatric colleagues for referring patients; Professor F. J. Ford, Associate Professor V. Schrire, and Dr. W. Beck for their encouragement and help; and Mrs. O. M. Cartwright for her assistance in the preparation of the manuscript.

### References

DePasquale, N. P., and Burch, G. E. (1963). The electrocardiogram, ventricular gradient and spatial vectorcardiogram during the first week of life. *Amer. J. Cardiol.*, **12**, 482.

Katz, L. N. (1946). *Electrocardiography*, 2nd ed., p. 139. Lea and Febiger, Philadelphia.

Keith, J. D., Rose, V., Braudo, M., and Rowe, R. D. (1961). The electrocardiogram in the respiratory distress syndrome and related cardiovascular dynamics. *J. Pediat.*, **59**, 167.

Macruz, R., Perloff, J. K., and Case, R. B. (1958). A method for the electrocardiographic recognition of atrial enlargement. *Circulation*, **17**, 882.

Nadas, A. S. (1963). *Pediatric Cardiology*, 2nd ed., p. 56. Saunders, Philadelphia and London.

Rudolph, A. M., Drorbaugh, J. E., Auld, P. A. M., Rudolph, A. J., Nadas, A. S., Smith, C. A., and Hubbell, J. A. (1961). Studies on the circulation in the neonatal period. The circulation in the respiratory distress syndrome. *Pediatrics*, **27**, 551.

Sutin, G. J., and Heese, H. de V. (1964). Electrocardiogram in idiopathic respiratory distress syndrome of newborn. *Lancet*, **2**, 532.

——, and Schrire, V. (1964). The electrocardiogram in the first two days of life. An interracial study . *Amer. Heart J.*, **67**, 749.

Usher, R. (1959). The respiratory distress syndrome of prematurity. I. Changes in potassium in the serum and the electrocardiogram and effects of therapy. *Pediatrics*, **24**, 562.

—— (1961). The respiratory distress syndrome of prematurity: clinical and therapeutic aspects. *Pediat. Clin. N. Amer.*, **8**, 525.

Walsh, S. Z. (1963). Evolution of the electrocardiogram of healthy premature infants during the first year of life. *Acta paediat.* (*Uppsala*), Suppl., **145**, 35.

*Arch. Dis. Childh.*, 1965, **40**, 406.

# FAT INFILTRATION IN THE TISSUES OF THE NEWBORN INFANT

BY

W. AHERNE

*From the Department of Pathology, Radcliffe Infirmary, Oxford*

(RECEIVED FOR PUBLICATION JANUARY 6, 1965)

Although there are many studies on the significance of fat droplets in parenchymal cells, few of them relate to the neonatal period. Scott (1961) found fat infiltration of the myocardium in infants who had been in respiratory distress. She associated this with other necropsy findings which suggested heart failure. Gruenwald (1949) observed fat vacuolation of the liver, more marked in the right lobe, together with other changes more clearly degenerative, in infants who had suffered prenatal hypoxia. Emery and Finch (1954), who were also interested in differences between the liver lobes, estimated chemically the fat content of the foetal and the neonatal liver, having first excluded as abnormal any specimen showing stainable fat droplets. They found a considerable variation in fat content, and a tendency for the right lobe to contain more after 24 hours of age. Inspection of their figures further suggests an increase in total mean fat content (based on dry weight) from 9% in the first 5 hours to 16% in the second day.

These authors have interpreted fat droplet infiltration as pathological. Dorkin and Weinberg (1949) observed more stainable fat in the neonatal human liver than they could attribute to any pathological cause, and concluded that its presence was a normal part of neonatal metabolism. If species differences do not invalidate comparisons, this view accords with experimental findings in newborn animals. Hard, Reynolds, and Winbury (1944) found a marked rise in the fat content of the guinea-pig liver during the last quarter of gestation. At term the level had reached 33-35% (dry weight). Immediately after birth this began to fall, like the liver glycogen level but less steeply, until the adult level of about 12% was attained in 3 to 4 days. Fat staining of the normal newborn rabbit liver (writer's observations) suggests a similar pattern of change.

It is now well known that tissue glycogen levels are high at term and are rapidly mobilized in the early neonatal period (Shelley, 1964). The possibility of changes in tissue fat content determined by birth prompted the following study.

## Material and Methods

The series comprised 69 infants, studied consecutively, of whom 7 were stillborn. Of the 62 liveborn infants about two-thirds were premature; all died in the first week of life. Causes of death need not be specified in detail; the necropsy findings were a representative cross-section of neonatal pathology. Nine of the infants came also into a trial of immediate feeding (Smallpeice and Davies, 1964); a few of these had been fed with expressed breast milk as early as 1-2 hours after delivery.

At necropsy, samples were taken of liver, myocardium, lung, kidney, diaphragm, rectus abdominis, and tibialis anterior. These tissues were mostly sectioned fresh on a Slee cryostat at 5$\mu$ and stained with Oil Red O. In a small proportion of cases stored formalin-fixed tissues were used, similarly cut and stained. Detailed histochemical analyses were made in a few representative cases, using Nile Blue Sulphate, periodic acid-Schiff, and Sudan Black B after acetone extraction. During the study 20 sets of samples were taken from older children for comparison.

In assessing the results the method of rank correlation was used. To test, for example, the correlation of tissue fat content with postnatal age, the procedure, in outline, was as follows. First, all the cases were ranked, with respect to each tissue separately, in descending order of fat droplet content as determined microscopically by visual assessment. A number was assigned to each case denoting its rank in each particular tissue series. Next, the cases were again ranked, now with respect to postnatal age in hours, in descending order of magnitude; again a number was assigned to each case denoting its rank. Finally, the tissue fat rank number was compared with the age rank number. Theoretically, perfect correlation would have been indicated by the coincidence of ranks; 1 with 1, 2 with 2, and so on. In practice the degree of correlation was obtained by means of Spearman's coefficient, and from this an estimate of the more widely used correlation coefficient, r, as described by Tippett (1952).

The ranked sequences also enabled comparisons to be made between one tissue and another, between premature and mature infants, and (in a more limited way) between one disease and another.

Chemical estimations of tissue carbohydrate levels were available in most cases, since a study of carbohydrate metabolism was made concurrently (Shelley, 1964).

## Results

**Liver and Muscle.** Sequential changes related to postnatal age were soon observed in samples of liver, myocardium, respiratory muscle (diaphragm, rectus abdominis), and skeletal muscle. Particular attention was therefore given to these tissues.

STILLBORN INFANTS. In the small group of stillborn infants examined, liver, myocardium, respiratory, and skeletal muscles were all devoid of fat droplets.

LIVEBORN INFANTS. In liveborn infants, especially in those of more than 30 weeks' gestation, fat droplet infiltration increased steadily with advancing postnatal age in liver, myocardium, respiratory, and skeletal muscles. This phenomenon appeared unrelated to the type of illness from which the infant had suffered. Infiltration reached maximum intensity at about 48 hours when, by and large, it was much greater than any seen in older children. After 48 hours the direct relation with postnatal age began to disappear: at 72 hours the intensity of fat infiltration was no greater than that at 48 hours, and it was often less. Too few cases were available to pursue the study beyond 72 hours.

TABLE 1

COEFFICIENTS OF CORRELATION BETWEEN TISSUE FAT DROPLET DENSITY AND POSTNATAL AGE TO 48 HOURS
(Gestation: 30 Weeks - Term)

| Tissue | Coefficient, r | Significance |
|---|---|---|
| Liver .. .. .. | 0·65 | $p < 0·01$ |
| Myocardium .. .. | 0·47 | $p < 0·01$ |
| Diaphragm .. .. | 0·66 | $p < 0·01$ |
| Rectus abdom. .. .. | 0·75 | $p < 0·01$ |
| Tibialis ant. .. .. | 0·52 | $0·05 < p < 0·02$ |

The correlation between fat content and age is shown numerically in Table 1. Typical histological appearances are shown in Figs. 1 to 3.

Fat droplets tended to appear earliest, and to be largest, in the liver. Infiltration began usually in the periportal cells. In muscle other than cardiac the droplets lay in parallel rows, mainly longitudinally, in relation to myofibrils. The intensity of infiltration was consistently greater in respiratory than in skeletal muscle; in 26 comparisons of diaphragm with tibialis anterior from the same case the diaphragm contained more fat in 22 instances. In general, however, the rate of fat infiltration, as judged by the rank achieved in the separate tissue series, was much the same in liver, myocardium, and muscle in any particular case. This is shown in Table 2, where pairs of ranked tissues are correlated.

TABLE 2

COEFFICIENTS OF CORRELATION BETWEEN FAT DROPLET DENSITY IN PAIRS OF TISSUES FROM THE SAME BODY

| | Liver | Myocardium | Diaphragm | Rectus Ab. |
|---|---|---|---|---|
| Liver .. .. | | | | |
| Myocardium .. | 0·62 | | | |
| Diaphragm .. | 0·74 | 0·69 | | |
| Rectus abdom. | 0·68 | 0·69 | 0·85 | |
| Tibialis ant. .. | 0·81 | 0·69 | 0·77 | 0·85 |

In each instance $p < 0·01$.

The intensity of fat infiltration at any particular postnatal age depended significantly on maturity, being clearly greater in the more mature infants.

The series contained too few dysmature infants for rigorous appraisal; however, one of the most strikingly infiltrated sets of tissues came from a dysmature infant who died at only 10 hours of age.

The relation of tissue fat content (estimated visually) and carbohydrate content (estimated chemically; Shelley, 1964) was inverse. It was not particularly close, however, and only appeared when the cases were broadly classified into four groups (3+, 2+, 1+, 0) according to fat content. A limited analysis of this topic is shown in Table 3.

**Other Tissues.** Samples of kidney showed some degree of fat droplet infiltration with advancing postnatal age, affecting mainly the proximal convoluted tubules. This was much less clear cut than in the tissues discussed above and was not actively studied. The lung was unique among the tissues sampled: here alone fat droplets (which appeared in the bronchiolar mucosa) were present in greater numbers in immature than in mature infants and did not

TABLE 3

RELATION OF FAT DROPLET CONTENT TO TOTAL CARBOHYDRATE CONTENT (POOLED CASES)

| Fat Content | Total Carbohydrate Content (mg./g. wet weight) | | |
|---|---|---|---|
| | Liver | Myocardium | Diaphragm |
| + + + | 2·2 | 9·9 | 1·3 |
| + + | 7·5 | 9·7 | 6·0 |
| + | 9·8 | 23·5 | 4·5 |
| 0 | 10·8 | 21·6 | 3·5 |

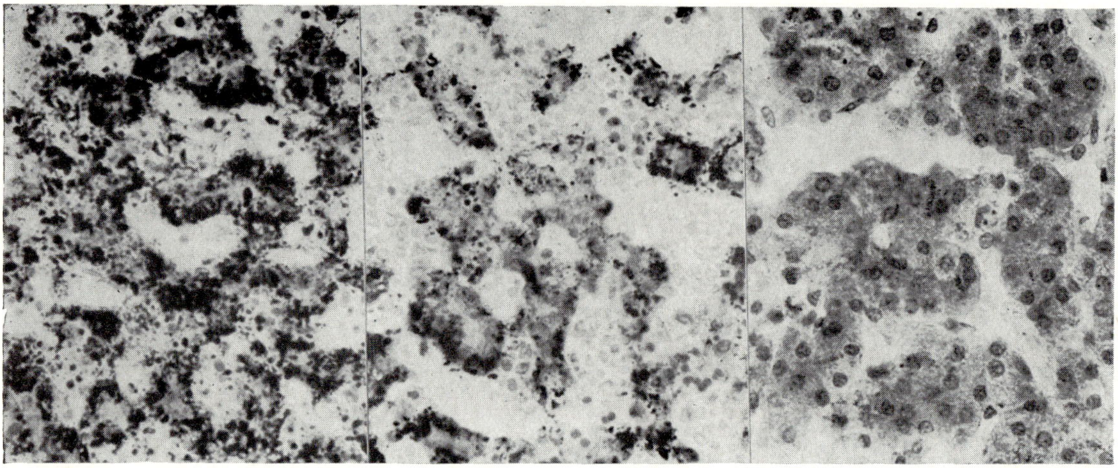

(a) (b) (c)
FIG. 1.—Liver parenchyma, showing (a) marked, (b) moderate, and (c) no fat infiltration. (Frozen section, Oil Red 0, Blue filter. × 243.)

change with age. Moreover, it was present here alone in stillbirths. These observations were not pursued further.

**Histochemical Analysis.** Differential staining showed that, in all cases examined, the droplets consisted of neutral fat.

## Discussion

In most cells fat is present in the form of a micellar dispersion (Dixon, 1958) and so cannot be demonstrated by fat soluble dyes. It is maintained in this form by phospholipid. Broadly, the conditions that determine its aggregation into droplets are these: deficiency of phospholipid, a block in utilization due to some lesion in the cell, or the delivery of fat in unusually large amounts to the normal cell.

The familiar fat infiltration of adult tissues can reasonably be explained in terms of phospholipid deficiency, as in malnutrition, or of katabolic block, as in prolonged anaemia, severe sepsis, or chemical intoxication. Not unnaturally, therefore, the pres-

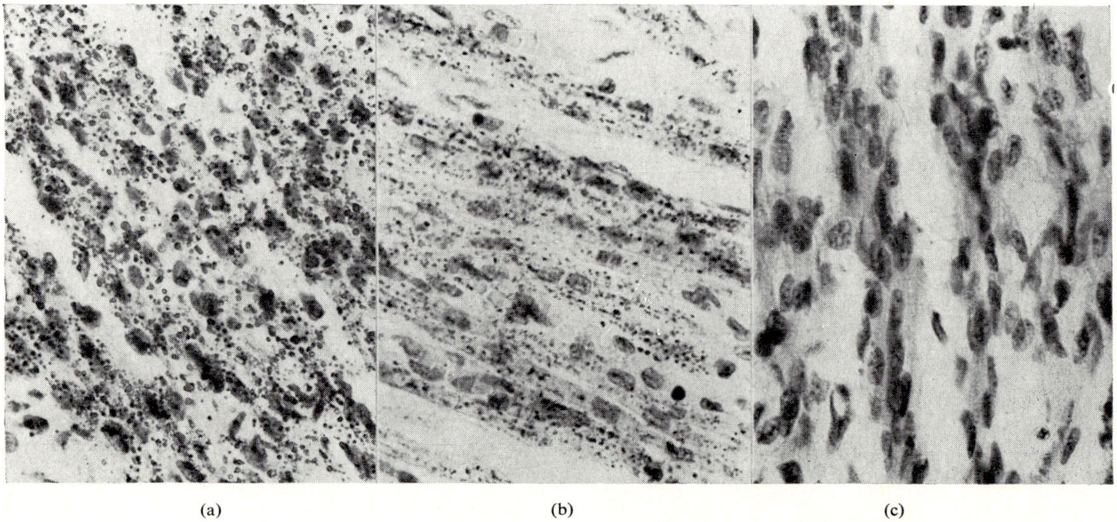

(a) (b) (c)
FIG. 2.—Myocardium, showing (a) marked, (b) moderate, and (c) no fat infiltration. (Frozen section, Oil Red 0. × 300.)

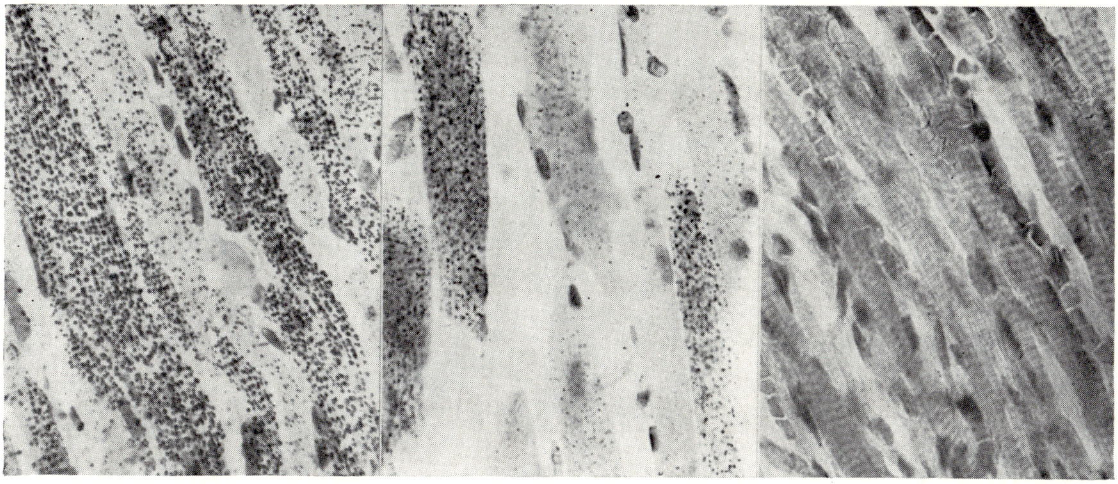

(a) (b) (c)

FIG. 3.—Diaphragm, showing (a) marked, (b) moderate, and (c) no fat infiltration. (Frozen section, Oil Red 0. × 300.)

ence of fat droplets is commonly regarded as an index of disease.

The present study suggests that it may be otherwise in the neonatal period. Whether the infant was fed within the first two hours or starved; whether it contracted a *Pseudomonas* septicaemia or not; whether it lingered 48 hours in respiratory distress or died suddenly of intraperitoneal haemorrhage did not seem to influence the intensity of droplet infiltration. This appeared to depend only on postnatal age. It is true that many infants had suffered prenatal or postnatal hypoxia, or both. And even those who died suddenly passed necessarily through an agonal phase. It is conceivable therefore that a defect of oxidative metabolism may usually have been present. However, a similar infiltration of droplets may be seen in the tissues of healthy newborn rabbits killed by decapitation and fixed without delay (Aherne and Hull, unpublished, 1964).

The question therefore arises whether fat may be delivered to the cell at an unusual rate or in unusual amounts in the neonatal period. Rafstedt (1955) found that all serum lipids were low at birth in man but soon rose rather steeply. This was accompanied by a marked change in the ratio of α- to β-lipoprotein. In the first four days the total serum lipids increased 80-90%; the increase in β-lipoprotein was more than 100%. The rate of lipid increase was greater in mature than in premature infants. It appeared uninfluenced by diet. Van Duyne and Havel (1959), in a briefer study, found that the level of plasma unesterified fatty acid (UFA) was low at birth in both man and lamb but rose rapidly within the first two hours, and was still rising at $6\frac{1}{2}$ hours after birth, when observations were discontinued. In one lamb experiment UFA had by then risen tenfold.

These observations may explain the correlation found in the present study between the degree of fat droplet infiltration and postnatal age. It seems reasonable to relate the number and size of droplets in parenchymal cells to the level of circulating lipid at the time of death. But in neither Rafstedt's study nor in that of Van Duyne and Havel did serum lipid rise unusually high. It is not clear, therefore, why droplet infiltration should be more striking than in older children. Moreover, Rafstedt observed a rise of serum lipid over several days, but in the present study fat droplet infiltration seemed at its most intense at 48 hours. It is possible that enzymes responsible for fat combustion have a low activity in the first day or so, and thereafter begin to cope with the increasing delivery of fat to the cell. But there is some evidence against this; it is established that the respiratory quotient falls to low levels in the early hours of life in man (Smith, 1945) and animal (Hard *et al.*, 1944). Indeed, Hard *et al.* concluded from their studies on the guinea-pig that, after the exhaustion of liver glycogen in the first few hours after birth, energy is derived mainly from the metabolism of fat for several days. It is also possible that the severe carbohydrate depletion in most infants of this series (see Shelley, 1964) may have decelerated fat breakdown. But this cannot have been true of the healthy fed newborn rabbits, where a similar droplet infiltration has been seen.

The present study can only be descriptive. A

simple explanation of the findings in terms of current morphological concepts does not emerge, and it is probable that experimental studies are needed. But it may be concluded that parenchymal fat droplet infiltration requires special interpretation when it is seen in the tissues of the newborn.


## Summary

Fat droplet infiltration was studied in parenchymal and muscular tissues of 62 liveborn infants who died from various causes in the first few days of life, and 7 infants who were stillborn. In liveborn infants fat droplets progressively infiltrated parenchymal and muscular tissues in the first 48 hours, irrespective of clinical state or mode of death. The intensity of infiltration in this period was directly related to postnatal age. After 48 hours the relation with age seemed to disappear: the study was not pursued beyond 72 hours. In stillborn infants fat was demonstrable only in the bronchiolar mucosa. The findings may be partly interpreted as reflecting progressive fat mobilization in the early hours of life.


I am grateful to Dr. A. H. T. Robb-Smith, Dr. G. S. Dawes, and Dr. D. Hull for their advice, to Mr. Ian Burns for technical assistance, and to Dr. T. Parry for the photomicrographs.

### References


Dixon, K. C. (1958). Fatty deposition: a disorder of the cell. *Quart. J. exp. Physiol.*, **43**, 139.

Dorkin, J. R., and Weinberg, T. (1949). Normal occurrence of histologically demonstrable fat in the liver of the newborn infant. *Arch. Path.*, **48**, 578.

Emery, J. L., and Finch, E. (1954). The fat and water content of the left and right liver before and after birth. *Arch. Dis. Childh.*, **29**, 242.

Gruenwald, P. (1949). Degenerative changes in the right half of the liver resulting from intra-uterine anoxia. *Amer. J. clin. Path.*, **19**, 801.

Hard, W. L., Reynolds, O. E., and Winbury, M. (1944). Carbohydrate, fat and moisture relationships in the pregnant, foetal and newborn guinea-pig. *J. exp. Zool.*, **96**, 189.

Rafstedt, S. (1955). Studies on serum lipids and lipoproteins in infancy and childhood. *Acta paediat.* (*Uppsala*), Suppl. 102, 44.

Scott, J. M. (1961). Fatty change in the myocardium of the newborn. *Brit. med. J.*, **2**, 1746.

Shelley, H. J. (1964). Carbohydrate reserves in the newborn infant. *ibid.*, **1**, 273.

Smallpeice, V., and Davies, P. A. (1964). Immediate feeding of premature infants with undiluted breast-milk. *Lancet*, **2**, 1349.

Smith, C. A. (1945). *The Physiology of the Newborn Infant*. Thomas, Springfield, Illinois.

Tippett, L. H. C. (1952). *The Methods of Statistics*, 4th ed., p. 274. Williams and Norgate, London.

Van Duyne, C. M., and Havel, R. J. (1959). Plasma unesterified fatty acid concentration in fetal and neonatal life. *Proc. Soc. exp. Biol.* (*N.Y.*), **102**, 599.

*Arch. Dis. Childh.*, 1965, **40**, 411.

# BIOCHEMICAL, PHARMACOLOGICAL, AND HISTOCHEMICAL STUDIES IN NEUROBLASTOMA

BY

P. P. ANTHONY, H. M. T. COLES, JOHN PRYSE-DAVIES, and LEONARD SINCLAIR
*From Westminster Children's Hospital and the Vincent Square Laboratories of Westminster Hospital*

(RECEIVED FOR PUBLICATION FEBRUARY 3, 1965)

In recent years there has been some interest in the autonomic effects produced by neural crest tumours and in their biochemical characteristics. Hypertension and diarrhoea have been reported in several cases in which there has also been an excessive excretion of catecholamines, their precursors, or metabolic products (Mason, Hart-Mercer, Millar, Strang, and Wynne, 1957; Isaacs, Medalie, and Politzer, 1959; Voorhess and Gardner, 1961; Käser and von Studnitz, 1961; Rosenstein and Engleman, 1963; Marsden, 1963). Most investigators have suggested that these substances have activated the smooth muscle of arterioles or the intestine to produce these effects. However, in other reported cases (Wilkins, 1957; Voorhess and Gardner, 1962) there has been no evidence of excessive secretion of adreno-medullary metabolites to account for these manifestations. Further, Rosenstein and Engleman (1963) and Sourkes, Denton, Murphy, Chavez, and Saint Cyr (1963) recorded cases with no symptoms referable to autonomically innervated structures but with significantly increased secretion of catecholamine derivatives.

This report concerns two cases of metastasizing neuroblastoma and the investigations undertaken upon them. Both had hypertension and in one this was associated with diarrhoea and convulsions. It is thought that the raised blood pressure in one case might be associated with the excessive production of catecholamines by the large tumour mass. In the other patient there is no evidence to indicate that the neuroblastoma produced abnormal amounts of catecholamine-like substances during the period of study or that these were responsible for severe hypertension and intractable diarrhoea.

## Methods

**Urinary Excretion of Catecholamines and Metabolites.** The combined and individual concentrations of noradrenaline and adrenaline were estimated in 24-hour collections of urine by a fluorometric method based on that of Weil-Malherbe and Bone (1957). 4-hydroxy-3-methoxymandelic acid (HMMA, formerly VMA) was determined by the spectrophotometric method of Pisano, Crout, and Abraham (1962). The concentration of 4-hydroxy-3-methoxyphenylacetic acid (homovanillic acid, HVA) was estimated by chromatography according to the method described by Robinson, Ratcliffe, and Smith (1959).

**Storage and Treatment of Tumour Tissue.** Blocks of each intra-abdominal tumour were removed within 20 minutes of death. Tissue for biochemical, pharmacological, and histochemical investigation was frozen immediately to $-70°$ C. using solid carbon dioxide and stored at this temperature until required. Some blocks used for immediate histochemical study were frozen directly on to microtome chucks for use with a cryostat.

Extracts of tumour tissues for biochemical determination of catecholamine concentrations and for pharmacological estimation of pressor substances were prepared by homogenization at 4° C. in 5% w/v trichloracetic acid using a Potter-Elvehjem hand homogenizer. The extracts for pharmacological study were further washed with diethyl ether to remove excess trichloracetic acid, as recommended by von Euler (1956).

Other tumour blocks were fixed immediately after removal from the body in neutral formalin and Helly's chromate fixative; these were paraffin-embedded and used for histological studies and examined for chromaffin cells.

**Determination of Catecholamine Concentrations in Tumour Tissue.** Extracts of weighed amounts of tumour tissue prepared as outlined above were investigated by the fluorimetric method used in the urine studies.

**Investigation of Pressor Substances in Tumour Tissue.** Washed extracts prepared as above were injected into the femoral vein of a dog anaesthetized with pentobarbitone, and arterial blood pressure was recorded directly via a cannula in the femoral artery (Dr. P. Cliffe). The effect of these extracts on the dog's blood pressure was compared with those obtained by injecting a standard noradrenaline solution, trichloracetic acid extracts of other tissues including a phaeochromocytoma, and saline extracts of the tumour and other tissues.

**Histochemical Investigation of Tumour Tissue.** Chromate fixation was used in an attempt to demonstrate chromaffin granules. The presence of noradrenaline was sought in 50$\mu$ cryostat sections fixed in formol calcium (Eränkö, 1955). The presence of ganglioneuromatous differentiation was investigated by enzyme histochemical means by studying non-specific esterase and cholinesterase activities in 15$\mu$ cryostat sections, using an azo dye coupling method and a modification of Gomori's acetylthiocholine technique respectively (details given by Pearse, 1960).

As monoamine oxidase plays an important role in the breakdown of adrenaline and noradrenaline in the tissues, the presence of this enzyme was also investigated. Employing the method of Glenner, Burtner, and Brown (1957) and 15$\mu$ cryostat sections of fresh tissue, tryptamine hydrochloride was used as the substrate, and activity was shown by the reduction of Nitro blue tetrazolium (Sigma Chemical Company). The specificity of this method was checked by using control sections pre-incubated for 30 minutes in 0·01 M Iproniazid (Marsilid, Roche Products) as a monoamine oxidase inhibitor.

## Case Reports

**Case 1.** M.V., a male infant, was delivered normally at full term on July 20, 1961, weighing 7 lb. (3,175 g.). The mother had not been ill nor had she taken any drugs during pregnancy. The child was admitted to Queen Mary's Hospital for Children, Carshalton, at the age of 1 year suffering from streptococcal tonsillitis and iron-deficiency anaemia. Two months later, aged 14 months, he was readmitted with fever and a history of anorexia, vomiting, and increasing pallor. A large, irregular mass was palpable in the left upper quadrant of the abdomen. The Hb had fallen to 38%, but no abnormal cells were detected in the peripheral blood film.

Shortly after his transfer to Westminster Children's Hospital, when aged 15 months, he developed a unilateral convulsion involving the right side of the face and body. This soon became generalized and continued for an hour despite vigorous anticonvulsant therapy. His blood pressure was noted at this time to be 180/110 mm.Hg. CSF was normal. A bone-marrow aspirate was reported by Dr. J. G. Humble to show the presence of abnormal cells resembling those from a metastatic neuroblastoma. Radiographs (Dr. F. Starer) showed a metastasis in the upper end of the right humerus and at the anterior end of the left eighth rib.

Further clinical features were a large subcutaneous haemangioma of the left buttock and some oedema of the left thigh which extended during four days to involve the left calf and upper portion of the right thigh. A saphenous venogram showed no evidence of obstruction of the left iliac or femoral veins but a lymphangiogram demonstrated dilatation of the lymphatics of the left foot and slow diffusion of dye, indicating lymph stasis in the left leg. Intravenous pyelography showed normal excretion by each kidney. At this time the blood urea was 26 mg./100 ml.

After consultation with Dr. K. A. Newton, treatment with cyanocobalamin 1 mg. intramuscularly thrice weekly and cyclophosphamide 20 mg. intravenously daily was commenced. Initially the tumour extended 3 in. (7·6 cm.) below the left costal margin in the mid-clavicular line and to a point in the right upper quadrant 2·5 in. (6·4 cm.) below the costal margin in the mid-clavicular line. During the first week of treatment it became much smaller, extending only 2 in. (5 cm.) downwards and across the abdomen only as far as the right mid-clavicular line. Simultaneously the haemangioma of the left buttock shrunk and became necrotic. The blood pressure, however, remained high (190/105 mm.Hg) and the Hb fell from 92 to 60%.

Treatment with cyclophosphamide was discontinued for one week. Six days after resuming the drug (i.e three weeks after admission) the child passed 8 loose green motions (see Fig. 1), and was pale with cold extremities and feeble, grunting respirations. On the following day the pallor was more marked and there was some abdominal distension with dullness in each flank.

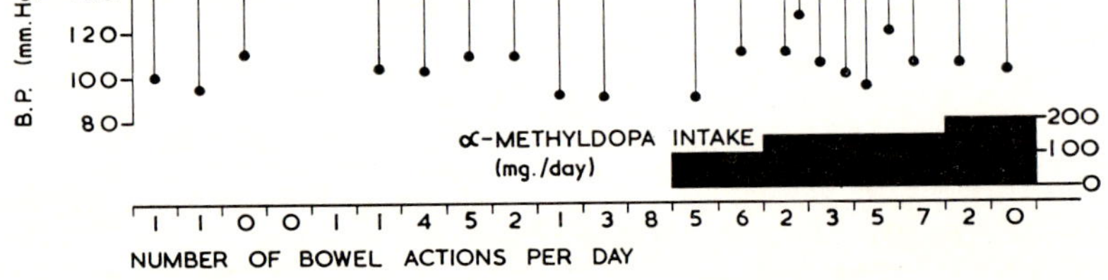


FIG. 1.—Case 1. The absence of an effect of α-methyldopa on blood pressure and bowel motility.

The Hb had fallen to 40% and he was thought to have had a retroperitoneal haemorrhage. After transfusion with 220 ml. fresh blood the Hb was only 48%. A further 170 ml. was given and the Hb rose to 74%. A fluctuant swelling now appeared at the anterior end of the left eighth rib. This became smaller during the next three days and the infant's general condition seemed to improve though the hypertension persisted.

In an attempt to reduce dopamine formation from dopa by the tumour and possibly thereby to diminish the diarrhoea as well as to mitigate the hypertension, treatment with α-methyldopa at a dosage of 100 mg./day was started two days after the onset of the diarrhoea (see Fig. 1). This was increased to 150 mg./day two days later and to 200 mg./day after a further four days. There was no fall in the blood pressure or decrease in the diarrhoea during the course of this therapy. On the day before death he was comatose and severely dehydrated. Repeated generalized convulsions could not be controlled with phenobarbitone and paraldehyde. Within 20 minutes of death (30 days from admission) necropsy was performed and a portion of the tumour removed for estimation of catecholamine content and pharmacological activity.

Necropsy (Dr. I. M. P. Dawson). The abdomen was protuberant and there was an area of scarring over the left buttock. A large lobulated tumour weighing approximately 670 g. (10% of the body weight) was found arising from the region of the left adrenal gland, carrying the spleen on the anterior surface, compressing the left lobe of the liver, the upper pole of the left kidney, and surrounding the aorta and the inferior vena cava. The cut surface was necrotic and no adrenal tissue could be identified. The only metastases found were in the right humerus and in the 8th left rib near the costal cartilage. The heart was very enlarged, weighing 54 g. and showing concentric left ventricular hypertrophy. No other cardiovascular changes were found. The kidneys appeared normal. There was evidence of an old retroperitoneal haemorrhage.

Histology. No adrenal tissue could be identified for certain. Much of the tumour was necrotic. The growth that remained consisted of loose sheets of round and oval cells, occasionally forming recognizable rosette structures with conspicuous fibrous and collagen framework. There was no evidence of conversion to ganglioneuroma. In sections of the kidney there were no vascular changes to suggest arterial hypertension.

**Case 2.** E.S. was 9 years, when in June 1963 he complained of nausea and pain in the right upper quadrant of the abdomen and was admitted to the London Jewish Hospital under the care of Dr. S. B. Dimson. There he was found to have an enlarged liver which was firm and palpable three fingers breadths below the right costal margin. The Hb was 70%. A bone-marrow biopsy showed evidence of round cell infiltration and a needle aspirate of the liver revealed infiltration with similar cells. An intravenous pyelogram demonstrated a centrally placed mass in the retroperitoneum displacing the right kidney laterally. The diagnosis at the time of transfer to the Westminster Children's Hospital, a month after first admission to hospital, was of an intra-abdominal neuroblastoma with metastasis. Just before this he had developed an evening fever, and his leucocyte count showed a few myelocytes and 2 normoblasts per 100 cells counted.

On admission to Westminster Children's Hospital in early August the liver had increased in size extending to the umbilicus and there was a palpable mass in the left para-aortic area. The blood pressure was 110/65 mm.Hg and Hb 60%. The only investigations of relevance at this time were the urinary excretion of HMMA (3·7 mg./24 hr.) and hydroxymethyl phenylacetic acid (14 mg./24 hr.). The serum lactic dehydrogenase was 5,000 units and the α-hydroxybutyric dehydrogenase 3,500 units (thought in retrospect to be due to tumour necrosis).

Within one week of admission his condition had deteriorated and the Hb had fallen to 54%. He was transfused with 1,200 ml. blood and given mustine hydrochloride 2·0 mg. intravenously daily. This induced nausea so was discontinued 2 days later and corticotrophin gel 20 units daily was substituted. During the ensuing week two estimations of 24-hour excretion of urinary catecholamines were 665 μg. and 590 μg., respectively. At this time he was normotensive and his clinical condition remained unchanged. By the end of August, however, he showed signs of inferior vena caval obstruction and had collapse/consolidation of the right lower lobe.

One week later his general state was worse, with Hb of 39%, platelet count of 600/c.mm., and 24-hour catecholamine excretion of 155 μg. Treatment was changed to prednisone 30 mg./day and he was transfused with 600 ml. packed cells. He appeared to improve but it was noted on the following day that his blood pressure had risen to 155/125 mm.Hg and his pulse rate had fallen from 100 to 70 per minute. The size of the abdominal mass had meanwhile increased and the liver had enlarged, extending to below the umbilicus.

Next morning the heart rate suddenly increased to 136 and he rapidly lapsed into unconsciousness, with frothing at the mouth and incontinence of urine and faeces. There was generalized muscular hypotonia and hyporeflexia, with conjugate deviation of the eyes to the right. The CSF pressure was over 300 mm. with a protein content of 40 mg./100 ml. There were 3 lymphocytes and more than 600 erythrocytes/c.mm. No abnormal cells were detected. The patient was treated with intravenous phentolamine and oral guanethidine but the hypertension and tachycardia persisted. The Hb fell to 28% and he was again transfused with 1,200 ml. packed cells. He continued to deteriorate and died at the end of September, less than four months from the onset of his illness.

Necropsy (Dr. J. Pryse-Davies). A preliminary necropsy was performed within 20 minutes of death in order to remove as freshly as possible specimens of the tumour from the abdomen for storage at −70° C. The necropsy was completed 10 hours later.

TABLE

COMPARISON OF CLINICAL FEATURES AND INVESTIGATIONS ON EACH PATIENT

| | Case 1 | Case 2 | |
|---|---|---|---|
| Autonomic effects present | Tachycardia, hypertension, and diarrhoea | Tachycardia, hypertension | |
| Response to phentolamine | Fall in blood pressure | No change | |
| Response to α-methyldopa | None | | |
| | In presence of hypertension | Before onset of hypertension | After onset of hypertension |
| Total daily urinary excretion of catecholamines (μg.) | 103 | 665 and 590 | 340 and 142 |
| Daily urinary excretion of HMMA (mg.) | 0·4 and 2·3 | — | 3·7 |
| Daily urinary excretion of HVA (mg.) | — | — | 14·0 |
| Concentration of catecholamines in tumour (wet weight) | Nil | — | 3·0 μg./g. |
| Effect of tumour extract on dog blood pressure | Nil | — | Rise |

The body was that of a wasted child with a protuberant abdomen due to a large retroperitoneal mass which pushed the liver forwards and was closely applied to the posterior wall of the abdomen enclosing the aorta and inferior vena cava. The left kidney was not affected but the right kidney was distorted, the pelvis being invaded but the cortex uninvolved though stretched around the growth. The tumour weighed 730 g. and measured 15 cm. in maximum diameter. The cut surface was reddish-pink in colour divided by some fibrous septa. Since the right adrenal gland was not identified it was presumed that the tumour had arisen from the right adrenal medulla or possibly from ganglionic tissue in this region. Metastases were present in the right parietal and visceral pleurae, in the pancreas, sternal, and femoral bone-marrow, in lymph nodes at the aortic arch and near the porta hepatis, in the skull at the lateral point of the greater wing of the right sphenoid bone and also the left parietal bone just lateral to the vertex.

HISTOLOGY. The tumour was composed of small round cells with scanty cytoplasm arranged in sheets but showing a few areas of classical rosette formation. There was a fair amount of necrosis and local haemorrhage. No evidence of hypertensive change was found in sections of the kidneys.

### Investigations

**Response to Phentolamine.** In Case 1 this was tested measuring systolic pressures only. The baseline level was 220 mm.Hg. One minute after 1 mg. of the drug intravenously it fell to 130 mm.Hg, rising again gradually to 155 mm.Hg. The response appears to be significant by the criteria of Soffer (1954).

In Case 2 there was no response to intravenous phentolamine 2 mg. initially, then 2 mg. hourly for 10 hours, and 3 mg. hourly for a further 5 hours. The blood pressure remained approximately 155/125 mm.Hg throughout.

**Excretion of Adreno-medullary Metabolites.** These are shown in the Table. In Case 1 the only complete 24-hour urine collection contained 103 μg. catecholamines. Few figures for the normal values at this age are available. Sourkes *et al.* (1963), using similar methods, give the range for combined adrenaline and noradrenaline excretion as 3 to 115 μg./24 hr. with a daily mean of 31 μg. The subject with the highest excretion in this series was a 13-month-old boy with supraventricular tachycardia. Voorhess and Gardner (1960) give a mean figure of less than 15 μg./24 hr. The excretion of catecholamines was much increased in Case 2. Initially they were 665, 590, and 340 μg./24 hr. and fell to 142 μg. terminally. The excretion of HMMA was within the normal range for each patient (M. Sandler and C. R. J. Ruthven, 1964, personal communication) and that of HVA was increased in Case 2 (14 μg./24 hr.).

**Response to α-Methyldopa.** This agent was tried in Case 1 (see Fig. 1). The dosage was increased from 100 mg. to 200 mg. over seven days. As can be seen there was no alteration in systolic blood pressure or amelioration of the diarrhoea. The drug was not used in Case 2.

**Biochemical and Pharmacological Investigations of Tumour Tissues.** An extract of the tumour in Case 1 was examined for the presence of catecholamine-like substances by Mr. C. R. J. Ruthven but none could be detected in stored material investigated 6 weeks after death. A similar extract from Case 2 was examined in the Vincent Square Laboratories of Westminster Hospital by Mr. B. Morris using the fluorimetric method. In this a total catecholamine concentration of 3·0 μg./g. wet tissue was found (2·4 μg. noradrenaline and 0·6 μg. adrenaline). The tumour weighed 730 g. Assuming a uniform distribution in the growth the total noradrenaline content was thus 1,750 μg. and that of adrenaline 438 μg.

The effects of extracts on the blood pressure of a dog were observed in each case. The tissues from the tumours had been stored for 6 months and 6 weeks, respectively. A similar extract was made of mouse kidney and a phaeochromocytoma; saline extracts of the tumour and mouse tissues were also examined. Each extract from Case 1 caused no significant rise of blood pressure when injected into an anaesthetized dog (Fig. 2a). The extract from the phaeochromocytoma (Fig. 3) and a standard noradrenaline solution (Fig. 2b) caused a sustained rise in pressure, while the mouse kidney and saline extracts of the tumour caused no alteration.

The injection of tumour extract from Case 2 produced a significant rise in femoral artery pressure which, by comparison with noradrenaline standards, indicated a

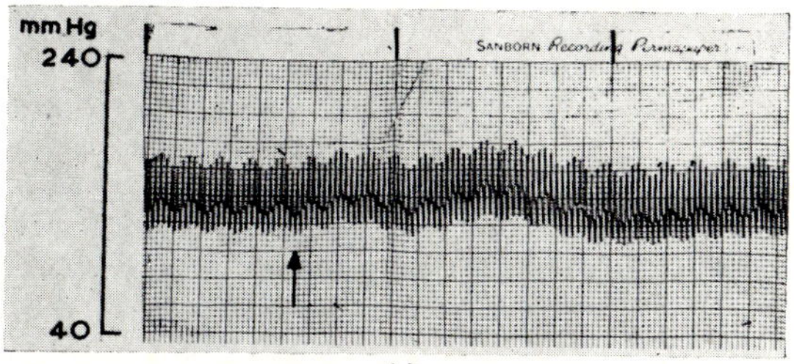


(a)

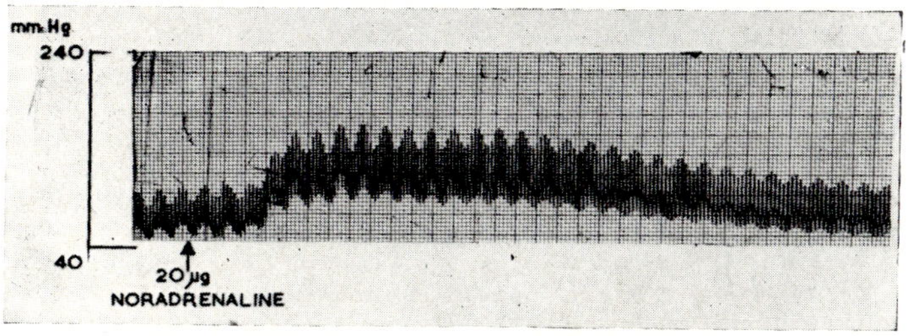


(b)

FIG. 2.—Effect on the femoral artery pressure of an anaesthetized dog of injecting (a) extract of tumour from Case 1—no effect (marker at top of recording equals 4 seconds); (b) 20 µg. noradrenaline.

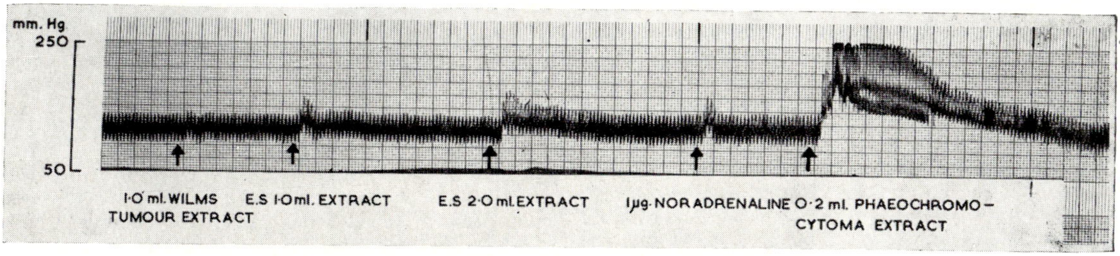


FIG. 3.—Effect of injecting extract of a Wilm's tumour, extract from tumour of Case 2 (E.S.), noradrenaline, and extract of a phaeochromocytoma on the femoral artery pressure of an anaesthetized dog. Marker at top of recording equals 20 seconds.

concentration in the tumour of 4 to 5 µg./g. weight of tumour. The phaeochromocytoma extract was still potent after storage of the tissue in the deep freeze for 7 months while an extract from a Wilm's tumour metastasis in liver caused no effect (Fig. 3).

**Histochemistry of Tumour Tissue.** Tissue fixed in Helly's fluid from both tumours did not show any evidence of chromaffin granules. Fluorescent microscopic techniques for noradrenaline were also negative in both cases. There was no evidence of selective non-specific esterase activity or of cholinesterase activity in either tumour. Monoamine oxidase activity was clearly demonstrated in freshly taken blocks from tumour in Case 2 in the cytoplasm of the small neoplastic cells throughout the sections: staining was completely inhibited in sections pre-incubated in iproniazid (Marsilid). Unfortunately this enzyme was not studied in tumour tissue from Case 1 at the time of removal from the body; no activity was detectable in blocks stored for 10 months at −70° C. During this period we have also investigated monoamine oxidase activity by this method in two Wilm's tumours with negative results.

## Discussion

The coincidence of diarrhoea, hypertension, and convulsions is quite uncommon in cases of adrenal neuroblastoma. In a recent review of the subject, Rosenstein and Engleman (1963) recorded but one instance in a series of 68 patients seen at Johns Hopkins Hospital between 1925 and 1962. Voorhess and Gardner (1961) had previously recorded one case and in the same year Smellie and Sandler described these manifestations in a child with a secreting intrathoracic ganglioneuroma. In the latter case, after the tumour had been removed, the diarrhoea subsided. This was also the result in a case reported by Stickler, Hallenbeck, and Flock

(1960), but in their patient it is of particular interest to note that, despite the relief of symptoms, the urinary excretion of excessive quantities of catecholamines persisted.

In all these patients the evidence indicated that there was an increased production of adrenal medullary metabolites. This was not so in our first case. The urinary excretion of catecholamines was thought to be at the upper limit of normal and that of HMMA within the normal range (M. Sandler and C. R. J. Ruthven, 1964, personal communication). The symptoms referable to the autonomic nervous system were not relieved by the administration of α-methyldopa; an extract of the tumour examined *post mortem* contained no catecholamines and had no effect on the blood pressure of an anaesthetized dog. Although the phentolamine test was positive, there is some doubt about the validity of this type of investigation (Pickering, 1955).

The accumulated evidence thus points to the conclusion that the hypertension and diarrhoea were not due to one of the series of compounds formed during the production or degradation of adrenaline and noradrenaline. Some of the points about these investigations, however, require more critical discussion.

Only a proportion of patients with neuroblastoma excrete excessive catecholamines. Bell (1963) and Voorhess and Gardner (1962) report several with normal or low excretions. In particular one case recorded by the latter investigators also had hypertension but, at necropsy, the growth had extensively invaded the kidneys, and it may have been that the urinary excretion of catecholamines was limited or the hypertension was nephrogenic. In Case 1 the urinary excretion of HMMA and catecholamines was not measured in relation to creatinine excretion, but there was never any evidence to indicate that renal function was sufficiently impaired to affect the excretion of monoamines significantly. The blood urea remained normal throughout except terminally, intravenous pyelography showed good elimination of the contrast material, and there was no post-mortem evidence of renal involvement.

As α-methyldopa is a competitive inhibitor of decarboxylase in tissues producing monoamines, it should theoretically have limited the production of dopamine from dopa and thus have blocked adrenaline, noradrenaline, and 5-hydroxytryptamine formation in the tumour. The lack of response could have been due to any of the following factors.

(1) The symptoms were not caused by these agents.

(2) The dose of α-methyldopa was insufficient.

(3) The tumour tissue was not penetrated by adequate concentrations of the drug.

It is impossible to be certain which of these was operative but, as regards the third, the tumour was very vascular and the blood supply to those parts that were metabolically active must have been good.

It may be, of course, that the agent produced by the tumour in Case 1 was not a catecholamine derivative. It could, for example, have been one of the kinins. An agent of this type may have been released by enzyme activators, such as proteases, produced by the tumour. A mechanism of this type might account for the unexplained diarrhoea reported by other workers, and further investigations on these lines may yet prove rewarding. It should be noted here that Birkenhäger (1963) has already reported a neuroblastoma in an adult male who had excessive excretion of 5-hydroxytryptophan derivatives in the urine.

There appears to be no doubt that the hypertension in Case 2 was related to the secretion of adrenergic agents from a tumour which was large and contained a significant amount of catecholamines, though less than some (Bell, 1963). It is also true that when the patient was first recognized to have a large growth with excessive catecholamine excretion his blood pressure was normal and the hypertension was sudden in onset. The rise in blood pressure occurred over two days, during which time he developed signs suggesting a cerebral metastasis. It appears that this was due either to a sudden secretion of catecholamine-like substances from the tumour tissue, or to the release of metabolically active metastasizing cells from the main tumour mass. This point should also be considered in relation to Case 1 where, though the primary tumour may not have been producing an active agent at the time of death, several of the metastases may have been doing so. Thus their pharmacological activity may have been overlooked in the post-mortem investigations.

The various factors discussed above in relation to the causes of hypertension and diarrhoea in these two children indicate the need for investigating the patient and the tumour by as many relevant methods as possible. Although the diagnosis of neuroblastoma may usually be made by routine clinical and pathological methods, a great deal more information about functional effects can be obtained by using the biochemical, pharmacological, and histochemical techniques reported in this paper. Enzyme histochemical studies of these tumours might well be developed further. Non-specific esterase and acetylcholinesterase should give an indication of ganglioneuromatous differentiation as recently suggested in work on carotid body tumours (Pryse-Davies, Dawson, and Westbury, 1964). Monoamine oxidase activity may also be of use in characterizing neuroblastoma cells, and it is interesting to speculate on the relation between catecholamine production and monoamine oxidase concentrations in such tumours.

## Summary

It has been assumed that the autonomic effects induced by neuroblastomata are always due to the production of catecholamine compounds. Two cases are reported with details of biochemical, pharmacological, and histochemical investigations. In one there was hypertension, and evidence suggested that this was due to the release of adrenaline and noradrenaline. In the other patient, who suffered both hypertension and diarrhoea, there was no evidence to indicate that the tumour was associated with excessive catecholamine activity, and it is postulated that another agent, not a catecholamine derivative, may have been produced by the tumour.

We wish to thank Dr. J. G. Humble, Dr. K. A. Newton, Mr. J. C. Ruthven, Dr. Merton Sandler, and Dr. J. H. Wilkinson for their co-operation, Dr. Ian Dawson for his constructive criticism, Dr. Percy Cliffe and the Department of Clinical Measurement, Westminster Hospital for invaluable help in the pharmacological work, and Dr. Peter Hansell and the Department of Medical Photography, Westminster Hospital for the preparation of the photographs. One of us (J.P-D) was in receipt of a grant from the British Empire Cancer Campaign.

### References

Bell, M. (1963). The clinical chemistry of neuroblastomas. In *West-European Symposia on Clinical Chemistry*, Vol. 2, ed. H. Varley and A. H. Gowenlock, p. 82. Elsevier, Amsterdam, London, and New York.

Birkenhäger, J. C. (1963). Metastasizing neuroblastoma with excretion of 5-hydroxyindoleacetic acid, serotonin and 5-hydroxytryptophan. *Acta med. scand.*, **174**, 621.

Eränkö, O. (1955). Distribution of adrenaline and noradrenaline in the adrenal medulla. *Nature* (*Lond.*), **175**, 88.

Euler, U. S. von (1956). *Noradrenaline: Chemistry, Physiology, Pharmacology and Clinical Aspects*, 1st ed., p. 62. Thomas, Springfield, Illinois.

Glenner, G. C., Burtner, H. J., and Brown, G. W., Jr. (1957). The histochemical demonstration of monoamine oxidase activity by tetrazolium salts. *J. Histochem. Cytochem.*, **5**, 591.

Isaacs, H., Medalie, M., and Politzer, W. M. (1959). Noradrenaline-secreting neuroblastomata. *Brit. med. J.*, **1**, 401.

Käser, H., and von Studnitz, W. (1961). Urine of children with sympathetic tumours. The excretion of 3-methoxy-4-hydroxy-mandelic acid. *Amer. J. Dis. Child.*, **102**, 199.

Marsden, H. B. (1963). Clinical and pathological features of neuroblastoma. In *West European Symposia on Clinical Chemistry*, Vol. 2, ed. H. Varley and A. H. Gowenlock, p. 71. Elsevier, Amsterdam, London, and New York.

Mason, G. A., Hart-Mercer, J., Millar, E. J., Strang, L. B., and Wynne, N. A. (1957). Adrenaline-secreting neuroblastoma in an infant. *Lancet*, **2**, 322.

Pearse, A. G. E. (1960). *Histochemistry: Theoretical and Applied*, 2nd ed. Churchill, London.

Pickering, G. W. (1955). *High Blood Pressure*, p. 404. Churchill, London.

Pisano, J. J., Crout, J. R., and Abraham, D. (1962). Determination of 3-methoxy-4-hydroxymandelic acid in urine. *Clin. chim. Acta*, **7**, 285.

Pryse-Davies, J., Dawson, I. M. P., and Westbury, G. (1964). Some morphologic, histochemical, and chemical observations on chemodectomas and the normal carotid body, including a study of the chromaffin reaction and possible ganglion cell elements. *Cancer* (*Philad.*), **17**, 185.

Robinson, R., Ratcliffe, J., and Smith, P. (1959). A screening test for phaeochromocytoma. *J. clin. Path.*, **12**, 541.

Rosenstein, B. J., and Engleman, K. (1963). Diarrhea in a child with a catecholamine-secreting ganglioneuroma: case report and review of the literature. *J. Pediat.*, **63**, 217.

Smellie, J. M., and Sandler, M. (1961). Secreting intrathoracic ganglioneuroma. *Proc. roy. Soc. Med.*, **54**, 327.

Soffer, A. (1954). Regitine and benodaine in the diagnosis of phoechromocytoma. *Med. Clin. N. Amer.*, **38**, 375.

Sourkes, T. L., Denton, R. L., Murphy, G. F., Chavez, B., and Saint Cyr, S. (1963). The excretion of dihydroxyphenylalanine, dopamine and dihydroxyphenylacetic acid in neuroblastoma. *Pediatrics*, **31**, 660.

Stickler, G. B , Hallenbeck, G. A., and Flock, E. V. (1960). Ganglioneuroblastoma associated with increased excretion of catecholamines. *Amer. J. Dis. Child.*, **100**, 634.

Voorhess, M. L., and Gardner, L. I. (1960). Catecholamine metabolism in neuroblastomas. *Lancet*, **2**, 651.

——, and —— (1961). Urinary excretion of norepinephrine, epinephrine and 3-methoxy-4-hydroxymandelic acid by children with neuroblastoma. *J. clin. Endocr.*, **21**, 321.

——, and —— (1962). Studies of catecholamine excretion by children with neural tumors. *ibid.*, **22**, 126.

Weil-Malherbe, H., and Bone, A. D. (1957). The estimation of catecholamines in urine by a chemical method. *J. clin. Path.*, **10**, 138.

Wilkins, L. (1957). *The Diagnosis and Treatment of Endocrine Disorders in Childhood and Adolescence*, 2nd ed., p. 254. Thomas, Springfield, Illinois.

*Arch. Dis. Childh.*, 1965, **40**, 418.

# THE EXCRETION OF 4-HYDROXY-3-METHOXY-MANDELIC ACID BY CHILDREN

BY

T. McKENDRICK* and R. W. H. EDWARDS

*From The Hospital for Sick Children, Great Ormond Street, London*

(RECEIVED FOR PUBLICATION NOVEMBER 9, 1964)

Much interest has been shown recently in the urinary excretion of 4-hydroxy-3-methoxy-mandelic acid (HMMA, but also known as VMA). It is accepted that its estimation may assist in the diagnosis of neuroblastoma and phaeochromocytoma, the high excretion usually found with these tumours being well above that possibly due to dietary constitutents, the stress of hospital admission, or recent operation. While most workers in describing methods or investigating clinical groups have included small numbers of normal subjects in order to define normal values of excretion, there have been no systematic studies of the excretion pattern in childhood. This paper records a study of 24-hour HMMA excretion in 132 normal children and in several small groups of children suffering from conditions that have been suspected of raising excretion rates of HMMA. In the series of children with proven neuroblastoma, as in those of most other workers, there are a few with normal HMMA excretion. Some of the non-pathological factors that might influence HMMA excretion have also been studied.

### Subjects and Methods

The following children provided 24-hour specimens of urine:

*Group 1:* 66 healthy children aged between 1 year 4 months and 15 years 6 months. They were normally active at home. The only restriction imposed was the avoidance of ice-cream and banana for the days before and during collection.

*Group 2:* 66 children in hospital, 54 of them were between 1 year 1 month and 15 years 10 months, the other 12 being less than 1 year. Though they were in hospital these subjects were active but probably less so than at home. Patients with acute or urinary infections, recent or imminent operation, or with any renal, endocrine, or metabolic disorder were excluded. The same dietary restrictions as in group 1 were applied.

*Group 3:* 20 children from group 1 provided a second specimen one year after the first.

*Group 4:* 21 patients aged from 4 months to 13 years 5 months who, though suspected of an adrenal tumour or neuroblastoma, were subsequently shown to have neither.

*Group 5:* 7 patients, all in hospital with hypertension from various causes. They were aged from 3 months to 12 years 4 months.

*Group 6:* 10 patients with tumours other than neuroblastoma, aged from 6 months to 11 years 5 months.

*Group 7:* 6 patients from whom neuroblastomata had previously been removed or had regressed. They were aged from 11 months to 13 years.

*Group 8:* 13 patients in whom a neuroblastoma was histologically proven. Their ages ranged from 5 months to 8 years.

From 8 subjects separate samples were collected for successive timed periods of 3 to 5 hours during 24 hours. All subjects passed between 5 and 7 specimens. Of the 8, 4 were in hospital but not in bed, and the other 4 were healthy normal subjects.

Successive 24-hour specimens for 1 day before and 3 days after a major operation were collected from 3 subjects. Similar collections were made from 5 subjects who consumed extra diet previously considered to interfere with HMMA estimation.

Urine was collected in polythene bottles containing 1 ml. 5 *N*-HCl per year of age of the child or proportionately less for the non-24 hour collections. Bottles were stored if necessary before analysis at 4° C. Analyses were performed in batches by the method of Pisano, Crout, and Abraham (1962). Each urine sample was analysed in duplicate with a blank and at least one recovery control of 25 $\mu$g. HMMA* in each batch (of 2 to 5 samples).

* Present address: Department of Child Health, Liverpool University, Alder Hey Children's Hospital, Liverpool 12.

* Supplied by Koch-Light Laboratories, Colnbrook, Bucks.

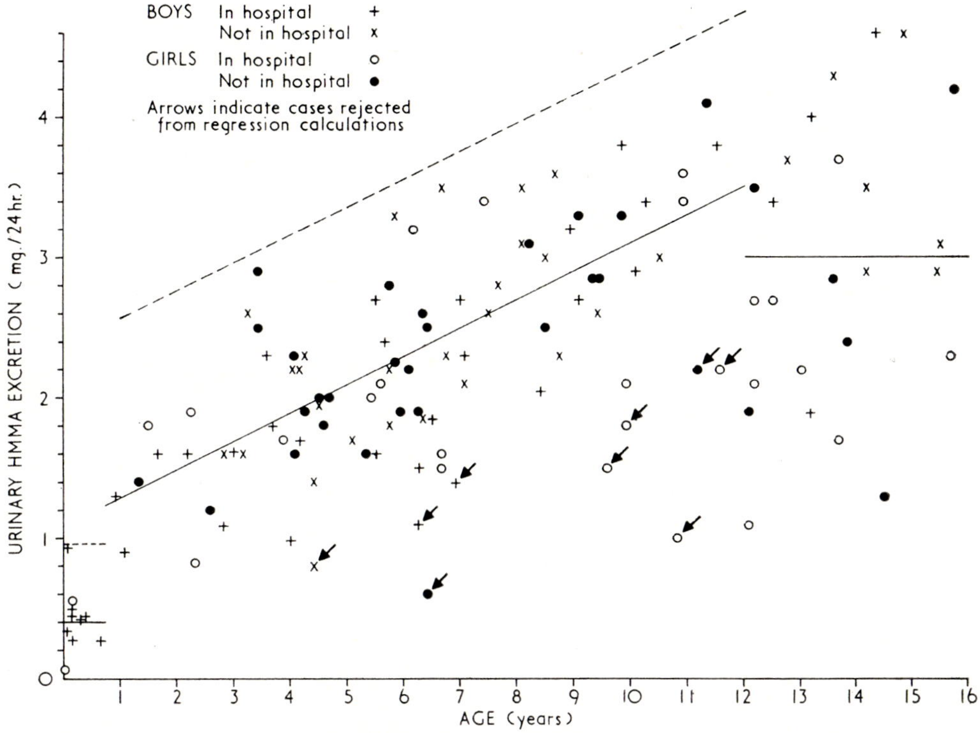


FIG. 1.—Scatter diagram relating 24-hour excretion of HMMA to age. The mean regression line between 1 and 11·9 years is drawn in ———, and 1% upper limit of confidence - - - - .
Children aged less than 1 year and those aged between 12 and 15·9 years were considered as separate groups. The average and 1% upper limit are shown in a similar manner to the regression line and its limit.

## Results

The mean recovery by periodate oxidation of aqueous HMMA 25 μg./ml. was 96·8 ± 3·8% (S.D.). From urine the mean recovery over the whole process was 84·8 ± 6·8% (S.D.) over 100 consecutive analyses.

The excretion of HMMA by healthy children and those in hospital (groups 1 and 2) is shown graphically in Fig. 1, where male and female, healthy and hospitalized children are separately designated. The regression of excretion on age was calculated for those aged 1 to 11·9 years (96 subjects in all); there were too few subjects below the age of 1 year, and those over the age of 12 showed much greater variation. The lowest points were not included in the calculation of the regression for it seemed likely that they represented incomplete collection or other abnormality; from 5 of 9 subjects thus 'eliminated' unusually small 24-hour urine specimens were received. With this elimination the numbers of points excluded by upper and lower 5% levels became equal.

The statistical test used to determine the significance of differences between subgroups of the children was based on a calculation of the regression data and then of the HMMA excretion at a standardized age. The age chosen was that of the average age of all the children and was termed the grand mean age. The average age of the children in each subgroup was very similar to the grand mean age so that no weighting due to age difference occurred. The calculated data is presented in Table 1.

The differences between the subgroups was tested using 't' values, but significance was not reached. This included a comparison of males and females, children in hospital and not in hospital, and those repeated after one year compared with their original values.

From the data of all the children the lines of regression and probability were calculated. Thus Fig. 1 shows the 1% line which is taken as the upper limit of normality. It is clear from Fig. 1 that the children aged less than 1 year were not proximate to the regression line. Their mean 24-hour HMMA excretion was 0·47 ± 0·33 mg. (SD) at 3 months of age.

TABLE 1

STATISTICAL DATA CALCULATED FROM HMMA EXCRETION OF NORMAL CHILDREN AGED 1 TO 11·9 YEARS

| Group | n | $\bar{x}$ | $\bar{y}$ | $\Sigma x$ | $\Sigma x^2$ | $\Sigma xy$ | $\Sigma y$ | Regression | | Calculated HMMA Excretion (mg./24 hr.) at grand mean age Y | Standard Deviation S |
|---|---|---|---|---|---|---|---|---|---|---|---|
| | | | | | | | | Slope (b) | Intercept | | |
| A: males | 25 | 6·28 | 2·44 | 156·99 | 1084·0126 | 403·196 | 61·10 | 0·199 | 1·20 | 2·41 | 0·48 |
| B: males in hospital | 23 | 5·99 | 2·24 | 137·74 | 1026·8590 | 350·447 | 51·50 | 0·208 | 0·99 | 2·27 | 0·56 |
| C: females | 25 | 6·02 | 2·37 | 130·41 | 1050·2780 | 392·982 | 59·35 | 0·247 | 0·89 | 2·41 | 0·24 |
| D: females in hospital | 14 | 6·52 | 2·24 | 91·22 | 741·2798 | 226·443 | 31·32 | 0·155 | 1·25 | 2·20 | 0·72 |
| Total in Groups A-D | 87 | 6·17(Y) | 2·34 | 536·36 | 3902·3794 | 1373·068 | 203·27 | 0·201 | 1·09 | 2·34 | 0·53 |
| E: Group 3 | 18 | 6·66 | 2·43 | 119·91 | 870·379 | 309·799 | 43·80 | 0·252 | 0·75 | 2·30 | 0·62 |

*Note*: n is the number of subjects in each group. Age is designated x and HMMA excretion y, $\bar{x}$ and $\bar{y}$ being the mean values. Y is grand mean. Results of 'outliers' indicated on Fig. 1 are not included in these calculations.
The significance of differences between the various pairs of HMMA values at the grand mean age (e.g. (A) and (C), and (B) and (D), (A) and (B) etc.) were tested using t = difference $(S_1^2/n_1 + S_2^2/n_2)^{-\frac{1}{2}}$ where $n_1$ and $n_2$ are the numbers of subjects in the groups compared and $S_1$ and $S_2$ are the standard deviations calculated for each group using $(n - 2)\ S = \Sigma\ (y - \bar{y})^2 - b^2\ \Sigma\ (x - \bar{x})^2$; b is the regression slope.

The relatively wide scatter shown in the children aged 12-15·9 years has made firm conclusions difficult. Study of the volumes of the girls' specimens received suggested that not all were complete 24-hour saves. The over-all average excretion was 3·05 ± 1·05 (SD; 25 subjects): that of the 11 boys was 3·54 ± 1·64 (SD) and of the girls 2·48 ± 1·43 (SD).

Brief clinical features and HMMA excretions of patients in groups 4 to 8 are shown in Tables 2 to 6. With the exception of children with neuroblastoma, none of these groups included any child with HMMA excretion above the 1% confidence limit of groups 1 and 2.

Of the 13 patients with neuroblastoma (all, as well as those of group 7 being proven histologically), 10

TABLE 2

PRINCIPAL FEATURES AND HMMA EXCRETION IN CHILDREN SUSPECTED OF HAVING NEUROBLASTOMA OR PHAEOCHROMOCYTOMA (GROUP 4)

| Patient | Sex | Age (yr.) | Clinical Features | Suspected Diagnosis | Duration of History (mth.) | HMMA Excretion (mg./24 hr.) | Conclusion |
|---|---|---|---|---|---|---|---|
| P.S. | M | 3/12 | Oedema, ascites, hypertension | Neuroblastoma | 2 | 0·22 | Protein-losing enteropathy |
| D.W. | F | 7/12 | Mass in left loin | Neuroblastoma | 3 | 0·7 | Urinary infection |
| S.W. | M | 10/12 | Failure to thrive; large liver and spleen | Neuroblastoma | 5 | 1·4 | Niemann Pick's disease |
| S.H. | F | 1 | Anaemia, high ESR and PUO | Neuroblastoma | 1 | 1·5 | Recovery but no diagnosis |
| C.M. | F | 1 1/12 | Failure to thrive, anaemia, abdominal swelling, sweating | Neuroblastoma | 7 | 0·32 | ? Protein-losing enteropathy |
| G.D. | M | 1 8/12 | Unusual seizures | Phaeochromocytoma | 12 | 1·1 | Epilepsy |
| N.H. | M | 2 1/12 | Large liver | Neuroblastoma | 1 | 0·75 | Cirrhosis |
| D.B. | F | 2 5/12 | Anaemia; glands in neck | Neuroblastoma | 2 | 1·1 | Infective adenitis |
| T.K. | M | 2 9/12 | Attacks of syncope ? hypoglycaemia | Phaeochromocytoma | 9 | 1·7 | Syncope |
| P.I. | M | 3 2/12 | PUO and large liver | Neuroblastoma | 2 | 0·6 | Leishmaniasis |
| D.H. | F | 5 1/12 | Failure to thrive; large liver | Neuroblastoma | 24 | 2·1 | Malnutrition |
| D.S. | M | 5 3/12 | Pain in back with oedema and limitation of movement | Neuroblastoma | ½ | 2·3 | Recovery; probably mild rheumatoid arthritis |
| C.P. | M | 5 3/12 | Attacks of fever, sweating, vomiting, and drowsiness | Phaeochromocytoma | 24 | 1·0 | Periodic syndrome |
| V.C. | F | 5 6/12 | Anaemia; decalcified vertebrae | Neuroblastoma | 9 | 2·1 | Leukaemia |
| P.F. | M | 7 6/12 | Right hemiparesis and hypertension | Phaeochromocytoma | ¾ | 2·8 | Post-op. thrombosis |
| B.R. | M | 8 8/12 | Fever; mass in abdomen | Neuroblastoma | ¼ | 1·5 | Nephritis |
| S.G. | F | 9 | Exophthalmos; hepatomegaly | Neuroblastoma | 1 | 2·3 | Not known |
| M.H. | F | 9 9/12 | Flexion spasm of the hip with tenderness in pelvis; abdominal pain | Neuroblastoma | 60 | 2·6 | Urinary infection |
| J.N. | M | 10 9/12 | Diarrhoea, abdominal pain, headaches, flushing | Phaeochromocytoma | 12 | 3·4 | Emotional problem |
| A.W. | M | 10 9/12 | Mentally subnormal, reputed to improve on cheese | Anomaly of amino acid metabolism | 129 | 2·9 | Not yet diagnosed |
| G.L. | M | 11 6/12 | Recurrent abdominal pain; hypertension on one occasion | Phaeochromocytoma | 3 | 3·2 | No organic lesion found |
| M.S. | M | 13 | Pain and tumour in right thigh | Neuroblastoma | 11 | 2·1 | Multiple malignant tumours; histology indefinite; no necropsy |
| A.L. | M | 13 6/12 | Loss of weight; mass in left loin | Neuroblastoma | 5 | 3·8 | Hydronephrosis |

TABLE 3

PRINCIPAL FEATURES AND HMMA EXCRETION IN CHILDREN WITH HYPERTENSION (GROUP 5)

| Name | Sex | Age (yr.) | Approximate Blood Pressure (mm.Hg) | Duration (mth.) | Cause | HMMA Excretion (mg./24 hr.) |
|---|---|---|---|---|---|---|
| G.H. | F | 3/12 | 125/90 to 180/120 | 3 | Coarctation of aorta | 0·30 |
| O.H. | M | 4/12 | 90/60 to 120/90 | ? 3 | ? Hypoplastic rt. kidney ? glomerulonephritis | 0·43 |
| A.H. | M | 7/12 | 120/80 to 170/130 | 1½ | ? Polyarteritis | 0·82 |
| G.W. | F | 5 6/12 | 190/50 | 12 | Chronic nephritis | 1·8 |
| D.M. | M | 9 | 150/80 to 200/140 | > 3 | Chronic pyelonephritis | 2·75 |
| P.C. | M | 11 | 160/120 | > 1½ | Chronic pyelonephritis | 3·2 |
| S.V. | F | 12 6/12 | 260/200 | 120 | Renal disease secondary to hypercalcaemia | 1·2 |

TABLE 4

HMMA EXCRETION IN CHILDREN WITH TUMOURS NOT ORIGINATING FROM SYMPATHETIC NERVOUS TISSUE (GROUP 6)

| Name | Sex | Age (yr.) | Tumour | HMMA Excretion (mg./24 hr.) |
|---|---|---|---|---|
| J.G. | M | 6/12 | Reticulum cell sarcoma | 0·51 |
| P.S. | M | 6/12 | Hepatoblastoma | 0·85 |
| A.N. | M | 10/12 | Reticulum cell sarcoma | 0·50 |
| J.W. | F | 4 6/12 | Lymphosarcoma | 2·2 |
| L.W. | F | 4 6/12 | Malignant hepatoblastoma | 2·9 |
| A.B. | M | 5 | Nephroblastoma | 1·6 |
| P.B. | M | 6 | Fibrosarcoma | 2·6 |
| M.M. | F | 9 | ? Angio-sarcoma | 3·0 |
| B.L. | M | 10 4/12 | Ganglioneuroma of coccyx | 1·5 |
| S.G. | M | 11 6/12 | | 4·0 |

TABLE 5

PRINCIPAL FEATURES AND HMMA EXCRETION IN CHILDREN FROM WHOM A NEUROBLASTOMA HAD BEEN REMOVED OR IN WHOM REGRESSION WAS CLINICALLY COMPLETE (GROUP 7)

| Name | Sex | Age at Examination (yr.) | Age at Diagnosis (yr.) | Site | Duration of History (mth.) | Present State | HMMA Excretion (mg./24 hr.) |
|---|---|---|---|---|---|---|---|
| T.G. | F | 1 7/12 | 8/12 | Mediastinum | 3 | Healthy | 0·20 |
| J.F. | F | 4 9/12 | 7/12 | Mediastinum | About 1 | Paraplegia | 1·8 |
| S.E. | F | 6 9/12 | 9/12 | Left loin | ½ | Healthy | 1·3 |
| C.L.* | F | 10 | 1 3/12 | Posterior mediastinum | 3 | Paraplegia | 0·32 |
| S.P.* | F | 11 6/12 | 9/12 | Upper mediastinum and neck | About 1 | Healthy | 3·7 |
| A.C. | F | 13 | 8 6/12 | Left leg and skull | 6 | Healthy | 2·3 |

* These patients were treated medically only because the tumours could not be removed.

TABLE 6

PRINCIPAL FEATURES AND HMMA EXCRETION IN 13 CHILDREN WITH NEUROBLASTOMA (GROUP 8)

| Patient | Sex | Age (yr.) | Clinical Features | Duration of History (mth.) | Abnormal I.V.P. | HMMA Excretion (mg./24 hr.) | Survival (mth.) |
|---|---|---|---|---|---|---|---|
| R.K. | F | 4/12 | Hepatomegaly | 3 | N.P. | 25 | > 6 |
| P.G. | M | 1 | Anaemia; multiple tumours | ¼ | N.P. | 63 | >15 |
| J.S. | M | 1 1/12 | Cranial mass | 1 | N.P. | 6·5 | ½ |
| G.W. | M | 1 2/12 | Sacral mass | 6 | N.P. | 1·3 | 9 |
| M.G. | M | 1 4/12 | Retroperitoneal mass | ½ | + | 5·3 | ¾ |
| J.W. | F | 1 4/12 | Anaemia; retroperitoneal mass | 12 | + | 16·0 | 14 |
| A.D. | M | 2 | Anaemia; limpness; retroperitoneal mass | ¾ | + | 1·1 | 1½ |
| L.S. | M | 2 6/12 | Anaemia; proptosis; retroperitoneal mass | 1/10 | + | 3·1 | 3 |
| P.M. | M | 3 9/12 | Anaemia and PUO; abdominal pain; bone secondaries | 3 | – | 27·5 | 14 |
| J.P. | F | 3 9/12 | Retroperitoneal mass | 2 | N.P. | 2·0 | 4 |
| P.E. | M | 6 | Paraplegia; pleural effusion; hepatomegaly | 24 | N.P. | 3·5 | 27 |
| B.G. | M | 7 | Anaemia and PUO | 1 | – | 102 | 7 |
| D.G. | M | 8 | Spinal compression; abdominal mass | 9 | – | 192 | 17 |

I.V.P. = intravenous pyelogram, + = abnormality demonstrated, — = normal, N.P. = 'not performed'.

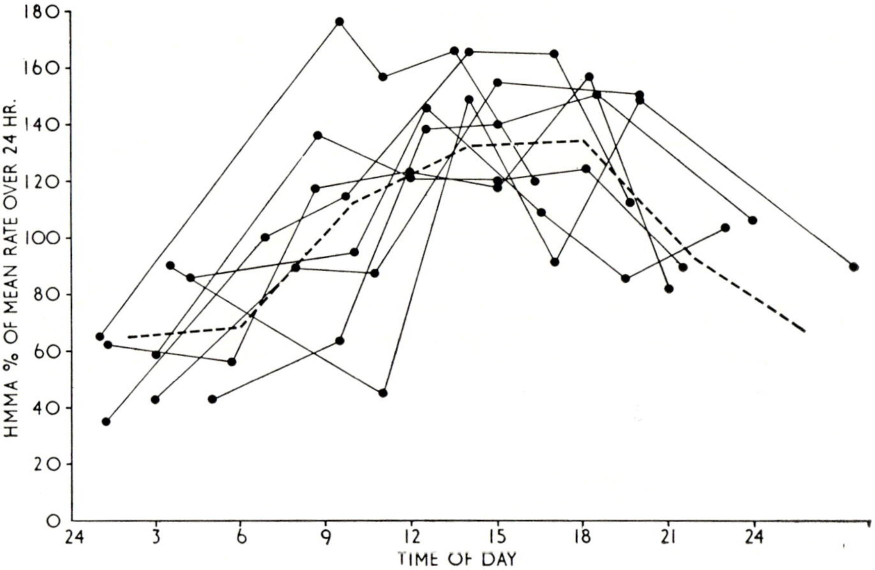


FIG. 2.—Rate of excretion of HMMA throughout 24 hours in 8 subjects, 7 aged between 1 year 4 months and 13 years, and 1 aged 37 years. Rates are plotted as percentage of mean rate over the 24 hours; all subjects produced between 5 and 7 specimens during this period. The curve joining average points was constructed by taking the average of rates of excretion interpolated at four-hourly intervals.

showed the expected high excretion; 3 (G.W., J.P., A.D.) showed a normal excretion, 1 of them showing this on three occasions (J.P.: 2·9, 1·0, and 1·3) but surgical intervention prevented repetition in the others. Two more had levels just inside (P.E.) or not far above (L.S.) the 1% confidence limits. In several patients, repeated estimations have been made during therapy: P.G. (over 9 months) showed 63, 55, 75, 48 mg./24 hr.; B.G. (over 7 months) showed 102, 187, 137, 116, 102, 147, 93, 128 mg./24 hr.; and J.W. (over 8 months) showed 16, 18, 31, 16 mg./24 hr.

Fig. 2 shows the changes in relative rate of HMMA excretion in 8 subjects over single 24-hour periods starting at midnight. In order to make the 8 sets of data comparable with each other the results of each set are plotted as a percentage of the mean rate shown over the whole 24-hour period. There is a very marked difference between day and night excretion rates, the average change being from about 65% of the over-all daily rate at 2·00 a.m. to 135% between 2·00 and 6·00 p.m.

Three patients were studied before and after major operations. The levels of successive 24-hour excretions are shown in Table 7. Chromatographic and some semi-quantitative methods of HMMA estimation may suffer interference from certain dietary constituents (Robinson, Ratcliffe, and Smith, 1959; Gitlow, Mendlowitz, Khassis, Cohen, and Sha, 1960; Mahler and Humoller, 1962). Substances containing vanillin, e.g. custard, ice-cream, and vanilla essence, and those such as banana and walnut which contain serotonin, noradrenaline, and dopamine have usually been excluded from diets. Five subjects consumed various quantities of these substances (as well as their normal diets) during the second of 3 or 4 successive daily 24-hour urine collections. The excretions of HMMA by these subjects are shown in Table 8. No increase was demonstrated in any subject.

## Discussion

First isolated by Armstrong, McMillan, and Shaw (1957), HMMA was shown by a study of the fate of tritium-labelled adrenaline and noradrenaline to be a major metabolite of these adrenal medullary secretions (LaBrosse, Axelrod, and Kety, 1958; Kopin, 1960). Most workers have studied the excretion of HMMA in relation to the diagnosis of phaeochromocytoma (e.g. Gitlow *et al.*, 1960), when adrenal medullary activity is known to be excessive, or of neuroblastoma (e.g. von Studnitz, Käser, and Sjoerdsma, 1963; Voorhess and Gardner, 1961). Attempts to study adrenal medullary response to stress by estimating serial HMMA excretion have been reported (Berman and Pettitt, 1961), and observations on other factors such as diurnal variation (Sunderman, Cleveland, Law, and Sunderman, 1960) and diet (Sandler and Ruthven, 1961) have been made.

TABLE 7

DAILY HMMA EXCRETION OF 3 PATIENTS BEFORE AND AFTER MAJOR OPERATION

| Patient | Sex | Age (yr.) | HMMA Excretion (mg./24 hr.) | | | |
|---|---|---|---|---|---|---|
| | | | Pre-operative | Post-operative | | |
| | | | | 1st day | 2nd day | 3rd day |
| C.A. | F | 4 | 1·6 | 1·1 | 1·1 | 1·0 |
| D.S. | M | 6 | 1·9 | 2·3 | 2·1 | |
| D.H. | F | 8 | 2·7 | 2·3 | 2·7 | 2·1 |

TABLE 8

DAILY HMMA EXCRETION BY SOME SUBJECTS BEFORE AND AFTER CONSUMPTION OF CERTAIN FOODS

| Subject | Sex | Age (yr.) | Dietary Extras | HMMA Excretion (mg./24 hr.) | | | |
|---|---|---|---|---|---|---|---|
| | | | | Pre-diet | Post-diet | | |
| | | | | | 1st day | 2nd day | 3rd day |
| I.M. | M | 6 | 5 bananas; 2 oz. ice-cream | 2·7 | 2·7 | 2·6 | 2·7 |
| R.S. | M | 8 | 5 bananas | 2·7 | 2·6 | 2·8 | |
| G.S. | M | 10 | 5 bananas | 2·7 | 2·7 | 1·8* | |
| V.E. | F | 19 | 6 bananas; 2 oz. walnuts | 4·3 | 3·8 | 3·9 | 3·4 |
| T.M. | M | 37 | 2 oz. walnuts; 4 oz. ice-cream | 5·8 | 6·0 | 5·4 | 5·3 |

* 12-hour daytime specimen only.

About a dozen methods of estimation have been described. The original method (Armstrong *et al.*, 1957) was by initial extraction with ethyl acetate, followed by two-dimensional chromatography, diazotization, and spectrophotometry; besides taking about 24 hours, this method requires dietary restriction to minimize interference from exogenous phenolic acids. The high voltage electrophoresis methods (von Studnitz and Hanson, 1959; Randrup, 1962) require expensive apparatus and may not always achieve clear separation of different phenolic acids. Low voltage electrophoresis (Klein and Chernaik, 1961) is a prolonged procedure. The diazotization methods of Woiwod and Knight (1961) and Gitlow *et al.* (1960) tend to give high results, probably because they are less specific. Similarly the colorimetric method using 4-chloro-*o*-phenylene-diamine and phosphoric acid (Fellman, 1963), though conveniently rapid, suffers interference from di-hydroxy-mandelic acid and p-hydroxy-mandelic acid, both of which are found in urine.

Several methods utilize the conversion of HMMA to vanillin as the basis of estimation. In the first of these (Sandler and Ruthven, 1959), initial extraction is by adsorption on to an anion exchange resin. This is followed by elution with ethyl acetate, evaporation to dryness, autoclaving with acid, and finally colorimetric estimation. The procedure is tedious and permits a recovery of 70% at best. Sunderman *et al.* (1960) used florisil adsorption for purification. Following extraction by ethyl acetate and back-extraction into potassium carbonate, HMMA is oxidized by ferricyanide to vanillin; the reaction, however, is less specific, allowing interference from dietary substances, and the terminal colorimetric estimation is sensitive to time, moisture, and temperature. The method described by Pisano *et al.* (1962) is rapid (less than 3 hours) and involves extraction with ethyl acetate, back-extraction into potassium carbonate, oxidation by sodium periodate, extraction of the resultant vanillin by toluene, and finally spectrophotometric estimation in potassium carbonate. This is the procedure we have employed.

In the present investigation a significant sex difference in HMMA excretion by normal children between the ages of 1 and 11·9 years was not observed. In this age-group there was a good linear relation between excretion and age.

In the first year of life, though the number of observations was small, the scatter was less and it was clear that the points were not co-linear with the older age-group. After the age of 12 years there was much greater variation, particularly in girls, and a sex difference previously reported in adults (Weise, McDonald, and LaBrosse, 1961; Georges and Whitby, 1964) was evident. The over-all average after the age of 12 was 3·05 ± 1·04 (SD) and is very similar to the adult level quoted by Ruthven (1963) of 3·7 ± 1·1 (SD) but is below that stated by Georges and Whitby (1964) of 5·45 ± 1·05 (SD).

The marked diurnal variation (from a minimum of 40% of the mean 24-hour rate to a maximum of 168% in one child) was much more pronounced than that reported by Weise *et al.* (1961). It is imperative to collect 24-hour samples, especially if excretion levels near the 1% 'borderline' are encountered. This variation also makes it difficult to study short-term physiological changes in adrenal medullary activities by serial estimations of HMMA excretion.

The constancy of results following ingested walnut, banana, and vanilla-flavoured ice-cream confirms that excreted HMMA is not of dietary origin and that dietary restriction is unnecessary when collecting urine for estimation by this method.

Residence in hospital *per se* produced no increase in HMMA excretion, but this observation must be qualified by the fact that no attempt was made to study excretion during the first day of admission; it is possible that the stress of admission might be associated with a temporary rise in HMMA excretion.

The failure to demonstrate a rise in excretion following operative stress is difficult to reconcile with the observations of Hunter, Marshall, and Oram (1963) that operation was followed by a large increase in adrenaline and noradrenaline excretion, and with the demonstration of LaBrosse, Axelrod, Kopin, and Kety (1961) that about 30-40% of injected adrenaline and noradrenaline could be recovered as HMMA within 48 hours. The latter workers showed that about 5% of injected adrenaline was excreted unchanged. The daily urinary excretion of adrenaline is quoted as 2-5 μg. and of noradrenaline as 25-50 μg. (von Euler, 1956). These figures suggest a daily production of about 0·5-1·0 mg. of these substances and if the metabolic pathways were the same this would produce about 0·2-0·4 mg. HMMA daily. Normal HMMA excretion (in adults) is about ten times this value. It may be that the very small increase that results from operative stress is hidden in the relatively larger amount of HMMA from other sources.

Of the 13 histologically proven neuroblastoma cases, 3 failed to show the significantly high HMMA excretion. Such normal excretion does not exclude the diagnosis. Rather does it indicate the need to estimate the homovanillic acid (HVA) excretion. This is unfortunately tedious, but may well be helpful, especially if histological diagnosis from biopsy material is uncertain (e.g. if necrosis is prominent). To the best of the authors' knowledge, patients with neuroblastoma do not have both normal HMMA and normal HVA excretion (M. Sandler, 1963, personal communication; Käser, Bettex, and von Studnitz, 1964).

All the children who remained free of clinical evidence of recurrence following successful surgical removal of neuroblastomata showed normal HMMA excretion. It remains to be seen whether a rise in urinary HMMA excretion precedes clinical effects if further tumours appear. Similarly, continuously high HMMA excretion during therapy provides an indication of the failure of therapy. With the known tendency of this tumour to go into remission, a fall in excretion in a single case might not necessarily indicate therapeutic success.

## Summary

The procedure of Pisano *et al.* (1962) for the determination of 4-hydroxy-3-methoxy-mandelic acid (HMMA, also known as VMA) has been employed to confirm the high excretion of this catecholamine metabolite in the urine of most children with neuroblastoma.

The urinary excretion of HMMA by 87 normal children was estimated. These children showed a linear regression of HMMA excretion against age within the limit 1 to 12 years of age. The upper 1% probability level of the regression was taken as the upper limit of normality in assessing the high excretions.

Residence of the children in hospital rather than at home, sex, the presence of tumours other than neuroblastomata, post-operative stress, and dietary factors have no effect on HMMA excretion.

A marked diurnal rhythm of HMMA excretion was demonstrated, making it imperative to perform the determinations only on complete 24-hour urine specimens.

We wish to thank the physicians and surgeons of The Hospital for Sick Children for allowing us to study their patients and Dr. M. D. Baber of the Edgware General Hospital for patient P.G.; Dr. B. E. Clayton for facilities in her department; Dr. C. O. Carter for help in designing the statistical analysis; Mr. R. Gardner and Miss A. Malone for some technical assistance; and the many normal subjects and their parents for producing the samples. One of us (R.W.H.E.) is in receipt of a grant from the Joint Research Board of The Hospital for Sick Children, and the Institute of Child Health.

### References

Armstrong, M. D., McMillan, A., and Shaw, K. N. F. (1957). 3-methoxy-4-hydroxy-mandelic acid, a urinary metabolite of norepinephrine. *Biochim. biophys. Acta (Amst.)*, **25**, 422.

Berman, M. L., and Pettitt, J. A. (1961). Urinary excretion of 3-methoxy-4-hydroxymandelic acid after several stress situations. *J. Lab. clin. Med.*, **57**, 126.

von Euler, U. S. (1956). *Noradrenaline*, p. 166. Thomas, Springfield, Illinois.

Fellman, J. H. (1963). Personal communication to C. R. J. Ruthven quoted in *The Clinical Chemistry of the Monoamines*, ed. H. Varley and A. H. Gowenlock, p. 40. Elsevier, Amsterdam.

Georges, R. J., and Whitby, L. G. (1964). Urinary excretion of metabolites of catecholamines in normal individuals and hypertensive patients. *J. clin. Path.*, **17**, 64.

Gitlow, S. E., Mendlowitz, M., Khassis, S., Cohen, G., and Sha, J. (1960). The diagnosis of pheochromocytoma by determination of urinary 3-methoxy, 4-hydroxymandelic acid. *J. clin. Invest.*, **39**, 221.

Hunter, R. B., Marshall, P. B., and Oram, F. J. (1963). Catechol amine excretion in normal persons and in cases of phaeochromocytoma. *Quart. J. Med.*, **32**, 225.
Käser, H., Bettex, M., and Studnitz, W. v. (1964). Further observations on the determination of catecholamine metabolites in tumours of sympathetic nervous system. *Arch. Dis. Childh.*, **39**, 168.
Klein, D., and Chernaik, J. M. (1961). Determination of urinary 3-methoxy-4-hydroxymandelic acid (vanillylmandelic acid) by paper electrophoresis. *Clin. Chem.*, **7**, 257.
Kopin, I. J. (1960). Technique for the study of alternative metabolic pathways: epinephrine metabolism in man. *Science*, **131**, 1372.
LaBrosse, E. H., Axelrod, J., and Kety, S. S. (1958). O-methylation, the principal route of metabolism of epinephrine in man. *ibid.*, **128**, 593.
——, ——, Kopin, I. J., and Kety, S. S. (1961). Metabolism of 7-$H^3$-epinephrine-d-bitartrate in normal young men. *J. clin. Invest.*, **40**, 253.
Mahler, D. J., and Humoller, F. L. (1962). A comparison of methods for determining catechol amines and 3-methoxy-4-hydroxymandelic acid in urine. *Clin. Chem.*, **8**, 47.
Pisano, J. J., Crout, J. R., and Abraham, D. (1962). Determination of 3-methoxy-4-hydroxymandelic acid in urine. *Clin. chim. Acta*, **7**, 285.
Randrup, A. (1962). Determination of urinary 3-methoxy-4-hydroxy-mandelic (vanilmandelic) acid by electrophoresis at low pH. *Scand. J. clin. Lab. Invest.*, **14**, 262.
Robinson, R., Ratcliffe, J., and Smith, P. (1959). A screening test for phaeochromocytoma. *J. clin. Path.*, **12**, 541.
Ruthven, C. R. J. (1963). The determination of metabolites of catecholamines by other techniques. In *The Clinical Chemistry of the Monoamines*, ed. H. Varley and A. H. Gowenlock, p. 39. Elsevier, Amsterdam.
Sandler, M., and Ruthven, C. R. J. (1959). Quantitative colorimetric method for estimation of 3-methoxy-4-hydroxymandelic acid in urine; value in diagnosis of phaeochromocytoma. *Lancet*, **2**, 114 and 1034.
——, and —— (1961). The estimation of 4-hydroxy-3-methoxymandelic acid in urine. *Biochem. J.*, **80**, 78.
von Studnitz, W., and Hanson, A. (1959). Determination of 3-methoxy-4-hydroxymandelic acid in urine by high voltage paper electrophoresis. *Scand. J. clin. Lab. Invest.*, **11**, 101.
——, Käser, H., and Sjoerdsma, A. (1963). Spectrum of catechol amine biochemistry in patients with neuroblastoma. *New Engl. J. Med.*, **269**, 232.
Sunderman, F. W., Jr., Cleveland, P. D., Law, N. C., and Sunderman, F. W. (1960). A method for the determination of 3-methoxy-4-hydroxymandelic acid ('vanilmandelic acid') for the diagnosis of pheochromocytoma. *Amer. J. clin. Path.*, **34**, 293.
Voorhess, M. L., and Gardner, L. I. (1961). Urinary excretion of norepinephrine, epinephrine and 3-methoxy-4-hydroxymandelic acid by children with neuroblastoma. *J. clin. Endocr.*, **21**, 321.
Weise, V. K., McDonald, R. K., and LaBrosse, E. H. (1961). Determination of urinary 3-methoxy-4-hydroxymandelic acid in man. *Clin. chim. Acta*, **6**, 79.
Woiwod, A. J., and Knight, R. (1961). The determination of 3-methoxy 4-hydroxy mandelic acid in urine. *J. clin. Path.*, **14**, 502.

*Arch. Dis. Childh.*, 1965, **40**, 426.

# IATROGENIC LESIONS IN BABIES FOLLOWING UMBILICAL VEIN CATHETERIZATION

BY

JEAN M. SCOTT

*From The Royal Maternity Hospital, Glasgow*

(RECEIVED FOR PUBLICATION OCTOBER 15, 1964)

During a study of babies with respiratory distress syndrome (RDS) and of the effects of intravenous bicarbonate and laevulose on glycogen reserves of the newborn (Scott, 1965), it was found that 2 babies developed complications arising out of treatment. One had an umbilical vein thrombosis with large pulmonary embolus. The other developed umbilical sepsis with a thrombophlebitis and pyaemia. It was, therefore, decided to carry out a more detailed examination of the vein and its branches in all future cases coming to necropsy in order to investigate the significance of these findings.

## Material and Methods

During the period under review 200 babies with RDS received bicarbonate and laevulose via the umbilical route (Hutchison, Kerr, Douglas, Inall, and Crosbie, 1964) and 92 of these came to necropsy: 35 belonged to the original series in which glycogen studies were made. Routine blocks were taken through the umbilicus after it had been carefully examined for evidence of sepsis. The umbilical vein and its branches within the liver were then opened longitudinally and the findings were noted. Serial transverse sections of the vessel, including adjacent liver substance, were taken in all cases where lesions existed, and in the latter part of the survey random blocks were selected, even in the absence of any gross pathology. Careful attention was also paid to pulmonary vessels and several blocks of lung were examined. In addition, routine blocks from other organs were also taken.

During the survey one Rhesus negative baby died following replacement transfusion, and this case was similarly examined, and older post mortem-material from 14 babies dying after replacement transfusion was reviewed.

## Results

In this department it has always been the custom to take a routine block of umbilicus at necropsy for microscopical examination. Thus any changes resulting from catheterization were immediately noticeable. These consisted of slight oedema of the wall of the vein and occasionally a diffuse mild polymorph infiltrate involving all coats. Frequently adventitial haemorrhages were also found. Babies who had had replacement transfusions showed similar features, but here the changes were not as marked as in those titrated with bicarbonate and laevulose. In the latter group an aseptic necrosis of the endothelium of the wall of the vein with subsequent fibrin deposition was also found. Remnants of nuclear material, staining black in H. and E. sections and positive for Feulgen, were occasionally seen in this fibrin or plastered against the wall of the vein. In the majority, this change remained localized to the umbilicus, but in 18 of the 92 babies examined, or approximately 20%, more extensive lesions were observed. Details of these are shown in the Table, where it can be seen that they fell into 4 main groups.

*Group I.* Cases 1 to 3 belonged to this group and in these babies changes similar to those noted in the umbilicus were seen in the umbilical vein and in its main branches within the liver substance (Fig. 1). There was no evidence of any thrombus formation, but small haemorrhages were frequent, around the vein, usually where one might have expected the tip of the catheter to lie.

*Group II.* Cases 4 to 9 were in this group and all had a spreading thrombosis of the umbilical vein and its main branches within the liver substance (Fig. 2). This was obvious on naked eye examination and most frequently the right branch, linking up with the portal vein, was the one involved. Haemorrhages in the vein wall and in the surrounding adventitial tissue were marked, and when serial blocks of the area were examined, it was found that in 4 instances (Cases 4, 5, 6, and 7) the thrombosis had spread further into portal tracts. A mid-zonal necrosis was present in Case 6 which lived for 146 hours (Fig. 3). This was obvious to the naked eye and involved both

TABLE

CHANGES IN UMBILICAL VEIN AND DEGREE OF SPREAD

| Case No. | Weight (g.) | Age (hr.) | Age (hr.) when catheterized | Catheter in (hr.) | Grade of Spread | Necropsy |
|---|---|---|---|---|---|---|
| 1 | 920 | 17 | 3 | 14 | I | Atelectasis, patchy HMD |
| 2 | 760 | 72 | 2 | 46 | I | Extreme prematurity, atelectasis |
| 3 | 1,160 | 168 | 3 | 48 | I | Coliform meningitis, HMD |
| 4 | 1,940 | 71 | 6 | 48 | II | Pneumonia, HMD, kernikterus |
| 5 | 2,060 | 52 | 5 | 47 | II | IVH, HMD |
| 6 | 1,220 | 146 | 4 | 64 | II | HMD umbilical vein thrombosis, hepatic necrosis, early pneumonia |
| 7 | 1,120 | 100 | 4 | 96 | II | IVH, HMD, pneumonia |
| 8 | 1,500 | 21 | 2 | 19 | II | IVHs, TT, HMD |
| 9 | 1,860 | 31 | 20 | 11 | II | HMD ? foetal blood loss; placenta praevia |
| 10 | 1,060 | 21 | 11 | 10 | III | ICH, TT |
| 11 | 1,660 | 58 | 3 | 55 | III | HMD, pulmonary embolus (large) |
| 12 | 1,100 | 34 | 4 | 30 | III | IVH, HMD |
| 13 | 2,180 | 121 | 28 | 93 | III | HMD, umbilical vein thrombosis, hepatic necrosis (mid-zonal), diabetic mother |
| 14 | 1,420 | 12 | 4 | 8 | III | IVHs, HMD |
| 15 | 2,460 | 33 | 25 | 8 | III | HMD |
| 16 | 920 | 96 | 6 | 47 | IV | Pyaemia, pneumonia, umbilical sepsis |
| 17 | 1,200 | 54 | 3 | 21 | IV | Pyaemia, umbilical vein thrombophlebitis, IVH |
| 18 | 2,120 | 94 | 35 | 59 | IV | Pyaemia, umbilical vein thrombophlebitis, HMD, early pneumonia |

HMD = hyaline membrane disease; IVH = intraventricular haemorrhage; ICH = intracranial haemorrhage; and TT = tentorial tear.

lobes. Case 7 was interesting: the baby was born at home and its cord had been dusted with powder; doubly refractile material was present both in the thrombus within the liver and in the block from umbilicus.

*Group III.* There were 6 cases (Cases 10 to 15) with pulmonary emboli. Apart from Case 11, the emboli were small and frequently multiple. They varied in age, some showing early organization. No related vascular upset, such as congestion or

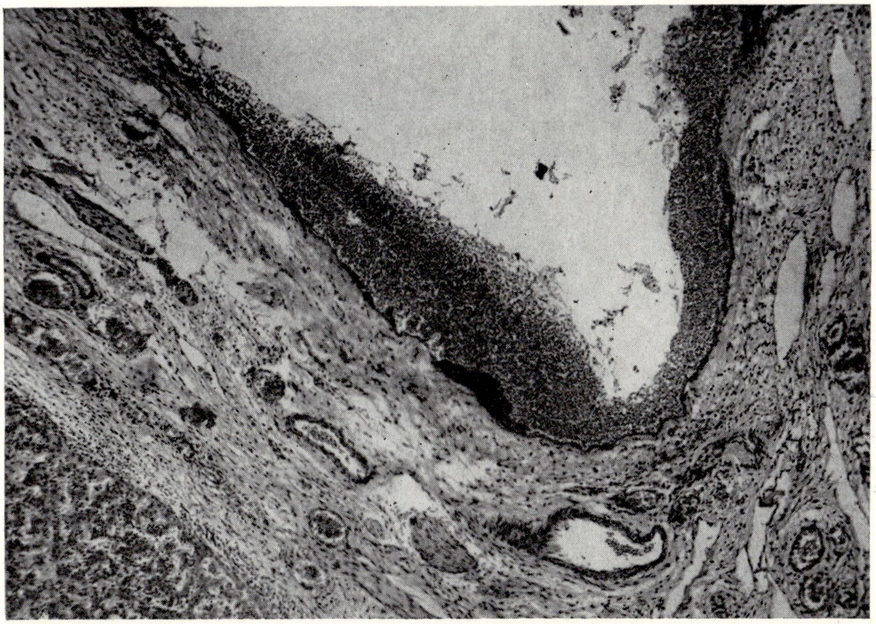

FIG. 1.—Major branch of umbilical vein within liver showing endothelial necrosis and blue-black mass, positive for Feulgen, plastered against wall of vein. (H. and E. × 66.)

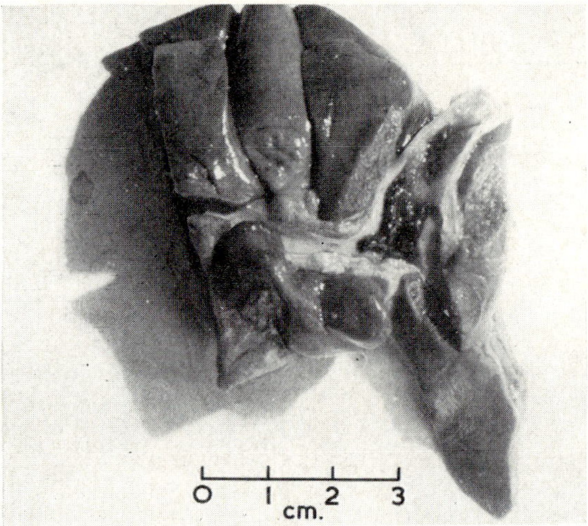


FIG. 2.—Umbilical vein opened longitudinally to show spreading thrombus.

haemorrhage, could be seen, and collapse was difficult to assess since resorption atelectasis due to the primary condition was so widespread. Thus diagnosis was not made until the lungs were examined microscopically.

In Cases 14 and 15, where the catheter had been *in situ* for only 8 hours, no thrombus was found in the umbilical vein. Case 15 was a late catheterization at 20 hours: this baby had been born at home and the cord dusted with powder; in one of the emboli doubly refractile material resembling hairs and a starch granule were found. All the other babies had umbilical vein thrombosis and Case 13 developed liver necrosis. As already stated a large pulmonary embolus was present in Case 11: this was recognized at necropsy, and clot filled a main branch of the left pulmonary artery and spread into the lung substance. No gross circulatory upset was evident.

*Group IV.* Infection developed in 3 (Cases 16, 17, and 18), where there was an umbilical vein phlebitis and septic emboli were seen within the liver and lung. In Case 16 an embolus had settled in the atrial appendage of the right atrium. At necropsy the whole appendage was distended with rather friable clot, and microscopically an inflammatory reaction could be seen spreading into the wall of the appendage.

Apart from one case of umbilical sepsis, thrombophlebitis, and septicaemia, none of the 15 Rhesus babies showed any of the above lesions. The case in which sepsis occurred was a late catheterization with replacement transfusion 24 hours after delivery outside.

**Discussion**

Routine examination of the umbilical vein in untreated babies dying with RDS or similar condition associated with marked venous congestion frequently reveals thrombus within the vein, but this is always

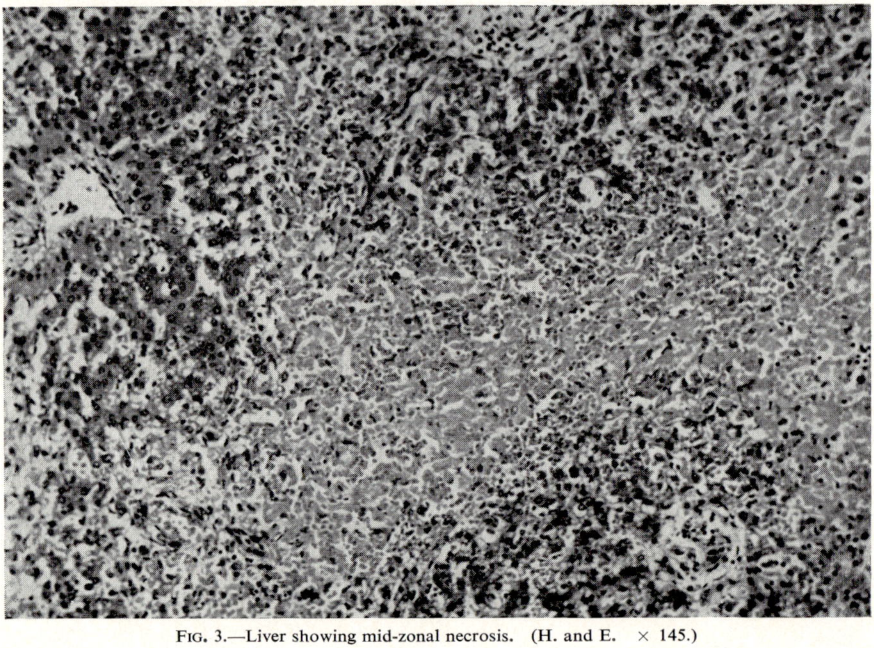

FIG. 3.—Liver showing mid-zonal necrosis. (H. and E. × 145.)

agonal in type and never adherent like the clot occurring in catheterized babies; nor is there evidence of haemorrhage or associated trauma as in the latter group.

Since all babies, including the Rhesus group, show changes at the level of the umbilicus and only a few develop more extensive lesions, it is doubtful if these local effects have any real significance. Any attempt to relate endothelial necrosis and its sequelae to bicarbonate and laevulose administration, as distinct from blood, would be unwise since the catheter was *in situ* considerably longer in titrated cases, and the question of continued trauma then arises.

Only 20% of the babies coming to necropsy showed lesions extending beyond the umbilicus. This figure should possibly be higher since only gross lesions were recorded in the first part of the survey, and hence no Group I cases were reported at that time. This in no way alters the picture however, for reference to the Table will show that it is very doubtful whether these Group I lesions have any real clinical significance. Two of the babies were extremely premature, under 1,000 g., and in the third which died of meningitis, there was no evidence to suggest that the umbilical route had been the portal entry for infection.

Of the remaining 15 cases in groups II, III, and IV, it can be seen that many of the babies died from other causes and it is doubtful whether the iatrogenic lesions influenced the ultimate course of events. There were, however, 6 cases where they apparently played a more significant part (Cases 6, 11, 13, 16, 17, and 18). Umbilical vein phlebitis and pyaemia accounted for three, umbilical vein thrombosis and liver necrosis for 2, and a large pulmonary embolus for the last. In all but one the catheter had been *in situ* for 47 hours or more, and the exception had an intraventricular haemorrhage that probably hastened death. When one considers, however, that during this period of survey 200 babies were treated and the mortality rate fell from 66 to 46% (Hutchison *et al.*, 1964) this number is relatively small. Though it did seem in these 6 cases that lengthy catheterization might carry an added risk it does not necessarily follow from this that the type or extent of lesion observed can be related to duration of catheterization. Too many other factors such as positioning of tip of catheter, possibility of local trauma, proportions of bicarbonate and laevulose used, and even tendency to thrombosis, are all involved. None the less, the pathological picture is clear; the earliest lesion consists of an aseptic endothelial necrosis, resulting in local and eventually spreading thrombosis involving the liver in certain cases. Embolism may well occur when fluids are being administered and, as these were given hourly, this would explain why emboli of various ages were seen in the lungs. More important still is the fact that these minor embolic episodes were 'silent' and the question arises whether any of the survivors suffered similarly. If so, it will be interesting to see whether any of these survivors subsequently develop signs of pulmonary abnormality such as has been reported in adults following thromboembolism by Wood (1956) and Emmanuel (1961).

## Summary

Of 200 babies treated with bicarbonate and laevulose via an umbilical vein catheter for respiratory distress syndrome, 92 came to necropsy. Complications arising from this form of therapy occurred in 20% of those that died, but in the majority of these other factors were responsible for death. Only in 6 instances was it felt that iatrogenic lesions could be regarded as immediate causes: 3 were cases of umbilical vein phlebitis and pyaemia; 2 had thrombosis and liver necrosis, and 1 had a large pulmonary embolus. The findings were compared with those seen in 15 Rhesus babies dying after replacement transfusion: amongst these there was only one case of umbilical vein phlebitis, and this was a late catheterization at 24 hours.

I would like to acknowledge the help and encouragement I have received from Dr. A. D. T. Govan. I am also grateful to Professor Hutchison for permission to study his case records and to Mr. Andrew Fraser and Mr. T. Pearston for photographic illustrations.

### References

Emmanuel, R. W. (1961). Pulmonary hypertension and mitral valvular disease in relation to anticoagulants. In *Symposium on Anti-coagulant Therapy*, ed. Sir G. W. Pickering, p. 271. Harvey and Blythe, London.

Hutchison, J. H., Kerr, M. M., Douglas, T. A., Inall, J. A., and Crosbie, J. C. (1964). A therapeutic approach in 100 cases of the respiratory distress syndrome of the newborn infant. *Pediatrics*, **33**, 956.

Scott, J. M. (1965). Histological observations on glycogen reserves of the foetus and newborn infant. *Arch. Dis. Childh.*, **40**, 317.

Wood, P. H. (1956). *Diseases of the Heart and Circulation*, 2nd ed. Eyre and Spottiswood, London.

*Arch. Dis. Childh.*, 1965, **40**, 430.

# BLOOD CHEMISTRY OF NORMAL FULL-TERM INFANTS IN THE FIRST 48 HOURS OF LIFE

BY

P. T. ACHARYA and W. W. PAYNE

*From the Department of Pathology, Queen Charlotte's Maternity Hospital, London*

(RECEIVED FOR PUBLICATION DECEMBER 4, 1964)

The intention was to study the changes in the composition of the blood in the newborn infant during the first 48 hours of life by taking capillary blood samples from the heel at frequent intervals and using a development of Sanz's (1957) ultramicro-technique for the analysis.

## Material and Methods

The subjects of the study were normal infants born in hospital of healthy mothers by normal delivery. The cord was clamped at once after birth. In a subsequent paper the effects of various abnormalities of birth are examined. *Sodium* and *potassium* were estimated by flame photometer in a dilution of 10 micro litres (μl.) in 5 ml. water; *chloride* by iodometric titration using silver iodate; *calcium* by adapting Wilkinson's EDTA titration method (1957) for 20 μl. serum; *total protein* by biuret using Natelson's (1957) technique; *urea* by a urease method modified from Archer and Robb (1925); *sugar* by a modification of Nelson-Somogy's (Natelson) using 10 μl.; *inorganic phosphorus* by an adaptation of Natelson's method; and *lactic acid* by adapting Barker and Summerson's (1941) method using 10 μl. serum. *Haematocrit* was estimated by using thin even bore heparinized capillary tubes. *Cell potassium* was estimated by taking 10 μl. whole freshly mixed blood in 5 ml. water, centrifuging, and estimating in the flame photometer.

The blood was taken from a heel using the technique described by Wilkinson (1960), but first covering the skin with sterile petroleum jelly and collecting in plastic tubing with a sealed end and a diagonally cut top containing 10 μl. of a heparin solution. Blood for sugar, phosphorus, and lactic acid was collected separately in a small tube containing fluoride and oxalate. A total of about 1 ml. was collected at 1, 2, 3 ,5, 7, 9, 11, 19, 24, 36, and 48 hours after birth. Cord blood was collected at birth from the umbilical vein. All estimations were performed in duplicate.

The results are shown in detail in a Ph.D. thesis by one of us (P.T.A.) accepted by the University of London (1962) and are here summarized.

Standard deviations have been calculated on the unjustified assumption of a normal distribution in all cases.

## Results

**Plasma Potassium.** Table 1 shows the mean and the range. It will be seen that the cord blood has a high value, 7·79 mEq/l., falling quickly at 1 hour and then slowly for the next 48 hours with a slight secondary peak at 3 hours. The most probable reason for the high cord value is the acute acidosis caused at birth by transient anoxia (James, 1960).

TABLE 1

PLASMA POTASSIUM CONCENTRATION (mEq/l.) OF NORMAL FULL-TERM INFANTS (PRESENT SERIES)

| Hours After Birth | Mean | Range | SD | No. of Determinations |
|---|---|---|---|---|
| Cord | 7·79 | 5·6–12·0 | ± 2·0 | 14 |
| 1 | 6·78 | 5·3–7·8 | ± 0·71 | 13 |
| 2 | 6·65 | 5·2–8·4 | ± 0·83 | 13 |
| 3 | 7·0 | 5·7–9·7 | ± 0·94 | 13 |
| 5 | 6·84 | 5·1–7·5 | ± 0·73 | 11 |
| 7 | 6·4 | 5·3–7·3 | ± 0·64 | 12 |
| 9 | 6·71 | 5·3–8·0 | ± 0·79 | 13 |
| 11 | 6·6 | 5·3–7·9 | ± 0·79 | 13 |
| 18 | 6·33 | 5·3–8·9 | ± 0·78 | 13 |
| 24 | 6·19 | 5·3–7·7 | ± 0·73 | 14 |
| 36 | 6·03 | 5·2–7·3 | ± 0·63 | 14 |
| 48 | 5·92 | 5·0–7·7 | ± 0·8 | 14 |

This causes an exchange transfer of $H^+$ ions from plasma with $K^+$ ions of the intracellular fluid of the RBC. Other writers have found levels in the cord blood both higher than ours, e.g. Widdowson and McCance (1956) 8·0 mg., Oliver, Demis, and Bates (1961) 9·1 mg.; and lower, e.g. Earle, Bakwin, and Hirsch (1951) 4·98 mg., Oberman, Gregory, Burke, Ross, and Rice (1956) 5·0 mg., and Österlund (1955) 5·1 mg. Only a few reports exist for the values during the next 48 hours, Overman, Etteldorf, Bass, and Horn (1951) found lower values. Pincus Gittleman, Saito, and Sobel (1956), in the first day of life, found values a little lower (5·4 mg.) and Usher (1959) 12-60 hour period found a mean of 6·01; Oliver *et al.* (1961) report a mean at 1 hour of 8·0 mg. and show a fall from the mean cord blood of 1·1 mg., compared with 1·0 in our series.

**Red Cell Potassium.** In only three normal infants was the RBC potassium estimated (Table 2), but the values show a fairly well-marked inverse relation to the changes in the level of the plasma potassium, suggesting that the changes are at least partly due to transfer to and from the cell to the plasma (these estimations were made following a discussion of the work with Professor R. A. McCance).

TABLE 2

RED CELL POTASSIUM CONCENTRATION (mEq/l.) OF FULL-TERM NORMAL INFANTS (PRESENT SERIES)

| Hours After Birth | Mean | Range | No. of Determinations |
|---|---|---|---|
| Cord | 99·6 | 97·0–102·0 | 3 |
| 1 | 103·0 | 97·0–109·0 | 3 |
| 3 | 100·3 | 99·0–101·0 | 3 |
| 5 | 103·6 | 103·0–105·0 | 3 |
| 7 | 106·0 | 101·0–112·0 | 3 |
| 12 | 100·3 | 100·0–102·0 | 3 |
| 18 | 102·6 | 101·0–104·0 | 3 |
| 24 | 105·0 | 100·0–108·0 | 3 |
| 36 | 108·3 | 101·0–112·0 | 3 |
| 48 | 107·0 | 100·0–114·0 | 3 |

**Plasma Sodium.** It will be seen from Table 3 that the mean cord plasma sodium is slightly higher than the mean adult level. There is a fall in the sodium occurring in nearly all subjects during the first 12 hours, which is shown in the mean value as occurring at 3 hours. This fall can be quite large—in one individual being as much as 31 mEq. After the fall the sodium level steadily rises to a level higher than the initial cord sodium. The results of other authors for cord blood vary: Overman *et al.* (1951) 134, Österlund (1955) 140, Widdowson and McCance (1956) 138, Oliver *et al.*, 139 mEq/l. Oliver *et al.* also estimated sodium at 1 hour and found a fall to 134 mEq/l. This fall cannot be due to loss of sodium in the urine, which is quite small during the first few hours of life, and the subsequent rise equally is not due to feeding, as in this series the policy was to give very little fluid in the first 24 hours and only a small increase in the second day. This increase in sodium has been attributed to loss of water which, if not replaced, leads to a degree of dehydration and an all round increase in the concentration of the blood constituents (Smith, 1959). The fall may be due to a transient fall in the circulating mineralo-corticoids or aldosterone, causing a temporary transfer of plasma sodium to the intracellular fluid.

TABLE 3

PLASMA SODIUM CONCENTRATION (mEq/l.) OF FULL-TERM NORMAL INFANTS (PRESENT SERIES)

| Hours After Birth | Mean | Range | SD | No. of Determinations |
|---|---|---|---|---|
| Cord | 146·78 | 126·0–166·0 | ± 8·1 | 14 |
| 1 | 145·38 | 122·0–153·0 | ± 8·23 | 13 |
| 2 | 145·5 | 121·0–155·0 | ± 8·42 | 14 |
| 3 | 142·0 | 109·0–159·0 | ± 10·4 | 14 |
| 5 | 143·57 | 124·0–156·0 | ± 7·2 | 14 |
| 7 | 143·49 | 130·0–153·0 | ± 5·8 | 14 |
| 9 | 144·93 | 130·0–159·0 | ± 4·1 | 14 |
| 11 | 146·2 | 132·0–159·0 | ± 5·6 | 14 |
| 18 | 145·5 | 132·0–159·0 | ± 7·3 | 14 |
| 24 | 146·42 | 131·0–156·0 | ± 6·5 | 14 |
| 36 | 147·78 | 134·0–160·0 | ± 6·9 | 14 |
| 48 | 148·7 | 139·0–162·0 | ± 4·3 | 14 |

**Plasma Chloride.** The changes in the chloride level are small and seem to bear no relation to the changes in the sodium level (Table 4), though large individual differences exist as shown by the wide range. Inspection of the individual curves shows that in the main there is not a great amount of variation during the whole 48 hours. Other authors' levels for cord blood are Overman *et al.*, 109, Österlund (1955) 97, Widdowson and McCance, 110, Kaiser and Goodlin (1958) 104, Oliver *et al.* (1961) 107 mEq/l.

TABLE 4

PLASMA CHLORIDE CONCENTRATION (mEq/l.) OF FULL-TERM NORMAL INFANTS (PRESENT SERIES)

| Hours After Birth | Mean | Range | SD | No. of Determinations |
|---|---|---|---|---|
| Cord | 103·28 | 98·0–110·0 | ± 4·63 | 14 |
| 1 | 102·53 | 90·0–110·0 | ± 5·68 | 13 |
| 2 | 98·3 | 81·0–106·0 | ± 7·5 | 13 |
| 3 | 101·07 | 83·0–114·0 | ± 7·0 | 13 |
| 5 | 100·71 | 90·0–111·0 | ± 5·19 | 13 |
| 7 | 104·3 | 94·0–117·0 | ± 6·1 | 13 |
| 9 | 101·56 | 83·0–115·0 | ± 7·41 | 14 |
| 11 | 102·46 | 82·0–114·0 | ± 7·34 | 13 |
| 18 | 103·46 | 87·0–114·0 | ± 7·28 | 13 |
| 24 | 105·57 | 98·0–119·0 | ± 6·1 | 14 |
| 36 | 102·43 | 92·0–114·0 | ± 7·24 | 14 |
| 48 | 102·78 | 93·0–112·0 | ± 7·14 | 14 |

**Blood Inorganic Phosphate.** The blood phosphorus level is higher in infants and growing children than in adults (Table 5). There is a small rise in phosphate level during the first few hours of life—possibly due to the utilization of glycogen and the liberation of the phosphate bound with glycogen in its initial formation. The later fall in phosphate is paralleled by a similar fall in calcium and may be due to deposition of calcium phosphate in the bones, but there are many factors causing variation in the phosphate level.

**Blood Urea.** The initial cord blood urea is largely determined by the maternal level. It will be

TABLE 5

BLOOD INORGANIC PHOSPHORUS CONCENTRATION (mg./100 ml.) OF FULL-TERM NORMAL INFANTS (PRESENT SERIES)

| Hours After Birth | Mean | Range | SD | No. of Determinations |
|---|---|---|---|---|
| Cord | 5·65 | 3·7–8·1 | ± 1·28 | 14 |
| 1 | 6·05 | 3·8–9·4 | ± 1·5 | 14 |
| 2 | 6·29 | 4·0–8·2 | ± 1·42 | 14 |
| 3 | 6·35 | 3·7–9·0 | ± 1·47 | 14 |
| 5 | 6·1 | 3·5–8·6 | ± 1·57 | 14 |
| 7 | 5·91 | 3·4–8·4 | ± 1·48 | 14 |
| 9 | 5·73 | 2·8–7·8 | ± 1·53 | 14 |
| 11 | 5·68 | 2·9–8·0 | ± 1·51 | 14 |
| 18 | 5·74 | 2·9–8·1 | ± 1·64 | 14 |
| 24 | 5·71 | 3·0–8·4 | ± 1·61 | 14 |
| 36 | 5·93 | 3·0–8·7 | ± 1·6 | 14 |
| 48 | 5·84 | 2·8–7·6 | ± 1·57 | 14 |

seen that the mean value falls during the first few hours of life and then slowly rises and finally stabilizes as the kidney begins to function (Table 6). The initial fall can be quite large in some subjects, up to 25 mg./100 ml. This cannot be explained by urinary secretion as this is almost nil during the first hours of life. It is probably due to utilization of urea for enzyme protein formation (Giordano, 1963; Houpt, 1963). The later rise is due to metabolism of tissue protein. The late rise in blood urea is recorded by McCance and Widdowson (1947, 1954, 1955). No record has been found of the initial fall.

TABLE 6

BLOOD UREA CONCENTRATION (mg./100 ml.) OF FULL-TERM NORMAL INFANTS (PRESENT SERIES)

| Hours After Birth | Mean | Range | SD | No. of Determinations |
|---|---|---|---|---|
| Cord | 29·37 | 21·0–40·0 | ± 7·3 | 13 |
| 1 | 29·71 | 18·0–62·0 | ± 10·4 | 12 |
| 2 | 24·3 | 6·0–36·0 | ± 8·1 | 13 |
| 3 | 25·7 | 7·0–41·0 | ± 9·3 | 13 |
| 5 | 27·45 | 8·0–34·0 | ± 6·6 | 13 |
| 7 | 27·6 | 5·0–41·0 | ± 9·7 | 13 |
| 9 | 28·52 | 6·0–58·0 | ± 12·2 | 13 |
| 11 | 32·29 | 8·0–63·0 | ± 11·8 | 13 |
| 18 | 33·45 | 9·0–63·0 | ± 11·9 | 13 |
| 24 | 31·84 | 7·0–69·0 | ± 12·9 | 13 |
| 36 | 32·53 | 13·0–77·0 | ± 14·0 | 13 |
| 48 | 30·76 | 13·0–68·0 | ± 12·9 | 13 |

**Blood Sugar.** The value of the blood sugar depends to some extent on the method of estimation. The method used here was for so-called 'true sugar', but it gives a higher result than the more specific glucose oxidase method by an average of 10 mg./100 ml. The difference represents other reducing sugars. The results show a level that is low by adult standards (Table 7). There is also a wide range, the lowest value being 29 mg. at 24 hours. There are also several high values, the highest being 144 mg. at 11 hours. These high values are sharp peaks and not a prolonged rise. There is a tendency for the blood sugar to fall often to quite low levels (30-40 mg.) during the 2-7 hours, with a final stabilizing between 50 and 60 mg. in the second day of life. These results are closely similar to those of Pederson (1952) and Farquhar (1954).

TABLE 7

BLOOD SUGAR CONCENTRATION (mg./100 ml.) OF FULL-TERM NORMAL INFANTS (PRESENT SERIES)

| Hours After Birth | Mean | Range | SD | No. of Determinations |
|---|---|---|---|---|
| Cord | 73·0 | 45·0–96·0 | ± 16·9 | 14 |
| 1 | 62·64 | 31·0–108·0 | ± 20·1 | 14 |
| 2 | 58·92 | 31·0–93·0 | ± 19·0 | 14 |
| 3 | 63·78 | 39·0–112·0 | ± 20·1 | 14 |
| 5 | 63·0 | 40·0–97·0 | ± 22·0 | 14 |
| 7 | 59·57 | 35·0–88·0 | ± 20·0 | 14 |
| 9 | 59·0 | 33·0–88·0 | ± 14·0 | 14 |
| 11 | 65·14 | 42·0–144·0 | ± 26·6 | 14 |
| 18 | 63·0 | 42·0–104·0 | ± 16·9 | 14 |
| 24 | 57·85 | 29·0–78·0 | ± 13·9 | 14 |
| 36 | 56·5 | 30·0–91·0 | ± 16·9 | 14 |
| 48 | 59·13 | 40·0–90·0 | ± 13·5 | 14 |

**Lactic Acid.** The high value in the cord blood is caused by two factors: the maternal blood lactate level is raised during labour and thus accounts for part of the increase (Table 8). The period of anoxia at birth accounts for the balance. As soon as the infant's blood is adequately oxygenated the lactic acid level begins to fall, but the rate of fall is slower than occurs in the adult, and the adult level of lactic acid (10 mg.) is not reached by all infants by the end of 2 days, though in the majority of infants it is.

TABLE 8

BLOOD LACTIC ACID CONCENTRATION (mg./100 ml.) OF FULL-TERM NORMAL INFANTS (PRESENT SERIES)

| Hours After Birth | Mean | Range | SD | No. of Determinations |
|---|---|---|---|---|
| Cord | 19·55 | 11·0–30·0 | ± 6·8 | 14 |
| 1 | 16·0 | 11·0–23·0 | ± 6·0 | 14 |
| 2 | 15·85 | 10·0–23·0 | ± 6·1 | 14 |
| 3 | 15·35 | 12·0–26·0 | ± 5·0 | 14 |
| 5 | 14·57 | 11·0–24·0 | ± 5·6 | 14 |
| 7 | 14·44 | 11·0–22·0 | ± 5·0 | 14 |
| 9 | 14·0 | 10·0–28·0 | ± 5·4 | 14 |
| 11 | 14·5 | 10·0–27·0 | ± 5·0 | 14 |
| 18 | 14·0 | 10·0–23·0 | ± 4·4 | 14 |
| 24 | 14·35 | 10·0–23·0 | ± 5·8 | 14 |
| 36 | 14·27 | 9·0–22·0 | ± 6·0 | 14 |
| 48 | 13·5 | 7·0–21·0 | ± 4·7 | 14 |

The level of the lactic acid is an index of the oxygenation, as anaerobic metabolism produces lactic acid.

Cord values for lactic acid have been reported by Hendricks (1957) 24, and Kaiser and Goodlin (1958) 21·6, but no record of the lactic acid during the first

48 hours has been found until Znamenáček and Přibylová (1964) who report values higher than ours.

**Total Plasma Protein.** The plasma protein level increases in the first hour (Table 9), due probably to loss of water from the plasma in the large calibre vein of the cord when compared with the plasma from the capillaries, as, with the changes of intravascular pressure in relation to tissue pressure caused by the alterations occurring at birth, the osmotic pressure of the plasma protein is insufficient to retain as much water as *in utero*. After this initial adjustment, the protein level is constant for the rest of the first 24 hours, but there is an increase in the second 24 hours, quite possibly due to the haemo-concentration seen in the sodium levels. The values reported show some variation: Denzer, Reiner, and Weiner (1939) 6·04, Rimington and Bickford (1947) 6·53, McMurray, Roe, and Sweet (1948) 6·0, Gairdner, Marks, Roscoe, and Brettell (1958) 6·5, Solomkin and Tauber (1959) 5·7, and Oliver *et al.* (1961) 6·4. Gairdner *et al.* reported a rise from 6·5 to 7·0 in 1 to 8 hours after birth, but Oliver *et al.* record a fall from 6·4 to 6·1 at the end of 1 hour. Graham, Wilson, Tsao, Baumann, and Brown (1951) record a steady fall from 6·12 at birth to 5·71 at 24 hours and Overman *et al.* a fall from 6·3 to 6·1 at 24 hours.

TABLE 9

TOTAL PROTEIN (PLASMA) CONCENTRATION (g./100 ml.) OF FULL-TERM NORMAL INFANTS (PRESENT SERIES)

| Hours After Birth | Mean | Range | SD | No. of Determinations |
|---|---|---|---|---|
| Cord | 6·13 | 4·8–7·3 | ± 0·67 | 10 |
| 1 | 6·77 | 5·8–8·1 | ± 0·73 | 9 |
| 2 | 6·52 | 5·8–7·9 | ± 0·56 | 6 |
| 3 | 6·73 | 5·7–8·4 | ± 0·6 | 9 |
| 5 | 6·61 | 5·6–8·5 | ± 0·63 | 9 |
| 7 | 6·6 | 5·5–7·7 | ± 0·7 | 10 |
| 9 | 6·84 | 5·7–7·9 | ± 0·56 | 6 |
| 11 | 6·6 | 5·6–8·0 | ± 0·66 | 9 |
| 18 | 6·63 | 5·8–8·2 | ± 0·68 | 9 |
| 24 | 6·78 | 5·9–7·7 | ± 0·72 | 10 |
| 36 | 6·93 | 5·9–8·2 | ± 0·73 | 10 |
| 48 | 7·17 | 6·0–8·5 | ± 0·76 | 10 |

**Packed Cell Volume.** This shows a short rise from cord to capillary at 1 hour and a slower rise up to 3 hours (Table 10). After this there is a steady fall, despite the haemo-concentration for the rest of the 48 hours (as mentioned above under Plasma Sodium).

As Gairdner *et al.* (1958) have shown, it is important to consider the size of the vessel from which the blood is taken. As a check, immediately after taking the cord blood at birth, capillary blood was collected from the heel in 3 babies. An interval of 5-10 minutes was inevitable between the time of collecting the two specimens, and the results of a full analysis are shown in Table 11.

It will be seen that the PCV is higher in all 3

TABLE 10

PACKED CELL VOLUME (%) OF FULL-TERM NORMAL INFANTS (PRESENT SERIES)

| Hours After Birth | Mean | Range | SD | No. of Determinations |
|---|---|---|---|---|
| Cord | 54·17 | 43·0–62·0 | ± 6·32 | 12 |
| 1 | 66·0 | 58·0–77·0 | ± 7·91 | 13 |
| 2 | 66·25 | 57·0–76·0 | ± 7·07 | 10 |
| 3 | 69·9 | 64·0–82·0 | ± 8·06 | 12 |
| 5 | 67·0 | 56·0–75·0 | ± 8·03 | 13 |
| 7 | 63·1 | 50·0–76·0 | ± 7·6 | 13 |
| 9 | 59·34 | 51·0–68·0 | ± 6·25 | 10 |
| 11 | 58·5 | 48·0–70·0 | ± 7·04 | 13 |
| 18 | 55·29 | 49·0–61·0 | ± 6·7 | 13 |
| 24 | 53·09 | 42·0–64·0 | ± 6·44 | 13 |
| 36 | 50·94 | 44·0–56·0 | ± 6·12 | 13 |
| 48 | 49·18 | 36·0–59·0 | ± 5·94 | 13 |

TABLE 11

COMPARISON OF SIMULTANEOUS DETERMINATIONS OF K, Na, PCV, TOTAL PLASMA PROTEIN, PLASMA CALCIUM, PLASMA MAGNESIUM, BLOOD UREA, BLOOD SUGAR, BLOOD INORGANIC PHOSPHATE, AND BLOOD LACTIC ACID: CONCENTRATIONS IN CORD BLOOD AND IN CAPILLARY BLOOD OBTAINED BY HEEL PRICK 5-10 MINUTES AFTER BIRTH

| | Infant No. | Cord Blood | Capillary Blood |
|---|---|---|---|
| Plasma potassium (mEq/l.) | 1 | 6·1 | 6·2 |
| | 2 | 5·5 | 5·5 |
| | 3* | 6·1 | 6·1 |
| Plasma sodium (mEq/l.) | 1 | 149·0 | 149·0 |
| | 2 | 151·0 | 150·5 |
| | 3* | 145·0 | 145·0 |
| PCV (%) | 1 | 58·5 | 69·0 |
| | 2 | 56·5 | 64·0 |
| | 3 | 56·0 | 63·0 |
| Total plasma protein (g./100 ml.) | 1 | 6·3 | 7·2 |
| | 2 | 5·85 | 6·7 |
| | 3* | 6·75 | 7·35 |
| Plasma calcium (mg./100 ml.) | 1 | 9·4 | 9·3 |
| | 2 | 9·55 | 9·6 |
| | 3* | 8·4 | 9·1 |
| Plasma magnesium (mg./100 ml.) | 1 | 1·31 | 1·53 |
| | 2 | 1·7 | 1·45 |
| | 3* | 1·8 | 2·04 |
| Blood urea (mg./100 ml.) | 1 | 33·0 | 32·2 |
| | 2 | 38·6 | 40·0 |
| | 3* | 31·5 | 74·4 |
| Blood sugar (mg./100 ml.) | 1 | 62·0 | 61·0 |
| | 2 | 65·0 | 64·0 |
| | 3* | 72·0 | 94·0 |
| Blood inorganic phosphate (mg./100 ml.) | 1 | 6·5 | 7·3 |
| | 2 | 5·3 | 6·2 |
| | 3* | 5·3 | 6·7 |
| Blood lactic acid (mg./100 ml.) | 1 | 22·0 | 37·5 |
| | 2 | 28·5 | 42·0 |
| | 3* | 42·0 | 51·0 |

* Delivered by forceps application.

cases by an average amount of 8·3%, against an increase of 11·8% between the average values in the cord and the 1-hour specimen. Thus the majority of the increase is due to the smaller diameter of the vessel. The other fraction of the increase, reaching a maximum at 3 hours, is due in all probability to a transfer of plasma from the vascular system to the interstitial fluid, often clinically apparent in a slight puffiness of the extremities and occasionally actual pitting oedema.

TABLE 12

PLASMA CALCIUM CONCENTRATION (mg./100 ml.) OF FULL-TERM NORMAL INFANTS (PRESENT SERIES)

| Hours After Birth | Mean | Range | No. of Determinations |
|---|---|---|---|
| Cord | 9·34 | 8·2–11·1 | 5 |
| 1 | 8·95 | 8·1–9·6 | 4 |
| 3 | 8·92 | 8·0–9·6 | 5 |
| 5 | 8·38 | 7·3–9·2 | 5 |
| 7 | 8·32 | 7·1–10·0 | 5 |
| 12 | 8·22 | 6·9–10·2 | 5 |
| 18 | 7·84 | 6·9–9·4 | 5 |
| 24 | 7·7 | 6·2–9·0 | 5 |
| 36 | 8·02 | 6·1–9·9 | 5 |
| 48 | 7·94 | 5·9–9·7 | 5 |

**Serum Calcium.** The technique used for estimation of calcium described by Wilkinson (1957) gives results averaging 0·8 mg. lower than the more usual oxalate method. There is a progressive fall of the calcium from birth till about 36 hours or occasionally longer (Table 12). This fall is not inversely connected with the level of phosphate as has been suggested, since for much of the time both fall together. It is more likely due to a temporary dysfunction of the parathyroids.

Values for calcium are given by Bakwin (1937) 11·0, Denzer *et al.* (1939) 11·53, Todd, Chuinard, and Wood (1939) 11·27, Bruck and Weintraub (1955) 10·59—all cord blood.

Bakwin records the level at intervals for the first 24 hours and finds a steady fall of 1·43 mg.

Denzer records results in the first and second days of life as 1·05 mg. less than his cord value. Todd also records a fall in the first 2 days of 1·34 mg.

## Discussion

This record of serial blood chemistry in infants is incomplete without the actual results for each age, but to record these either in tables or graphically would result in too unwieldy a paper. Those interested can consult the original thesis of P.T.A. in the University of London.

To appreciate the hourly variations, in Figs. 1 and 2 the means of all the estimations have been collected together. In these infants the factor of a variable intake is absent, as the total intake in the first 48 hours was very low, so that the variations in the composition of the plasma should represent

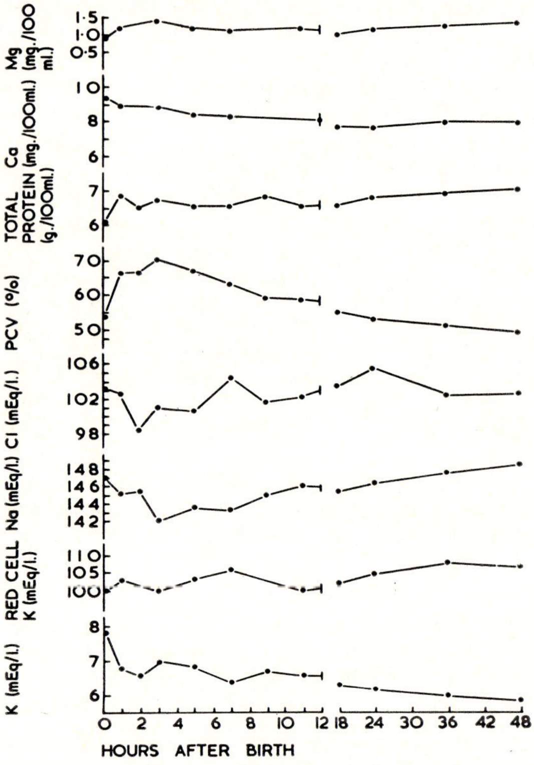


FIG. 1.—Mean values, over first 48 hours of life, of potassium, sodium, chloride, PCV, total protein, calcium, and magnesium.

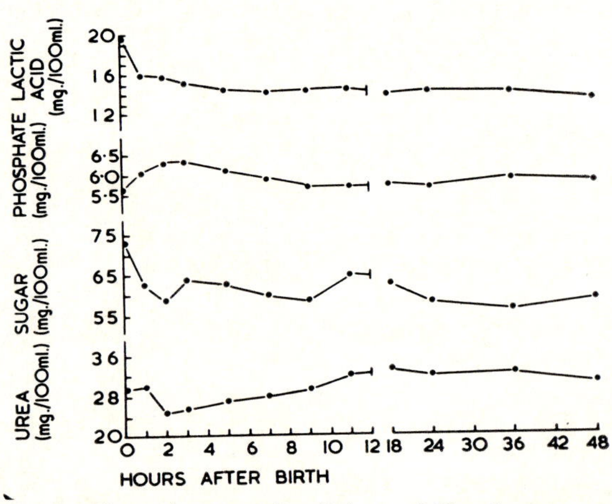


FIG. 2.—Mean values, over first 48 hours of life, of urea, sugar, inorganic phosphorus, and lactic acid.

endogenous events occurring within the child, and an endeavour has been made to explain these in terms of known biochemical responses to the stimuli resulting from the events of birth and adaptation to independent existence. Not enough is known, however, to enable a clear picture of the causes of these changes to be made. In a subsequent paper, changes due to unphysiological situations will be reported.

## Summary

The changes in the plasma sodium, potassium, chloride, phosphate, urea, sugar, lactic acid, calcium, total protein and packed cell volume during the first 48 hours of life have been reported and briefly discussed.

It is a pleasure to acknowledge the help given us by Professor J. H. Pinkerton, Dr. A. White Franklin, and Dr. A. P. Norman, and the ward sisters and staff, especially Sister Penrice and Sister Fairbrother, and to Dr. B. C. Mukerji for technical help. We are indebted to the Board of Governors of the Hospital for a grant enabling this work to be done, and to the M.R.C. for a personal grant to one of us (P.T.A.).

### References

Archer, H. E., and Robb, G. D. (1925). The tolerance of the body for urea in health and disease. *Quart. J. Med.*, **18**, 274.

Bakwin, H. (1937). Pathogenesis of tetany of the new-born. *Amer. J. Dis. Childh.*, **54**, 1211.

Barker, S. B., and Summerson, W. H. (1941). The colorimetric determination of lactic acid in biological material. *J. biol. Chem.*, **138**, 535.

Bruck, E., and Weintraub, D. H. (1955). Serum calcium and phosphorus in premature and full-term infants. *Amer. J. Dis. Child.*, **90**, 653.

Denzer, B. S., Reiner, M., and Weiner, S. B. (1939). Serum calcium in the newborn. *Amer. J. Dis. Child.*, **57**, 809.

Earle, D. P., Bakwin, H., and Hirsch, D. (1951). The plasma potassium level in the newborn. *Proc. Soc. exp. Biol.* (*N.Y.*), **76**, 756.

Farquhar, J. W. (1954). Control of the blood sugar level in the neonatal period. *Arch. Dis. Childh.*, **29**, 519.

Gairdner, D., Marks, J., Roscoe, J. D., and Brettell, R. O. (1958). The fluid shift from the vascular compartment immediately after birth. *ibid.*, **33**, 489.

Giordano, C. (1963). Use of exogenous and endogenous urea for protein synthesis in normal and uremic subjects. *J. Lab. clin. Med.*, **62**, 231.

Graham, B. D., Wilson, J. L., Tsao, M. U., Baumann, M. L., and Brown, S. (1951). Development of neonatal electrolyte homeostasis. *Pediatrics*, **8**, 68.

Hendricks, C. H. (1957). Studies on lactic acid metabolism in pregnancy and labor. *Amer. J. Obstet. Gynec.*, **73**, 492.

Houpt, T. R. (1963). Urea utilization by rabbits fed a low-protein ration. *Amer. J. Physiol.*, **205**, 1144.

James, L. S. (1960). Acidosis of the newborn and its relation to birth asphyxia. *Acta paediat.* (*Uppsala*), **49**, Suppl. 122, 17.

Kaiser, I. H., and Goodlin, R. C. (1958). Alterations of pH, gases and hemoglobin in blood and electrolytes in plasma of fetuses of diabetic mothers. *Pediatrics*, **22**, 1097.

McCance, R. A., and Widdowson, E. M. (1947). Blood-urea in the first nine days of life. *Lancet*, **1**, 787.

——, and —— (1954). The influence of events during the last few days *in utero* on tissue destruction and renal function in the first two days of independent life. *Arch. Dis. Childh.*, **29**, 495.

——, and —— (1955). Protein catabolism and renal function in the first two days of life in premature infants and multiple births. *ibid.*, **30**, 405.

McMurray, L. G., Roe, J. H., and Sweet, L. K. (1948). Plasma protein studies on normal newborn and premature infants. *Amer. J. Dis. Child.*, **75**, 265.

Natelson, S. (1957). *Microtechniques of Clinical Chemistry: for the Routine Laboratory.* Thomas, Springfield, Illinois.

Oberman, J. W., Gregory, K. O., Burke, F. G., Ross, S., and Rice, E. C. (1956). Electrophoretic analysis of serum proteins in infants and children. I. Normal values from birth to adolescence. *New Engl. J. Med.*, **255**, 743.

Oliver, T. K., Jr., Demis, J. A., and Bates, G. D. (1961). Serial blood-gas tensions and acid-base balance during the first hour of life in human infants. *Acta paediat.* (*Uppsala*), **50**, 346.

Österlund, K. (1955). A comparative investigation of the concentration of certain electrolytes in maternal and cord blood. *Ann. Paediat. Fenn.*, Suppl. 4.

Overman, R. R., Etteldorf, J. N., Bass, A. C., and Horn, G. B. (1951). Plasma and erythrocyte chemistry of the normal infant from birth to two years of age. *Pediatrics*, **7**, 565.

Pederson, J. (1952). *Diabetes and Pregnancy. Blood Sugar of Newborn Infants During Fasting and Glucose Administration.* Danish Science Press, Copenhagen.

Pincus, J. G., Gittleman, I. F., Saito, M., and Sobel, A. E. (1956). A study of plasma values of sodium, potassium chloride, carbon dioxide, carbon dioxide tension, sugar, urea, the protein base-binding power, pH, and haematocrit in prematures on the first day of life. *Pediatrics*, **18**, 39.

Rimington, C., and Bickford, J. A. (1947). Pre- and post-natal development in immunity. Serum-albumin and serum-globulin levels in maternal and cord bloods of premature infants. *Lancet*, **1**, 781.

Sanz, M. C. (1957). Ultramicro methods and standardization of equipment. *Clin. Chem.*, **3**, 406.

Smith, C. A. (1959). *The Physiology of the Newborn Infant*, 3rd ed. Thomas, Springfield, Illinois.

Solomkin, M., and Tauber, W. F. (1959). A study of constituents of the bloods of mother and infant at birth. *Conn. Med.*, **23**, 141.

Todd, W. R., Chuinard, E. G., and Wood, M. T. (1939). Blood calcium and phosphorus in the newborn. *Amer. J. Dis. Child.*, **57**, 1278.

Usher, R. (1959). The respiratory distress syndrome of prematurity. I. Changes in potassium in the serum and the electrocardiogram and effects of therapy. *Pediatrics*, **24**, 562.

Widdowson, E. M., and McCance, R. A. (1956). The effect of development on the composition of the serum and extra-cellular fluids. *Clin. Sci.*, **15**, 361.

Wilkinson, R. H. (1957). A micro-method for serum calcium and serum magnesium. *J. clin. Path.*, **10**, 126.

—— (1960). *Chemical Micromethods in Clinical Medicine.* Charles C. Thomas, Springfield, Illinois.

Znamenáček, K., and Přibylová, H. (1964). Some parameters of respiratory metabolism in the first 3 days after birth. *Acta paediat.* (*Uppsala*), **53**, 241.

*Arch. Dis. Childh.*, 1965, **40**, 436.

# THE EFFECT OF ABNORMAL BIRTH ON BLOOD CHEMISTRY DURING THE FIRST 48 HOURS OF LIFE

BY

W. W. PAYNE and P. T. ACHARYA
*From the Department of Pathology, Queen Charlotte's Maternity Hospital, London*

(RECEIVED FOR PUBLICATION DECEMBER 4, 1964)

This study arose out of a plan to examine the changes in blood chemistry during the first 48 hours of life. No attempt was made to select cases and it was only later on, when it was found that the results varied with the manner of birth, that the normal group (Acharya and Payne, 1965) was separated. The remainder were grouped into (1) forceps delivery and prolonged difficult delivery, (2) planned caesarean section, (3) maternal toxaemia (with caesarean section), (4) maternal diabetes, (5) infants showing symptoms of respiratory distress syndrome, and (6) deaths. With so many groups the numbers in each are small, and therefore no attempt was made to calculate standard deviations of the mean. For comparison of groups, however, the mean values have been calculated. The same technique and methods have been used throughout, except that only 10 specimens of blood (instead of 12) have been collected over 48 hours, because occasionally the baby's heels became rather tender. No trouble occurred after the reduction in number of pricks. The cord was clamped at once after birth.

Fig. 1 shows the mean values for the infants from groups 1 (6 cases), 2 (4 cases), and 3 (6 cases), the mean normal values (Acharya and Payne, 1965) and the mean of 4 infants with respiratory distress

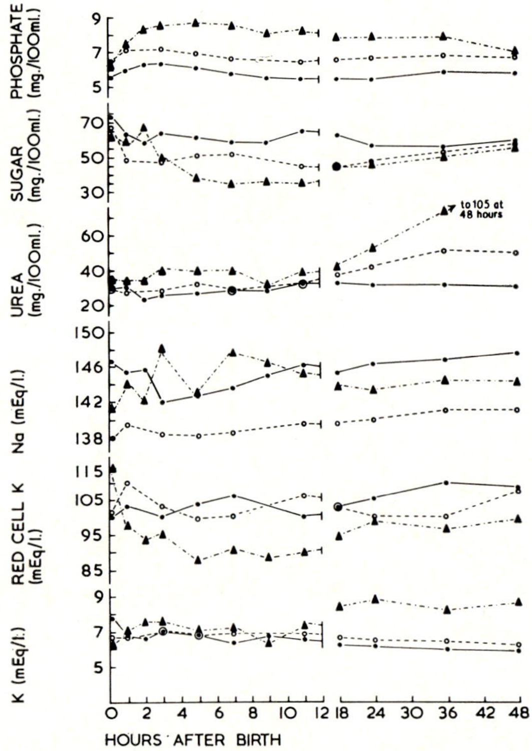


(a)

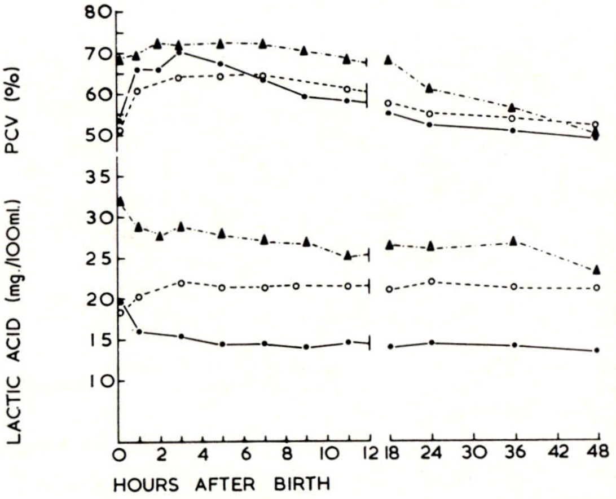


(b)

FIG. 1a and 1b.—Mean values in normal infants (●), infants delivered by stressful obstetric procedures (○), and infants with respiratory distress who survived 48 hours (▲). (a) Plasma and red cell potassium, plasma sodium, blood urea, sugar, and phosphate. (b) Lactic acid and PCV.

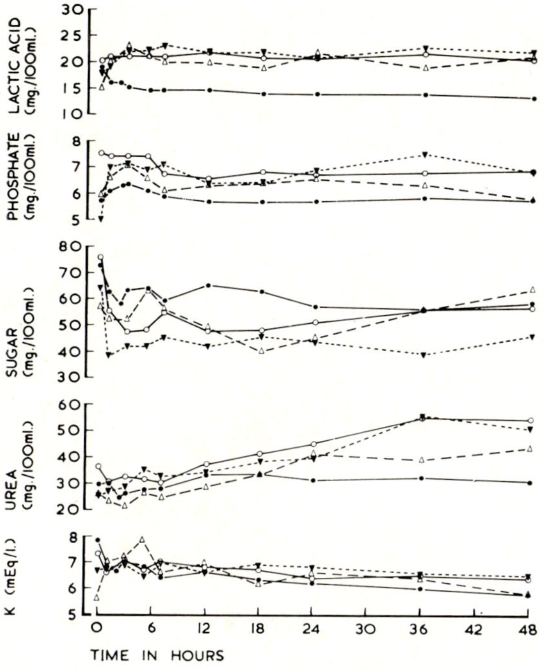


FIG. 2.—Mean values in caesarean section (△), maternal toxaemia (▼), forceps delivery (○), and normal delivery (●), of plasma potassium, urea, sugar, phosphate, and lactic acid.

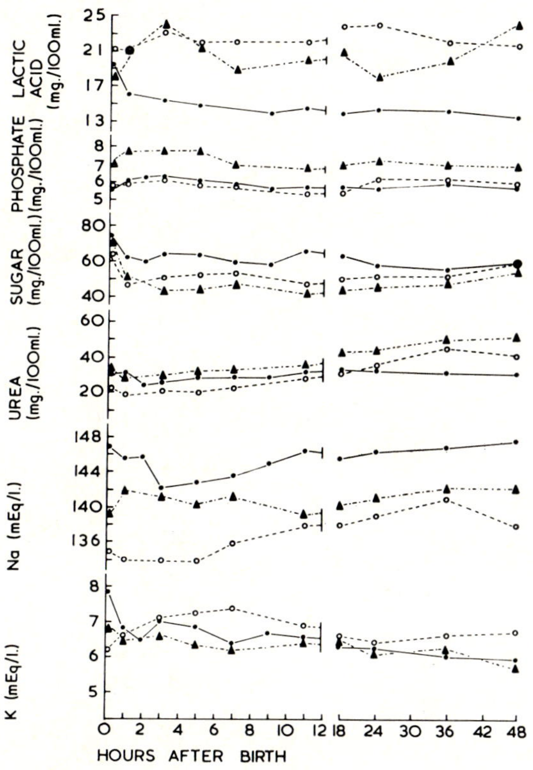


FIG. 3.—Comparison of mean values between normally born infants (●), infants stressfully born but clinically normal (○), and infants stressfully born with peripheral cyanosis (▲).

syndrome (RDS) who survived the first 48 hours of life.

The serum potassium shows no change in the first 12 hours but, as has also been reported by Usher (1959), it rises in the later period (18-48 hours) in the 4 cases of RDS. In contrast the serum sodium in the stressfully born infants, groups 1, 2, and 3, is lower for the whole period but in RDS shows no well-marked change. Blood urea shows no change in the first 12 hours but in the 18 to 48-hour period the values in the groups 1, 2, and 3 are significantly higher than normal, and in RDS are much higher than in both normal and groups 1, 2, and 3. Sugar, after the first 3 hours, falls to lower levels in groups 1, 2, and 3 and in RDS; but by the end of 48 hours there is no material difference in the three groups. The inorganic phosphorus shows a small increase in groups 1, 2, and 3 and a well-marked increase in RDS. Lactic acid is persistently raised for the whole 48 hours in groups 1, 2, and 3. In RDS the initial value is very high but subsequently there is a small but steady decrease, though it is still high at 48 hours. The packed cell volume is raised in RDS and remains high until 36 hours of age.

In Fig. 2 the potassium, phosphorus, urea, sugar, and lactic acid levels are shown for each of the three groups 1, 2, and 3 together with the normal. It will be seen that on the whole the three groups resemble each other and differ from the normal, except that the blood urea in the caesarean section group shows less change.

As many of the group 1 infants born with stress were clinically quite normal, in Fig. 3 a comparison has been made between these infants and the remainder. In the infants who were not quite normal clinically the most frequent abnormality was cyanosis of hands and feet, and this symptom has been used to characterize the group. The *clinically normal* stressed group shows a lower sodium, a smaller rise in urea, and a smaller fall in sugar than the *cyanosed* group. The lactic acid values are not significantly different, but the cyanosed group has a much higher phosphorus level than the clinically normal group where the phosphorus level does not differ from that of the normal control group.

In Fig. 4 the results from 4 infants born by caesarean section to diabetic mothers are shown.

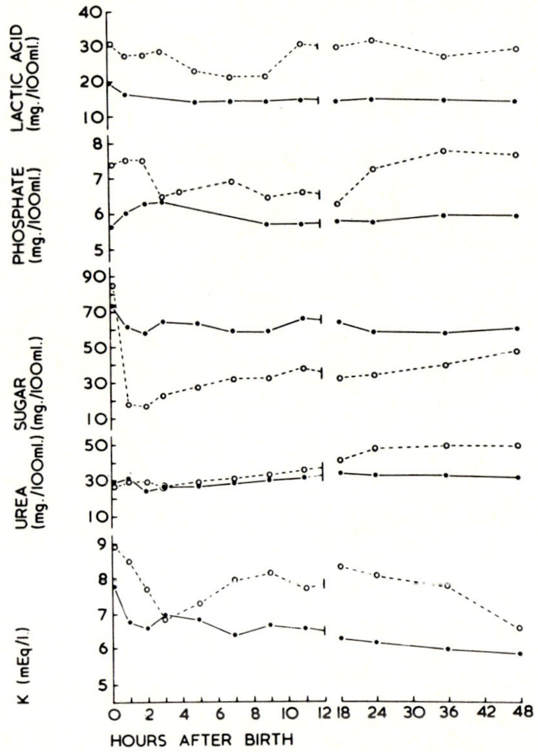


FIG. 4.—Comparison of normally born infants (●) and infants born of diabetic mothers (○).

They show similar departures from normal as in the previous groups, but the fall in blood sugar is much greater and the rise in potassium is also greater.

In Fig. 5a and b the values obtained in 4 fatal cases of RDS are shown individually, together with the normal. It will be seen that the same type of change already recorded is present to a greater degree.

## Discussion

Many factors are involved in the determination of the actual level of a given substance in the blood and our present knowledge is insufficient to give adequate explanations for all the changes observed.

The known variants at birth which could affect the blood composition can be grouped into 5 categories: (1) circulatory; (2) respiratory; (3) hormonal; (4) metabolic; and (5) environmental.

**Circulation Factors.** At birth the pulmonary circulation has to be established, and this entails the opening up of a large capillary bed. Owing to the physical factors involved in a flow of fluid containing small particles (Gairdner, Marks, Roscoe, and Brettell, 1958), a layer of plasma free from particles becomes adherent to the walls of the capillaries. This is equivalent to removing a part of the plasma of the blood and causes the PCV to increase—which happens within a few minutes.

Failure to close the ductus will lead to some blood by-passing the lungs and thus to a lowering of the oxygen saturation of the arterial blood even if the lungs are fully expanded: if expansion is only partial the blood circulating through the unexpanded parts will remain venous in character and will also lower the arterial oxygen saturation. Pathological conditions in the lungs at birth may also reduce gas exchange. Hypoxia produces incomplete combustion of the acid break-down products of carbohydrate metabolism, of which lactic acid is by far the largest individual component. This decreases the *p*H and bicarbonate by causing a metabolic acidosis proportional to the degree of hypoxia.

As a result of the acidosis there will be a transfer of H ions from plasma into cells, with a balancing transfer of K from cell to plasma as shown by the increase in plasma K in acidosis.

With regard to the high phosphorus values found, in anoxia, the only source of energy for essential body functions lies in the anaerobic breakdown of glucose to lactic acid. This gives some energy at the expense of increased metabolic acidosis. With the exhaustion of available carbohydrate, the individual cells become unable to maintain their functional stability, the so-called 'sodium pump' fails and the necessary electrical potentials on cell surfaces become discharged. The mitochondria of the cell, 'the power houses', discharge all their available active P and become disorganized; and if oxygen is not soon available the adenosine triphosphate (ATP) breaks down into its constituent parts, which escape into the circulation and cause an increase in the phosphorus, amino acids, and pentoses (McShan, Potter, Goldman, Shipley, and Meyer, 1945; Migone, 1962). This is an irreversible event and, though some organs of the body more richly endowed at birth with glycogen may survive, these cells will die, and if vital to the body, the end-result will be death to the baby. These changes are similar to those found in experimental irreversible shock, and it is suggested that the terminal stages of death in infants suffering from RDS are those of shock.

The various hormones are known to influence the chemistry of the body. The hormonal situation of the newborn is difficult to assess. *In utero* the foetus is not independent of its mother in its control of its endocrine glands, and, though all the necessary glands exist and are capable of activity, there is suggestive evidence that the maternal endocrine

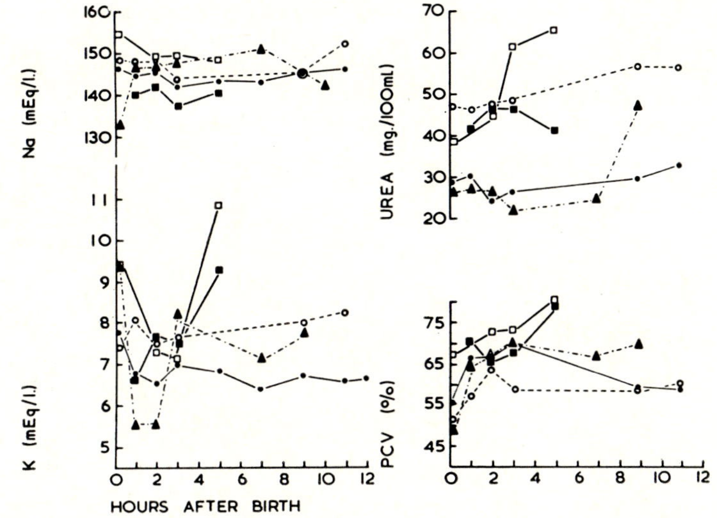


(a)

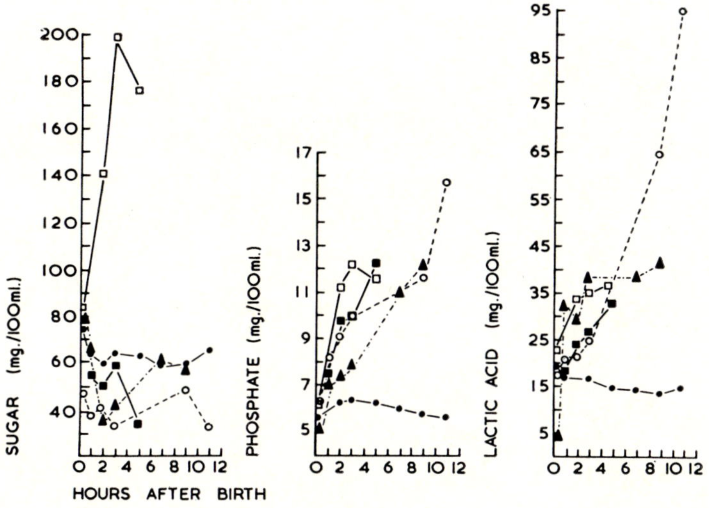


(b)

FIGS. 5 (a and b).—Blood changes in 4 infants who died with respiratory distress (○, ▲, □, ■), compared with average normal infant (●).

secretions enter the foetal circulation (Migeon, 1961) and to some extent inhibit the foetal gland activity. An additional complication is due to the existence of a large foetal zone in the suprarenal whose function is still unknown. It atrophies at birth and is replaced by adult type of cells which are present in small amounts in the foetal gland. The metabolism of the adrenal hormones is different in the newborn, and the urinary steroids are very different from the usual adult pattern (Cathro, Birchall, Mitchell, and Forsyth, 1963). Examination of the urine does not give as much information about the activity of the suprarenal gland as later on in life, but there is evidence that the neonatal suprarenal will respond to stimulation (Klein, 1955) by ACTH or by stressful situations.

The infant's parathyroids may also be affected by the high output of maternal parathyroid hormone required for the liberation of stored calcium by the mother during the last 2 months of pregnancy, when the calcium requirements of the foetus greatly exceed the maternal intake. Though at birth the calcium level in the cord blood is normal, there is a fairly constant fall in the neonatal calcium level during the next 24-48 hours (Acharya and Payne, 1965) but only occasionally a fall low enough to cause tetany. At the same time, the blood inorganic phosphate level is high when the urinary phosphate excretion is low, suggesting an effect of low level of parathormone in the renal tubules (Smith, 1959).

**Metabolic Effects.** Since from the moment of birth the infant becomes responsible for its own energy needs, and is indeed using energy in amounts varying with its environment, it has to rely on its stores of energy-producing substances; it will be many hours before its alimentary canal will be able to supply its daily needs. The main stores of energy are glycogen (Shelley, 1964) and fat (Widdowson and Spray, 1951) and a full-term infant is well endowed with both. Not all organs of the body can store energy, and so the infant will have to keep the levels of circulating energy producing substances at a level high enough for their needs. The biggest organ requiring energy is the brain, and the nerve cells do not appear to be able to utilize fat but need carbohydrate or its metabolites lactic and pyruvic acid. The mechanisms for the maintenance of a suitable level are similar to those of the adult, e.g. adrenaline and possibly glucocorticoids; but a bigger stimulus appears to be needed to bring the blood sugar up to a safe level. It seems that in the first few days of life the metabolism of the infant can maintain itself at a lower level of blood sugar than in the child or adult, but sometimes there is a difficulty in maintaining even this low level and the efforts needed may cause symptoms such as 'jitteriness', possibly a side-effect of the action of adrenaline, or actual fits, which are probably a 'final demand note' from the brain to the tissues. Fits will force the muscles to give up some of their carbohydrate stores in the form of lactic acid. Excess ACTH may also be called forth to increase the glucocorticoids, with probably also an increased mineralocorticoid effect as shown by alteration in the sodium potassium levels.

Muscles can use their stored glycogen as a source of energy, even in the absence of oxygen, but with adequate oxygen they will use free fatty acids equally as well. Normally the level of fuel is kept as constant as possible (Randle, Garland, Hales, and Newsholme, 1963) and there is an inverse relation between free fatty acid and glucose. This relation is, however, not maintained in the presence of extra insulin or adrenaline or corticoids.

In the stressed infants and in infants with low food stores, the need for fuel, and also increased corticoid secretion, leads to protein breakdown giving rise to increased blood amino acids and ultimately to increased urea production. Some of the amino acids can be turned into glucose and used as such, and it is possible that the cerebral cells can use unaltered amino acids as a source of energy. Apart from breakdown of protein in response to stress, in the absence of protein food the level of amino acid will need to be maintained to enable cell regeneration and growth to occur, and this can only be done by robbing Peter to pay Paul—i.e. less important proteins, such as serum albumin and skeletal muscle tissue, will be broken down in order to build up essential proteins. It has also been shown (Giordano, 1963) that urea can be utilized as a source of nitrogen for the non-essential amino acids—the need for essential amino acids will demand tissue protein breakdown until an adequate intake is achieved.

**Conclusions.** In the light of the preceding discussion, it is possible to guess at the causes of the variations that occurred.

The variations in potassium and sodium over the 48 hours tend to be reciprocal, but the actual levels of potassium are affected by the *p*H, by glycogen utilization, and by tissue breakdown. Sodium variations are affected only by the element of concentration due to loss of water, and the low values can most simply be related to the level of mineralocorticoids. Urea does not materially change during the first 12 hours, and no difference between normal and stressed groups occurs, but from 18 hours onward the greater the stress the higher is the urea and this can only be due to a greater amount of tissue breakdown. With sugar the difference between the normal and the stressed groups is most marked in the more stressed, but this difference gets less during the second day. This may well be due to gluconeogenesis from tissue protein, as the increase of urea occurs at this time. The rise in the phosphate could be due to $CO_2$ retention (Cordier and Piery, 1955), to liberation from the cell when glycogen is broken down to glucose, or to tissue breakdown. However, this last factor is not a likely cause since there is no increase in the blood phosphate in the second 24 hours at a time when tissue breakdown is at a maximum and, indeed, its highest level is during the earliest hours of life when glycogen is being used most rapidly.

The lactic acid level shows the most striking differences. In all the stressed groups, the level is higher throughout the whole 48 hours, except at birth when the level is also high in the normals. The two most common causes for a high lactic acid are low oxygen levels and muscular exercise. As there was no observable difference in muscular activity between the difficult labour group and the normally born group, the probable cause of the continued rise in lactic acid is a lack of oxygen, due to some shunting in the circulation; to a failure of the lungs to effect gaseous exchange in the RDS group; or to some degree of peripheral stasis, which would be shown as cyanosis of the extremities, as actually seen in about half of the stressed cases and in none of the normal cases. However, if the stressed group is divided into those with and those without cyanosis (see Fig. 3), it will be seen that those with no cyanosis had, in fact, a slightly higher lactic acid level, so peripheral stasis is probably not a cause of raised blood lactic acid.

A study of the changes in the blood chemistry of the 4 fatal cases of RDS shows a similar, but greater, departure from the normal as in the stressed group (Fig. 5a and b).

The potassium rises terminally in all, but not to a level that is lethal in the newborn infant, who seems to tolerate much higher potassium levels than older children and adults. The blood urea rises earlier but has not time to become very high. Sodium shows no material change. The most striking changes are in the sugar, which is low in 3 and very high in 1, in the phosphorus which rises rapidly, and in the lactic acid which also is very high.

Can any treatment reverse these changes? Up to the present, in the similar changes in animal experimental shock, there is no way in which fully developed shock can be corrected, but prevention by various techniques has had more success. It is by studying this aspect of the treatment of severe RDS that improved results may be obtained.

## Summary

A group of infants, born by forceps or caesarean section, of normal or toxaemic or diabetic mothers, was studied in respect of the variation in the blood levels of sodium, potassium, chloride, glucose, urea, inorganic phosphate, lactic acid, and total plasma protein during the first 48 hours of life. The results were compared with those from normal newborn infants, and certain differences were found. Two other groups of babies suffering from the respiratory distress syndrome, one group of those who recovered, the other of those who died, were also studied, and similar but greater differences noted.

It is a pleasure to acknowledge the help given us by Professor J. H. Pinkerton, Dr. A. White Franklin, and Dr. A. P. Norman, and the ward sisters and staff, especially Sister Penrice and Sister Fairbrother, and to Dr. B. C. Mukerji for technical help. We are indebted to the Board of Governors of the Hospital for a grant enabling this work to be done, and to the Medical Research Council for a personal grant to one of us (P.T.A.). Our thanks are also due to Professor J. P. M. Tizard, Dr. J. A. Davis, and Dr. J. W. Scopes for much help in the preparation of this paper.

### References

Acharya, P. T., and Payne, W. W. (1965). Blood chemistry of normal full-term infants in the first 48 hours of life. *Arch. Dis. Childh.*, **40**, 430.

Cathro, D. M., Birchall, K., Mitchell, F. L., and Forsyth, C. C. (1963). The excretion of neutral steroids in the urine of newborn infants. *J. Endocr.*, **27**, 53.

Cordier, D., and Piery, Y. (1955). Influence de l'anoxie, de l'asphyxie et de l'hypercarbie sur la teneur en phosphore inorganique du plasma du rat. Relations entre la phosphatémie et l'absorption intestinale des phosphates minéraux. *J. Physiol. (Paris)*, **47**, 147.

Gairdner, D., Marks, J., Roscoe, J. D., and Brettell, R. O. (1958). The fluid shift from the vascular compartment immediately after birth. *Arch. Dis. Childh.*, **33**, 489.

Giordano, C. (1963). Use of exogenous and endogenous urea for protein synthesis in normal and uremic subjects. *J. Lab. clin. Med.*, **62**, 231.

Klein, R. (1955). Adrenal function in infants and children, p. 31. Report of 13th M. & R. Pediatric Research Conference, Columbus, Ohio.

McShan, W. H., Potter, Van R., Goldman, A., Shipley, E. G., and Meyer, R. K. (1945). Biological energy transformations during shock as shown by blood chemistry. *Amer. J. Physiol.*, **145**, 93.

Migeon, C. J. (1961). The endocrine function of the newborn. In *Ciba Foundation Symposium on Somatic Stability in the Newly Born*, ed. G. E. W. Wolstenholme and M. O'Connor, p. 215. Churchill, London.

Migone, L. (1962). In *Shock: Pathogenesis and Therapy*, ed. D. K. Brock, p. 76. Springer, Berlin.

Randle, P. J., Garland, P. B., Hales, C. N., and Newsholme, E. A. (1963). The glucose fatty-acid cycle. Its role in insulin sensitivity and the metabolic disturbances of diabetes mellitus *Lancet*, **1**, 785.

Shelley, H. J. (1964). Carbohydrate reserves in the newborn infant. *Brit. med. J.*, **1**, 273.

Smith, C. A. (1959). The *Physiology of the Newborn Infant*, 3rd ed, p. 392. Blackwell, Oxford.

Usher, R. (1959). The respiratory distress syndrome of prematurity. I. Changes in potassium in the serum and the electrocardiogram and effects of therapy. *Pediatrics*, **24**, 562.

Widdowson, E. M., and Spray, C. M. (1951). Chemical development *in utero*. *Arch. Dis. Childh.*, **26**, 205.

*Arch. Dis. Childh.*, 1965, **40**, 442.

# NORMAL/TRISOMY 13-15 MOSAICISM IN TWO INFANTS

BY

A. D. BAIN, J. INSLEY, D. M. DOUGLAS, I. K. GAULD, and H. A. SCOTT

*From the Department of Pathology, Royal Hospital for Sick Children, Edinburgh, and the Departments of Pathology and Child Life and Health, The University, Edinburgh*

(RECEIVED FOR PUBLICATION OCTOBER 21, 1964)

It is generally accepted that there is a recognizable clinical syndrome associated with trisomy for one of the 13-15 group of chromosomes. The clinical features of this trisomic syndrome were first described by Patau, Smith, Therman, Inhorn, and Wagner (1960). In a recent paper Smith, Patau, Therman, Inhorn, and DeMars (1963) described a series of 7 cases and reviewed 7 others. The majority of the infants were either stillborn or died in early infancy with cardiac or cerebral malformations.

It is perhaps surprising that only three instances of mosaicism for trisomy 13-15 have been reported (Warkany, Rubinstein, Soukup, and Curless, 1962; Beçak, Beçak, and Schmidt, 1963). The two infants described in this paper show some of the features associated with trisomy 13-15 and have a proportion of their cells trisomic for a 13-15 chromosome.

### Case Reports

**Case 1.** A female infant, birth weight 8 lb. 1½ oz. (3,670 g.), was born at 41 weeks' gestation after a normal pregnancy. The father and mother, both aged 22, were well and unrelated.

At birth the infant was limp, breathed poorly, but responded to simple resuscitation. The following abnormal features were noted: small receding chin (Fig. 1), central cleft of soft palate extending to junction with hard palate, and port wine stain over occiput extending down over the upper part of the neck. *Right hand:* flexion of middle and ring fingers; the forefinger was flexed over the middle finger; the little finger was long and curved inwards at the junction of the proximal and middle phalanx. *Left hand:* the little finger was long and flexed inwards at the terminal phalangeal joint. The feet were large and flat but not rocker-bottomed. The eyes, lips, and skull were normal.

The infant was lethargic, did not suck, and during the first 24 hours frequently regurgitated. Twelve hours after birth she had frequent apnoeic cyanotic attacks, followed later by generalized convulsions. She died 44 hours after birth.

Necropsy revealed further abnormalities. The heart was slightly enlarged; there was a large abnormally patent foramen ovale; a small high interventricular septal defect; a large ductus arteriosus; there was no coarctation of the aorta. There was a defect in the anterior part of the falx. The brain showed poorly developed olfactory nerves but no other macroscopical abnormality. The uterus was large and septate. There was no renal or urinary tract abnormality. Buccal and bladder smears showed normal sex chromatin.

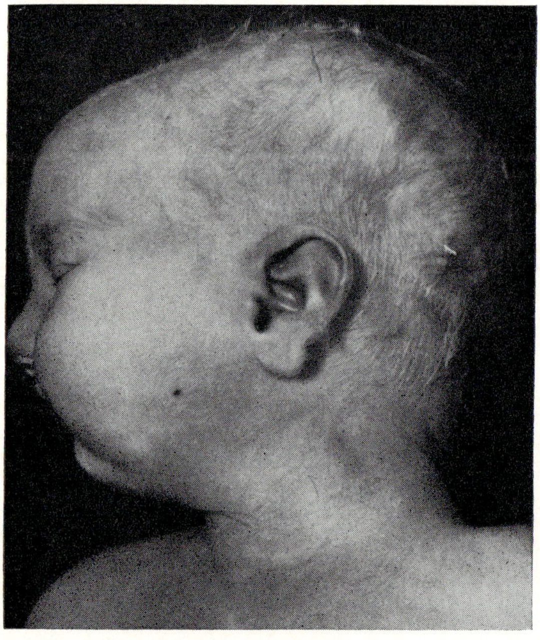

FIG. 1.—Appearance of Case 1.

**Case 2.** A male infant, birthweight 8 lb. 14 oz. (4,024 g.), was born at 42 weeks' gestation following surgical induction of labour. Moderate hypertension was noted in the fifth month of pregnancy, but this did not progress. The mother, aged 29 years, the father, aged 33 years, and two brothers, aged 5½ and 3½ years, were well. The parents were not related.

The infant was slow to breathe at birth. Subsequently he fed poorly with increasing breathlessness. The features were those seen in Fig. 2. The head was big in

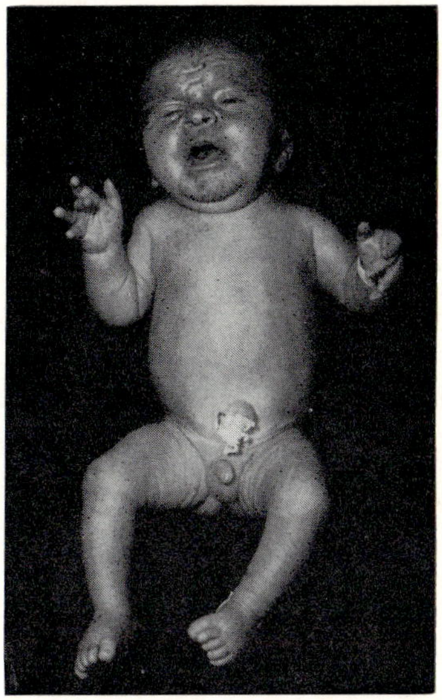

FIG. 2.—Appearance of Case 2.

comparison with the trunk, occipito-frontal circumference was 14·25 in. (36 cm.); the features were coarse; the forehead sloped backwards and the skin was grossly wrinkled; the ears were low-set. The hands showed flexion deformities of the right middle fingers and to a lesser extent of the other fingers; there was ulnar deviation of both hands, the left more than the right. The nipples were set widely apart. The heart was enlarged with a short grade II systolic murmur audible in the pulmonary area and just audible at the back of the neck. A chest radiograph confirmed cardiac enlargement. The eyes, lips, palate, and feet were normal.

Cardiac failure was diagnosed and the infant was digitalized. He died after a series of cyanotic attacks at the age of 6 weeks.

Necropsy revealed considerable cardiac enlargement particularly involving the left ventricle which showed pronounced hypertrophy of its walls. There was a subaortic stenosis; the aortic valve and the aorta were normal. The anterior part of the falx cerebri was fenestrated. The brain showed no macroscopical abnormality. There was no abnormality of the kidneys and urinary tract. Bladder and buccal smears were negative for sex chromatin.

### Chromosome Analysis

Satisfactory chromosome preparations were obtained from peripheral blood in Case 2, using a modification of the technique of Moorhead, Nowell, Mellman, Battips, and Hungerford (1960). In Case 1, the infant died shortly after admission to hospital and only post-mortem studies could be carried out. For this purpose lymphocyte cultures were prepared from thymus and spleen using the technique of Bain and Gauld (1964).

In both cases a proportion of cells showed 47 chromosomes, the extra one being in the 13-15 group (Fig. 3). The results are summarized in the Table.

Chromosomes were examined from the peripheral blood of each of the parents of both infants and were found to be normal.

TABLE

| | No. of Chromosomes | | | | | |
|---|---|---|---|---|---|---|
| | <45 | 45 | 46 | 47 | 48 | >48 |
| Case 1 { Thymus | — | — | 23 | 8 | — | — |
| Case 1 { Spleen | — | — | 12 | 21 | — | — |
| Case 2 .. .. | — | 1 | 36 | 14 | — | — |

### Discussion

These infants presented clinical features which bore some resemblance to those described for the fully developed trisomy 13-15 syndrome. They were unlike the three previously recorded cases of mosaicism involving an extra 13-15 chromosome.

The clinical features usually associated with trisomy 13-15 are as follows: anomalies of the eyeball; polydactyly and/or fixed finger flexion; deformed or low-set ears; cleft palate; deformities of the external genitalia and/or undescended testes in the male and septate uterus in the female; various heart defects; gross deformity of the brain; hare-lip; haemangiomata, and simian palm creases. Most survivors were judged to be mentally retarded and deaf. Many suffered recurrent apnoeic or convulsive episodes.

One infant, however (Marshall, Newnham, Rawstron, Ellis, and Stevens, 1964), who presented most of these features, was found to have a normal karyotype.

The two mosaics described here did not fully conform to the pattern of a 13-15 trisomy. The disproportionately large head, the coarse facies, and deep wrinkling of the brow present in Case 2 are not recognized features of the syndrome. Both infants, however, showed fixed finger flexion and congenital heart disease, indication sufficient to warrant chromosome investigation.

The three previously reported cases with this form of mosaicism were all males. In that described by Warkany *et al.* (1962) there was fixed finger flexion; deformities of the toes; absent patellae; and asymmetry of the face and legs together with speech and motor defects. In this case there was unexplained heart failure but congenital heart disease was never proved. The other two males, who were unrelated, had generalized congenital analgesia and mild mental retardation (Beçak *et al.*, 1963).

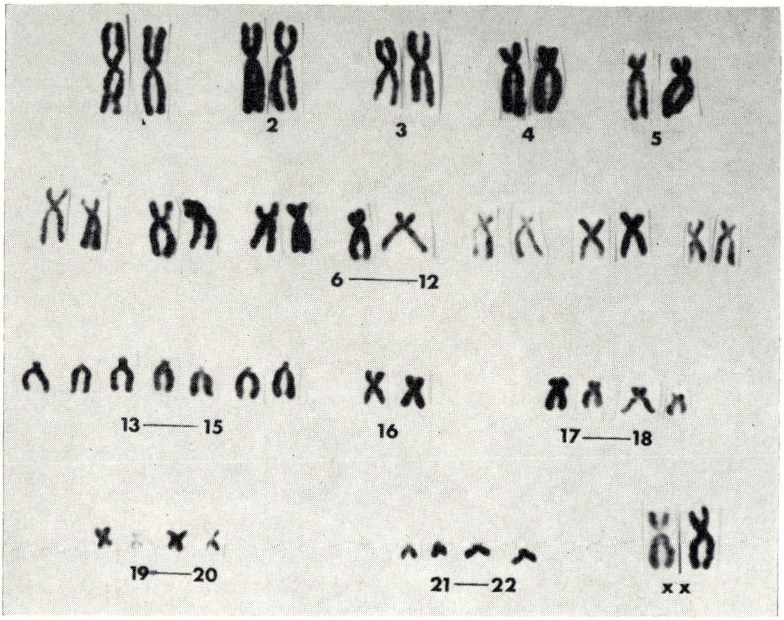


(a)

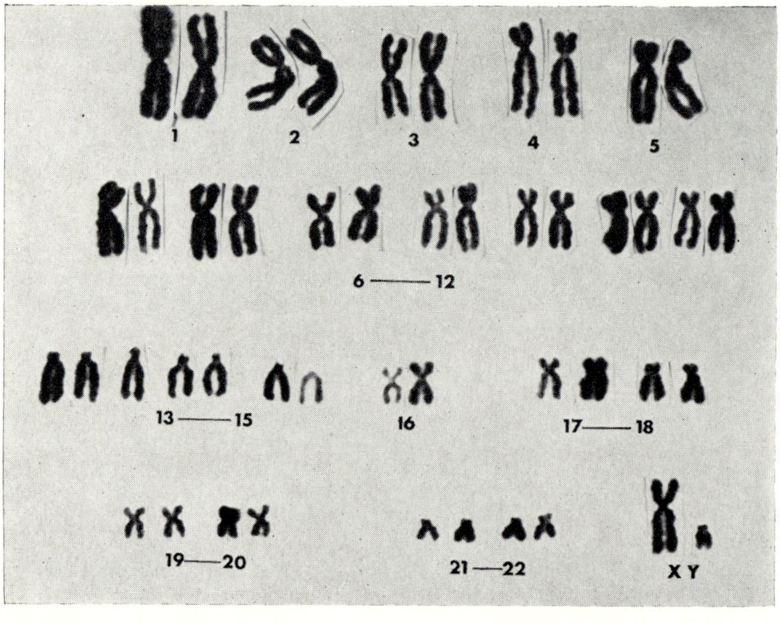


(b)

FIG. 3.—(a) 13-15 chromosomes from Case 1 (thymus), and (b) Case 2 (blood).

**Summary**

Two cases of trisomic mosaicism for chromosomes 13-15 are reported. Each showed some of the features of trisomy 13-15 and both died in early infancy.

This work was supported by a grant from the Distillers Company Ltd., to the University of Edinburgh, and by the Board of Management, Royal Hospital for Sick Children, Edinburgh.

REFERENCES

Bain, A. D., and Gauld, I. K. (1964). The use of thymus and spleen in the demonstration of chromosomes post mortem in foetuses and infants. *Brit. J. exp. Path.*, **45**, 530.

Beçak, W., Beçak, M. L., and Schmidt, B. J. (1963). Chromosome trisomy of group 13-15 in two cases of generalised congenital analgesia. *Lancet*, **1**, 664.

Marshall, R., Newnham, R. E., Rawstron, J. R., Ellis, J. R., and Stevens, L. J. (1964). Features of 13-15 trisomy syndrome with normal karyotype. *ibid.*, **1**, 556.

Moorhead, P. S., Nowell, P. C., Mellman, W. J., Battips, D. M., and Hungerford, D. A. (1960). Chromosome preparations of leukocytes cultured from human peripheral blood. *Exp. Cell Res.*, **20**, 613.

Patau, K., Smith, D. W., Therman, E., Inhorn, S. L., and Wagner, H. P. (1960). Multiple congenital anomaly caused by an extra autosome. *Lancet*, **1**, 790.

Smith, D. W., Patau, K., Therman, E., Inhorn, S. L., and DeMars, R. I. (1963). The $D_1$ trisomy syndrome. *J. Pediat.*, **62**, 326.

Warkany, J., Rubinstein, J. H., Soukup, S. W., and Curless, M. C. (1962). Mental retardation, absence of patellae, other malformations with chromosomal mosaicism. *ibid.*, 61, 803.

*Arch. Dis. Childh.*, 1965, **40**, 446.

# BRITISH PAEDIATRIC ASSOCIATION

**Proceedings of the Thirty-sixth Annual Meeting**

The Annual Meeting of the British Paediatric Association was held in Scarborough from April 21 to 24, 1965.

The following members of the Association were present:

*Honorary Members:* F. M. B. Allen, Sir George Godber, S. K. Guthrie, P. Henderson, A. R. Macgregor, Sir Alan Moncrieff, W. W. Payne, B. E. Schlesinger, Sir Wilfrid Sheldon, and Cicely D. Williams.

*Corresponding Member:* R. McIntosh.

*Ordinary Members:* A. G. V. Aldridge, E. C. Allibone, I. M. Anderson, H. Angelman, J. D. Andrew, J. Apley, G. C. Arneil, M. W. Arthurton, R. Astley, M. D. Baber, R. G. G. Barry, T. E. D. Beavan, E. M. Belton, A. C. Blandy, A. Bogdan, J. P. Bound, B. D. Bower, T. A. Brand, R. W. Brookfield, R. J. K. Brown, M. F. G. Buchanan, J. H. Burkinshaw, D. Burman, E. A. J. Byrne, A. H. Cameron, W. A. B. Campbell, W. H. P. Cant, C. O. Carter, A. E. Claireaux, P. R. Clay, B. E. Clayton, E. N. Coleman, D. G. Cottom, E. C. R. Couper, S. D. M. Court, P. J. N. Cox, E. M. Creak, K. W. Cross, V. M. Crosse, A. A. Cunningham, J. G. Dathan, J. A. Davis, W. M. Dennison, M. E. Disney, R. H. Dobbs, S. P. Dundon, M. Eastwood, M. Egan, F. M. R. Elgood, H. L. Ellis, R. W. B. Ellis, J. W. Farquhar, G. V. Feldman, H. V. L. Finlay, J. O. Forfar, R. M. Forrester, A. W. Franklin, M. S. Fraser, M. J. L. Frazer, A. A. H. Gailey, D. M. T. Gairdner, W. F. Gaisford, B. Gans, D. H. Garrow, J. M. Garvie, H. McC. Giles, E. Goldblatt, G. R. Griffith, L. Haas, E. W. Hart, C. C. Harvey, J. D. Hay, J. L. Henderson, W. Henderson, J. P. Heycock, E. E. Hill, A. Holzel, T. H. Hughes-Davies, J. L. P. Hunter, J. H. Hutchison, K. Hugh-Jones, R. S. Illingworth, R. J. Isaac, A. D. M. Jackson, R. H. Jackson, U. James, S. E. M. Jarvis, H. Everley Jones, L. F. Jones, M. C. Joseph, A. J. Keay, K. R. Keay, M. M. Kerr, C. W. Kesson, G. M. Komrower, B. M. Laurance, D. N. Lawson, J. Luder, P. MacArthur, D. Macaulay, A. M. MacDonald, R. I. Mackay, M. M. McLean, B. McNicholl, T. P. Mann, W. J. Matheson, R. M. Mayon-White, R. A. Miller, R. G. Mitchell, J. N. Montgomery, D. C. Morley, D. Morris, M. B. Morris, J. H. Moseley, P. D. Moss, G. H. Newns, T. C. Noble, A. P. Norman, T. E. Oppé, J. N. O'Reilly, A. P. M. Page, C. G. Parsons, D. Pickering, J. W. Platt, B. W. Powell, L. J. Prosser, R. J. Pugh, J. P. R. Rees, I. D. Riley, E. G. G. Roberts, K. B. Rogers, J. Rubie, J. Sakula, T. R. Savage, L. G. Scott, O. Scott, R. A. Shanks, J. D. Sheward, M. J. Simpkiss, K. Simpson, W. C. Smallwood, R. E. Smith, R. W. Smithells, A. L. Speirs, J. M. Stansfeld, R. E. Steen, J. K. Steward, D. G. H. Stone, W. P. Sweetnam, James Thomson, John Thomson, D. C. Thursby-Pelham, J. J. Tillie, J. P. M. Tizard, W. M. L. Turner, C. Upjohn, D. G. Vulliamy, C. B. M. Warren, A. G. Watkins, B. W. Webb, R. G. Welch, I. G. Wickes, R. Wigglesworth, A. W. Wilkinson, H. P. Williams, D. A. J. Williamson, M. J. Wilmers, S. G. F. Wilson, O. H. Wolff, B. Wolman, B. S. B. Wood, B. Woodhead, T. Wright, W. F. Young, S. Yudkin, R. B. Zachary.

*Newly-elected Members:* I. M. Cullum, P. Davies, V. Dubowitz, M. Dynski-Klein, A. W. Ferguson, N. T. Jaco, C. S. Livingstone, E. McKay, N. M. Mann, S. Mason, S. Russell, W. H. Schutt, C. H. M. Walker, P. Wallis.

The following were present as guests of the Association: Dr. Henry Barnett, Sir George Godber, Mr. G. J. Piller, and Dr. Cicely Williams.

The following attended the meeting as guests of members of the Association:

A. Adiao, R. H. Alway, R. Asfour, F. N. Bamford, D. Barltrop, H. Barrie, B. Bayes, R. Chamberlain, G. W. Chance, R. Evans, W. Gottfried, M. Griffiths, D. R. Harvey, D. Holdaway, D. Hull, O. N. Jayaswal, E. Jones, M. Lawrence, B. Leonard, B. Lepshitz, S. Lewis, J. McAinsh, T. McKendrick, V. Marrian, H. Marwick, J. Meredith, B. J. Naidoo, G. Pampiglione, R. Pearce, D. Pickering, A. Piesowicz, J. Perez del Pulgar, R. Roberts, D. C. Robinson, P. Rowlands, D. Rush, P. Russell, I. B. Sardharwalla, J. Shackleton, W. Shakespeare, B. Smith, C. Sohn, G. P. Solimano, L. Stimmler, T. Takeuchi, E. Tempany, S. M. Tucker, G. C. Turner, R. H. R. White, R. K. Whitmore, Y-M Yang. The three Heinz Fellows for 1965 were present: Dr. A. E. Dugdale, Mr. A. McKellar, and Dr. P. T. Wei.

The Annual General Meeting was held on Thursday, April 22, 1965, with the President, Professor Wilfrid Gaisford, in the chair.

The Minutes of the last meeting, which had been published in the *Archives of Disease in Childhood*, were received and approved.

Election of Officers. The following were elected:

President: Professor R. W. B. Ellis.

President-Elect: Professor A. G. Watkins.

Honorary Treasurer: Professor J. D. Hay.

Honorary Secretary: Dr. T. E. Oppé.

Members of Council 1965-68: Dr. E. W. Hart,

Dr. J. B. Heycock, Professor R. G. Mitchell, Dr. B. S. B. Wood.

Honorary Members: Professor Wilfrid Gaisford, Dr. Cécile Asher, Dr. E. M. Creak, Dr. V. M. Crosse, Dr. D. Taylor.

Ordinary Members: Dr. Iris M. Cullum (Boston), Dr. Pamela Davies (Oxford), Dr. M. Dawkins (London), Dr. V. Dubowitz (Sheffield), Dr. Martha Dynski-Klein (London), Dr. A. W. Ferguson (Bedford), Dr. E. G. Fox (Glasgow), Dr. L. A. Hawkins (Doncaster), Dr. N. T. Jaco (Truro), Dr. J. D. Kershaw (Colchester), Dr. C. S. Livingstone (Dewsbury), Dr. Joan B. T. Logan (Belfast), Dr. E. McKay (Aberdeen), Dr. N. M. Mann (Manchester), Dr. S. Mason (London), Dr. E. P. G. Michell (London), Dr. Patricia Mortimer (London), Dr. Sheenah Russell (Dumfries), Dr. W. H. Schutt (Edinburgh), Dr. C. H. M. Walker (Dundee), Dr. Patricia Wallis (London).

The Honorary Treasurer's report and statement of accounts for 1964-65 were received and approved and the auditors reappointed for the following year.

The report of the Council was received and approved and is printed below.

**Report of the Council, 1964-65**

1. Obituaries. The Association has suffered the loss of two Original Members—C. McNeil and A. E. Naish, J. J. Mason Brown, an Honorary Member, and A. F. Hartmann and André Thomas, Corresponding Members.

2. Distinctions. The Council has noted with great pleasure the distinction of a Knighthood which has been conferred on Professor Alan Moncrieff, an Honorary member and past President.

3. Council Membership. The membership of the Council during 1964-65 has been: Professor Wilfrid Gaisford, Dr. G. C. Arneil, Dr. P. T. Bray, Dr. Beryl Corner, Professor R. W. B. Ellis, Dr. J. W. Farquhar, Dr. A. A. H. Gailey, Dr. R. R. Gordon, Dr. E. W. Hart, Professor J. D. Hay, Dr. W. Henderson, Dr. B. Laurance, Dr. T. P. Mann, Dr. A. P. Norman, Dr. T. E. Oppé, Sir Wilfrid Sheldon, Dr. R. W. Smithells, Professor O. H. Wolff, and Dr. S. Yudkin. *Observers*. The Council has been greatly indebted to Dr. Roma Chamberlain, Ministry of Health, and Dr. T. K. Whitmore, Department of Education and Science, for their assistance to Council.

4. Meetings. Council has met on four occasions since its last report: on June 13, 1964, November 7, 1964, February 13, 1965, and April 3, 1965.

5. In addition to receiving reports from Standing and sub-committees, the following matters were considered:

6. Policy Matters concerning internal administration of Association.

*Resignations*. Council has received resignation from membership from Dr. F. F. Kane, Dr. D. N. Nicholson, Dr. M. Capes, and Dr. T. N. Fisher.

*Heinz Fellows of the British Paediatric Association*. Dr. A. E. Dugdale (Brisbane), Mr. A. MacKellar (Perth), and Dr. P. T. Wei (Hong Kong) have been awarded "A" Fellowships for 1965 and will be attending the Annual Meeting at Scarborough.

*James Spence Medal*. The James Spence Medal for 1965 has been awarded to Dr. Cicely Williams in recognition of her outstanding contributions in the field of tropical paediatrics. Dr. Williams will be the guest of the Association at Scarborough and the medal will be presented at the Annual Dinner.

*Rules of the Association*. Council has given consideration to the problems of overseas membership, Honorary membership, and regional representation on Council. Certain alterations to the Rules of the Association are proposed by Council and will be included on the agenda of the Annual General Meeting.

*Faculty of Paediatrics or Academic Body*. Arising from a memorandum from Professor Hubble and a recommendation from the Standing Committee on Education, Council has on several occasions discussed the possible establishment of an academic body. At the February meeting Council accepted the desirability of establishing an academic body within the framework of the Association to be responsible for matters relating to paediatric education and the advancement of paediatric knowledge. Professor R. W. B. Ellis, Professor D. V. Hubble, and Dr. T. E. Oppé are members of a working party which is considering the detailed functions of an academic body; an appropriate title; the integration of the body within the administrative framework of the B.P.A.; the cost of maintaining such a body; and ways in which the cost can be met. Council awaits a further report of the working party and will keep members informed on the progress of this scheme.

*Special Committee on Medical Education of the General Medical Council*. The Association has been invited to submit a memorandum on the place of paediatrics in the undergraduate curriculum, in preregistration house appointments, and postgraduate education.

Council believes that this is one of the most important matters that have arisen in recent years and has set up a special *ad-hoc* sub-committee to consider the matter and to prepare a memorandum. The President, Dr. F. S. W. Brimblecombe, Dr. E. W. Hart, Professor J. D. Hay, Professor D. V. Hubble, Professor J. H. Hutchison, Dr. B. M. Laurance, Dr. T. E. Oppé (Secretary), Dr. R. C. MacKeith, and Dr. G. Neligan have been invited to serve.

Council has chosen the topic 'Paediatrics in the undergraduate curriculum' for the evening discussion at Scarborough.

Dr. T. E. Oppé will be glad to hear from any members wishing to communicate with the *ad-hoc* sub-committee (Dr. T. E. Oppé, Paediatric Unit, St. Mary's Hospital, London W.2).

*Memoranda Published by the Association*. Council has decided that members should be provided with a list of the memoranda which have been produced by the Association during the past five years. This will be sent out with the handbook each year.

7. Discussions with the Ministry of Health.

*Medical Statistics of the Ministry of Health*. The first census of children and adolescents in hospital on June 24, 1964, is still being analysed by the Ministry statisticians. The date for the second census will not be decided until the first analysis has been completed.

*Conference on Maternity Services*. At the invitation of the Chief Medical Officer, the Association was represented by Sir Wilfrid Sheldon and Dr. F. S. W. Brimblecombe at a discussion on the Maternity Services. There was full discussion of the implications of 48-hour discharge and the possible increase in children's ward admissions which might result from this. Representations were made to the Ministry requesting that paediatricians should be included in any discussions when a 48-hour discharge scheme was considered in an area.

*Care of Children with Meningomyeloceles.* Sir George Godber wrote to the President expressing concern on this problem and inviting the Association to nominate representatives to serve on a committee to consider this matter. Dr. R. W. Smithells and Dr. R. H. Forrester represented the Association and reported that the meeting had been useful and that the Ministry recognized the size and extent of the problem and believed that the best solution was the enhancement of existing facilities. The problem of how this could best be done had been referred to the Standing Medical Advisory Committee of the Ministry, and further information as to their decisions was awaited.

*Notification of Infectious Disease.* The Ministry sought the opinion of the Association regarding the desirability of continuing notification of ophthalmia neonatorum. The Council decided to advise that notification of ophthalmia neonatorum was unnecessary; that the regulations should be amended; and that notification should be confined to cases of gonococcal ophthalmia.

*Senior Registrar Establishment—Platt Review Committee Report.* On the invitation of the Royal College of Physicians, the President and the Honorary Secretary attended a meeting at the Ministry of Health to consider the Senior Registrar establishment in paediatrics. The establishment was reviewed in the light of vacancies due to death, retirement, and the creation of new consultant posts advocated in the Platt Review Committee Report. The total increase in the Senior Registrar establishment recommended to fill these vacancies appeared to be three or four extra posts.

*Safety Measures in Nursing Children in Hospital.* Following the death of two children attributed to the use of restrainers, the Ministry called a meeting to consider safety measures in the nursing of children in hospital, with especial reference to the use of restrainers. Dr. Trevor Mann and the Secretary represented the Association. A draft report of the recommendations drawn up by the Committee was submitted to Council and approved. The Ministry will publish the memorandum. Further meetings will be held to consider the design of beds and cots for use in children's units.

*'Battered Baby' Syndrome.* Sir George Godber wrote to the President saying that he had been informed that the Accidents in Childhood Committee was to consider the problem of 'the battered baby'. Sir George offered the fullest co-operation of the Ministry in this matter. This offer was gratefully received and referred to the Accidents in Childhood Standing Committee to assist in their consideration of the problem.

8. STANDING COMMITTEES OF THE ASSOCIATION.

*Mental Health*—No report.

*Nursing.* The General Nursing Council has informed the Nursing Committee that it is not its intention at present to close the Sick Children's Nurses' Register. The G.N.C. also stated its requirement of occupied beds to permit the use of a hospital as a training school for the R.S.C.N. qualification. This figure was lower than had previously been stated and will permit the majority of children's hospitals to continue as training schools. With the permission of the G.N.C. this document was circulated to all members for their information.

Through our representation in Scotland and Ulster, similar assurances were obtained from the Nursing Councils in Scotland and Northern Ireland, respectively.

*Standing Joint Committee with the Royal College of Obstetricians and Gynaecologists.* This Committee, which has not met for a number of years, has been revived and has met to discuss the responsibilities and status of the paediatrician in the care of newborn infants. The paediatric staffing and sessional requirements for the care of the newborn and special care units have also been discussed. At present only a draft report has been submitted and is still under review.

*Accidents in Childhood.* The problem of the 'battered baby' has occupied the time of the Committee during this year. A memorandum is in preparation outlining the way in which this problem should be handled. The Committee is also preparing a memorandum on Accidents in Childhood which it is hoped will be accepted for publication in the medical press.

*Paediatric Nomenclature.* The Committee has worked throughout the year reviewing and revising the International Classification of Disease and the Cardiff Classification of paediatric conditions.

*Heinz Fellowship Committee.* As reported elsewhere in this document, Heinz Fellowships for 1965 have been awarded. Messrs. H. J. Heinz have generously increased their total award from £2,500 to £3,000 per annum in order that the same number of awards may be made each year, despite the increased cost of travel and maintenance.

*Hospitals Committee.* An interim report has been received.

*Education Committee.* 'Careers in Paediatrics', a report prepared by the Education Committee, was published in the *Archives of Disease in Childhood.*

A further report suggested the establishment of an academic body and this is mentioned elsewhere in this document. Other matters concerning paediatric education are still under consideration by Council.

*Overseas Committee.* No report is yet available. The response to the questionnaire was very disappointing and only 25 replies were received. These are still being analysed and a report is awaited.

*Standing Committee for Scotland.* A Standing Committee for Scotland has been set up 'to represent the B.P.A. in discussion of matters of paediatric interest and importance in Scotland with the Department of Home and Health'.

Professor J. O. Forfar, Professor J. L. Henderson, Professor J. H. Hutchison, Dr. P. MacArthur, Professor R. G. Mitchell, and Dr. James Thomson have been invited to serve.

9. AD-HOC COMMITTEES.

*Hypercalcaemia Sub-committee.* The report of the Committee has been published in the *British Medical Journal* (June 27, 1964, **1**, 1659-1661).

*Ad-hoc Sub-committee on Register of Handicapped Children in Scotland.* The Principal Medical Officer, Scottish Department of Home and Health, invited the Association to submit comments on his proposed scheme for a Register of Handicapped Children. Council invited the Professors of Child Health in Scotland to submit a memorandum. This was gratefully acknowledged by the Principal Medical Officer who then asked whether a Scottish Committee was available for the direct reference of such problems. It is from this concept that the Standing Committee for Scotland has grown.

10. REPRESENTATIVES OF THE ASSOCIATION ON OTHER BODIES.

*British Committee for the Scientific Study of Mental Deficiency.* Professor J. P. M. Tizard has resigned and has been replaced by Dr. G. Komrower.

*National Bureau for Co-operation in Child Care.* Dr. A. White Franklin has been appointed as the representative of the Association.

*Medical Commission on Accident Prevention.* Dr. V. Smallpeice represents the Association.

11. CORRESPONDENCE WITH OTHER ASSOCIATIONS OR OFFICIAL BODIES.

*Mother Care for Children in Hospital Committee.* Correspondence has been exchanged with the M.C.C.H. Committee concerning the visiting of children in hospital, and paediatric teaching.

*Central Midwives Board—Definition of the Lying-in Period.* The Central Midwives Board has been undertaking a revision of its rules and has requested the opinion of the Association regarding its definition of the lying-in period. Council submitted comments on the draft definition and expressed the hope that the term 'lying-in period' would give place to 'postnatal period' as quickly as legislation permitted. The suggested definition which was put forward was: 'Lying-in period (or postnatal period) means a period after the end of labour during which the continued attendance of the midwife in the interests of the mother and child is necessary.'

*General Register Office—modification of death certificate in the perinatal period.* The Registrar General set up a small committee to consider whether the death certificate in the perinatal period could be modified to give more information. The Association was invited to nominate a representative, and Dr. N. Butler was appointed to serve. No report is yet available.

*Medical Examination for Adoption.* Dr. Everley Jones asked Council to reconsider the problem of the medical examination of children for adoption. Professor Illingworth raised the question of the necessity for serological tests for syphilis in children who were to be adopted. Council considered these problems and learnt that the National Conference of Societies Registered for Adoption had a medical sub-committee (which included three B.P.A. members) which was considering these problems. An exchange of correspondence with the National Conference of Societies Registered for Adoption led Council to decide to defer further consideration of these problems until the report of the medical sub-committee was available.

*Play Needs of Children in Hospital.* The Save the Children Fund has set up a committee to consider the play needs of children in hospital. Dr. D. Morris has represented the Association at a preliminary meeting.

12. OTHER MATTERS CONSIDERED BY COUNCIL.

*Visit to Finland.* Twenty members of the Association were the guests of the Finnish Paediatric Association in August 1964, and visited Helsinki and Turku. The Association presented a Visitors Book to the Finnish Paediatric Association as a memento of a memorable visit and wonderful hospitality.

*Children's Medical and Surgical Center, Baltimore.* Dr. A. White Franklin represented the Association at the dedication exercises of the Center and presented a Visitors Book as a gift from the Association.

*International Paediatric Association.* Bulletins from the I.P.A. have been circulated to all members and information concerning the International Paediatric Congress in Tokyo.

*Donald Paterson Prize Essay.* The Prize Essay for 1966 has been advertised in the medical press. Members are reminded to bring this to the notice of possible candidates.

Council recommended alterations to the Rules of the Association as follows:

*Rule 2.* Council proposed that the rule shall be amended to read: 'It shall consist of Ordinary Members, Honorary Members and those Corresponding Members appointed before 1962. Ordinary Members at the time of nomination shall be actively engaged in the practice or teaching of paediatrics or in paediatric research. In addition individuals who have contributed to the advancement of paediatrics in the allied specialties may be nominated for Ordinary Membership, but election of these will be on a restricted basis and maintain a balance between the specialties. Nominations for election to Honorary Membership shall be restricted to Ordinary Members on their retirement, and to individuals in the United Kingdom or Overseas, whom the Association wishes to honour. Retirement from active practice shall not debar an individual from continuing as an Ordinary Member of the Association.'

*Rule 3.* Council proposed the following addition to the rule: 'Observers from the Ministry of Health and such other bodies as Council may from time to time deem advantageous shall be invited to attend meetings of Council and Annual General Meetings.'

*Rule 4.* Council proposed that the last paragraph shall be altered to read: 'No candidate may be proposed for election to these offices unless his or her name, duly proposed and seconded, has been submitted to the Secretary at least three months before the Annual Meeting.'

*Rule 11.* Council proposed that in paragraph 3 '. . . to the Secretary before the Annual Meeting' shall be altered to '. . . to the Secretary at the Annual Meeting' and that 'Scrutineers shall be appointed by the General Meeting' shall be altered to 'Scrutineers shall be appointed at the General Meeting'.

*Rule 12.* Council proposed that the first line shall be altered to read: 'Scientific communications should be spoken . . .'

*Rule 14.* Council proposed that 'Their names shall be entered in a book provided for the purpose' shall be changed to read 'Their names shall be entered on the attendance sheets provided for the purpose'.

*Rule 16.* Council proposed that Rule 16 shall be deleted from the Rules of the Association.

These alterations were approved by the meeting.

The President then declared the Annual General Meeting closed.

**Scientific Sessions**

Scientific Sessions were held in the Royal Hotel, Scarborough, on April 22 and 23 and the following communications were presented:

A. W. WILKINSON (London). 'Giant Haemangio-lymphangioma.' In this condition there is at birth extensive enlargement of one or more limbs and sometimes part of the trunk due to a congenital obstruction of lymphatic drainage. The subcutaneous tissue is largely replaced by fibrous tissue surrounding cystic spaces filled with lymph. This is associated with haemangiomatous staining of the skin. The enlargement of the limb is progressive and may be associated with excessive growth in length of the bones in the affected area.

The clinical features, histological appearances, and surgical management were described and illustrated.

C. H. M. WALKER, introduced by PROFESSOR J. L. HENDERSON (Dundee). 'Partial Perfusion for Neonatal Respiratory Distress.' A system has been devised for partial perfusion of newborn infants with respiratory distress. Extracorporeal flow and volume are regulated by a weight-servo electronic control so that the patient is maintained at $\pm$ 5 g. of the starting body-weight. The data from 97 puppy experiments demonstrate the value of careful weight control, accurate pre-perfusion temperature, and biochemical monitoring. Histological sections reveal the importance of haemodilution of the perfusate blood. This system has proved capable of sustaining life in totally apnoeic infants and of providing well-controlled haemodialysis in newborn infants with renal failure.

D. M. T. GAIRDNER (Cambridge). 'Acid-base Changes Following Exchange Transfusion with Citrated Blood.' The electrolyte in A.C.D. blood consists of 2 parts of trisodium citrate to 1 part of citric acid, and forms a buffered system with a blood *p*H of about 6·7. Transfusion therefore leads to (1) an immediate metabolic *acidosis*, which is followed by (2) a metabolic *alkalosis* as the citrate is metabolized to bicarbonate. The rates at which these two effects operate vary in different babies, and determine how severe is the acidosis that develops initially, and at what stage acidosis is replaced by alkalosis.

The blood *p*H, $Pco_2$, bicarbonate, and citrate levels were measured in 17 babies during and following exchange transfusion. There was a marked difference in the handling of citrate between babies of less than 1 day old, who tended to develop a more or less severe metabolic acidosis, and those of a few days old, who metabolized citrate fast enough to neutralize the citric acid transfused.

After transfusion a marked alkalosis developed in all the babies, which was sustained for at least 3 days. The correction of this alkalosis could be hastened by adding NaCl to the feeds, showing that the slow correction was partly due to the low Cl intake of babies fed milk. Adding $NH_4Cl$ to feeds further hastened the correction of the alkalosis.

The practical implications of both the initial acidosis and the later alkalosis were discussed.

B. J. LEONARD, introduced by DR. B. M. LAURANCE (Derby) 'White Cell Alkaline Phosphatase in the Developing Foetus.' Because of the consistently low or absent activity of alkaline phosphatase in the neutrophils in myeloid leukaemia, the development of this enzyme in the white cells in the foetus and in the newborn has been investigated. The results of a cytochemical technique for demonstrating this enzyme have been made in 84 normal adults, 59 full-term infants, and 239 premature infants as young as to the 27th week. Normal full-term infants have values from 4-9 times the normal adult level. The same high phosphatase activity was seen in prematurity, the enzyme appearing very early in intrauterine life. Approximately 15% of normal full-term infants and 15% of premature infants do not show this increase in white cell alkaline phosphatase activity. Some of these develop jaundice in the newborn period and require replacement transfusions. This jaundice is not associated with any blood group incompatibility between the mother and infant but is always associated with an absence or considerable reduction in white cell alkaline phosphatase activity. The values are as low as in leukaemic white cells.

These findings are compared with the white cell alkaline phosphatase activity in collagen disorders, pregnancy, and following the administration of steroids in normal and leukaemic patients.

A. MACKELLAR (Perth, Western Australia), Heinz Fellow. 'Mycobacterial Lymphadenitis in Childhood.' A study was made of approximately 32 patients with the following aims. (a) To show that in Western Australia, as in many other countries, mycobacterial lymphadenitis in childhood is due mainly to anonymous strains. (b) To describe the clinical features, histology, and bacteriology, with special reference to the value of double Mantoux testing. (c) To discuss the management.

CICELY D. WILLIAMS (London). 'Populations and Paediatrics.' Problems of over-population are attracting a great deal of attention both in the developed and in the less-developed countries. There is some danger that by reducing the birth rate many people will believe that malnutrition is reduced, and that the quality of a population is thereby automatically improved.

More attention to the social aspects of paediatrics will enable paediatricians and other doctors to advise governments and communities with respect to policies in child care.

R. H. JACKSON (Newcastle upon Tyne). 'Tuberous Sclerosis in Childhood.' In recent years 12 children have been diagnosed in the Department of Child Health,

Newcastle, as having tuberous sclerosis. In addition, an assessment has been made of all cases occurring in children throughout the region. The main clinical features are described: these include convulsions, mental retardation, enlarged kidneys, phakomata in the fundi, and skin lesions. Illustrations of the eye and skin lesions will be shown. Tuberous sclerosis is not commonly diagnosed in childhood, and it is felt that a wider knowledge of its clinical presentation in infancy and early childhood would lead to earlier and more frequent diagnosis.

G. Pampiglione, introduced by Dr. A. E. Claireaux (London). 'Some Neurophysiological and Neuropathological Observations in 'Infantile Spasms'.' The reports on the post-mortem findings in patients with the syndrome of infantile spasms are few. Fewer still are the patients in whom an adequate clinical and neurophysiological documentation could be carried out during the course of the disease. The present contribution is based on observations made on 9 children who had been admitted to The Hospital for Sick Children and whose brains became available for post-mortem examination. No lesions could be recognized in 3 patients. The possible relationship of the gross lesions found in the remaining 6 was discussed in relation to some of the neurophysiological findings.

M. Laurence, introduced by Professor A. G. Watkins (Cardiff). 'Survey of Major Central Nervous System Abnormalities in South Wales.' Exhaustive ascertainment of all the cases of major central nervous system malformation (anencephaly, spina bifida, cranium bifidum, and congenital hydrocephalus) that occurred in the South Wales mining valleys and the Vale of Glamorgan between 1956 and 1962 showed the area to have probably the highest central nervous system malformation rate in the world with 10 per 1,000 births. There were in addition very marked local differences in the incidence between 3/1,000 and 14/1,000 births. In order to find the possible factors responsible for these variations and therefore perhaps their causes, and to obtain some genetic and family risk data, the affected families and their controls were interviewed. Some of these results, and the implications for the community, were presented.

E. M. Creak (London). 'Some Aspects of Mental Handicap Studied in the 'Thousand Families Survey'.' Observations recorded for 15 years on randomly selected children (The Thousand Families survey) should provide information likely to aid our understanding of mental subnormality. These records were, therefore, scanned for severely subnormal children (3), children in E.S.N. schools (10), and a group of 20 others whose level of intelligence, tested within the survey, seemed no higher than that of the 10 in E.S.N. schools.

Particular attention was directed towards the early developmental history. Findings suggest that mental subnormality, sufficient to cause severe school difficulty, may not be manifest until the demands created by school attendance bring it to light. Reasons for this and the outcome to date in these three groups of children were discussed.

R. H. R. White, introduced by Dr. P. R. Evans (London). 'The Pathology of the Nephrotic Syndrome.' Percutaneous renal biopsy has been performed on 60 children with the nephrotic syndrome during the past two years. Lesions seen by optical microscopy have been classified as *proliferative* and *non-proliferative*, and divided according to severity into grades I (minimal changes), II (moderate), and III (severe). Specimens from some patients in grades II and III show features suggesting a post-streptococcal aetiology. Macroscopic haematuria, hypertension, and azotaemia at the time of onset have little diagnostic significance but, with one exception, macroscopic haematuria only occurred in grade III patients, in which it was associated with renal insufficiency. Proteinuria is less selective with proliferative than non-proliferative lesions and is least selective in grade III patients.* Grade I patients generally respond well to steroid therapy, grade II patients more often show residual proteinuria, and grade III patients respond poorly. Of 18 patients who had repeat renal biopsies, 6 out of 7 with persistent proteinuria had static or progressive lesions.

E. Tempany, introduced by Dr. A. P. Norman (London). 'Peptic Ulceration in Childhood.' Peptic ulceration in childhood is a subject that has received scant attention in the past. During the past decade approximately 50 cases have been seen at The Hospital for Sick Children. In these the diagnosis has been made either by radiological evidence of ulceration, or in some cases, in infancy, the diagnosis was made at necropsy. In this latter group histological evidence confirmed that the ulceration was neither terminal nor resulted from autolysis.

The case notes were reviewed with reference to family history of peptic ulceration, the duration and severity of symptoms, and the response to treatment.

Sir George Godber (London). 'The Development of Paediatric Services.'

George Frederic Still Memorial Lecture. The lecture was delivered on April 22 by Dr. Henry Barnett (New York). 'Paediatric nephrology: the scientific study of the kidneys and their diseases in infants and young children.'

Evening Discussion. A discussion on 'Paediatrics in the undergraduate curriculum' was held on the evening of Thursday, April 22. The topic was opened with papers by Dr. John Apley, Dr. A. White Franklin, and Professor J. H. Hutchison, and followed by general discussion.

The Ulster Cup competition was held at Ganton Golf Club on Friday, April 23, and was won by Dr. B. McNicholl.

The Annual Dinner was held on the evening of Friday, April 23, with the President, Professor Wilfrid Gaisford, in the chair. The James Spence Medal for 1965 was presented to Dr. Cicely Williams.

---

* Cameron, J. S.. and White, R. H. R. (1965). *Lancet*, **1**, 463.

# BOOK REVIEWS

**The Children's Hospital Medical Vade-Mecum,** 5th ed. (Paper back—6s.; loose-leaf—12s. 6d.) Birmingham: The Children's Hospital. 1964.

If a camel is a horse designed by a committee, this is a camel of the fifth generation which is not only very useful as a beast of burden but is also slim and compact.

The hardest decision to make in a compilation of this sort is what to leave out. Not everybody would have included all the items found in it, but none will dispute that what is included is up to date, intensely useful and practical, crisply set out, and admirably high-lighted. For housemen and undergraduates it brings together many details not readily available in standard textbooks. The range is stimulatingly wide: normal data of development and of investigations; techniques and apparatus; special conditions at various stages of childhood; diets, milks, and other foods; drugs and antibacterials.

The outline of 'what to do' and 'how to do it' is admirable. There might be argument about the jugular veins as a site of choice for the inexperienced in obtaining blood, but this would be clarified under tuition; the dose of digoxin for infants in heart failure could be increased, but how gratifying to see that this common condition is emphasized. I should like to see a short introduction by the distinguished head of the department on 'when to do it and when *not* to do it', to counter attitudes like those recently expressed in a foreign book in which one read that a child seldom enters hospital or is seen by a paediatrician without having blood taken for tests of some sort. Not in Birmingham, one can be certain.

A section on when to take radiographs might be added, not for the Birmingham graduates, who do not need it, but for those many others who wisely acquire this booklet.

It is a measure of its success that, unassuming though it is, this little compilation stimulates constructive criticism. Perhaps the most sincere tribute that can be paid to the latest generation of compilers is to suggest that it should be adopted nationally by other children's hospitals and medical schools.

**Recent Advances in Paediatrics,** 3rd ed. Edited by DOUGLAS GAIRDNER. (Pp. viii + 349; 86 figures + tables. 60s.) London: J. & A. Churchill. 1965.

The third edition of this notably successful series has been eagerly awaited and its publication will now be warmly welcomed. So many new developments in paediatrics have occurred in the past seven years that the editor has had a rich selection of topics from which to choose, and he has shown superb judgement, for the 15 topics about which the contributors have written reflect truly the main growing points of paediatrics in recent years. A particularly pleasing feature is the fact that all of the contributors have been actively engaged in the study of their subject and, consequently, much original work, hitherto unpublished, is incorporated in the articles along with a judicious and ample selection of the work of others. The importance, in a book of this kind, of providing a guide to further reading is emphasized by the inclusion of over 1,200 references—a most valuable feature.

Eleven of the 15 chapters are by British authors, the others being by contributors from Sweden, Australia, and Uganda. The first 4 chapters by Dawes, Karlberg and Celander, Gairdner, and Drillien respectively are devoted to the very important and rapidly developing field of circulatory and respiratory physiology and pathology in the newborn and the effect of disturbances at that crucial time on the later development of the child. Then follow two chapters on specific biochemical disorders of the newborn, the first by Neligan on idiopathic hypoglycaemia, that fascinating entity which has only recently achieved more general recognition, and the second by J. W. Farquhar who has written a most authoritative review on the influence of maternal diabetes on foetus and child.

There are three excellent chapters concerned with important aspects of growth, the mysteries of which are attracting much more intensive and well-merited research than hitherto: chromosomal abnormalities by Baikie of Melbourne, disorders of growth by Hubble, and that puzzling aberration 'obesity' by Wolffe. Kwashiorkor, about which much has been written in recent years, is thoroughly reviewed by the late R. F. A. Dean who was himself in the van of progress until his death just before the publication of this book. He has stressed the unexpectedly important part which carbohydrate metabolism is now known to play in this gross nutritional disorder.

The chapter on aspects of cancer in childhood by the late Martin Bodian is of particular interest, for the past ten years of his life were mainly devoted to the study of cancer in childhood and this is an analysis of his massive collection of cases and meticulously careful observations. His colleague, Barbara Ockenden, prepared his draft for publication. The huge total of 1,168 neoplasms verified at Great Ormond Street Hospital in the last 37 years are classified and reviewed.

Steroid treatment in asthma, which tends to be abused and must be supervised with great care, is discussed by Norman; and the technique and value of renal biopsy are reviewed by Black and White who are themselves leading authorities on the subject. Finally, Macnab, in the two concluding chapters, has reviewed the striking advances which have been achieved in the past few years in the understanding and management of hydrocephalus and spina bifida cystica in infancy.

**Postgraduate Courses in Pediatrics. Vol. 15. Leberkrankheiten beim Kind.** Edited by E. Rossi. (Pp. ii + 84; 13 figures + 16 tables. sFr./DM.15.) Basel: S. Karger. 1965.

This Swiss paper-back presents a brief and uneven review of liver disease in childhood. Six chapters are in German and one in French.

Vest's account of bilirubin metabolism is lucid but becomes less so when dealing with the (admittedly confusing) eponymous and often familial types of jaundice. Much the same ground is covered by the French contributor who does, however, give some idea of the relative frequency of liver disease, particularly in early childhood. Even so, the rarer and rarest types of jaundice remain a jumble.

By far the best contribution is Richterich's chapter on liver cell physiology and the physiological basis, specificity, significance, and limitations of liver function tests.

The account of needle biopsy scarcely does justice to a most valuable procedure.

Mangold's comprehensive but haphazard list of childhood cirrhosis may be a boon to examination candidates who possess a photographic memory.

The chapter on serum hepatitis is satisfactorily adequate. The final contribution, in railway-timetable style, on the definition, aetiology, and treatment of hepatic coma appears to have been an editorial afterthought.

The bibliography of one of the chapters is arranged neither numerically nor alphabetically—most infuriating. Another chapter has no bibliography at all. The booklet is well printed but badly bound, and has no index.

**Practical Paediatrics.** By Don Hilson. (Pp. 462; 28 figures + 16 diagrams. 84s.) London: Staples Press. 1964.

Dr. Hilson's book is unusual. From its title it is evidently intended as a practical guide rather than an academic text, and on the cover it is stated that 'it should be particularly valuable as a practical aid to the graduate in the paediatric ward, and to the family practitioner in his day-to-day work'. To this end it is written in the style of a tutorial, with direct instructions and many tabulated lists. The aims of the book are high, but perhaps Dr. Hilson has underestimated the difficulties of attaining them. It is one thing to talk to a small group of students on selected topics, but another matter to record this in cold print and at the same time to extend the topics to cover virtually the whole field of paediatrics. It is doubtful if our greatest teachers—men like Robert Hutchison—would have succeeded, but then they would not have tried. The loose phrase which may pass unnoticed in extempore speech is laid bare to cold analysis; the ambiguity which can be corrected by simple question and answer at the end of a seminar remains unresolved. Unfortunately the book abounds in careless phrases, and one fears that careless writing points to muddled thinking. What can one make of a paragraph such as this?—

> 'Give Thyroid extract B.P. commencing with 15 mgs. or grs. $\frac{1}{4}$, or use thyroxine sodium 0·025 mgs. daily gradually increasing the dosage to just short of toxicity. This produces diarrhoea, irritability, loss of weight and tachycardia in infancy, and in addition in older children, palpitations, sweating and fainting. This must be continued for life.'

To detail the many faults would be too great a task for a short review. In view of the immense amount of work that has gone into the preparation of this book, I feel deeply sorry to have to say that because of its inaccuracies and because of the bad example of its thought and writing I should not like it to be read by any of my students.

**Asian Pediatrics.** The Scientific Proceedings of the First All-Asian Congress of Pediatrics New Delhi, January 1961. Edited by Sisir K. Bose and A. K. Dey. (Pp. xx + 476; illustrated. 160s.) London: Asia Publishing House. 1965.

This volume comprises the Scientific proceedings of the first All-Asian Congress of Pediatrics held in New Delhi in 1961.

It contains contributions under the following headings: nutrition; the gastro-intestinal system; infectious diseases; the respiratory system; the cardiovascular system; the haemopoietic system; the genito-urinary system; the skin; the nervous system; social pediatrics; growth and development; and miscellaneous. There are 140 contributors.

**The Adolescent in Psychotherapy.** By Donald J. Holmes. (Pp. xviii + 337. 67s. 6d.) London: J. & A. Churchill. 1964.

In the author's opinion empiricism is still superior to theory in the day-to-day practice of psychiatry. Many a psychiatrist observing his internist colleagues may think that this applies fairly widely in their domain too. Dr. Holmes succeeds remarkably well in presenting clinical material and technical subtleties (inevitably difficult for the non-psychiatrist) lucidly and in well-disciplined language. Indeed, what he has to say should be of real value to the general clinician who is interested in helping difficult adolescents to grow up as persons.

The book is in 3 parts. Part 1, which is much the longest, is probably more relevant than Parts 2 and 3 to those wanting to learn more of adolescents, adolescence, the interaction between adult and adolescent, and psychotherapeutic processes.

Part 2, which deals with certain aspects of individual psychotherapy, and Part 3, which discusses residential treatment, are of less immediate concern to those who are not psychiatrists or psychologists.

The book is not one into which the reader can profitably merely dip: it merits careful reading by paediatricians at any rate to the end of Part 1, and by junior psychiatrists from the beginning to the end. These young people between the 12th and 18th years of life who are no longer children nor yet adults can be very rewarding patients, and Dr. Holmes has performed a useful service in giving us this book. It is a pity that it is rather costly.

**Endokardfibrosen. Klinik-Therapie-Pathologie.** By RUDOLF WENGER. (Pp. viii + 206; 42 figures + 14 tables. DM. 30.) Stuttgart: Georg Thieme. 1964.

In a monograph of 200 pages and including 700 references, Dr. Wenger endeavours to give us a synoptic work on the whole range of endocardial fibroses. About half of the book deals with primary endocardial fibroelastosis of infancy and childhood, the remainder with fibroelastosis in adolescence and adult life, endomyocardial fibrosis, parietal fibroplastic endocarditis, and endocardial fibrosis in the carcinoid syndrome and in sclerodermia.

This study is based on 800 published cases of childhood fibroelastosis to which the author adds 34 cases of his own or referred to him by his colleagues. His main aims are to demonstrate that fibroelastosis is not limited to infancy and early childhood but that there exist transitional types of the disease encountered at puberty and in adults, and that there are links between primary congenital and secondary acquired forms. A schematic presentation shows the interrelation of these pathological manifestations. Though each aspect of primary fibroelastosis is discussed extensively, in the end the profusion of detail leaves the reader with a somewhat blurred picture, in the same way as comprehensive bibliographical reviews which contain contradictory opinions on a particular subject.

The appended 34 brief case histories of childhood fibroelastosis are recorded without critical personal evaluation. From the clinical point of view the presence of organic heart murmurs is regarded as compatible with the diagnosis, while a number of authors stipulate absence of such bruits as a diagnostic criterion.

The rapid accumulation of medical knowledge has also overtaken this book in spite of the author's obvious effort to be up to date. Thus the diagnostic significance of the mumps antigen skin test, which seems to be a most useful procedure, has missed its entry into its pages. Though a considerable section of the monograph is concerned with conditions unlikely to occur in childhood, its exhaustive discussion of the problem of fibroelastosis makes it very interesting reading, especially for the paediatric cardiologist and all those that are engaged in research into the various facets of endocardial fibroses.

As one might expect, the production of the book by the Georg Thieme publishing company of Stuttgart is of a high standard. Paper, print, and reproduction of the black and white photographs are excellent.

**Blutkrankheiten im Kindesalter. Postgraduate Courses in Pediatrics.** Edited by E. ROSSI. Vol. 11-12: (Pp. 158; illustrated; 48s.) Basel and New York: S. Karger. 1964.

Among the 8 small volumes edited since 1961 by Ettore Rossi as postgraduate courses in paediatrics, this is one of the most instructive. It contains 9 articles, 7 in German and 2 in French, reviewing not only the progress so far achieved in the study of blood diseases in childhood but also spotlighting the haematological problems still to be solved. The difficulties facing the research worker engaged in the study of leukaemias in the young are presented in a masterly way. A stimulating discussion deals with the various aspects of lymphocytosis and lymphopenia. On one condition the author puts a great deal of emphasis and regrets that only very few paediatricians are aware of its existence, namely 'chronic constitutional neutropenia with lymphocytosis'. It occurs from early infancy up to the age of 3 years, predisposes to infections of the upper respiratory tract, hyperthermia, and recurrent bouts of pyrexia. The children prone to the disorder are described as of 'partially allergic, partially degenerative and partially dyscranial constitution'. The reviewer felt that because of the rather nebulous nature of the syndrome and/or its description, most paediatricians might justifiably plead ignorance.

Somewhat disconcerting also are the author's views on the value of the Paul Bunnel test in infectious mononucleosis, to which he accords only a 10% diagnostic reliability.

The chapters on metabolic disorders of the red cells, mechanisms of haemolysis, aplastic anaemia, structural defects of human haemoglobin, as well as on the development of the red cells and the relationship to the anaemias are well written and illuminating.

The references are well selected and up to date, except for the chapter on thrombocytopenias where they have been omitted.

The section on the function of the platelets is well documented.

One further minor omission occurs in the discussion of steroid therapy of thrombocytopenic purpura where the initial dose is given as 3 mg./kg. bodyweight but no mention is made of the type of steroid recommended.

In spite of the few criticisms, this is an excellent survey of paediatric haematology and could profitably be read by any paediatrician.

*Arch. Dis. Childh.*, 1965, **40**, 455.

# CYSTS ARISING IN THE RENAL CORPUSCLE

## A MICRODISSECTION STUDY

BY

THELMA J. BAXTER

*From the Department of Pathology, University of Melbourne, Melbourne, Victoria, Australia*

(RECEIVED FOR PUBLICATION OCTOBER 20, 1964)

Cysts of various organs have always attracted attention, if only because of their space-occupying character. In recent times their generally innocuous nature and apparently incidental appearance in many conditions have caused them to be relatively ignored. Nevertheless, apart from their morphological dominance in some conditions, they raise many questions of fundamental nature and importance.

An interesting feature of the published material dealing with polycystic kidneys has been the large amount written on causation and mode of formation, with almost complete absence of precise information as to their structure and tissue relations.

This is largely due to the difficulty in obtaining such information, though more gross and imprecise observations are easily made. One of the best methods of gaining detailed data at present available is microdissection. Amongst the infrequent published results in which this technique is used are those of Greene (1922), Lambert (1947), Bialestock (1956, 1958, 1960), Oliver (1960), Baxter (1961a, b), Paatela (1961), and Osathanondh and Potter (1964).

From these it is apparent that there is a wide range in the distribution of cysts in the nephron and that a study of a large series of cases is necessary to elucidate many of the basic problems. The present paper gives a preliminary statement on some of these cases.

### Material and Methods

The specimens were obtained at necropsy from 5 infants, of whom 4 were stillborn and 1 survived for six days after birth, as well as 1 from a child of 4 years.

The condition was bilateral in the 6 cases, and, in the first 5, cysts were predominantly corpuscular (glomerular) in origin, while in the sixth renal corpuscles and tubules were equally involved.

The relevant information is given in the Table. Case 6 resulted from the third pregnancy of a mother whose first had been normal. This was followed by twins, one of whom died soon after delivery. Post-mortem examination of this infant showed that the kidneys had appearances similar to the specimen from the case here reported.

Four normal kidneys (that is, those showing neither gross nor histological abnormality), two from babies of 37 weeks' gestation, one at 40 weeks' gestation, and one from

TABLE

RELEVANT DATA FROM SIX CASES SHOWING CYSTS OF THE RENAL CORPUSCLE

| Case | Sex | Period of Gestation (wk.) | Size of Specimen | Congenital Anomalies | Post-mortem Findings |
|---|---|---|---|---|---|
| 1 | Female | 37 (stillborn) | Portion only received | Right hare-lip and cleft palate; left talipes; congenital heart with hypoplastic aortic arch; gall-bladder absent; uterus duplex | — |
| 2 | Female | 48 (lived 4 yr.) | 4·5 × 3 × 1·6 cm. | Hypoplastic kidneys, each weighing 19 g. | — |
| 3 | Male | 36/52 (stillborn) | 3·7 × 2·2 × 2·0 cm. | Hydrocephalus; enlarged thyroid; ascites; mobile caecum | Body of abnormal appearance, weighed 3,290 g. |
| 4 | Female | 39/52 (lived 6 days) | 4·2 × 2·5 × 2·1 cm. | Gross talipes | Sub-dural haemorrhage; partial atelectasis |
| 5 | Not stated | 40/52 (stillborn) | Portion only received | Not stated | — |
| 6 | Not stated | 40/52 (stillborn) | Portion only received | Enlarged + + + cystic kidneys; combined weight 400 g. | — |

a child aged 3½ years (attempts to procure renal tissue from a 4-year-old child proved unsuccessful) were obtained for comparison.

The renal tissue was fixed in formol-saline. Appropriate pieces were removed for histological examination. Small tissue wedges were cut and macerated with concentrated hydrochloric acid in accordance with the technique described by Oliver, MacDowell, and Tracy (1951). After maceration was complete, the tissue was washed in water until the immersing fluid gave a constant *p*H reading when it was concluded that equilibrium had been established. Microdissection technique followed the procedures employed in previous publications (Baxter, 1959, 1960, 1961a, b). The photographs obtained are of unstained microdissected material.

## Results

**Macroscopical Appearances.** In polycystic renal disease, the kidneys range in gross form from those in which there are minute spaces in the parenchyma (Case 3), to those where the renal substance is replaced by a large mass of scattered or closely-packed thin-walled cysts of various sizes (Case 6).

The external appearance may be normal or there may be large cysts projecting from the surface and thus the over-all organ is much larger than usual. Since corpuscles occur in the cortex, cysts arising from these are more prominent here. A common observation is of numerous small cystic spaces occurring under the capsule. These give a faint granular semi-translucent appearance to the capsule and subcapsular zone (Case 1). At times it has a finely sago-like character.

On sagittal section, cysts of various sizes are scattered through the cortex and the general distribution may not be specially characteristic. However, in typical cases numerous minute cysts give the cortex a somewhat porous impression with a layer of tiny cysts immediately beneath the capsule (Cases 3 and 6). Occasionally the outer rim has a scalloped form due to slightly larger cysts projecting on the surface (Case 5).

In size the cysts may be barely discernible to the naked eye, or pinhead in size, or range from these to examples 2 or more cm. in diameter (Cases 2 and 4). Many cysts of similar size may be grouped together but frequently those of different diameters are intermingled.

The cyst wall is usually thin so that the colour of the contents is apparent. This may be watery, opalescent, or more or less deeply pigmented. Some of the older cysts have thick walls.

Typical cysts of corpuscular origin are confined to the cortical zone and do not extend below the cortico-medullary junction. Nevertheless, there is sometimes involvement of some of the tubules. It is not practicable to distinguish the later stages of the two types of cyst, and occasionally a few are found in the medullary zone. The extreme example is the mixed type (Case 6) in which corpuscles and tubules are approximately equally involved.

**Histological Appearances.** It is important to appreciate that material examined microscopically shows the smallest cysts and therefore attention is directed largely to these; only parts of the walls of larger cysts are viewed and described.

Most of the cysts do not show specially differentiating features. The thin wall has a thin fibrous capsule and is lined by a single layer of cells, usually cuboidal but which may be columnar or flattened. Infrequently, the cells are multi-layered. The contents are homogeneous and lightly staining.

Some cysts have a small glomerular tuft. These range from slightly dilated but otherwise normal corpuscles, through small cysts with well-defined though rudimentary tufts, to those in which the tuft, though still recognizable, has almost completely disappeared (Fig. 1).

Occasionally more than one tuft is present (Fig. 2). In some it seems reasonable to deduce from the pattern that the tuft has become divided into two parts. In others the mechanism of development is not apparent. Very rarely three tuft remnants may be seen.

In the above examples the type of cyst is beyond question. However, many cysts show no such evidence of their nature or origin, and in some of these either their relation to the proximal convoluted tubule or the nature of their vascular supply may still give a clue to their character. Nevertheless, many of the cysts have no feature that would distinguish them out of hand from cysts of the tubules. Their association with indubitable corpuscular cysts may suggest their probable nature and origin. The following features were observed in the renal tissue.

(a) Capsule.—This was intact, normal in appearance, and stripped easily in Cases 1, 2, and 3, but was considerably thickened in Cases 4, 5, and 6.

(b) Cortex.—The subcapsular cortex was remarkable for the number of renal corpuscles with dilated capsular spaces (Cases 2 and 3), many of which attained cystic proportions (Cases 1 and 4). The cortical parenchymal elements were not reduced to any extent in Cases 1 and 3, but in Cases 2, 4, 5, and 6 there was considerable reduction. In certain areas of these sections the parenchyma was reduced to a few cystic remnants which were encircled by connective tissue. In Cases 5 and 6 the entire sections consisted of a meshwork of connective tissue containing cystic spaces and small blood vessels both of

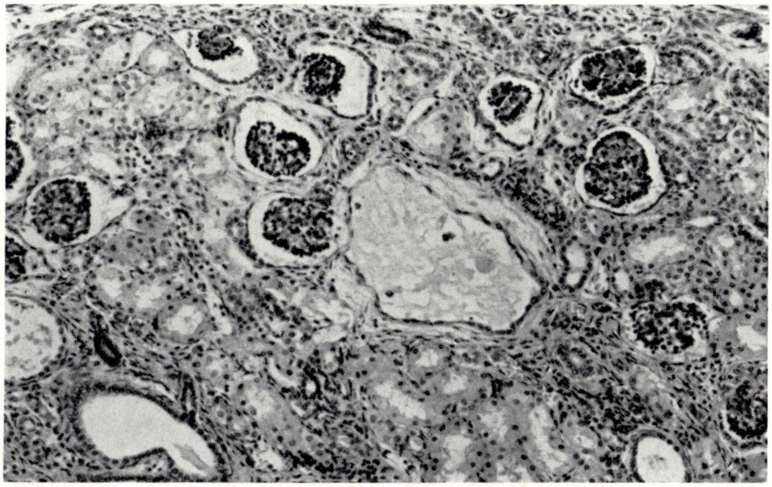

FIG. 1.—Low-power photomicrograph showing renal corpuscles (glomerular tufts being of different sizes) and dilated tubules (Case 4). (Haematoxylin and eosin. × 100.)

which were more numerous and larger in Case 6 than in Case 5.

In some of the larger cystic corpuscles hyperplasia, resulting in a heaping up of the lining layer of cells, from 2-3 cells (Cases 1 and 4) up to 5 cells deep (Case 5), was observed.

There was considerable variation in the size and shape of the glomerular tuft of the cystic renal corpuscles. The tuft was sometimes quite large, either filling the capsule (Cases 3 and 4) or surrounded by a well-defined capsular space (Cases 1, 2, and 4). At other times it was small, shrunken, and attached to one side of a large cystic space (Cases 1 and 6). The glomerulus was rounded or digitate in shape (Case 4) and occasionally two tufts were present within the once cystic capsule (Cases 1, 2, and 6). In the largest cysts the glomerular tufts were no longer present.

In addition to the large renal corpuscles in the cortex of Case 3, there was an active subcapsular (nephrogenic) zone in which renal corpuscles and tubules in various stages of maturation appeared.

(c) MEDULLA.—Changes in the parenchymal elements of the medulla ranged from very slight (Case 3) to gross (Case 5). In Case 4 there was slight reduction in the parenchymal elements accompanied by proliferation of connective tissue elements, and occasional tubules showed dilatation; but in

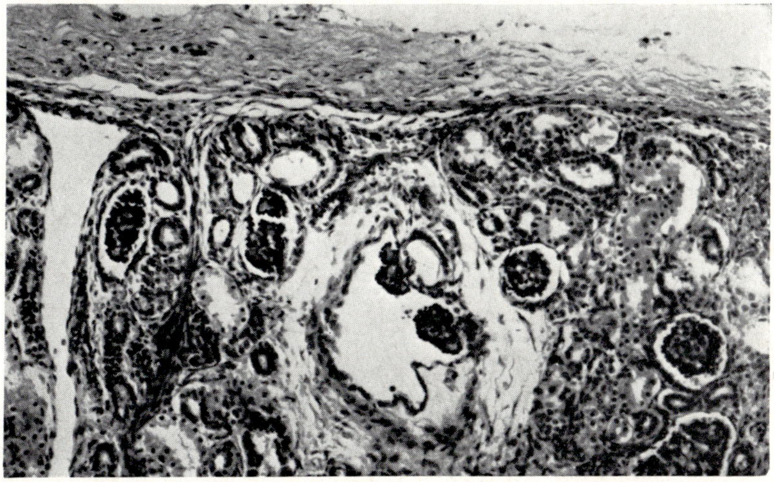

FIG. 2.—Low-power photomicrograph of subcapsular cortex demonstrating a cystic renal corpuscle encircled by connective tissue and containing two tufts (Case 1). (Haematoxylin and eosin. × 100.)

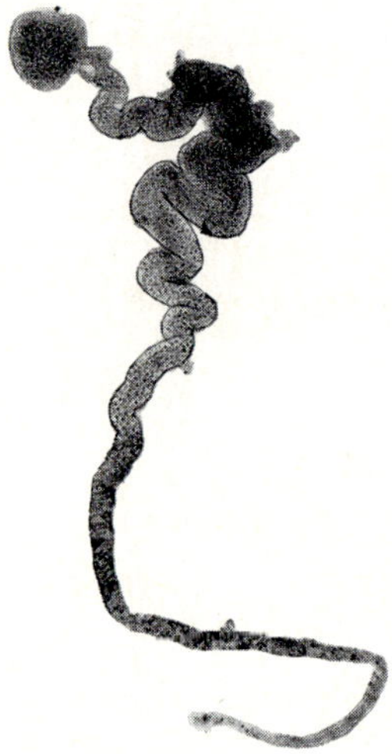

FIG. 3.

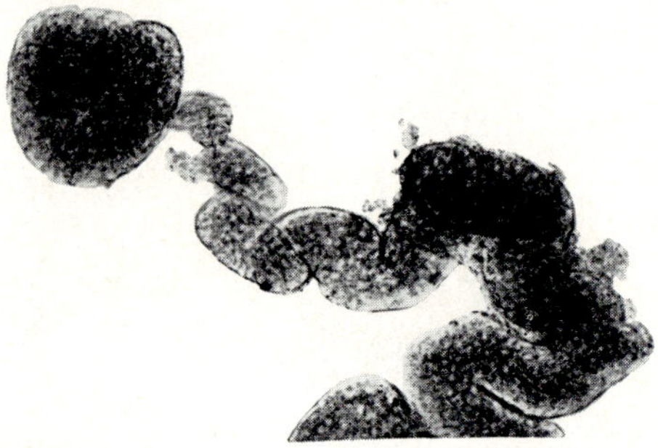

FIG. 4.

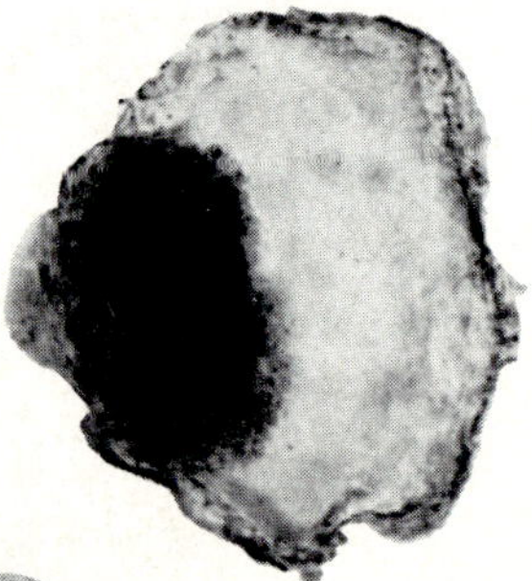

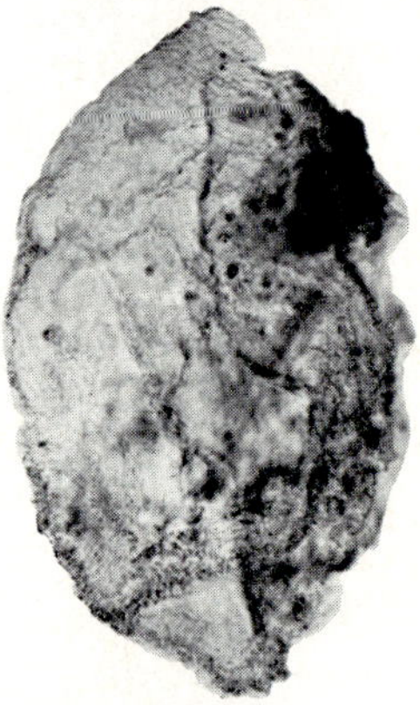

FIG. 7.

FIG. 6 (centre)

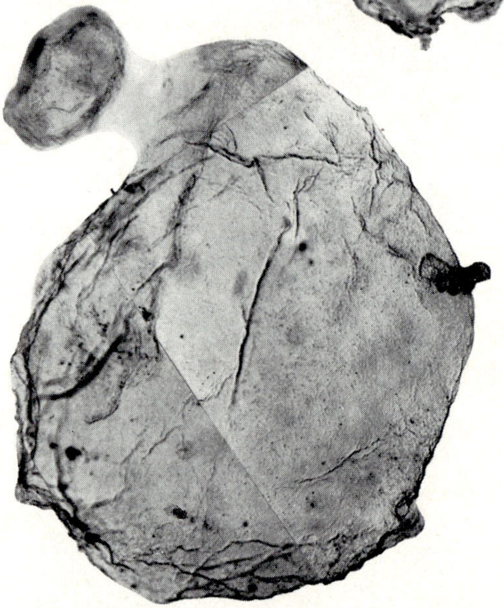

FIG. 5.

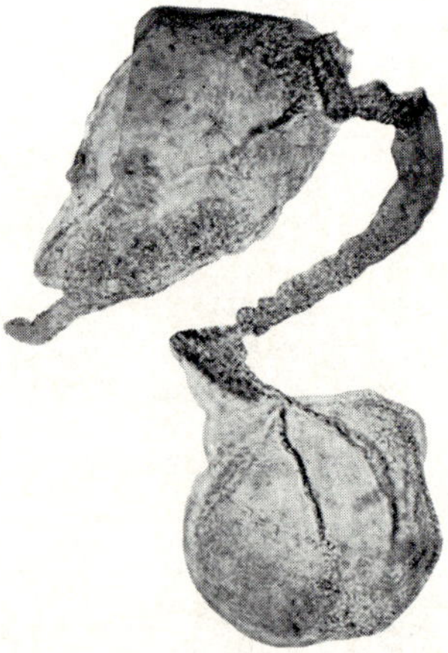

FIG. 10.

FIG. 3.—Proximal convoluted tubule from a long-loop nephron showing an enlarged renal corpuscle and over-all tubular dilatation (Case 4). (× 32.) Renal corpuscle, 211 μ diameter; tubule diameter range, 25-112 μ.

FIG. 4.—Low-power enlargement of renal corpuscle and first coils of the proximal tubule (Fig. 3). The renal corpuscle is attached to the tubule by a slender segment. (× 75.)

FIG. 5.—Large cyst with small, insignificant tubular connexion, and a small cyst. Glomerular tufts were not observed in either cyst (Case 6). (× 32.) Large cyst, 2,160 × 1,850 μ; small cyst, 250 × 160 μ.

FIG. 6.—Corpuscular cyst (372 × 310 μ) with obvious glomerular tuft (Case 2). (× 105.)

FIG. 7.—Corpuscular cyst (645 × 435 μ) dissected from subcapsular cortex with small tuft situated at the upper pole (Case 1). (× 72·5.)

FIG. 10.—Cystic renal corpuscle with obvious glomerular tuft and thickened arteriole, attached to a short proximal tubule which terminates in a cyst (Case 6). (× 81.) Renal corpuscle, 446 × 250 μ; tubule diameters range, 25-50 μ; cyst, 310 × 235 μ.

Case 1 there were regions where a few isolated cystic tubules existed in large expanses of connective tissue. In other cases (Nos. 2, 5, and 6) there was quite remarkable reduction of the parenchyma, but many of the medullary tubules exhibited active hyperplasia of the cell linings (Case 6). In these instances the medulla was reduced to a few cystic elements or sometimes only minute structures were present (Cases 1, 2, 5, and 6).

Scattered areas of haemorrhage were present (Cases 1, 2, and 4) and cellular infiltrations were seen in all cases. The latter consisted mainly of small round cells but included plasma cells, occasional polymorphonuclear leucocytes, macrophages, and numerous fibroblasts.

(d) Blood Vessels.—Some of the vessels were thin walled and sinusoid in character (Case 5) but many showed medial thickening (Cases 4, 5, and 6).

**Microdissection Studies.** Examination of tissue during microdissection provides evidence of topographical and spatial relations not available by other means. The emphasis on smaller cysts in histological studies applies, in considerable measure, here also. However, since it is the smaller examples that are closest to normal structures, both in their own architecture, with preservation, at least in part, of the glomerular tuft, and in the relation and frequent attachment to the tubular system, this has significant advantages. The various forms of small cysts, with their clear gradations to the larger ones, provide reasonable presumptive evidence of the mode of development of this group from the normal corpuscle. Moreover, during dissection the intermediate-sized cysts are visualized even though their precise topographical relations and connexions are not recognizable.

The smallest cysts are slightly dilated corpuscles (Figs. 3 and 4); there are all gradations between these and large, even colossal, cysts (Fig. 5). The degree of distension is apparent when we consider that the diameter (in figures) is related to the cube root of the cyst volume. A cyst twice the diameter is eight times the size of the normal renal corpuscle.

In the small cysts a glomerular tuft is clearly distinguishable. Its size varies considerably (Figs. 6 and 7); in the smallest, whose diameter exceeds that of the normal corpuscle only slightly, it may occupy most of the cavity (Fig. 8). With increasing cyst size, the relative volume of the tuft becomes less and even disproportionately so and gradually disappears (Fig. 9). Though usually single, it or its remnants may be double or multiple. The larger cysts are morphologically indistinguishable from others, and this is where microdissection is specially valuable in demonstrating topographical relations and connexions with the tubules and blood vessels.

The wall of the cyst is thin but it becomes thicker with enlargement and, presumably, with increasing age. Often the large cysts collapse and become more or less crenated and folded.

The distribution of the cysts conforms with that already mentioned above. They occur in the cortex and are usually more numerous in the subcapsular zone. During dissection, cysts and cyst groups become separated from the tissue mass as the superficial tissue is removed. In the foetus they are associated with groups of developing corpuscles (Case 3).

A communication with the proximal convolution is found in most of the small cysts. Larger cysts have a much narrower connexion (Fig. 5). In accordance with a general phenomenon, the larger the cyst the smaller and more delicate this junction. As the cyst enlarges, the link becomes elongate and tenuous. In still larger cysts no communication is found.

The proximal convolution, with which the cyst communicates, may be part of a complete nephron, but, at times, atrophy of parts of the tubule has occurred leaving only residual segments, and the cyst then communicates with a short blindly-ending loop of the tubule or may terminate in a cyst (Fig. 10).

The blood vessels supplying the small cysts correspond closely with those of the normal corpuscle and this usually applies to cysts retaining a tuft or tuft remnants. Frequently the efferent vessel is considerably thickened and is often of dimensions comparable with the afferent arteriole, which demonstrates, at times, an obvious vessel of Ludwig. In larger examples the blood supply of the wall is less clearly defined and does not approximate to any normal blood supply of the corpuscle.

Changes in the Tubules. The two normal forms of nephron, the long loop and short loop, are found, but in most cases the difference between these is greater than usual (Cases 3, 4, and 6; Fig. 11).

Changes in a nephron may be of two kinds, occurring separately or together.

(i) Dilatation occurs either along the whole or most of the tubule, to a different degree in different parts, or as a single swelling or multiple localized distensions in different parts, constituting cysts. These may be few in number or, infrequently, numerically equal to the corpuscular type cysts (Case 6).

Their tubular character and origin is apparent when they are part of, and continuous with, the tubule. With enlargement, as in the case of the corpuscular cysts, their attachment may become

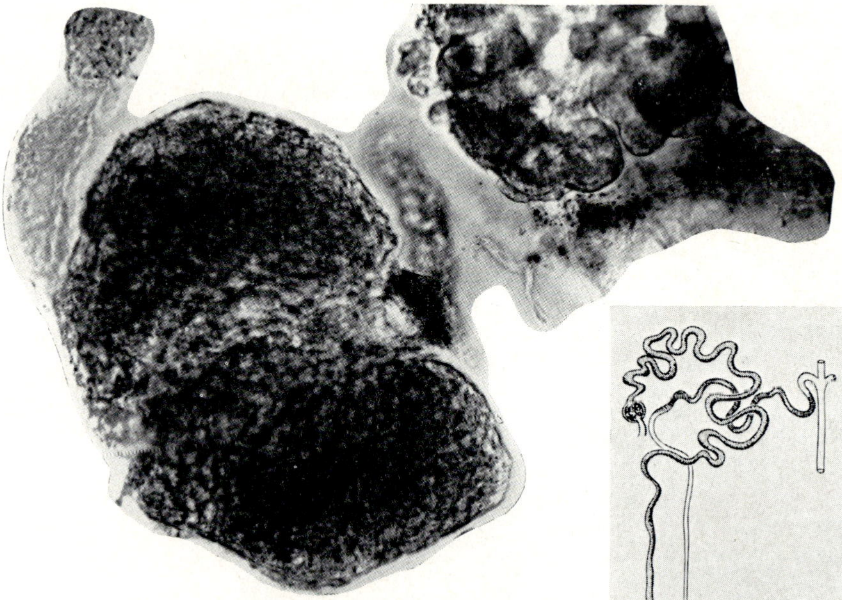

FIG. 8.—Enlarged renal corpuscle, 470 × 350 μ (reniform shape), with a thickened efferent arteriole branching to neighbouring coils of a proximal convoluted tubule (Case 2). (× 140.)

smaller until this is a stalk which is elongate and thin. This gradually withers and disappears. At this stage the origin of the cyst becomes indeterminate.

Associated with the enlargement of the tubule or part of it there is an increase in the number of lining cells. It is apparent that some hyperplasia of parenchymal elements must have occurred. These localized areas of hyperplasia may be associated with the production of numerous diverticula (Fig. 12).

(ii) Atrophy of parts of the tubule is demonstrated by the occurrence of blindly-ending tubular segments separated from adjacent portions of the same nephron. Sometimes almost the whole nephron has disappeared (Cases 1, 3, 4, and 6).

Corpuscles and small cysts communicate with short (Fig. 13) (or long) segments of the proximal convolution. This segment may have a normal diameter or may be dilated.

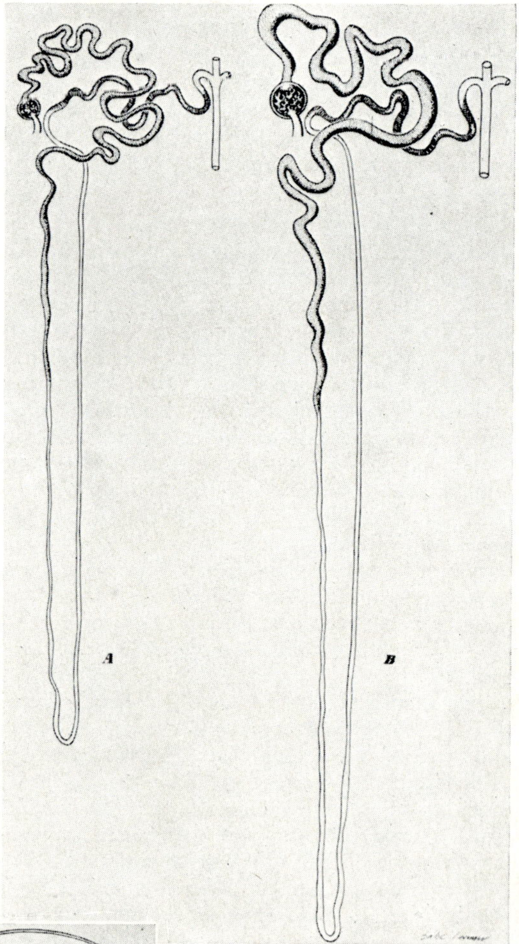


FIG. 11.—Diagrammatic representation of (A) normal long loop nephron and (B) corresponding nephron from Case 4. The abnormal nephron shows a cystic renal corpuscle and dilatation of all tubular elements as well as an increase in length.

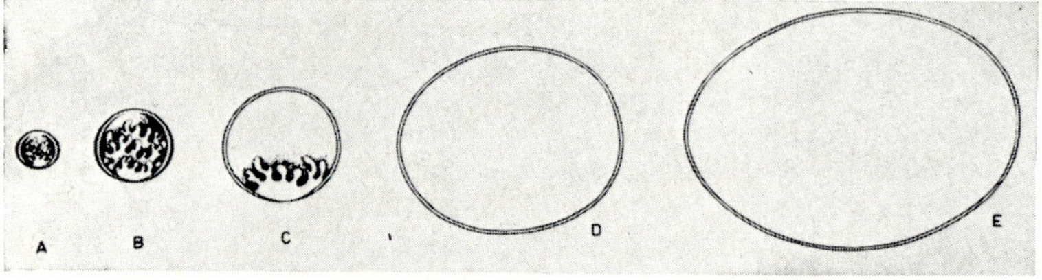


FIG. 9.—Diagrammatic representation of the range of cyst size observed in Case 4. (A) represents a normal renal corpuscle, (B-E) the range of cysts (without tubular connexions).

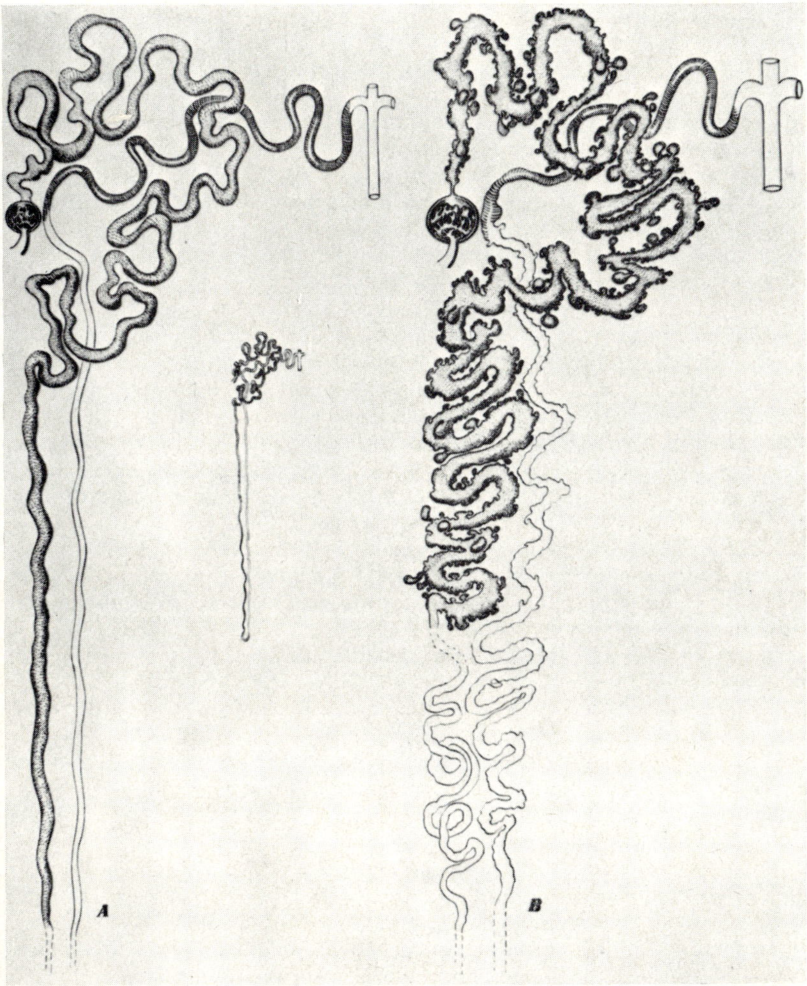


FIG. 12.—Diagrammatic representation of (A) the normal long loop nephron (upper region, insert, one-sixth size) and (B) the corresponding nephron from Case 2. The abnormal nephron shows increase in corpuscular size and over-all dilatation of all tubule components. There is hyperconvolution of the proximal convoluted tubule as well as convolution in the descending and ascending limbs of Henle's loop. Diverticula of considerable size occur profusely in the proximal convoluted tubule.

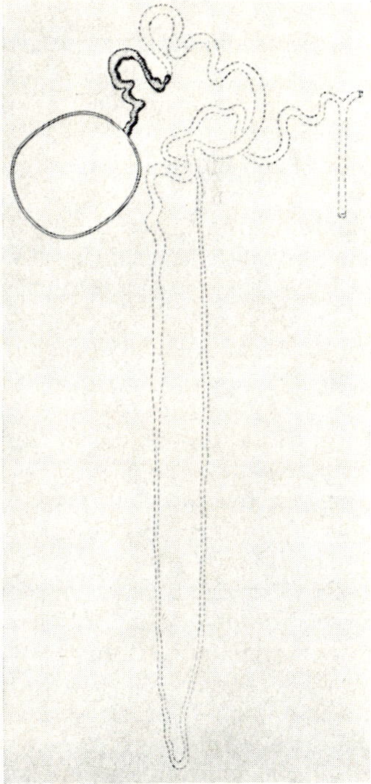

FIG. 13.—Diagrammatic representation of an incomplete unit. This consists of a large cystic renal corpuscle with a short, blindly-ending attached tubule (Case 4).

On the other hand, occasional aglomerular nephrons or segments were found, showing that atrophy also affects some of the corpuscles (Cases 1, 3, and 6).

### Discussion

It has long been thought that cysts arise in some part of the nephron and that different parts can be involved. However, it is only relatively recently that reasonably precise information has been available and, even yet, this is small in amount. Cysts of the corpuscle or the tubule are recognized, but much more detailed knowledge is required.

The gross appearances and the distribution of cysts are commonly so similar in different types that distinction can be made only on histological study. Moreover, it is in only a proportion (the smaller and early forms) that significant differences are found.

When these have been established it is then possible to recognize differentiating features in some previously indeterminate types and to suggest the probable origin of others. Thus, even on macroscopic examination, it is now reasonable to deduce that cysts, confined to the cortical region and especially when they are accumulated in the subcapsular zone, are probably predominantly corpuscular in type. On microscopical examination, the nature and origin of some tuftless cysts will be indicated by their relation and attachment to a proximal convolution, while in others the form of the supplying vessels or the close association with groups of undoubted corpuscular cysts may strongly suggest the corpuscular origin.

This emphasizes the importance of microdissection amongst the technical methods employed. It provides demonstration of spatial relations and attachments to adjacent nephron components not otherwise obtainable. Furthermore, it gives a view of structures which, because low-power magnifications of tissue units are used, is intermediate between macroscopic and ordinary histological study.

It needs to be appreciated that, during microdissection, the larger cysts become separated, gradually migrate, and are removed from the field. Thus most attention is given to the small structures and those still in contact with, or part of, the nephron. All the measurements made during dissection are, therefore, confined to this group. In order to obtain a complete over-all picture, it is necessary to add these to the measurements of larger cysts.

The important feature of the smaller cysts is the tuft. Double tufts occur reasonably often. As a cyst enlarges, the tuft becomes distorted and, with lateral spreading, it sometimes becomes separated into two parts. Whether multiple tufts are merely an extension of such a process or arise in some other way is not apparent. Small tuft remnants must be distinguished from the papillary developments in the wall that are occasionally observed. These do not have the complex vascular structure of tuft components.

In all cases there are some changes in the remainder of the nephron. It is obvious that changes are not strictly nor precisely localized to one single component of the nephron. It is remarkable that effects, from whatever agents, can apparently be predominantly localized to one small segment; however, in all cases it is apparent that the factors responsible for the alteration are acting, in some measure, on the whole nephron.

Changes in the corpuscle are, on the one hand, in the direction of dilatation of the capsule (with a necessarily associated hyperplasia of the lining cells) and, on the other, atrophy resulting in a complete disappearance of a corpuscle, giving rise to an aglomerular nephron.

Similar changes occur in the tubules. Dilatation and hyperplasia may be diffuse or localized to certain parts of the nephron. Not unnaturally, such changes are more obvious in cases where tubule irregularities are comparable in degree with those of the corpuscle (as in the typical mixed type of cysts—Case 6) than in predominantly corpuscular cystic organs. These tubular cysts appear to fall into groups according to the specific region especially involved, but this question belongs more properly to the consideration of tubular cysts. What is important is that cysts may be localized to one zone and that tubules of normal diameter may be present above and below the cyst.

Atrophy and hypoplasia also occur. Parts of the nephron shrink and disappear. This leaves incomplete units, with blind ends, and these may be dilated (or even cystic) or may be normal in diameter. At other times the unit may terminate in a diverticulum or a connective tissue tuft.

The corpuscle or cyst is therefore in communication with either a complete nephron or a short blindly-ending portion of the proximal convolution or longer nephron component. Where this is grossly distended, the corpuscle or cyst communicates with a tubular cyst. More frequently, however, there is a thin tubule uniting the corpuscular cyst with another cyst lower down in the nephron. This has an important bearing on the explanation of the mode of development of these renal cysts.

The hypotheses proposed fall into two main groups:

(i) The older ones, in general, have a fundamentally mechanical basis. Obstruction to some part of the tubule, due to inflammation, with stricture development or compression, or to a 'failure of union' of the nephrogenic zone, with the outgrowth from the Wolffian duct, implies a localized area above which dilatation should occur. The localization of cysts to one region, such as the crest of Henle's loop, and the normal tubule between this and the corpuscle shows that the simple hypothesis depending, presumably, on hydrodynamic factors alone is quite inadequate.

(ii) Recent investigations show that the factors responsible are usually of another (chemical) kind and are much more complex than was originally envisaged. Not only has the importance of metallic ions been shown to be significant in the adult, but the concept of complex chemical substances (organizers) in the foetus has opened up a new field. In addition, there are indications that tissue inter-relations, with the action of physicochemical or physical factors, also play an important role.

These factors are still insufficiently understood to

allow us to allocate any specific processes to these tissue changes, but the maintenance of an organoid and complicated structure in itself demonstrates the complexity of the factors involved. At the same time, this alters our outlook and enables us to assess critically the mechanical views that have imposed unsubstantiated philosophical notions on morphology and pathology.

Thus, though we begin simply with a study of the structural features of these cysts, this provides information that has an important bearing on concepts of cyst development.

### Conclusions

Cysts of corpuscular type and form comprise a group that can be distinguished from tubular cysts.

In a series of 25 cases, they constituted almost a quarter (6 cases). In this group, corpuscular cysts usually predominate (5 cases) but were found to be mingled with an equal number of tubular cysts in one case (Case 6). They occur in the cortex and may predominate in the subcapsular zone.

Small cysts contain tufts or tuft remnants and are often still attached to the proximal convoluted tubule. Larger cysts may be recognizable by their relation to the tubule or association with undoubted corpuscular cysts; but still larger ones are usually indistinguishable from the larger tubular cysts.

Changes are found also in the tubules. Diffuse or localized dilatations accompanied by hyperplasia occur and cysts are found along the tubule. Localized areas of hyperplasia may result in the formation of diverticula.

Retrogressive changes are also associated with the proliferative activity. Corpuscles disappear and aglomerular nephrons are seen. Atrophy of parts of the tubules results in incomplete segments of different parts of the nephron.

These observations show that mechanical factors, implicit in older hypotheses (such as, for example, the 'failure of union' proposition), are insufficient to explain the data. The cysts develop from the action of complex factors which, though producing maximal effects at certain sites, affect the tissue as a whole.

My grateful thanks are extended to the following pathologists for providing the material and the relevant clinical details for this investigation: Dr. Hans Bettinger of the Royal Women's Hospital (Cases 1 and 4) and Dr. Elsie Abrahams, Queen Victoria Memorial Hospital, both of Melbourne (Cases 3 and 5); Dr. R. D. K. Reye, Royal Alexandra Hospital for Children, Sydney (Case 2), and particularly Professor R. A. Willis, U.K., for Case 6 which excited special interest.

### References

Baxter, T. J. (1959). Early nephron changes: a microdissection study. *Aust. Ann. Med.*, **8**, 35.

—— (1960). Cortisone-induced renal changes in the rabbit: a microdissection study. *Brit. J. exp. Path.*, **41**, 140.

—— (1961a). Morphogenesis of renal cysts. *Amer. J. Path.*, **38**, 721.

—— (1961b). Observations on a polycystic kidney by microdissection. *Aust. N.Z. J. Surg.*, **31**, 115.

Bialestock, D. (1956). The morphogenesis of renal cysts in the stillborn studied by micro-dissection technique. *J. Path. Bact.*, **71**, 51.

—— (1958). Microdissection study of nephrons and cysts from an infant with pyelonephritis. *Aust. Ann. Med.*, **7**, 93.

—— (1960). Morphogenesis of unilateral multicystic kidney in childhood. *ibid.*, **9**, 53.

Greene, C. H. (1922). Bilateral hypoplastic cystic kidneys. *Amer. J. Dis. Child.*, **24**, 1.

Lambert, P. P. (1947). Polycystic disease of the kidney. *Arch. Path.*, **44**, 34.

Oliver, J. (1960). Microcystic renal disease and its relation to 'infantile nephrosis'. *Amer. J. Dis. Child.*, **100**: 312.

——, MacDowell, M., and Tracy, A. (1951). The pathogenesis of acute renal failure associated with traumatic and toxic injury. Renal ischemia, nephrotoxic damage and the ischemuric episode. *J. clin. Invest.*, **30**, 1307.

Osathanondh, V., and Potter, E. L. (1964). Pathogenesis of polycystic kidneys. *Arch. Path.*, **77**, 459.

Paatela, M. (1961). Renal microdissection studies in congenital nephrotic syndrome. *Ann. Paediat. Fenn.*, **7**, 155.

*Arch. Dis. Childh.*, 1965, **40**, 464.

# CYSTS ARISING IN THE RENAL TUBULES

## A MICRODISSECTION STUDY

BY

THELMA J. BAXTER

*From the Department of Pathology, University of Melbourne, Melbourne, Victoria, Australia*

(RECEIVED FOR PUBLICATION OCTOBER 23, 1964)

The variety of the appearances and distribution of renal cysts shows the necessity for accumulating a large body of basic morphological knowledge before they can be properly understood. As yet relatively little precise information is available, though some microdissection studies have already been made on cystic kidneys by Greene (1922), Bialestock (1956, 1960), Paatela (1961), and Osathanondh and Potter (1964), and of cysts associated with infantile nephrosis or microcystic renal disease by Oliver (1960), Giles, Pugh, Darmady, Stranack, and Woolf (1957), Fetterman and Feldman (1960), and Paatela (1961, 1963).

These cysts show a wide variety of forms in regard to size, shape, and relation to the tubules which, in a group of reasonably comparable examples, can be recognized as being stages in the evolution of the larger (presumably older), well-developed forms.

The group of cases studied appears to give some indication of the general features and, though this investigation can be regarded as only preliminary, the information obtained indicates directions for further inquiry.

### Material and Methods

The specimens were obtained *post mortem* from 18 cases and, in one instance (Case 25), by surgical removal. With this exception the condition was bilateral in all cases and covered a range from a foetus of 30-32 weeks' gestation to a child aged 7 years. The relevant details are given in Table 1.

Eight normal kidneys covering the age range of the cases were microdissected in order to establish normal nephron dimensions for comparison with the cystic tissue.

The kidneys were fixed in formol saline. Tissue was set aside for histological examination and wedges were cut and macerated with concentrated hydrochloric acid in accordance with the technique described by Oliver, MacDowell, and Tracy (1951). At the completion of maceration the tissue was washed and microdissected in a manner similar to that employed previously (Baxter, 1961, 1965). The photographs (Figs. 9-20) are of unstained microdissected material.

### Results

**Macroscopical Appearances.** Some of the kidneys are normal in size (Cases 12 and 13) or, sometimes, even smaller than usual (Cases 7, 8, 9, 10, 17, 21, 22, 23, 24). When enlarged, this is due to the presence of numbers of relatively large cysts replacing the renal tissue (Cases 14, 15, 16, 18, 19, 25). These cysts may occur diffusely through the organ or be localized to certain zones or areas. Relatively few obvious, large, cysts may be scattered throughout the tissue, but, on more detailed examination, numerous small cysts give the tissue a honeycomb appearance. Though cysts may occur in the subcapsular region, here a predominance of corpuscular cysts (Baxter, 1965) is not seen; cysts occur throughout both cortex and medulla.

Cysts may be 2-3 cm. or larger in diameter (occasional ones as large as the rest of the kidney) but many of them are small averaging 1 mm. in diameter. The method of examination (naked eye, with a lens, or by microdissection) determines the range that attracts most attention, and it is important that, to obtain an adequately comprehensive view, all three methods be integrated.

The distribution of cysts is usually uniform throughout the renal substance, but those nearer the surface, for simple physical reasons, may become larger and so dominate the remainder (Case 25). The parenchyma is usually compressed and may atrophy, though its total volume may be only slightly reduced.

Cysts are commonly spherical though small cysts in the medulla often have a linear form conforming with the general character of the surrounding tubules. The walls are thin but are increasingly thicker and fibrous with enlargement of the cyst.

TABLE 1

GENERAL FEATURES OF NINETEEN CASES OF CYSTIC KIDNEYS

| Case No. | Sex | Period of Gestation (wk.) or Age | Size of Specimen (cm.) | Congenital Anomalies | Necropsy | Size of Cysts (diameter in mm.) |
|---|---|---|---|---|---|---|
| 7 | M | 37 | L—2 × 1 × 0·5 R—solitary cyst | Renal facies; talipes (bilateral) | Bladder thick walled; ureter and urethra dilated | Not visible in left kidney |
| 8 | F | 40 (lived one day) | 2·5 × 2 × 0·6 | — | Small bowel atresia | < 1·0 |
| 9 | M | 40 (lived 3½ wk.) | 4 × 2·2 × 1·2 L—6 g. R—4 g. | — | Early pneumonia | < 1·0 |
| 10 | M | 7 mth. | 3·2 × 2 × 1·2 | — | Ureters tortuous; one showed constriction 3 cm. from origin | 0·5-3 |
| 11 | F | 7 mth. | Portion received | Polycystic disease of liver and pancreas | Gross left ventricular hypertrophy | 0·5-2 |
| 12 | F | 7 yr. | 13 × 5·5 × 5 | Polycystic disease of liver | Obstructive biliary cirrhosis; splenomegaly | 0·5-6 |
| 13 | F | 7 mth. | 9 × 3·2 × 3·2 | Polycystic disease of liver | Acute cholangitis | 0·5-1·5 |
| 14 | M | 39 | Enlarged; combined weight, 1,360 g. | Patent ductus arteriosus; cystic disease of liver and pancreas | Body weighed 5 kg. gross oedema; lungs atelectatic | 0·5-3 |
| 15 | — | 40 | Enlarged (portion received) | — | Partial atelectasis | 0·5-1·5 |
| 16 | F | 40 (lived one day) | 11 × 6 × 5; combined weight, 450 g. | Cystic dilatation of bile-ducts | Bilateral pneumothorax and partial atelectasis | 0·5-1·5 |
| 17 | F | 7 wk. | R—2·6 × 1·8 × 0·8 L—3 × 2 × 1 | Renal facies; well-developed urachus | — | 0·5-1·0 |
| 18 | M | 30-32 | Enlarged (portion received) | Head, feet, external genitalia; ventricular septal defect | Body oedematous, weighed 1,880 g. | 0·5-1·0 |
| 19 | M | 36 | 12 × 8 × 5; combined weight—540 g. | Widespread defects of face, limbs, and CNS | — | 0·5-1·0 |
| 20 | — | 40 | Portion received | Information not available | | < 1·0 |
| 21 | M | 36 | 3 × 1·0 × 0·5 | Renal facies; inversion of feet; megaureters | Subdural haemorrhage | 0·5-10·0 |
| 22 | M | 34-36 | 2 × 1·4 × 0·6 | Bilateral talipes; vesico-urachal fistula | Bilateral pneumothorax; atelectasis | 3·0-7·0 |
| 23 | M | 40 | 2·5 × 0·8 × 0·6; combined weight—5 g. | Renal facies | Pneumothorax; interstitial emphysema | 0·5-2·0 |
| 24 | F | 37 (lived 7 days) | 8 × 5 × 2·5 | Turner's (Albright's) syndrome | Pneumonia | 5-20 |
| 25 | M | 4 wk. | 7·0 × 5·9 × 3·2 | Unilateral cystic kidney (surgical specimen) | | 1·0-55·0 |

**Microscopical Appearances.** The cysts have a connective tissue layer wall, thin and tenuous in the smaller examples. Between these, the parenchyma is relatively normal (Fig. 1). The septa between larger cysts has less parenchyma and more connective tissue (Figs. 2 and 3). Frequently the older cysts are completely encircled by connective tissue.

The lining is a layer of cuboidal cells, commonly flattened and occasionally stratified in larger cysts, and sometimes columnar in smaller ones (Fig. 4). The cysts do not show special features and the lining does not correspond specifically with that of a component of the nephron. Blood vessels range from capillaries and sinusoids to thickened larger vessels.

Cellular infiltrations were present in all cases. Small round cells predominated, but plasma cells, polymorphonuclear leucocytes, macrophages, and numerous fibroblasts were also present.

**Microdissection Studies.** Dissection of the softened tissue gives a group of tubules that are gradually separated. These may be normal, shrunken, or dilated. The various regions are recognized by continuity with other parts (corpuscle or Henle's loop) or by their convoluted or straight character. Where possible, the various parts are retained in continuity and so are easily recognized. A diffuse enlargement of tubules is often present and diverticula are frequently prominent.

Nephron length may be normal (Fig. 5) or may be increased. This occurs with greater convolution (Cases 9 and 10) in some zones, or increased length of Henle's loop. In other cases, diminution of

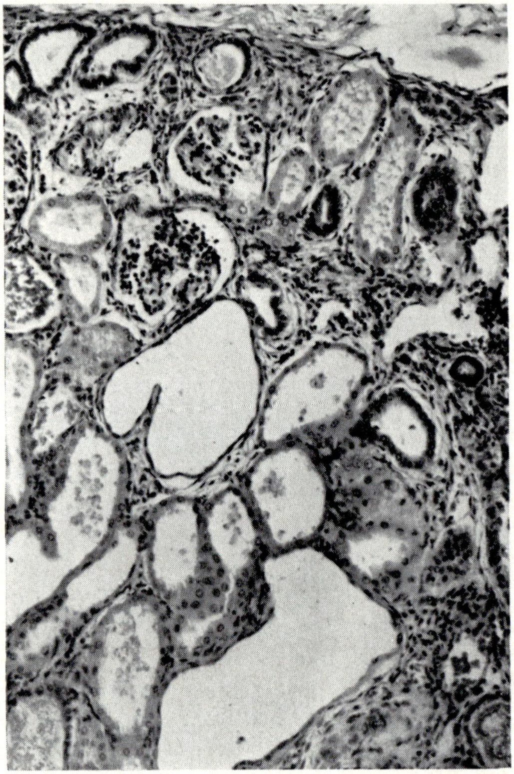

FIG. 1.—Low-power photomicrograph of renal cortex, showing a single renal corpuscle and mild cystic dilatation of tubules (Case 9). (Haematoxylin and eosin. × 100.)

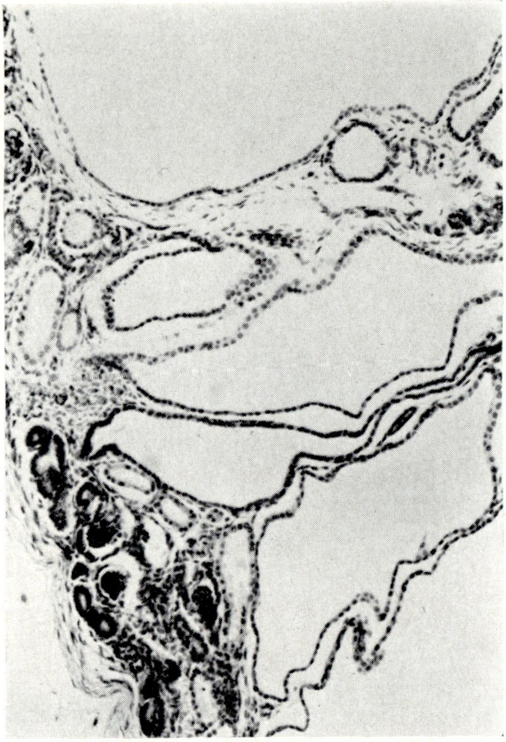

FIG. 2.—Low-power photomicrograph of capsule and subcapsular cortex, showing the subcapsular rim of parenchyma and a nephrogenic zone. The wide cystic spaces are lined by well-defined cells (Case 20). (Haematoxylin and eosin. × 100.)

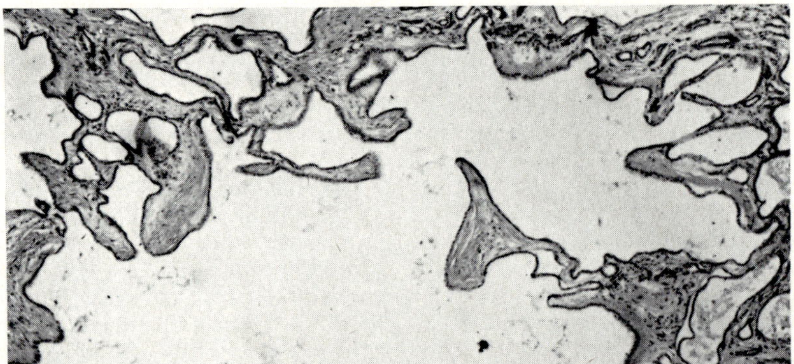

FIG. 3.—Low-power photomicrograph of large tubular cysts at the cortico-medullary junction (Case 12). (Haematoxylin and eosin. × 40.

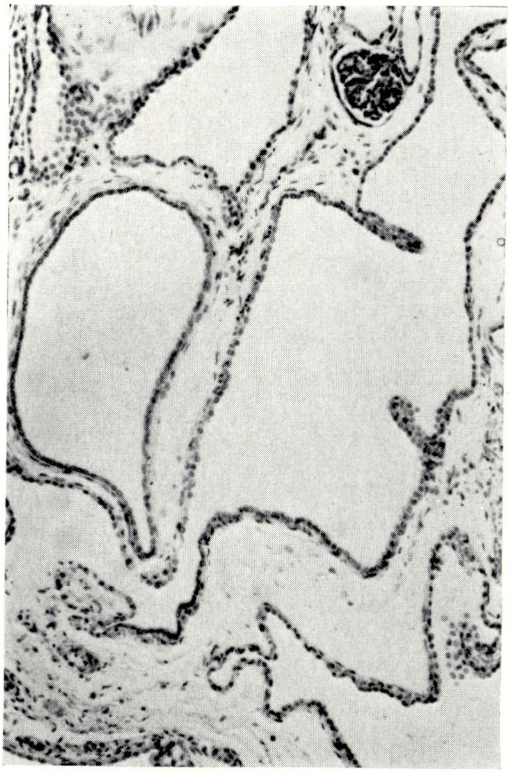

FIG. 4.—Low-power photomicrograph of tubular cysts showing well-differentiated epithelial lining cells (Case 20). (Haematoxylin and eosin. × 100.)

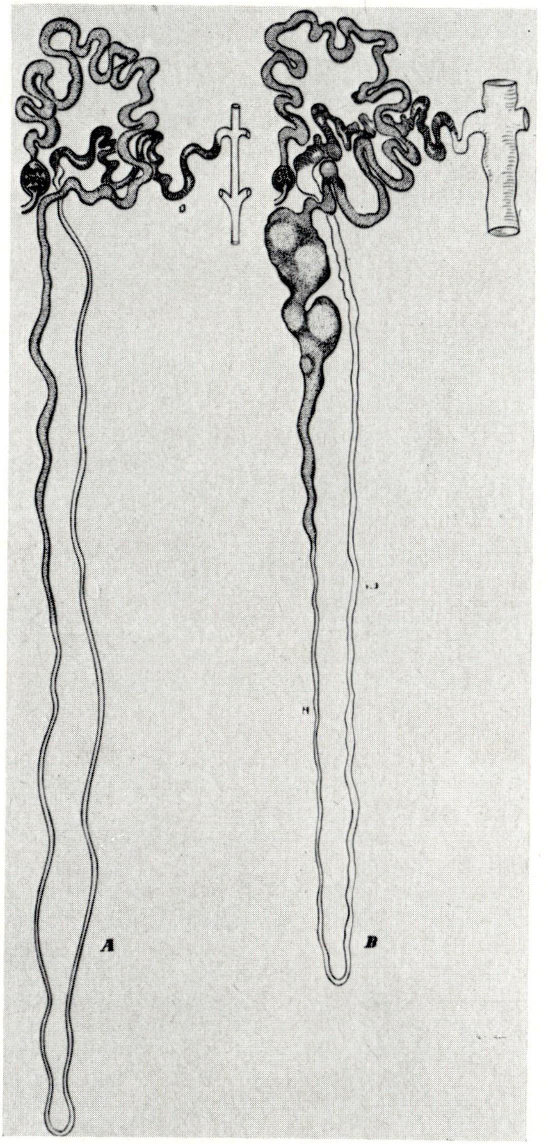


FIG. 5.—Diagrammatic representation of (A) normal long loop nephron and (B) the corresponding nephron from Case 11. There is a decrease in corpuscular size and all tubular components exhibit dilatation. Localized cysts are present in the proximal convoluted tubule and there is slight localized dilatation at the junction of the apex of the ascending limb of Henle's loop with the distal convoluted tubule. The collecting tubules show dilatation to a gross degree.

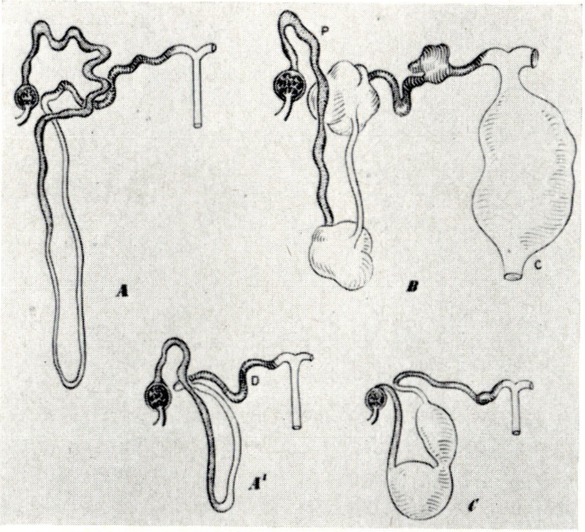


FIG. 6.—Diagrammatic representation of (A) and (A[1]), the normal short loop nephrons, and (B) and (C), the corresponding nephrons from Case 18. (B) shows an increase in corpuscular size and slight dilatation of all nephron components as well as localized cystic dilatation. These occur at both the crest and apex of Henle's loop, in the distal convoluted tubule and in the collecting tubules. The descending limb of Henle is absent and there is considerable reduction in length. With the diminutive unit (C), there is slight reduction in corpuscular size and there are localized cystic dilatations involving the major portions of the nephron. At the crest of Henle's loop a large cyst is present and this opens to another cystic structure which involves almost the entire ascending limb of Henle. Cysts in the distal convoluted and collecting tubules were not observed in these diminutive units.

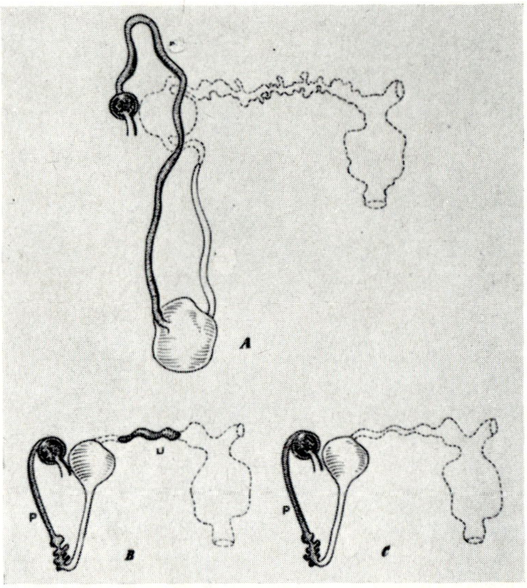


FIG. 7.—Diagrammatic representation of the range of incomplete nephrons observed in Case 14. (A). a short loop unit, shows the ascending limb of Henle's loop ending blindly just before the usual site of the localized cyst (observed in complete units). (B) and (C) represent two examples of diminutive type showing a persistence of the units as far as the localized cyst at the apex of the ascending limb of Henle's loop, while in (B) there also persists an isolated remnant of distal convoluted tubule.

length and diameter is found to be due to atrophy or relative 'failure of development' (Fig. 6).

Though the parts of the nephron may differ greatly in diameter, it is commonly a continuous structure. Sometimes only localized segments (referred to as 'incomplete units') are found. These have smooth blindly-ending extremities (Fig. 7). It is assumed that these arise where atrophy of the segments has resulted in their disappearance. A corpuscle may be absent and we then have an aglomerular nephron or proximal convolution (Fig. 8).

Cysts are found in relation to all parts of the tubule and may be either attached to or, though in close proximity, completely separated from the nephron.

They occur in various forms.

(i) A localized fusiform dilatation of part of a tubule, the cyst being in continuity with this and its cavity communicating with the tubule lumen above and below it. Though it commonly tapers at each end, the junction may be abrupt.

(ii) An eccentric enlargement of the tubule, the cyst thus projecting from one side of it. The larger examples expand and the communication with the lumen, at first wide, becomes gradually narrower. In some cases, the cyst is attached by a relatively narrow stalk.

(iii) Diverticula are usually small but, particularly where they are numerous, some are large. These resemble closely the cysts of the preceding group.

The attachment of these varies considerably in size: while it is long and narrow, with a negligible lumen in some, others have a longer, thinner, and even a tenuous union, and still others are quite separate from the tubule.

Cysts occur in complete nephrons and are found also in isolated segments or 'incomplete units'. It is noteworthy that even where there is complete obstruction of the tubule, dilatation is not necessarily present.

Cysts may be multiple or single. When multiple there may be several in one zone or they may be in widely separated regions: for example, in the proximal convoluted tubule and the collecting tubule (Fig. 5).

Cysts occur most frequently at certain specific sites; the repetition of this in different cases indicates a clear pattern of behaviour. There are naturally minor differences between different cases but the over-all agreement and conformity to type is a striking phenomenon and the important contribution of this study. The observations are given in Table 2, but in addition some special features deserve comment and are now discussed.

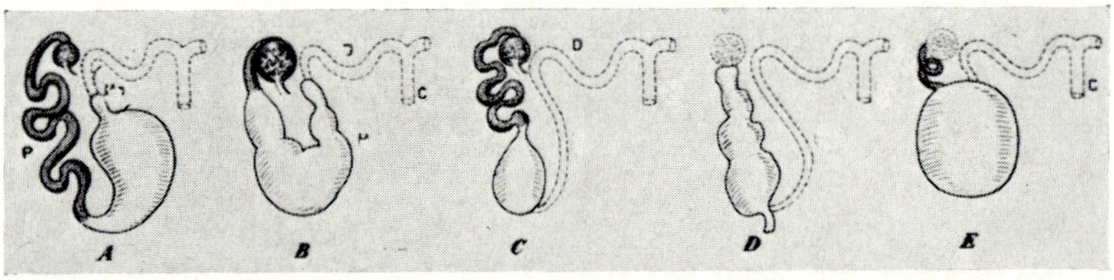


FIG. 8.—Diagrammatic representation of the range of incomplete nephrons observed in Case 25. (A) represents a small renal corpuscle attached to a well-convoluted proximal tubule. This passes to a cystic structure occupying almost the entire length of the ascending limb of Henle's loop. It terminates in a small dilatation close to the apex of the limb. (B) represents a large renal corpuscle attached to a short proximal tubule opening into a large cystic structure occupying the whole of the unit from the proximal tubule through to a region close to the apex of the ascending limb. (C) represents a proximal convoluted tubule (with attached renal corpuscle) terminating blindly in a small cyst. (D) and (E) represent aglomerular units, (D) consisting of a cystic tubule extending from the proximal tubule through the crest of Henle's loop where it terminates in a small diverticulum, and (E) a round cystic unit to which is attached a short tubule.

TABLE 2

LOCATION OF CYSTS, INCIDENCE OF DIFFUSE DILATATION, AND INCOMPLETE UNITS IN 19 CASES OF POLYCYSTIC KIDNEY

| Case No. | Location of Cyst | | | | | Diffuse Dilatation | Incomplete Units |
|---|---|---|---|---|---|---|---|
| | Proximal Convoluted Tubule | Crest of Henle's Loop | Apex of Henle's Loop (junction with distal tubule) | Distal Convoluted Tubule (DCT) | Collecting Tubule (CT) | | |
| 7 | — | — | —* | — | — | + | + |
| 8 | — | — | C | — | — | — | — |
| 9 | C | — | C | — | C | + | + |
| 10 | C | — | C | — | C | + | — |
| 11 | C | — | C | C | C | + | — |
| 12 | — | — | — | C* | C* | — | — |
| 13 | — | — | C | C | C | † (DCT only) | — |
| 14 | —* | C | C | —* | C | — | + |
| 15 | C* | C | — | —* | C | — | — |
| 16 | — | C | — | — | C | † (CT only) | + |
| 17 | —* | — | C | C | C | + | — |
| 18 | — | C | C | C | C | — | + |
| 19 | — | C | — | C | C | — | + |
| 20 | C | — | — | — | C | + | + |
| 21 | — | C | — | — | — | — | + |
| 22 | — | — | C | — | — | — | + |
| 23 | — | — | — | — | C | † (CT only) | — |
| 24 | — | — | — | — | C | † (DCT only) | + |
| 25 | — | — | — | — | — | — | + * |
| No. of cases .. | 5 | 6 | 9 | 6 | 14 | 10 | 11 |

C = Cysts. * Diverticula present. † Diffuse dilatation and incomplete units present.

A diffuse readily observable dilatation of tubules was found in 10 examples (over one-half of the cases). If less obvious distension were included, the proportion would be higher; those of about twice the normal diameter or above were arbitrarily placed in the 'dilated' group. Several zones were commonly affected, but in two cases dilatation was confined to the collecting system. Incidentally, in one of these, in addition to cysts in this region, there were cysts at the crest of Henle's loop where no diffuse dilatation occurred. Thus cysts may or may not be associated with diffuse tubular dilatation.

Cysts are commonest in the collecting tubules and least frequent in the proximal convoluted tubule and ascending limb of Henle's loop. In this group they were not found in either corpuscles or the descending limb of Henle's loop.

Cysts of the proximal convoluted tubule occurred five times in this series (Fig. 9). In every case there were cysts also in the collecting tubules, but otherwise no special feature was observed. Diverticula were associated in one of these cases. Cysts arose in any part of the convolution, but in a given case they were found localized to a specific zone. In two of the cases segregated tubular segments were present and cysts were found in some of these.

The descending limb of Henle was commonly dilated, and was then not demarcated clearly from the proximal convolution; consequently it was not practicable to determine its precise limits.

The crest of Henle's loop was the site of cysts in six examples (a third of the cases, Figs. 10 and 11). Though commonly single, the cyst was sometimes double. Being relatively large and sharply delimited from the very narrow tubule, it presented an arresting appearance. Diverticula were prominent in one case (Case 14).

The ascending limb was frequently diffusely dilated but could be recognized since it was delimited by the crest and the apex of the loop (Fig. 12). Isolated tubular segments were commonly found. Though cysts did not occur along the length of this portion, diverticula were seen occasionally and, in one case, were numerous and large. On the other hand cysts occurred often at the distal extremity.

The junction of the ascending limb of Henle and the distal convoluted tubule was one of the commonest sites of cyst formation, cysts being found here in 9 cases (Figs. 13 and 14). The cysts were single or multiple, clearly delimited from the communicating tubule, and often occurred at the junction. When they were found on either the loop or convolution side of the junction they extended for only a short distance along the tubule. Occasional detached lengths in this unit contained a cyst. Most cysts of the junction were associated with cysts of the collecting tubules.

Cysts of the distal convoluted tubules were seen in 6 cases. Single or multiple, they occurred at various places in the convolution. Some were found in sequestered segments of the tubule. They were commonly, though not invariably, associated with cysts of the junction or of the collecting tubules.

Cysts of the collecting tubules were the most

FIG. 9

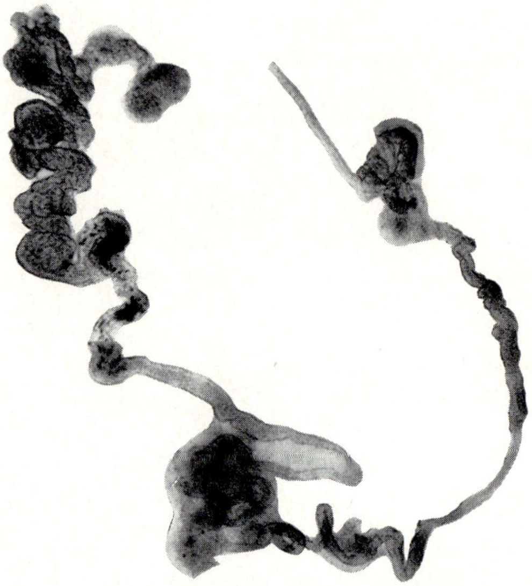

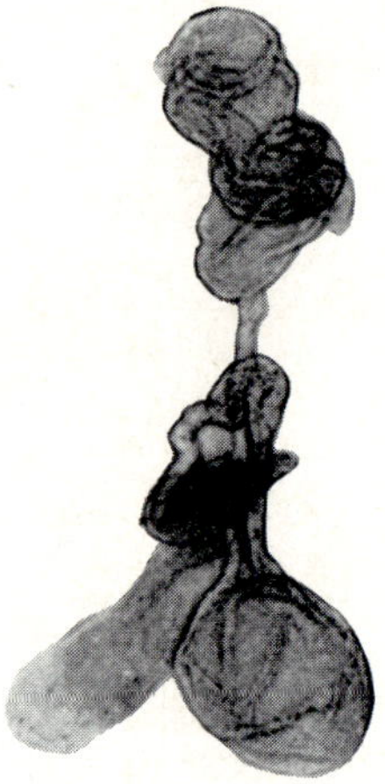

FIG. 10

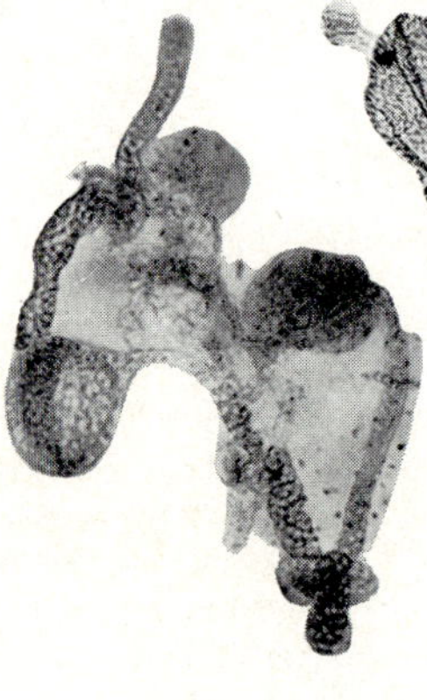

FIG. 13

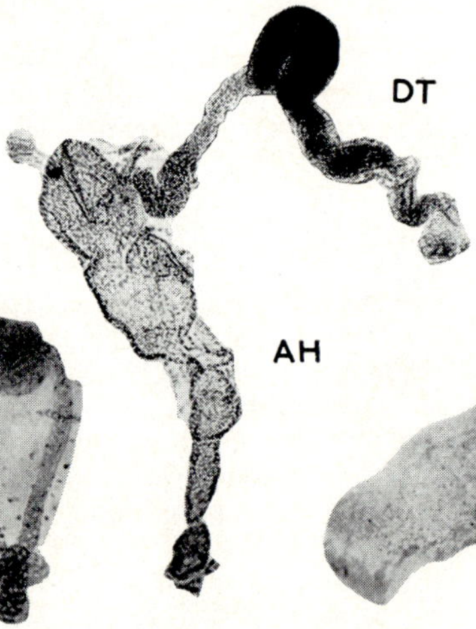


FIG. 12

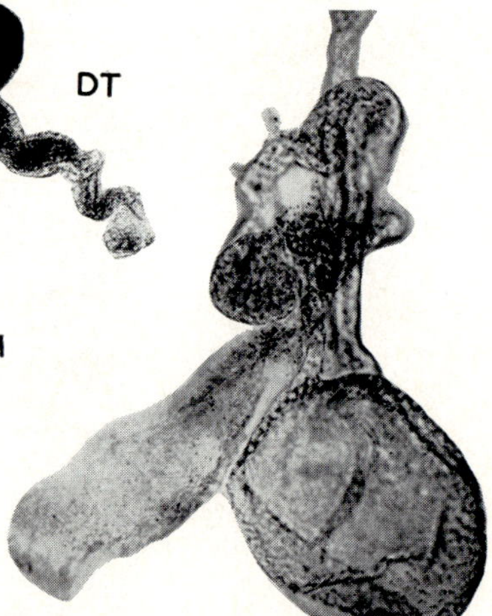

FIG. 11

FIG. 9.—Low-power montage of typical short loop nephron from Case 10. There is slight increase in corpuscular size and over-all dilatation of all components as well as localized cysts in the proximal convoluted tubule. The crest of Henle's loop shows coiling and convolution of the ascending limb. (× 46.) Renal corpuscle, 260 × 160 μ; diameter ranges proximal convoluted tubule, 37-225 μ; of Henle's loop, descending limb, 25-50 μ; of ascending limb, 30-87 μ; and distal convoluted tubule, 30-74 μ; the nephron length, 14·9 mm.

FIG. 10.—Nephron, diminutive type from Case 18, showing localized cysts at the crest of Henle's loop and in the collecting tubule into which the short distal convoluted tubule opens. (× 70.) Renal corpuscle, 100 × 87 μ; diameter range of proximal convoluted tubule, 25-37 μ. The cyst at crest of Henle's loop 285 × 260 μ. The diameter ranges of ascending limb of Henle's loop, 25-31 μ; of distal convoluted tubule, 25-31 μ; and of collecting tubule, 125-200 μ; the cyst length, 430 μ; and the nephron length, 1·4 mm.

FIG. 11.—Low-power photomicrograph to show more clearly the renal corpuscle and adjacent tubules of Fig. 10. (× 110.)

FIG. 12.—Ascending limb of Henle's loop (Case 17), showing over-all dilatation which is maximal at the junction of the limb with the distal convoluted tubule. Dark material is deposited within the lumen of the distal tubule, diameter range, 37-198 μ. (× 66.) AH = ascending limb of Henle's loop; DT = distal convoluted tubule.

FIG. 13.—Nephron, diminutive type (Case 14), showing coiling of the tubule at the crest of Henle's loop and a localized cyst at the apex of the limb at its junction with the distal convoluted tubule. (× 105.) Renal corpuscle, 125 × 87 μ; diameter ranges of proximal convoluted tubule, 12-44 μ; of ascending limb of Henle's loop, 19-44 μ; and of distal convoluted tubule, 25-44 μ. The cyst, 112 × 112 μ; and nephron length, 1·9 mm.

FIG. 14

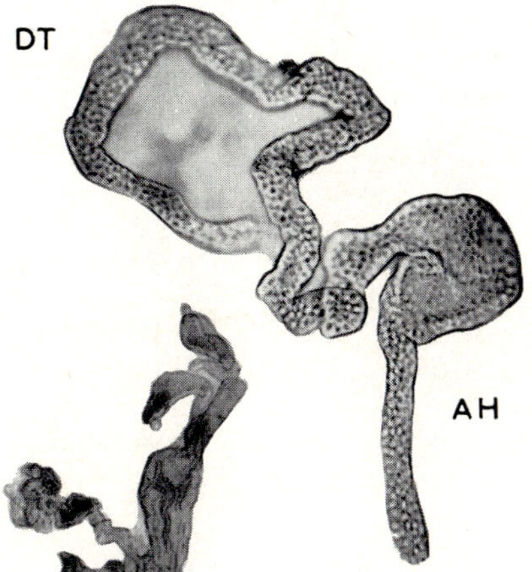


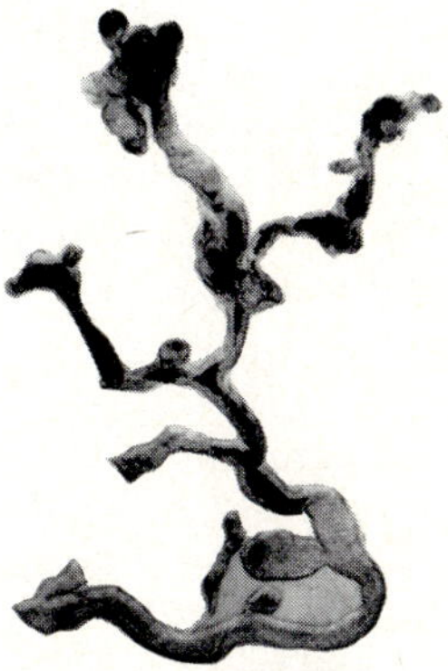

FIG. 15

FIG. 16

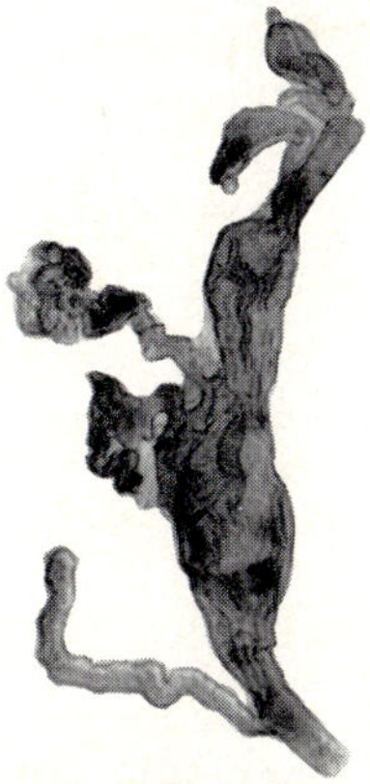

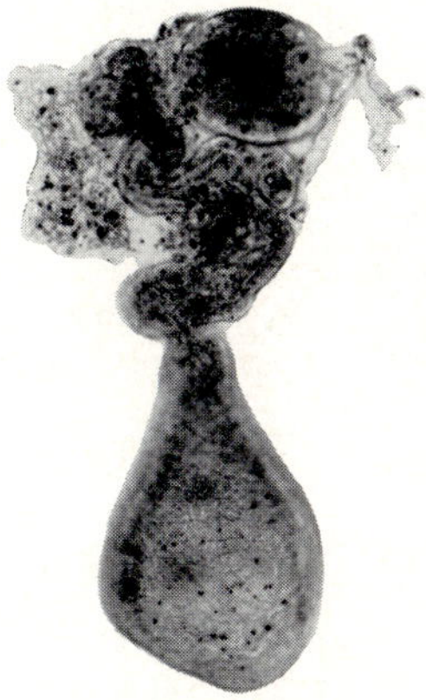

FIG. 19

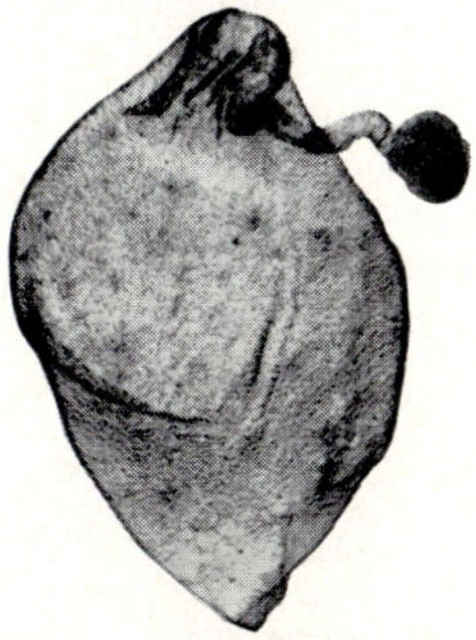

FIG. 17

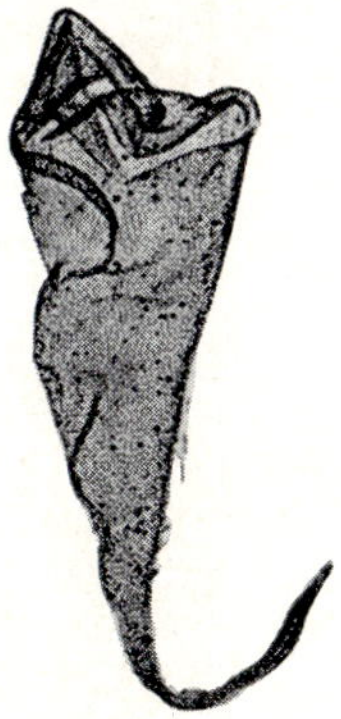

FIG. 20

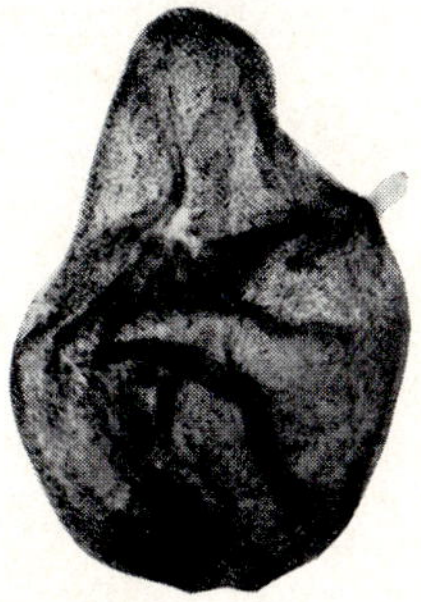

FIG. 18

FIG. 14.—Apex of the ascending limb of Henle's loop and its junction with the distal convoluted tubule showing a prominent localized cystic dilatation (Case 8). (× 120.) AH = ascending limb of Henle's loop; DT = distal convoluted tubule. Diameter ranges of ascending limb of Henle's loop, 25-100 μ; and of distal convoluted tubule, 30-60 μ.

FIG. 15.—Collecting tubule and branches showing numerous cysts and diverticula along their course. A variety of shapes is exhibited here (Case 12). (× 60.)

FIG. 16.—Montage showing a cystic collecting tubule with branches. Each of the top branches appears to terminate blindly in a small diverticulum. (× 46.) Diameter ranges of main trunk, 87-275 μ; and of branches, 25-124 μ.

FIG. 17.—Large cone-shaped cyst from Case 20. This is characteristic of the grossly cystically dilated collecting tubules found in this kidney. (× 50.) Diameter range, 48-350 μ; attached tubule, 12-25 μ.

FIG. 18.—Proximal convoluted tubule terminating in a cystic dilatation. The arterioles are clearly seen (Case 25). (× 140.) Renal corpuscle, 100 × 87 μ; proximal convoluted tubule, diameter range, 25-50 μ; cyst, maximum diameter, 136 μ, minimum diameter, 50 μ.

FIG. 19.—Short proximal convoluted tubule opening into a massive cyst. The cyst had a fine tubular connexion which was disrupted during dissection. This terminated blindly (Case 18). (× 56.) Renal corpuscle, 160 × 125 μ; proximal tubule, diameter range, 31-62 μ; cyst, maximum diameter, 650 μ.

FIG. 20.—Small cyst with insignificant tubular connexion. This was dissected free from enmeshing connective tissue and its origin was quite obscure (Case 19). (× 90.) Cyst, 590 × 410 μ; tubule diameter, 12 μ.

common, occurring in 14 cases. These showed a wider range of features than those in other parts. The cysts, either single or multiple, were spherical, ovoid, or flask-shaped, at times pedunculated, and occurred in all parts of the collecting tubule (Figs. 15, 16, and 17). Diverticula were prominent in one case (Case 12).

Cysts were accompanied either by diffuse dilatation of tubules (in one case this being confined to the collecting tubules), or their shrinkage and partial disappearance resulted in incomplete elements that were either isolated segments or blindly-ending portions of tubule in continuity with the main tree.

Incomplete units were found in 10 cases (Figs. 18 and 19). In most instances their position, relation to other parts of the nephron, and size and conformation enabled them to be assigned to their appropriate segment; only in 2 (Cases 19 and 21) was the majority of the various components and structures insufficiently characteristic to prevent their origin being recognized (Fig. 20). In one of these there were many diverticula attached to portions of tubules of indeterminate lineage (Case 21).

## Discussion

Renal cysts, which arise from the parenchyma, may occur in any part of the nephron and it is customary to divide them into two groups: glomerular and tubular. The former have been discussed previously (Baxter, 1965).

Tubular cysts are the more common and were found in 19 cases of the present series of 25. One example, not included here but already referred to (Baxter, 1965), was of a mixed type. These tubular cysts, occurring in all parts of the nephron, show a wide range of appearance and relation to adjacent structures. The naming of cysts as 'tubular' is merely a simple and very elementary designation. The recognition of the different forms and sites is the significant contribution of microdissection to the study of these cysts.

That the tubular cysts show such a wide variety of characteristics is important not only from the viewpoint of simple morphology but also because these have such an important bearing on current views of their origin and mode of formation.

Although the cysts are necessarily circumscribed and thus involve localized segments of the nephron, there is practically invariably involvement of the whole unit. This is a feature that cannot be demonstrated readily by ordinary histological methods but can be shown clearly in microdissection material, especially when this is carefully and precisely measured and the measurements are compared with those of corresponding normal structures.

Two pathological processes, hyperplasia and hypoplasia, are both evident. Increase in the amount of tissue with cellular proliferation is apparent in the cysts, in that, apart from stratification of cells or papillary developments, there is clearly a greater number of cells lining the increased area of the cyst wall. It is shown also in the increase in the nephron components between the cysts, with the elongation of some tubules and their frequent dilatation.

On the other hand hypoplasia and even atrophy of parts of the tissue occur in some areas and is in some cases a predominant feature with loss of most of the nephron structure. This is well shown by the disappearance of lengths of a nephron and the occurrence of segments of tubule which end blindly and do not necessarily communicate in any way with a nephron. That the two processes are frequently closely associated is demonstrated by the dilatation (with a typical epithelial lining) of some of these segments and the occurrence of cysts in them.

At first sight, when only a few cases have been studied, the cysts appear to be scattered haphazardly along the nephron. When further cases are studied, however, it becomes clear that there are, in most, some well-defined patterns of distribution of the cysts. In some cases cysts are localized to one area but, more often, they occur in more than one part of the tubule and may sometimes be consistently present in widely separated areas, such, for example, as the junction of the ascending limb of Henle's loop with the distal convoluted tubule, and the collecting tubule. Cases 7, 23, and 25 did not conform to the well-defined cyst patterns shown in the other kidneys investigated but showed a generalized dilatation of the tubules and a relatively random distribution of cysts. In this respect these cases were similar to that described by Bialestock (1956). When cysts occur in incomplete and isolated segments their general location is similar to that found in the complete nephron.

The factors responsible for these changes are complex and far from being understood. Some are clearly of a general nature, as indicated by the involvement, in some measure, of the whole of the nephron and a large proportion of those present. At the same time, there are also local factors to explain the remarkable localization of maximal change in many cases. The repetition of patterns in different cases is an indication of a frequent regional activity of some factors. Some of these have already been envisaged but there are certainly others that are still unknown and, what is more important, the interaction of these various agents and processes is still obscure.

Although several of these patterns of distribution of cysts have been demonstrated in these cases, it is apparent that, with the investigation of further examples, still others will be found. This present study, therefore, is to be regarded as a preliminary to more complete examination of a larger group of cases.

## Conclusions

Cysts of the tubular type are the common form found in the kidney and were present in about three-quarters (19) of a series of 25 cases.

They occur throughout the whole renal substance. Small cysts are scattered throughout the parenchyma, but some typical types, such as occur in the sponge kidney, constitute unique subgroups. They occur in the cortex but do not show the distinctive predominantly subcortical distribution of corpuscular cysts.

Cysts are commonly round or ovoid on section, but elongated structures lying between and in line with the parallel tubules in the midzone are often a prominent feature.

They occur as diffuse or localized dilatations in various parts of the tubule.

Some zones of the tubule are commonly involved so that specific sites recur in different cases, thus providing definite sub-types of tubular cysts.

The cysts from different parts of the nephron are essentially similar in appearance, so that, at present, they are to be distinguished principally by their association with some special part of the nephron.

Cyst formation is, usually of necessity, associated with proliferative cellular activity. However, retrogressive changes also occur, as shown by the presence of aglomerular nephrons and, following atrophy and disappearance of parts of the tubule, incomplete, blindly-ending segments.

Detailed observations such as these have an important bearing on hypotheses of aetiological factors determining the formation of the cysts.

My grateful appreciation for providing the material and relevant clinical details for this work is extended to the following pathologists: Dr. Elsie Abrahams, Queen Victoria Memorial Hospital (Cases 7, 9, 16, 17, 18, 20, 22, 24, and 25) and Drs. Hans Bettinger and H. Attwood of the Royal Women's Hospital (Cases 19 and 23) of Melbourne; Dr. R. D. K. Reye, Royal Alexandra Hospital for Children, Sydney (Cases 8, 10, 11, 12, and 13); Dr. Allan Pound, Brisbane (Case 14 and 21) and Dr. Thomas Pullar, Palmerston North, New Zealand (Case 15).

### References

Baxter, T. J. (1961). Morphogenesis of renal cysts. *Amer. J. Path.*, **38**, 721.

—— (1965). Cysts arising in the renal corpuscle. A microdissection study. *Arch. Dis. Childh.*, **40**, 455.

Bialestock, D. (1956). The morphogenesis of renal cysts in the stillborn studied by micro-dissection technique. *J. Path. Bact.*, **71**, 51.

—— (1960). Morphogenesis of unilateral multicystic kidney in childhood. *Aust. Ann. Med.*, **9**, 53.

Fetterman, G. H., and Feldman, J. D. (1960). Congenital anomalies of renal tubules in a case of 'infantile nephrosis'. *Amer. J. Dis. Child.*, **100**, 319.

Giles, H. McC., Pugh, R. C. B., Darmady, E. M., Stranack, F., and Woolf, L. I. (1957). The nephrotic syndrome in early infancy: a report of three cases. *Arch. Dis. Childh.*, **32**, 167.

Greene, C. H. (1922). Bilateral hypoplastic cystic kidneys. Report of a case simulating chronic diffuse nephritis in a girl three years of age. *Amer. J. Dis. Child.*, **24**, 1.

Oliver, J. (1960). Microcystic renal disease and its relation to 'infantile nephrosis'. *ibid.*, **100**, 312.

——, MacDowell, M., and Tracy, A. (1951). The pathogenesis of acute renal failure associated with traumatic and toxic injury. Renal ischemia, nephrotoxic damage and the ischemuric episode. *J. clin. Invest.*, **30**, 1307.

Osathanondh, V., and Potter, E. L. (1964). Pathogenesis of polycystic kidneys. *Arch. Path.*, **77**, 459.

Paatela, M. (1961). Renal microdissection studies in congenital nephrotic syndrome. Preliminary report. *Ann. Paediat. Fenn.*, **7**, 155.

—— (1963). Renal microdissection in infants with special reference to the congenital nephrotic syndrome. *ibid.*, **9**, Suppl. 21.

*Arch. Dis. Childh.*, 1965, **40**, 474.

# INTERMITTENT POSITIVE PRESSURE RESPIRATION AS A TREATMENT IN SEVERE RESPIRATORY DISTRESS SYNDROME*

BY

M. DELIVORIA-PAPADOPOULOS, H. LEVISON, and P. R. SWYER

*From the Research Institute of the Hospital for Sick Children, and the Department of Paediatrics, University of Toronto*

(RECEIVED FOR PUBLICATION NOVEMBER 30, 1964)

Since the initial work of Donald and Lord (1953) and Donald, Kerr, and MacDonald (1958), there have been several reported survivals of infants with the respiratory distress syndrome (RDS) treated by assisted ventilation (Benson, Celander, Haglund, Nilsson, Paulsen, and Renck, 1958; Stahlman, Young, and Payne, 1962; Delivoria-Papadopoulos and Swyer, 1963; Heese, Wittmann, and Malan, 1963). Previous work in our unit (Delivoria-Papadopoulos and Swyer, 1964) demonstrated the possibility of reversing at least temporarily the biochemical changes of terminal asphyxia in patients dying with RDS.

The purpose of this study was to gain further information regarding criteria for initiating assisted ventilation and its technique in relation to the clinical features and course of the disease.

## Material and Methods

The diagnosis of RDS in the 20 infants in this study was based on the usually accepted clinical (Dunham, 1961) and radiological (Peterson and Pendleton, 1955) criteria.

Previous experience of assisting ventilation, begun only after repeated resuscitative attempts by bagging had failed, yielded only 1 survivor out of 19 (Delivoria-Papadopoulos and Swyer, 1964). In our present series assisted ventilation was started as soon as it was obvious that mask bagging would be ineffective in restoring sustained respiration. Thus infants did not deteriorate over many hours as in our previous series. Even so, 8 were in cardiac arrest and 16 were severely bradycardic (<60/min.). All had the biochemical picture of profound hypoxaemia and hypoventilation when first intubated and ventilated. Their clinical and biochemical data are summarized in Table 1. The gestational ages, birth weights, and clinical details are given in Table 2. The infants were intubated with Cole's endotracheal tubes, No. 10-16 according to the baby's size, and intermittent positive pressure respiration (IPPR) was given with the Bird Mark VIII ventilator equipped with the minimal dead space (0·28 ml.) infant circle (S. Segal, 1963, personal communication). Pressures used in severely ill infants were of the order of 30-35 cm. $H_2O$. With improvement in the clinical and biochemical condition, pressures could be gradually reduced to 15-18 cm. $H_2O$. It was necessary also to increase pressures temporarily after airway suction. Respiratory rates were maintained between 50 and 70/min., using automatic triggering if the infant did not spontaneously breathe at these rates. Regulation within these ranges was made by clinical judgement of the degree of expansion of the infant's chest, the infant's colour, activity, and response to stimuli. The '40% air mix' on the ventilator was selected, though it is likely that oxygen percentages

* Supported in part by a grant from the Department of National Health and Welfare, Ottawa, Canada, and in part by a grant-in-aid from the Banting Research Foundation.

TABLE 1

CLINICAL AND BIOCHEMICAL STATUS OF INFANTS AT THE START OF IPPR

| Clinical Signs | | | Acid-Base Balance | | | $PaO_2$ in 100% $O_2$ |
|---|---|---|---|---|---|---|
| Respiration | Heart | Colour | *p*H | $PaCO_2$ | B.B. (p)* | |
| Arrest, < 3/min., or gasping | Arrest or <60/min. | Central + peripheral cyanosis in 100% $O_2$ | <6·80 | >120 mm. Hg | <25 mEq/l. | <30 mm. Hg |

* Plasma buffer base.

TABLE 2

CLINICAL DETAILS OF TWENTY INFANTS WITH RESPIRATORY FAILURE TREATED WITH IPPR

| Case No. and Sex | | Birth Weight (kg.) | Gestation (wk.) | Complications of Pregnancy or Delivery | Mode of Delivery | Age at Onset of IPPR (hr.) | Total Hours on Ventilator | Age at Death (hr.) |
|---|---|---|---|---|---|---|---|---|
| *Group I* | | | | | | | | |
| 1 | M | 1·4 | 32 | Footling breech | Vaginal | 8 | 101 | 109 |
| 2 | M | 1·0 | 26 | Toxaemia, breech | Vaginal | 6 | 37 | 43 |
| 3 | F | 3·4 | 37 | Uncontrolled diabetes, thrombophlebitis | Caesarean | 6 | 33 | 39 |
| 4 | F | 1·7 | 30 | — | Vaginal | 6 | 82 | 88 |
| 5 | F | 3·7 | 35 | Uncontrolled diabetes | Caesarean | 7 | 132 | 139 |
| 6 | M | 2·0 | 30 | Placenta praevia | Vaginal | 4 | 109 | 113 |
| 7 | F | 1·7 | 32 | Precipitous delivery | Vaginal | 6 | 18 | 24 |
| *Group II* | | | | | | | | |
| 8 | F | 2·0 | 34 | — | Vaginal | 40 | 126 | 166 |
| 9 | M | 3·3 | 36 | Uncontrolled diabetes | Vaginal | 35 | 112 | 147 |
| 10 | M | 2·5 | 36 | — | Vaginal | 36 | 12 | 48 |
| 11 | M | 1·2 | 32 | Surgical removal ureteral calculi | Vaginal | 50 | 59 | 109 |
| 12 | M | 1·3 | 36 | Twin pregnancy | Caesarean | 62 | 8 | 70 |
| 13 | F | 1·6 | 34 | Placenta praevia | Vaginal | 27 | 244 | 271 |
| 14 | M | 2·6 | 36 | — | Caesarean | 47 | 48 | Lived |
| 15 | M | 2·8 | 39 | Disproportion | Caesarean | 52 | 324 | Lived |
| 16 | M | 2·3 | 32 | Uncontrolled diabetes, toxaemia | Caesarean | 28 | 72 | Lived |
| 17 | F | 1·8 | 33 | Premature rupture membrane | Vaginal | 49 | 156 | Lived |
| 18 | M | 3·5 | 40 | Severe birth asphyxia | Vaginal | 30 | 48 | Lived |
| 19 | M | 3·1 | 36 | Placenta praevia | Caesarean | 42 | 192 | Lived |
| 20 | M | 2·2 | 36 | — | Caesarean | 41 | 96 | Lived |

averaging 60 or more resulted (Fairley and Britt, 1964). The adequacy of alveolar ventilation so obtained was checked by periodic $PaCO_2$ measurements (Figs. 2 and 3). Following intubation and initiation of IPPR, a low tracheostomy was performed (Fearon, 1962; Fearon, Smith, Delivoria-Papadopoulos, Levison, and Swyer, 1964) within 12 hours to facilitate the maintenance of a clear airway. All infants had serial arterial blood gas and chemical studies after admission, immediately before and after IPPR, and at 3- to 6-hour intervals for the first two days, then at 8- to 12-hour intervals. After the 6th day on the ventilator, blood acid-base determinations were done daily. In 14 infants the umbilical artery was catheterized with a No. 5 French polyvinyl tube filled with heparinized saline. On removal of the catheters blood was sampled by femoral artery puncture. All infants received 10% glucose intravenously (65 ml./kg./day) and sodium bicarbonate by slow syringe injection according to the estimated base deficit. Blood transfusion was given (in 11 infants) in the presence of a haematocrit below 38%. Electrocardiogram, heart rate, respiratory rate, and colonic and environmental temperatures were monitored. Blood *p*H was measured by glass electrode (Astrup, Jørgensen, Siggaard Anderson, and Engel, 1960), $CO_2$ content by means of Kopp-Natelson gasometer (Natelson, 1951), $P_{CO_2}$ by the Severinghaus electrode (Severinghaus and Bradley, 1958), and $P_{O_2}$ by the Clark electrode (Severinghaus and Bradley, 1958) after a 15-minute period of breathing 100% $O_2$ on the ventilator. Plasma buffer base was derived from the Singer-Hastings nomogram (Singer and Hastings, 1948). All measurements were made at 38° C., and no correction was made for the infant's body temperature.

## Results

The infants were divided into two groups according to the duration of the clinical course from birth to cardio-respiratory failure. Group I (7 infants) had a short clinical course before failure (4-8 hours). The mean age at failure and start of IPPR was 7 hours (Fig. 1 and Table 2). Death occurred after an average of 72 hours on the ventilator. Necropsy revealed hyaline membrane disease (HMD) in every case.

Group II (13 infants) had a longer clinical course (28-52 hours) from birth to respiratory failure. The mean age at acute decompensation and start of IPPR was 40 hours. The mean ventilator time was 132 hours (Fig. 1 and Table 2). Of the 13 infants, 6 died; necropsy revealed HMD in all. Complications are summarized in Table 3. Klebsiella pneumonia was treated with Cephalosporin C. While all fatal cases had post-mortem evidence of HMD, additional intractable infection and technical problems associated with airway maintenance were the final cause of death in 6 patients in Group II. The technical aspects of IPPR and tracheostomy have been discussed in another communication (Fearon *et al.*, 1964). Seven infants were weaned off the ventilator and with one exception were apparently mentally and physically normal at 22, 18, 14, 13, 10, and 7 months of age, though more prolonged follow-up is being carried out. One infant (Case 18) is retarded but had a traumatic delivery.

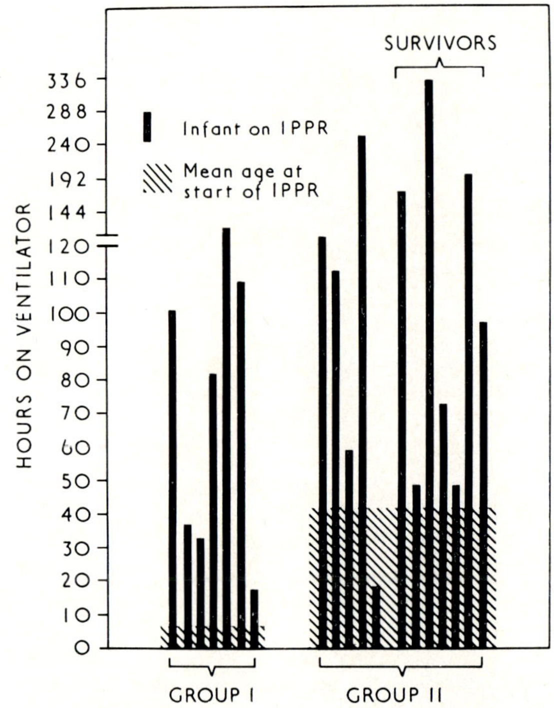


FIG. 1.—Duration of positive pressure ventilation in Group I (initiated at a mean age of 7 hours) compared with Group II (initiated at a mean age of 40 hours).

It is of interest that 2 of the 7 survivors had cardiac arrest which yielded to external cardiac massage combined with the assisted ventilation.

Representative examples of the biochemical course for Groups I and II are given in Figs. 2 and 3.*

* A Table giving serial biochemical data for each patient will be forwarded on request by one of the authors (P.R.S.).

## Discussion

There was a clear difference between the two groups clinically and biochemically. In Group I, where the short clinical course from birth to cardiorespiratory failure indicated a more severe disease, IPPR applied at the onset of acute decompensation improved the condition only temporarily. Though the respiratory and metabolic acidoses were both corrected within 6 hours, subsequent deterioration set in after a variable interval from 24 to 139 hours (Fig. 2).

The infants in Group II seemed at first to be as severely ill as those in Group I judging by the physical examination, retraction score, radiographs, and biochemical status. However, they were able to maintain reasonable compensation for the degree of hypoventilation and kept their acid-base balance within limits compatible with life for at least 24 hours by maximal muscular respiratory effort, though additional bicarbonate buffer was given as required to repair deficits (Case 19, Fig. 3). The immediate cause of their failure before IPPR was begun seemed to be neuromuscular exhaustion rather than overwhelming lung disease.

Compared to Group I, the infants of Group II improved much faster on IPPR. Respiratory acidosis was restored to normal within the first hour and the metabolic acidosis treated with buffers was maintained within normal limits throughout the course of IPPR.

The $PaO_2$ levels in Group I, while breathing 100% oxygen, showed an early but poorly maintained improvement and by 36 hours were falling once more. In contrast, Group II patients showed a steady improvement in $PaO_2$ to reach normal levels by the fourth day on the ventilator (Fig. 4), indicating a reduction in the large A-a gradient characteristic of the acute stage of the disease (Nelson, Prod'hom, Cherry, Lipsitz, and Smith, 1963; Strang and

TABLE 3

MEDICAL AND TECHNICAL COMPLICATIONS IN TWENTY INFANTS TREATED WITH IPPR

| Complications in 13 Fatal Cases | | | | Complications in 7 Survivors | | | |
|---|---|---|---|---|---|---|---|
| Technical | No. of Infants | Medical | No. of Infants | Technical | No. of Infants | Medical | No. of Infants |
| Tube in right main bronchus | 12 | Klebsiella pneumonia | 7 | Tube in right main bronchus | 6 | Klebsiella pneumonia | 4 |
| Tube in left main bronchus | 3 | Erythroblastosis foetalis | 2 | Tube in left main bronchus | 1 | Unknown pneumonia | 1 |
| Subcutaneous tube displacement | 4 | Intracerebral haemorrhage | 3 | Obstructive secretions | 7 | Pneumothorax | 1 |
| Leak past tracheostomy tube | 6 | Haemorrhagic disease of newborn | 1 | Subcutaneous tube displacement | 3 | Anaemia | 5 |
| Obstructive secretions | 13 | Pneumothorax | 3 | Leak past tracheostomy tube | 7 | Hyperbilirubinaemia | 1 |

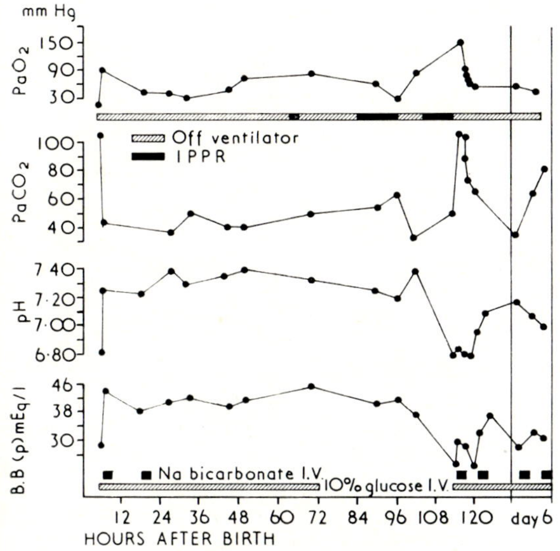


FIG. 2.—Biochemical course of infant (Case 5, Group I) from the start of intermittent positive pressure respiration at 7 hours of age until death on day 6. B.B.(p) = plasma buffer base.

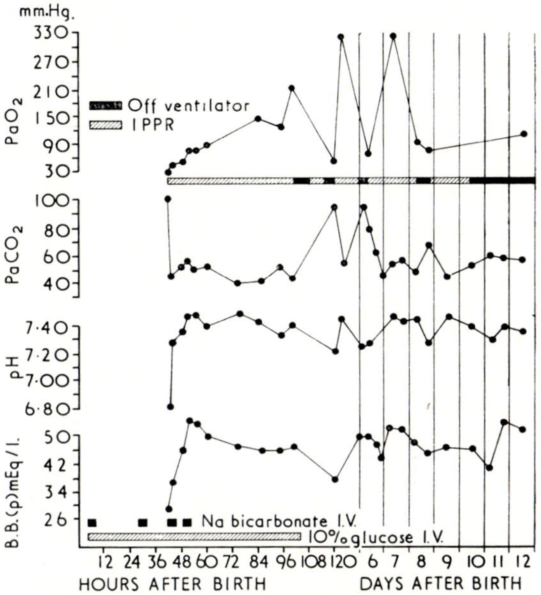


FIG. 3.—Biochemical course of infant (Case 19, Group II) from the start of intermittent positive pressure respiration at 42 hours of age (lived).

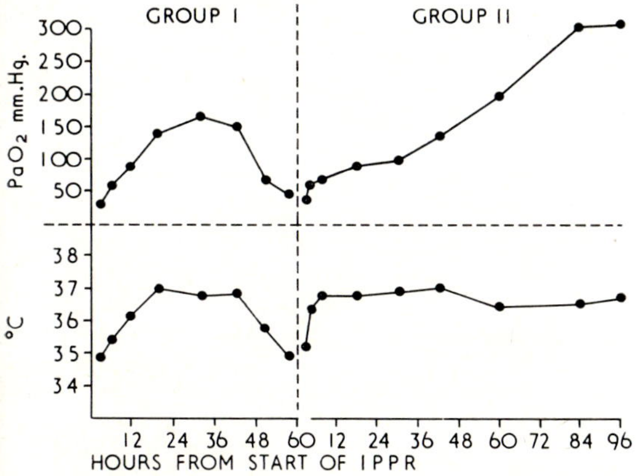


FIG. 4.—Mean arterial oxygen tensions after breathing 100% oxygen for 15 minutes, and colonic temperatures of 4 infants in Group I and 8 infants in Group II during positive pressure ventilation.

MacLeish, 1961; Warley and Gairdner, 1962). The effects of continued exposure to the relatively high oxygen percentages delivered by the ventilator (even with the '40% air mix') are unknown but may be harmful (Robertson, Tunell, and Rudhe, 1964). Improvements in ventilator design permitting graded reduction in oxygen concentrations are desirable.

Since in Group I the mean time on the respirator was relatively short (72 hours, Fig. 1, Table 2), the technical and medical complications associated with IPPR were not as prevalent as with the infants of Group II who required ventilation for longer periods (up to 14 days).

Our results suggest that when respiratory failure occurs after, rather than before, 24 hours of age, there is a better chance of survival with assisted ventilation. The patients who suffer respiratory failure within the first 24 hours after birth (Group I) have probably severe progressive pulmonary disease, and IPPR merely prolongs, rather than saves, life.

In Group II, it seemed that there was minimal progression of pulmonary changes, thus permitting survival by applying IPPR 'as an extra respiratory muscle' which alleviated neuromuscular exhaustion, and thus allowed a relatively normal acid-base balance to be maintained and possibly prevented further pulmonary collapse.

No infant weighing less than 1,800 g. at birth survived in either group.

It is pertinent here to make some general remarks on the management of ventilators in the treatment of respiratory failure in such cases. According to Didier and Helmholz (1964) the problems with infants 'seem to increase exponentially as patient size diminishes'. This is certainly our own experience and any success with this method is completely dependent on continuous well-trained, experienced nursing and medical supervision, with 24-hour facilities for biochemical determinations. Infants undergoing assisted ventilation must never be left alone. Maintenance of adequate airflow into the lungs is crucial, and a breakdown of less than 5 minutes will reduce an infant in relatively good condition to a moribund state. For any hope of success a suitable organization for intensive care incorporating the above principles is essential.

## Conclusion

Our results suggest that if infants over 1,800 g. with failing respiration after 24 hours of age are placed on IPPR, and before a damaging degree of metabolic acidosis has developed, approximately one-half will survive with our present methods.

On the basis of our experience we suggest that assisted ventilation should be instituted as soon as any three of the following five indications are present (Table 4).

TABLE 4

INDICATIONS FOR ASSISTED VENTILATION

| Clinical | | | Biochemical | |
|---|---|---|---|---|
| Respiratory Rate | Heart Rate | Colour | $PaCO_2$ | $PaO_2$ |
| <30/min. or >120/min. | <80/min. or >160/min. | Generalized cyanosis in 100% $O_2$ | >80 mm. Hg | <40 mm. Hg while breathing 100% $O_2$ |

If further work confirms our results, a decrease in mortality in infants over 1,800 g. could be anticipated. While approximately 40% of our mortality from RDS in this exclusively referral hospital takes place in infants weighing over 1,800 g. at birth (Hanley, Braudo, and Swyer, 1963), it is probable that this represents only about 5% of the over-all mortality from RDS in the population at large. Thus we suggest that assisted ventilation should only be considered in centres where special facilities can be concentrated.

## Summary

Twenty infants dying from acute cardio-respiratory failure due to respiratory distress syndrome were ventilated by intermittent positive pressure respiration.

Of these 20, 7 died at less than 24 hours of age and IPPR merely prolonged life; 13 died at more than 24 hours of age; and 7 survived, 6 as yet having no evidence of neurological damage.

Criteria are suggested for the selection of patients for IPPR.

The needs of an organization carrying out assisted ventilation in infants are discussed.

We thank Dr. C. E. Snelling and other members of the staff of the Hospital for Sick Children for their help and encouragement, Dr. B. Fearon for surgical advice and for performing tracheostomies, Dr. S. H. Jackson for biochemical advice, the nursing staff of the premature nursery, Mr. D. McIntosh for technical help, and Miss C. MacLennan for secretarial assistance.

We acknowledge the help of Dr. Peter Fleming in the management of Klebsiella pneumonia with Cephalosporin C; we also thank Glaxo Laboratories of Canada and England for supplies of Cephalosporin C.

REFERENCES

Astrup, P., Jørgensen, K., Siggaard Anderson, O., and Engel, K. (1960). The acid-base metabolism: A new approach. *Lancet*, **1**, 1035.

Benson, F., Celander, O., Haglund, G., Nilsson, L., Paulsen, L., and Renck, L. (1958). Positive-pressure respirator treatment of severe pulmonary insufficiency in the newborn infant. A clinical report. *Acta anaesth. scand.*, **2**, 37.

Delivoria-Papadopoulos, M., and Swyer, P. R. (1963). An experimental study of the possibility of reversing the biochemical changes of terminal hyaline membrane disease by assisted ventilation. Program and abstracts. Soc. for Pediatric Research, 33rd Annual Meeting, p. 33. (Abstr. *J. Pediat.*, **63**, 733.)

——, —— (1964). Assisted ventilation in terminal hyaline membrane disease. *Arch. Dis. Childh.*, **39**, 481.

Didier, E. P., and Helmholz, H. F., Jr. (1964). Principles in the selection and use of mechanical ventilators and assisters. *Med. Clin. N. Amer.*, **48**, 867.

Donald, I., Kerr, M. M., and MacDonald, I. R. (1958). Respiratory phenomena in the newborn. Experiments in their measurement and assistance. *Scot. med. J.*, **3**, 151.

——, and Lord, J. (1953). Augmented respiration: Studies in atelectasis neonatorum. *Lancet*, **1**, 9.

Dunham, E. C. (1961). *Premature Infants*, 3rd ed., ed. W. M. Silverman, pp. 231-235. Hoeber, New York.

Fairley, H. B., and Britt, B. A. (1964). The adequacy of the air-mix control in ventilators operated from an oxygen source. *Canad. med. Ass. J.*, **90**, 1394.

Fearon, B. (1962). Acute laryngotracheobronchitis in infancy and childhood. *Pediat. Clin. N. Amer.*, **9**, 1095.

——, Smith, C., Delivoria-Papadopoulos, M., Levison, H., and Swyer, P. R. (1964). The idiopathic respiratory distress syndrome in the newborn. *Ann. Otol. (St. Louis)*, **73**, 1082.

Hanley, W. B., Braudo, M., and Swyer, P. R. (1963). Neonatal respiratory distress: experience at the Hospital for Sick Children, Toronto 1960-1961. *Canad. med. Ass. J.*, **89**, 375.

Heese, H. D., Wittmann, W., and Malan, A. F. (1963). The management of the respiratory distress syndrome of the newborn with positive-pressure respiration. *S. Afr. med. J.*, **37**, 123.

Natelson, S. (1951). Routine use of ultramicro methods in the clinical laboratory. *Amer. J. clin. Path.*, **21**, 1153.

Nelson, N. M., Prod'hom, L. S., Cherry, R. B., Lipsitz, P. J., and Smith, C. A. (1963). Pulmonary functions in the newborn infant: the alveolar-arterial oxygen gradient. *J. appl. Physiol.*, **18**, 534.

Peterson, H. G., Jr., and Pendleton, M. E. (1955). Contrasting roentgenographic pulmonary patterns of the hyaline membrane and fetal aspiration syndromes. *Amer. J. Roentgenol.*, **74**, 800.

Robertson, B., Tunell, R., and Rudhe, U. (1964). Late stages of pulmonary hyaline membranes of the newborn. *Acta paediat. (Uppsala)*, **53**, 433.

Severinghaus, J. W., and Bradley, A. F. (1958). Electrodes for blood $pO_2$ and $pCO_2$ determination. *J. appl. Physiol.*, **13**, 515.

Singer, R. B., and Hastings, A. B. (1948). An improved clinical method for the estimation of disturbances of the acid-base balance of human blood. *Medicine (Baltimore)*, **27**, 223.

Stahlman, M., Young, Wm., and Payne, G. (1962). Studies of ventilatory aids in hyaline membrane disease. Program and abstracts. Soc. for Pediatric Research, 32nd Annual Meeting. p. 12. (Abstr. *Amer. J. Dis. Child.*, **104**, 526.)

Strang, L. B., and MacLeish, M. H. (1961). Ventilatory failure and right-to-left shunts in newborn infants with respiratory distress syndrome. *Pediatrics*, **28**, 17.

Warley, M. A., and Gairdner, D. (1962). Respiratory distress syndrome of the newborn—principles in treatment. *Arch. Dis. Childh.*, **37**, 455.

*Arch. Dis. Childh.*, 1965, **40**, 480.

# BLOOD VOLUME AND HAEMATOCRIT STUDIES IN RESPIRATORY DISTRESS SYNDROME OF THE NEWBORN

BY

J. A. INALL, M. M. BLUHM* MARGARET M. KERR, T. A. DOUGLAS, C. S. HOPE, and J. H. HUTCHISON

*From the Departments of Child Health and Biochemistry, University of Glasgow*

(RECEIVED FOR PUBLICATION FEBRUARY 18, 1965)

The observation that a raised venous pressure appears to be of benefit to newborn babies with respiratory distress (Bonham Carter, Bound, and Smellie, 1956) led Bound, Harvey, and Bagshaw (1962) to assess the effect of delayed clamping of the umbilical cord of premature babies. In that investigation it was concluded that the placental transfusion was responsible for the lower incidence of respiratory distress in those premature babies where clamping of the cord was delayed. It occurred to us that these observations might have a common basis in some abnormality of the blood volume in those babies who develop the respiratory distress syndrome (RDS). While we were studying a therapeutic approach to RDS (Hutchison, Kerr, Douglas, Inall, and Crosbie, 1964), we took the opportunity to measure the blood volumes of 17 babies. A group of 20 normal premature babies was also studied by the same technique. This paper describes the results of these studies.

The criteria previously described for the diagnosis of severe idiopathic respiratory distress (Hutchison *et al.*, 1964) were common to all cases. These were (1) respiratory grunting; (2) tachypnoea over 60 per minute after the first hour; (3) marked and persistent sternal, subcostal, and intercostal recession during inspiration; (4) cyanosis when breathing air; and (5) characteristic radiographic changes, i.e. diffuse reticulogranular mottling in the lung fields and an 'air bronchogram'.

## Material and Methods

The blood volumes were measured at times varying from 2½ to 9 hours after birth. 13 of the 17 babies with RDS had birth weights below 2·5 kg. The 20 'normal' babies were healthy newborns with a birth weight of less than 2·5 kg. In 16 the blood volumes were measured within 9 hours of birth. Although the time of cord clamping was not accurately recorded, the policy in the hospital was such that few, if any, of the babies that were studied would have had the cord clamping delayed.

**Haematocrits.**—These were determined in a microhaematocrit centrifuge (Hawksley Ltd., London).

**Blood volumes** were estimated by an isotope dilution technique using $^{131}I$ radioiodinated human serum albumin (RIHSA) obtained from Radiochemical Centre, Amersham, England. The radioactivity was measured in a scintillation counter (Isotope Developments Ltd.). 30 minutes before the injection of the radioiodinated albumin, 1 mg. potassium iodide was given intravenously to minimize the possible uptake of $^{131}I$ by the thyroid gland.

**Preparation of RIHSA for Injection.**—The RIHSA was diluted with sterile water so that the final solution contained 0·5 μc $^{131}I$/ml.; 1% stable HSA was added as carrier.

**Measurement of Quantity Injected.**—The quantity administered was determined by counting the syringe before and after the injection. For this purpose, the syringe was placed into a plastic adapter, thus achieving a constant spatial relation between radioactivity and detector (Fig. 1).

Since the blood samples were diluted to 3 ml. with water and counted in a plastic vial, it was necessary to derive the factor relating the activity of 1 ml. RISHA in the syringe adapter to 1 ml. diluted to 3 ml. and counted in a plastic vial. This factor was determined experimentally and used throughout the investigation.

**Technique of Injection and Sampling.**—The RIHSA was injected into a scalp vein through a polythene catheter attached to a needle. After completion of the injection the syringe was refilled through a three-way tap with 20% fructose solution and this also was injected through the catheter and needle. Blood samples were taken from an umbilical catheter 5, 15, and 30 minutes after the initial injection.

Haematocrits were measured on each sample in

* Present address: Radiotherapy Department, North Middlesex Hospital, Silver Street, Edmonton, London N.18.

duplicate, and for radioactivity 1 ml. of whole blood was diluted with 2 ml. water and counted in a plastic vial in the scintillation counter. A semilogarithmic plot of activity against time enabled the zero time activity to be determined by extrapolation.

The whole blood volume was obtained by dividing the counts injected by the activity of the zero time sample:

$$\text{i.e. } \frac{\text{Actual counts/100 sec. injected}}{\text{Counts/ml. whole blood/100 sec.}} = \frac{\text{Whole blood}}{\text{volume (ml.).}}$$

In certain cases plasma was prepared and this was counted instead of the whole blood. However, this procedure requires the removal of a greater volume of blood from the baby and for this reason whole blood was preferred. It should be stated that RIHSA measures plasma volume directly, the red cell volume and total blood volume being inferred on the assumption that the packed cell volume of the blood sample is the same as the whole body haematocrit. We know, of course, that this is not so in adults, but correction factors for premature infants of different weights and gestation periods are not available. We do not think that our assumption invalidates our subsequent arguments.

## Results

The data for the normal babies are shown in Table 1 and for the babies with RDS in Table 2. It will be seen that the mean value for the blood volume of the normal babies was 107 ml./kg., and 94 ml./kg. for the babies with RDS, but the difference is not statistically significant ($p > 0 \cdot 1$). The results of the haematocrit estimations show a mean figure of 58% for the normal babies and 48% for the babies with RDS, and this is statistically a highly significant difference ($p < 0 \cdot 01$).

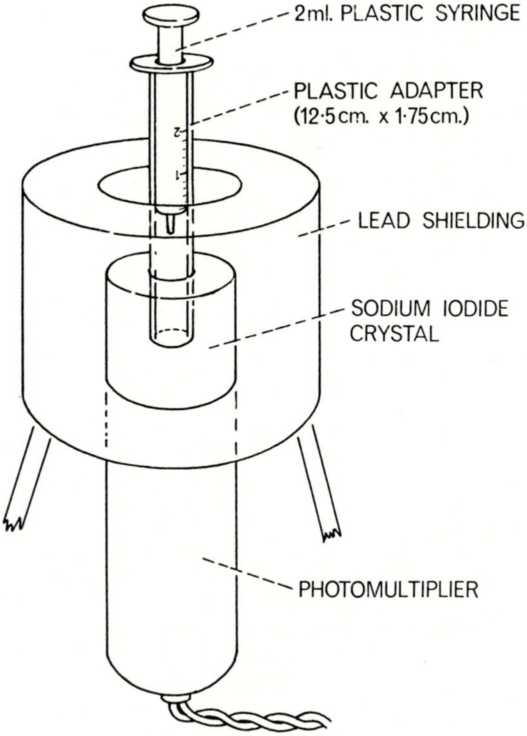


FIG.—Illustration of plastic syringe and adapter in IDL scintillation counter.

TABLE 1

DETAILS OF NORMAL BABIES

| Case No. | Weight (kg.) | Age (hr. min.) | Blood Volume (ml.) | Blood Volume (ml./kg.) | Haematocrit (%) |
|---|---|---|---|---|---|
| 1 | 2·29 | 1 25 | 224 | 97·7 | 63 |
| 2 | 1·78 | 7 25 | 188 | 105·5 | 65 |
| 3 | 1·97 | 8 45 | 175 | 88·7 | 50 |
| 4 | 1·18 | 15 55 | 206 | 115·6 | 74 |
| 5 | 2·23 | 6 — | 198 | 88·7 | 50 |
| 6 | 1·41 | 7 55 | 145 | 102·8 | 63 |
| 7 | 1·76 | 7 35 | 227 | 128·9 | 63 |
| 8 | 2·15 | 8 40 | 294 | 136·7 | 53 |
| 9 | 1·94 | 6 30 | 216 | 111·2 | 62 |
| 10 | 2·02 | 5 15 | 230 | 113·9 | 68 |
| 11 | 2·38 | 16 45 | 245 | 102·9 | 56 |
| 12 | 1·55 | 13 30 | 142 | 91·6 | 45 |
| 13 | 2·08 | 7 5 | 266 | 127·7 | 42 |
| 14 | 1·98 | 8 — | 272 | 137·4 | 64 |
| 15 | 2·33 | 5 30 | 235 | 100·8 | 48 |
| 16 | 1·84 | 18 — | 227 | 123·3 | 59 |
| 17 | 2·05 | 8 — | 196 | 95·5 | 49 |
| 18 | 1·76 | 2 5 | 186 | 105·6 | 61 |
| 19 | 1·73 | 8 50 | 172 | 99·4 | 61 |
| 20 | 1·63 | 6 30 | 102 | 62·5 | 66 |
| Mean . . . . . . | 1·93 | | 207·3 | 106·8 | 58·1 |
| SD . . . . . . | 0·259 | | 45·58 | 17·87 | 8·30 |
| SEM . . . . . . | 0·059 | | 10·46 | 4·09 | 1·90 |

TABLE 2

DETAILS OF BABIES WITH RESPIRATORY DISTRESS SYNDROME

| Case No. | Weight (kg.) | Age (hr. min.) | Blood Volume (ml.) | Blood Volume (ml./kg.) | Haematocrit (%) |
|---|---|---|---|---|---|
| 1 | 1·81 | 3 40 | 198 | 109·3 | 44 |
| 2 | 2·58 | 3 55 | 250 | 96·8 | 48 |
| 3 | 2·34 | 4 10 | 210 | 89·7 | 61 |
| 4 | 1·75 | 7 25 | 158 | 90·2 | 47 |
| 5 | 2·09 | 4 40 | 214 | 102·3 | 53 |
| 6 | 1·31 | 4 10 | 158 | 120·6 | 41 |
| 7 | 3·04 | 8 55 | 240 | 78·7 | 48 |
| 8 | 1·04 | 3 40 | 94 | 90·3 | 34 |
| 9 | 2·23 | 5 30 | 222 | 99·5 | 44 |
| 10 | 2·22 | 2 55 | 204 | 91·8 | 56 |
| 11 | 2·01 | 4 50 | 176 | 87·5 | 45 |
| 12 | 2·62 | 6 35 | 229 | 87·2 | 53 |
| 13 | 2·08 | 6 25 | 206 | 98·9 | 47 |
| 14 | 1·95 | 5 40 | 194 | 99·3 | 56 |
| 15 | 1·72 | 6 — | 152 | 88·3 | 48 |
| 16 | 1·68 | 3 30 | 140 | 83·3 | 47 |
| 17 | 2·67 | 4 10 | 222 | 83·0 | 46 |
| Mean .. .. .. | 2·07 | | 192·2 | 93·9 | 48·1 |
| SD .. .. .. | 0·49 | | 39·48 | 10·12 | 6·135 |
| SEM .. .. .. | 0·123 | | 9·87 | 2·53 | 1·534 |

## Discussion

Assessment of the blood volume, its alterations in the immediate postnatal period, and the factors involved in such alterations in the normal newborn have been made by a number of workers. Some have also made conjectures as to the relation of such changes to the development of RDS. These alterations in blood volume could be of clinical importance if delayed clamping of the umbilical cord, which results in a placental transfusion, can prevent the development of RDS (Bound *et al.*, 1962).

The various studies of the blood volume of the newborn infant have produced somewhat conflicting results. Gairdner, Marks, Roscoe, and Brettell (1958) and Clark and Gairdner (1960) have suggested that there is a diminution in the blood volume in the first 2 hours of life due to an outward shift of plasma fluid. On the other hand, Sisson and Whalen (1960) have demonstrated an increase in the blood volumes which they suggest is derived from blood in a storage space such as the liver. However, it does seem certain that a placental transfusion as a result of delay in clamping the cord will be followed by an increase in the blood volume of the baby, and that this increase persists for up to 4 hours (De Marsh, Windle, and Alt, 1942; Usher, Shephard, and Lind, 1963). Some of these writers suggest a possible relation between the various blood volume changes and RDS, but Usher *et al.* (1963) reported that no abnormality of respiration developed in any of their cases, irrespective of the time of clamping the cord. Steele (1962) has suggested from his studies that the blood volume might best be kept in the low normal range for premature babies, and Taylor, Bright, and Birchard (1959) showed more abnormal respiratory signs in those babies receiving a placental transfusion.

Our mean figure of 94 ml./kg. for babies with RDS is not statistically different from the mean of 107 ml./kg. for the control series of premature babies. These values are close to those of the full-term normal babies described by Mollison, Veall, and Cutbush (1950), some of whom had received a placental transfusion, and to those of Usher *et al.* (1963), where cord clamping was delayed. We have, therefore, found no characteristic deviation of the blood volume in RDS. On the other hand, the haematocrit does show a significant deviation.

Most published values for the range of haematocrit in the full-term newborn are in the papers already noted, where the estimation was a necessary part of the technique of blood volume determination. An average normal figure of 50% is noted for the cord blood. Gairdner *et al.* (1958) record a rising haematocrit in the first hours of life in 30 of 39 babies, predominantly of average birth weight and without delay in cord clamping. Although exact figures are not given, in a typical case discussed, a change from 53% to 61% is noted as being average. The authors suggest a plasma shift into extravascular spaces including the pulmonary alveoli, with a possible contribution to the development of RDS. Usher *et al.* (1963) have in contrast shown that changes in the haematocrit are dependent on the time of clamping the cord. They noted that 16 cord haematocrits gave an average of 48% and they use this as the normal for all cases studied. Where the clamping of the cord was delayed, there was an increase in the haematocrit to a mean of 59% at 30 minutes and 64% at 4 hours, but when the cord was clamped immediately a level of 48% persisted. Neither group showed any tendency to develop respiratory distress, but none of the babies was below 2·5 kg. birth weight. Babies with a low birth weight were specifically studied by Pincus, Gittleman, Saito, and Sobel (1956), though their samples were of capillary blood. They showed uncorrected haematocrit figures with an average of 58%, and it can be assumed that the venous haematocrit would have been lower. Blanc and Lermontoff (1961) gave figures of over 60% for babies weighing 1·0-2·0 kg. and up to 24 hours of age. Our figures for the babies with RDS show a mean value of 48%, which contrasts with most other published results for babies who were not in respiratory distress, and when the difference from the value of 58% in our normal premature is considered it is found to be statistically significant ($p < 0 \cdot 01$).

Certain things seem to follow from this observed low figure in the distressed babies. First, if, as De Marsh *et al.* (1942) and Usher *et al.* (1963) have each separately indicated, the haematocrit is a function of the volume of the placental red cell transfusion, these babies with a low haematocrit might be inferred to have been deprived of this transfusion and this could be taken to support the thesis that such a transfusion tended to prevent the development of respiratory distress. We know that the majority of these babies did in fact have the cord clamped early. Furthermore, Redmond, Isana, and Ingall (1965) have recently demonstrated that the placental transfusion may be related to the infant's first breaths and initial pulmonary aeration, rather than to the time interval between delivery and clamping of the umbilical cord; and a delay in the onset of respiration is common in infants who subsequently develop RDS. On the other hand the total blood volumes in our cases with RDS fall within the high ranges that Usher *et al.* (1963) described in their patients with delayed clamping of the cord, and they were not significantly different from the blood volumes of premature infants who did not develop RDS.

Secondly, such low values for the haematocrit in our cases with RDS are certainly not compatible with the sometimes expressed but inadequately investigated belief that babies with RDS have an increased haematocrit. Danks and Stevens (1964) have recently described a baby where polycythaemia caused late respiratory distress which responded well to a 'dextrose exchange transfusion'. They mention that certain groups of babies may carry a particular risk of respiratory distress due to haemoconcentration, but it is clear that in the majority of babies with idiopathic RDS a high haematocrit is not found. Finally, if these babies with RDS have a total blood volume in the range of normal premature babies, as our results seem to indicate, and yet have a low haematocrit and hence a low circulating red cell volume, it is possible that the circulating red cell volume may have diminished during the development of the distressed state or as a consequence thereof. We have no evidence to indicate where the missing red cells have gone. The constant necropsy finding of intense pulmonary congestion, sometimes associated with haemorrhage, might suggest sequestration of the red cells in the lungs, and such an occurrence might explain, in part at least, the respiratory difficulty which these infants experience.

## Summary

The blood volumes and haematocrit values were measured in 17 infants with the idiopathic respiratory distress syndrome and in 20 unaffected infants with a birth weight of less than 2·5 kg. Cord clamping was not delayed in these infants.

The mean figure for blood volume in babies with RDS (94 ml./kg.) was not statistically different from the mean of 107 ml./kg. for the unaffected babies ($p > 0 \cdot 1$). The haematocrit estimations showed a mean of 48% for babies with RDS and 58% for the unaffected babies, which is a highly significant difference ($p < 0 \cdot 01$).

The low values for the haematocrit in our cases of RDS contrast with the sometimes expressed belief that such babies have a high haematocrit. They may indicate sequestration of the red cells in the lungs and this might be related in some degree to the respiratory distress.

Part of the expenses of this study was met by a grant from the Scottish Hospitals Endowments Research Trust.

### References

Blanc, W. A., and Lermontoff, T. (1961). Hematocrit values in premature infants. In *Dunham's Premature Infants*, ed. W. A. Silverman, 3rd ed., p. 542. Hoeber Medical Division, New York.

Bonham Carter, R. E., Bound, J. P., and Smellie, J. M. (1956). Mean venous pressures in the first hours of life. *Lancet*, **2**, 1320.

Bound, J. P., Harvey, P. W., and Bagshaw, H. B. (1962). Prevention of pulmonary syndrome of the newborn. *ibid.*, **1**, 1200.

Clark, A. C. L., and Gairdner, D. (1960). Postnatal plasma shift in premature infants. *Arch. Dis. Childh.*, **35**, 352.

Danks, D. M., and Stevens, L. H. (1964). Neonatal respiratory distress associated with a high haematocrit reading. *Lancet*, **2**, 499.

De Marsh, Q. B., Windle, W. F., and Alt, H. L. (1942). Blood volume of newborn infant in relation to early and late clamping of the umbilical cord. *Amer. J. Dis. Child.*, **63**, 1123.

Gairdner, D., Marks, J., Roscoe, J. D., and Brettell, R. O. (1958). The fluid shift from the vascular compartment immediately after birth. *Arch. Dis. Childh.*, **33**, 489.

Hutchison, J. H., Kerr, M. M., Douglas, T. A., Inall, J. A., and Crosbie, J. C. (1964). A therapeutic approach in 100 cases of the respiratory distress syndrome of the newborn infant. *Pediatrics*, **33**, 956.

Mollison, P. L., Veall, N., and Cutbush, M. (1950). Red cell and plasma volume in newborn infants. *Arch. Dis. Childh.*, **25**, 242.

Pincus, J. B., Gittleman, I. F., Saito, M., and Sobel, A. E. (1956). A study of plasma values of sodium potassium, chloride, carbon dioxide, carbon dioxide tension, sugar, urea and the protein base binding power pH, and haematocrit in prematures on the first day of life. *Pediatrics*, **18**, 39.

Redmond, A., Isana, S., and Ingall, D. (1965). Relation of onset of respiration to placental transfusion. *Lancet*, **1**, 283.

Sisson, T. R. C., and Whalen, L. E. (1960). The blood volume of infants. III. Alterations in the first hours after birth. *J. Pediat.*, **56**, 43.

Steele, M. W. (1962). Plasma volume changes in the neonate. *Amer. J. Dis. Child.*, **103**, 10.

Taylor, P. M., Bright, N. H., and Birchard, E. L. (1959). The effect of immediate versus delayed clamping of the umbilical cord on mortality and respiratory rates of the newborn infant. *Amer. J. Dis. Child.*, **98**, 649.

Usher, R., Shephard, M., and Lind, J. (1963). The blood volume of the newborn infant and placental transfusion. *Acta paediat. (Uppsala)*, **52**, 497.

*Arch. Dis. Childh.*, 1965, **40**, 485.

# THE METABOLIC ERROR IN PRIMARY HYPEROXALURIA*

BY

T. D. R. HOCKADAY, J. E. CLAYTON, and L. H. SMITH, JR.†

*From Department of the Regius Professor of Medicine, the Radcliffe Infirmary, Oxford, U.K., and the Endocrine Unit, the Massachusetts General Hospital, Boston, U.S.A.*

(RECEIVED FOR PUBLICATION MAY 28, 1964)

Knowledge of the incidence of a disease in successive generations of a family has value beyond the basis it provides for prediction of the health of future generations. Should the incidence suggest inheritance according to simple Mendelian rules, the disease probably has its origin in abnormality of a single genetic particle, though this has never been directly demonstrated. Garrod (1908) linked the occurrence of metabolic errors with the inheritance of Mendelian characteristics. Abnormalities inherited according to Mendelian laws were shown to result from inactivity of a single enzyme, first in moulds (Beadle and Tatum, 1941) and later in human disease (e.g. deficiency of erythrocyte diaphorase in one type of methaemoglobinaemia (Gibson, 1948)). Alteration of only one amino acid in a protein is sufficient to cause disease, as in the haemoglobinopathy of sickle-cell anaemia (Ingram, 1957).

In the many common diseases with a familial tendency that are, at least partially, genetically determined (e.g. essential hypertension, diabetes mellitus, schizophrenia), simple Mendelian rules do not apply, and summation of the actions of several genes has been evoked. In seeking the mechanisms through which inherited flaws are manifest, it seems simpler to study conditions with clear-cut Mendelian inheritance despite their rarity.

The evidence that 'primary hyperoxaluria' is inherited as a Mendelian recessive characteristic will be discussed, and taken as the foundation for a search for an enzymatic fault. All patients with apparently similar metabolic abnormalities will not necessarily have the same metabolic defect, nor will all alterations in one enzyme protein be identical or have the same effect on function. Thus, in the glycogenoses, excess of liver glycogen may be associated with any one of four different enzyme deficiencies (Cori, 1957), and at least five different single amino acid abnormalities of haemoglobin are known. At present only those cases of inherited disease that occur within one family can be considered identical in origin.

### The Clinical Condition and its Inheritance

Primary hyperoxaluria (Archer, Dormer, Scowen, and Watts, 1957) or oxalosis (Ying Chou and Donohue, 1952) is a rare and serious disease, which usually presents before the age of 10 years and often causes death from renal failure before the age of 20. It is characterized by excessive deposition of calcium oxalate in the kidneys, recurrent calcium oxalate stones in the urinary tract, excessive urinary excretion of oxalate not caused by excessive ingestion of oxalate, and the finding at necropsy of calcium oxalate crystals throughout the body. None of these abnormalities alone is pathognomonic of the disease, since each occurs in conditions other than primary hyperoxaluria, as has been discussed by Hockaday, Clayton, Frederick, and Smith (1964). On the other hand, the presence of all three abnormalities is not essential in the diagnosis of primary hyperoxaluria. In the absence of any critical *in vitro* test, this is best illustrated by members of a sibship of whom some show all the classical features and some do not. Dr. E. G. Hall has kindly given permission for reference to a further member, born in 1962, of family No. 4 of Hall, Scowen, and Watts (1960). This child was in renal failure in his first month and died in his first year, yet never had renal calculi despite renal and bony oxalate deposits. Four of his sibs, who also had hyperoxaluria, had recurrent oxalate calculi.

The boy, a mongol of birth weight 6 lb. 9 oz. (2,976 g.), was admitted to hospital at the age of 1 month because of a 3-day history of 'convulsions'—in fact, tetany. The

* Based on the Donald Paterson Prize Essay, 1964, by one of us (T.D.R.H.)

† Present address: Chief of Medicine, San Francisco Center of the University of California Medical School, San Francisco, California, U.S.A.

blood urea was 115 mg./100 ml. and the serum calcium 7·6 mg./100 ml. Urinary excretion of oxalate was around 50 mg./24 hr. The blood urea concentration rose to 250 mg./100 ml., but later he improved slowly and the blood urea decreased. On radiological examination the kidneys had a uniformly increased density but did not contain calculi. At the age of 7 months the boy died at home from aspiration of food. At necropsy the kidneys were rather small and had a smooth surface. There were no calculi but both cortex and medulla were speckled with minute gritty granules. Histological examination showed deposits of oxalate throughout the kidneys and scattered in the bones, but little evidence of oxalate elsewhere.

The first proven case of primary hyperoxaluria was in a 7-year-old girl troubled by urinary calculi since the age of 2 years (Newns and Black, 1953). Apart from this first measurement of the abnormally high urinary excretion of oxalate, this case was important because the patient's elder brother had died at 8½ years from renal failure consequent to multiple calcium oxalate stones and another sib had died shortly after premature birth. Aponte and Fetter (1954), in a report of 3 brothers, 2 of whom were identical twins, described the first cases to show all the features now thought typical of the disease. Thereafter 'primary hyperoxaluria' and 'oxalosis' were generally considered to be the same condition.

Inheritance of primary hyperoxaluria as a recessive characteristic is based upon 16 families in which sibs were affected (Buri, 1962; Hockaday *et al.*, 1964). The most extensive surveys of urinary oxalate excretion by the relatives of patients (Archer, Dormer, Scowen, and Watts, 1958b; Scowen, Watts, and Hall, 1959) showed abnormally high values in some sibs, but never in parents or other relatives. Likewise, no parent has had a medical history typical of primary hyperoxaluria, though parents or other close relatives may have had renal stones in middle age. Parental consanguinity has been reported in four cases.

The following brief description of two patients and their families, previously reported only in summary (Hockaday *et al.*, 1964), provides additional evidence that primary hyperoxaluria is inherited as a Mendelian recessive characteristic.

### Case Reports

**Case 1.** J.M., a 13-year-old girl, had passed gravel in her urine and had had slight haematuria when less than 1 year old. These symptoms, together with flank and abdominal pain, had recurred frequently. Despite repeated urinary infections, recently controlled by continual antibiotic treatment, the girl is healthy, of normal size, and menstruates regularly. Her urinary oxalate excretion varied from 200 to 240 mg./24 hr. (the upper limit of normal is 60 mg./24 hr.).

Her parents, not consanguineous, have had 6 other children. One healthy daughter, age 23, is married with a healthy child, and one son age 7 is healthy. A 4½-year-old boy, though physically healthy, is mentally retarded. One son died age 7 years, after pain, vomiting, fever, haematuria, and the passage of gravel had begun in his second year. A kidney removed at operation shortly before his death contained many deposits of calcium oxalate. Another son died at 13 years and a daughter died at 5½ years; both had had abdominal pain, haematuria, and passage of gravel since infancy. The parents are healthy and without evidence of disease of the urinary tract.

**Case 2.** T.S., an 18-year-old college student, has had recurrent urinary calculi since the age of 9. In the past she had had episodes suggestive of renal colic, more frequently dull pain in both renal angles, and episodes of urinary frequency and nocturia. Although she has been relatively free of symptoms during the past 2 years, radiological examination has shown stones in both kidneys. Her urinary excretion of oxalate was 190 and 230 mg./24 hr. on two separate occasions. She is a normally developed girl and no abnormalities were found on abdominal examination, except for tenderness on palpation posteriorly over the left renal angle.

The girl has 6 sibs, 4 of whom are healthy. A 6-year-old brother has had recurrent renal stones, and both he and another brother age 5 years have increased urinary excretion of oxalate. The parents, from unrelated families, are healthy and have no history of renal disease.

Claims that primary hyperoxaluria is inherited as a dominant trait are based on study of a few families only. The evidence has consisted of slight increase of urinary oxalate excretion by relatives in previous generations (Shepard, Krebs, and Lee, 1958), of the occurrence of renal stones in previous generations, but without hyperoxaluria or a typically severe clinical course (McLaurin, Beisel, McCormick, Scalettar, and Herman, 1961), or of case histories in which death from uraemia and increased urinary excretion of oxalate went with other features suggestive of a primary renal disorder (Lagrue, Laudat, Meyer, Sapir, and Milliez, 1959; Dempsey, Forbes, Melick, and Henneman, 1960).

No consistent abnormality has yet been detected in the parents of patients, who are presumed heterozygous for the condition.

### Metabolic Investigations

Neither increased alimentary absorption nor decreased destruction of oxalate is likely to be the cause of oxalosis and primary hyperoxaluria. Archer, Dormer, Scowen, and Watts (1958a) showed that patients absorbed oxalate normally. Injected $^{14}C$-labelled oxalate can be almost completely recovered from urine and does not contribute to expired carbon dioxide (Elder and Wyngaarden, 1960), which indicates that oxalate is metabolically inert in humans.

Increased formation of oxalate within the body, the result of the postulated enzyme defect, seems a more probable mechanism of the disease. The only known precursor of oxalate is glyoxylate (Fig. 1), though carbon atoms 1 and 2 of ascorbic acid may be converted to oxalate without prior formation of glyoxylate (the results of Atkins, Dean, Griffin, Scowen, and Watts (1963) agree with this possibility). Possible precursors of glyoxylate are glycollate, glycine, and $\gamma$-hydroxy-$\alpha$-ketoglutarate, a metabolite of hydroxyproline (Goldstone and Adams, 1962). Since increased urinary excretion of glycollate is as characteristic of the disease as is hyperoxaluria (Frederick, Rabkin, Ritchie, and Smith, 1963), deficient conversion of glyoxylate to glycollate cannot be its cause. Also, $\gamma$-hydroxy-$\alpha$-ketoglutarate may be metabolized more readily by way of malate than by decomposition to glyoxylate and pyruvate (Payes and Laties, 1963). The evidence for the formation of glyoxylate from glycine comes from *in vitro* experiments, in which high concentrations of glyoxylate were used (Nakada and Weinhouse, 1953). Because such concentrations inhibit tissue respiration the findings may apply only to tissues with such an abnormal metabolism. Other experiments have demonstrated that glycine is an important precursor of oxalate *in vivo*. Crawhall, de Mowbray, Scowen, and Watts (1959a) and Crowhall, Scowen, and Watts (1959b), in studies of two hyperoxaluric patients, showed that the proportion of urinary oxalate formed from glycine was normal in both.

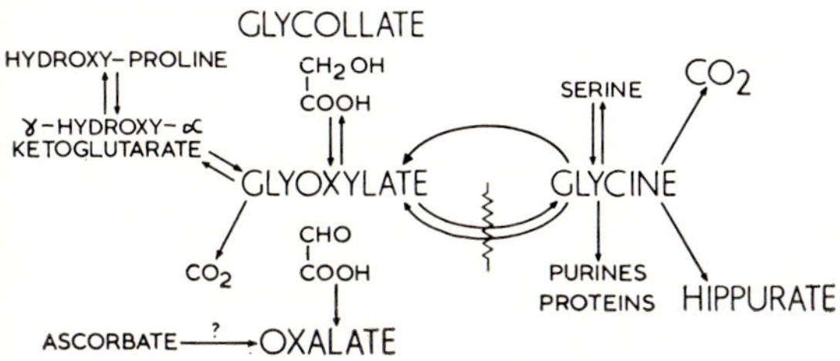


FIG. 1.—Major pathways of glyoxylate metabolism and oxalate synthesis in mammals.

Many transaminase enzymes are present in both mitochondria and the cytoplasmic sap (Baudhuin, Beaufay, Rahman-Li, Sellinger, Wattiaux, Jacques, and de Duve, 1964). The equilibrium position for the reversible interconversions of glycine and glyoxylate catalysed by transaminase enzymes is strongly in favour of glycine, but glycine oxidase (Ratner, Nocito, and Green, 1944) catalyses an irreversible formation of glyoxylate.

The mode of oxidation of glyoxylate to carbon dioxide is uncertain, though one reaction involves glutamate or $\alpha$-ketoglutarate; its exact mechanism is unknown (Nakada and Sund, 1958; Crawhall and Watts, 1962a). Glycine is sometimes assumed to be oxidized principally via glyoxylate, but conversion of glyoxylate to carbon dioxide after transamination to glycine is equally possible. Glyoxylate and glycollate are readily converted to glycine *in vivo* in rats (Weinhouse and Friedmann, 1951) and in pigeons (Weissbach and Sprinson, 1953), and glycine may be oxidized to carbon dioxide mainly by reactions involving serine, pyruvate or hydroxy-pyruvate, $\delta$-amino-laevulinic acid, or amino acetone, but not glyoxylate.

The metabolism of glyoxylate, by mitochondria from liver biopsy specimens from hyperoxaluric patients, was normal in its conversion to glycine, oxalate, and carbon dioxide (Crawhall and Watts, 1962b). In contrast, Frederick *et al.* (1963), after they injected $^{14}C$-carboxyl-labelled glyoxylate intravenously, recovered much less isotopic carbon dioxide from patients than from normal subjects.

## Our Recent Findings

The results of our recent studies on the defective metabolism in primary hyperoxaluria are summarized in this section according to the type of measurement made.

The time-honoured method used for metabolic investigations is the measurement of the amount of a substance excreted in the urine of a subject both under normal conditions and after administration of a possible precursor in large amount. Urinary glyoxylate concentration had not been measured previously by a quantitative method. Using the principle of isotope dilution, a method was developed for the measurement of urinary glyoxylate (Hockaday, Frederick, Clayton, and Smith, 1965). Patients with primary hyperoxaluria excreted more glyoxylate in the urine than did normal children (Hockaday *et al.*, 1964), in line with previous findings for oxalate and glycollate. The significance of the values obtained for glyoxylate is uncertain because the reactivity of glyoxylate with a number of compounds in urine makes it likely that the amount of glyoxylate in voided urine is not the same as that of urine in the renal calyces.

The effect of the ingestion of large amounts of ascorbic acid, glycine, or 1-hydroxyproline on the urinary excretion of glyoxylate, glycollate, and oxalate was observed in both healthy subjects and in patients with primary hyperoxaluria (Table 1). A change was seen only after 1-hydroxyproline (200 mg./kg.), when urinary excretion of glyoxylate and

TABLE 1

URINARY EXCRETION OF OXALATE, GLYOXYLATE, AND GLYCOLLATE AFTER ORAL ADMINISTRATION OF GLYCINE AND HYDROXYPROLINE IN PRIMARY HYPEROXALURIA

| | Oxalate (μ mole/hr.) | | | Glycollate (μ mole/hr.) | | | Glyoxylate (μ mole/hr.) | | |
|---|---|---|---|---|---|---|---|---|---|
| | Normal | Patient 1 | Patient 2 | Normal | Patient 1 | Patient 2 | Normal | Patient 1 | Patient 2 |
| *Glycine, 400 mg./kg.* | | | | | | | | | |
| Before dose .. .. .. | 15 | 48 | 162 | 30 | 59 | 244 | 0·43 | 0·24 | 0·78 |
| After dose, 0-3 hr. .. .. | 19 | 52 | 116 | 52 | 96 | 119 | 0·68 | 0·36 | 0·51 |
| 3-6 hr. .. .. | 17 | 73 | 113 | 70 | 56 | 106 | 0·92 | 0·34 | 0·62 |
| 6-9 hr. .. .. | 12 | 47 | 110 | 61 | 179 | 124 | 0·64 | 0·23 | 0·52 |
| *1-Hydroxyproline, 200 mg./kg.* | | | | | | | | | |
| Before dose .. .. .. | 21 | 55 | 120 | 39 | 68 | 106 | 0·35 | 0·15 | 0·48 |
| After dose, 0-3 hr. .. .. | 32 | 91 | 121 | 238 | 253 | 172 | 1·26 | 0·92 | 0·33 |
| 3-6 hr. .. .. | 23 | 94 | 106 | 272 | 402 | 139 | 1·35 | 0·51 | 0·69 |
| 6-9 hr. .. .. | 29 | 90 | 127 | 174 | 386 | 298 | 1·01 | 0·61 | 0·12 |

*N.B.* Patient 1 is Case 2 (age 11 years) of Frederick *et al.* (1963) and Patient 2 is their Case 1 (age 14 years) when some impairment of renal function (blood urea nitrogen = 34 mg./100 ml.) was already evident.

After 3 g. ascorbic acid, urinary excretion of oxalate, glyoxylate, and glycollate was unchanged in both a patient and his mother.

glycollate (but not oxalate) increased. Previously, repeated observations had shown that urinary oxalate excretion is unchanged by large amounts of glycine or ascorbic acid (Elder and Wyngaarden, 1960).

A second method of investigation is to follow the entry into various metabolites of an isotopic carbon atom from a compound concerned in oxalate metabolism. After intravenous injection of carboxyl-labelled $^{14}C$-glycollate, the entry of $^{14}C$ into expired carbon dioxide and urinary oxalate and glycollate showed the same difference between hyperoxaluric patients and control subjects as when $^{14}C$-glyoxylate had been injected: there was a low recovery of $^{14}C$ in carbon dioxide and increased recovery in urinary oxalate and glycollate. The urinary glyoxylate of patients also contained more $^{14}C$ than that of control subjects. Urinary hippurate and glycine, like carbon dioxide, contained less $^{14}C$ when collected from patients than from healthy subjects or even the parent of a patient (Table 2, Fig. 2). The patients showed no evidence of renal failure (blood urea nitrogen concentrations and creatinine clearances were normal).

This decreased recovery of injected $^{14}C$ as urinary hippurate and glycine from patients compared with controls was confirmed for $^{14}C$-carboxyl-labelled glyoxylate on its intravenous infusion for 6 hours, instead of the single, rapid injection used in previous studies (Frederick *et al.*, 1963). Observations on expired carbon dioxide were made hourly during the last 3 hours of the infusion, when an approximately steady state had been reached, and these (as well as measurements on urine for 24 hours from the start of the infusion) are listed in Table 3 and illustrated in Fig. 3. The pattern in patients of decreased recovery of isotope as urinary hippurate and glycine, as well as respiratory carbon dioxide, was maintained, as was the increase in isotope found as urinary glycollate, glyoxylate, and oxalate.

These observations on urinary hippurate and glycine strongly suggest a defect in the conversion of glyoxylate to glycine in primary hyperoxaluria. They can be easily reconciled with the observations

TABLE 2

RECOVERY OF RADIOACTIVITY AFTER INTRAVENOUS INJECTION OF SODIUM GLYCOLLATE, $CH_2OH \cdot {}^{14}COONa$
(1μ mole/kg. body weight and 20 μc. given to each)

| Subjects | Percentage Recovery of Administered Radioactivity in Two Periods (Time in Hr.) | | | | | | | | | | | % Recovery Admini-stered |
|---|---|---|---|---|---|---|---|---|---|---|---|---|
| | Expired $CO_2$ | Urinary Oxalate | | Urinary Glyoxylate | | Urinary Glycollate | | Urinary Hippurate | | Urinary Glycine | | |
| | 0–2 | 0–2 | 2–24 | 0–2 | 2–24 | 0–2 | 2–24 | 0–2 | 2–24 | 0–2 | 2–24 | Counts |
| Normal .. .. | 22·3 | 0·7 | 0·11 | 0·07 | 0·05 | 1·8 | 0·14 | 3·5 | 0·53 | 0·11 | 0·02 | 29·3 |
| Normal 2 .. .. | 14·2 | 1·1 | 0·14 | 0·11 | None | 2·7 | 0·05 | 1·4 | 0·51 | 0·15 | 0·06 | 19·4 |
| Heterozygote .. | 20·5 | 1·1 | 0·07 | 0·16 | None | 2·8 | 0·13 | 5·8 | 0·42 | 0·15 | 0·15 | 31·3 |
| Patient 1 (L.E.) .. | 2·1 | 3·8 | 13·7 | 0·45 | 0·14 | 9·5 | 27·0 | 0·18 | 0·08 | 0·01 | 0·02 | 57·0 |
| Patient 2 (D.M.) .. | 3·0 | 4·4 | 11·0 | 0·08 | 0·09 | 14·9 | 20·1 | 0·39 | 0·35 | 0·01 | 0·02 | 54·4 |

L.E. was an 8-year-old girl and D.M. was a 5-year-old boy. Both have had recurrent urinary oxalate calculi since the age of 2-3 years and have increased urinary excretion of oxalate. Though both had renal calculi on radiographs, there was no significant impairment of renal function in either.

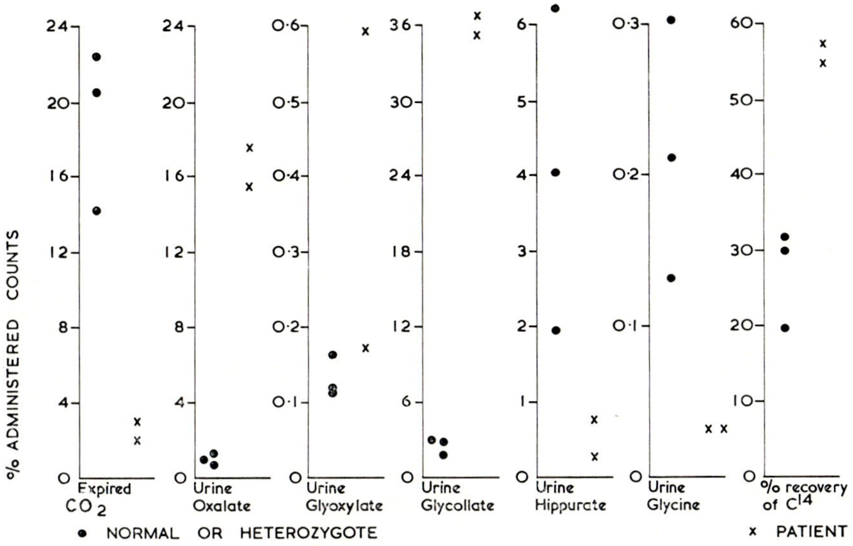


FIG. 2.—Metabolism of carboxyl-labelled glycollate-$^{14}C$ in man. The recovery is shown of injected $^{14}C$ in respiratory $CO_2$ (2 hours), 5 urinary compounds (24 hours), and these 6 compounds combined after rapid intravenous injection of sodium glycollate (1μmole/kg. body weight).

suggesting impaired conversion of glyoxylate to carbon dioxide only if it is accepted that glyoxylate is converted to carbon dioxide primarily via glycine. It must be emphasized that the specific activities of the excreted labelled compounds were not measured.

The third and most crucial method of investigation is the *in vitro* demonstration of defective metabolism by tissue from a patient, The hypothesis of defective conversion of glyoxylate to glycine is not new and has been tested *in vitro* with tissue from patients. Neither Shepard, Krebs, Lee, and Johnson (1960) nor Crawhall and Watts (1962b) found any abnormality in transamination. However, a defect in the conversion of glyoxylate to glycine might be difficult to detect because of the number of enzymes that can catalyse this reaction. In studies of rat liver, Nakada (1964) recently reported the purification of a specific glyoxylate-glutamate transaminase confined to the cytoplasmic sap and different from the main mitochondrial glutamate transaminases. The mitochondria are also the main site of ω-transaminase, for which ornithine is the most reactive donor (Meister, 1954; Peraino and Pitot, 1963), while the greater part of the alanine and aspartate-aminotransferase activity is in the cell sap (Baudhuin *et al.*, 1964). Transamination

TABLE 3

RECOVERY OF $^{14}C$ IN URINE ON INTRAVENOUS INFUSION OF SODIUM GLYOXYLATE† ($CHO \cdot C^{14}OONa$) FOR 6 HOURS

† (1μ mole/kg. body weight and 25 μc. given to both)

| Subject | Times (hr.) | % Urinary Counts Recovered As | | | | | % Urine Counts Recovered | % Administered Counts Recovered in Urine |
|---|---|---|---|---|---|---|---|---|
| | | Oxalate | Glyoxylate | Glycollate | Hippurate | Glycine | | |
| Heterozygote .. | 0–3 (Infusion) | 61·6 | 4·7 | 8·4 | 0·50 | 0·045 | 75·0 | 44·2 |
| | 3–4 (Infusion) | 54·7 | 2·7 | 11·8 | 0·44 | 0·042 | 69·7 | |
| | 4–5 (Infusion) | 65·6 | 3·8 | 25·1 | 0·37 | 0·080 | 95·1 | |
| | 5–6 (Infusion) | 76·1 | 0·9 | 7·7 | 0·63 | 0·071 | 85·4 | |
| | 6–8 | 64·6 | 0·3 | 6·3 | 0·49 | 0·089 | 71·9 | |
| | 8–10 | 69·4 | 0·6 | 5·5 | 4·91 | 0·014 | 80·4 | |
| | 10–12 | 64·6 | 0·4 | 4·4 | 0·80 | 0·003 | 70·2 | |
| | 12–23 | 59·9 | 1·6 | Zero | 0·39 | Zero | 61·9 | |
| Patient (J.M.) .. | 0–3 (Infusion) | 58·0 | 22·5 | 18·3 | 0·18 | 0·004 | 99·0 | 57·2 |
| | 3–4 (Infusion) | 68·4 | 34·9 | 13·2 | 0·12 | 0·004 | 116·6 | |
| | 4–5 (Infusion) | 63·0 | 24·4 | 26·2 | 0·06 | 0·010 | 113·7 | |
| | 5–6 (Infusion) | 43·8 | 11·1 | 21·0 | 0·02 | 0·004 | 75·9 | |
| | 6–8 | 48·8 | 10·0 | 16·9 | 0·03 | 0·020 | 75·7 | |
| | 8–10 | 56·4 | 2·3 | 14·4 | 0·08 | 0·011 | 73·2 | |
| | 10–12 | 38·0 | 1·5 | 50·8 | 0·41 | 0·007 | 90·7 | |
| | 12–21 | 29·4 | Zero | 22·2 | 0·24 | 0·006 | 51·8 | |

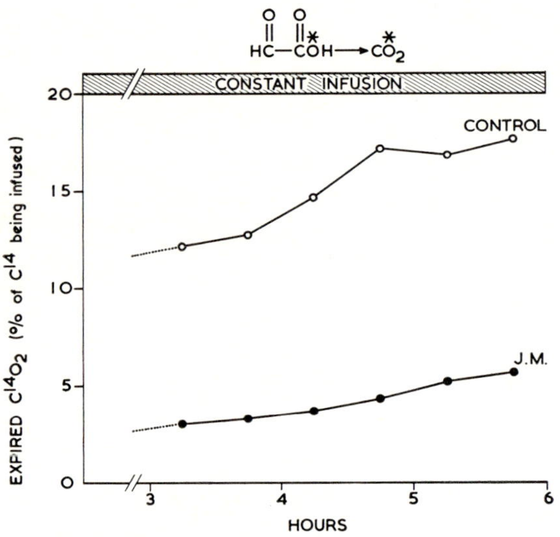


FIG. 3.—Metabolism of carboxyl-labelled glyoxylate-$^{14}C$ in man. Its conversion to respiratory $^{14}CO_2$ is expressed as percentage of isotope being infused during the collection period, and is compared in a patient with primary hyperoxaluria and in her mother. One $\mu$ mole/kg. body weight of glyoxylate was infused throughout a 6-hour period (from Hockaday *et al.* (1964) with permission of the publishers).

may also be associated with deamidation, as when glutamine or asparagine is the donor (Meister, Sober, Tice, and Fraser, 1952).

Attempts to demonstrate defective glycine formation from glyoxylate *in vitro* have so far been unsuccessful. Enzymatic transamination of glyoxylate was not found in intact erythrocytes, nor haemolysates, intact or sonicated leucocytes, or plasma. A cytoplasmic glyoxylate-glutamate transaminase in human liver exhibits similar characteristics to those recently described for this enzyme in rat liver (Nakada, 1964). In a single study this enzymatic activity was normal in liver obtained *post mortem* from a typical patient with primary hyperoxaluria (tissue obtained with the help of Dr. O. Wrong). The transamination reactions that convert glyoxylate to glycine are being studied at present, and this work must be extended to all the transaminase enzymes active with glyoxylate.

## Treatment

The primary aim of understanding the pathogenesis of a disease is to provide a basis for treatment. Admittedly identification of the protein, abnormality of which underlies a metabolic error, has rarely, as yet, been followed by an improvement in methods of treatment. Two possible ways of treating hyperoxaluria are to increase the urinary solubility of oxalate and to manipulate metabolism so that the amount of oxalate formed in the body and the amount excreted in the urine are reduced. Apart from avoidance of foods with a particularly high oxalate content (e.g. spinach, tomato, rhubarb, chocolate, coffee, and tea) and drinking a large volume, dietary measures are not likely to help. A low protein diet does not reduce urinary oxalate.

Because vitamin B6 provides a co-factor for glyoxylate-glycine transamination and for the interconversion of glycine and serine, and because hyperoxaluria is found in B6-deficient animals (Gershoff, Faragalla, Nelson, and Andrus, 1959), pyridoxine treatment has been tried for hyperoxaluria, though B6 deficiency in infants is not accompanied by clinical or biochemical evidence of hyperoxaluria (Scriver and Hutchison, 1963). However, B6 supplements, either alone or combined with folic acid, have had no consistent effect on either urinary oxalate excretion or on the clinical course of hyperoxaluria. A number of other agents, including ascorbic acid, *d*-glutamate, and histidine, have been given, also without apparent effect. A reduction in urinary oxalate has often followed ingestion of sodium benzoate (Archer *et al.*, 1958a; Daniels, Michels, Aisen, and Goldstein, 1960), but the improvement lasted for only two weeks despite continued treatment. Presumably the increased conversion of glycine to hippurate associated with excess benzoate provokes a compensatory hypertrophy of mechanisms producing glycine. This idea is supported by the 'rebound' to unusually high levels of urinary oxalate excretion that occurs immediately administration of benzoate ceases.

## Summary

The clinical features of primary hyperoxaluria are recurrent renal calculi and nephrocalcinosis in the young. Inheritance of this condition as a Mendelian recessive characteristic prompts search for a defective enzyme in patients with this disease.

The metabolism of oxalate and glyoxylate is reviewed briefly, together with previous metabolic observations on patients with hyperoxaluria.

The detailed results are given of the recovery of $^{14}C$ as expired carbon dioxide and urinary oxalate, glyoxylate, glycollate, glycine, and hippurate after intravenous injection of carboxyl-labelled glycollate or glyoxylate. There was less $^{14}C$ in carbon dioxide, glycine, and hippurate from the patients than from normal subjects or parents of patients.

These results suggest defective transamination of glyoxylate to glycine in patients with primary hyperoxaluria. No support for this belief has come from preliminary observations *in vitro* with blood cells and liver tissue from patients.

No satisfactory treatment of this condition has been found, though the usual symptomatic treatment for oxalate calculi should be given.

### References


Aponte, G. E., and Fetter, T. R. (1954). Familial idiopathic oxalate nephrocalcinosis. *Amer. J. clin. Path.*, **24**, 1363.

Archer, H. E., Dormer, A. E., Scowen, E. F., and Watts, R. W. E. (1957). Primary hyperoxaluria. *Lancet*, **2**, 320.

——, ——, ——, and —— (1958a). The aetiology of primary hyperoxaluria. *Brit. med. J.*, **1**, 175.

——, ——, ——, and —— (1958b). Observations on the possible genetic basis of primary hyperoxaluria. *Ann. hum. Genet.*, **22**, 373.

Atkins, G. L., Dean, B. M., Griffin, W. J., Scowen, E. F., and Watts, R. W. E. (1963). Primary hyperoxaluria; the relation between ascorbic acid and the increased urinary excretion of oxalate. *Lancet*, **2**, 1096.

Baudhuin, P., Beaufay, H., Rahman-Li, Y., Sellinger, O. Z., Wattiaux, R., Jacques, P., and de Duve, C. (1964). Tissue fractionation studies. 17. Intracellular distribution of monoamine oxidase, aspartate aminotransferase, alanine aminotransferase, D-amino acid oxidase and catalase in rat-liver tissue. *Biochem. J.*, **92**, 179.

Beadle, G. W., and Tatum, E. L. (1941). Genetic control of biochemical reactions in neurospora. *Proc. nat. Acad. Sci.* (*Wash.*), **27**, 499.

Buri, J-F. (1962). L'oxalose. *Helv. paediat. Acta*, **17**, Suppl. 11.

Cori, G. T. (1957). Biochemical aspects of glycogen deposition diseases. *Mod. Probl. Pädiat.*, **3**, 344.

Crawhall, J. C., de Mowbray, R. R., Scowen, E. F., and Watts, R. W. E. (1959a). Conversion of glycine to oxalate in a normal subject. *Lancet*, **2**, 810.

——, Scowen, E. F., and Watts, R. W. E. (1959b). Conversion of glycine to oxalate in primary hyperoxaluria. *ibid.*, **2**, 806.

——, and Watts, R. W. E. (1962a). The metabolism of glyoxylate by human- and rat-liver mitochondria. *Biochem, J.*, **85**, 163.

——, and —— (1962b). The metabolism of (1-$^{14}$C) glyoxylate by the liver mitochondria of patients with primary hyperoxaluria and non-hyperoxaluric subjects. *Clin. Sci.*, **23**, 163.

Daniels, R. A., Michels, R., Aisen, P., and Goldstein, G. (1960). Familial hyperoxaluria. *Amer. J. Med.*, **29**, 820.

Dempsey, E. F., Forbes, A. P., Melick, R. A., and Henneman, P. H. (1960). Urinary oxalate excretion. *Metabolism*, **9**, 52.

Elder, T. D., and Wyngaarden, J. B. (1960). The biosynthesis and turnover of oxalate in normal and hyperoxaluric subjects. *J. clin. Invest.*, **39**, 1337.

Frederick, E. W., Rabkin, M. T., Ritchie, R. H., Jr., and Smith, L. H., Jr. (1963). Studies on primary hyperoxaluria. I. *In vivo* demonstration of a defect in glyoxylate metabolism. *New Engl. J. Med.*, **269**, 821.

Garrod, A. E. (1908). The Croonian lectures on inborn errors of metabolism. *Lancet*, **2**, 1, 73, 142, 214.

Gershoff, S. N., Faragalla, F. F., Nelson, D. A., and Andrus, S. B. (1959). Vitamin $B_6$ deficiency and oxalate nephrocalcinosis in the cat. *Amer. J. Med.*, **27**, 72.

Gibson, Q. H. (1948). The reduction of methaemoglobin in red blood cells and studies on the cause of idiopathic methaemoglobinaemia. *Biochem. J.*, **42**, 13.

Goldstone, A., and Adams, E. (1962). Metabolism of $\gamma$-hydroxyglutamic acid. I. Conversion to $\alpha$-hydroxy-$\gamma$-ketoglutarate by purified glutamic-aspartic transaminase of rat liver. *J. biol. Chem.*, **237**, 3476.

Hall, E. G., Scowen, E. F., and Watts, R. W. E. (1960). Clinical manifestations of primary hyperoxaluria. *Arch. Dis. Childh.*, **35**, 108.

Hockaday, T. D. R., Clayton, J. E., Frederick, E. W., and Smith, L. H., Jr. (1964). Primary hyperoxaluria. *Medicine* (*Baltimore*), **43**, 315.

——, Frederick, E. W., Clayton, J. E., and Smith, L. H., Jr. (1965). Studies on primary hyperoxaluria. II. Urinary oxalate, glycolate, and glyoxylate measurement by isotope dilution techniques. *J. Lab. clin. Med.*, **65**, 677.

Ingram, V. M. (1957). Gene mutations in human haemoglobin: the chemical difference between normal and sickle cell haemoglobin. *Nature* (*Lond.*), **180**, 326.

Lagrue, G., Laudat, M. H., Meyer, P., Sapir, M., and Milliez, P. (1959). Oxalose familiale avec acidose hyperchlorémique secondaire. *Sem. Hôp. Paris*, **35**, 2023.

McLaurin, A. W., Beisel, W. R., McCormick, G. J., Scalettar, R., and Herman, R. H. (1961). Primary hyperoxaluria. *Ann. intern. Med.*, **55**, 70.

Meister, A. (1954). Enzymatic transamination reactions involving arginine and ornithine. *J. biol. Chem.*, **206**, 587.

——, Sober, H. A., Tice, S. V., and Fraser, P. E. (1952). Transamination and associated deamidation of asparagine and glutamine. *ibid.*, **197**, 319.

Nakada, H. I. (1964). Glutamic-glycine transaminase from rat liver. *ibid.*, **239**, 468.

——, and Sund, L. P. (1958). Glyoxylic acid oxidation by rat liver. *ibid.*, **233**, 8.

——, and Weinhouse, S. (1953). Studies of glycine oxidation in rat tissues. *Arch. Biochem.*, **42**, 257.

Newns, G. H., and Black, J. A. (1953). A case of calcium oxalate nephrocalcinosis. *Gt Ormond Str. J.*, **5**, 40.

Payes, B., and Laties, G. G. (1963). The enzymatic conversion of $\gamma$-OH-$\alpha$-ketoglutarate (HKG) to malate: a postulated step in the cyclic oxidation of glyoxylate. *Biochem. biophys. Res. Commun.*, **13**, 179.

Peraino, C., and Pitot, H. C. (1963). Ornithine-delta-transaminase in the rat. I. Assay and some general properties. *Biochim. biophys. Acta* (*Amst.*), **73**, 222.

Ratner, S., Nocito, V., and Green, D. E. (1944). Glycine oxidase. *J. biol. Chem.*, **152**, 119.

Scowen, E. F., Watts, R. W. E., and Hall, E. G. (1959). Further observations on the genetic basis of primary hyperoxaluria. *Ann. hum. Genet.*, **23**, 367.

Scriver, C. R., and Hutchison, J. H. (1963). The vitamin $B_6$ deficiency syndrome in human infancy: biochemical and clinical observations. *Pediatrics*, **31**, 240.

Shepard, T. H., Krebs, E. G., and Lee, L. S. (1958). Studies on familial oxalosis. *Amer. J. Dis. Child.*, **96**, 490.

——, ——, ——, and Johnson, M. L. (1960). Primary hyperoxaluria. III. Nutritional and metabolic studies in a patient. *Pediatrics* **25**, 1008.

Weinhouse, S., and Friedmann, B. (1951). Metabolism of labeled 2-carbon acids in the intact rat. *J. biol. Chem.*, **191**, 707.

Weissbach, A., and Sprinson, D. B. (1953). The metabolism of 2-carbon compounds related to glycine. I. Glyoxylic acid. *ibid.*, **203**, 1023.

Ying Chou, L., and Donohue, W. L. (1952). Oxalosis: possible "inborn error of metabolism" with nephrolithiasis and nephrocalcinosis due to calcium oxalate as the predominating features. *Pediatrics*, **10**, 662.

*Arch. Dis. Childh.*, 1965, **40**, 492.

# LACTIC ACIDOSIS WITH NECROTIZING ENCEPHALOPATHY IN TWO SIBS

BY

HELEN E. WORSLEY, R. W. BROOKFIELD, J. S. ELWOOD*, R. L. NOBLE, and W. H. TAYLOR†

*From the Royal Liverpool Children's Hospital, and the Department of Chemical Pathology, Liverpool*

(RECEIVED FOR PUBLICATION FEBRUARY 8, 1965)

The plasma lactate concentration is raised physiologically, during muscular exertion, and sometimes in diseases associated with demonstrable hypoxaemia, such as peripheral circulatory failure, severe shock, acute bronchial asthma, and obstructive emphysema. The plasma lactate level is also significantly raised in respiratory alkalosis arising from primary hyperventilation, and often in metabolic alkalosis. When there is alkalosis, there is usually no hypoxaemia, and the plasma concentration of pyruvate, the immediate precursor of lactate, is also proportionally raised. Gevers and Dowdle (1963) have shown that alkaline conditions stimulate the glycolytic rate *in vitro* of rat liver and kidney slices and that the effect is exerted at a stage or stages proximal to the dehydrogenation of triosephosphate.

A distinction has thus been drawn (Huckabee, 1961) between the alkalotic and the hypoxaemic group, for in the latter 'excess' lactate, relative to pyruvate, is found. 'Excess' lactate is defined as,

$$(Ln-Lo)-(Pn-Po)\ (Lo/Po),$$

where Ln and Pn are the actual values of lactate and pyruvate, respectively, and Lo and Po, the expected respective normal values.

Recently, a syndrome of lactic acidosis has been described (Huckabee, 1961; Daughaday, Lipicky, and Rasinski, 1962) in patients who have 'excess' lactate but apparently no hypoxaemia. The patients show hyperpnoea, dyspnoea, and metabolic acidosis, and have a poor prognosis. They present with a variety of diseases including poliomyelitis, gastric ulcer, coronary thrombosis, pneumonia, and non-ketotic diabetic acidosis.

This paper describes two brothers who presented with identical clinical features of hyperpnoea, progressive ataxia, mental deterioration, loss of scalp hair, and convulsions, and who each showed, at necropsy, degenerative changes in the central nervous system. One of the brothers was investigated biochemically and found to have a severe lactic acidosis, apparently of primary origin.

## Methods

Blood pyruvate was estimated by the method of Friedemann and Haugen (1943), plasma lactate by that of Hullin and Noble (1953), and blood glucose by a glucose oxidase method (Marks, 1959). Chromatography of plasma organic acids was carried out by the procedures described by Smith (1960).

## Case Reports

**Case 1.** A boy aged 17 months was referred to the out-patient department of the Royal Liverpool Children's Hospital on August 16, 1960, by Dr. J. Lawson. Six weeks previously, a few hours after an injection of poliomyelitis vaccine, there had been twitching of both sides of his body and one week previously he had begun to stagger. Hitherto he had walked well. The parents were alarmed because 7 years earlier an elder male sib (Case 2) had developed similar symptoms and had died. On examination the child appeared to be perfectly normal, but 9 days later, because the mother was convinced of the similarity of the symptoms to those of the dead child, admission was arranged.

The birth weight had been 7 lb. (3,175 g.) and the delivery normal. He first stood at 10 months, walked at 13 months, and spoke simple words at 16 months. He had had measles and rubella. His height was 33 in. (84 cm.) and his weight 27 lb. 14 oz. (12·6 kg.). Physical examination again revealed no abnormality except that he appeared to walk with rather a wide base. In other respects examination of the nervous system yielded negative results. The plantar responses were flexor in type and the optic discs were normal.

During the next three weeks he developed a slight intention tremor, his gait became frankly unsteady and there were episodes of hyperventilation. The rate of respiration was increased and the depth very much so. He usually sat with his body leaning forward and with his head thrown slightly backward. He kept his mouth closed. He did not seem to be greatly distressed and

* Present address: Department of Pathology, Altnagelvin Hospital, Londonderry, N. Ireland.

† Correspondence about this paper should be addressed to W. H. Taylor, Dept. of Chemical Pathology, United Liverpool Hospitals, Ashton Street, Liverpool 3.

continued to look about him, but he made no attempt to speak or to play. These episodes occurred spontaneously at rest and lasted for up to four hours. When hyperventilation was frequent, incoordination increased and he had difficulty in feeding himself. From time to time there were coarse spontaneous movements as well as an intention tremor. These involved all the limbs and the head and, on occasion, resembled a convulsion except that consciousness was not lost and the child was still able to drink. There was no tachycardia and his blood pressure remained normal. When hyperventilation was prolonged, his extremities were noted to be cold, cyanosed, and slightly oedematous. Rapid fluctuations in weight were not fully accounted for by variations in food intake.

*Investigations.* The haemoglobin concentration was 78% (11·6 g./100 ml.) of normal and the leucocytes numbered 8,000/c.mm., 67% being lymphocytes. The serum sodium, potassium, and protein levels were normal, but the plasma chloride level was often raised and varied from 102 to 115 mEq/l. The plasma bicarbonate was low, varying from 12 to 19 mEq/l. The urine contained a trace of protein and its *p*H varied from 5·5 to 6·5 with low or absent bicarbonate. The serum phosphate level was low for a child of his age, being 3·3-4·0 mg./100 ml. Liver function tests were normal. That the hyperventilation and lowered plasma bicarbonate arose from a metabolic acidosis was indicated by the acid urine and by estimations of the blood *p*H. A value of *p*H 7·36 was obtained at a time when the plasma bicarbonate was 19 mEq/l., and another of *p*H 7·28 when the plasma bicarbonate was 13 mEq/l. The serum glutamate-oxaloacetate and glutamate-pyruvate transaminase levels were raised, varying, respectively, from 185 to 360 units/100 ml. (normal, 23-107) and from 195 to 600 units/100 ml. (normal, 22-110).

The CSF had a normal protein content (40 mg./100 ml.), and was under normal pressure. Dr. J. Rees Roberts reported that the electroencephalogram showed paroxysmal activity which was generalized and consistent with cerebral injury. An intravenous pyelogram pointed to normal structure and function. The skull and bony skeleton were radiologically normal, except that the bone-age was estimated to be only 6-12 months.

The cause of the acidosis was next elucidated. Diabetes mellitus was excluded because the fasting blood sugar (95 mg./100 ml) and the glucose tolerance curve were normal and the urine was free from ketone bodies. The plasma ketonic acid concentration was normal (20 mg./100 ml.). Chromatography of the urine revealed a generalized aminoaciduria, but the plasma amino acid nitrogen level was not raised, nor was the plasma amino acid distribution unusual. Indoxyl sulphate, tryptophan, and indolyl acetic acid were present in the urine in normal amounts. Chromatography of the plasma for organic acids revealed no abnormal constituents, but it was noted that the spot for lactic acid developed quickly and appeared dense. The plasma lactate level was then estimated quantitatively on two occasions when the patient was fasting, and not in a hyperpnoeic attack. High values of 30·5 mg./100 ml. and 38·7 mg./100 ml. were obtained, compared with the normal range of 6-18 mg./100 ml. and with a value of 10·5 mg./100 ml. for a normal fasting control. The blood pyruvate level was raised, values of 2·1 and 2·4 mg./100 ml. being found. The calculation for 'excess' lactate gave a value of + 0·33 mEq/l., thus revealing no significant excess. During a hyperpnoeic attack the plasma lactate rose to 54 mg./100 ml. (6·0 mEq/l.).

It was concluded that the patient suffered from a persistent lactic acidosis, exacerbations of which were responsible for the hyperpnoeic episodes. Associated with this was a renal aminoaciduria, and possibly phosphaturia, and a progressive lesion of the central nervous system.

PROGRESS. The patient died 7 months after his first admission. His decline was progressive but with intermissions. He found it increasingly difficult to maintain his balance, even when sitting. The muscle tone appeared reduced, but the tendon jerks could still be elicited. The plantar responses became extensor. During the early stages of his illness he appeared in no way retarded, and often showed persistence in attempting to compensate for his lack of coordination. As time went on, increasing tremor impaired his movements and he was no longer able to feed himself. The periods of hyperventilation were more frequent and prolonged, and the associated twitching was often so severe as to resemble a convulsion. He drooled constantly, his skin became dry, and his hair began to fall out. His vision deteriorated and he was found to have developed bilateral primary optic atrophy. Ultimately he could not sit without support, was withdrawn from his surroundings, and stared vacantly or slept.

During these months, he was treated with antibiotics on numerous occasions because of intermittent respiratory infections, and with a vitamin B complex, containing aneurine, riboflavine, nicotinamide, and pyridoxine. The muscle twitchings were to some extent controlled by chloral hydrate. He was also given alkalinizing agents, at first sodium bicarbonate, and later sodium citrate. Although these partially corrected the acidosis biochemically, the clinical symptoms were not improved and the hyperpnoeic attacks persisted. At a later stage in the illness and in an attempt to inhibit the excess lactate production, sodium fluoride was given in a dosage of 6 mg. daily. An initial improvement was noted. The patient became more interested in his surroundings and attempted to play, to feed himself, and to stand. Yet the bouts of hyperpnoea persisted and the plasma lactate, after three weeks, was still high (41·4 mg./100 ml.). The fluoride was discontinued because of uncertainty as to its efficacy and in order to assess the effect of its withdrawal. His condition deteriorated further and 6 days later he died, being then 25 months old.

NECROPSY FINDINGS. The fundus of the stomach was adherent to the diaphragm over an area 3 cm. in diameter. Here the stomach wall, especially the mucosa, was thin and atrophic, but no ulceration had occurred. A gradual transition to normal was noted between this area and the adjacent normal mucosa. Histological examination showed the mucosa and muscularis to be thin and

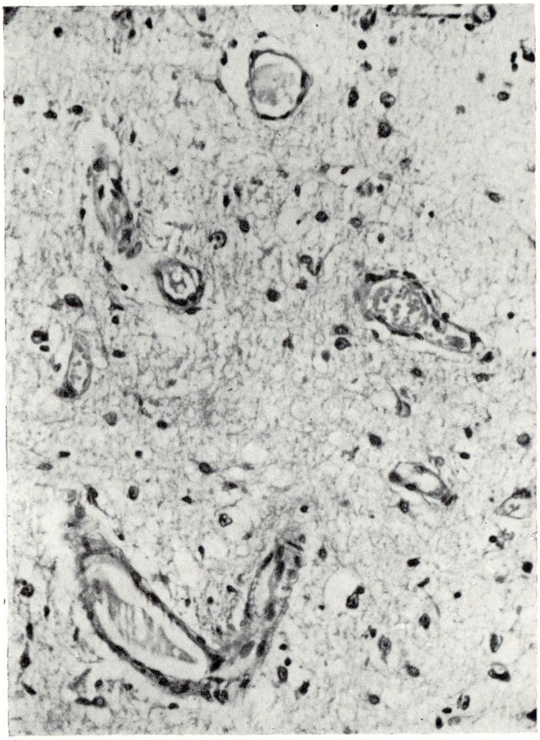

FIG. 1.—Mid-brain of Case 1 (H. and E. × 140.) Dilatation and hyalinization of capillaries in peri-aqueductal formatio reticularis.

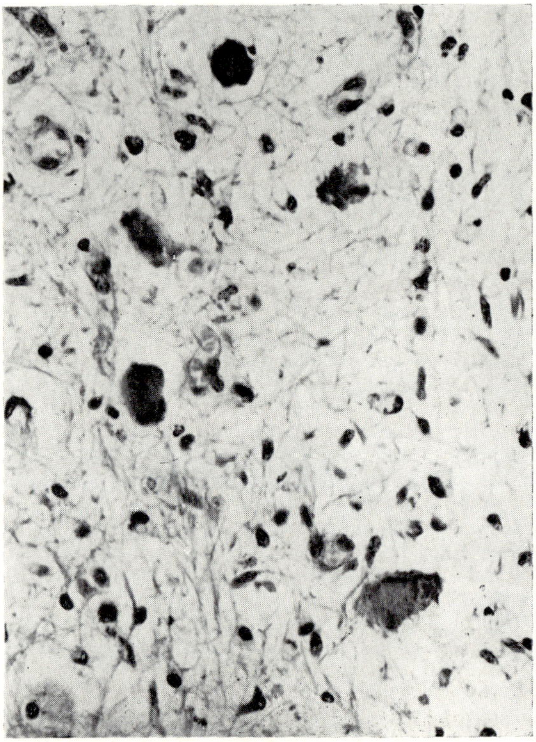

FIG. 2.—Medulla of Case 1. (H. and E. × 140.) Edge of cystic lesion in medial olivary nucleus showing vascularization and occasional fat-laden phagocyte. Note relative sparing of neurones and little gliosis.

slightly hyalinized but otherwise normal in structure in the adherent area.

After fixation, no striking macroscopic abnormality was seen in the brain and spinal cord. There was only slight prominence of the capillaries and doubtful sponginess of the white matter of the cerebellum. The other organs examined were normal.

*Histological examination of the brain.* In both the grey and white matter, symmetrical but non-systematized areas of degeneration of brain substance were present, in which surviving axons formed a loose network enmeshing remaining neurones. Fat-laden phagocytes were present near active lesions. Inflammatory cells were absent, and microglial and astrocytic activity was not a prominent feature, though occasionally present. There was loss of intensity of myelin staining with occasional globules of free fat and 'ballooning' of the myelin sheath, so that a clear zone appeared between it and the axon. This appearance we have called 'fenestration'. Such areas were devoid of significant gliosis.

Prominent, dilated, and engorged capillary blood vessels, with some hyalinization of their walls, accompanied this degeneration of the parenchyma and often covered a greater area than it. There was, however, little endothelial proliferation or capillary budding. This appearance we have called 'vascularization' (Fig. 1).

In general, neuronal bodies showed few degenerative changes.

The tractus gracilis and cuneatus, at the level of the decussation of the pyramids in the *medulla*, showed vascularization and demyelination with abundant fat-laden phagocytes. Cyst formation had occurred in these demyelinated areas. Similar changes were observed in the medial lemniscus at the level of the olive (Fig. 2). Advanced vascularization was evident in the formatio reticularis, especially about the central canal, the nuclei cuneatus and gracilis, the cranial nuclei XII, X, IX, and V, and to a lesser extent in the olivary, dorsal, and medial olivary nuclei. Some loss of neurones was discernible in these nuclei.

In the *pons*, less marked demyelination and vascularization had occurred in the medial lemniscus than in the medulla. Advanced vascularization had occurred in the formatio reticularis and the cranial nuclei VIII, VII, VI, and V. These nuclei also showed some loss of neurones, with degenerative changes in those neurones remaining. The adjacent white matter showed fenestration.

In the *mid-brain* the caudal limit of the red nucleus was mildly vascularized, and the white matter of the rubro-

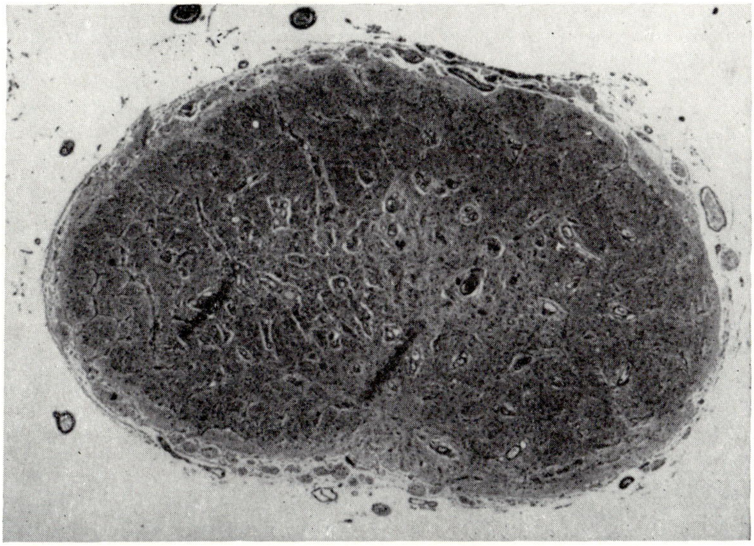

FIG. 3.—Optic nerve (H. and E. × 30.) of Case 1. Severe vascularization and demyelination of central part.

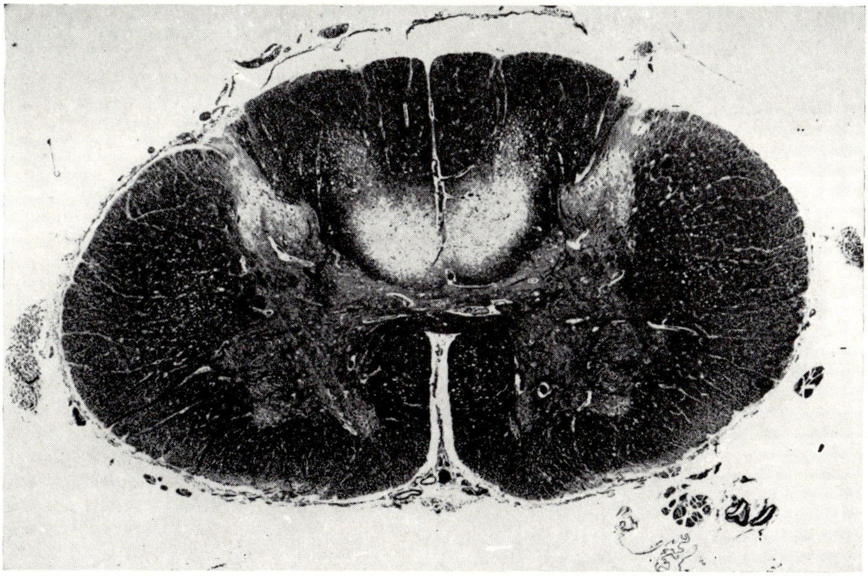

FIG. 4.—Thoracic spinal cord of Case 1. (Loyez. × 10.) Demyelination of posterior white columns.

spinal tract, the superior cerebellar peduncle, and the medial longitudinal bundle was fenestrated. At this level the medial lemniscus was normal. Vascularization, loss of pigment, and mild degenerative changes were observed in the substantia nigra.

Advanced vascularization, some astrogliosis, and moderate neuronal degeneration had occurred in the tegmentum, throughout the formatio reticularis, the inferior, and superior colliculi, and the external geniculate bodies, and in cranial nucleus IV. Neuronal loss and vascularization involved the whole of each corpus mamillarium, and the remaining neurones showed degenerative changes.

In the *cerebrum*, vascularization was evident in the caudate, anterior, and lateral thalamic nuclei, and to a lesser extent in the putamen and medial thalamic nuclei;

degenerative changes in the neurones, however, were sparse. The cerebral cortex and white matter of the hemispheres were essentially normal.

Reduction in number and marked degenerative changes in the Purkinje cells, and some vascularity and minor degenerative changes in the neurones of dentate nucleus were the only abnormalities seen in the *cerebellum*.

The *optic nerves* were severely vascularized and their central parts demyelinated (Fig. 3).

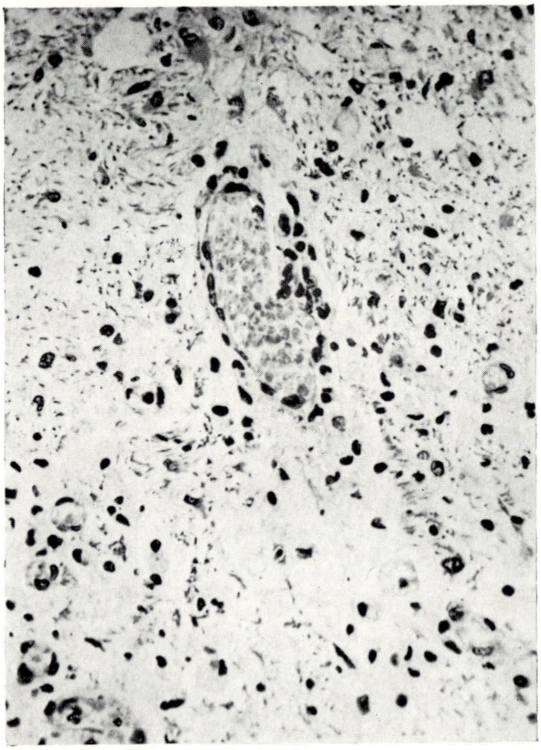

FIG. 5.—Thoracic spinal cord of Case 1. (H. and E. × 300.) Demyelinated zone showing vascularization, some fat-laden phagocytes, but little gliosis.

*Histological examination of spinal cord.* Symmetrical lesions, detectable at most levels but maximal in upper thoracic and lower cervical segments, can be grouped as follows.

(a) Vascularization of the grey commissure and bases of the posterior horns. The anterior horns and remainder of the posterior horns were only involved in the upper thoracic segments, and at these levels only were minor degenerative changes noted in the anterior horn cells.

(b) At all levels, part of the lateral white columns, i.e. the spino-cerebellar and lateral cortico-spinal tracts and to a lesser extent the anterior spino-cerebellar tract, showed fenestration of the myelin.

(c) The most striking lesions were in the posterior columns (Fig. 4). In lumbar segments, vascularity and fenestration of myelin were apparent. In the lower thoracic segments, vascularity, demyelination, and some microglial proliferation were noted in about one-third of the posterior columns adjacent to the grey commissure. This lesion became more severe on ascending the cord and was maximal in upper thoracic and lower cervical segments, where abundant fat-laden phagocytes and free fat globules were also present, but there was surprisingly little gliosis (Fig. 5). At upper cervical levels only a small band of vascularization and demyelination passed through the central area of each posterior column, forming a V-shaped lesion with its apex between the posterior fissure and the grey commissure.

**Case 2.** The elder male sib of Case 1, the firstborn child of the family, was brought to the Royal Liverpool Children's Hospital on October 25, 1952. He was then 19 months old. Delivery had been normal and his weight at birth was 8½ lb. (3,855 g.). There was a history of muscular twitching between the ages of 3 to 10 months. Attacks had occurred approximately weekly, and each lasted for a few minutes. There was no tonic phase, but the child appeared to lose consciousness. From the age of 10 to 14 months, there were no further attacks, but thereafter episodes of twitching recurred, once more at about weekly intervals. He started to walk at the age of 14 months, and it was noticed that he was unsteady and fell easily. There had been no other illness.

Physical examination in the out-patient department showed a flabby child who appeared to be mentally retarded. The gait was unsteady and there was a tendency to fall backwards. Muscle tone and motor power seemed normal. The tendon reflexes were brisk and the plantar responses were flexor.

After admission to hospital, skull radiographs showed that there was no bony change or abnormal calcification. The electroencephalogram showed a moderate amount of delta activity, but the record was considered to be within the limits of the normal for his age. The CSF protein content was normal at 15 mg./100 ml. The haemoglobin concentration was 88% (13·0 g./100 ml.) and the white cells numbered 7,000 per c.mm. with a normal differential distribution. There was only one attack of twitching while he was in hospital. In it there were jerking movements of the right arm, trunk, and head; he did not react to stimuli and though sitting up he appeared to be unconscious. The twitching lasted for about 30 seconds and recurred about 5 minutes later.

He was seen to be hyperpnoeic for the first time when he attended at the out-patient department on February 3, 1953. There was mild bronchitis but no other change in the physical signs. Plasma electrolyte examinations revealed a raised serum sodium and chloride of 161 and 115 mEq/l., respectively, while the plasma bicarbonate was low at 15 mEq/l. The urine *p*H was 6. There was no proteinuria, but a small amount of reducing substance was observed.

He was readmitted to hospital on March 24, 1953. Hyperventilation was now occurring frequently. His nutritional state remained good. He was very unsteady and could not stand, but sat without support and rocked to and fro. The left plantar response was doubtful, but otherwise the physical signs were unchanged. There were several attacks of twitching lasting up to half an hour. An air encephalogram was normal. The CSF was again normal.

At an out-patient attendance on April 21, 1953, it was noted that his hair had been falling out. On May 12, he was referred to the Neurological Department of the Royal Southern Hospital and was admitted for further study. Hyperventilation was still a marked feature, but it caused no distress. The deep reflexes were very brisk and this time both plantar reflexes were extensor. The optic discs were a little pale: vision appeared to be normal. He was drowsy and inattentive. Biochemical investigations revealed a low plasma bicarbonate of 15·5 mEq/l. and a urinary *p*H of 5·5. Glucose was demonstrated in the urine on one occasion, and amino acid chromatography suggested a generalized aminoaciduria.

He was treated with an alkaline mixture containing potassium citrate and sodium bicarbonate. There was temporary clinical amelioration with some diminution of the hyperventilation, but there was no improvement in drowsiness. Fourteen days after this last admission he collapsed and died.

At necropsy, the lungs, heart, abdominal organs, kidneys, and brain were macroscopically normal. Histological examination of the kidney and brain revealed no abnormality at the time. New sections were cut 8 years later and were examined in the light of the findings from Case 1. The majority of these sections showed a normal brain, but in the midbrain there was vascularity and some neuronal degeneration of the reticular formation in the region of the aqueduct. The dentate nucleus showed marked neuronal degeneration and some demyelination of the white matter.

### Other Members of the Family

The resting plasma lactate levels of the mother, father, and sister of the two patients were normal, being respectively 9·2, 13·2, and 12·0 mg./100 ml. Both parents belonged to quite large family groups. There had been no early deaths in either group and no relatives had had illness in any way resembling that of the two children who are the subjects of this study.

### Lactic Acid Formation by the Erythrocytes

Erythrocytes produce lactate readily by glycolysis from glucose, and much of the resting plasma lactate is thought to derive from this source. Since the resting plasma lactate level was raised in Case 1, the formation of lactate by the patient's erythrocytes was studied *in vitro*.

Heparinized blood was allowed to glycolyse, both in an atmosphere of nitrogen and in oxygen, in a Warburg apparatus at 37° C. The rates of disappearance of glucose and formation of lactate were compared with those of blood from a normal control subject (aged 36 years). The oxygen uptake was also measured. The results are shown in Table 1. They indicate that after 105 minutes the blood glucose of the normal subject had been converted more or less quantitatively to lactic acid, both aerobically and anaerobically, for 41·5 mg. of glucose yielded 49·7 mg. and 44·7 mg. of lactic acid, respectively. There was thus an apparent 'non-glucose' lactate production of 3·2 mg./100 ml. anaerobically, a value that is within the limits of experimental error. Aerobically, the oxygen uptake in 105 minutes was 3,133 μl./100 ml. blood. Assuming that glucose was katabolized oxidatively, this uptake represents a glucose loss of 4·2 mg./100 ml. The apparent aerobic 'non-glucose' lactate production was thus 49·7 − (41·5 − 4·2) = 12·4 mg./100 ml. This is outside the limits of experimental error.

In the patient, on the other hand, a considerable anaerobic 'non-glucose' lactate production was revealed. Thus in 105 minutes only 12·5 mg. glucose/100 ml. were katabolized anaerobically but 31·0 mg. lactate/100 ml. were formed, — an excess of 18·5 mg./100 ml. The oxygen uptake was 1,733 μl./100 ml. blood, equivalent to the katabolism of 2·3 mg. glucose/100 ml. The lactate concentration of the blood increased aerobically by 33·5 mg./100 ml. and the glucose concentration fell by 14·3 mg./100 ml. The apparent aerobic non-glucose lactate production was thus 33·5 − (14·3 − 2·3) = 21·5 mg./100 ml. The formation of 'non-glucose' lactate, both aerobically and anaerobically, in the patient, was thus greatly in excess of that of the control.

The oxygen uptake of the blood of the patient was roughly the same as that of the control in terms of red cell content, being, respectively, 1,733 μl./100 ml. with

TABLE 1

AEROBIC AND ANAEROBIC FORMATION OF LACTIC ACID IN THE BLOOD OF CASE 1, AFTER INCUBATION AT 37° C. FOR 105 MINUTES

| | Blood Glucose (mg./100 ml.) | | | Blood Lactate (mg./100 ml.) | | | Haematocrit % | Oxygen Uptake (μl./100 ml.) | Lactate Production (mg./100 ml.) per 1% Haematocrit in | |
|---|---|---|---|---|---|---|---|---|---|---|
| | Initial | After Incubation in $N_2$ | After Incubation in $O_2$ | Initial | After Incubation in $N_2$ | After Incubation in $O_2$ | | | $N_2$ | $O_2$ |
| Control | 43<br>40 | 0<br>0 | 0<br>0 | 12·3 | 57 | 62 | 48 | 3,133 | 0·93 | 1·03 |
| Case 1 | 34<br>32·5 | 19<br>22·5 | 19 | 28·5 | 59·5 | 62 | 28 | 1,733 | 1·11 | 1·20 |

a corrected haematocrit of 28% and 3,133 µl./100 ml. with a corrected haematocrit of 48%. The rate of anaerobic katabolism of glucose was, however, slower in the patient's blood per volume of red cells than in the control, being 12·5 mg./100 ml. in 105 minutes with a haematocrit of 28% compared with at least 41·5 mg./100 ml. with a haematocrit of 48% in the control. Of the total blood glucose available for katabolism in the patient, relatively more was in the plasma, 72% as against 52% when compared with the normal control, so that the diminished rate of glucose katabolism might be related to the necessity for the plasma glucose to enter the relatively small number of cells. On the other hand the rate of lactate production by the patient's cells, anaerobically, was 19% greater per unit volume of red cells than that of the control and 17% greater aerobically. However, as all the glucose of the normal subject was katabolized, his true rate of lactate production might have been higher.

In order to confirm that the patient's erythrocytes were forming lactate more readily than normal erythrocytes, the experiment set out in Table 2 was carried out, using a second normal subject (aged 33 years). The erythrocytes from each subject were

TABLE 2

PRODUCTION OF LACTIC ACID, ANAEROBICALLY, BY THE ERYTHROCYTES OF CASE 1, COMPARED WITH THOSE OF NORMAL CONTROL

| Incubation Mixture | Lactic Acid Content (mg./100 ml.) | | |
|---|---|---|---|
| | Before Incubation | After Incubation | Difference |
| Patient's cells, 3 ml.<br>Patient's plasma, 3 ml. | 22·7 | 43·3 | 20·6 |
| Control cells, 3 ml.<br>Control plasma, 3 ml. | 13·2 | 31·0 | 17·8 |
| Patient's cells, 3 ml.<br>Control plasma, 3 ml. | 12·8 | 32·6 | 19·8 |
| Control cells, 3 ml.<br>Patient's plasma, 3 ml. | 23·0 | 40·6 | 17·6 |
| Patient's cells, 3 ml.<br>Patient's plasma, 3 ml.<br>DL-alanine = 50 mg./100 ml. | 22·7 | 44·3 | 21·6 |

separated from the plasma, washed in isotonic saline, and incubated with each plasma separately, under the same conditions at 37° C. for 85 minutes. Differences of *p*H and bicarbonate concentration in the two samples of plasma appeared not to affect the rate of lactate production, for the patient's cells formed lactate equally rapidly with each plasma, and so did the erythrocytes of the control subject. However, the patient's cells produced 17% more lactate than did the control cells from the patient's plasma, and 11% more from the control plasma. It should be noted that the patient's resting lactate level was again raised.

These experiments, taken together, indicate that the patient's erythrocytes formed lactate more rapidly than did those of two normal subjects, but that not all of this lactate came from glucose. In an attempt to ascertain what other substances than glucose might be converted to lactate, the patient's cells were also incubated with DL-alanine, but a significant increase in lactate formation did not occur.

Subsequently it has been possible to repeat the experiment of Table 2 in a female patient aged 22 years complaining of muscular weakness, who had a high resting plasma lactate (75·5 mg./100 ml.) without recurrent attacks of acidosis or hyperpnoea. The cause of this hyperlactataemia is, as yet, unknown. The normal control was a woman of similar age. The patient's erythrocytes formed lactate at a rate identical with those of the control subject. It is unlikely, therefore, to be the general rule that the erythrocytes in hyperlactataemia produce lactate more rapidly than do normal erythrocytes. The aetiological significance of the increased rate of lactate production by the erythrocytes of Case 1 is thereby enhanced.

## Discussion

**Biochemical Features.** Though there is no direct evidence of lactic acidosis in Case 2, the similar clinical presentation of the two cases, the similar biochemical findings, the similar clinical course, including loss of scalp hair, and the parents' early recognition of the onset of the disease in Case 1, combine to suggest very strongly an identical and, therefore, familial condition. Neither parent, nor a female sib born between the two brothers, appear to be affected.

The differential diagnosis, biochemically, is essentially between primary lactic acidosis, and respiratory alkalosis from primary hyperventilation. The evidence supports the former diagnosis, for in both patients the urine was acid at rest and during the hyperpnoeic attacks, and in Case 1 the blood *p*H became more acid as the lactate level rose during hyperpnoea. In respiratory alkalosis both the blood and urinary *p*H would be expected to become more alkaline. Furthermore in neither patient did necropsy reveal any lesion in the brain that could specifically be held responsible for a primary hyperventilation syndrome.

The attacks of hyperpnoea seemed to arise, therefore, from intermittent sudden increases in lactic acid concentration in the plasma. The ataxia, hypotonia, and muscular tremor were present when there was little or no hyperpnoea, and did not result from hyperpnoea, though they were exacerbated by it. They thus represent a second feature of the syndrome, associated with the diffuse cerebral and cerebellar lesions. A third feature is the renal aminoaciduria and low serum phosphate. The occasionally raised plasma chloride must also be explained. It seems that the over-all acidosis was partly caused by lactate accumulation and partly also by chloride. In the absence of dietary loading of chloride, this hyperchloraemia is probably also a renal manifestation; though an acid urine was secreted, it seems as if the kidneys were not able to compensate fully for the increased lactic acid load, so that chloride was retained in exchange for lactate. Just as in renal acidosis of infants, the kidneys cannot cope with a normal anionic load, and hyperchloraemia ensues.

The *in vitro* studies upon glycolysis established that the patient's erythrocytes produced lactate more quickly than did those of two normal subjects, but that much of this lactate did not come from glucose. There are two possible explanations for this. The lactate might be formed from other substances than those of the glycolytic sequence, or there may be in the patient's erythrocytes an unusual distribution of intermediate compounds of the glycolytic sequence. Because of the raised amounts of transaminases in the plasma, the possibility that amino acids might act as lactate precursors was investigated, but the addition of alanine to the patient's erythrocytes *in vitro* (Table 2) did not significantly increase the yield of lactate. Furthermore, the patient's serum did not contain sufficient amino acids to account quantitatively for the 'non-glucose' lactate production. The key to the problem almost certainly lies in the specificity of the glucose oxidase method for blood glucose. By this method the patient's fasting blood glucose value was low (33 mg./100 ml.), but by copper reduction methods, the fasting blood 'sugar' was normal (60 to 95 mg./100 ml.). The former method does not estimate the phosphorylated hexoses of the glycolytic sequence (glucose-6-phosphate, fructose-6-phosphate and fructose 1 : 6 diphosphate), but the latter method does. The second hypothesis, that in the patient a greater proportion of the total blood 'sugar' exists as hexose phosphates, rather than as glucose, would thus account for, (a) the 'non-glucose' lactate production, (b) the increased rate of lactate production demonstrated *in vitro*, and (c) the low true glucose level in the blood. The smaller but significant 'non-glucose' lactate production of normal subjects would also be explained as arising from the amounts of hexose phosphates present normally.

On this hypothesis the plasma pyruvate concentration should also be raised and this was found to be the case. The value for 'excess' lactate depends very much on the level of 'expected' value that is assumed. In our patient the 'excess' lactate was $+ 0\cdot33$ mEq/l. which is not significant. Even if the higher values of American workers for Po and their lower values for Lo were used, the highest possible value for 'excess' lactate would be only $+ 2\cdot8$ mEq/l. This eliminates hypoxia as a cause of the raised lactate level, and suggests a rate of production of pyruvate greater than its rate of utilization, with its subsequent conversion to lactate.

There is no evidence to show that tissues other than erythrocytes contributed to the lactic acidosis, though the precipitation of a prolonged hyperpnoeic attack by mild exertion suggests that glycolysis in muscle might also have taken place at a faster rate than normal.

Only one infant with primary lactic acidosis has been described previously (Hartmann, Wohltmann, Purkerson, and Wesley, 1962). The patient was a female mongol who presented at the age of 2 months with attacks of 'heavy breathing', muscular weakness, and failure to gain weight. During the attacks she sometimes became unconscious, with laryngeal and bronchiolar spasm and asphyxial convulsions. Investigation showed that the resting plasma lactate was raised and that during the attacks there was severe acidaemia with the lactate concentration rising as high as $18\cdot0$ mEq/l. (162 mg./100 ml.). There was also a hyperchloraemia. The attacks responded to treatment with sodium bicarbonate, calcium gluconate, and magnesium sulphate. The authors have investigated the aetiology of the lactic acidosis in some detail and have excluded circulatory failure, glycogen storage disease, and aneurine deficiency. They demonstrated an increased rate of glycolysis of heparinized whole blood, but have been unable to define the metabolic lesion more closely. Their patient is clearly very similar to our patients in many respects, but differs in that she is female, mongoloid, and slowly losing the metabolic abnormality. Nor did she exhibit the neurological lesions and the renal tubular defect.

**Neurological Features.** The striking vascularity of the lesions in Case 1 cannot be due to closer approximation of capillaries as a result of disappearance of the neural parenchyma, since it was often present in areas in which the normal structure was still recognizable. That the necrosis is dependent on an antecedent vascular abnormality is unlikely in view of the persistence of neurones in areas of gross destruction. The relative absence of gliosis may result from degenerative processes overtaking neuroglial formation as well as the parenchyma, as is seen in rapidly advancing cases of subacute combined degeneration of the cord. In more chronic cases, or following therapeutic arrest of the disease, gliosis is the rule.

The published material suggests that the condition of 'necrotizing encephalopathy' described by Leigh (1951), Feigin and Wolf (1954), Richter (1957), Ule (1959), Reye (1960), and Tuthill (1960) is similar to the neurological manifestations of Case 1. Of 15 reported cases in infants, 11 were in males, and 4 in females. Tuthill (1960) describes twin boys, both of whom were affected, and 2 of Feigin and Wolf's cases were sibs. In Reye's case an older female sib had died at 2 years from a similar illness, and in Richter's Case 3, the child's mother, herself a physician, stated that her brother had died at 13 months from a disease which she considered similar to that of her son. In 6 of the reported cases there were one or more normal sibs.

The ages at death of the reported cases ranged from 7 months to 4½ years, with a mean of 21 months. The onset of symptoms varied from birth to 2 years, failure of mental and nervous development was prominent, and difficulty in deglutition and inability to sit or stand were frequent presenting symptoms. Motor weakness was present in 11, with ataxia in 6; 5 had defective pupillary reflexes, 4 were blind, and 4 were deaf. Cranial nerve palsies were common. In all, respiratory difficulties were present and often led to death. Convulsions were common. Symmetrical lesions were constantly found in the mesencephalic tegmentum, pons, and medulla; other sites were not constantly involved. Cord involvement was present in 5: in 4 of these there were severe changes in the posterior columns, especially the tractus gracilis, which increased on ascent and maximally involved the thoracic and cervical regions. Significantly, in none were the corpora mamillaria involved. These symmetrical lesions are of similar structure to those in our case.

The superficial similarity of the lesions to those of Wernicke's encephalopathy tempts one to incriminate an abnormality of aneurine metabolism. Some authors (Feigin and Wolf, 1954; Tuthill, 1960; Ule, 1959) have regarded necrotizing encephalopathy as the morphological equivalent in infants of Wernicke's encephalopathy, but the involvement of the substantia nigra and the invariable sparing of the corpora mamillaria and absence of haemorrhage distinguish the two conditions. In our cases the corpora mamillaria were severely involved, the substantia nigra was affected, and haemorrhage was absent.

It is, however, not justifiable to assume that a particular morphological picture represents only one pathogenesis. It may well be that the appearance in these cases is the response of the immature nervous system to a variety of toxic effects; for example, carbon monoxide poisoning in man and animals, and poisoning by quinoline derivatives in monkeys, both result in symmetrical necrotic lesions similar in morphology and distribution to those of 'necrotizing encephalopathy' (Richter, 1957).

Among all reports cited, the only hint of a metabolic abnormality was in Case 1 of Feigin and Wolf (1954). In this child, as in both of ours, a persistently low plasma bicarbonate was found (in a personal communication from Feigin, the $CO_2$ combining power was stated to be 10·6 mEq/l.).

**Effects of Fluoride.** The connexion between the biochemical abnormalities and the neurological features remains obscure. If the hypothesis of enhanced glycolysis with a dynamic excess of phosphorylated hexoses is correct, fluoride ought to help correct the metabolic abnormality and improve the clinical features. This happened to only a small extent, but it is arguable that the dose of fluoride was too small. Certainly if we were to see further examples of this metabolic abnormality, we would wish to observe the effect of fluoride in higher dosage and would recommend such a trial to others.

## Conclusion

Our patients appear to afford the first-described example of familial lactic acidosis in infancy. The association with necrotizing encephalopathy indicates that lactate metabolism should be investigated in all patients in whom the latter diagnosis is made. The role of fluoride in treatment should be explored further.

## Summary

Two brothers are described who presented during the second year of life with ataxia, muscle twitching, and intermittent hyperpnoea at rest. The condition progressed, with mental deterioration, loss of scalp hair, and death after about 6 months.

One child had widespread, symmetrical, degenerative lesions of the brain and spinal cord resembling those previously described in infants with 'necrotizing encephalopathy'. The histological lesions in the second child were similar, but not so marked, nor so widespread.

The intermittent hyperpnoea of one child, and possibly of both, resulted from spontaneous increases of lactic acid in the blood. The erythrocytes were able to form lactic acid by glycolysis at a rate faster than those of two normal subjects. It is suggested that the proportion of phosphorylated hexoses to free glucose in the blood may have been raised, thus partly accounting for the increased glycolytic rate.

There was also a renal aminoaciduria and a lowered serum phosphate concentration.

This is believed to be the first description of familial lactic acidosis in young children.

We wish to acknowledge the help given to us by Dr. R. R. Hughes, Dr. C. A. St. Hill, Dr. J. Lawson, Dr. J. Rees Roberts, Dr. R. W. Evans, Dr. D. Boulter, and the members of the laboratory staff who assisted with the biochemical and histological investigations. J.S.E. acknowledges gratefully a grant for technical assistance from the Research Fund of the Board of Governors of the United Liverpool Hospitals.

### References

Daughaday, W. H., Lipicky, R. J., and Rasinski, D. C. (1962). Lactic acidosis as a cause of nonketotic acidosis in diabetic patients. *New Engl. J. Med.*, **267**, 1010.

Feigin, I., and Wolf, A. (1954). A disease in infants resembling chronic Wernicke's encephalopathy. *J. Pediat.*, **45**, 243.

Friedemann, T. E., and Haugen, G. E. (1943). Pyruvic acid. II. The determination of ketoacids in blood and urine. *J. biol. Chem.*, **147**, 415.

Gevers, W., and Dowdle, E. (1963). The effect of pH on glycolysis *in vitro*. *Clin. Sci.*, **25**, 343.

Hartmann, A. F., Wohltmann, H. J., Purkerson, M. L., and Wesley, M. E. (1962). Lactate metabolism: studies of a child with a serious congenital deviation. *J. Pediat.*, **61**, 165.

Huckabee, W. E. (1961). Abnormal resting blood lactate. *Amer. J. Med.*, **30**, 833, 840.

Hullin, R. P., and Noble, R. L. (1953). The determination of lactic acid in microgram quantities. *Biochem. J.*, **55**, 289.

Leigh, D. (1951). Subacute necrotising encephalomyelopathy in an infant. *J. Neurol. Neurosurg. Psychiat.*, **14**, 216.

Marks, V. (1959). An improved glucose-oxidase method for determining blood, C.S.F. and urine glucose levels. *Clin. chim. Acta*, **4**, 395.

Reye, R. D. K. (1960). Subacute necrotising encephalomyelopathy. *J. Path. Bact.*, **79**, 165.

Richter, R. B. (1957). Infantile subacute necrotizing encephalopathy with predilection for the brain stem. *J. Neuropath. exp. Neurol.*, **16**, 281.

Smith, I. (1960). *Chromatographic and Electrophoretic Techniques*, Vol. 1. Heinemann, London.

Tuthill, C. R. (1960). Der morphologische Wernicke-Komplex in frühem Kindesalter (Familiäre Erkrankung bei 7 Monate alten Zwillingen.) *Arch. Psychiat. Nervenkr.*, **200**, 520.

Ule, G. (1959). Über eine der Wernickeschen Pseudoencephalitis entsprechende Encephalopathie bei Kindern. *Virchows Arch. path. Anat.*, **332**, 204.

*Arch. Dis. Childh.*, 1965, **40**, 502.

# INFANTILE NEUROAXONAL DYSTROPHY*

BY

L. CROME* and S. D. V. WELLER

*From the Queen Mary's Hospital for Children, Carshalton, Surrey, and the Children's Hospital, Sydenham, London*

(RECEIVED FOR PUBLICATION DECEMBER 11, 1964)

One of the imperfectly understood neuropathological changes is formation of so-called 'spheroids' or 'spheroid bodies' ('Schollen'—in the German literature). These structures are usually roundish homogeneous or faintly granular bodies measuring up to a 100 μ in diameter. They are believed to be focal distensions of axis cylinders, dendrites, or parts of cell bodies, though their direct continuity with neuroplasm is often not demonstrable. They are more frequent in formations of grey matter than of white matter. The presence of occasional spheroids is not unusual in a variety of diverse conditions, such as encephalitis, diabetes, heart failure, carbon monoxide poisoning, and cerebral arteriosclerosis. However, in a few recorded cases spheroids were sufficiently numerous to dominate the morphological picture. Some of these patients were infants or children showing a somewhat uniform clinical picture and pattern of encephalopathy, so that they could have been cases of the same disease or syndrome. This condition has been designated infantile neuroaxonal dystrophy by Cowen and Olmstead (1963) who have reviewed the previous reports and fully described 2 new cases.

The total of recorded cases is only 9 . The onset of the disease occurred between 2 and 3 years, and the age at death ranged from 3 to 13 years. There were 8 girls among the patients. 2 were identical twins and another 2 pairs were sibs. Cowen and Olmstead distinguished an infantile from a 'late infantile' form of the condition, the latter being of later onset, having a more prolonged course, and being, perhaps, a variant of Hallervorden-Spatz disease.

The condition was first described by Seitelberger (1952), and later reports include those by Seitelberger (1954), Rabinowicz and Wildi (1957), Gross, Kaltenbäck, and Uiberrack (1957), Seitelberger and Gross (1957), and, as stated already, Cowen and Olmstead. The pathological findings have been described in only 3 cases. Another case of late infantile Hallervorden-Spatz disease has been recently described by Seitelberger, Gootz, and Gross (1963).

The emerging clinical picture is of apparently normal early development followed by a somewhat abrupt onset of slowly progressive motor and mental disability. However, early development may not be really normal and some of the children are stated to have been definitely mentally backward before the onset of other signs. The children then cease to stand or walk, become hypotonic, and may show strabismus and dysphagia. Blindness, and possibly deafness, develops in most cases. Some of the older children may show spasticity, involuntary movement, flexion deformity, and extensor spasms. Epilepsy was present in two instances. Microcephaly was specifically noted in 2 cases but cannot be excluded in most of the others. The signs and symptoms are of progressive dementia and paralysis. No specific laboratory findings have been reported, and it is hence unlikely that the condition could be diagnosed with any certainty unless previously established in an affected sib.

Histologically, spheroids are found in all parts of the central nervous system, being particularly numerous in the tegmentum of the brain-stem and posterior horns of the spinal cord. Their shape, tinctorial properties, and histochemical features have been studied very fully. It has been established that they contain protein in combination with complex lipids, some of which may be glycolipids. A small amount of polysaccharides may also be present. As a rule, the spheroids do not provoke any cellular reaction, but many show such evidence of regression and dissolution as uneven density, fissuring, and vacuolation of the cytoplasm. Some disappear entirely leaving empty spaces. Another feature of the condition is the occurrence of a somewhat characteristic pattern of associated pathological changes, the chief of which are cerebellar atrophy and sclerosis, accumulation of lipid and gliosis in the striatum, and degeneration of the optic pathway and of some of the long tracts in the brain-stem and spinal

* Part of the histological work was paid for by a grant, made by the National Society for Mentally Handicapped Children.

cord, i.e. the pyramidal, spinocerebellar, spinothalamic, and the gracile and cuneate fasciculi. Cowen and Olmstead have also observed accumulation of somewhat similar adventitious material to that contained in the spheroids in enlarged cells of the germ centres of the spleen and lymph glands and in some of the Kupffer cells in the liver. In 2 of the older cases (Gross *et al.*, 1957; Seitelberger *et al.*, 1963) there was deposition of pigment, as in Hallervorden-Spatz disease, in the globus pallidus and red zone of the substantia nigra.

The pathogenesis of the above-mentioned changes is obscure but the available data suggest the operation of some congenital enzymopathy with, perhaps, an autosomal recessive pattern of inheritance.

Spheroids are known to occur fairly constantly in Hallervorden-Spatz disease, and Seitelberger has, therefore, suggested that infantile neuroaxonal dystrophy is an early non-pigment forming variant of that disease. This concept is not fully accepted by Cowen and Olmstead.

We record below two further familial cases, apparently the first to be recognized in the United Kingdom.

## Case Reports

**Case 1.** This girl, born October 28, 1951, was admitted to hospital at 10 months with feeding difficulties. She was mentally backward and had had several *grand mal* seizures. In hospital she continued having *petit mal* attacks for which she was given troxidone ('tridione'). Shortly after admission she developed pertussis from which she never fully recovered. The leucocyte counts ranged from 10,000 to 54,000 with, in general, an equal proportion of lymphocytes and neutrophil polymorphs A radiograph showed pulmonary atelectasis of the right lower lobe. One specimen of urine, among many, showed a reduction to Benedict's solution, but a glucose tolerance test was normal. The serum calcium was 10·6 mg./100 ml. The stool trypsin was on the low side of normal. A urine chromatogram on June 18, 1952, was reported upon by Professor C. E. Dent as follows: 'A pretty normal glycine pattern of amino-acid excretion; there was a slight excess of cystine and lysine, which could suggest that the child was a heterozygote for cystinuria but it would otherwise be of no particular significance.'

Her skin was dry and, in view of the neurological peculiarities, vitamin B deficiency was suspected. She was, therefore, given a large dose of vitamin B complex without any noticeable change in her condition. She died aged 1 year from bronchopneumonia, which was confirmed at necropsy. It is recorded that other somatic organs showed no significant change, and that the brain was normal. However, the brain was not examined by a neuropathologist and no neural material was kept for subsequent re-examination or histological study.

The following sections stained with haematoxylin and eosin have been preserved and were kindly made available for the present study: one each of the lung, lymph node, liver, and 2 of the kidney. The section of the lung showed a combination of bronchopneumonia, collapse, and inhalation pneumonia. The lymph node showed sinus catarrh. The cells of the germ centres were not enlarged and contained no adventitious material of the kind described by Cowen and Olmstead. One of the renal sections showed normal structure; the other presented a necrotic area surrounded by granulation tissue within a compressed rim of the renal cortex.

**Case 2.** This child was born on September 24, 1961, 10 years after his sister (Case 1 above). The family have had no other children. He was admitted to hospital at 6 months, having become rather 'jerky' during the previous fortnight; he would catch his breath and the head and arms would then jerk forward. The frequency of these episodes had increased, and at the time of admission they were recurring in thrice daily series. When he was younger it was noticed that following a feed he would become quite blue and stiff with both arms held forward, the legs shaking and the eyes staring. This would last about 10 minutes. He would then bring up some wind after which he would appear to recover.

On admission his Hb was 74% (Haldane); WBC, 13,000/c.mm. The urine was normal. The CSF contained 5 white cells per c.mm., chiefly lymphocytes, and 200 RBC's. The chlorides were 785 mg.; sugar, 60 mg.; and protein, 50 mg./100 ml. The electroencephalogram showed 'multiple discharging areas'.

He was put on phenobarbitone, gr. ¼ t.d.s., and was given a course of prednisone. This made little difference to the severity and frequency of the fits and involuntary movements, and the steroid was therefore stopped. He was discharged from hospital after three weeks. At home, the jerks became continuous. He had several severe chest infections, the last of which led to his death at 18 months.

The post-mortem examination (Dr. C. Hunter-Craig) revealed an acute respiratory infection. The liver showed slight mottling of its surface. Histologically, the lungs presented a mixed pattern of bronchopneumonia, collapse, and catarrhal pneumonia, and the liver showed a pattern of cellular vacuolation and oedema. No other somatic tissues have been preserved for histological examination.

The brain weighed 810 g. (average normal for the age, 1,026 g.). The cerebellum together with the brain-stem weighed 50 g. The brain was symmetrical and the pattern of the gyri was normal. The cerebellum was small and indurated. The vermis was particularly small not reaching the level of the inferior part of the cerebellar tonsils. The degree of myelination appeared to be consistent with the age of the child. The cut surface of the cerebellum showed absence of the normal demarcation between the cortex and white matter in the folia and generalized sclerosis (Fig. 1) of the white matter. Pallor and some blurring of the structural pattern was present at all levels of the basal parts of the brain-stem.

Blocks of the frontal, parietal, temporal, and occipital

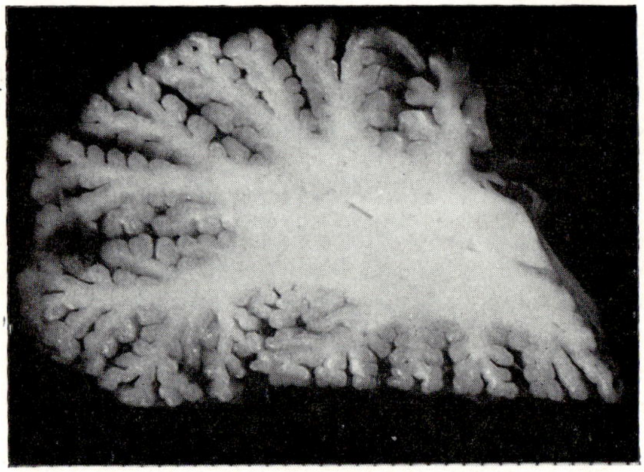

FIG. 1.—The cut surface of the cerebellum.

lobes, the midbrain, pons, medulla, and cerebellum were embedded in celloidin and sections subsequently stained with HVG, PTAH, cresyl violet, by the Heidenhain method for myelin and the Holzer method for fibrous glia. Blocks of the optic nerves, basal ganglia, medulla, upper part of the cervical spinal cord and cerebellum were used for frozen sections which were stained for fat, with PAS, by the Kulschitsky-Pal method for myelin and by silver impregnation methods. Blocks of the occipital and frontal lobes, cerebellum, pons, and the lowermost available portion of the medulla were also embedded in paraffin and sections stained with luxol fast blue for myelin, by the Holzer method, and the Bodian method for axis cylinders. The paraffin sections were also stained with H and E, HVG, PAS, and luxol fast blue.

The most obvious histological changes were observed in the medulla and the cerebellum.

The dorso-lateral parts of the medullary tegmentum showed areas containing numerous spheroids (Fig. 2). These varied in diameter from about 10 to 80 $\mu$. Some were contiguous, imparting a somewhat honeycombed appearance to the affected area. Others were separated from each other by neural tissue. A few had coalesced to form larger structures (Fig. 3), while the presence of many empty spaces in the affected areas indicated corresponding disappearance of spheroids. With most of the stains the spheroids presented a nearly homogeneous or faintly granular appearance. Many showed regressive changes, being pale, fissured, vacuolated, or fragmented. Only the central portions were demonstrable in the case of some spheroids. In general, then, the staining properties were those of hyalinized, degenerating, or 'dissolving' protein. Some of the spheroids were partly or wholly

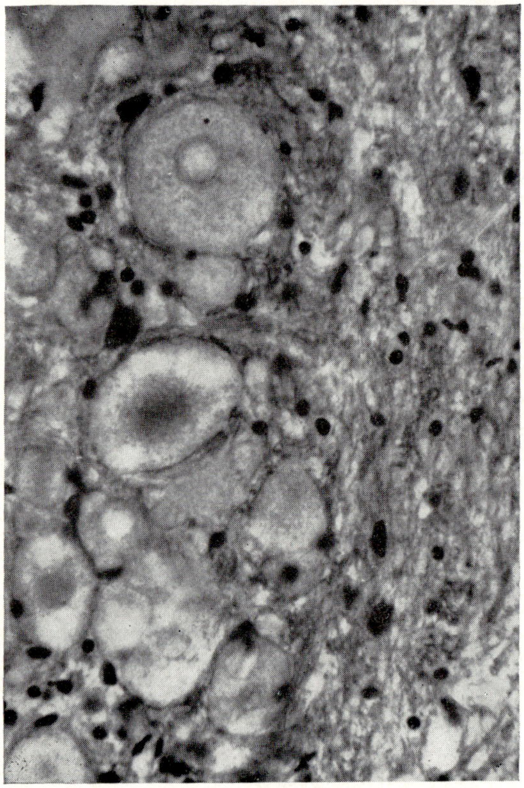

FIG. 2.—'Spheroids' in the dorso-lateral part of the medullary segmentum. (HVG $\times$ 380.)

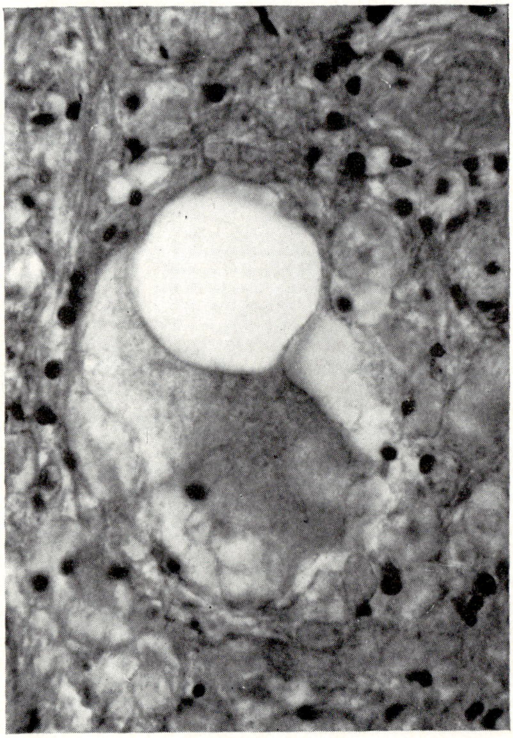

FIG. 3.—Coalescence and regressive changes of the spheroids. (HVG $\times$ 380.)

argyrophil by the Bielschowsky method. Only a very occasional spheroid stained faintly with PAS, and none was sudanophil with the fat stains. The tissue around the spheroids showed no marked cellular reaction, though occasional glial cells could be seen flattened against the margins of some of them, and a few microglial clusters were also present in areas affected by spheroid formation. Some of the smaller spheroids were very inconspicuous and many were not identifiable with certainty. It is, therefore, probable that isolated spheroids, particularly in formations other than the medulla, were not recognized. In fact, only few spheroids were observed outside the medulla. These were situated in the tegmentum of the pons, the midbrain, the caudate nucleus, and the thalamus.

Besides the spheroids, and perhaps not specially related to them, there were a number of reactive microglial clusters grouped around particles of degenerating neural material both in the white and grey matter. Most of these glial clusters were seen in the medulla, but some were present in the tegmentum and the basal areas at other levels of the brain-stem. Fine fibrillary gliosis was also widespread throughout the brain-stem, particularly its basal portions. This gliosis was accentuated around the ventricles, the aqueduct, and the periphery of the brain-stem. The nuclear formations in the brain-stem had lost some neurones, especially in areas containing the spheroids, but the most marked neuronal loss with corresponding astrocytic overgrowth was present in the inferior olives, particularly their dorsal folds. The dorsal accessory olives were entirely devoid of neurones. Sections of the most caudal part of the medulla stained by the Holzer method showed generalized fibrous gliosis in all but their central portions (Fig. 4).

The cerebellum displayed generalized atrophy and sclerosis affecting all its layers (Fig. 5). Although this change was severe everywhere, some parts showed greater involvement than others. The relatively best preserved parts were the cerebellar tonsils. The molecular layer of the cerebellum was shrunken and gliotic. Both the Purkinje and granular cell layers were severely depleted and there was proliferation of Bergmann glia. The axis cylinders of a few of the surviving Purkinje cells showed cigar-shaped or torpedo-like dilatations, and it is noteworthy that their staining resembled closely that of the spheroids. The cerebellar white matter showed pallor of myelin staining and heavy fibrous gliosis. Some neuronal loss was present in the dentate nuclei, though these formations were in a better state of preservation than other parts of the cerebellum.

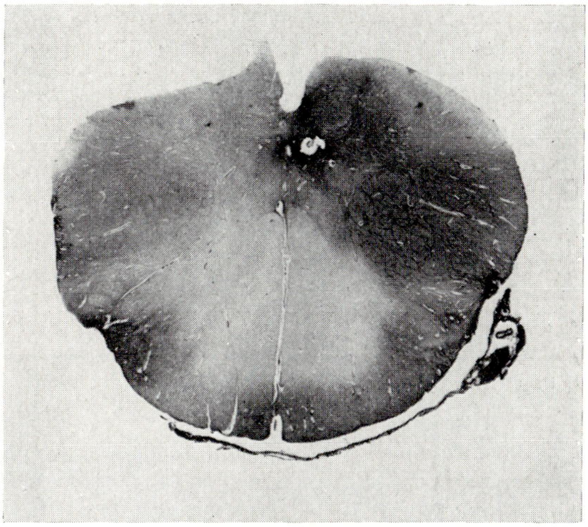

FIG. 4.—Lowermost part of the medulla. (Holzer. × 7.)

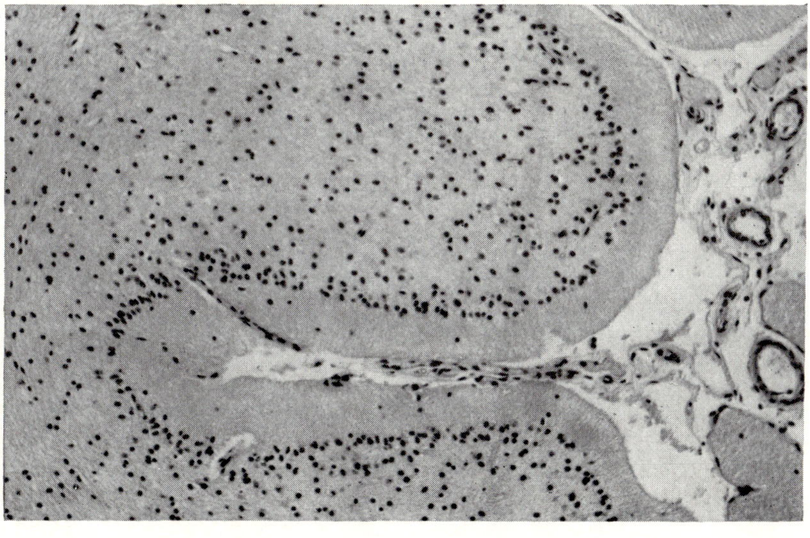

FIG. 5.—Cerebellum showing atrophy of all layers. (H and E × 170.)

TABLE

NEUROCHEMICAL FINDINGS (PROFESSOR J, N. CUMINGS)

| | Frontal Lobe and Cerebellum (g./100 g. tissue) | | | | | | | |
|---|---|---|---|---|---|---|---|---|
| | Cerebral White Matter | | Normal for Age | Cerebral Cortex | | Normal for Age | Cerebellum | |
| | Wet | Dry | | Wet | Dry | | Wet | Dry |
| Total phospholipid .. | 4·50 | 18·00 | 20 | 2·60 | 14·4 | 18 | 1·80 | 12·50 |
| Total cholesterol .. .. | 3·00 | 12·00 | 13 | 0·95 | 5·70 | 6 | 0·93 | 5·80 |
| Esterified cholesterol .. | 0 | 0 | 0 | 0 | 0 | 0 | 0 | 0 |
| Total cerebroside .. .. | 2·10 | 8·40 | 14 | 0·28 | 1·60 | 5 | — | — |
| Total hexosamine .. .. | — | 0·41 | 0·4 | — | 0·61 | 0·7 | — | 0·39 |
| Neuraminic acid .. .. | — | — | — | — | 0·21 | 0·35 | — | — |
| Water (%) .. .. .. | 75·0 | | 76 | 82·1 | | 85 | 84·1 | |

*Thin layer chromatography:* *White matter* shows a loss of cerebroside but a normal phospholipid pattern.
*Cortex:* ganglioside pattern normal.

Marked focal astrocytic gliosis with neuronal loss was also present in the basal ganglia, particularly the ventrolateral thalamic nuclei. A few microglial clusters were seen in the globus pallidus. No iron deposit or pigment was demonstrable in any part of the basal ganglia and the substantia nigra contained only the expected minimal quantity of pigment. Only a small quantity of sudanophil material was present around a few of the blood vessels in the striatum.

The meninges were normal. The cerebral cortex showed terminal oedema and unevenness of neuronal staining. Some nerve cells had faded almost entirely, appearing as 'ghost cells'. Definite neuronal loss was ascertainable at the troughs of some of the cerebral sulci. The white matter of the centrum semi-ovale presented widespread fine fibrillary gliosis. The staining of myelin throughout the central nervous system was somewhat pale but the pattern of myelination was probably consistent with the age of the patient. Fat staining showed only slight accumulation of brightly sudanophil granules, and attempts to demonstrate an excess of PAS positive material in the neuronal cytoplasm were unsuccessful. Some of the larger neurones did contain a small quantity of PAS positive material, but this was probably well within normal limits.

The optic nerves and tracts showed a seemingly normal state of myelination and no ascertainable loss of axis cylinders. Only a doubtful overgrowth of fibrous astrocytes was demonstrable at the periphery of the optic nerve.

The spinal cord was not available for examination. The neurochemical findings are given in the Table.

## Comment

The over-all similarity of the present case to those previously described as infantile neuroaxonal dystrophy is impressive and it is probable that the elder child had the same condition. The present cases are the youngest on record, and it seems likely that the disease had commenced at, or soon after, birth. This early onset and rapid course explain, perhaps, some of the unusual features. Blindness had apparently not developed and the optic pathway showed only minor anatomical abnormality. The deposition of spheroids was restricted almost entirely to the medulla. The striatum showed only minimal changes while the thalamus was much more extensively involved. No excess of pigment was present in any examined part of the brain, but this should, perhaps, not be expected in a child of 18 months, even if the condition were related to Hallervorden-Spatz disease. The present data thus add little to the problem of the relation of infantile neuroaxonal dystrophy to that disease, an issue fully considered by Cowen and Olmstead.

The neurochemical findings were non-specific. The loss of cerebrosides in the white matter with a normal phospholipid pattern could possibly be explained by the presence of fine fibrous gliotic tissue and a relative deficiency of myelin in the sampled material.

It has been suggested by Seitelberger that the condition is a form of lipidosis. There is nothing to support this view in the present cases.

In a recent communication, Sung (1964) reported the presence of spheroids within the gracile and cuneate nuclei, and within the nucleus of the descending tract of the trigeminal nerve in each of the 6 cases of mucoviscidosis examined by him. Citing experimental work, he suggested that the change might be due to vitamin E deficiency. Sung's description and illustrations leave, perhaps, some doubt as to the exact similarity of the lesions, particularly in number and distribution, to those presented above. Moreover, the associated cerebellar changes, as in infantile neuroaxonal dystrophy, are not mentioned by him. Nevertheless, since it is known that some spheroids can occur in a variety of conditions, there is no reason to assume that infantile neuroaxonal dystrophy is always identical in origin.

## Summary

A sister and her brother died at 12 and 18 months, respectively, with mental retardation, paralysis, and epilepsy. The brain of the second child was examined neuropathologically. Allowing for certain divergences, the changes were those of infantile neuroaxonal dystrophy. The condition was almost certainly congenital in the present patients who died at an earlier age than any of the previously recorded ones. The sister was probably suffering from the same disorder.

We are greatly indebted to Professor J. N. Cumings for the neurochemical analysis of the material, and to Professor C. E. Dent for permission to quote his findings. Dr. John Keall has kindly placed the brain of Case 2 and the remaining histological preparations at our disposal.

## References

Cowen, D., and Olmstead, E. V. (1963) Infantile neuroaxonal dystrophy. *J. Neuropath. exp. Neurol.*, **22**, 175.

Gross, H., Kaltenbäck, E., and Uiberrack, B. (1957). Über eine spätinfantile Form der Hallervorden-Spatzschen Krankheit. I. Mitteilung: Klinisch-anatomische Befunde. *Dtsch. Z. Nervenheilk.*, **176**, 77.

Rabinowicz, Th., and Wildi, E. (1957). Spastic amaurotic axonal idiocy. A familial juvenile form of a lipo-glyco-proteidic thesaurismosis including a pallidal siderosis. In *Cerebral Lipidoses*, ed. J. N. Cumings, p. 34. Van Bogaert, Oxford.

Seitelberger, F. (1952). Eine unbekannte Form von Infantiler Lipoid-speicher-Krankheit des Gehirns. In *Proc. 1st int. Congr. Neuropath., Rome, 1952*, vol. 3, p. 323. Rosenberg & Sellier, Turin.

—— (1954). Eine eigenartige Stoffwechselerkrankung der Ganglienzellen im Zentralnervensystem. In *Proc. 5th int. neurol. Congr., Lisbon, 1953*, vol. 3, p. 484. Lisbon.

——, and Gross, H. (1957). Über eine spätinfantile Form der Hallervorden-Spatzschen Krankheit. II. Histochemische Befunde; Erörterung der Nosologie. *Dtsch. Z. Nervenheilk.*, **176**, 104.

——, Gootz, E., and Gross, H. (1963). Beitrag zur spatinfantilen Hallervorden-Spatzschen Krankheit. *Acta neuropath. (Berl.)*, **3**, **16**.

Sung, J. H. (1964). Neuroaxonal dystrophy in mucoviscidosis. *J. Neuropath. exp. Neurol.*, **23**, 567.

*Arch. Dis. Childh.*, 1965, **40**, 508.

# THE INSULIN-GLUCOSE TOLERANCE TEST IN PITUITARY GROWTH RETARDATION

BY

OLAV TRYGSTAD

*From the Paediatric Research Institute, University Hospital, Rikhospitalet, Oslo, Norway*

(RECEIVED FOR PUBLICATION JANUARY 14, 1965)

The differential diagnosis of growth retardation has become of great importance in the past few years, since human growth hormone (HGH) treatment has become available to patients with pituitary dwarfism. The diagnosis of low birthweight dwarfism (Black, 1961) is usually easy, but before puberty the differentiation of constitutionally retarded growth (Wilkins, 1957) from pituitary dwarfism may be very difficult. The insulin tolerance test has proved, in our experience, a useful supplement to other tests in the selection of patients for HGH treatment, despite the contrary conclusions of some other workers (Colombo, Richterich, Rossi, and Feinsmith, 1962). In this paper we give our experience with the insulin-glucose test, comparing its usefulness with that of other tests of endocrine function.

## Material and Methods

During the past two years the insulin tolerance test has been carried out on 22 patients between 6 and 19 years of age who were diagnosed as having pituitary growth retardation. Of these, 13 are now receiving continuous treatment with HGH; 9 have been treated for more than a year with good response, their height increments ranging from 7 to 13 cm. during the first year of treatment.

During the same period insulin tolerance tests have also been carried out on 12 patients in whom the diagnosis of constitutional growth retardation has been made, and on 15 control patients without hormonal or metabolic disorders, and of the same age distribution.

The insulin tolerance tests were carried out after the patients had been in hospital for at least three days on a moderately high carbohydrate diet. Patients with pituitary failure are known to be hypersensitive to insulin, which often causes a considerable decrease in blood sugar, followed by a very slow return to normal levels. Even when adrenaline or glucagon are injected the blood sugar rises only slowly. The usual insulin tolerance test may, therefore, be hazardous in these patients. For a standardized test without reduction of the insulin dose when insulin hypersensitivity is suspected, we have preferred the less dangerous insulin-glucose tolerance test (Engel and Scott, 1950).

Crystalline glucagon-free insulin, 0·1 I.U./kg. body weight is given intravenously. The insulin is diluted 1 : 10 in saline. 30 minutes after the insulin injection or when the first significant symptoms of hypoglycaemia appear, whichever is the earlier, the child is given oral glucose 1·75 g./kg. (in apple juice). Capillary blood for sugar determination was obtained in this series at 0, 20, 30, 45, 60, 90, 120, 150, and 210 minutes after the insulin injection, but as no significant differences between the groups were found after the administration of glucose, the test may be ended at 60 minutes. Blood sugar determinations were performed by the method of Hagedorn, Halström, and Jensen (1935).

During the first 30 minutes the child is observed closely for signs of hypoglycaemia: if these occur a blood specimen must be obtained and glucose given immediately, intravenously in severe cases. In our series of patients with pituitary dwarfism, we observed significant hypoglycaemic signs in one patient (A.S.); oral glucose was given at 25 minutes and the signs rapidly subsided.

The insulin-glucose tolerance test is less time consuming than the ordinary insulin tolerance test, where the child has to be observed closely for hypoglycaemic signs for at least an hour after insulin injection. Furthermore, with the ordinary dosage, severe hypoglycaemia often occurs in patients with pituitary hypofunction, so that the test may have to be performed more than once, after starting with one-third the usual dose.

## Results

Table 1 shows the mean results of the insulin-glucose tolerance tests in the groups described. Table 2 gives further details about the tests performed on the patients with pituitary dwarfism in whom the diagnosis had been proved by response to HGH treatment over a period of more than a year.

In the normal child the blood sugar drops to about 50% of the initial fasting value in 15 to 20 minutes (Colombo *et al.*, 1962). A fall below 50% is usually said to indicate an abnormal insulin tolerance (Williams, 1962), but this is not in accord with our experience. Table 3 presents the numbers of patients in whom the test was 'abnormal' by this

TABLE 1

RESULTS OF INSULIN-GLUCOSE TOLERANCE TESTS

| | No. | Blood Sugar Concentrations After (minutes) Mean ± SD | | | | | | | | | Maximum Decrease | |
|---|---|---|---|---|---|---|---|---|---|---|---|---|
| | | 0 | 20 | 30 | 45 | 60 | 90 | 120 | 150 | 210 | % | SD |
| Controls .. .. .. | 15 | 94 ± 9 | 45 ± 6 | 60 ± 13 | 114 | 142 | 168 | 157 | 138 | 91 | 52 | ± 6·5 |
| Constitutional dwarfism | 12 | 92 ± 16 | 41 ± 11 | 55 ± 13 | 102 | 131 | 157 | 147 | 117 | 91 | 55 | ± 7·5 |
| Pituitary dwarfism, HGH treated more than 1 year | 9 | 88 ± 15 | 53 ± 14 | 42 ± 11 | 94 | 127 | 149 | 136 | 118 | 91 | 52 | ± 15·5 |
| Pituitary dwarfism ? .. | 13 | 93 ± 15 | 55 ± 14 | 45 ± 12 | 97 | 120 | 153 | 155 | 146 | 111 | 53 | ± 9·5 |

TABLE 2

RESULTS OF INSULIN-GLUCOSE TOLERANCE TESTS IN 9 PATIENTS SHOWING GOOD RESPONSE TO TREATMENT WITH HGH FOR MORE THAN A YEAR

| Patient | Age (yr.) | Height Increment | | Blood Sugar Concentration After (minutes) | | | | | | | | | Maximum Decrease (%) |
|---|---|---|---|---|---|---|---|---|---|---|---|---|---|
| | | Before Treatment (cm./yr.) | On Treatment (cm./mth.) | 0 | 20 | 30 | 45 | 60 | 90 | 120 | 150 | 210 | |
| A.S. | 12½ | 9/5 | 24/36 | 90 | 48 | 25* | 107 | 136 | 210 | 154 | 141 | 106 | 72 |
| C.S. | 9½ | 6/4½ | 28/36 | 115 | 58 | 31 | 94 | 151 | 155 | 206 | 131 | 76 | 73 |
| A.S.F. | 9 | 23/6 | 16/27 | 95 | 44 | 38 | 100 | 140 | 164 | 125 | 86 | 94 | 60 |
| T.V. | 16 | 25/9 | 14/24 | 78 | 57 | 44 | 86 | 117 | 130 | 107 | 101 | 105 | 44 |
| T.H.S. | 12½ | 15/7½ | 11/24 | 57 | 47 | 42 | 63 | 115 | 129 | 132 | 154 | 80 | 26 |
| T.R.M. | 8½ | 11/5½ | 9/15 | 76 | 32 | 46 | 72 | 76 | 72 | 68 | 105 | 86 | 58 |
| R.E. | 19 | 28/9½ | 9/13 | 93 | 72 | 47 | 97 | 127 | 193 | 171 | 150 | 101 | 49 |
| K.V. | 6 | 6/1½ | 7/12 | 97 | 80 | 67 | 107 | 154 | 125 | 117 | 82 | 78 | 31 |
| O.L. | 10 | 16/4 | 7/12 | 90 | 41 | 39 | 117 | 123 | 173 | 140 | 109 | 97 | 56 |
| Mean: ± SD | 11½ | 2·65/1 | 7½/12 | 88<br>15·2 | 53<br>14·4 | 42<br>11·1 | 94<br>16·2 | 127<br>21·9 | 149<br>37·7 | 136<br>37·0 | 118<br>25·4 | 91<br>11·5 | 52<br>15·5 |

* 25-minute blood sample (hypoglycaemic symptoms).

TABLE 3

MAGNITUDE OF BLOOD SUGAR DECREASE DURING INSULIN-GLUCOSE TOLERANCE TEST

| | Blood Sugar Decrease of | |
|---|---|---|
| | > 50% (No.) | > 60% (No.) |
| Controls .. .. .. .. .. .. | 9/15 | 2/15 |
| Constitutional dwarfism .. .. .. | 9/12 | 4/12 |
| Pituitary dwarfism, HGH treated .. | 5/9 | 2/9 |
| Pituitary dwarfism ? .. .. .. | 8/13 | 3/13 |

TABLE 4

NUMBER OF CASES SHOWING DECREASE IN BLOOD SUGAR BETWEEN 20 AND 30 MINUTES

| | No. |
|---|---|
| Controls .. .. .. .. .. .. | 0/15 |
| Constitutional dwarfism .. .. .. .. | 0/12 |
| Pituitary dwarfism, HGH treated .. .. .. | 8/9 |
| Pituitary dwarfism ? .. .. .. .. | 12/13 |

criterion, showing that there was no difference between the groups. 6 patients in whom pituitary function was presumed to be normal showed a fall in blood sugar to below 40% of the initial fasting value.

During the first 20 minutes the decrease in blood sugar concentration after insulin injection seemed to be slightly greater in children with normal pituitary function than in those with hypopituitarism. The difference, however, is not statistically significant (p between 0·05 and 0·025).

Table 4 and the Figure show the numbers of patients in each group where the lowest blood sugar value was recorded not in the 20-minute but in the 30-minute sample. None of the controls or the patients with constitutional growth retardation had lower blood sugar values in the 30-minute than in the 20-minute sample. Two of the controls had the same concentration in the 20- and 30-minute samples, perhaps because the lowest level was reached between the two blood samples.

The change in blood sugar concentration between the 20- and the 30-minute sample is significantly different when compared with the controls in both groups of pituitary dwarfism ($p < 0{\cdot}001$). The group with constitutional dwarfism shows no difference from the controls ($p = 0{\cdot}9$-$0{\cdot}8$).

Only two patients originally diagnosed as pituitary dwarfs had an increase in blood sugar from the 20-minute sample to the 30-minute sample. Both these patients had normal metyrapone tests, and there may be some doubt about the diagnosis. One of them (T.R.M.) was born with a grave foetal

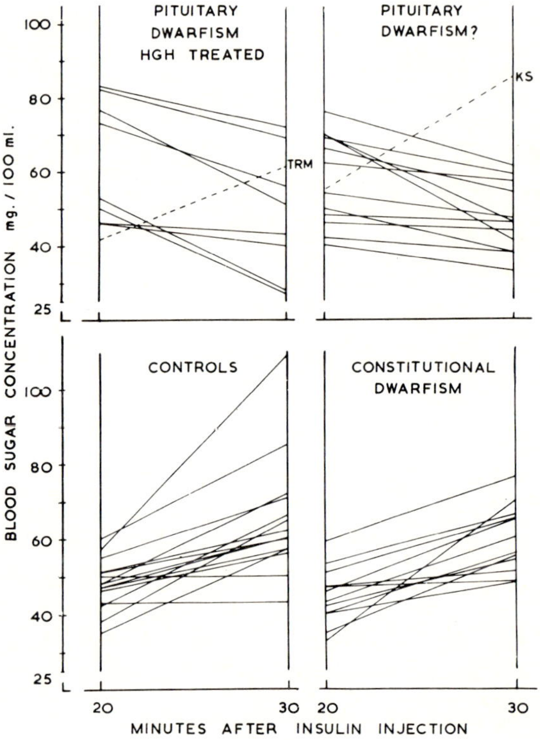


FIG.—Change in blood sugar concentration between 20 and 30 minutes after insulin injection in four groups of cases: proven pituitary dwarfism, unproven pituitary dwarfism, normal controls, and constitutional dwarfism. Broken lines indicate the two suspected pituitary dwarfs with normal insulin-glucose tolerance tests (see text). The blood-sugar concentrations are calculated after adjusting the fasting level to 100 mg./100 ml.

asphyxia. He may possibly have a low birth weight dwarfism, because he and a younger sister had an intrauterine growth retardation, though he has grown 9 cm. in 17 months on HGH treatment, having grown only 9 cm. in the course of the previous 42 months. The other (K.S.) may also be suffering from constitutionally retarded growth and adolescent development, but because of his extreme shortness (137 cm. at 17 years) the effect of HGH was tried. However, the response has not been very striking after 8 months of treatment (height increment 4 cm.).

We, therefore, regard the insulin-glucose tolerance test as abnormal when the blood sugar curve shows a continuous decrease until glucose is given.

## Discussion

In childhood the differentiation of pituitary dwarfism from constitutional growth retardation is difficult, the diagnosis resting upon a number of features, none of which are pathognomonic.

The early diagnosis of pituitary dwarfism is important now that HGH treatment can be offered. In untreated cases our experience is the same as Kaplan's (1964), that the bone age of the pituitary dwarfed child increases with time more than does height age, so that the prognosis concerning the final height likely to be achieved with HGH therapy deteriorates with time.

The previous view (Daughaday, 1962) that pituitary growth retardation generally starts after the second year of life, is usually not familial, and is predominantly seen in boys, does not accord with our experience (Trygstad and Seip, 1964), and we regard these features as of little diagnostic value. Immunological methods for plasma HGH determinations do not as yet seem to be decisive in the diagnosis of pituitary dwarfism. Large and rapid variations in plasma HGH concentration occur during the day (Hunter, and Greenwood, 1964) and the values found in normal controls and in hypopituitarism overlap (Utiger, Parker, and Daughaday, 1962). Plasma HGH determinations after insulin hypoglycaemia may prove to be a more useful test.

The activity of the different pituitary hormones should be evaluated by the available tests. Though most pituitary dwarfs do not mature sexually, this is not always true (Antonin, 1961). The corticotrophin and thyrotrophin reserves may also be normal, so that the possibility of an isolated HGH deficiency must be considered.

Table 5 shows the main criteria on which we base the differential diagnosis between constitutional and pituitary growth retardation.

Table 6 shows the results in two other tests we have studied. The urinary excretion of 17-ketogenic steroids (17-KGS) has proved of no diagnostic value in our patients, all four groups having the same mean daily excretion of 17-KGS.

The metyrapone test, however, provides good evidence of the pituitary corticotrophin reserve. Metyrapone, 70-100 mg./kg. body weight, is given orally in 6-10 doses during 24 hours. This substance blocks cortisol synthesis, and the blood concentration of its precursor, 11-β hydroxycortisol (compound 'S'), therefore increases. With a normal pituitary, therefore, there is increased corticotrophin secretion and increased compound 'S' formation. The increase in urinary excretion of compound 'S' (THS) after metyrapone is interpreted as normal when it exceeds 1 mg./24 hr. and the increase of urinary 17-KGS excretion exceeds 100%.

The metyrapone test has been carried out in 18 patients provisionally diagnosed as pituitary dwarfism. Of these, 12 showed an abnormal and 6 a normal response. One of the latter had a craniopharyngioma with growth retardation during the past four years, and a height increment of only 2 cm. during the past two years. In this patient the insulin-glucose tolerance test was abnormal, indicating a pituitary failure. Of the patients in Table 2 T.R.M. and R.E. had normal tests, A.S. had 300%, and T.V. 100% increase in urinary 17-KGS excretion.

None of our pituitary dwarfs have had hypoglycaemic episodes, and there are no significant differences in the fasting blood sugar levels between the groups (Table 1).

Hypoglycaemia induced by insulin is probably chiefly due to the increased peripheral uptake of glucose. The return of blood glucose concentration to normal levels may depend on several factors: (i) increased glucose release by the liver, (ii) decreased sensitivity of the peripheral tissue to insulin, e.g. caused by the increased growth hormone secretion evoked by the hypoglycaemia, (iii) an increase in the level of insulin inhibitors or antagonists, and (iv) gradual inactivation of the injected insulin.

The hypersensitivity to insulin in hypopituitarism and secondary adrenal insufficiency may be caused by changes in some or all of these factors, but we do not know which factor is most important.

Recently it has been demonstrated that insulin-induced hypoglycaemia will produce an abrupt rise in the level of HGH in plasma (Hunter and Greenwood, 1964; Roth, Glick, Yalow, and Berson, 1964). Insulin and growth hormone seem to interact and behave like a new hormone that does not stimulate either glucose or free fatty acid uptake by the peripheral tissues (Zierler and Rabinowitz, 1963). Luft and Cerasi (1964) suggest that the biological activity of circulating insulin may be masked by increased amounts of an insulin inhibitor elicited by the growth hormone.

A number of years ago Young (1938) demonstrated that injections of anterior pituitary extracts in rabbits made the animals more resistant to the hypoglycaemic effect of insulin. Our own unpublished observations demonstrate that HGH treatment of pituitary dwarfs tends to restore the insulin-glucose tolerance test to normal. The insulin tolerance test is generally considered to be a test of corticotrophin—adrenal reserve, but it may perhaps be a more specific test for the somatotrophic function of the pituitary.

TABLE 5

DIFFERENTIATION OF CONSTITUTIONAL FROM PITUITARY GROWTH RETARDATION

| Diagnostic signs | Constitutional Dwarfism | Pituitary Dwarfism |
|---|---|---|
| Familial occurrence | Often | At times |
| Growth retardation since birth | At times | At times |
| Growth velocity after third year | 3-5 cm./yr. | 1-4 cm./yr. |
| Puberty | Late | Usually absent |
| Bone age retardation | Moderate | Severe |
| Serum P, inorganic | Normal | Often low |
| Serum total cholesterol | Normal | Often high |
| Serum protein-bound iodine | Normal | Often low |
| Metyrapone test | Normal | Often abnormal |
| Insulin-glucose tolerance test | Normal | Often abnormal |

TABLE 6

URINARY EXCRETION OF 17-KETOGENIC STEROIDS AND RESULTS OF METYRAPONE TEST

| | Mean Age* (yr.) | Mean Daily Excretion of 17-KGS in Urine (mg.) | Abnormal Metyrapone Response |
|---|---|---|---|
| Normals | 10·2 (6-14) | 2·9 | 0/9 |
| Constitutional growth retardation | 9·9 (6-18) | 3·3 | 0/12 |
| Pituitary dwarfism, HGH treated | 11·5 (6-19) | 3·0 | 7/9 |
| Pituitary dwarfism ? | 10·6 (6-18) | 3·0 | 5/9 |

* The four groups were matched for age, except that all 9 children in the normal control group, being pre-pubertal, were less than 14 years.

The test was performed on 12 patients diagnosed as constitutional growth retardation and on 15 normal controls with the same age distribution as the pituitary dwarfs; all 27 had a normal test.

In interpreting the insulin-glucose test, the decrease in blood sugar between 20 and 30 minutes best differentiated the group of pituitary dwarfs.

In this study the insulin-glucose tolerance test proved a better diagnostic aid than the metyrapone test.

**Summary**

The insulin-glucose tolerance test was performed on 22 patients diagnosed as pituitary dwarfism: in 9 of them the diagnosis had been confirmed by a growth response to human growth hormone. Only 2 patients had a normal test, and the diagnosis was doubtful in these.

The author wishes to extend his thanks to Drs. T. M. Chalmers, Addenbrooke's Hospital, Cambridge; J. Jervell, Biochemical Institute, University of Oslo; and M. Seip, Paediatric Department, University Hospital, Oslo for advice.

REFERENCES

Antonin, J. M. F. (1961). Hypothalamo—hypophysärer Zwergwuchs mit spontaner Pubertät. *Helv. paediat. Acta*, **16**, 267.
Black, J. (1961). Low birth weight dwarfism. *Arch. Dis. Childh.*, **36**, 633.
Colombo, J. P., Richterich, R., Rossi, E., and Feinsmith, B. (1962). Die diagnostische Bedeutung der Insulinbelastung. *Ann. paediat. (Basel)*, **199**, 110.
Daughaday, W. H. (1962). In *Textbook of Endocrinology*, by R. H. Williams, 3rd ed., pp. 51-53. W. B. Saunders, Philadelphia.
Engel, F. L., and Scott, J. L. (1950). The insulin-glucose tolerance test. A modified procedure for the detection of hypoglycemia

unresponsiveness in pituitary and adrenal insufficiency. *J. clin. Invest.*, **29**, 151.

Hagedorn, H. C., Halström, F., and Jensen, N. (1935). Hurtige metoder til bestemmelse av blodsukker ved kaliumferricyanid. *Hospitalstidende*, **78**, 1193.

Hunter, W. M., and Greenwood, F. C. (1964). Studies on the secretion of human-pituitary-growth hormone. *Brit. med. J.*, **1**, 804.

Kaplan, S. A. (1964). *Growth Disorders in Children and Adolescents*, p. 69. Thomas, Springfield, Illinois.

Luft, R., and Cerasi, E. (1964). Effect of human growth hormone on insulin production in panhypopituitarism. *Lancet*, **2**, 124.

Roth, J., Glick, S. M., Yalow, R. S., and Berson, S. A. (1964). The influence of blood glucose on the plasma concentration of growth hormone. *Diabetes*, **13**, 355.

Trygstad, O., and Seip, M. (1964). Hereditary pituitary dwarfism treated with human growth hormone. *Acta paediat. (Uppsala)*, **53**, 527.

Utiger, R. D., Parker, M. L., and Daughaday, W. H. (1962). Studies on human growth hormone. I. A radioimmunoassay for human growth hormone. *J. clin. Invest.*, **41**, 254.

Wilkins, L. (1957). *The Diagnosis and Treatment of Endocrine Disorders in Childhood and Adolescence*. Blackwell Scientific Publications, Oxford.

Williams, R. H. (1962). *Textbook of Endocrinology*, 3rd ed., p. 621. W. B. Saunders, Philadelphia.

Young, F. G. (1938). The identity and mechanism of action of the glycotropic (anti-insulin) substance of the anterior pituitary gland. *Biochem. J.*, **32**, 1521.

Zierler, K. L., and Rabinowitz, D. (1963). Roles of insulin and growth hormone, based on studies of forearm metabolism in man. *Medicine (Baltimore)*, **42**, 385.

*Arch. Dis. Childh.*, 1965, **40**, 513.

# BLOOD 5-HYDROXYTRYPTAMINE LEVELS IN THE NEWBORN

BY

MEENA HAZRA*, SYLVIA BENSON, and M. SANDLER†

*From the Bernhard Baron Memorial Research Laboratories and Institute of Obstetrics and Gynaecology, Queen Charlotte's Maternity Hospital, London*

(RECEIVED FOR PUBLICATION DECEMBER 18, 1964)

During the course of a long-term investigation, still in progress, designed to shed light on the observation of Pare, Sandler, and Stacey (1960) that certain children with mental handicap have high blood 5-hydroxytryptamine (5HT) concentrations, some data on levels in normal newborn infants were obtained which seem to be worthy of record.

## Method

Whole-blood 5HT levels were measured by the method of Contractor (1964) with the following modifications. (a) Capillary blood obtained from the heel with minimal squeezing was used instead of venous blood. It had previously been established in four normal adults that 5HT levels in capillary and venous blood drawn simultaneously were in close agreement.
(b) The procedure was scaled down to allow the use of 1 ml. blood instead of 2 ml. and carboxymethylcellulose columns were reduced in height from 10 to 5 cm. These changes inevitably reduced the sensitivity of the procedure and increased the error of the method from $\pm$ 5% to $\pm$ 36%, but as the observed changes in blood levels in each age-group were greater than this margin of error, they were considered to be significant.

Platelets were counted by the method of Dacie and Lewis (1963).

## Results

Samples of capillary blood were taken from normal full-term infants at 1 day and 1 week of life while in Queen Charlotte's Hospital; follow-up samples were subsequently obtained at 4-6 weeks, 12 weeks, and 24 weeks while at home, though some infants were not accessible for the later samples. Results are shown in the Table.

Values were low at birth but then rose to reach a peak at 4-6 weeks, there being a highly significant difference between mean values at these periods despite the wide scatter of individual concentrations. There was a significant drop at 12 weeks, after which levels remained constant.

The mean platelet count on day 1 was 166,000 $\pm$ 25,000 (S.D.) per c.mm. and did not change significantly throughout the investigation.

## Discussion

Although it has previously been established that circulating 5HT levels are low at birth, no detailed study of changes in concentration during the first six months of life has hitherto been published. Taking the difference of method into account, values determined by Mitchell and Cass (1959) in umbilical venous blood (12 $\pm$ 12 mμg./ml.) are not dissimilar from those described here. It is not possible to compare our findings with those of Grasso, Bianchi, Crosti, and Ermacora (1961), however, for though they found significantly low levels in the newborn period, they expressed their results in terms of concentration per $10^9$ platelets.

The cause of these low values remains speculative.

* Present address: Department of Paediatrics, Civil Hospital, Ahmedabad, India.

† Requests for reprints should be sent to M. Sandler.

TABLE

WHOLE BLOOD 5-HYDROXYTRYPTAMINE LEVELS (mμg./ml.) FROM BIRTH TO 24 WEEKS OF AGE

| | 1 day | 1 week | 4-6 weeks | 12 weeks | 24 weeks |
|---|---|---|---|---|---|
| Mean $\pm$ S.D. .. .. .. | 21 $\pm$ 13 | 53 $\pm$ 38 | 162 $\pm$ 64 | 110 $\pm$ 62 | 115 $\pm$ 76 |
| Number of subjects .. .. | 27 | 26 | 24 | 18 | 16 |
| p .. .. .. .. .. .. | $< 0{\cdot}001$ (1 day–1 week) | $< 0{\cdot}001$ (1 week–4-6 weeks) | $< 0{\cdot}05$ (4-6 weeks–12 weeks) | Not significant (12 weeks–24 weeks) | |

It is generally agreed that circulating 5HT is bound almost wholly to blood platelets. The present data, however, show platelet counts to lie within the normal adult range (Dacie and Lewis, 1963). There does not appear to be any defective uptake of 5HT by platelets deriving from cord blood (Stacey, 1965), despite a limited experiment implying the contrary by Mitchell and Cass (1959). Enhanced breakdown of 5HT, though theoretically possible, is unlikely, for monoamine oxidase, the enzyme largely responsible for its inactivation, is decreased during the newborn period both in the human (Epps, 1945) and in the rat (Shimizu and Morikawa, 1959; Nachmias, 1960; Karki, Kuntzman, and Brodie, 1962). Endogenous release of 5HT from viable platelets has never been demonstrated under physiological conditions, though some exchange of radio isotopically labelled aminc has been noted in patients with the carcinoid syndrome (Zucker, Hellman, and Zumoff, 1964), and alkaline extracts of various tissues can provoke such release *in vitro* (Toh, 1956; Giarman, Potter, and Day, 1960).

In certain experimental animals, brain 5HT levels are low at birth (Kato, 1960; Nachmias, 1960; Karki *et al.*, 1962; Smith, Stacey, and Young, 1962; Hsia, Nishimura, and Brenchley, 1963), though there is some species variation (Pepeu and Giarman, 1962). If this finding can be extrapolated to man, there exists the likelihood of defective synthesis of 5HT in early life. In common with some other enzyme systems (Driscoll and Hsia, 1958), 5-hydroxytryptophan decarboxylase, which elaborates 5HT from its precursor amino acid, has a decreased activity during the newborn period in several species, though this reduction varies very much with the tissue (Huang, Tannenbaum, and Hsia, 1960; Smith *et al.*, 1962; Karki *et al.*, 1962; Hsia *et al.*, 1963). Bennett and Giarman (1964), however, indicate that defective tryptophan 5-hydroxylation is more likely to be responsible for low 5HT levels encountered in the newborn rat.

Mitchell and Cass (1959) formed the impression that an increase in blood 5HT content occurs rather abruptly at 16-20 weeks of age, but as their contention was based on 8 single estimations in different children, it is not possible to attach much significance to their findings. The considerably larger series reported here shows that a rise to adult levels (Contractor, 1964) occurs gradually and is maximal by the 4-6th week of life. As discussed above, its cause is presumably connected with the maturation of enzyme systems at the site of synthesis and is independent of platelet number. Stacey and Young (1964) have shown in the newborn guinea-pig that platelet 5HT level rises in parallel to, and thus probably derives from, intestinal 5HT content. It does not seem too unlikely that a similar connexion may exist in the human infant.

Though it was not practicable to measure 24-hour urinary output of the major metabolite of 5HT, 5-hydroxyindoleacetic acid, in our series, because of difficulties in collection of specimens, the data of other workers (Serra, 1958; Rappallini and Murtagh, 1962) suggest that, expressed per kilogram body weight, there is a low rate of 5HT synthesis in the newborn period, which rises to approximately adult levels after 1 month (Serra, 1958). While this finding mirrors our own observations, their work might usefully be repeated using more precise analytical methods.


## Summary

Whole blood 5-hydroxytryptamine (5HT) levels, determined in a series of normal full-term infants, were low at birth (21 $\pm$ 13 mμg./ml.) but rose to adult concentrations (162 $\pm$ 64 mμg./ml.) by 4-6 weeks of life, though blood platelet counts remained unchanged. These findings are likely to be connected with the maturation of enzymes responsible for 5-hydroxytryptamine synthesis.



This work was supported by a generous grant from the National Society for Mentally Handicapped Children who defrayed the salaries of M.H. and S.B.

We are grateful to Dr. A. White Franklin and Dr. A. P. Norman for allowing us to examine their patients, to Miss Glenda Hale for carrying out platelet counts, and to the mothers of the infants tested whose willing co-operation made the investigation possible.


### References


Bennett, D. S., and Giarman, N. J. (1964). Schedule of appearance of serotonin (5-HT) and associated enzymes in developing rat brain. *Pharmacologist*, **6**, 171.

Contractor, S. F. (1964). The estimation of 5-hydroxytryptamine in human blood. *Biochem. Pharmacol.*, **13**, 1351.

Dacie, J. V., and Lewis, S. M. (1963). *Practical Haematology*, 3rd ed., p. 61. Churchill, London.

Driscoll, S. G., and Hsia, D. Y.-Y. (1958). The development of enzyme systems during early infancy. *Pediatrics*, **22**, 785.

Epps, H. M. R. (1945). The development of amine oxidase activity by human tissues after birth. *Biochem. J.*, **39**, 37.

Giarman, N. J., Potter, L. T., and Day, M. (1960). Release of 5-hydroxytryptamine and histamine from neoplastic mast cells by alkaline tissue extracts. *Experientia (Basel)*, **16**, 492.

Grasso, E., Bianchi, P., Crosti, P. F., and Ermacora, E. (1961). The pathogenesis of haemorrhages in newborn babies. Experimental observations of the platelet serotonin. *Panminerva med.*, **3**, 49.

Hsia, D. Y.-Y., Nishimura, K., and Brenchley, Y. (1963). Mechanisms for the decrease of brain serotonin. *Nature (Lond.)*, **200**, 578.

Huang, I., Tannenbaum, S., and Hsia, D. Y.-Y. (1960). Development of 5-hydroxytryptophan decarboxylase activity in rat kidney. *ibid.*, **186**, 717.

Karki, N., Kuntzman, R., and Brodie, B. B. (1962). Storage synthesis, and metabolism of monoamines in the developing brain. *J. Neurochem.*, **9**, 53.

Kato, R. (1960). Serotonin content of rat brain in relation to sex and age. *ibid.*, **5**, 202.

Mitchell, R. G., and Cass, R. (1959). Histamine and 5-hydroxytryptamine in the blood of infants and children. *J. clin. Invest.*, **38**, 595.

Nachmias, V. T. (1960). Amine oxidase and 5-hydroxytryptamine in developing rat brain. *J. Neurochem.*, **6**, 99.

Pare, C. M. B., Sandler, M., and Stacey, R. S. (1960). 5-Hydroxyindoles in mental deficiency. *J. Neurol. Neurosurg. Psychiat.*, **23**, 341.

Pepeu, G., and Giarman, N. J. (1962). Serotonin in the developing mammal. *J. gen. Physiol.*, **45**, 575.

Rappallini, C., and Murtagh, J. J. (1962). La serotonina y el acido 5-hidroxindolacetico en el recien nacido. *Sem. méd.* (*B. Aires*), **121**, 1239.

Serra, U. (1958). L'eliminazione urinaria dell'acido 5-idroxindol acetico in bambini normali. *Fol. endocr.* (*Roma*), **11**, 410.

Shimizu, N., and Morikawa, N. (1959). Histochemical study of monoamine oxidase in the developing rat brain. *Nature* (*Lond.*), **184**, 650.

Smith, S. E., Stacey, R. S., and Young, I. M. (1962). 5-hydroxytryptamine and 5-hydroxytryptophan decarboxylase activity in the developing nervous system of rats and guinea-pigs. In *Proc. 1st int. pharmacol. Meeting*, vol. 8, *Pharmacological Analysis of Central Nervous System*, p. 101. Pergamon Press, Oxford.

Stacey, R. S. (1965). Clinical aspects of cerebral and extracerebral 5-hydroxytryptamine. In *5-Hydroxytryptamine and Related Indolealkylamines*. (*Heffter's Handbuch der experimentellen Pharmakologie*, *Vol.* 19, ed. V. Erspamer), p. 744. Springer, Berlin.

——, and Young, I. M. (1964). Concentration of 5-hydroxytryptamine in the small intestine and platelets of the developing guinea pig. *Biochem. Pharmacol.*, **13**, 129.

Toh, C. C. (1956). Release of 5-hydroxytryptamine (serotonin) and histamine from platelets by tissue extracts. *J. Physiol.* (*Lond.*), **133**, 402.

Zucker, M. B., Hellman, L., and Zumoff, B. (1964). Rapid disappearance of $C^{14}$-labeled serotonin from platelets in patients with carcinoid syndrome. *J. Lab. clin. Med.*, **63**, 137.

*Arch. Dis. Childh.*, 1965, **40**, 516.

# BIOCHEMICAL STATUS OF HEALTHY PREMATURE INFANTS IN THE FIRST 48 HOURS OF LIFE

BY

J. YU, W. W. PAYNE, A. IFEKWUNIGWE, and J. STEVENS

*From the Nuffield Neonatal Research Unit, Institute of Child Health, Hammersmith Hospital, London*

(RECEIVED FOR PUBLICATION DECEMBER 4, 1964)

The development of satisfactory ultramicro-methods of biochemical analysis has made it possible to carry out repeated estimations in newborn infants. At the same time, advances in knowledge of the biochemical aspects of disease processes, on which so much modern therapy is based, make it necessary to acquire a knowledge of normal values.

Serial studies of the blood chemistry of term infants have already been published (Acharya and Payne, 1965). In this paper we report similar studies on healthy premature infants in whom simultaneous measurements of a number of biochemical values were repeated at timed intervals over the first 48 hours of life.

## Material and Methods

**Routine Baby Care.** All the babies in this study were nursed in incubators heated to between 31·6 and 33·3° C., depending on birth weight. Extra oxygen was given even in the absence of respiratory distress in the very small premature babies, if breathing was very periodic or if the deep body temperature fell (Hill, 1961).

Most of the babies were starved for the first 12 hours of life. Feeding was begun with one feed of water followed subsequently by full strength 'pooled' expressed breast milk. Babies with birth weights below 2,000 g. were started on 4 ml. three-hourly and babies weighing from 2,000-2,500 g. on 6 ml. three-hourly, daily increments of 32 ml./kg. day being made. In general, babies weighing less than 1,700 g. were tube fed, the tube being repassed for each feed.

**Sampling Techniques.** The babies in this series were selected because of their normal clinical progress without reference to the biochemical findings.

The total number studied was 31, of whom 6 were less than 1,500 g. and 25 between 1,500 and 2,500 g. Of the latter group 9 were males and 16 were females.

Blood specimens were obtained from an umbilical arterial catheter, at 1, 3, 6, 9, 12, 18, 24, 36, and 48 hours. In many of the babies born in the hospital, specimens of cord blood were collected. As the cycle of collections began at varying times during the day, there was no fixed relation between sampling and feeding times; however, the caloric intake of the premature infants during the first 24 hours was negligible, being between 17-26 calories.

Whole blood, 1·3 ml., was collected into a heparinized 2 ml. syringe; 0·2 ml. was immediately placed into a fluoride tube for glucose, phosphate, and lactate determination and placed in a refrigerator; 0·1 ml. was taken for *p*H, $Pco_2$, and bicarbonate estimation, and the remainder was centrifuged. The plasma was removed at once and refrigerated at 4° C. until the remaining estimations could be performed. The catheter was kept patent with heparinized saline.

**Laboratory Methods.** *p*H was determined using an E.I.L. meter with replaceable electrode system. $Pco_2$ and standard bicarbonate were derived from a modified E.I.L. equilibration unit (Stevens and Lanning, 1964).

Sodium and potassium were estimated with an E.E.L. flame photometer; chloride by a titrimetric method using mercuric nitrate and ethanolic diphenyl carbazone; urea by Fearon's method using diacetyl monoxime; and phosphorus with the molybdic method of Fiske and Subbarow (1925). The amount of fluoride is critical because if the concentration exceeds 40 mg./100 ml. it interferes with the phosphorus estimation, yielding low results.

The estimation of blood glucose by a modification of the method of Marks (1959), using glucose oxidase, was performed within 12 hours of collection.

Calcium and magnesium were estimated by a flame photometer (Alcock and MacIntyre, 1960); lactate by the method of Barker and Summerson (1941); pentose by Bial's method (Green, Stoner, and Bielschowsky, 1949); and amino acids by the method of Danielson (1933). The biuret method of Kingsley (1939) and Gornall, Bardawill, and David (1949) was used for protein estimation.

## Results

The results are illustrated in Figs. 1-5.

***p*H.** *p*H levels in cord blood were low with a mean of 7·23 in premature infants of birth weight less than 1,500 g. They rose rapidly with the establishment of respiration to normal newborn levels.

Rather unexpectedly, the smaller premature infants attained acid-base balance more rapidly than the bigger infants. The smaller infants reached a *p*H 7·30 by 1 hour as compared with 3 hours in larger female babies and 4 hours in male babies. These larger male infants continued to lag behind and often needed 48 hours to reach a *p*H 7·40. Of the 6 premature babies who were less than 1,500 g. at birth, 5 reached a *p*H 7·40 by 12 hours.

**$Pco_2$.** Male babies greater than 1,500 g. had the highest $Pco_2$ of the population studied. The $Pco_2$ of these babies remained between 30 mm. and 40 mm. Hg during the first 48 hours of life. The mean values for infants less than 1,500 g. fell between that of the heavier males and the females who, with values from 25-35 mm.Hg, were lowest.

The trend in all these groups showed a slow fall from the maximum level seen in the cord blood.

**Standard Bicarbonate.** The standard bicarbonate is a simple and fair estimate of metabolic acidosis. In well, premature infants, standard bicarbonate levels confirmed the rapid establishment of acid-base homeostasis suggested by a study of *p*H levels. Up to the first 6 hours of life, the smaller premature infants again had slightly higher values than larger infants, reaching a standard bicarbonate value of 20 mEq/l. by 3 hours.

In infants over 1,500 g. the over-all mean value for the male during this period was greater than that for the female by 1·8 mEq/l.

The rise in bicarbonate lagged slightly behind the rise of blood *p*H.

**Lactic Acid.** There was a wide range in serum lactate levels, in general those babies with the more difficult deliveries having the higher values. The mean lactate level in the cord blood of infants greater than 1,500 g. was 33 mg./100 ml. and this fell quickly to 21 mg. at 3 hours, after which the fall was more gradual, not reaching 15 mg. until 48 hours.

During this time, the lactate levels of the smaller infants remained higher than those of the heavier ones.

**Sodium.** The range of cord sodium levels in premature babies was wide. Those babies under 1,500 g. tended to have higher levels (142-163 mEq/l.) which remained higher than the mean for those babies heavier than 1,500 g. throughout the 48 hours of study. The larger babies showed cord levels 116-142 with a mean of 132·4 mEq/l. No prenatal factors influencing the cord level could be found, nor did the cord levels seem to affect or indicate later progress.

Over the first 48 hours, the serum sodium slowly rose in all babies so that at 48 hours it was 5·0-5·5 mEq/l. higher than the lowest level reached at 1-3 hours.

**Potassium.** Serum potassium levels in cord blood were high by adult standards, ranging from 5·0-10·2 mEq/l. By 1 hour the level had fallen, after which one-half of the babies showed a gradual and continuous fall over the next 48 hours, whereas in the remainder the serum $K^+$ again rose slowly to reach a maximum at 18-36 hours.

After 24 hours the mean values for the lower weight group were above those for the higher, being 5·6 and 5·8 mEq/l. at 24 and 36 hours as compared with 4·6 and 4·4 in the heavier group.

**Chloride.** The serum chloride values in premature infants were within the normal adult range of 96-106 mEq/l. throughout the 48-hour period of study. In general, there was a gradual rise of 2-8 mEq/l. in individual cases over this time. The mean values for small premature infants remained below those for infants heavier than 1,500 g. at birth.

There was no correlation between chloride levels and PCV, nor between the chloride concentration and the clinical state of the baby.

**Serum Calcium.** Calcium levels in the cord blood of premature infants were high, mean 5·3 mEq/l. The calcium levels then fell to a minimum of 4·3 mEq/l. at 18-24 hours before rising again. The smaller premature infants of less than 1,500 g. birth weight showed a similar trend, but their mean values were lower than those of heavier babies. In the smaller weight group, many individual low values such as 3·2-3·5 mEq/l. were seen in apparently well and asymptomatic babies.

**Serum Magnesium.** The trends in serum magnesium levels were very similar to those of serum calcium, with a high cord level, a subsequent fall, and then recovery. The minimum levels seemed somewhat earlier, however, 12-18 hours. The smaller premature infants had lower magnesium levels than the heavier ones in the first 24 hours. At 12-18 hours, the mean was 1·3 mEq/l. as compared with 1·5 in the babies over 1,500 g., and at 48 hours 1·8 mEq/l., compared with 1·6.

**Blood Inorganic Phosphate.** There was a wide range in the inorganic phosphate levels of premature infants from 3·0-7·4 mg./100 ml. These levels did not correlate with the weights of the babies, or with any known factors operating at the time of birth. In

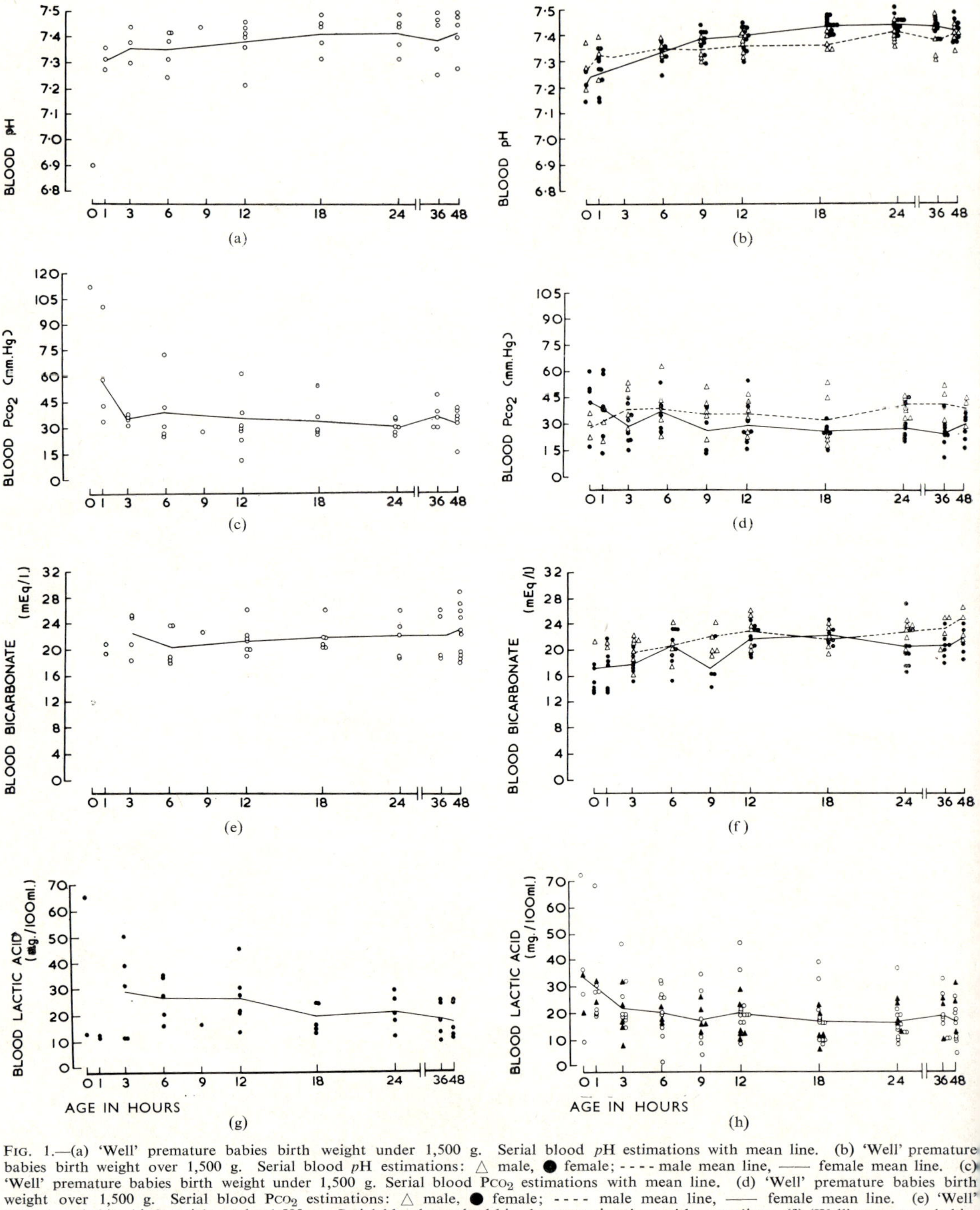


FIG. 1.—(a) 'Well' premature babies birth weight under 1,500 g. Serial blood *p*H estimations with mean line. (b) 'Well' premature babies birth weight over 1,500 g. Serial blood *p*H estimations: △ male, ● female; - - - - male mean line, —— female mean line. (c) 'Well' premature babies birth weight under 1,500 g. Serial blood $Pco_2$ estimations with mean line. (d) 'Well' premature babies birth weight over 1,500 g. Serial blood $Pco_2$ estimations: △ male, ● female; - - - - male mean line, —— female mean line. (e) 'Well' premature babies birth weight under 1,500 g. Serial blood standard bicarbonate estimations with mean line. (f) 'Well' premature babies birth weight over 1,500 g. Serial blood standard bicarbonate estimations: △ male, ● female; - - - - male mean line, —— female mean line. (g) 'Well' premature babies birth weight under 1,500 g. Serial blood lactic acid estimations with mean line. (h) 'Well' premature babies birth weight over 1,500 g. Serial blood lactic acid estmations: ▲ male, ○ female; with mean line of both.

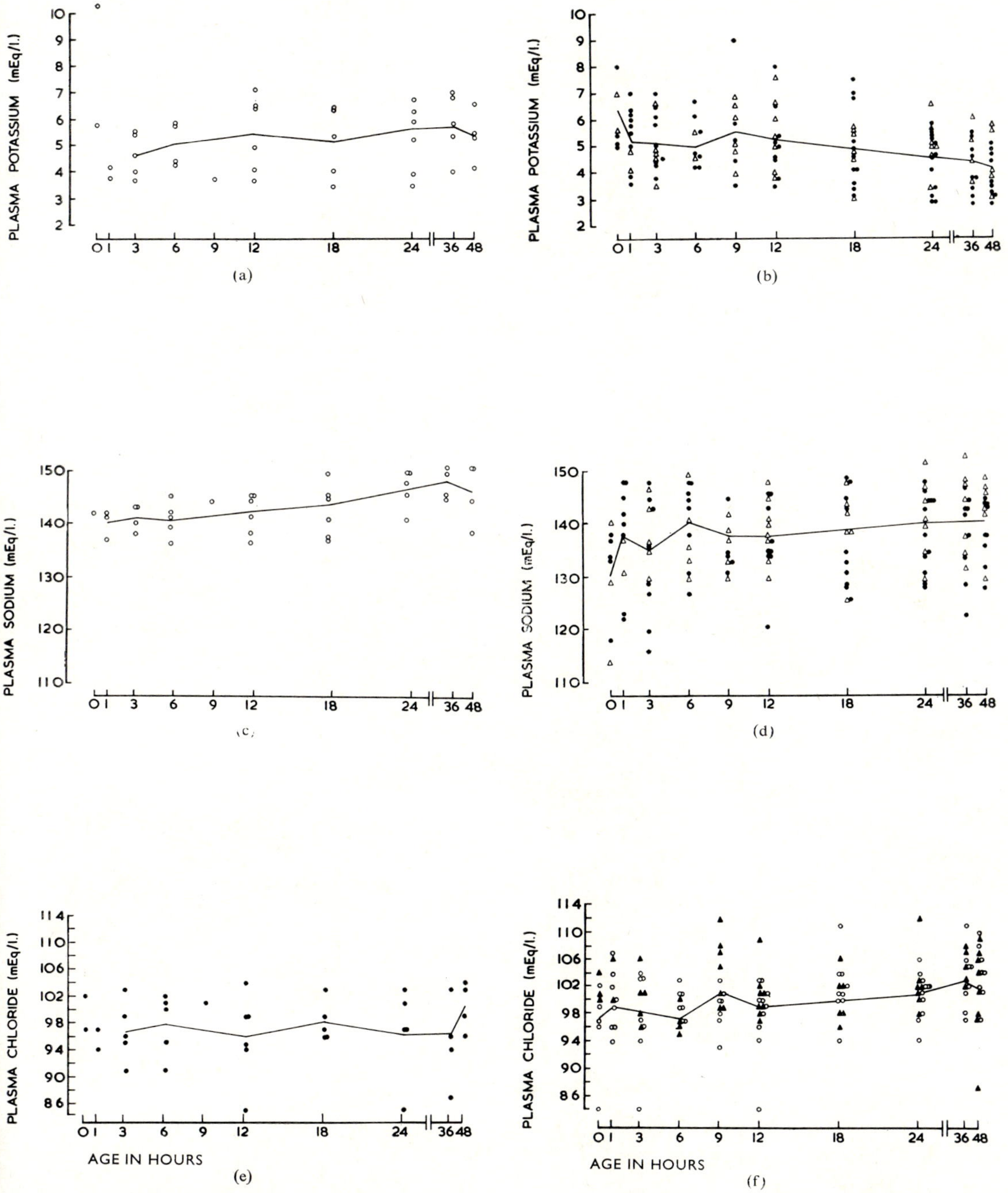


FIG. 2.—(a) 'Well' premature babies birth weight under 1,500 g. Serial plasma potassium estimations with mean line. (b) 'Well' premature babies birth weight over 1,500 g. Serial plasma potassium estimations: △ male, ● female; with mean line of male and female. (c) 'Well' premature babies birth weight under 1,500 g. Serial plasma sodium estimations with mean line. (d) 'Well' premature babies birth weight over 1,500 g. Serial plasma sodium estimations: △ male, ● female; with mean line of male and female. (e) 'Well' premature babies birth weight under 1,500 g. Serial plasma chloride estimations with mean line. (f) 'Well' premature babies birth weight over 1,500 g. Serial plasma chloride estimations: ▲ male, ○ female; with mean line of both.

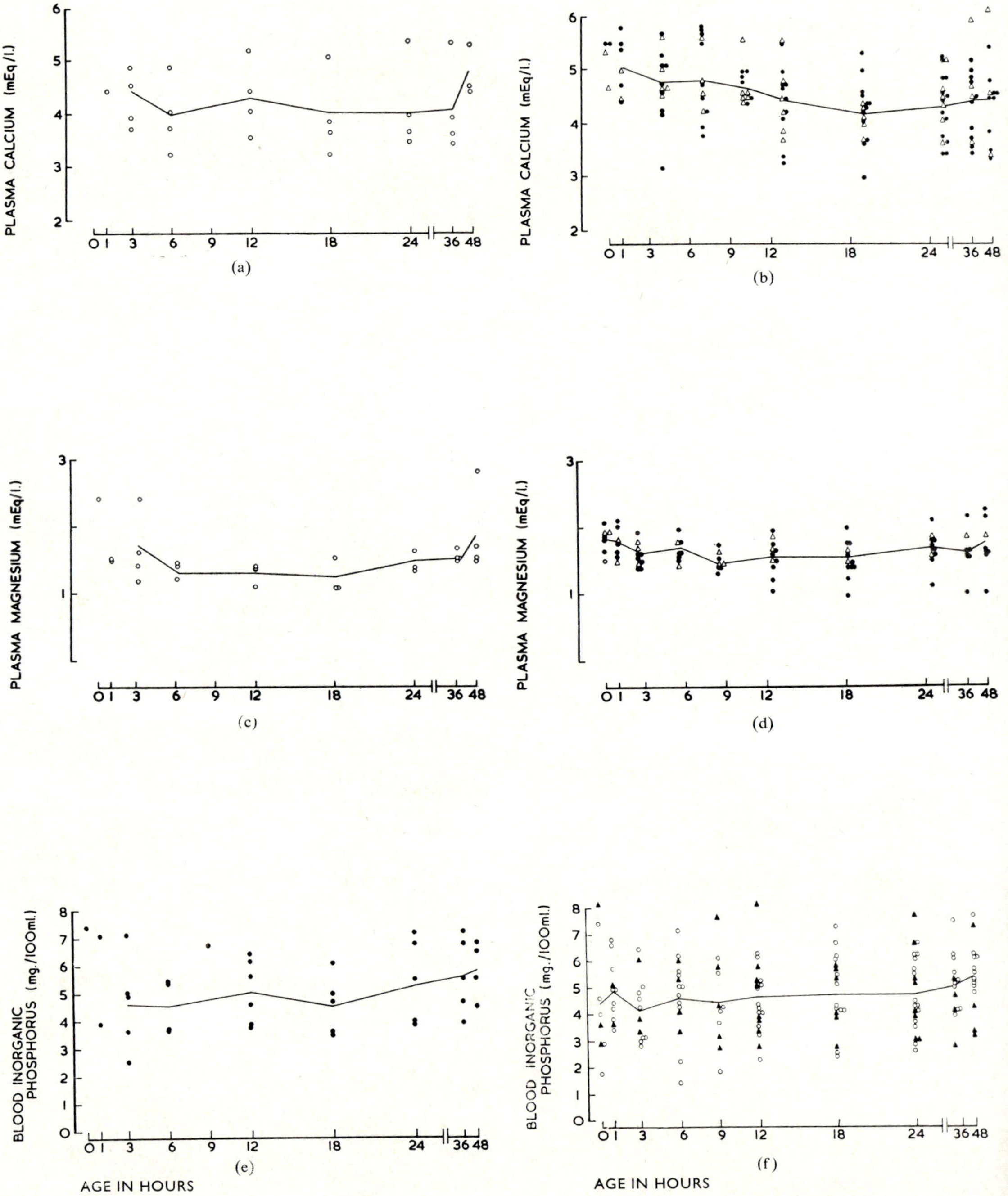


FIG. 3.—(a) 'Well' premature babies birth weight under 1,500 g. Serial plasma calcium estimations with mean line. (b) 'Well' premature babies birth weight over 1,500 g. Serial plasma calcium estimations: △ male, ● female; with mean line of male and female. (c) 'Well' premature babies birth weight under 1,500 g. Serial plasma magnesium estimations with mean line. (d) 'Well' premature babies birth weight over 1,500 g. Serial plasma magnesium estimations: △ male, ● female; with mean line of male and female. (e) 'Well' premature babies birth weight under 1,500 g. Serial blood inorganic phosphorus estimations with mean line. (f) 'Well' premature babies birth weight over 1,500 g. Serial blood inorganic phosphorus estimations: ▲ male, ○ female; with mean line of both.

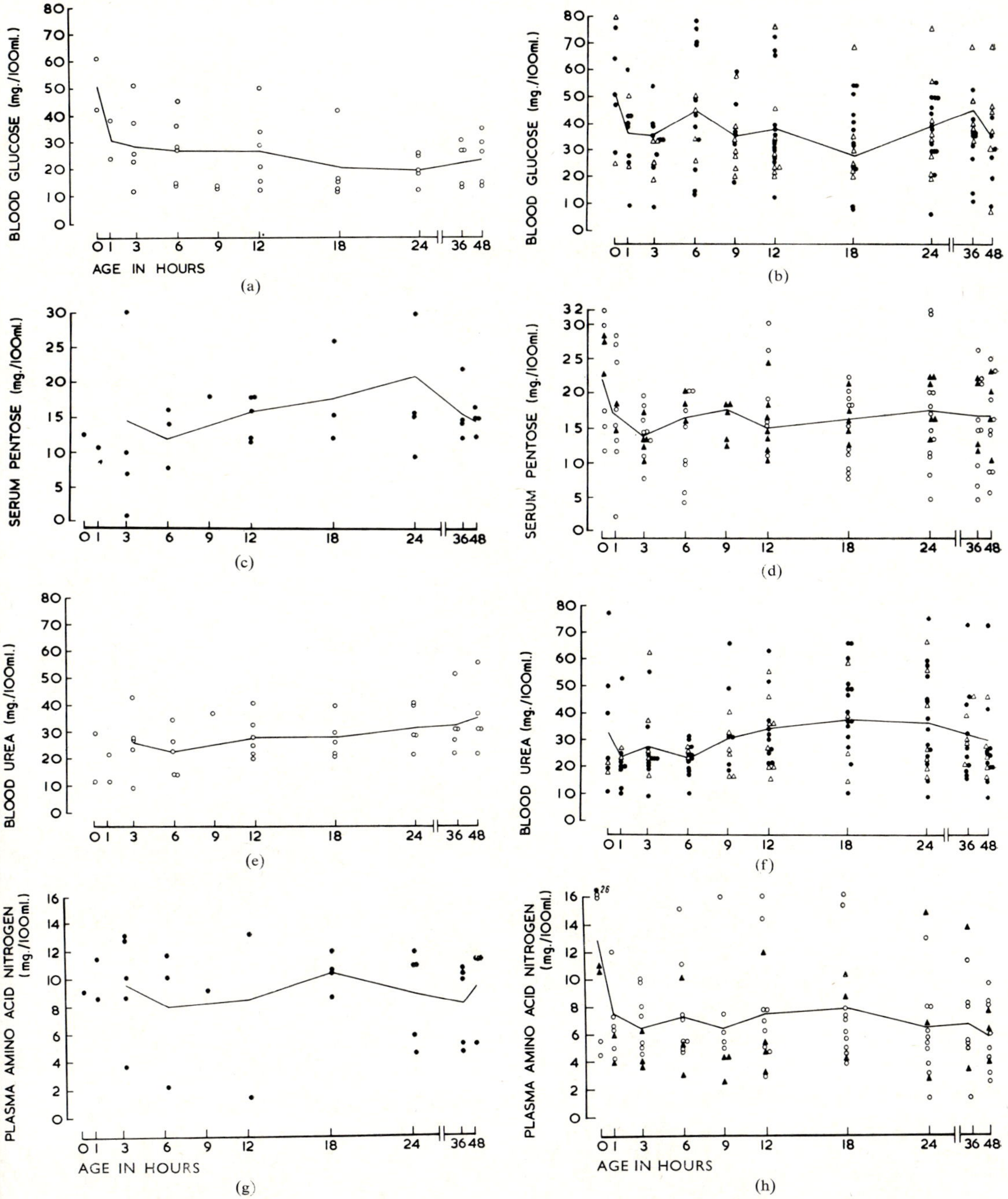


FIG. 4.—(a) 'Well' premature babies birth weight under 1,500 g. Serial blood glucose estimations with mean line. (b) 'Well' premature babies birth weight over 1,500 g. Serial blood glucose estimations: △ male, ● female; with mean line of male and female. (c) 'Well' premature babies birth weight under 1,500 g. Serial serum pentose estimations with mean line. (d) 'Well' premature babies birth weight over 1,500 g. Serial serum pentose estimations: ▲ male, ○ female; with mean line of both. (e) 'Well' premature babies birth weight under 1,500 g. Serial blood urea estimations with mean line. (f) 'Well' premature babies birth weight over 1,500 g. Serial blood urea estimations: △ male, ● female; with mean line of male and female. (g) 'Well' premature babies birth weight under 1,500 g. Serial plasma amino acid nitrogen estimations with mean line. (h) 'Well' premature babies birth weight over 1,500 g. Serial plasma amino acid nitrogen estimations: ▲ male, ○ female; with mean line of both.

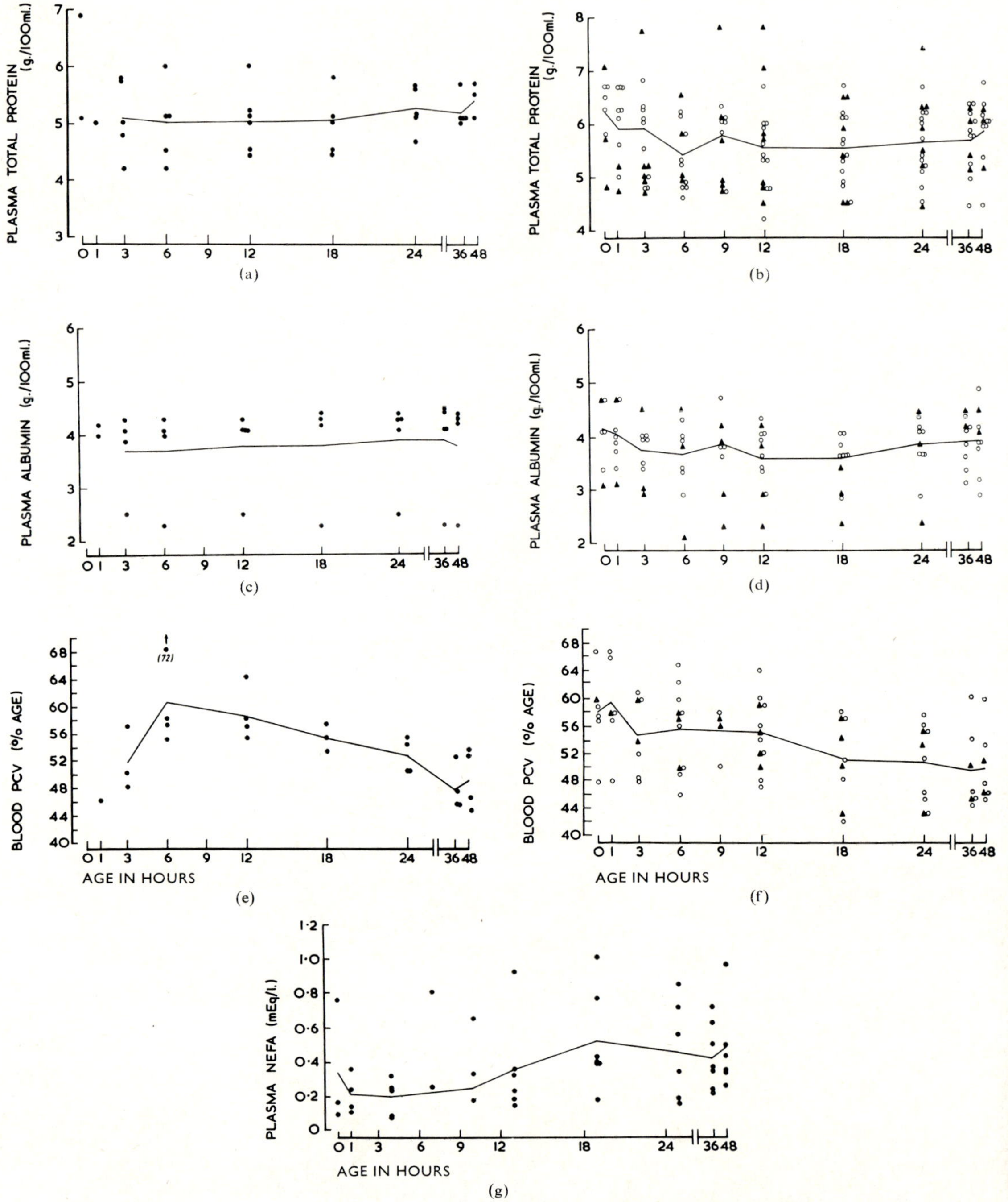


FIG. 5.—(a) 'Well' premature babies birth weight under 1,500 g. Serial total protein estimations with mean line. (b) 'Well' premature babies birth weight over 1,500 g. Serial total protein estimations: ▲ male, ○ female; with mean line of both. (c) 'Well' premature babies birth weight under 1,500 g. Serial plasma albumin estimations with mean line. (d) 'Well' premature babies birth weight over 1,500 g. Serial plasma albumin estimations: ▲ male, ○ female; with mean line of both. (e) 'Well' premature babies birth weight under 1,500 g. Serial packed cell volume estimations with mean line. (f) 'Well' premature babies birth weight over 1,500 g. Serial packed cell volume estimations: ▲ male, ○ female; with mean line of both. (g) 'Well' premature babies. Serial non-esterified fatty acid estimations with mean line.

general there was an upward trend during the period of study, so that at 48 hours the serum phosphate was higher than at 24 hours. This peak coincided with the establishment of adequate feeding.

Individual babies maintained their phosphate levels within a narrow range of 1-2 mg./100 ml. over the first 2 days.

**Glucose.** Low glucose levels by adult standards have often been demonstrated in well newborn infants. In our small group of well premature infants weighing less than 1,500 g. every infant had a blood glucose level of 20 mg./100 ml. or less at some time during the first 48 hours. These levels usually reached their lowest values from 24-48 hours.

The larger premature infants had significantly higher glucose levels throughout the study period, the means falling between 35 and 45 mg./100 ml. A fall during the second 24-hour period was not seen in these bigger infants.

**Urea.** Cord blood urea values were within the normal adult range but dropped within the first 6 hours of life. There was then a gradual rise over the next 36-48 hours after which a further fall occurred. This occurred at about 24 hours in babies larger than 1,500 g. but at 48 hours in smaller ones. The normal range over the 48 hours was 10-40 mg./100 ml., with considerable variation from baby to baby. The trends in urea were preceded by similar trends in amino acid values.

**Amino Acid Nitrogen.** The mean values for amino acid nitrogen were higher in the smaller premature infants than in the heavier ones, the range being 7·9-10·2 mg./100 ml. as compared with 5·4-7·5 mg./100 ml. Individual values up to 16·2 mg./100 ml. were seen in well infants.

As with urea values, there was a fall during the first 3-6 hours, then a gradual rise up to 18 hours, then a further fall. These trends preceded the similar changes seen in the blood urea levels.

**Pentose.** There was a wide range in pentose levels in newborn infants from 2 to 43 mg./100 ml., mean values varying from 13·7 to 22·8 mg./100 ml. In the small number studied, there was no obvious difference between the small and large premature infants. The pentose range in individual babies tended to remain within narrow limits.

**Serum Albumin and Globulin.** The serum albumin did not vary with birth weight, the means over the first 48 hours ranging from 4·1 to 3·5 g./100 ml. Babies heavier than 1,500 g. showed a transient fall in albumin levels at 12-18 hours.

A similar fall was noted in the levels of total globulins, but here there was a difference in the two weight groups; the mean cord level in babies less than 1,500 g. was 1·4 g./100 ml. while that of the heavier babies was 2·0 g.

## Discussion

There are no strictly comparable published reports giving the results of serial multiple biochemical estimations on the premature newborn infant over the first 48 hours of life. Our results show that in individual babies a wide range of values may be compatible with a normal clinical progress, but that the levels of each substance studied generally follow a trend over the 48 hours which is common to a particular group of infants. Many babies, particularly those less than 1,500 g., may have biochemical values generally regarded as pathological without showing any symptoms. Whether these values are within the 'physiological range', or whether small infants lack the ability to react to them, one cannot say. The biochemical changes seen in symptomatic newborn babies will be reported shortly.

**Acid-base Balance.** The immediate problems of extrauterine survival concern respiration and acid-base balance. In the normal adult, acid-base homeostasis is achieved by renal conservation of base with ammonia production, by various buffer systems, and by elimination of carbon dioxide from the lungs. During the first hours of life, renal mechanisms in newborn infants are functioning poorly and at capacity (McCance and von Finck, 1947) and so play little part in acid-base balance.

The trend of the mean *p*H in babies of less than 1,500 g. rises more rapidly than that of heavier babies during the first 6-12 hours of life. Almost all the smaller babies show periodic breathing during this time, which has been shown to produce an overall greater ventilation than regular respiration; premature infants with periodic breathing have also been shown to have significantly higher *p*H values than those with regular breathing (Chernick, Heldrich, and Avery, 1964); and over this period the fall in $Pco_2$ is steeper in smaller babies. Of the three groups studied here, it is interesting to note that the male infants heavier than 1,500 g. achieve acid-base balance significantly later than females of corresponding weight.

The standard bicarbonate of premature infants stabilizes at a lower level than normal term infants.

The periodic breathing and the resultant hyperventilation may represent attempts by the immature baby to maintain adequate oxygenation in the face of possible diffusion deficiencies (Stahlman, 1957), ventilatory deficiencies, and vascular shunts (James and Burnard, 1961). Such a relative hypoxia would explain the higher lactate levels and lower standard bicarbonate levels found in the smaller premature infants. The oxygen tension of well premature infants is about 60-80 mm.Hg (J. M. Gupta, 1964, personal communication) and at the lower limits approaches the critical level for lactate production (Huckabee, 1958).

**The Parathyroid and Homeostasis.** Hormones from the parathyroid have long been known to control calcium and phosphorus metabolism, but their importance in magnesium homeostasis has only recently been investigated (MacIntyre, 1963; MacIntyre, Boss, and Troughton, 1963).

The early trends in serum calcium have been described in newborn term infants by Acharya and Payne (1965) and similar findings have been found in this study. The magnesium values reported are, we believe, the first serial estimations in premature infants. Our levels are generally higher than those of other authors using colorimetric methods, but lie largely within the adult limits defined by Alcock and MacIntyre (1960) using the same spectrophotometric method.

Many hypotheses have been suggested to explain the fall in serum calcium and magnesium after the first 24 hours of life, including that of parathyroid hypofunction. A recent report of neonatal fits associated with hypomagnesaemia (Davis, Harvey, and Yu, 1965) presents evidence to suggest that there is a transient deficiency in parathyroid activity during the first days of life and that this may result in low levels of calcium and magnesium as found. This deficiency may be demonstrated by the introduction of cows' milk feedings with its added phosphate load.

In this small series, there was no correlation between calcium and phosphorus levels and the values for the two weight groups did not differ significantly. In both groups the level of inorganic phosphorus rose slowly during the 48 hours, a finding already reported by Bruck and Weintraub (1955). This trend probably results from the dietary phosphate load and the diminished parathyroid activity.

Perhaps the most significant feature shown by these routine studies is that low levels of calcium, e.g. 3·2 mEq/l. and magnesium 1·0 mEq/l., may exist in babies who are well and asymptomatic and that such apparently pathological levels may not be the cause of the symptoms that are sometimes attributed to an isolated low reading.

**The Electrolytes and Body Water.** In premature infants there is a wide range of values for serum sodium and potassium levels. The higher levels are seen in the smaller premature infants and in those exposed to birth stress. The serum sodium level tends to rise slowly over the first 48 hours, presumably as a result of dehydration. The heavier infants over this time show a slow fall in serum potassium from levels that are high by adult standards. These early high levels may exist as a consequence of the acidaemia associated with birth (James, 1960) and glycolysis, their subsequent fall indicating the achievement of acid-base balance and a homeostatic endeavour to maintain ionic balance with sodium.

There is a positive correlation between serum sodium and chloride levels as in adults. The levels of sodium and chloride do not correlate with the changes in packed cell volumes in the small sample obtained, suggesting that haemo-concentration and dilution are occurring independently of changes in the concentration of the extracellular fluid. Any movements between the intra- and extracellular fluids must depend on the cellular sodium and potassium 'pumps'. Little is known about the control of ionic movement in extra renal tissue, but it is likely that steroids influence other cell membranes in addition to those of the nephron cells. Since preliminary results in babies suggest that the adrenal cortex can respond to stress with an increased production of cortisol (W. W. Payne, 1964, unpublished data), it is conceivable that changes in serum electrolytes in well premature infants may be partly steroid dependent.

Another major factor in the distribution of extracellular fluid is capillary permeability. The capillary walls of newly born premature babies leak protein (Usher, 1961), and this movement into tissue fluids may contribute to the transient fall of total serum proteins.

**Energy and Substrates.** Hypoglucosaemia and its clinical correlates have received much attention recently, and serial values for blood glucose in the newborn are well documented. The trends over the first 24 hours of life are similar in our findings to those of other authors (Baens, Lundeen, and Cornblath, 1963; Ward, 1953) with a rapid fall from cord levels of over 50 mg./100 ml. to levels below 35 mg., subsequently. Of our small group of clinically normal babies weighing less than 1,500 g. at birth, all had blood glucose levels less than 20 mg./100 ml. at some time during the first 24 hours of life. Such levels may be in part a reflection of the diminished liver glycogen stores that are found in extremely immature infants (Shelley, 1964): only a carefully designed long-term project will show whether these babies are in fact 'well'.

The high amino acid nitrogen values seen in these small babies may result from the need to revert to gluconeogenesis as an energy source until adequate feeding is established. As one might expect if there were protein katabolism, the rise in blood urea lags slightly behind the rise in amino acid nitrogen. After 24 hours the urea level in babies greater than 1,500 g. begins to fall, while that of the smaller babies continues to rise slowly. It is likely that in the second 24 hours of life babies less than 1,500 g. are still receiving inadequate calories by mouth and with smaller initial food stores need to utilize body protein as an energy source.

Insufficient data had been collected to comment on fat metabolism, the last 7 infants only having been studied. From the scanty data, it appears that the non-esterified fatty acid (NEFA) levels in newborn infants lie in the adult range. Of the 7 infants, 2 were less than 1,500 g. at birth and their NEFA levels at 48 hours were 0·38 and 0·27 mEq/l. as compared with a range 0·46-1·15 in the 5 heavier infants. The general trend upwards in NEFA levels is in agreement with the values reported by Van Duyne and Havel (1959) for NEFA levels in normal mature newborn infants.

## Summary

Serial chemistry over the first 48 hours of life is reported in 31 premature infants. The pattern of changes in individual parameters of sodium, potassium, chloride, *p*H, $Pco_2$, bicarbonate, glucose, pentose, lactate, urea, amino acids, magnesium, calcium, phosphorus, non-esterified fatty acid, and proteins is reported.

Small premature infants achieve acid-base balance following the acidaemia of birth with remarkable rapidity. Other homeostatic mechanisms are, however, slower to function, as is shown by the relative hypocalcaemia and hypomagnesaemia seen at 18-24 hours.

The low glucose levels and the evidence of heightened gluconeogenesis suggest a lack of stored glycogen and fat reserves.

The absence of symptoms in the presence of high potassium, low sugar, low calcium, and low magnesium levels is noted as a characteristic of the newborn and particularly the premature infant.

We would like to thank the Nuffield Foundation and the Sir William Coxen Trust for providing the facilities for this work, Professor J. P. M. Tizard, Dr. J. A. Davis, and the late Dr. M. J. R. Dawkins for their help in the preparation of this paper, and Professor J. P. M. Tizard and Dr. J. A. Davis for access to their patients. We are specially indebted to the Ward Sisters, M. S. Castle, S.R.N., M. Pinder, S.R.N., and J. James, S.R.N., for their great help in the handling of the children.

A part of this was incorporated in a thesis for M. D. London by A.I.

### References

Acharya, P. T., and Payne, W. W. (1965). Blood chemistry of normal full-term infants in the first 48 hours of life. *Arch. Dis. Childh.*, **40**, 430.

Alcock, N., and MacIntyre, I. (1960). Interrelation of calcium and magnesium absorption. *Biochem. J.*, **76**, 19P.

Baens, G. S., Lundeen, E., and Cornblath, M. (1963). Studies of carbohydrate metabolism in the newborn infant. VI. Levels of glucose in blood in premature infants. *Pediatrics*, **31**, 580.

Barker, S. B., and Summerson, W. H. (1941). The colorimetric determination of lactic acid in biological material. *J. biol. Chem.*, **138**, 535.

Bruck, E., and Weintraub, D. H. (1955). Serum calcium and phosphorus in premature and full-term infants. *Amer. J. Dis. Child.*, **90**, 653.

Chernick, V., Heldrich, F., and Avery, M. E. (1964). Periodic breathing of premature infants. *J. Pediat.*, **64**, 330.

Danielson, I. S. (1933). Amino acid nitrogen in blood and its determination. *J. biol. Chem.*, **101**, 505.

Davis, J. A., Harvey, D. R., and Yu, J. S. (1965). Neonatal fits associated with hypomagnesaemia. *Arch. Dis. Childh.*, **40**, 286.

Fiske, C. H., and Subbarow, Y. (1925). The colorimetric determination of phosphorus. *J. biol. Chem.*, **66**, 375.

Gornall, A. G., Bardawill, C. J., and David, M. M. (1949). Determination of serum proteins by means of the biuret reaction. *ibid.*, **177**, 751.

Green, H. N., Stoner, H. B., and Bielschowsky, M. (1949). The effect of trauma on the pentose content of the plasma in animals. *J. Path. Bact.*, **61**, 101.

Hill, J. R. (1961). The physics and physiology of the development of homoeothermy. In *Ciba Foundation Symposium on Somatic Stability in the Newly Born*, ed. G. E. W. Wolstenholme and M. O'Connor, p. 156. Churchill, London.

Huckabee, W. E. (1958). Relationships of pyruvate and lactate during anaerobic metabolism. III. Effect of breathing low-oxygen gases. *J. clin. Invest.*, **37**, 264.

James, L. S. (1960). Acidosis of the newborn and its relation to birth asphyxia. *Acta paediat.* (*Uppsala*), **49**, Suppl. 122, 17.

——, and Burnard, E. (1961). Biochemical changes occurring during asphyxia at birth and some effects on the heart. In *Ciba Foundation Symposium on Somatic Stability in the Newly Born*, ed. G. E. W. Wolstenholme and M. O'Connor, p. 75. Churchill, London.

Kingsley, G. R. (1939). The determination of serum total protein, albumin, and globulin by the biuret reaction. *J. biol. Chem.*, **131**, 197.

McCance, R. A., and von Finck, M. A. (1947). The titratable acidity, *p*H, ammonia and phosphates in the urines of very young infants. *Arch. Dis. Childh.*, **22**, 200.

MacIntyre, I. (1963). Magnesium metabolism. In *Sci. Basis Med. Ann. Rev.*, p. 216.

——, Boss, S., and Troughton, V. A. (1963). Parathyroid hormone and magnesium homoeostasis. *Nature* (*Lond.*), **198**, 1058.

Marks, V. (1959). An improved glucose-oxidase method for determining blood, C.S.F. and urine glucose levels. *Clin. chim. Acta*, **4**, 395.

Shelley, H. J. (1964). Carbohydrate reserves in the newborn infant. *Brit. med. J.*, **1**, 273.

Stahlman, M. T. (1957). Pulmonary ventilation and diffusion in the human newborn infant. *J. clin. Invest.*, **36**, 1081.

Stevens, J. F., and Lanning, K. (1964). Micro $Pco_2$ equilibration unit. *Lancet*, **2**, 447.

Usher, R. H. (1961). The metabolic changes in respiratory distress syndrome of prematurity seen as a failure of somatic compensations for asphyxia. In *Ciba Foundation Symposium on Somatic Stability of the Newly Born*, ed. G. E. W. Wolstenhome and M. O'Connor. Churchill, London.

Van Duyne, C. M., and Havel, R. J. (1959). Plasma unesterified fatty acid concentration in fetal and neonatal life. *Proc. Soc. exp. Biol.* (*N.Y.*), **102**, 599.

Ward, O. C. (1953). Blood sugar studies in premature babies. *Arch. Dis. Childh.*, **28**, 194.

*Arch. Dis. Childh.*, 1965, **40**, 526.

# THE JEJUNAL MUCOSA IN KWASHIORKOR*

BY

DAVID BURMAN
*From Derbyshire Children's Hospital, Derby*

(RECEIVED FOR PUBLICATION DECEMBER 21, 1964)

The 'tissue paper' intestine of patients with severe kwashiorkor is well known to tropical pathologists and it is usually considered to involve all coats of the intestinal wall. However, histological study of the small gut mucosa in man has been very difficult until the advent of peroral biopsy (Shiner, 1956). This paper reports a series of 17 infants with kwashiorkor whose jejunal mucosa was studied after peroral biopsy.

## Material and Methods

The patients studied were all in the Children's Ward of King George VI Hospital, Nairobi, in February and March 1963. They were all under the age of 3 years and all presented with the clinical picture of kwashiorkor as described by Trowell, Davies, and Dean (1954a). They all had marked wasting, oedema, dyspigmentation of the hair, and the typical dermatosis.

Jejunal biopsies were performed by a technique already described (Burman, 1963) using an adult Crosby capsule (Crosby and Kugler, 1957). The specimens were examined with the dissecting microscope before sections were cut. The sections were stained with haematoxylin and eosin and by the periodic acid-Schiff (PAS) technique.

All haematological investigations were carried out on venous samples using sequestrene as the anticoagulant. The haemoglobin content was measured by the cyan-methaemoglobin method and the packed cell volume by the Hawksley microhaematocrit.

The serum folate was measured as *L. casei* activity using the technique of Baker, Herbert, Frank, Pasher, Hutner, Wasserman, and Sobotka (1959) as modified by Chanarin and Berry (1964). The total serum proteins and the serum globulin were estimated with an auto-analyser using the methods of Stevens (1959) and Glenn (1965), respectively. The sera for these estimations were separated as soon as possible and kept in a deep freeze, or in $CO_2$ snow, until the estimations were performed at St. Mary's Hospital.

## Results

Studies were carried out on 17 patients. Their ages, sex, weight, serum proteins, haematological

* This work was undertaken while holding a Heinz Fellowship administered by the British Paediatric Association and the Nuffield Foundation.

DETAILS OF 17

| Case No. | Sex | Age (mth.) | Weight (kg.) | Serum Proteins (g./100 ml.) | | Haemo-globin (g./100 ml.) | PCV (%) | MCHC (%) | Bone-marrow | Serum Folate (mμg./ml.) | As… Co… |
|---|---|---|---|---|---|---|---|---|---|---|---|
| | | | | Total | Albumin | | | | | | |
| 1 | M | 36 | 9·5 | 4·3 | 1·7 | 7·0 | 24·5 | 28·6 | NB | 25·0 | |
| 2 | F | 24 | 6·4 | 3·7 | 1·6 | 8·0 | 32 | 25 | NB | 6·0 | Dy… |
| 3 | F | 12 | 4·08 | 5·6 | 2·8 | 8·0 | 29·5 | 27·1 | NB | 2·5 | M… |
| 4 | F | 18 | 6·8 | 4·1 | 2·2 | 9·4 | 33 | 28·5 | NB | 8·0 | |
| 5 | M | 12 | 5·89 | 4·7 | 2·7 | 5·3 | 18 | 29·4 | MB | 13·5 | Dy… |
| 6 | M | 18 | 6·8 | 7·8 | 3·8 | 7·6 | 29·5 | 25·8 | MB | 12·5 | |
| 7 | M | 30 | 8·6 | 6·4 | 2·0 | 9·7 | 32·5 | 29·8 | NB | 7·5 | M… |
| 8 | F | 30 | 6·8 | 3·8 | 1·5 | 9·5 | 33·5 | 28·4 | NB | 6·5 | |
| 9 | M | 12 | 7·7 | 3·2 | 1·6 | 10·3 | 36·5 | 28·2 | NB | 4·0 | |
| 10 | F | 13 | 6·8 | 5·4 | 3·0 | 6·4 | 22·5 | 28·4 | NB | 10·0 | |
| 11 | F | 18 | 7·7 | 6·2 | 3·6 | 10·5 | 38·0 | 27·6 | — | 14·5 | |
| 12 | M | 24 | 10·9 | 3·7 | 1·9 | 11·0 | 40·0 | 27·5 | NB | 6·0 | |
| 13 | M | 18 | 6·4 | 4·7 | 2·6 | 9·7 | 33·0 | 29·4 | — | 7·5 | |
| 14 | F | 13 | 5·9 | 4·6 | 2·7 | 10·3 | 34 | 30·3 | NB | 6·0 | M… |
| 15 | F | 18 | 7·3 | 5·5 | 3·1 | 3·0 | 13 | 22·1 | — | 14·5 | M… |
| 16 | F | 12 | 6·8 | 5·7 | 3·4 | 8·0 | 30 | 26·7 | — | 7·5 | |
| 17 | M | 14 | 6·4 | 2·8 | 1·0 | 7·5 | 27 | 27 | NB | 30·0 | |

NB, normoblastic; MB, m…

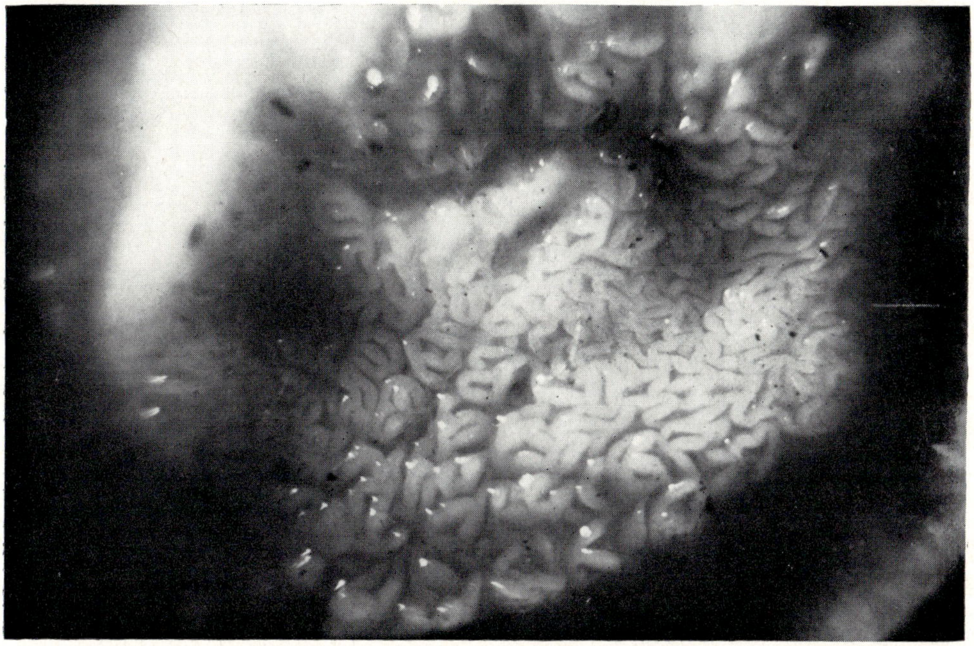

FIG. 1.—The dissecting microscope appearances of Case 3 showing ridges. (× 13.)

findings, and findings in the jejunal mucosa are given in Table 1. The dissecting microscope appearances are classified by a system whereby ++++ are distributed between ridges, leaves, and fingers after inspection of the whole specimen. Fingers are defined as projections where the cross-section is roughly circular. Ridges are projections where the largest cross-sectional diameter is at least 10 times the smallest (Baker, Mathan, and Cherian, 1963), and leaves lie between these two. The method is only semi-quantitative and Fig. 1 shows the dissecting microscope appearances of Case 3. The same technique was applied to 15 specimens obtained from infants aged 1 to 3 years who were investigated for a variety of gastro-intestinal symptoms in England. None of these infants had coeliac disease, fibrocystic disease of the pancreas, dysentery, or other disease of the small gut, and, for the purpose of this paper, they

ASHIORKOR

| Jejunal Mucosa | | | | | | | Comment |
|---|---|---|---|---|---|---|---|
| Dissecting Microscope | | | Histology | | | | |
| s | Leaves | Fingers | Villi | Cellular Infiltration of Substantia Propria | Brush Border | Epithelial Cells | |
| + | | | B | + + + | N | I | |
| | + + + + | | N | + + + | N | N | |
| + | | | N | + + + | N | I | |
| | + + | | N | + + + | N | I | |
| + | | | N | + + + | N | I | |
| + | | | N | + + | N | N | Lymphoid follicle |
| | + | + | B | + + + | N | N | Some villi tongue shaped |
| | + + + + | | B | + + + + | N | I | |
| | + | + | B | + + + | N | I | |
| + | | | B | + + + + | N | I | |
| | + + | | N | + + + | N | I | |
| + | | | N | + + + | N | I | Lymphoid follicle |
| | + + + + | | B | + + + + | N | I | |
| | + + + + | | B | + + + | N | I | |
| + | | | N | + + + | N | N | |
| | + + + + | | B | + + + | N | I | |
| + | | | N | + + + + | N | I | |

N, normal; I, irregular.

TABLE 2

DISSECTING MICROSCOPE APPEARANCES OF JEJUNAL MUCOSA IN PATIENTS WITH KWASHIORKOR COMPARED WITH NORMAL CHILDREN

| | No. of Patients | Villous Type (%) | | |
|---|---|---|---|---|
| | | Ridges | Leaves | Fingers |
| Normal | 15 | 5 | 48 | 47 |
| Kwashiorkor | 17 | 59 | 38 | 3 |

TABLE 3

CELLULAR INFILTRATION OF SUBSTANTIA PROPRIA OF JEJUNAL MUCOSA IN PATIENTS WITH KWASHIORKOR COMPARED WITH NORMAL CHILDREN

| | Degree of Cellular Infiltration | | | | Total |
|---|---|---|---|---|---|
| | + | ++ | +++ | ++++ | |
| No. normal | 5 | 14 | 1 | | 20 |
| No. with kwashiorkor | | 1 | 12 | 4 | 17 |

are considered to be normal. Table 2 compares the dissecting microscope appearances of these two groups of children, and it can be seen that leaves are common in both groups, but fingers are found in most 'normal' children and are very uncommon in infants with kwashiorkor. Ridges are the predominant villous type in kwashiorkor but are distinctly rare in the English children.

In the sections of the mucosa, the villi were either tall and slender, similar to those normally found, or were broader than usual (Fig. 2). The characteristic type of villus seen in each section is tabulated in Table 1. Broad villi were predominant in 8 specimens but there was no correlation with the dissecting microscope appearances. The width of the villi in section presumably depends upon whether the majority of the leaf or ridge-shaped villi were cut transversely or longitudinally.

The cellular infiltration of the substantia propria was assessed by a semi-quantitative method from + to ++++. The sections were assessed at the same time as 20 English infants of the same age who were considered normal. Each section was assessed on at least two occasions with consistent results. The two groups of children are compared in Table 3 and it can be seen that the children with kwashiorkor have a greater cellular infiltrate than the normal group. The cells of the substantia propria are lymphocytes, plasma cells, eosinophils, and polymorphs. There was no relation between the degree of cellular infiltration and the presence of dysentery.

The superficial epithelial cells appeared normal in

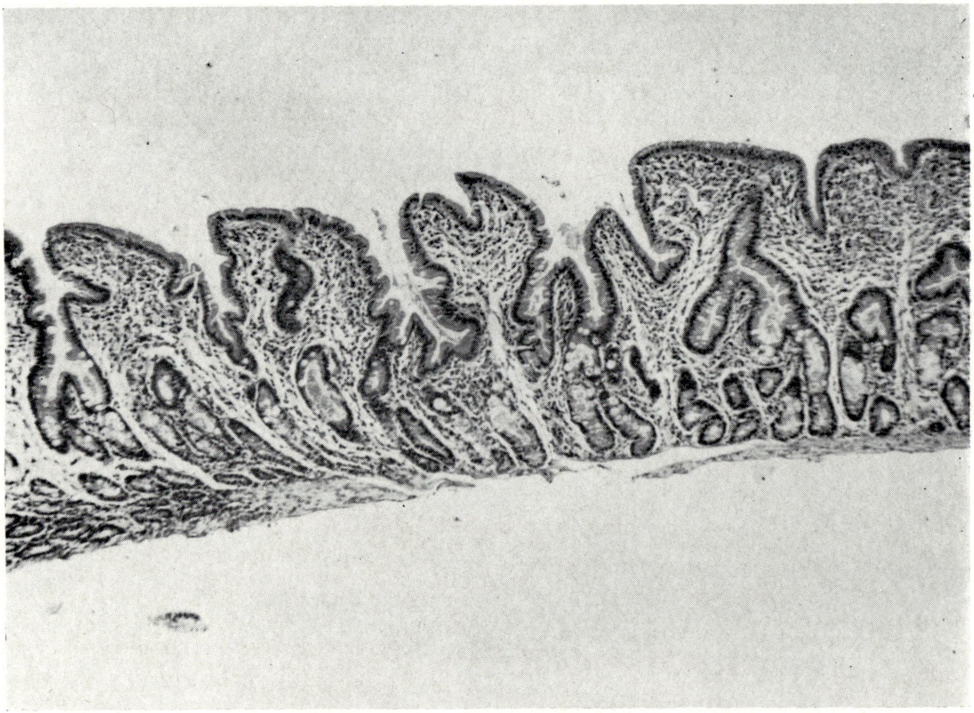

FIG. 2.—Section of jejunal mucosa from Case 7 showing broad villi but normal epithelium. (H and E × 96.)

4 patients, but in the other 13 they were abnormal. They were shorter than usual with an average height about three-quarters of that of cells at the tip of a normal villus. Their nuclei, instead of being basal and arranged in neat rows with regular size, shape, and staining properties, were irregular in all these respects and the epithelium was infiltrated with lymphocytes (Fig. 3). The goblet cells, which vary considerably in normal patients, appeared normal in size and number. The Paneth cells in the crypts also appeared normal with normal granules.

The brush border was studied in sections stained with both the H and E and the PAS techniques and in all cases the brush border was normal (Fig. 4).

**Discussion**

The typical jejunal mucosa in patients with kwashiorkor consists of villi in the shape of ridges and leaves with an increased cellular infiltrate of the substantia propria. The superficial epithelial cells show some shortening with irregular nuclei but a normal brush border. There is an increased lymphocytic infiltration in the epithelium. These changes are very similar to those found by Sprinz, Sribhibhadh, Gangarosa, Benyajati, Kundel, and Halstead (1962) in a third of Thai people from a low socio-economic group. That the abnormality of the epithelium is typical of patients with kwashiorkor is supported by the fact that 2 of the 4 specimens with normal epithelium were from 2 of the 4 patients whose serum albumin was over 3 g./100 ml. One of these, Case 15, had a very low haemoglobin (3·0 g./100 ml.) and presumably this was the cause of the oedema in this child. Of the 4 with a normal epithelium, 2 had malaria, another had dysentery, and the fourth had a megaloblastic bone-marrow. One of them, Case 6, was the only one in the whole series where the cellular infiltration of the substantia propria was assessed as only ++. The patients with a normal epithelium thus appear to differ from the majority of patients studied in one or more respects, though all were diagnosed clinically as kwashiorkor.

The brush border of the normal epithelial cell has been shown under the electron microscope to consist of large numbers of microvilli which increase the absorptive area of the gut by a factor of approximately 20 (Spencer, 1961). In kwashiorkor, the brush border appears normal, but obviously electron microscopic studies are urgently needed to confirm this. The normality of the Paneth cells reported

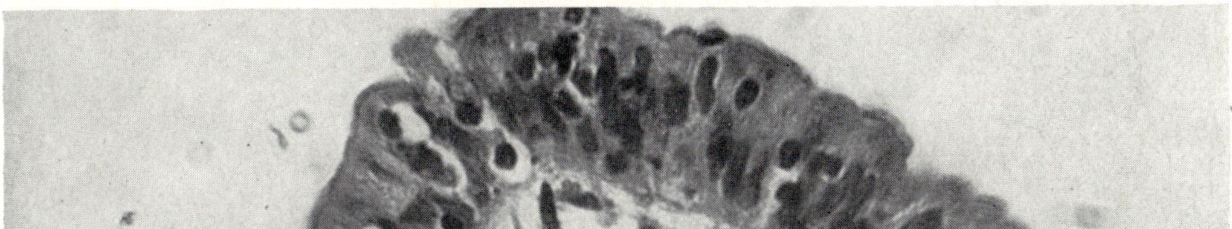

FIG. 3.—A high power view of villous epithelium from Case 1 showing irregular nuclei with lymphocytic infiltration. (H and E × 720.)

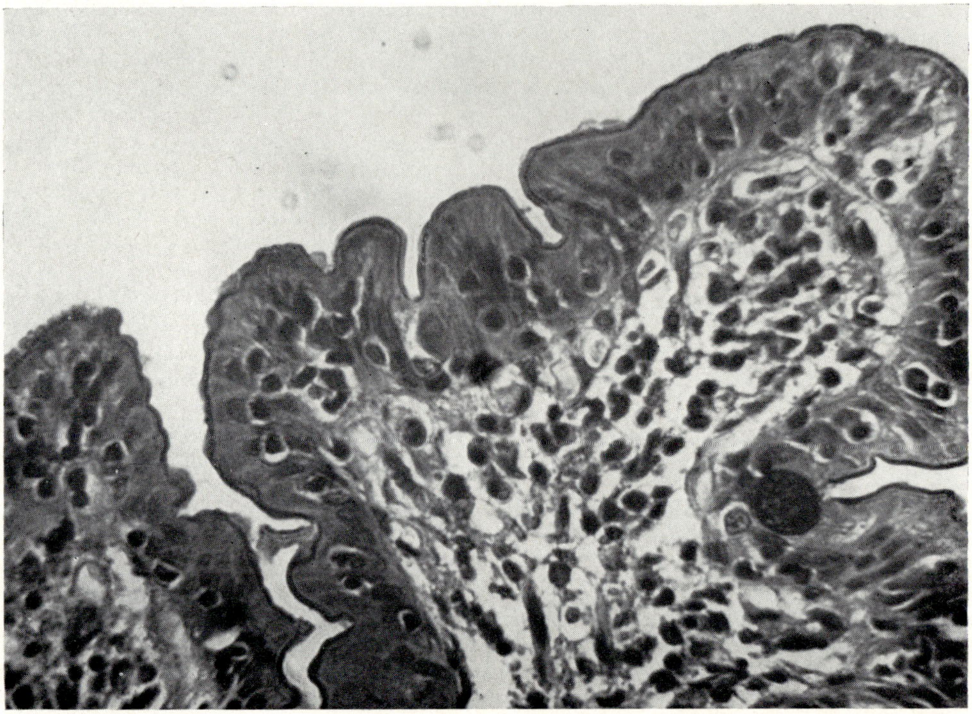

FIG. 4.—A high power view of villous epithelium from Case 1, showing a normal brush border. (PAS. × 720.)

here is contrary to their reduction in size and lack of granularity described by Trowell, Davies, and Dean (1954b).

The group of children available as controls were English or West Indian children living in London, and clearly specimens of jejunal mucosa from African children who have not got kwashiorkor are needed. This is particularly so in the case of the dissecting microscope appearances. A similar picture was seen in 21 older patients with hookworm disease in Mombasa, Kenya (Burman, 1965), and J. P. Stanfield (1964, personal communication) has found the changes to persist 5 months after the treatment of kwashiorkor was started. Baker, Ignatius, Mathan, Vaish, and Chacko (1962) have been unable to find any correlation between xylose and fat excretion and villous architecture. They also found that the villi of normal Southern Indians were entirely leaves, ridges, and convolutions, though stillborn foetuses from the same population had only finger-shaped villi. A similar difference between the villous architecture in the foetus and the adult has been noted in rats (Baker *et al.*, 1963) and in long-nosed bandicoots (van Lennep, 1962). The presence of ridge-shaped villi in the jejunal mucosa of patients with kwashiorkor cannot be considered specific and, in two cases in the present series, only ridges were seen with the dissecting microscope when the histology was quite normal. Ridges and leaves may well be present in the majority of Africans, though Booth (1962) described finger-shaped villi in a small group of African controls in Kampala, unless they were malnourished, had pancreatic steatorrhoea, or suffered from severe hookworm infestation.

The changes in the intestinal mucosa in kwashiorkor are thus relatively minor and cannot be described as complete atrophy. They are not sufficient to account for the steatorrhoea which is usually found (Gillman and Gillman, 1951). These biopsies were taken from the upper jejunum, and Passmore (1947) points out that the intestinal atrophy is most marked in the terminal ileum. It is thus possible that major changes lower down the small gut may have been missed.

The haematological findings in this series of patients were very similar to those found by Kondi, MacDougall, Foy, Mehta, and Mbaya (1963) in patients with kwashiorkor and marasmus on admission to the same ward in Nairobi. The two series are compared in Table 4. The serum folate

TABLE 4

HAEMATOLOGICAL FINDINGS IN PRESENT SERIES COMPARED WITH THOSE FOUND BY KONDI *ET AL.* (1963)

| | No. of Patients | Haemoglobin (g./100 ml.) | | PCV (%) | | MCHC (%) | | Megaloblastic Bone-marrow |
|---|---|---|---|---|---|---|---|---|
| | | Mean | Range | Mean | Range | Mean | Range | |
| Present series .. .. | 17 | 8·3 | 3·0–11·0 | 29·9 | 13–40 | 27·6 | 22–30 | 2 = 12% |
| Kondi and others .. | 47 | 9·0 | 4·2–12·0 | 30·0 | 15–37 | 30·0 | 24–37 | 5 = 11% |

levels recorded here differ from those found by Kondi and her colleagues. In 6 of her 7 cases, the serum folate was low and in one it was abnormally high. In the present paper, 9 had a level below 8 mμg./ml. which was the lowest figure recorded by Chanarin and Berry (1964) in 28 normal English adults. Of the 8 patients with a normal serum folate, 6 were the only 6 with haemoglobins below 6 g./100 ml., and 2 were the only 2 with megaloblastic bone-marrows. From these data, it seems unlikely that folic acid deficiency is the main cause of either the severe anaemia or the megaloblastic erythropoieses present on admission in patients with kwashiorkor. The dissecting microscope appearances of the jejunal mucosa in patients with a low and normal serum folate are compared in Table 5. Those

TABLE 5

DISSECTING MICROSCOPE APPEARANCES OF JEJUNAL MUCOSA IN PATIENTS WITH KWASHIORKOR RELATED TO SERUM FOLATE LEVELS

| Serum Folate | No. of Patients | Villous Type (%) | | |
|---|---|---|---|---|
| | | Ridges | Leaves | Fingers |
| Normal .. .. | 8 | 88 | 12 | 0 |
| Low .. .. | 9 | 33 | 61 | 6 |

with a normal serum folate have virtually all ridge-shaped villi, whereas this type of villus accounts for only one-third of the total when the serum folate is low. If the ridged mucosa is a more severe stage of abnormality than leaves (Booth, Stewart, Holmes, and Brackenbury, 1962), then the abnormal dissecting microscope appearances in kwashiorkor cannot be due to folic acid deficiency. Of the 4 specimens which showed normal epithelial cells, only 2 had a low serum folate, so that this finding also does not appear to be related to folic acid.

## Summary

Jejunal biopsies were carried out on 17 patients with kwashiorkor. The specimens had ridge or leaf-shaped villi with increased cellularity of the substantia propria. The epithelial cells are short with irregular nuclei. This change does not appear to be related to folic acid deficiency.

I am very grateful to Dr. J. R. Harries for permission to study patients under his care. Dr. Henry Foy provided facilities at the Wellcome Trust Research Laboratories, Nairobi, and was extremely helpful in arranging this visit as well as providing excellent advice on all aspects of the investigation. Dr. I. Chanarin kindly performed the estimations of serum *L. casei* activity and Dr. B. Houghton the serum protein estimations.

REFERENCES

Baker, H., Herbert, V., Frank, O., Pasher, I., Hutner, S. H., Wasserman, L. R., and Sobotka, H. (1959). A microbiologic method for detecting folic acid deficiency in man. *Clin. Chem.*, **5**, 275.

Baker, S. J., Ignatius, M., Mathan, V. I., Vaish, S. K., and Chacko, C. C. (1962). Intestinal biopsy in tropical sprue. In *Intestinal Biopsy. Ciba Foundation Study Group No. 14*, ed. G. E. W. Wolstenholme and M. P. Cameron, p. 84. Churchill, London.

——, Mathan, V. I., and Cherian, V. (1963). The nature of the villi in the small intestine of the rat. *Lancet*, **1**, 860.

Booth, C. C. (1962). Discussion. In *Intestinal Biopsy. Ciba Foundation Study Group No. 14*, ed. G. E. W. Wolstenholme and M. P. Cameron, p. 102. Churchill, London.

——, Stewart, J. S., Holmes, R., and Brackenbury, W. (1962). Dissecting microscope appearances of intestinal mucosa. *ibid.*, p. 2.

Burman, D. (1963). Celiac disease. I. Diagnosis by jejunal biopsy. *Clin. pediat.* (*Philad.*), **2**, 581.

—— (1965). The jejunal mucosa in hookworm disease. In preparation.

Chanarin, I., and Berry, V. (1964). Estimation of serum *L. casei* activity. *J. clin. Path.*, **17**, 111.

Crosby, W. H., and Kugler, H. W. (1957). Intraluminal biopsy of the small intestine; the intestinal biopsy capsule. *Amer J. dig. Dis.*, **2**, 236.

Gillman, J., and Gillman, T. (1951). *Perspectives in Human Nutrition.* p. 188. Grune and Stratton, New York.

Glenn, J. H. (1965). Turbidimetric method for the determination of serum globulin using the autoanalyzer. *J. clin. Path.*, **18**, 131.

Kondi, A., MacDougall, L., Foy, H., Mehta, S., and Mbaya, V. (1963). Anaemias of marasmus and kwashiorkor in Kenya. *Arch. Dis. Childh.*, **38**, 267.

Passmore, R. (1947). Mixed deficiency diseases in India: a clinical description. *Trans. roy. Soc. trop. Med. Hyg.*, **41**, 189.

Shiner, M. (1956). Duodenal biopsy. *Lancet*, **1**, 17.

Spencer, R. P. (1961). Microvilli and intestinal surface area; an evaluation. *Gastroenterology*, **41**, 313.

Sprinz, H., Sribhibhadh, R., Gangarosa, E. J., Benyajati, C., Kundel, D., and Halstead, S. (1962). Biopsy of small bowel of Thai people. *Amer. J. clin. Path.*, **38**, 43.

Stevens, D. L. (1959). *Technicon Handbook.*

Trowell, H. C., Davies, J. N. P., and Dean, R. F. A. (1954a). *Kwashiorkor*, p. 69. Edward Arnold, London.

——, ——, and —— (1954b). *ibid.*, p. 150.

van Lennep, E. W. (1962). The histology of the mucosa of the small intestine of the long-nosed bandicoot. *Acta anat.* (*Basel*), **50**, 73.

*Arch. Dis. Childh.*, 1965, **40**, 532.

# EFFECT OF UNDERNUTRITION IN EARLY LIFE ON PHYSICAL AND MENTAL DEVELOPMENT

BY

VERA CABAK and R. NAJDANVIC
*From the Paediatric Clinic, Sarajevo, Yugoslavia*

(RECEIVED FOR PUBLICATION AUGUST 14, 1964)

It was pointed out by Trowell, Davis, and Dean (1954) that, 'Nothing is known about the completeness of recovery from severe kwashiorkor', and this is to a large extent still true. An increase in the body weight is admittedly a sign of recovery, and indeed a very important criterion of it, but unless the final weight and height attained are also known it is impossible to say whether it has been complete. The experiments on animals give some information about this problem. McCance and Widdowson (1962) showed that the body weights of rats undernourished during suckling never reached those of their controls in spite of subsequent unlimited food. Undernutrition for the first six months of life can also affect the final stature of cockerels (Pratt and McCance, 1961), but this has not been found to be true of all species and for these differences references should be made to Aron (1911), Moulton, Trowbridge, and Haigh (1921), Jackson (1925), Clarke and Smith (1938), Crichton, Aitken, and Boyne (1959), and McCance (1962). The extent of the undernutrition and the age at which it affects the animal are also certainly important (Widdowson and McCance, 1963).

Even less is known about the mental than about the physical development of children after a period of undernutrition (Stoch and Smythe, 1963; Graham, 1964). Attention has been drawn to defects in their ability to learn a language (Waterlow, Cravioto, and Stephen, 1960), which is one of the most important ways of estimating the intelligence of a child (Stevanović, 1937). Jersild (1955) has stated that, 'A positive relationship is usually found between language ability and mental ability.' Many authors, moreover (Porter, 1895a, b; Boas, 1940; Tanner, 1955), have found that children who are physically advanced for their age score higher in mental tests than those who are less mature, but of the same chronological age. Lat, Widdowson, and McCance (1960) showed this to be true also of rats.

## Material and Methods

Children were selected from the records who had been admitted for malnutrition (marasmus) to the Hospital for sick children in Sarajevo between 1951 and 1957. Though slight oedema was present in a few, there were no other signs of kwashiorkor. Their ages at the time were between 4 and 24 months. At the time of admission they had all been 27% or more below the correct weight for their age, according to the tables of Lust, Pfaundler, and Husler (1953). Children suffering from chronic diseases such as tuberculosis or diseases of the central nervous system were excluded from the investigation and, for financial reasons, only children from the town of Sarajevo were invited to attend. This restricted the numbers and, for various reasons, some did not come, so that finally only 36 children were available. The history of the health and development of these children after discharge was taken, the body weight and height were measured, the intelligence was tested by Binet-Simon scale as adapted by Stevanović (1937), and finally their grade at school was recorded. At the time of the follow-up assessment their ages were between 7 and 14 years. The parents of these children were mainly unskilled and skilled workers, but about one-third was drawn from the professions or were army officers.

## Results

Fig. 1 shows the deficits in the expected weight for age at the time of admission plotted against the age. Most of the cases were less than 12 months old and all the most serious were below this age.

The body weights of these children at the time of interview are shown in Fig. 2 in comparison with the weights of the healthy schoolchildren of Sarajevo (Jelisavčić-Mihal, 1961). More of the children were below the standard curve at 7 or 8 years of age than later, but the mean values and the standards were not significantly different at any age by the 't' test.

Fig. 3 shows the heights of the 36 children, also in comparison with local standards. The results are similar to those for weights.

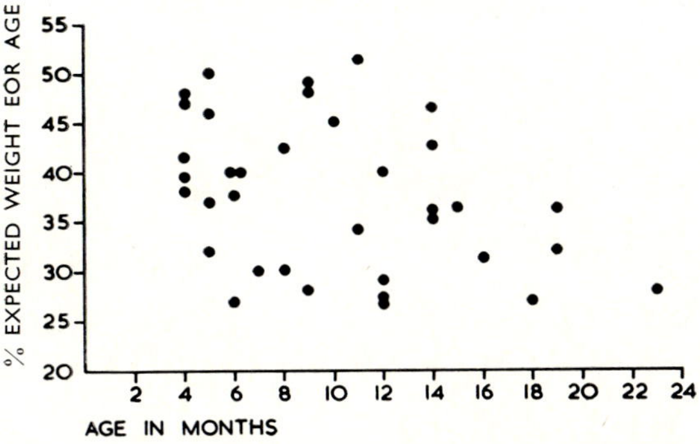


FIG. 1.—Deficit in body weight of the undernourished children, expressed as a percentage of the weight to be expected at that age, plotted against their age on admission.

The results of the intelligence tests are shown in Fig. 4. Only 18 were within the normal IQ limits (91-110), 12 were 'stupid', with IQs between 71 and 90, and the remaining 6 children had IQs of 70 or below. None showed an IQ greater than 110. In other words, half the children were below the limit of normal intelligence, and this difference between normal and subnormal intelligence was highly significant by the Kolmogorov Smirnov test ($p = 0{\cdot}01$).

There are no local standards for the dispersion of the intelligence quotient, so the present results have been compared with those for Serbian children (Stevanović, 1957). Of the Serbian children, 21% were below normal intelligence as against 50% of the previously undernourished children, and 32% of the Serbian children were above the range of the undernourished children. The mean IQ of the undernourished series was 88, in contrast to 101 for children from Mostar, 80 miles from Sarajevo, and 109 for children from Beograd. It is well known that socio-economic factors influence the IQ but even if all the undernourished children had come from families of 'non-qualified' workers their IQ was below the mean value of 93 for this group.

No correlation was found using the Spearman test (Siegel, 1956) between the age of the children when they were ill and undernourished and their subsequent

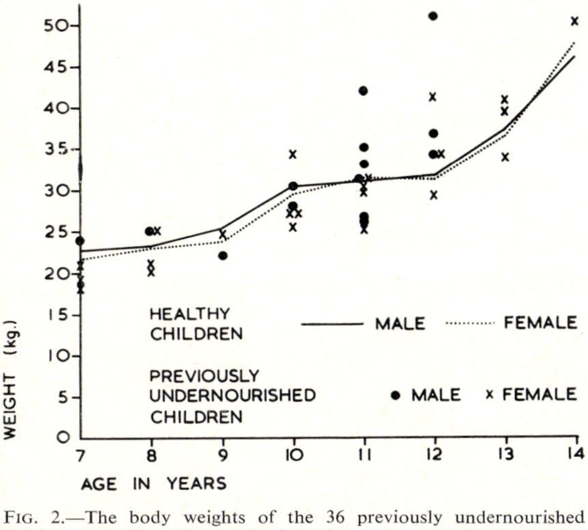


FIG. 2.—The body weights of the 36 previously undernourished children when they attended for interview compared with the weights of healthy schoolchildren in Sarajevo.

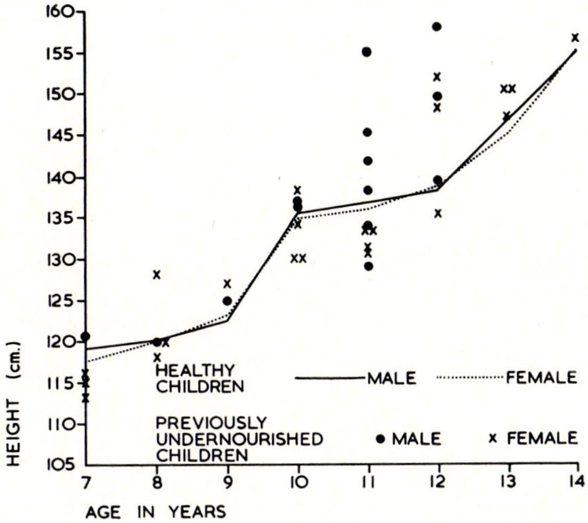


FIG. 3.—The heights of the 36 previously undernourished schoolchildren when they attended for interview compared with the heights of healthy schoolchildren in Sarajevo.

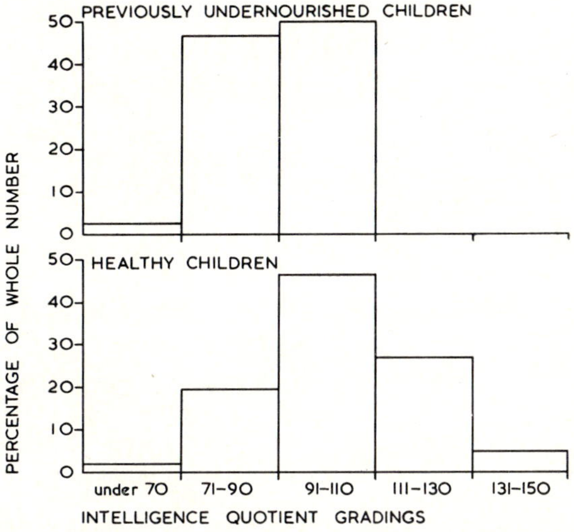


FIG. 4.—The distribution of quotients of intelligence shown by the 36 undernourished children compared with the standards established for Serbian children.

mental development and IQ. A correlation, however, was found between the deficit in the expected weight for age on the original admission and the IQ on subsequent re-examination. The school grades of these children were in good agreement with their rating by IQ tests, and this confirms the experience of others.

## Summary

Serbian children who had been seriously undernourished in infancy were found at school-age to have normal physical characteristics but subnormal mental capacity.

I am grateful to Dr. E. Serstnev for his assistance with the statistical analysis of the results and to Dr. L. Skoric for help in the appraisal of the results of the intelligence tests. Professor R. A. McCance encouraged me to write this paper, and advised and helped me over its presentation. I would like to thank him for all he has done.

### References

Aron, H. (1911). Nutrition and growth. *Philipp. J. Sci. B.*, **6**, 1.

Boas, F. (1940). *Race, Language and Culture.* MacMillan, New York.

Clarke, M. F., and Smith, A. H. (1938). Recovery following suppression of growth in the rat. *J. Nutr.*, **15**, 245.

Crichton, J. A., Aitken, J. N., and Boyne, A. W. (1959). The effect of plane of nutrition during rearing on growth, production, reproduction and health of dairy cattle: 1. Growth to 24 months. *Anim. Prod.*, **1**, 145.

Graham, G. (1964). *Diet and Bodily Constitution. Ciba Foundation Study Group No. 17*, p. 11. J. & A. Churchill, London.

Jackson, C. M. (1925). *The Effects of Inanition and Malnutrition Upon Growth and Structure.* J. & A. Churchill, London.

Jelisavčić-Mihal, M. (1961). Prilog antropometrijkom ispitivanju školske omladine. *Biltin Rep. Z. za Zdrav. zaštitu br.*, 1-2, 78.

Jersild, T. A. (1955). *Child Psychology*, 4th ed., p. 417. Staples Press, London.

Lat, J., Widdowson, E. M., and McCance, R. A. (1960). Some effects of accelerating growth: III. Behaviour and nervous activity. *Proc. roy. Soc. B*, **153**, 347.

Lust, F., Pfaundler, M. von, and Husler, J. (1953). *Krankheiten des Kindesalters.* Urban & Schwarzenberg, Munich.

McCance, R. A. (1962). Food, growth, and time. *Lancet*, **2**, 621, 671.

——, and Widdowson, E. M. (1962). Nutrition and growth. *Proc. roy. Soc. B*, **156**, 326.

Moulton, C. R., Trowbridge, P. F., and Haigh, L. D. (1921). Studies in animal nutrition: 1. Changes in form and weight on different planes of nutrition. *Res. Bull. Mo. agric. Exp. Sta.*, **43**, 73.

Porter, W. T. (1895a). The physical basis of precocity and dullness. *Trans. Acad. Sci. St Louis*, **6**, 161.

—— (1895b). The relation between the growth of children and their deviation from the physical type of their sex and age. *ibid.*, **6**, 233.

Pratt, C. W. M., and McCance, R. A. (1961). Severe undernutrition in growing and adult animals: 6. Changes in the long bones during the rehabilitation of cockerels. *Brit. J. Nutr.*, **15**, 121.

Siegel, S. (1956). *Nonparametric Statistics: for the Behavioral Sciences.* McGraw Hill, New York.

Stevanović, B. (1937). *Merenje Inteligencije.* Ed. Drag. Gregorić, Belgrade.

—— (1957). *Pedagoška psihologija.* Ed. Naučna Knjiga, Belgrade.

Stoch, M. B., and Smythe, P. M. (1963). Does undernutrition during infancy inhibit brain growth and subsequent intellectual development? *Arch. Dis. Childh.*, **38**, 546.

Tanner, J. M. (1955). *Growth at Adolescence.* Blackwell, Oxford.

Trowell, H. C., Davis, J. N. P., and Dean, R. F. A. (1954). *Kwashiorkor*, p. 225. Edward Arnold, London.

Waterlow, J. C., Cravioto, J., and Stephen, J. M. L. (1960). Protein malnutrition in man. *Advanc. Protein Chem.*, **15**, 131.

Widdowson, E. M., and McCance, R. A. (1963). The effect of finite periods of undernutrition at different ages on the composition and subsequent development of the rat. *Proc. roy. Soc. B*, **158**, 329.

*Arch. Dis. Childh.*, 1965, **40**, 535.

# INFANTILE HYPERCALCAEMIA AND CARDIOVASCULAR LESIONS

## EVIDENCE, HYPOTHESIS, AND SPECULATION

BY

ERIC N. COLEMAN

*From the Royal Hospital for Sick Children, Glasgow, and the University Department of Child Health, Glasgow*

(RECEIVED FOR PUBLICATION DECEMBER 30, 1964)

Since the recognition of the benign and severe forms of infantile hypercalcaemia (Lightwood, 1952; Fanconi, Girardet, Schlesinger, Butler, and Black, 1952), circumstantial evidence has assigned a causal role to vitamin D ingested by infants peculiarly sensitive to that substance. The disease failed to disappear, though its incidence declined, after the vitamin $D_2$ content of infant foods and vitamin concentrates had been reduced (Stewart, Mitchell, Morgan, Lowe, and Thomson, 1964; British Paediatric Association Report, 1964). It accounted for the admission of 39 infants to the Royal Hospital for Sick Children, Glasgow, during 1956-57 at the height of its incidence, but of only 13 during 1962-63. All but one of these 13 patients lived outside the city (10) or on its periphery (2), a situation contrasting with the recent incidence of infantile rickets in the area (Arneil and Crosbie, 1963), which has been largely confined to the central districts of the city.

Children poisoned with a massive dose of vitamin D may sustain damage to the cardiovascular system (Hjelt, Tähkä, and Hallman, 1956), and it is quite logical to expect similar effects in a disease acknowledged as qualitatively identical. Cardiovascular lesions have indeed been reported in infantile hypercalcaemia, and while their inconstancy and variety are notable they represent a serious aspect of the disease deserving close attention.

### Electrocardiographic and Clinical Findings

An abnormal contour of the ST-T complex in the bipolar limb leads was reported in 14 of 24 patients suffering from infantile hypercalcaemia (Coleman, 1959), but further experience and the use of praecordial leads have shown the incidence to be higher. Indeed 12 of the 13 patients admitted to hospital during 1962-63 demonstrated the abnormality; no electrocardiographic examination was made of the remaining patient. The abnormal pattern bears little resemblance to that usually attributed to hypercalcaemia and may persist longer than the elevation of serum calcium. Instead of the Q-T interval ($QT_c$) being short and reflecting a short S-T interval, it is of average duration because the shortened S-T interval is masked by a broad T wave; this has a flattened or notched summit and is usually tall. The abnormal T wave is typically present not only in bipolar leads I and II, but also in unipolar leads from V4 to V6 (Fig. 1). Furthermore even in bipolar leads with apparently normal T wave summits the waves can be shown to be of significantly greater length than in healthy infants (Coleman, 1961).

Of the 13 patients with infantile hypercalcaemia during 1962-63, 4 gave transient electrocardiographic evidence of left ventricular hypertrophy. Three

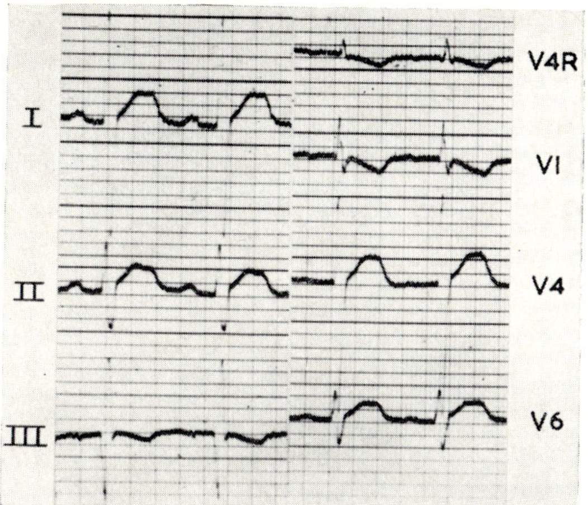


FIG. 1.—Infantile hypercalcaemia. Broad plateau T waves in leads I, II, V4, and V6.

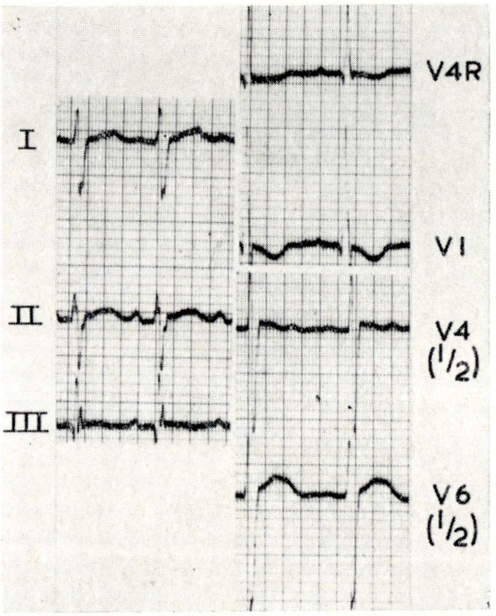


FIG. 2.—Infantile hypercalcaemia and pulmonary stenosis. V4 and V6 recorded at half-standard amplitude. Right ventricular hypertrophy and abnormal T waves (II and V6).

others had systemic hypertension which was most pronounced in the single patient who suffered from the disease in its severe form. This patient, from his first attendance when 5 months old, had a systolic murmur at the pulmonary area and by 18 months physical signs characteristic of pulmonary valve stenosis, with electrocardiographic evidence of right ventricular hypertrophy (Fig. 2). Cardiac catheterization confirmed the diagnosis; the right ventricular pressure was 45/0 mm. Hg, but the systolic pressure gradient of 30 mm. Hg over the pulmonary valve was regarded as insufficient to justify surgical treatment. None of these patients died.

**Experimental Findings**

Because the electrocardiographic changes were so specific and might result from a myocardial lesion, the possibility of a specific lesion caused by vitamin D was examined after its administration in large doses to young rabbits.

Vitamin $D_3$ in arachis oil was given by mouth to 9 rabbits, vitamin $D_2$ in arachis oil was given to 9 rabbits, and there were 9 controls. The rabbits belonged to 6 litters, and the administration of vitamin D was carried out within 10 days and completed by the age of 6 weeks. The dosage per g. body weight was from 100 to 770 international units of vitamin $D_3$ and from 40 to 420 units of vitamin $D_2$. Where possible they were allowed to survive to 4, 8, or 40 weeks after the beginning of the experiment, but 7 that had received vitamin D died, and another had to be killed earlier than planned.

An aortic lesion was present in every rabbit given vitamin D, but in none of the controls. In most the lesions were widespread, but the thoracic aorta was most severely affected (Fig. 3). The inner half of the media was affected and in some instances there was intimal thickening. The least severe lesions were the most cellular, with many fibroblasts and macrophages. The elastic fibres were distorted or even disrupted and between the elastic laminae

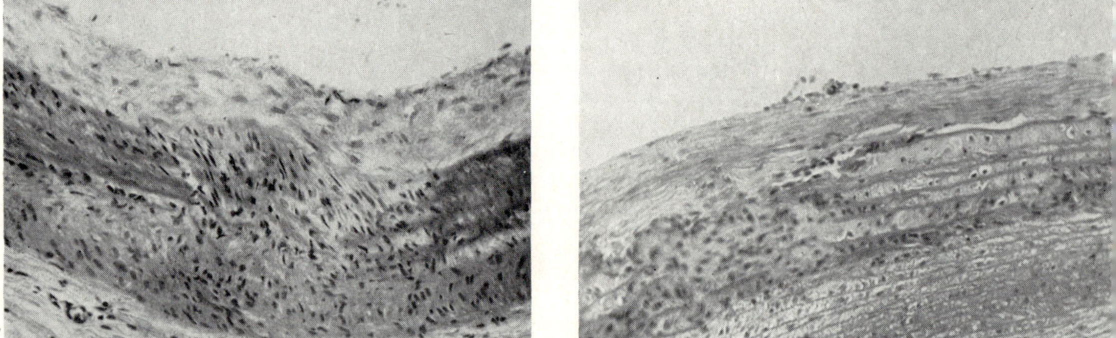

(a) (b)

FIG. 3.—Rabbit thoracic aorta. Longitudinal sections. (H. and E. × 150.) (a) Early lesion. Thickened intima. Elastic laminae straightened, thickened, and disrupted. Fibroblast proliferation. (b) Severe lesion showing in addition cartilage formation and proliferation of fibroblasts and macrophages.

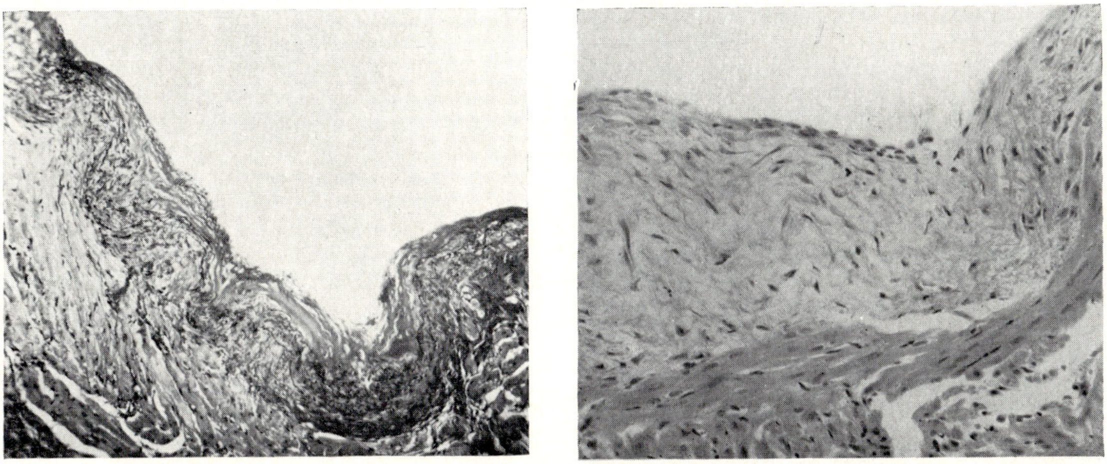

(a) (b)

FIG. 4.—Rabbit left atrial wall. (a) Subendocardial fibrous tissue proliferation; collagenous layer and deeper fibroelastic layer. (Verhoeff-van Gieson. × 67.) (b) Another example. Fibrous tissue proliferation overlying normal muscle. (H. and E. × 275.)

muscle cells were destroyed. Here calcium deposition was often suggested by staining reactions; cartilage had formed in 2 instances and bone in one instance.

Two died in congestive heart failure ($D_2$ 347 units/g.; $D_3$ 103 units/g.); histology of the heart revealed no focal lesion but hypertrophy of muscle fibres and severe aortic wall lesions. Four others ($D_2$ 230 units/g., 40 units/g.; $D_3$ 770 units/g., 660 units/g.) had focal myocardial lesions which in 3 consisted of periarterial muscle fibre necrosis with staining reactions suggesting the presence of calcium, and, in relation to dead muscle fibres, a cellular reaction consisting of macrophages, fibroblasts, and multinucleate giant cells. In the fourth rabbit ($D_2$ 40 units/g.) focal lesions were present at some distance from the arterial branches and consisted of a patchy loss of muscle fibres with replacement by granulation tissue in which were macrophages, eosinophils, and occasional giant cells, but without evidence of calcium deposition. The rabbit that became ill and had to be killed 6 weeks after the administration of vitamin D ($D_2$ 40 units/g.) was the only one in which coronary artery lesions were detected; there was distortion and disruption of the internal elastic lamina, thickening of the intima, and narrowing of the media.

In 10 rabbits that had received vitamin D there were lesions immediately subjacent to the mural endocardium of the left ventricle, left atrium, or right ventricle ($D_2$ 40-420 units/g.; $D_3$ 100-770 units/g.). Immediately beneath the endocardium there was a collagenous layer containing only a few fibroblasts; in some there was a deeper and substantially thicker layer of fibroelastic tissue which sometimes surrounded islands of muscle cells (Fig. 4).

Serum calcium levels in excess of those of the control animals (10-11·5 mg./100 ml.) were found as long as 32-38 weeks after the administration of vitamin $D_2$ or $D_3$ had ceased (12·9-14·1 mg./100 ml.).

## Discussion

The wide but inconstant array of cardiovascular lesions reported in a relatively few cases of infantile hypercalcaemia has included left ventricular or biventricular myocardial hypertrophy, myocardial fibrosis, or calcification, valvular endocardial lesions including fibrosis and calcification, lesions of the intima and inner media of arteries including the coronaries, and peripheral systemic and pulmonary arterial stenosis (Schlesinger, Butler, and Black, 1956; Joseph and Parrott, 1958; Lamy, Nezelof, Fauré, Jammet, and Aussannaire, 1958; Rashkind, Golinko, and Arcasoy, 1961; Bonham Carter and Sutcliffe, 1964).

**Aortic Lesions.** Black and Bonham Carter (1963) have described aortic supravalvar stenosis in a child thought to have suffered from severe infantile hypercalcaemia. Histological features in the aorta were thickening of the media with fibrosis and some deficiency of both muscle and elastic tissue, a circular ridge of fibrous tissue, and, distal to this stricture, intimal thickening with atheromatous change. There was fibrous thickening of the aortic valve.

The lesions in rabbits reported here indicate the susceptibility of the aortic media and intima in one mammalian species to damage by vitamin D. Extensive examination of the controls failed to reveal any vestige of the spontaneous aortic lesion known to occur in some laboratory rabbits (Kesten, 1935). The histological pattern of the experimental lesion seems to resemble that of the human lesion described by Black and Bonham Carter (1963), and therefore lends support to the concept of a causal relation between infantile hypercalcaemia and aortic supravalvar stenosis on the assumption that the former disease is causally linked with vitamin D activity.

**Endocardial Lesions.** The experimental lesion immediately subjacent to the mural endocardium has no exact counterpart in infantile hypercalcaemia. The only endocardial lesion detected during 1962-63 in the hospital in association with infantile hypercalcaemia was pulmonary stenosis confirmed by cardiac catheterization. The same association occurred in a male infant of 6 months who died of the severe type of infantile hypercalcaemia in 1954. In addition to advanced renal medullary calcinosis necropsy revealed pale, thickened, rigid, but discrete, pulmonary valve cusps in a valve ring of average size, these appearances being due to the presence of oedematous fibrillary collagen within the cusps (Fig. 5).

This pulmonary valve lesion may have its parallel in the aortic valve lesion mentioned by Black and Bonham Carter (1963).

The fibroelastic form of the experimental lesion is reminiscent of congenital endocardial fibroelastosis, and like that disease affects principally the left heart chambers. Endocardial fibroelastosis remains of uncertain aetiology. It has no recognized connexion with infantile hypercalcaemia or vitamin D, but its known association with congenital cardiovascular malformations is so inconstant (Forfar, Miller, Bain, and Macleod, 1964) that other or additional causal factors are likely. The experimental lesion indicates decisively that a form of endocardial fibroelastosis may be caused by a toxic substance, but since the human disease usually presents in the earliest weeks of life (Forfar *et al.*, 1964) its occurrence then seems to require the transplacental passage of the toxic substance. Not only has transmission through the placenta been claimed for vitamin D (Decio and Alamanni, 1956), but the early appearance of the striking clinical features of severe infantile hypercalcaemia suggests the likelihood of prenatal intoxication in some instances. The lesion of congenital endocardial fibroelastosis may not be confined to the endocardium, but may, as in the case of infantile hypercalcaemia, occasionally include myocardial fibrosis or calcification and coronary artery lesions (Blumberg and Lyon, 1952; Thomas, Lee, McGavran, and Rabin, 1956). Curiously, the hospital incidence of endocardial fibroelastosis proven at necropsy, as of infantile hypercalcaemia diagnosed clinically, has declined since 1958 when measures had been taken and the reasons publicized for reducing the vitamin $D_2$ intake of infants (Table).

TABLE
NUMBER OF CASES DURING FIRST YEAR OF LIFE

| Disease | 1954–58 | 1959–63 |
|---|---|---|
| Infantile hypercalcaemia .. .. | 61 | 24 |
| Endocardial fibroelastosis .. .. | 19 | 10 |

Outside the cardiovascular system, however, severe infantile hypercalcaemia and endocardial

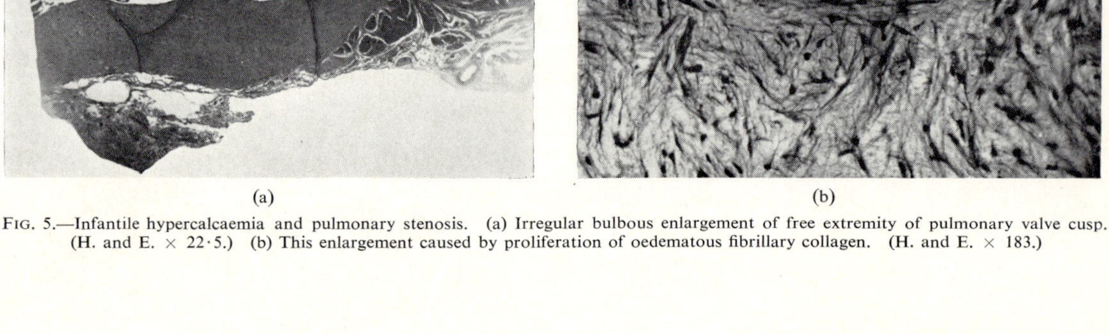

(a) (b)

FIG. 5.—Infantile hypercalcaemia and pulmonary stenosis. (a) Irregular bulbous enlargement of free extremity of pulmonary valve cusp. (H. and E. × 22·5.) (b) This enlargement caused by proliferation of oedematous fibrillary collagen. (H. and E. × 183.)

fibroelastosis are quite dissimilar, and an attempt to reconcile these as effects of a single intrauterine toxic agent relies on the concept that the quality of teratogenic effect depends on the dose of the agent and the timing of its application during embryogenesis.

**Myocardial Lesions.** The infrequency of myocardial and coronary artery lesions in the experimental material would not suggest the probability of a high incidence in infantile hypercalcaemia, though in that disease similar lesions have been found at necropsy (Rashkind *et al.*, 1961). It is evident, however, that no conclusion is possible as to the relative amounts of vitamin D required in different species to produce similar lesions and especially in relation to a disease dependent for its existence on hypersensitivity.

The electrocardiographic features of infantile hypercalcaemia, which are of such constancy as to be of diagnostic value, are caused neither by hypercalcaemia nor by any generalized electrolyte disturbance. Quinidine intoxication may temporarily produce prominent and broad T waves, and a lengthened Q-T interval (Sagall, Horn, and Riseman, 1943), indicating the increased refractory period of the ventricular myocardium. In infantile hypercalcaemia the abnormal shape of the ST-T complex in leads I, II, and V4 to V6 outlasts the hypercalcaemic phase of the disease, and it is tempting to suggest that it signifies left ventricular myocardial damage. In children poisoned with massive doses of vitamin $D_2$ a closely similar ST-T pattern has been described (Jelke, 1946; Skatvedt, 1947; Hjelt *et al.*, 1956), and the possibility exists that a specific toxic effect is exerted on myocardial metabolism by vitamin D or some related toxic sterol, or that a specific pattern of myocardial damage is caused by such a substance. Correlation of electrocardiographic pattern with myocardial pathology was reported in one child who died of classical vitamin D poisoning; the T waves had been tall and broad and the myocardium showed periarterial necrosis and fibrosis (Hjelt *et al.*, 1956).

The search for left ventricular lesions of a type that could cause electrocardiographic signs such as these included the myocardial fibrosis of uncertain pathogenesis found as a rare accompaniment of fibrocystic disease of the pancreas (Kintzen, 1950; Feer, 1952; Powell, Newman, and Hooker, 1957; Nezelof and Lancret, 1959), for McGiven (1962) described a child in whose published electrocardiogram the ST-T complexes of lead I, V4, and V5 were closely similar if not identical with those described here. In the only other reported electrocardiogram (Nezelof and Lancret, 1959) the T waves were also abnormal. The characteristic lesion affects principally the left ventricular myocardium and consists of muscle fibre degeneration, and replacement by fibrous tissue. Endocardial fibroelastosis has been twice reported (McGiven, 1962; Nezelof and Lancret, 1959). Nezelof and Lancret (1959) did not mention diet or medication but vitamin D had been given in all other instances. Nephrocalcinosis was present in both patients whose renal histology has been reported; this would, according to Shanks and MacDonald (1959), argue the occurrence at some time of hypercalcaemia. Rickets is virtually unknown in fibrocystic disease of the pancreas but extra vitamin D is customarily added to the diet as it is in coeliac disease. It seems possible that there could exist in fibrocystic disease a compensatory mechanism for the conservation of vitamin D and accordingly that toxic effects of overdosage might readily occur.

In regard to the absence of calcification in this cardiac lesion and other lesions ascribed to vitamin D, it is evident from animal feeding experiments (Gillman and Gilbert, 1956), as from some cardiac lesions in infantile hypercalcaemia (Rashkind *et al.*, 1961), and from the natural history of nephrocalcinosis associated with infantile hypercalcaemia (Shanks and MacDonald, 1959), that calcification is neither a primary nor an invariable feature of these lesions.

**Prognosis.** Spontaneous healing and complete repair have been reported by Gillman and Gilbert (1956) in relation to a wide range of cardiovascular lesions induced in the rat with vitamin $D_2$. There is no reason to suppose that human cardiovascular lesions similarly produced would behave differently, provided that the toxic stimulus were removed. No conclusion is possible from the present experimental material, because of the apparent long persistence of vitamin D effect as judged from serum calcium levels.

## Summary and Conclusions

In infantile hypercalcaemia (infantile hypersensitivity to vitamin D) the high incidence of transient changes in the ST-T complex of the left praecordial electrocardiogram suggests a high incidence of transient damage to the left ventricular myocardium.

Vitamin D given in high dosage to young rabbits causes lesions of the aortic wall, of the mural endocardium (fibroelastosis), and occasionally of the myocardium.

The possibility exists that congenital endocardial fibroelastosis and the myocardial lesion of fibrocystic disease of the pancreas are related to vitamin D.

The persistence of infantile hypercalcaemia and

the possibility of residual cardiovascular lesions is disquieting. Where infantile rickets and infantile hypercalcaemia coexist in different parts of the same community as they do in south western Scotland, it may prove impracticable to eliminate one without increasing the incidence of the other, and in such circumstances it is impossible to evade making a responsible inquiry into the nature of residual effects and their relative importance.

I thank Professor J. H. Hutchison and Dr. R. A. Shanks for access to the clinical material, Dr. A. M. MacDonald for advice on histology, the Departments of Biochemistry and Radiology at the Royal Hospital for Sick Children, and Messrs. W. Mason and J. Devlin for the illustrations. I am indebted to Professor Hutchison for criticism of the manuscript.

## References

Arneil, G. C., and Crosbie, J. C. (1963). Infantile rickets returns to Glasgow. *Lancet*, **2**, 423.

Black, J. A., and Bonham Carter, R. E. (1963). Association between aortic stenosis and facies of severe infantile hypercalcaemia. *ibid.*, **2**, 745.

Bonham Carter, R. E., and Sutcliffe, J. (1964). A syndrome of multiple arterial stenosis, in association with the severe form of idiopathic hypercalcaemia. *Arch. Dis. Childh.*, **39**, 418.

Blumberg, R. W., and Lyon, R. A. (1952). Endocardial sclerosis. *Amer. J. Dis. Child.*, **4**, 291.

British Paediatric Association Report (1964). Infantile hypercalcaemia, nutritional rickets, and infantile scurvy in Great Britain. *Brit. med. J.*, **1**, 1659.

Coleman, E. N. (1959). Electrocardiographic changes in idiopathic hypercalcaemia of infancy. *ibid.*, **2**, 467.

—— (1961). Electrocardiography in idiopathic hypercalcaemia and other cation disorders of childhood. M.D. Thesis, Glasgow University.

Decio, R., and Alamanni, V. (1956). Il passaggio transplacentare delle vitamine A, E, $D_2$ somministrate alla madre per via venosa. *Minerva ginec.*, **8**, 381.

Fanconi, G., Girardet, P., Schlesinger, B., Butler, N., and Black, J. (1952). Chronische Hypercalcämie, kombiniert mit Osteosklerose, Hyperazotämie, Minderwuchs und kongenitalen Mißbildungen. *Helv. paediat. Acta.*, **7**, 314.

Feer, W. (1952). Xerophthalmie und Myokardschaden bei Pankreasfibrose. *Schweiz. med. Wschr.*, **82**, 102.

Forfar, J. O., Miller, R. A., Bain, A. D., and Macleod, W. (1964). Endocardial fibroelastosis. *Brit. med. J.*, **2**, 7.

Gillman, J., and Gilbert, C. (1956). Calcium, phosphorus and vitamin D as factors regulating integrity of the cardiovascular system. *Exp. Med. Surg.*, **14**, 136.

Hjelt, L., Tähkä, H., and Hallman, N. (1956). Chronic hypercalcaemia and vitamin D in early childhood. II. Post-mortem studies. *Ann. Paediat. Fenn.*, **2**, 75.

Jelke, H. (1946). Über D-Vitamin-Vergiftung. *Acta med. scand.*, Suppl. **170**, 345.

Joseph, M. C., and Parrott, D. (1958). Severe infantile hypercalcaemia with special reference to the facies. *Arch. Dis. Childh.*, **33**, 385.

Kesten, H. D. (1935). Early incidence of spontaneous medial degeneration ("arteriosclerosis") in the aorta of the rabbit. *Arch. Path.*, **20**, 1.

Kintzen, W. (1950). Zystische Pankreasfibrose kombiniert mit Myokardfibrose. *Int. Z. Vitamin.-forsch.*, **22**, 273.

Lamy, M., Nezelof, C., Fauré, C., Jammet, M. L., and Aussannaire, M. (1958). La forme sévère de l'hypercalcemie idiopathique (à propos de deux observations anatomo-cliniques). *Arch. franç, Pédiat.*, **15**, 1001.

Lightwood, R. (1952). Idiopathic hypercalcaemia with failure to thrive: nephrocalcinosis. *Proc. roy. Soc. Med.*, **45**, 401.

McGiven, A. R. (1962). Myocardial fibrosis in fibrocystic disease of the pancreas. *Arch. Dis. Childh.*, **37**, 656.

Nezelof, C., and Lancret, P. (1959). Lésions de fibrose myocardique au cours de la maladie fibro-kystique du pancreas. *Arch. franç. Pédiat.*, **16**, 1035.

Powell, L. W., Jr., Newman, S., and Hooker, J. W. (1957). Cystic fibrosis of the pancreas complicated by myocardial fibrosis. *Virgina med. Mth.*, **84**, 178.

Rashkind, W. J., Golinko, R., and Arcasoy, M. (1961). Cardiac findings in idiopathic hypercalcemia of infancy. *J. Pediat.*, **58**, 464.

Sagall, E. L., Horn, C. D., and Riseman, J. E. F. (1943). Studies on the action of quinidine in man. I. Measurement of the speed and duration of the effect following oral and intramuscular administration. *Arch. intern. Med.*, **71**, 460.

Schlesinger, B. E., Butler, N. R., and Black, J. A. (1956). Severe type of infantile hypercalcaemia. *Brit. med. J.*, **1**, 127.

Shanks, R. A., and MacDonald, A. M. (1959). Nephrocalcinosis infantum. *Arch. Dis. Childh.*, **34**, 115.

Skatvedt, M. (1947). A case of D-vitamin intoxication *Ann. paediat. (Basel)*, **168**, 148.

Stewart, W. K., Mitchell, R. G., Morgan, H. G., Lowe, K. G., and Thomson, J. (1964). The changing incidence of rickets and infantile hypercalcaemia as seen in Dundee. *Lancet*, **1**, 679.

Thomas, W. A., Lee, K. T., McGavran, M. H., and Rabin, E. R. (1956). Endocardial fibroelastosis in infants associated with thrombosis and calcification of arteries and myocardial infarcts. *New Engl. J. Med.*, **255**, 464.

*Arch. Dis. Childh.*, 1965, **40**, 541.

# ACCESSORY LOBE OF LIVER PRESENTING THROUGH A CONGENITAL DEFICIENCY OF ANTERIOR ABDOMINAL WALL

BY

GEORGE JOHNSTONE

*From Muhimbili Hospital, Dar es Salaam, Tanzania*

(RECEIVED FOR PUBLICATION JANUARY 4, 1965)

Abnormalities of the liver, though varied, are rare, are of little clinical importance, rarely require treatment, and are usually discovered at necropsy. The case about to be described confutes the latter statements, because the abnormality was obvious at birth and required treatment. Meckel (1822) reported several cases of accessory lobes of the liver. Jacquemet (1896) and Forni (1915) reviewed the published material. Cullen (1925) in an exhaustive review mentioned 91 cases. This article deals with an African child born with an accessory lobe of the liver projecting through a hiatus in the upper anterior abdominal wall. In addition the child had solitary dextrocardia and two nipples on the left side.

### Case Report

On October 21, 1963, a female African child was seen 5 hours after birth with a bluish-red sausage-like mass projecting through a gap in the left lower thoracic region (Fig. 1). It appeared between two nipples, of which one was slightly higher and the other considerably lower than the right nipple. There was granulation tissue at the lower end of the gap through which the mass projected (Fig. 2). There was no bleeding or discharge and the mass could be reduced within the integuments. It was not possible to say from where it was arising nor from which cavity. The site of the gap and the colour of the mass gave rise to the erroneous impression that this was herniated collapsed lung tissue. The heart was displaced to the right side. The child otherwise appeared to be healthy.

**Operation.** At operation on October 23, the mass was reduced and it was seen that the edges of the gap were fused and that there were exuberant granulations at the lower end. An incision was made over the lower ribs to include the edges of the gap. The pleural cavity was opened and a normal inflated lung was found. The pleural cavity was closed and the original incision extended downwards as an upper paramedian incision. The abdominal cavity was entered and the mass was found to be projecting from the antero-superior border of the left lobe of the liver (Fig. 3). The mass, which was broader at the base than at the tip, was approximately 5 cm. long by 2 cm. broad at the base. The outer layer was continuous with the surface of the liver but there was a marked colour change between the liver and the pro-

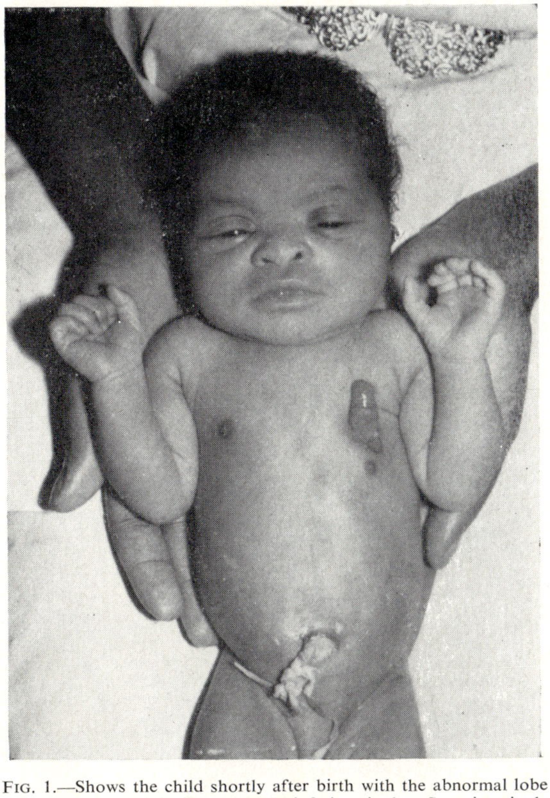

FIG. 1.—Shows the child shortly after birth with the abnormal lobe projecting on the left side above the inferior nipple. Superior nipple obscured.

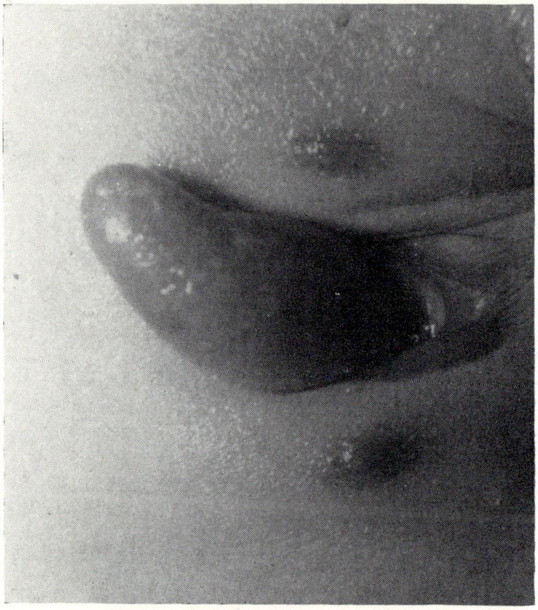

FIG. 2.—The liver projection has moved medially. Both nipples shown, also the exuberant granulation tissue at the lower end of the hiatus.

jection. The mass was transfixed, ligated at its base, and then excised. No other abnormalities of the liver were discovered. The wound was closed in layers.

**Post-operative.** A chest radiograph 3 days after operation showed that the left lung was expanded and that the heart was still on the right side.

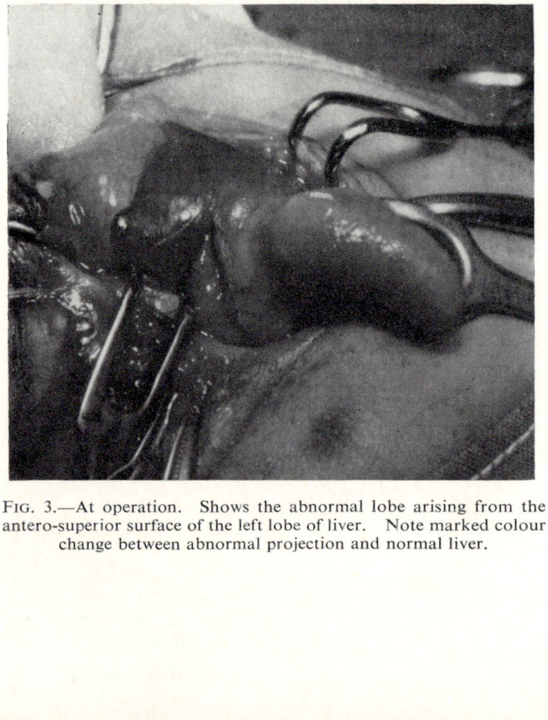

FIG. 3.—At operation. Shows the abnormal lobe arising from the antero-superior surface of the left lobe of liver. Note marked colour change between abnormal projection and normal liver.

**Histology.** Sections of the tissue showed an outer layer of necrosis with a deeper layer of granulation tissue. Deep to this again there was recognizable normal liver tissue with a polymorph infiltration which gradually lessened in the depths of the tissue.

The post-operative convalescence was uneventful and the child was discharged with a well-healed wound on November 2, 1963. She was readmitted on November 20, 1963. A barium meal with follow-through showed that there were no abnormalities of rotation of the gut. Electrocardiograms were inconclusive. The child was again seen at 7 months of age. Chest radiograph showed persistent dextrocardia (Fig. 4). The child's general condition was good (Fig. 5). She measured 24 in. (61 cm.) in length and weighed 12 lb. 3 oz. (5·5 kg.). There was a depression of the chest wall at the site of incision, and both left nipples were smaller than the one on the right side. The sclerotics were a light china blue but there was no evidence of cyanosis.

## Discussion

The child when first seen was 5 hours old, and despite the abnormalities her general condition was good. The bluish-red mass projected upwards and towards the left from the gap in the left hypochondrium. It was mobile and easily reduced within the body cavity. Difficulty in diagnosis arose because of the site and the colour. Intra-abdominal examination was kept to a minimum, but if it had been more extensive then there is little doubt that an accurate diagnosis could have been made.

No explanation for this abnormal projection from an apparently otherwise normal liver can be given. As the result of occupying an abnormal position and being outside the normal habitat of the liver the surface was necrotic, but the deeper tissues were protected by the formation of granulation tissue. The granulation tissue had spread on to the normal liver surface but stopped abruptly at a line where the liver was protected from external influences. There was a marked colour change at the junction of the abnormal projection with the liver.

The liver, in the developing embryo, occupies most of the space of the upper abdominal cavity. At the 35 mm. stage it is approximately 10% of the body weight. After this the growth rate diminishes, the left lobe growing more slowly than the right, so that at birth the liver is only 5% of the body weight (Hamilton, Boyd, and Mossman, 1962). The left lobe is directly related to the anterior abdominal wall in a small area of the epigastrium in the left substernal angle (Hollinshead, 1956). This abnormal projection would therefore be in direct contact with the developing anterior abdominal wall. The somatopleure is very thin and transparent. Thickening starts dorsally and advances ventrally until in the late embryonic period there is only a

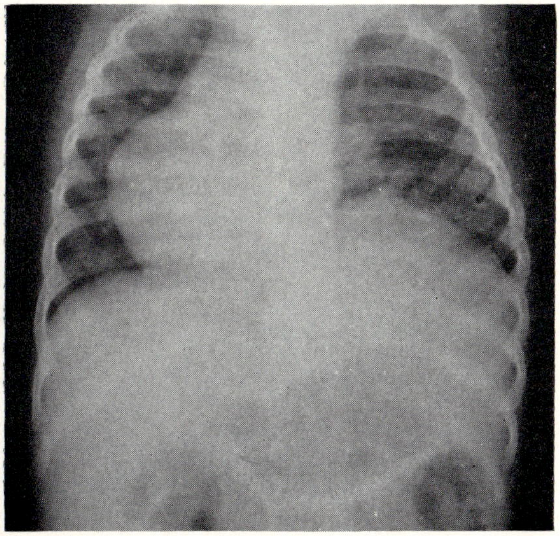

FIG. 4.—Chest radiograph of May 22, 1964, shows persistent dextrocardia.

broad diamond-shaped transparent area around the attachment of the umbilical cord (Hamilton *et al.*, 1962). As the hiatus in the child's anterior abdominal wall had fused edges one can only presume that the abnormal lobe of liver perforated and projected through the somatopleure and thus prevented the development and ultimate fusion of the elements of the anterior abdominal wall.

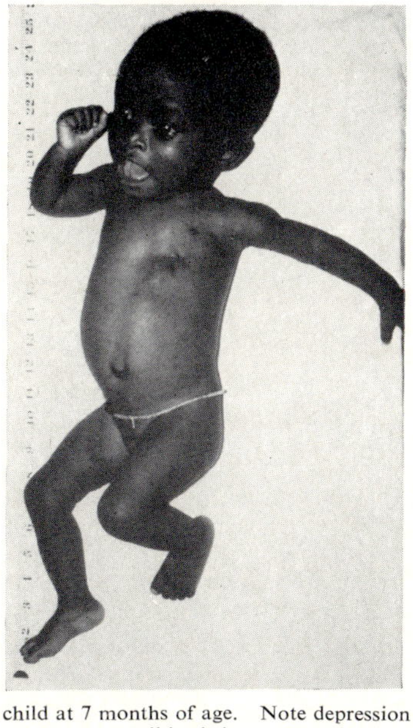

FIG. 5.—The child at 7 months of age. Note depression at centre of well-healed scar.

Though the gap in the anterior abdominal wall is directly attributable to the abnormal lobe of liver, there appears to be no relation between these abnormalities, the dextrocardia, and the multiple nipples. The nipples were left pending future developments and elective surgery.

The dextrocardia appears to be the rare variety of isolated congenital dextrocardia in which the other viscera are in the normal position. This variety is usually associated with grave cardiac anomalies. The latter have not, so far, been found in this child.

Anomalies in the size and shape of the liver are common but accessory lobes less so. Abnormalities are usually discovered at necropsy or, occasionally, at operation. Cullen (1925) listed the abnormalities as (1) diminution in size of one or more lobes, (2) hypertrophy of one or more lobes, (3) marked furrowing, (4) marked lobulation, (5) Riedel's lobe, (6) thoracic displacement of the liver through a congenital deficiency in the diaphragm, (7) accessory lobes, either attached directly to the liver by hepatic tissue or by a mesentery, (8) part of the liver appearing in an amniotic hernia, (9) accessory lobes arising from the gall-bladder, and (10) liver tissue embedded in the suprarenal gland.

Messing and Ashley-Montagu (1932) reported the absence of the left lobe, and Wakefield (1899) reported a congenital malformation with absence of the Spigellian lobe, rudimentary quadrate and left lobes, and an enlarged right lobe. Chouke (1932) reported an anomalous lobe of the liver. All these were discovered at necropsy. Friedman, Solis-Cohen, and Levine (1947) made a radiological diagnosis of an accessory lobe arising from the superior surface of the right lobe of the liver by means of a diagnostic pneumoperitoneum.

Riedel's lobe is the commonest abnormality of the liver. Thoracic displacement of the liver through a congenital gap in the diaphragm is usually incompatible with life, and where part of the liver appears in an amniotic hernia resection of part of the liver may be necessary before the abdominal contents can be reduced.

Accessory lobes of the liver are subdivided into (1) those attached to the liver by a pedicle of liver tissue and (2) those connected to the liver by a mesentery (Cullen, 1925). For their viability it is essential that accessory lobes have a hepatic artery, hepatic vein, portal vein, and a bile-duct. They usually communicate through the liver but occasionally they have made systemic connexions outside of the liver. The case reported had a sessile attachment to the antero-superior border of the left lobe of the liver and presumably had the necessary arteries, veins, and duct. The accessory lobes arising from the gall-bladder may be attached either by a pedicle or a mesentery.

Accessory lobes of the liver are of little clinical importance because they are usually situated on the deep surface of the liver, cause no disturbance, and do not require to be removed. However, the case being reported required treatment because of the exteriorization of the abnormal lobe and the gap in the upper abdominal wall. In Inglis' (1911) case the accessory lobe was palpable during life, appeared to expand and pulsate, but as it caused no pain or discomfort was left alone, and its nature was only discovered at necropsy. Cullen (1925) reported a case with recurrent epigastric pain, nausea, vomiting, and faintness, where at operation the fibrous pedicle of an accessory lobe from the right lobe of the liver had undergone strangulation due to twisting of the pedicle.

Calori's (1880) case had supernumerary digits on the right foot and in the case quoted by Cullen (1925), where liver tissue was found embedded in one of the suprarenals, there were congenital cardiac abnormalities. The present case has a supernumerary nipple on the left side and there is radiological evidence of isolated dextrocardia but so far congenital defects of the heart have not been detected and the child remains well.

## Summary

The case of a newborn child with an accessory lobe of the liver, a hiatus of the anterior abdominal wall, isolated dextrocardia, and multiple nipples is presented. The development of the liver and abdominal wall is considered and the available published material on abnormalities of the liver is reviewed. The significance of isolated dextrocardia is mentioned, and it is noted that liver abnormalities are usually only discovered at necropsy.

I wish to thank Dr. W. J. Maelor Evans, Chief Medical Officer, Ministry of Health, Tanzania, for his permission to publish this article and Dr. G. Rutledge for referring the patient. I also wish to express my thanks and appreciation to Drs. P. Grech, M. T. Maletnlema, Eccles, and G. A. S. Kombe for their help, and Dr. J. Hamerton for the photographs.

### References

Calori, L. (1880). Sulla coesistenza di un' eccessiva divisione del fegato e di qualche dito soprannumerario nelle mani o nei piedi. *Mem. R. Accad. Bologna*, **2**, 335.

Chouke, K. S. (1932). A note on an anomalous lobe of the liver. *Anat. Rec.*, **53**, 177.

Cullen, T. S. (1925). Accessory lobes of the liver. An accessory hepatic lobe springing from the surface of the gallbladder. *Arch. Surg.*, **11**, 718.

Forni, G. (1915). Contributo allo studio del cosidetto fegato accessorio. *Boll. Sci. med.*, 3, 106.

Friedman, P. S., Solis-Cohen, L., and Levine, S. (1947). Accessory lobe of the liver and its significance in roentgen diagnosis. *Amer. J. Roentgenol.*, **57**, 601.

Hamilton, W. J., Boyd, J. D., and Mossman, H. W. (1962). *Human Embryology*, 3rd ed., pp. 241, and 420-421. W. Heffer, Cambridge.

Hollinshead, W. H. (1956). *Anatomy for Surgeons*, Vol. 2, p. 317. Cassell, London.

Inglis, J. P. P. (1911). Extra extrinsic hepatic lobe. *Polyclinic*, **15**, 9.

Jacquemet, M. (1896). Considérations sur les anomalies du foie et des voies bilaires. Thèse de Lyon.

Meckel, J. F. (1822). *Tabulae Anatomico-Pathologicae*, Fasc. III., p. 14, Tabula XXIV. I. F. Gleditsch, Leipzig.

Messing, A., and Ashley-Montagu, M. F. (1932). A note on a case of complete absence of the left lobe of the liver in man. *Anat. Rec.*, 53, 169.

Wakefield, P. A. (1899). Congenital malformation of the liver: absence of the lobus Spigelii, rudimentary quadrate and left lobes, with enlargement of the right lobe. *J. Anat.* (*Lond.*), 33, 50.

*Arch. Dis. Childh.*, 1965, **40**, 545.

# DIVERTICULUM OF THE LEFT VENTRICLE

## REPORT OF A CASE

BY

EL-SAYED EL-AKKARI, M. KAMAL BADR EL-DIN, and A. SAMIR KASSEM

*From the Faculty of Medicine, Alexandria University, Alexandria, U.A.R.*

(RECEIVED FOR PUBLICATION JANUARY 5, 1965)

Congenital diverticulum of the left ventricle of the heart is considered to be a rare malformation. Up to 1958, Keith, Rowe, and Vlad could only collect 13 cases from the published reports. Successful operations had been recorded by Roessler (1944), Skapinker (1951), Potts, DeBoer, and Johnson (1953), and Mustard, Duckworth, Rowe, and Dolan (1958).

The purpose of this paper is to present the clinical angiocardiographic, surgical, and pathological data in an infant with congenital diverticulum of the left ventricle of the heart.

### Case Report

A boy aged 4 days was admitted to the hospital on February 2, 1964, presenting with a pulsating mass inside a huge ventral hernia. He had been born at full term, the product of a normal gestation and spontaneous delivery. Parents were first cousins.

*Physical examination* revealed a non-cyanotic infant, in no distress, weighing 3,700 g. There was no clubbing of the fingers or toes. The respiratory rate was 40 a minute, and the pulse rate was 130 a minute. The radial and femoral pulsations were normal. The blood pressure in the right arm was 75/50 mm.Hg.

*Clinical examination* of the heart revealed no praecordial bulge. The apex was in the 5th left intercostal space, one finger's breadth inside the nipple line. There were no other pulsations over the praecordium and there were no thrills. Auscultation revealed a soft systolic murmur, grade 2/6, heard maximally over the lower part of the sternum and down over the pulsating mass.

*Abdominal examination* revealed a huge ventral hernia extending from the xiphoid process to the umbilicus (Fig. 1). The skin covering it was thin and deeply pigmented. The hernia was bulging through a huge defect in the anterior abdominal wall, and at the upper part of the hernia a pulsating tubular mass ($3 \times 1 \cdot 5$ cm.) was seen protruding out just below the xiphisternum. Its pulsations were synchronous with those of the heart, and firm pressure on it provoked extrasystoles.

The liver was not enlarged and the spleen was not palpable.

*Radiography* revealed that the soft tissue shadow of the pulsating mass was continuous with the cardiac shadow (Fig. 2).

*Electrocardiogram* revealed right axis deviation, and vertical heart, the praecordial leads showing evidence of right and left ventricular hypertrophy.

Operation was postponed for about three weeks because of mild umbilical sepsis. During this time there was an increase in the size both of the ventral hernia and of the pulsating mass. The infant was operated on at the age of 1 month, the operation being done under general anaesthesia with fluothane, nitrous oxide, and oxygen. Exploration was performed through a hockey-stick thoraco-abdominal incision extending from the left nipple through the 5th intercostal space down to the xiphoid process and extending in the middle line to the umbilicus. Dissection of the upper part of the hernia revealed the presence of a diverticulum of the heart which was covered by pericardium only on its anterior surface. The diverticulum was bulging through a defect between the two slips of the diaphragm arising from the xiphoid process. The ventral hernia was covered with a peritoneal sac independent from the diverticulum.

Operative angiography revealed the continuity of the diverticular cavity with that of the left ventricle. It also demonstrated the simultaneous opacification of the aorta and the pulmonary artery. The pericardial covering was dissected from the diverticulum, and a Potts clamp was applied to its base at its junction with the left ventricle. During the application of the clamp the electrocardiogram revealed a temporary bradycardia with evident S-T change which returned to normal after removal of the clamp. The diverticulum was excised and the base was stitched by interrupted mattress suture; the endocardium was closed; the muscle coat was sutured in another layer; the clamp was released and the sutures were made water-tight. The defect in the diaphragm was easily closed by interrupted silk sutures. The chest was closed leaving a drain. The electrocardiogram showed changes in the S-T segment when the diverticulum was cut, and these

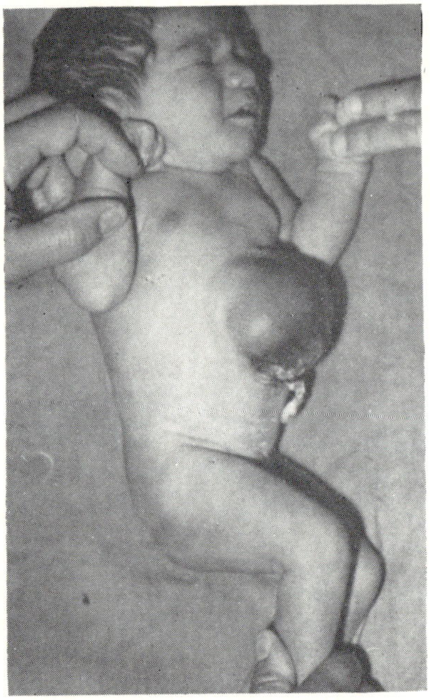

FIG. 1.—A huge ventral hernia with a pulsating tubular mass in its upper part.

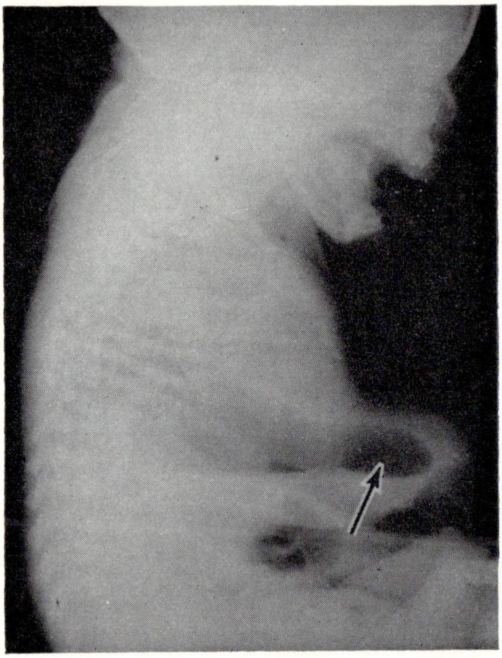

FIG. 2.—Lateral radiograph showing the soft tissue shadow of the diverticulum (arrow) to be continuous with the cardiac shadow.

persisted throughout the rest of the operation. Apart from these changes the beats were regular and the voltage was normal. Reduction of the contents of the ventral hernia as a test for distress did not produce any further change in the cardiogram, and this encouraged us to proceed with hernial repair at the same time. The sac was excised and abdominal exploration did not reveal any gastro-intestinal anomaly. The contents were reduced and the defect in the anterior abdominal wall was closed.

Half an hour after the end of the operation, which passed smoothly, sudden ventricular fibrillation developed and the child died soon afterwards.

**Necropsy.** Apart from the diverticulum the heart revealed a huge ventricular septal defect in the membraneous part measuring about 12 mm. in diameter.

Histological examination of the diverticulum revealed that the main bulk of the diverticular wall was made up of cardiac muscle fibres arranged in all directions in which neither Purkinje fibres nor nodal tissue was seen. The framework was made up of connective tissue rich in elastic fibres, and the diverticulum was lined with endothelium. The outside covering was a serous membrane with subpericardial connective tissue rich in fat cells and containing numerous blood vessels.

## Comment

In this case, apart from the presence of a true congenital cardiac diverticulum, there were other congenital abnormalities, namely, defects in the basilar pericardium, and in the ventral portion of the diaphragm, and a huge defect in the anterior abdominal wall. The association of these congenital anomalies confirms the suggestion of Potts *et al.* (1953) that the condition is primarily due to some abnormality of the septum transversum. This latter normally gives rise to the basilar portion of the pericardium, the ventral leaf of the diaphragm, and the ventral cephalic part of the abdominal wall (Politzer and Sternberg, 1930; Margulies, 1945). During development the epicardium of the cardiac loop fuses to the ventral leaf of the septum transversum, and as the latter descends the attached epimyocardium is pulled ventrally and caudally and a true congenital diverticulum results.

The high mortality in the reported infants who were not corrected by surgery warranted early operation. Although this was completed successfully, ventricular fibrillation set in soon afterwards and the child died.

It seems advisable to manage this type of case in two stages, first to excise the diverticulum and later to deal with the ventral hernia. The correction of the latter in the same stage may put too much strain on the heart, especially in the presence of intracardiac defects.

REFERENCES

Keith, J. D., Rowe, R. D., and Vlad, P. (1958). *Heart Disease in Infancy and Childhood*, p. 599. Macmillan, New York.

Margulies, L. (1945). Omphalocele (amniocele): its anatomy and etiology in relation to hernias of umbilicus and the umbilical cord. *Amer. J. Obstet. Gynec.*, **49**, 695.

Mustard, W. T., Duckworth, J. W. A., Rowe, R. D., and Dolan, F. G. (1958). Congenital diverticulum of the left ventricle of the heart. *Canad. J. Surg.*, **1**, 149.

Politzer, G., and Sternberg, H. (1930). Über die Entwicklung der ventralen Körperwand und des Nabelstranges beim Menschen. *Z. Anat. Entwickl.-Gesch.*, **92**, 279.

Potts, W. J., DeBoer, A., and Johnson, F. R. (1953). Congenital diverticulum of the left ventricle. *Surgery*, **33**, 301.

Roessler, W. (1944). Erfolgreiche operative Entçernung eines ektopischen Herzdivertikels an einem Neugeborenen. *Dtsch. Z. Chir.*, **258**, 561.

Skapinker, S. (1951). Diverticulum of the left ventricle of the heart. *Arch. Surg.*, **63**, 629.

*Arch. Dis. Childh.*, 1965, **40**, 548.

# THE CAUSES OF CONGENITAL CLUB FOOT

BY

EVA D. ALBERMAN

*From the Paediatric Research Unit, Guy's Hospital Medical School, London*

(RECEIVED FOR PUBLICATION JANUARY 4, 1965)

. . . 'I devoted much attention to the nature of these distortions, from the circumstance of my being afflicted with Talipes in the left foot.'

*William Little* (1839)

Hippocrates was the first to suggest that permanent crippling can follow abnormal intrauterine pressure. More recently, Browne (1936) has been the foremost exponent of the view that this is a major cause of congenital club feet. The theory had first been challenged in the early 19th century by the authors of several very detailed studies on the condition. Little (1839) felt that the variety of deformities found in club feet could not be accounted for by the pressure theory, or by the theory of arrested foetal development, as suggested by von Walther (1833). Little, like Guérin (1839), considered that as in club foot of postnatal onset, congenital talipes is due to muscle paralysis or spasm. Adams (1873) also inclined towards this 'dynamic' theory, but thought that in some cases, particularly of talipes calcaneous or calcaneovalgus, the origin was mechanical distortion.

All authors acknowledge the strong family history in about one-tenth of patients with foot deformities, and the frequent coexistence of other congenital defects. Ehrenfried (1912) found associated anomalies in 13·4% of the 232 cases he investigated. Crabbe (1960) in a review of 172 patients with congenital talipes found associated congenital defects in 11·2%. He pointed out that mechanical compression could not account for the significant increase of anomalies such as arachnodactyly, cleft palate, webbing of the toes, and sacral agenesis, which are probably faults in mesenchymal differentiation. Wynne-Davies (1964) has recently reported the results of family studies on 635 patients with club feet, and also concluded that defective formation of connective tissue was an important aetiological factor.

Previous investigations have been carried out on patients attending orthopaedic clinics, so that babies with associated lethal malformations or those with very slight deformities have been excluded. A study of all babies with foot deformities noted in a consecutive series of births gives an estimate of the incidence of each type, together with associated anomalies, and an indication of any predisposing factors in pregnancy.

In the following account, the birth and antenatal records of 170 babies with foot deformities delivered at Queen Charlotte's Maternity Hospital during the years 1958 to 1961 are compared with those of a control series.

## Method

The birth records of 170 babies noted to have foot deformities at birth in Queen Charlotte's Maternity Hospital during the years 1958 to 1961 were studied and relevant details abstracted. Similar details were abstracted from a control series of 170 births immediately preceding them in the labour ward register.

All babies born at this hospital are examined by the obstetric house surgeon and are referred to the paediatrician if any abnormality is found. Classification of the deformities was made on the basis of the description in the records. The patients were placed into the following categories: talipes equinovarus, talipes calcaneovalgus, metatarsus varus, and a fourth class of mixed or other clinical types. Patients with deformities of which the clinical description was not sufficiently detailed to allow classification were included in the latter group. Table 1 gives the numbers in each clinical group.

Among the 170 cases were 3 pairs of sibs born at Queen Charlotte's during the period of the study. Both of one pair suffered from talipes equinovarus, both of the second were described as having 'talipes' and were in the 'other' group, and one of the third pair had metatarsus varus while her sib was in the 'other' group. There were, therefore, 3 less mothers than there were patients with foot deformities, 167 compared with 170 controls. Only one of each of the 5 pairs of twins in the series had been affected. Two had been like sex pairs but in both the placenta was considered to be binovular in type, and it is, therefore, probable that all 5 pairs were dizygotic.

TABLE 1
NUMBERS OF TWINS AND SINGLETONS IN CLINICAL CATEGORIES

| Clinical Category | Talipes Equinovarus | Talipes Calcaneovalgus | Metatarsus Varus | Mixed or Other | All | Controls |
|---|---|---|---|---|---|---|
| Singletons | 36 | 32 | 34 | 63 | 165 | 169 |
| Twins | 0 | 0 | 0 | 5 | 5 | 1 |
| All | 36 | 32 | 34 | 68 | 170 | 170 |

Only information available from the records was considered, and family histories were those obtained as a routine at the booking visit. The length of gestation was calculated from the recorded date of the first day of the last menstrual period.

The tests of significance used were the $\chi^2$ test using fourfold tables and Yates' correction, the difference between proportions, and Student's 't' test for the difference between means. A 5% level of probability or less was accepted as statistically significant.

## Results

**The Incidence of Foot Deformities.** The 170 babies in this study were derived from 12,048 births which included 466 stillbirths and neonatal deaths. This gave an incidence of 14·1 babies recorded as having foot deformities in 1,000 births. The incidence of each clinical type is given in Table 2.

TABLE 2
INCIDENCE OF CLINICAL TYPES IN TOTAL BIRTHS

| Clinical Type | Incidence per Thousand Total Births (Nos. in brackets) |
|---|---|
| Talipes equinovarus | 3·0 (36) |
| Talipes calcaneovalgus | 2·7 (32) |
| Metatarsus varus | 2·8 (34) |
| Mixed and 'others' | 5·6 (68) |
| All | 14·1 (170) |

**The Mothers.** The mothers of the cases were recorded as having slightly, though not significantly, more congenital malformations. Four mothers had had operations for congenital malformations. One who had bunions and flat feet had undergone surgery at the age of 11 years, two others had had a congenital dislocation of the hips, and the fourth had had torticollis. No record of any foot deformity was found in these last three patients. Antepartum diagnosis of uterine malformations was slightly more common amongst the mothers of the affected babies, but the excess was not significant.

No significant difference was found between the mean maternal age of the propositi and that of the controls. Although the proportion of primiparae amongst the mothers of the propositi was consistently higher than that in the controls, this excess was significant only in the group with talipes calcaneovalgus, in which three-quarters of the babies had been firstborn compared with just over one-half of the controls ($p < 0\cdot05$).

These findings are set out in detail in Table 3.

**Pregnancy and Delivery.** Table 4 gives some details of the pregnancies and deliveries of the cases and controls. There were few differences between these, the only difference of statistical significance being the longer mean period of gestation of babies

TABLE 3
MEAN MATERNAL AGE, PRIMIPARITY, AND CONGENITAL DEFECTS OF THE MOTHERS

| | Talipes Equinovarus | Talipes Calcaneovalgus | Metatarsus Varus | Mixed or 'Other' | Controls |
|---|---|---|---|---|---|
| Mean maternal age (yr.) (No. known in brackets) | 27·2 (35) | 26·8 (32) | 27·2 (34) | 26·6 (68) | 26·2 (170) |
| Per cent. primiparae | 61·1 | 75·0 | 55·9 | 57·3 | 51·8 |
| Congenital malformations | Flat feet and bunions at 11 years<br>Bicornuate uterus | Congenital dislocation of hips—arthrodesis | Congenital pulmonary stenosis<br>Arcuate uterus | Dysplasia of the hip—'shelf' operation<br>Torticollis<br>Double vagina and uterus | Bunions<br>Spondylolisthesis<br>Cleft palate<br>Uterus arcuformis<br>?? Bicornuate uterus |
| | 2 in 35 mothers 5·7% | 1 in 32 mothers 3·1% | 2 in 34 mothers 5·9% | 3 in 67 mothers 4·5% | 5 in 170 mothers 2·9% |

TABLE 4

PREGNANCY AND DELIVERY

| | Talipes Equinovarus | | | | Talipes Calcaneovalgus (32) | | Metatarsus Varus (34) | | Others (68) | | Controls (170) | |
|---|---|---|---|---|---|---|---|---|---|---|---|---|
| | With Associated Defect (12)* | | Without Associated Defect (24)* | | | | | | | | | |
| | No. | % | No. | % | No. | % | No. | % | No. | % | No. | % |
| Attempted version (failed and successful) | 2 | (17) | 2 | (8) | 2 | 6 | 0 | 0 | 7 | 10 | 29 | 17 |
| Breech delivery | 4 | (33) | 0 | (0) | 1 | 3 | 0 | 0 | 3 | 4 | 5 | 3 |
| Caesarean section | 0 | (0) | 0 | (0) | 0 | 0 | 4 | 12 | 4 | 6 | 9 | 5 |
| Mean length of gestation (wk.) | 39·5 (2 unknown) | | 39·1 (4 unknown) | | 39·7 (2 unknown) | | 40·9 (2 unknown) | | 40·0 (4 unknown) | | 39·8 (11 unknown) | |

* Where there are fewer than 30 cases the percentages are given in parentheses.

TABLE 5

PROPORTION OF BOYS AND MEAN BIRTH WEIGHT OF BABIES

| Clinical Type | No. | Mean Birth Weight (lb.) | Boys | |
|---|---|---|---|---|
| | | | No. | % |
| Talipes equinovarus (with associated defect) | 12 | 6·8 (1 unknown) | 8 | (67) |
| Talipes equinovarus (without associated defect) | 24 | 7·2 | 14 | (58) |
| Talipes calcaneovalgus | 32 | 6·7 | 11 | 34 |
| Metatarsus varus | 34 | 7·7 | 14 | 41 |
| Mixed or 'other' | 68 | 7·0 | 30 | 44 |
| Controls | 170 | 7·3 | 83 | 49 |

Where there are fewer than 30 cases the percentages are given in parentheses.

with metatarsus varus, over a week longer than that of the controls ($p < 0{\cdot}05$). Also in this group more than 1 in 10 babies were delivered by caesarean section, twice as many as in the controls, but this difference is not statistically significant. The proportion of breech delivery among babies with foot deformities was slightly, but again not significantly, higher than among the controls.

**The Babies.** In Table 5 are set out the mean birth weights and the proportion of boys in the cases and the controls.

An excess of boys was found among all babies with talipes equinovarus, in the proportion of 1·6 to 1. In contrast, an excess of girls was found in the other types of foot deformities, most marked among the babies with talipes calcaneovalgus, in whom the proportion was 1·9 to 1.

The mean birth weight of most groups of babies with foot deformities was very similar to that of the controls, when allowance was made for length of gestation, birth order, and sex ratio. The one exception was the group of babies with talipes equinovarus associated with other malformations, in which the mean birth weight was lower than that of controls of similar gestational age.

More associated defects were reported in the babies with foot deformities than might have been expected in comparison with the controls. In the latter, a congenital defect was noted in 16 out of 170 babies (9·4%). Defects other than those of the feet were noted in 12 (33%) of the talipes equinovarus group, 7 (22%) of the talipes calcaneovalgus group, 8 (24%) of the metatarsus varus group, and 8 (12%) of the remaining babies with foot deformities. The defects are listed in Table 6.

**Congenital Defects in Older Sibs.** In all, the control babies had a total of 140 older sibs. Of these, 5 (3·6%) were known to have had severe congenital malformations (Table 7). The babies with talipes equinovarus had 30 older sibs and 4 (13·3%) had had severe malformations, significantly more than in the controls ($p < 0{\cdot}05$). In order to determine whether a history of malformations in older sibs was confined to propositi who themselves had malformations other than of the feet, the group of talipes equinovarus patients was divided into those in whom this was the sole apparent defect, and those in whom it was associated with any other malformation. The 12 propositi with associated defects had only 3 older sibs between them, and of these one had died with hydrocephalus and spina bifida. The remaining 24 without associated defects had 27 older sibs; of these 2 had died with central nervous system malformations, and one had

TABLE 6
ASSOCIATED ANOMALIES

| Case No. and Sex | Associated anomalies | Survival |
|---|---|---|
| *Talipes Equinovarus* (36)—33% incidence | | |
| 1 M | Hydrocephalus and lumbar meningomyelocele, paralysis of lower limbs; anterior dislocation of knees | |
| 2 F | Hydrocephalus; meningomyelocele; Arnold-Chiari malformation; congenital dislocation of hip | Died |
| 3 M | Potter's facies; hydrocephalus; meningomyelocele; Arnold-Chiari malformation; renal agenesis; congenital dislocation of hip | Died |
| 4 F | Oxycephalic appearance (later developed pyloric stenosis and died with hydrocephalus) | Died |
| 5 M | Small pilonidal sinus | |
| 6 M | Small pilonidal sinus | |
| 7 F | Slightly crooked face | |
| 8 M | Asymmetrical head | |
| 9 M | R. leg hyperflexed, ankle by R. ear; cauliflower ears; constriction ring at base of penis | |
| 10 M | Tibial recurvatae; four toes on each foot | |
| 11 F | Marked capillary naevus on forehead | |
| 12 M | Umbilical hernia | |
| *Talipes Calcaneovalgus* (32)—22% incidence | | |
| 13 F | Suspicion of pilonidal sinus | |
| 14 F | Asymmetrical head; small occipital lump | |
| 15 F | Asymmetrical face: nose to left, jaw to right. ? 3rd fontanelle | |
| 16 M | Compression—left ear applied to left shoulder | |
| 17 M | Branchial cleft sinus | |
| 18 F | Vascular naevus of abdomen | |
| 19 M | Abnormal nose, ears, eyes; limited knee extension; short fleshy neck; micrognathos; microphallus; atresia or coarctation of aorta; cor biloculare; diaphragmatic hernia, pulmonary hypoplasia | Died |
| *Metatarsus Varus* (34)—24% incidence | | |
| 20 F | Two accessory nipples right ear | |
| 21 M | Hypospadias; accessory auricle right ear | |
| 22 F | Accessory auricle left ear | |
| 23 M | Pilonidal sinus; small penis | |
| 24 F | 'Mongoloid but not mongol' | |
| 25 M | Congenital heart defect | |
| 26 M | Bulging right parietal region | |
| 27 F | Umbilical hernia | |
| *Mixed or Others* (68)—12% incidence | | |
| 28 M | Deep sacrococcygeal pit | |
| 29 M | Bilateral aural tags | |
| 30 F | Torticollis | |
| 31 F | Torticollis | |
| 32 M | Dysplasia of hip (familial); mild hypospadias | |
| 33 F | Bilateral simple cataract | |
| 34 M | Abnormality of whole of right leg and pelvis; inguinal hernia (later developed medulloblastoma) | |
| 35 M | Exomphalos; cleft palate and lip; malrotation of heart; stenosis of pelvi-ureteral junction | Stillbirth |
| *Controls* (170)—9·4% incidence | | |
| 36 F | Capillary naevus upper lip, and tip and bridge of nose | |
| 37 M | Accessory auricle of ear | |
| 38 F | All joints lax; small angioma | |
| 39 M | Large fontanelle and wide sutures | |

TABLE 6 (*continued*)

| Case No. and Sex | Associated anomalies | Survival |
|---|---|---|
| 40 M | Mild hypertelorism and small lump on forehead | |
| 41 M | Club hand; horseshoe kidney | Stillbirth |
| 42 F | ? Pilonidal sinus | |
| 43 F | Capillary haemangioma; left upper lid and centre of forehead | |
| 44 M | Heart murmur (later ? mild pulmonary stenosis) | |
| 45 M | Renal hypoplasia; bilateral inguinal herniae | Died at 4 mth. |
| 46 F | Congenital heart disease | |
| 47 M | ? Mucous tag in mouth | Died at 1 yr. |
| 48 M | L. lateral fontanelle; pedunculated tumour on right little finger | |
| 49 M | Webbing of 2nd and 3rd toes | |
| 50 F | Sternomastoid swelling (later found to have spastic paraplegia) | |
| 51 F | Umbilical hernia | |

congenital heart disease. This proportion with malformations, 3 in 27 (11%), was over three times as large as that in the control group, though the difference no longer reached the 5% level of significance.

There were 2 patients of particular interest in the group. One mother who had a bicornuate uterus had first a stillbirth with iniencephaly and then a baby with apparently uncomplicated talipes equinovarus. A second mother, who had had a myomectomy for the removal of 25 fibroids and had many remaining fibroids, had borne a child with talipes equinovarus who had died with hydrocephalus, followed by a baby with apparently uncomplicated talipes equinovarus.

No congenital malformations had been reported amongst the older sibs of babies with metatarsus varus or talipes calcaneovalgus, but in the remaining group of mixed and 'other' cases, 5 out of 51 previous sibs (9·8%) had had foot deformities. No foot deformities had been recorded among older sibs of the controls.

## Discussion

**Incidence.** The incidence of foot deformities in this series of hospital births was 14·1 per 1,000 total births. This is a little higher than the incidence reported in a recent series of hospital births (Marden, Smith, and McDonald, 1964), in which the incidence of equinovarus, severe calcaneovalgus, and severe metatarsus adductus deformities together was 8·2 per 1,000. However, the latter series did not include any stillbirths, and it is likely that the present series includes more mild deformities.

In the present series there were 5 times as many twins among the affected babies as among the controls. While this difference was not statistically significant, this slight excess was similar to that

TABLE 7

MALFORMATIONS IN OLDER SIBS

| | Talipes Equinovarus | Talipes Calcaneo-valgus | Metatarsus Varus | Mixed or 'Other' | Controls |
|---|---|---|---|---|---|
| No. of all older sibs | 30 | 20 | 23 | 51 | 140 |
| Congenital malformations recorded | Hydrocephalus and spina bifida<br>* ? Hydrocephalus; talipes (died)<br>Iniencephaly<br>Congenital heart disease | — | — | * Talipes<br>* Talipes<br>Talipes<br>Talipes<br>Talipes | Anencephaly and spina bifida<br>Anencephaly<br>Achondroplasia<br>'Progressive spinal atrophy'<br>'Congenital malformation'; ? type |
| Total incidence (%) .. .. | 13·3 | — | — | 9·8 | 3·6 |

* Included in series.

found by Ehrenfried (1912) in a series of patients with a foot deformity.

**Clinical Types.** It is clear that the term congenital club foot comprises a heterogeneous group of conditions. There are three main clinical types: talipes equinovarus, talipes calcaneovalgus, and metatarsus varus. Within these are several sub-groups with differing clinical associations and, apparently, of different aetiology. The findings in the three main groups will be discussed separately.

**Talipes Equinovarus.** Malformations of the central nervous system are the major deformity in many babies with equinovarus, and in these it seems probable that the foot deformity is caused by a defect in the nerve supply to the lower limbs. In the present series an overt neurological malformation was found in 4 out of 36 babies born with talipes equinovarus. In 2 further patients with apparently uncomplicated talipes equinovarus, the history of a previous sib with a lethal malformation of the central nervous system was also suggestive of a neurological basis for the foot deformity.

Although there were no examples in this series, it is clear from the published material that congenital club foot may be associated with neurological defects other than hydrocephalus and spina bifida. It has been described in association with spastic diplegia (Ingram, 1964), with bulbar palsy (Graham, 1964), and Möbius' syndrome (congenital facial diplegia) (Evans, 1955). However, Evans suggested that in Möbius' syndrome the defect may be a congenital deficiency of the muscles rather than nuclear agenesis. Talipes equinovarus has also been described in association with undoubted skeletal or muscular defects. Case 10 (Table 6) is an example of an equinovarus deformity associated with tibiae recurvatae and 4 toes on each foot. There is also a well-recognized association between talipes and arthrogryposis.

Wynne-Davies (1964) in a painstaking survey of 163 patients with talipes equinovarus and their relatives found that there was an excess of associated malformations which could be attributable to a hereditary defect of connective tissue. A significant excess of the patients she examined had a generalized joint laxity, and she suggested that this laxity had increased the susceptibility of the foetus to intra-uterine forces. In the present series also, the finding that at least two mothers of babies with equinovarus had uterine malformations suggested that intra-uterine pressure had played some part in causing the deformity.

Equinovarus deformities of the feet, often together with facial malformations, have been described in cases of oligohydramnios, both in those with renal agenesis (Potter, 1961) and in those secondary to other causes (Bain, Smith, and Gauld, 1964). In this series, Case 9 with talipes equinovarus (Table 6), in which there had been a 7-week history of ruptured membranes, is an example of such an association. No entirely satisfactory explanation of the mechanism of the foetal deformation has yet been put forward, though it is usually attributed to 'uterine pressure' (Bain *et al.*, 1964). Drachman and Coulombre (1962) found that experimental immobilization of chick embryos was followed by the development of limb deformities and suggested that immobilization might also cause joint deformities in the human foetus.

In this, as in all previous series, boys with talipes equinovarus have exceeded girls in the ratio of about 2 to 1 (Little, 1839; Adams, 1873; Wynne-Davies, 1964). Moreover, Wynne-Davies found that male relatives of female patients are at particular risk. This apparent male susceptibility to equinovarus is intriguing in view of the high incidence of talipes equinovarus reported in patients found to have an XYY sex chromosome constitution. In 11 patients with this constitution, selected for study because of mental, genital, or familial defects, 2 were said to have talipes equinovarus (K. E. Buckton, J. A. Bond, and J. A. McBridge, 1962, personal communication; Castilla and Breg, 1963; Court Brown, Harnden, Jacobs, Maclean, and Mantle, 1964; Fraccaro, Davies, Glen Bott, and Schutt, 1962; Hustinx and Val Olphen, 1963; St. M. Milcu, I. Negoescu, M. Garoiu, I. Iliescu, M. Augustin, and C. Maximilian, 1963, personal communication; Ricci and Malacarne, 1964; Sandberg, Ishihara, Crosswhite, and Koepf, 1963; Vignetti, Capotorti, and Ferrante, 1964). In a further unpublished case (Paediatric Research Unit, H2599/359) bilateral calcaneovarus and flexion deformities of the knees were found. In patients with XXYY constitution a high proportion of skeletal malformations has also been described (Robinson, Miller, Dill, and Kamburoff, 1964), including 2 with talipes equinovarus (Barr, Carr, Soltan, Wiens, and Plunkett, 1964; Muldal, Ockey, Thompson, and White, 1962). It is noteworthy that the presence of a Y chromosome appears to increase the risk of specifically a varus deformity, while, it will be shown below, females are more likely to develop a valgus deformity.

**Talipes Calcaneovalgus.** Features of the group with talipes calcaneovalgus in this series were an excess of girls and an excess of firstborn children, findings similar to those described by Wynne-Davies (1964). Her suggestion that there was an aetiological connexion between this condition and congenital dislocation of the hip was borne out by the finding that in two babies in this series, one with calcaneovalgus and the other with a 'valgus' deformity, the mothers had suffered from congenital dislocation of the hips.

Wynne-Davies found that among patients with talipes calcaneovalgus, as among those with equinovarus, there was an excessive number with generalized joint laxity. Carter and Wilkinson (1964) suggested that in congenital dislocation of the hips an adverse uterine posture superimposed on a generalized joint laxity and a shallow acetabulum could cause the dislocation. They considered that generalized joint laxity was either familial or a temporary hormonal-induced condition in newborn girls. This hormonal-induced laxity could account for the excess of girls with congenital dislocation of the hip. It seems possible that analogous factors predispose to talipes calcaneovalgus; a combination of unduly lax ligaments, slightly abnormal articular surfaces, and unusual uterine forces. Wynne-Davies suggested that the tight abdominal musculature found in primiparae may explain the apparent increase in risk to firstborn children.

However, in the group of calcaneovalgus, as in equinovarus, there is evidence for the existence of at least one aetiological sub-group. Calcaneovalgus feet have been described in 10 out of 23 babies with $E_1$ trisomy (Polani, 1964), and the clinical features of one patient in the present series (Case 19, Table 6) would be consistent with such a diagnosis. Polani found that in this condition hypertonus was often present and hydramnios was common, features that seem to rule out the possibility that intrauterine pressure played a part in causing the deformity. Moreover, he noted that in all 12 cases in which the hips had been examined, abduction had been limited, and in two they had been dislocated. Two-thirds of the cases of $E_1$ trisomy had been girls. The similarity of these features to those in the uncomplicated cases of talipes calcaneovalgus provoke further speculation about the aetiology of the condition, but as yet the connexion between the deformity and abnormalities of the chromosomes is obscure.

**Metatarsus Varus.** In the group of patients with metatarsus varus the high incidence of associated malformations, including congenital heart disease, hypospadias, and aural tags, suggested a defect arising early in foetal development. Nevertheless in this group there is a raised incidence of postmaturity, a condition in which a decrease in liquor amnii is said to occur (Walker, 1954), again a hint that mechanical distortion *in utero* may play some part in causing the condition.

## Conclusions

The findings in the present study, as in that by Wynne-Davies (1964), confirm the complexity of factors that interact to produce congenital deformities of the feet. Methods that will help unravel the aetiology of these conditions are further intensive family studies of patients with different clinical types, and the study of more generalized congenital defects in which the foot deformity may be subsidiary to other malformations.

## Summary

Among babies born in Queen Charlotte's Maternity Hospital during the years 1958 to 1961, there were 170 with foot deformities, an incidence of 14·1 per 1,000 total births.

A study of birth histories suggested that in many of the babies the deformity had resulted from the interaction of abnormal environmental and hereditary factors. However, the predisposing causes in the different clinical types appeared to differ. Associated neurological malformations were often found in babies with talipes equinovarus, and a family history of central nervous system malformations was unduly common. No such associations were found in babies with talipes calcaneovalgus, but there were indications that the condition was related in some way to congenital dislocation of the hips.

The apparent susceptibility of males to talipes equinovarus and females to talipes calcaneovalgus is discussed in the light of their reported association with anomalies of chromosome constitution.

I am most grateful to the Board of Governors of Queen Charlotte's Hospital, and Dr. White Franklin and Dr. Norman for allowing me to study their cases. I am also indebted to Miss Terry, the Records' Officer, for her help, Professor Polani for many helpful suggestions, and to the Cytogenetic Staff of the Paediatric Research Unit for the chromosome analysis of Case H2599/359.

The work was supported by the Spastics Society.

### References

Adams, W. (1873). *Club Foot. Its Causes, Pathology and Treatment*, p. 217. Churchill, London.

Bain, A. D., Smith, I. I., and Gauld, I. K. (1964). Newborn after prolonged leakage of liquor amnii. *Brit. med. J.*, **2**, 598.

Barr, M. L., Carr, D. H., Soltan, H. C., Wiens, R. G., and Plunkett, E. R. (1964). The XXYY variant of Klinefelter's syndrome. *Canad. med. Ass. J.*, **90**, 575.

Browne, D. (1936). Congenital deformities of mechanical origin. *Proc. roy. Soc. Med.*, **29**, 1409.

Carter, C., and Wilkinson, J. (1964). Persistent joint laxity and congenital dislocation of the hip. *J. Bone Jt Surg.*, **46-B**, 40.

Castilla, E. E., and Breg, W. R. (1963). The XYY sex chromosome constitution. The National Foundation Mammalian Cytogenetics Conference, Sept. 26-28, 11.

Court Brown, W. M., Harnden, D. G., Jacobs, P. A., Maclean, N., and Mantle, D. J. (1964). Abnormalities of the sex chromosome complement in man. *Spec. Rep. Ser. med. Res. Coun. (Lond.)*, **305**, 107.

Crabbe, W. A. (1960). Aetiology of congenital talipes. *Brit. med. J.*, **2**, 1060.

Drachman, D. B., and Coulombre, A. J. (1962). Experimental club-foot and arthrogryposis multiplex congenita. *Lancet*, **2**, 523.

Ehrenfried, A. (1912). The occurrence and etiology of club-foot. *J. Amer. med Ass.*, **59**, 1940.

Evans, P. R. (1955). Nuclear agenesis. Möbius' syndrome: the congenital facial diplegia syndrome. *Arch. Dis. Childh.*, **30**, 237.

Fraccaro, M., Davies, P., Glen Bott, M., and Schutt, W. (1962). Mental deficiency and undescended testis in two males with XYY sex chromosomes. *Folia hered. path. (Milano)*, **11**, 211.

Graham, P. J. (1964). Congenital flaccid bulbar palsy. *Brit. med. J.*, **2**, 26.

Guérin, J. (1839). *Mémoire sur les Variétés Anatomiques du Pied-bot Congénital.* Cinquième Mémoire sur les Difformités du Système Osseux. Au Bureau de la Gazette Medicale, Paris.

Hustinx, T. W. J., and Val Olphen, A. H F. (1963). An XYY chromosome pattern in a boy with Marfan's syndrome. *Genetica*, **34**, 262.

Ingram, T. T. S. (1964). *Paediatric Aspects of Cerebral Palsy*, p. 243. E. & S. Livingstone, Edinburgh and London.

Little, W. J. (1839). *A Treatise on the Nature of Clubfoot and Analogous Distortions*, pp. xli & 23. W. Jeffs, London.

Marden, P. M., Smith, D. W., and McDonald, M. J. (1964). Congenital anomalies in the newborn infant, including minor variations. *J. Pediat.*, **64**, 357.

Muldal, S., Ockey, C. H., Thompson, M., and White, L. L. R. (1962). "Double male"—a new chromosome constitution in the Klinefelter syndrome. *Acta endocr. (Kbh.)*, **39**, 183.

Polani, P. E. (1964). Chromosome anomalies. *Ann. Rev. Med.*, **15**, 93.

Potter, E. L. (1961). *Pathology of the Fetus and the Infant.* Year Book Medical Publishers, Chicago.

Ricci, N., and Malacarne, P. (1964). An XYY human male. *Lancet*, **1**, 721.

Robinson, G. C., Miller, J. R., Dill, F. J., and Kamburoff, T. D. (1964). Klinefelter's syndrome with the XXYY sex chromosome complex. *J. Pediat.*, **65**, 226.

Sandberg, A. A., Ishihara, T., Crosswhite, L. H., and Koepf, G. F. (1963). XYY genotype: report of a case in a male. *New Engl. J. Med.*, **268**, 585.

Vignetti, P., Capotorti, L., and Ferrante, E. (1964). XYY chromosomal constitution with genital abnormality. *Lancet*, **2**, 588.

Walker, J. (1954). Foetal anoxia. *J. Obstet. Gynaec. Brit. Emp.*, **61**, 162.

Walther, P. F. von (1833). *System der Chirurgie*, vol. 1, p. 344. G. Reimer, Berlin. (Cited by Little, 1839, p. xli.)

Wynne-Davies, R. (1964). Family studies and the cause of congenital club foot. *J. Bone Jt Surg.*, **46-B**, 445.

*Arch. Dis. Childh.*, 1965, **40**, 555.

# INCUBATOR-BORNE *PSEUDOMONAS PYOCYANEA* INFECTION IN A NEWBORN NURSERY

BY

DINAH BARRIE

*From the Department of Clinical Microbiology, Louis Jenner Laboratories, St. Thomas's Hospital and Medical School, London*

RECEIVED FOR PUBLICATION JANUARY 18, 1965)

In recent years, *Pseudomonas pyocyanea* and other Gram-negative bacteria have appeared more frequently as important pathogens. This has followed the effective antibiotic treatment of infections due to most other organisms and is also related to the increasing use of certain equipment which may become readily contaminated and which is difficult to sterilize. The problem is particularly serious in the neonatal period.

A small outbreak occurred in the premature baby unit of this hospital. During a period of three weeks, 4 babies were involved, of which the first, and most seriously affected, died. The aim of the present account is to re-emphasize the pathogenicity of *Ps. pyocyanea*, to describe the investigation and control of such an outbreak, and to suggest a routine for decontaminating incubators and other equipment.

## Case Reports

**Case 1.** This baby, weighing 940 g. (2 lb. 1 oz.), was born after spontaneous premature labour at 29 weeks' gestation. He developed respiratory distress and was treated in an incubator with oxygen, penicillin, streptomycin, and intravenous dextrose. He improved initially, but by the ninth day his weight had fallen to 700 g. (1 lb. 8 oz.) and frequent apnoeic attacks developed. Dextrose was again given intravenously with ampicillin and methicillin. On the following day he had a generalized pustular rash and a purulent discharge from one eye. The bacteriological findings (see Table 1) showed a widespread *Ps. pyocyanea* infection. Intramuscular colomycin was started but his condition worsened rapidly and he died after only one dose had been given.

TABLE 1

BACTERIOLOGICAL RESULTS OF CASE 1

| Day | Source | Results |
|---|---|---|
| 1 | Skin | Sterile |
| 10 | Pharynx | Very heavy growth of *Ps. pyocyanea* |
| 10 | Eye | Heavy growth of *Ps. pyocyanea* |
| 12 | Skin | Moderate growth of *Ps. pyocyanea* |
| 12 | Ankle | Scanty growth of *Ps. pyocyanea* |
| 12 | Skin | Heavy growth of *Ps. pyocyanea* |

**Case 2.** This baby, weighing 1,160 g. (2 lb. 9 oz.), was born after spontaneous premature labour at 27 weeks' gestation, and was resuscitated by endotracheal intubation and lung inflation. He was nursed in an incubator, and prophylactic penicillin and streptomycin were given. He made good progress until the eighth day when he developed conjunctivitis and an inflamed umbilicus, which was treated with erythromycin and novobiocin while awaiting the bacteriological findings. These (see Table 2) indicated a mixed infection with *Streptococcus faecalis*, *Ps. pyocyanea*, and *Staph. aureus*. However, both infections cleared without further treatment and he made a complete recovery.

TABLE 2

BACTERIOLOGICAL RESULTS OF CASE 2

| Day | Source | Result |
|---|---|---|
| 7 | Eye | Mixed organisms including heavy growth of *Strep. faecalis* |
| 7 | Umbilicus | Scanty growth of *Ps. pyocyanea*, scanty growth of *Staph. albus*, and moderate growth of *Strep. faecalis* |
| 7 | Stool | No pathogens isolated |
| 20 | Umbilicus | Single colony of *Ps. pyocyanea*, scanty growths of *Staph. aureus*, and *Strep. faecalis* |
| 31 | Eye | Sterile |

**Case 3.** This baby, a twin weighing 1,135 g. (2 lb. 8 oz.), was born by forceps delivery at 29 weeks' gestation. He developed respiratory distress and was treated in an incubator with oxygen, penicillin, streptomycin, and intravenous dextrose. On the fourth day, he was lethargic and jaundiced, and the umbilicus appeared inflamed. A course of erythromycin and novobiocin was started but was changed to intramuscular colomycin when the bacteriological findings became available (see Table 3). The umbilicus was cleaned with hydrogen peroxide and sprayed with 'Polybactrin' (a solution con-

TABLE 3

BACTERIOLOGICAL RESULTS OF CASE 3

| Day | Source | Result |
|---|---|---|
| 4 | Umbilicus | Heavy growth of 2 types of coliform organism |
| 7 | Umbilicus | Scanty growth of *Ps. pyocyanea* |
| 11 | Umbilicus | Sterile |
| 11 | Stool | No pathogens isolated |
| 12 | Umbilicus | Sterile |
| 18 | Umbilicus | Sterile |
| 19 | Stool | No pathogens isolated |
| 21 | Stool | Scanty growth of *Ps. pyocyanea* |
| 25 | Stool | Scanty growth of *Ps. pyocyanea* |
| 29 | Stool | Scanty growth of *Ps. pyocyanea* |
| 38 | Stool | No pathogens isolated |

taining neomycin, polymyxin B, and bacitracin). Despite troublesome diarrhoea due to colomycin, his general condition improved and he recovered completely.

**Case 4.** This baby, weighing 1,800 g. (4 lb.), was born by breech delivery at 35 weeks' gestation, the membranes having ruptured 12 days previously. Respiration was established after intubation and lung inflation. He was nursed in an incubator, and prophylactic penicillin and streptomycin were given. Apart from marked jaundice with a maximum serum bilirubin level of 19 mg./100 ml. on the fifth day, his progress was satisfactory. In the course of investigating the outbreak, he was found to have a symptomless umbilical colonization with *Ps. pyocyanea*, which rapidly cleared after spraying with Polybactrin.

## Method

After the third case of *Ps. pyocyanea* infection had occurred, cultures were taken from all the babies in the nursery, the incubator, respirator, water manometer used in resuscitation, suction apparatus, scales, taps, hand disinfectant dispensers, unused disposable napkins, rubber bands used for cord occlusion, rubber tubing, and many other items in the nursery and labour wards. Swabs were first moistened in peptone water and were inoculated onto blood agar plates incubated aerobically at 37° C. overnight. *Ps. pyocyanea* was identified by its typical colonies, odour, and Gram stain characteristics. The cytochrome oxidase test was used only if the organism did not fulfil these criteria. The antibiotic sensitivity pattern was determined for each specimen.

## Results

All four incubators were contaminated with *Ps. pyocyanea* (see Table 4). The contamination occurred mainly on the plastic sleeves and was not found in the water of the humidifying reservoir. After cleaning the sleeves with soap and water and hypochlorite solution (Milton* 1:80), the organism was still present and sterile cultures were obtained only by completely removing all sleeve rims and steeping them in the hypochlorite solution.

Swabs taken from parts of the Bird respirator, which had been used to resuscitate the first baby, were sterile, but a moderate growth of *Ps. pyocyanea* was obtained from the face mask. The organisms were also isolated from two out of three resuscitation devices in the labour wards and the nursery; contamination was confined to the water and no organisms were recovered from the tubing. A blood agar plate was held at the position of the endo-

* Milton (Milton Pharmaceuticals Ltd.) is a proprietary preparation containing 1% sodium hypochlorite. A dilution of 1:80, giving 125 parts per million of hypochlorite, was used throughout.

TABLE 4

BACTERIOLOGICAL FINDINGS OF INCUBATORS

| Source | Case 1* | Case 2 | Case 3 | Case 4 |
|---|---|---|---|---|
| Water reservoir | — | Heavy growth of coliforms | Scanty growth of coliforms | Sterile |
| Humidity exit | Sterile | Sterile | Sterile | Sterile |
| Sleeves | Sterile | — | Moderate growth of *Ps. pyocyanea* | Moderate growth of *Ps. pyocyanea* |
| Walls | — | Single colony of *Ps. pyocyanea*, scanty growth of coliforms | Sterile | — |
| Tray | Sterile | — | — | Scanty growth of *Staph. albus* |
| Napkin exit port | — | Heavy growth of coliforms | Sterile | — |
| After cleaning incubators with Milton 1:80 | | | | |
| Sleeves | Heavy growth of *Ps. pyocyanea* | Moderate growth of *Ps. pyocyanea*, scanty growth of yeasts | Scanty growth of *Ps. pyocyanea* | Moderate growth of *Ps. pyocyanea* |
| Walls | Scanty growth of *Ps. pyocyanea* | Sterile | Sterile | Sterile |
| After sleeves removed and cleaned with Milton 1:80 | Sterile | Sterile | Sterile | Sterile |

* This incubator had already been cleaned and returned into general circulation.

tracheal tube and the device was operated for two minutes, but no organisms could be demonstrated despite an estimated 2·5 million *Ps. pyocyanea* organisms per ml. of water. This was as expected since the water column is used as a safety device for applying positive pressure, and there is no direct contact between the water and the patient.

Swabs of all other items were mostly sterile or had scant growths of non-pathogens.

**Discussion**

There are a disturbing number of reports of colonization and infection of newborn infants by *Ps. pyocyanea* (Geppert, Baker, Copple, and Pulaski, 1952); Hoffman and Finberg, 1955); Asay and Koch, 1960). Laursen (1962) found that nasal contamination with *Ps. pyocyanea* occurred in 9% of infants in the premature nursery but in less than 0·3% of normal infants nursed with their mothers. Among the infants from whom *Ps. pyocyanea* was recovered, 90% had had oxygen therapy, almost invariably in incubators.

Common reservoirs of infection in nursery outbreaks include humidifiers, storage bottles, taps, wash-basins, and even the water used for bathing the infants' eyes. Sever (1959), in a bacteriological survey of the water in incubators and of storage bottles, found gross contamination with mean bacterial counts of up to 15,000 organisms per ml. which included *Esch. coli*, *Alcaligenes faecalis*, *Achromobacter*, *Staph. aureus*, *Ps. pyocyanea*, yeasts, and fungi.

Kresky (1964) found a 55% colonization rate of babies by Gram-negative organisms. She devised a scheme for cleaning and disinfecting nursery equipment, using 1% Povidone iodine, as a result of which colonization of babies was reduced to 4·5%, and contamination of equipment was virtually eliminated.

Experimental work on the influence of relative humidity on various organisms has shown different effects on survival. A relative humidity of 95-98% at 37° C. allows an actual increase in the number of viable staphylococci, whereas a 55% relative humidity appeared to be the least favourable for their survival (McDade and Hall, 1963). However, Gram-negative organisms, such as *Esch. coli* and *Serratia marcescens*, have been similarly studied by Davis and Bateman (1960) who found moisture inhibitory to both, a relative humidity of 93% being more so than 75%, 11%, or dry air. On the basis of the influence of humidity on the survival of organisms, Silverman (1964) has suggested that premature infants should be nursed at a relative humidity of only 50%.

In the outbreak under review, management was directed first towards the immediate treatment of affected babies and those at risk, and secondly to the long-term problem of eliminating bacterial contamination of equipment, especially incubators. Affected babies were isolated, handling was reduced to a minimum, liberal use was made of sterile disposable gloves, special attention was paid to the incubator sleeves, and the unit was closed to further admissions. The major problem was that of cleaning and sterilizing incubators. These are now used extensively for nursing not only premature infants but also many sick infants, suffering from known infections such as gastro-enteritis and pneumonia. Fumigation with formalin vapour would seem the simplest, but its disadvantage is that prolonged airing is needed before re-use, and that it cannot sterilize the outer surfaces; the probable route of spread from incubator to incubator was by direct inoculation from the hands and arms of the attendants.

The plastic sleeves on the latest models of incubators have been replaced by sliding or hinged doors, though previous models are being used extensively. Fixed port doors are still vulnerable to bacterial contamination and require even more careful attention than removable parts.

Certain incubator manufacturers recommend the addition of antiseptics such as benzalkonium chloride to the water in the humidity reservoir. Objections to this are first that contamination, which was found to be centred on the plastic sleeves, would be unaffected by this manœuvre; in addition it is now well known that some organisms not only survive but actually multiply in many antiseptics.

In the scheme to be presented, hypochlorite solution (Milton 1:80), which already holds a time-honoured place in sterilizing feeding bottles and teats, was chosen for the incubators. Since the scheme has been in operation, no further infections with *Ps. pyocyanea* have occurred and bacteriological spot checks have shown treated incubators to be free from pathogens.

**Summary**

Four cases of *Ps. pyocyanea* infection in a premature nursery are described. A bacteriological survey showed the organisms to be present in the incubators, especially the sleeves. A practical scheme is outlined for eliminating such contaminants from incubators.

I am grateful to Dr. D. G. Cottom for permission to report cases under his care, and to Dr. Mark Ridley for helpful comments.

REFERENCES

Asay, L. D., and Koch, R. (1960). Pseudomonas infections in infants and children. *New Engl. J. Med.*, **262**, 1062.

Davis, M. S., and Bateman, J. B. (1960). Relative humidity and the killing of bacteria. I. Observations on *Escherichia coli* and *Micrococcus lysodeikticus*. *J. Bact.*, **80**, 577.

Geppert, L. J., Baker, H. J., Copple, B. I., and Pulaski, E. J. (1952). Pseudomonas infections in infants and children. *J. Pediat.*, **41**, 555.

Hoffman, M. A., and Finberg, L. (1955). Pseudomonas infections in infants associated with high-humidity environments. *ibid.*, 46, 626.

Kresky, B. (1964). Control of Gram-negative bacilli in a hospital nursery. *Amer. J. Dis. Child.*, **107**, 363.

Laursen, H. (1962). Incidence of Pseudomonas aeroginosa and other gram-negative rods in newborn infants. *Acta obstet. gynec. scand.*, **41**, 254.

McDade, J. J., and Hall, L. B. (1963). An experimental method to measure the influence of environmental factors on the viability and the pathogenicity of *Staphylococcus aureus*. *Amer. J. Hyg.*, 77, 98.

Sever, J. L. (1959). Possible role of humidifying equipment in spread of infections from the newborn nursery. *Pediatrics*, **24**, 50.

Silverman, W. A. (1964). Diagnosis and treatment: use and misuse of temperature and humidity in care of the newborn infant. *ibid.*, 33, 276.

# Appendix

The following scheme, duplicated on a single sheet, accompanies all incubators. A detailed description of the cleaning procedure is given on one side for the guidance of the nursing staff. The reverse side is in the form of a certificate which is intended to ensure that the full cleaning procedure has been carried out. An incubator is not used again until such a certificate has been completed and signed.

## CLEANING PROCEDURE FOR INCUBATORS

### Part I

(Normally completed in the Ward)

Incubators are often needed urgently. To ensure proper working order and to prevent infection being conveyed from one baby to the next, it is important that the following procedure be carried out meticulously after each baby and that Part I of the Certificate is completed.

1. Enter the details of the last baby nursed in the incubator in the special history card for that incubator. This makes it possible to trace the sources of cross-infection.
2. Empty the water from the humidity reservoir by inverting the perspex filler on the front panel.
3. Remove the sleeves, wash them with soap and water, and then steep in Milton 1 : 80 solution for 1 hour. When the incubator is in use, this should be done daily as the sleeves are an important source of contamination and cross-infection.
4. Clean the perspex hood with warm water, soap, and 1% cetrimide.
(IMPORTANT: Perspex is destroyed by ether, acetone, and chloroform, and these must NEVER be used for removing stains. Adhesive plaster marks can be removed with spirit or 'Zoff'.)
5. Clean the mattress with warm water, soap, and 1% cetrimide. (NOTE: Never stick pins into the mattress when changing napkins. This perforates the waterproof cover and is a cause of cross-infection. If you see any perforations of the cover, discard and put on a new one.)
6. Using warm water, soap, and 1% cetrimide, clean the entire interior.
7. Boil any rubber tubing used.

### Part II

(Normally completed by the Surgical Equipment Store)

1. Remove power unit.
2. Fill lower deck tanks with Milton solution 1 : 80 and leave for 1 hour.
3. Remove sleeve rims and steep rims and sleeves in Milton solution 1 : 80 for one hour.
4. Remove dirty filter and replace with a clean filter.
5. Wipe all parts (head, upper deck, humidity vent, mattress, cupboard, power unit, and flex) with Milton solution 1 : 80.
6. Air the incubator in a clean place. If an infant with a known infection has been nursed in the incubator, it should be aired for 24 hours, and, whenever possible, cleared by the Bacteriology Laboratory before re-use.

NOTE:
If the incubator is to be used for a new case without first being returned to the Surgical Equipment Store for sterilization, then all the routine steps carried out by them should be carried out on the Ward.

INCUBATOR CERTIFICATE

1. Incubator history card entry made ☐
2. Water emptied ☐
3. Sleeves washed and sterilized ☐
4. Hood cleaned ☐
5. Mattress cleaned ☐
6. Rubber ring, upper and lower decks cleaned ☐

This incubator has been cleaned as above, prior to sterilization

Signed.................................. Date..................

1. Power unit removed ☐
2. Tanks sterilized with Milton ☐
3. Sleeves and rims sterilized with Milton ☐
4. Filter replaced ☐
5. All parts cleaned with Milton ☐
6. Incubator aired ☐

This incubator has been cleaned with Milton as above, and is now ready for use.

Signed.................................. Date..................

*Immediately before use in the Ward*

1. Wipe over
2. Fit sleeves
3. Fill humidity reservoir with sterile distilled water
4. Warm up

When a baby needs prolonged incubator care, the incubator should be changed weekly.

*Arch. Dis. Childh.*, 1965, **40**, 560.

# HAND, FOOT, AND MOUTH DISEASES

BY

S. R. MEADOW*

(RECEIVED FOR PUBLICATION MARCH 25, 1965)

Hand, foot, and mouth disease is being recognized more often, and it is becoming clear that it is mainly a disease of children. The association of mouth ulcers, and vesicles of the feet and hands, with Coxsackie group A viruses has been found in many centres, most often with the A type 16 virus, but sometimes with A types 5 and 10. Because of the mild nature of the disease and its sporadic outbreaks, one observer rarely sees many cases, hence a description of a series of 69 cases seen in general practice may be of value.

Hand, foot, and mouth disease was occurring in many parts of Britain in the second half of 1963: it was reported in Buckinghamshire, Swindon, and Bristol (Crow, Warin, and Wilkinson, 1963), and Aberdeen, Durham, and London (Lipp, 1963; Tattersall, 1963; Meadow, 1963; Abrahams, 1963). In Banbury, Oxfordshire, many cases were appearing. To be certain that these belonged to a clinical entity, complete virology studies would have been needed, whereas only limited virus studies were feasible. Therefore the outbreak was investigated mainly from a clinical and epidemiological approach. From this it became clear that the 69 cases fell into two clinical series, X and Y.

The larger group, series X, consisted of 51 cases originating in one of three outbreaks, and was made up of persons with one or more of the three well-described signs: mouth ulcers, foot vesicles, and hand vesicles. A further group of 18 patients (series Y) had only mouth lesions and these were of a slightly different character from those of series X. At first it seemed likely that series Y had hand, foot, and mouth disease, as infected persons do not necessarily have hand and foot lesions. However, on following up contacts, all cases of series Y could be traced to one of two original sources, but not to any of the 51 cases in the larger series, X. Furthermore the clinical pattern in series Y, and the mouth lesions, were recognizably different from those of hand, foot, and mouth disease. Series X, the 51 cases of hand, foot, and mouth disease, will be described first.

### Hand, Foot, and Mouth Disease (Series X)

**Clinical Features.** In the Banbury, Oxfordshire, area, there was an epidemic illness during September and October 1963. The illness was mild, only half of the patients consulting a doctor, and ran a course of under 10 days, regressing spontaneously.

AGE INCIDENCE. Amongst 51 cases the age distribution was: 0-5 years, 24; 5-10 years, 10; 10-20 years, 2; 20-40 years, 15.

The small number in the 10-20 years group reflects the fact that the families infected had young children but few members in their teens.

SEX INCIDENCE. There were 30 male and 21 female cases.

MOUTH ULCERS. These were present in all 51 and were often preceded for one or two days by a feeling of malaise, sore throat, and sore mouth. Vesicles appeared, 3-6 mm. in diameter (Fig. 1a), some of them regressing and some bursting rapidly, leaving small shallow oval grey ulcers with a hyperaemic border. In some cases the original vesicles were seen to originate as tiny red macules, and were painful. They occurred in most areas of the mouth except on the posterior pharynx. They were rare on the tonsils and common on the tongue, buccal mucosa, palate, and gums. In 40 cases there were from 1 to 7 ulcers, and 11 had more than 8 ulcers.

HAND LESIONS. In 43 cases there were vesicular lesions which were usually noticed 1 to 2 days after the mouth lesions. They began as red macules (Fig. 1b), gradually becoming vesicular. Some enlarged to form a flaccid superficial blister 3-10 mm. in diameter, containing clear fluid; others remained deeper and smaller. The majority remained oval in shape. They occurred most often on the lateral borders of the proximal phalanges of the fingers and the ulnar borders of the palm. The usual number was two to five, though three small children had a

* Formerly general practitioner, Banbury, Oxfordshire. Present address, Guy's Hospital, London S.E.1.

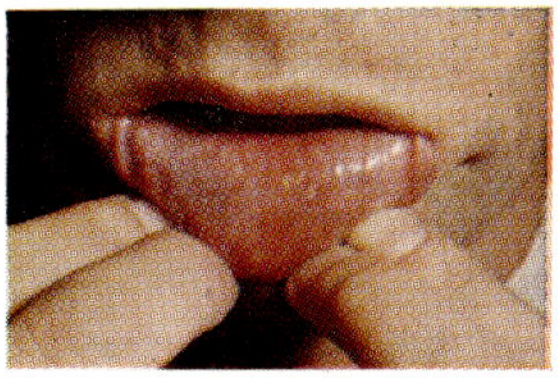

FIG. 1a.—Ulcers on buccal mucosa of the lower lip.

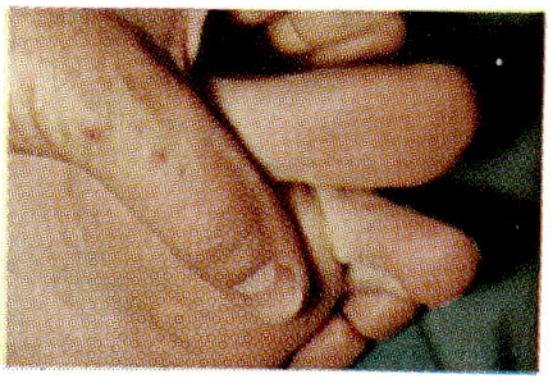

FIG. 1b.—Small papules on the dorsum of the thumb; a large flaccid blister on the under surface of the second toe was also present.

profuse eruption of tiny palmar blisters. The siting of the blisters seemed related to trauma, blisters being common around rings and on the medial palmar border of those who wrote a lot. They did not irritate and subsided gradually, leaving behind a small red spot.

FOOT LESIONS (Fig. 2a and b). These were present in 17 cases, and uncommon in young children: of 23 children under the age of 3, only 4 had foot lesions. The blisters had the same characteristics as the hand lesions. They were usually present on the toes of women who wore tight shoes; otherwise they tended to be sited on the lateral borders of the feet.

BUTTOCK RASH. This was present in 23 cases, including every recorded case under the age of 3. It was seen on about the third day of the illness, beginning as a scattered red rash of distinct macules and papules, most of which became vesicles. The vesicular stage lasted a few hours only, until a maculo-papular appearance was resumed.

GENERAL SYMPTOMS. There was malaise and marked anorexia in 40 cases. Most of the adults had no general symptoms. There was a pyrexia of up to 101° F. (38·3° C.) in only 3 cases; and the rest were afebrile. When blood counts were done, there was either a normal white cell count or a slight leucocytosis.

OTHER FEATURES. In 30 cases there was redness of the ear-drums, subsiding within 3 days. One housewife had a maculo-papular rash of the knees. One child had vesicles on the shoulders.

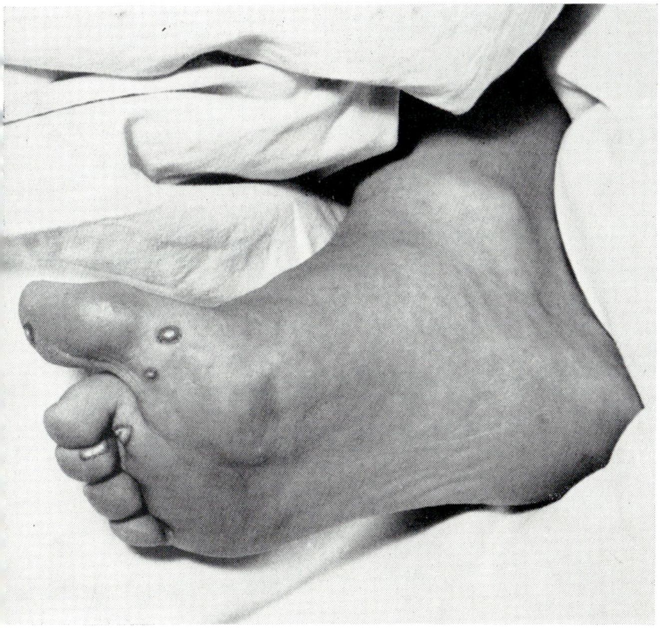

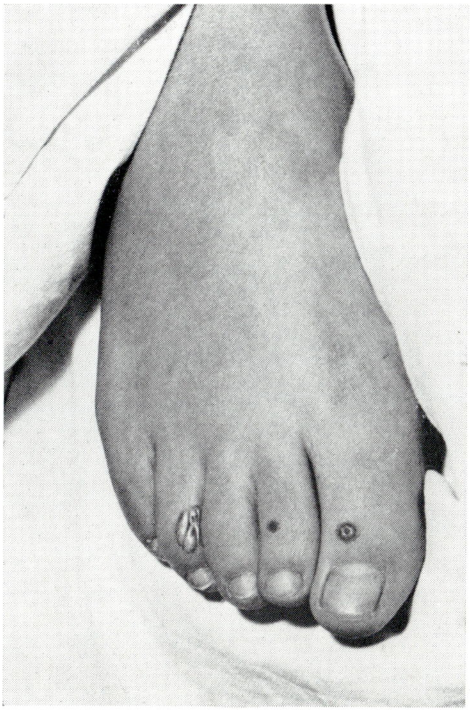

FIG. 2a and b.—Typical vesicular foot lesions.

SEQUELAE. One girl developed an attack of asthma. There were no other complications. No abnormality was found in 20 cases reviewed 3 months after the illness.

**Epidemiology.** Banbury is a country town of 20,000 inhabitants in North Oxfordshire. All the cases lived within 5 miles of the town centre. Over a period of two months there were three outbreaks in the area to which all cases could be traced. It was most infectious within individual households, usually occurring in more than half the members, beginning in the young children. In the community as a whole it was not very infectious, and it was seen to affect families on one side of a road and not the other, or only the families whose children played much together. For instance, in one village road of modern semi-detached houses, 6 families out of a row of 7 houses had the illness, while none of those on the other side of the road or farther along it caught the infection.

The disease affected all social classes. The higher incidence of adults (33%) in this series than in the 1957 Toronto outbreak (20%) (Robinson, Doane, and Rhodes, 1958) or the 1959 Birmingham outbreak (12%), described by Alsop, Flewett, and Foster (1960), is probably due only to the closer follow-up of contacts.

The incubation period was 2 to 5 days. As an example of the epidemiological pattern the dates on which individual members of neighbouring families A, B, C, D, E, and F were affected are shown below in Table 1 (italics denote adults).

TABLE 1

| Date (September 1963) | | | | | | | | |
|---|---|---|---|---|---|---|---|---|
| 1st | 2nd | 3rd | 4th | 5th | 6th | 7th | 8th | 9th |
| B | | C | *E* | *F* | | D | *D* | *A* |
| B | | C | F | A | | | | |
| | | *B* | F | | | | | |
| | | | D | | | | | |

**Virology.** Primary isolation was attempted at the Public Health Laboratory, Oxford, in monkey kidney and amnion tissue cultures and by inoculation into newborn mice. Specimens from seven different patients included two specimens of vesicle fluid, two of faeces, and five faucial swabs.

Dr. F. O. MacCallum isolated Coxsackie A 16 virus from one of the specimens, a vesicle on a child's finger. This was isolated in monkey kidney tissue culture. Although primary inoculation into newborn mice failed to yield the virus, the positive tissue culture when inoculated into newborn mice produced typical paralysis. Dr. MacCallum obtained similar results from a member of the Radcliffe Infirmary staff who caught the illness. The virus isolated from the child was neutralized by a convalescent serum from the Radcliffe patient, who in turn neutralized Coxsackie A 16 virus.

Serological investigations were performed on 5 adults, but the tests were unfortunately very incomplete. The results for Coxsackie A 16 virus were as follows.

Case 1: 4th-day and also 4th-week serum positive at more than 1 : 40
Case 2: 6th-day serum negative at 1 : 10
Case 3: 11th-day serum negative at 1 : 10
Case 4: 12th-day serum positive at 1 : 10
Case 5: 12th-day serum negative at 1 : 10

The results on Cases 2, 3, 4, and 5 are inconclusive because of the absence of tests later than the 12th day. The result in Case 1 is surprising, as it suggests past and not present infection with the virus. This patient had all the clinical manifestations of hand, foot, and mouth disease and had been in contact with other cases.

**Course.** The disease was self-limiting. Most children were off colour for only 5 days, all were normal within 10 days. Treatment did not affect the duration of the illness.

### Mouth Disease (Series Y)

Eighteen cases of an infectious illness with characteristic mouth lesions were seen. Contact with other cases of the disease was common, while there was no apparent contact with any of the cases in series X. These people had a recognizable clinical illness which ran true to type and which differed from hand, foot, and mouth disease and other ulcerative conditions of the mouth in several ways.

It resembled hand, foot, and mouth disease only in its age incidence and incubation period: it differed in that the sufferers were more ill and that half had a fever of 100° to 101° F. (38° C.). No hand, foot, or buttock lesions appeared, and the mouth lesions differed from those of hand, foot, and mouth disease. When starting they looked like Koplik's spots, usually on the buccal mucosa. As the spots enlarged they became ragged grey-yellow ulcers, from two to ten in number. They had a predilection for the fraenum of the tongue and the median raphe of the hard palate. They did not appear on the posterior pharynx nor on the anterior pillar of the fauces. There was no associated gingivitis. In addition to the ulcers, red petechiae were present on the palate, similar to those that are seen in glandular fever. Spontaneous recovery occurred within a week.

**Laboratory Investigations.** Swabs of the mouth lesions in two patients yielded no virus. Neutralization tests with the sera of one patient showed her to be infected with Coxsackie A 16 virus, serum on the third day being negative at 1 : 10, and in the sixth week positive at more than 1 : 80. Blood counts of 7 patients showed white cell counts between 6,000 and 11,000. Paul Bunnell test on five patients was negative.

The contrasting features of the two types of cases are shown in Table 2.

TABLE 2
FEATURES OF TWO TYPES OF CASES

| | Series X | Series Y |
|---|---|---|
| No. of cases .. .. | 51 | 18 |
| Hand vesicles .. .. | 85% (43) | None |
| Foot vesicles .. .. | 33% (17) | None |
| Mouth ulcers .. .. | 100% (51) | 100% (18) (starting as 'Koplik's) |
| Palate petechiae .. .. | None | 89% (16) |
| Degree of illness .. .. | Mild | Moderate |
| Fever .. .. | 5% (3) | 50% (9) |
| Buttock rash .. .. | 45% (23) | None |
| Rash elsewhere .. .. | 4% (2) | None |

## Discussion

The 51 cases in series X of hand, foot, and mouth disease showed the characteristics of the 24 cases described by Alsop *et al.* (1960) in Birmingham in 1959. In Banbury, Coxsackie A type 16 virus was isolated from a specimen of vesicle fluid: the Birmingham outbreak was also associated with Coxsackie A type 16 virus. Like those cases and in contrast with both the 1957 Toronto disease (Robinson *et al.*, 1958) and the 1959 California outbreak (Magoffin, Jackson, and Lennette, 1961) general symptoms were slight and general body rash absent.

A buttock rash was recorded in 4 of the 24 Birmingham cases and in 4 out of 16 cases seen at a preparatory school in Buckinghamshire (Brown, Wright, and Ogden, 1964). In the present series the buttock rash occurred in each of the 23 cases occurring in children under the age of 3, while foot lesions were rare in this age-group. The site of the vesicles appears to be related to trauma: on hands and feet they develop in areas subject to friction. It is suggested that the buttock rash should be recognized as a feature of hand, foot, and mouth disease in young children.

When the cases of mouth ulceration in series Y presented, it seemed sensible to consider them as variants of hand, foot, and mouth disease, and a watch was kept for the full disease in their contacts. This did not occur and it seemed that this was a different clinical entity (Table 2). Not only was the natural history and appearance of the mouth ulcers different, but it was epidemiologically distinct. It was a mild infectious illness which could have been a very mild herpetic stomatitis, though there was no apparent herpetic stomatitis prevalent in the area, and it was not associated with gingivitis or adenopathy. Moreover herpes virus is comparatively easy to demonstrate, while the Coxsackie A virus may be more difficult. The lesions of herpangina (Coxsackie A types 2, 4, 5, 6 and 10) are characteristically on the anterior pillar of the fauces and not on the gingival or buccal mucosa, as in this mouth disease.



Full virology and serology studies might have elucidated the problem, but were difficult to arrange in a busy country general practice. However, the one conclusive piece of virological evidence in series Y suggested infection also with Coxsackie A type 16 virus: the series of cases was followed up without any developing peripheral vesicles, so that this finding was unexpected. The different disease picture presumably resulted from an alteration in the virus rather than an alteration in the host. This is possible, for it is becoming apparent that viruses indistinguishable by present techniques may be associated with more than one disease. Coxsackie A type 5 is an example; formerly associated with classical herpangina, it has been isolated from 7 cases of hand, foot, and mouth disease by Flewett, Warin, and Clarke (1963).

A further difficulty is that similar clinical pictures can be produced by different organisms. In particular, the mouth seems very limited in its response to viral infections. Ulcerative mouth lesions occur in many infections including varicella, Echo types 4, 9, and 16, infectious mononucleosis, herpes simplex, and any one of six or more different Coxsackie group A viruses (Bedson, Downie, MacCullum, and Stuart-Harris, 1961). Hand, foot, and mouth disease has now been shown to be associated with three different types of Coxsackie group A viruses: type 16 (Robinson *et al.*, 1958), type 10 (Clarke, Morley and Warin, 1964), and type 5 (Flewett *et al.*, 1963).

It is likely that hand, foot, and mouth disease is more common than its documentation suggests. When a patient presents with a sore throat, the physician does not examine his toes or even his fingers. During the 12 months subsequent to this outbreak 3 further sporadic cases have been encountered in different parts of the country.

## Summary

An outbreak of hand, foot, and mouth disease is described, involving 51 cases. In addition to the hand vesicles, foot vesicles, and mouth ulcers, children under the age of 3 had a characteristic rash on the buttocks. There was some evidence that Coxsackie A type 16 virus was the causal agent.

A similar though clinically distinct disease is described, characterized by Koplik's type spots leading to mouth ulceration, petechiae on the soft palate, and general illness.

I am grateful to the Public Health Laboratory at Oxford for the virology studies, and in particular to Dr. F. O. MacCallum for the patience with which he received a succession of often inappropriate specimens, and for advice. I thank my former partners in Banbury for bringing cases to my notice. Guy's Hospital Medical School financed the publication of the photographs.

### References

Abrahams, A. H. (1963). Hand, foot, and mouth disease. *Brit. med. J.*, **2**, 1473.

Alsop, J., Flewett, T. H., and Foster, J. R. (1960). 'Hand-foot-and-mouth disease' in Birmingham in 1959. *ibid.*, **2**, 1708.

Bedson, S., Downie, A. W., MacCallum, F. O., and Stuart-Harris, C. H. (1961). *Virus and Rickettsial Diseases of Man*, 3rd ed. Edward Arnold, London.

Brown, J. M., Wright, J. A., and Ogden, W. S. (1964). Hand, foot, and mouth disease. *Brit. med. J.*, **1**, 58.

Clarke, S. K. R., Morley, T., and Warin, R P. (1964). Hand, foot, and mouth disease. *ibid.*, **1**, 58.

Crow, K. D., Warin, R., and Wilkinson, D. S. (1963). Hand, foot, and mouth disease. *ibid.*, **2**, 1267.

Flewett, T. H., Warin, R. P., and Clarke, S. K. R. (1963). Hand, foot, and mouth disease associated with Coxsackie A5 virus. *J. clin. Path.*, **16**, 53.

Lipp, K. L. (1963). Hand, foot, and mouth disease. *Brit. med. J.*, **2**, 1473.

Magoffin, R. L., Jackson, E. W., and Lennette, E. H. (1961). Vesicular stomatitis and exanthem. *J. Amer. med. Ass.*, **175**, 441.

Meadow, S. R. (1963). Hand, foot, and mouth disease. *Brit. med. J.*, **2**, 1473.

Robinson, C. R., Doane, F. W., and Rhodes, A. J. (1958). Report of an outbreak of febrile illness with pharyngeal lesions and exanthem: Toronto, summer 1957—isolation of group A Coxsackie virus. *Canad. med. Ass. J.*, **79**, 615.

Tattersall, P. H. (1963). Hand, foot, and mouth disease. *Brit. med. J.*, **2**, 1473.

*Arch. Dis. Childh.*, 1965, **40**, 565.

# DENTAL MANIFESTATIONS OF PSEUDOHYPOPARATHYROIDISM

BY

G. MacL. RITCHIE
*From the University College Hospital Dental School, London*

(RECEIVED FOR PUBLICATION FEBRUARY 23, 1965)

Pseudohypoparathyroidism is a metabolic disease caused by a disturbance in the peripheral action of parathormone. Clinically the disease is similar to idiopathic hypoparathyroidism.

Characteristically the patients are dwarfed in stature, thick set, and obese, having round faces and greasy skin. There is considerable reduction in the length of the 3rd and 4th fingers and toes and dimpling of the corresponding knuckles when the fist is clenched. Mentally these patients are slightly retarded.

Radiographs show that the 3rd and 4th metacarpals and metatarsals are short. Epiphysial closure is in advance of age, and there are patches of soft tissue calcification and ectopic ossification, usually in the thighs. Radiating striae of calcification of the basal ganglia are also described as a frequent finding.

Investigation of the clinical pathology shows that the calcium level is low, resulting in tetany in the untreated case, and the inorganic phosphorus level is raised.

Biopsies have shown that the parathyroid glands are normal or even slightly hyperplastic, and no phosphate diuresis follows administration of the hormone.

### Case Reports

Four cases of this disease have been studied and the dental findings are presented. In two the family history is of considerable interest.

**Case 1.** This was a stockily built little boy of 10 years, with broad jaws and chin, depressed root of nose, and eyes set widely apart. The skull exhibited frontal bossing and the fingers and toes were short and stubby. Gait was slow and rolling, and he was unable to run. Mental development was slightly retarded but he was a placid and amiable child.

Radiographically the metacarpals and metatarsals were short and there were scattered areas of soft tissue calcification but no calcification of the basal ganglia.

The following blood levels were present: serum calcium 8·3 mg./100 ml., serum phosphorus 8·2 mg./100 ml., and alkaline phosphatase 10 King Armstrong units/100 ml.

*Family History.* There was no family history of mental defect, epilepsy, or abnormal physical features. Normal pregnancy was terminated at 39 weeks by caesarean section, but at 10 weeks it was noted that the child was 'odd' looking and had a marked micrognathia. He had two older brothers both of whom were normal.

At 10 years the following teeth were present in the mouth:

$$\frac{\text{C B 1} \mid \overset{2}{\text{1 3}}}{\text{321} \mid \text{12C 4}}$$

The deciduous teeth had been lost early due to caries. The incisors were a dull dark yellow colour and were grossly hypoplastic. Both upper lateral incisors were missing, or the right one may have been present as a very reduced tooth. The first molars on the right side were just beginning to erupt. The pulps of all the teeth were large, and there was considerable calcification present especially in the lower incisors.

Radiographically the enamel layer was thin and hypoplastic, and both lower first molars had very thin roots. Both upper lateral incisors, upper right second premolar, and lower right first premolar were missing.

**Case 2.** This was a 16-year-old girl with the typical clinical and radiographic features of the disease; intellectually she was rather slow and fell into the dull average range.

The serum calcium level was 8·5 mg./100 ml., serum phosphorus 4·5 mg./100 ml., and the alkaline phosphatase 7·9 King Armstrong units/100 ml.

*Family History.* Both parents were alive and well: The mother, who was short in stature and of dull intelligence but otherwise normal, had given birth to six previous children all of whom were girls. Two, in addition to this patient, survived and are well and three died from convulsions on the day of birth.

*Dental Investigation.* The following teeth were missing at 16 years: $\frac{6 \mid 2\ 4\ 6.}{6 \mid \ \ 56}$ The $\frac{4 \mid}{5 \mid}$ had never developed and the lower premolars and canines were very hypoplastic.

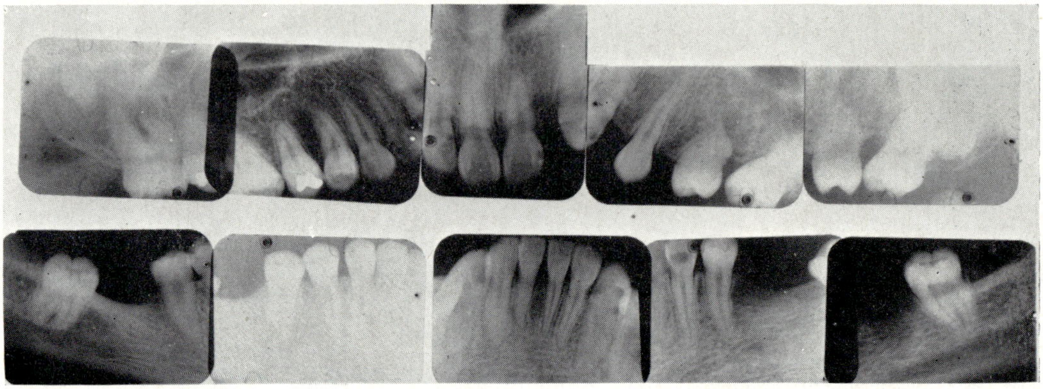

FIG. 1.—Case 2. Intra-oral radiographs at 18 years show several missing teeth, including 8/8, and the premolars have short stubby roots. The enamel is thin and the pulps large with considerable calcification.

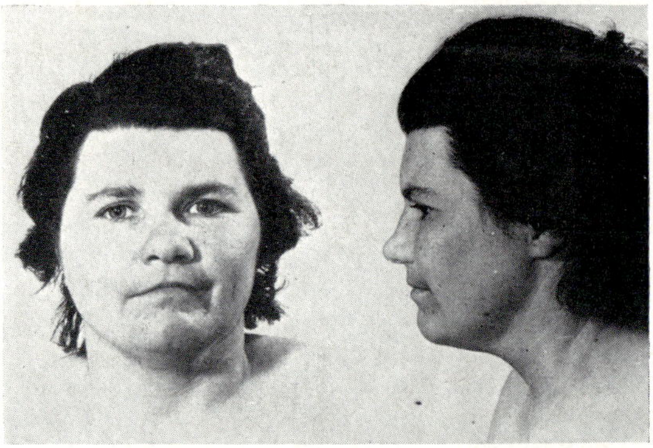

FIG. 2.—Case 3. Typical facial appearance in pseudohypoparathyroidism, with frontal bossing and short wide jaws.

The teeth were dull white in colour and many were carious. Radiographically, 8|8 were missing and the upper premolars had short stubby roots. All the teeth had thin enamel especially the lower incisors. The pulps, which were large, contained considerable amounts of calcified material (Fig. 1).

**Case 3.** This girl had developed mild symptoms of tetany at 6 years of age following operation for an acute mastoid infection.

At 18 years she presented with all the typical physical and radiographic features of the disease including bowing of the tibia, frontal bossing (Fig. 2), slight mental retardation, and calcification of the basal ganglia on skull radiography.

The serum calcium level varied between 6·0-6·6 mg./100 ml., the serum phosphorus was 4·24-6·8 mg./100 ml., and the alkaline phosphatase 2·7-6·9 King Armstrong units/ 100 ml.

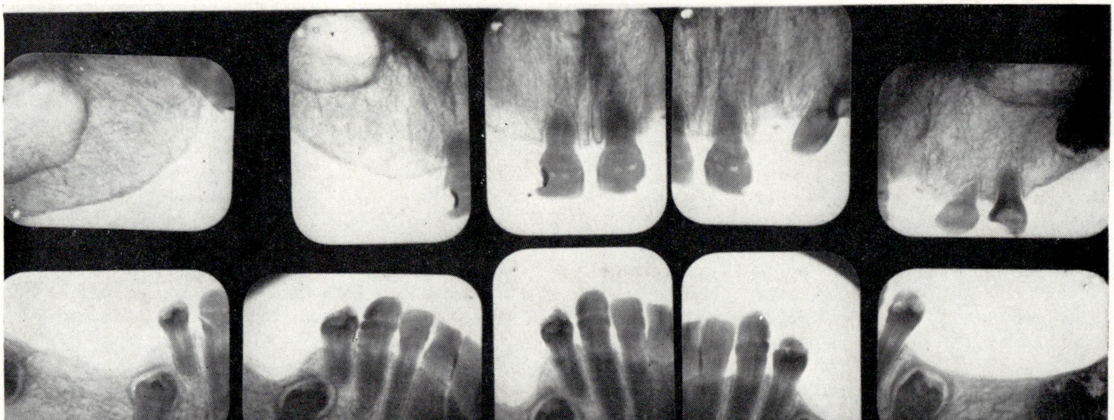

FIG. 3.—Case 3. Radiographs at 29 years show several unerupted posterior teeth, the crowns and roots of which are small. Here also the enamel is thin and pulps are large and calcified.

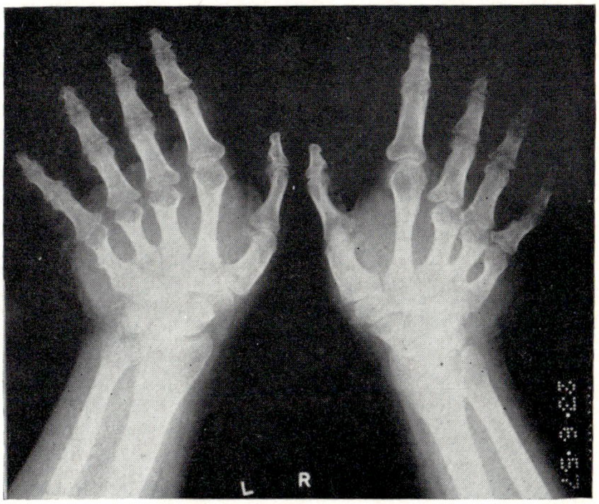


FIG. 4.—Case 4. Radiograph shows reduction in length of all the metacarpals.

In this case there was no significant family history.

A dental report at this age noted that the lower first premolars, and all the first and second molars were unerupted. The second molars showed no proper root formation (Fig. 3). The following teeth were present at 29 years. 8 | , but only the lower six
87 4321 | 1234 78
front teeth were erupted. These teeth were dull white in colour with bands of pitted hypoplasia. The crowns and roots of all these teeth were small and the enamel was thin. The pulps were large and extensively calcified.

**Case 4.** This girl was diagnosed as having pseudohypoparathyroidism when she was 10 years old. She was short in stature, obese, round faced, and the bridge of her nose was flat. The limbs, hands, and fingers were characteristically short and she was mentally retarded. Radiographic examination revealed characteristically short metacarpals and metatarsals (Fig. 4), spur formation of the tibia, and scattered soft tissue calcification of the basal ganglia, though this was apparent 10 years later.

The serum calcium level was 4·5 mg./100 ml., and the serum phosphorus 10 mg./100 ml. at 10 years of age.

*Family History.* Both parents were alive and well, but there was a history of epilepsy on the father's side of the family, though he was not affected himself. There was a remarkable physical resemblance between mother and daughter. The mother was short in stature with characteristic shortness of the 3rd and 4th metacarpals (Fig. 5) and metatarsals, soft tissue calcification, and spurs on the tibia. She has had four other children all of whom died at birth or were stillborn. One of four children herself she was the only one with the characteristic deformities. She had lost all her own teeth early in life.

*Dental Investigation.* The teeth present at 24 years were as follows: 7 5 3 | 78. These teeth were well
7 54 | 345 7
formed but had small clinical crowns, except for the canines. The incisors were lost due to paradontal disease, and these were small teeth also.

### Summary of Dental Findings

The clinical findings in these cases of pseudohypoparathyroidism are similar to those reported in cases of idiopathic hypoparathyroidism, and may be summarized as follows.

(1) Teeth dull white in colour with hypoplastic pit-

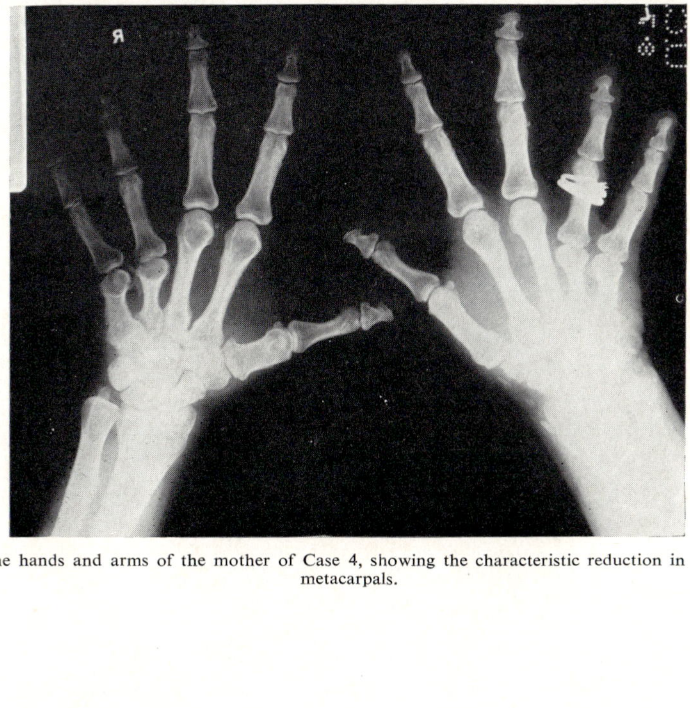

FIG. 5.—Radiograph of the hands and arms of the mother of Case 4, showing the characteristic reduction in length of the 3rd and 4th metacarpals.

ting. (2) Crowns are small and the roots are often short with blunt ends. (3) The enamel is thin and the pulp chambers large, often nearly occluded by calcified deposits. (4) In some cases there may be many unerupted teeth. (5) A full complement of teeth is not always developed, premolars being the teeth most usually missing. (6) The teeth are lost early due to caries. (7) The jaws are short and wide in all cases.

## Treatment

These cases have been treated with vitamin D and A.T.10: this has resulted in an improvement in the general medical condition, and attacks of tetany have been avoided. The tooth substance laid down after the initiation of this treatment appears normal, though no improvement takes place in that already laid down and calcified.

Hypoplastic teeth are prone to caries and regular dental inspection is advisable, with the importance of oral hygiene stressed. The use of topical fluorides and fluoride toothpastes may assist in reducing the incidence of caries.

Orthodontic treatment may be necessary to correct a malocclusion, and a careful radiographic watch should be kept for the possible development of dentigerous cysts where unerupted teeth are present.

## Dental Histology

The histology of the dental tissues during the time of the metabolic upset shows certain abnormalities (Figs. 6 and 7). The dentine had an irregularly calcified matrix, indicated by the mottled pattern of dark spheres on a lighter staining background with haematoxylin and eosin staining. There was normal scalloping of the amelodentinal junction, but the tubules exhibited sharp bends near the pulpal and amelodentinal junctions. The cementum was thick, cellular, and cartilage-like, with what appeared to be vascular channels in the deeper layers extending into the dentine. The canalized area appeared to be less well calcified compared with the surrounding tissues. Most pulps were largely occluded by a calcified tissue which exhibited a series of whorl patterns (Fig. 8). The canalization was similar to that reported by Humphreys (1939) and Sunde and Hals (1961). This, however, occurred in the most recently formed dentine nearest the pulp in patients who were suffering from idiopathic hypoparathyroidism. Similar canalization was produced experimentally in parathyroprivic rats by Schour, Chandler, and Tweedy (1937).

## Review of Reported Cases

Relatively few cases of pseudohypoparathyroidism

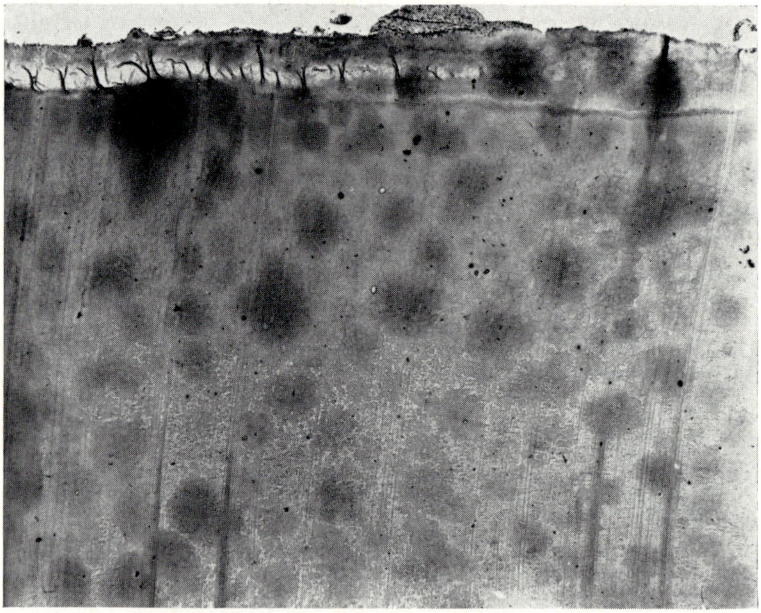

Fig. 6.—Decalcified longitudinal section of an incisor tooth, showing a mottled pattern in the dentine, a thick cartilage like cementum, and what appears to be vascular canals. (H. and E. × 25.)

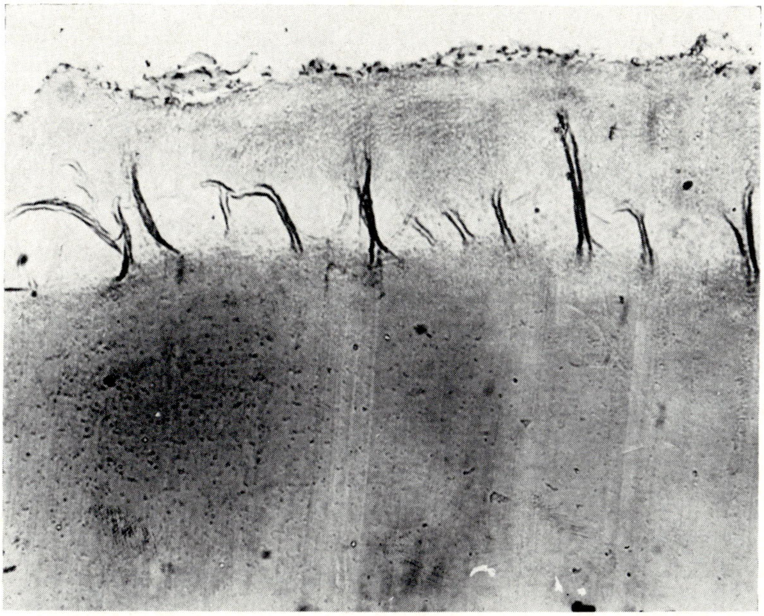

FIG. 7.—Section showing the typical appearance of the 'vascular canals' in higher magnification. (× 90.)

have been reported and most of these contain little or no reference to the state of the dental tissues. Mackler, Fouts, and Birsner (1952) reported two interesting cases of familial disease, and noted that there were many unerupted teeth and those that were erupted were notched. Prentice (1954) reported a case in which the few remaining teeth were hypoplastic, malformed, and misplaced. Peterman and

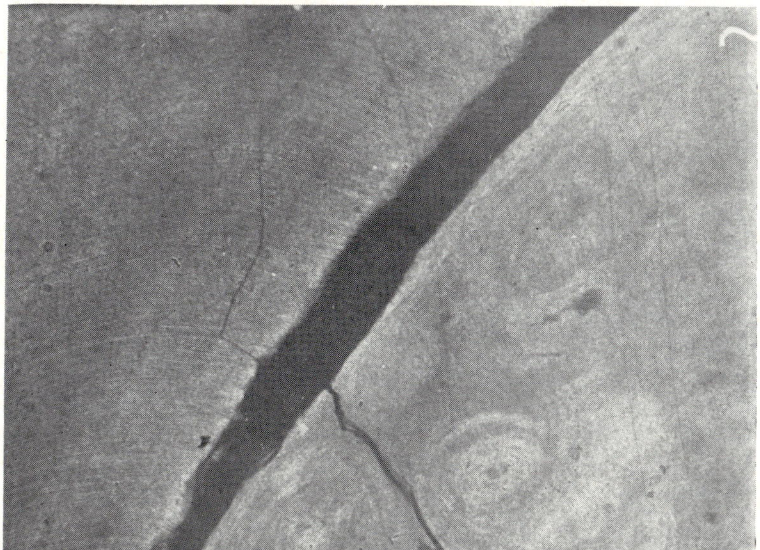

FIG. 8.—Microradiograph of a ground longitudinal section of incisor tooth, showing a natural pattern of curvature of the dentinal tubules and an interesting whorl pattern of the calcified mass in the pulp. (× 75.)

Garvey's (1949) case had incisors with short roots, and the second premolars were missing. Among the findings in a case reported by Moehlig and Gerisch (1950) were enamel hypoplasia and non-eruption of several teeth, and poorly-formed teeth with lack of proper root formation of the second molars. Non-eruption of the first molars and lower first premolars was reported by de Mowbray, Llewellyn Smith, and Symonds (1954). Trevathan (1961) described the dental manifestations of a case in some detail. The incisors were conical and had thin enamel. The first premolars and deciduous upper canines had short roots and many teeth were unerupted. One of the cases reported by Elrick, Albright, Bartter, Forbes, and Reeves (1950) was totally edentulous at 12 years.

There have been several reviews of cases of idiopathic hypoparathyroidism, notably by Drake, Albright, Bauer, and Castleman (1939), Sutphin, Albright, and McCune (1943), Lovestedt (1950), Steinberg and Waldron (1952), and Hinrichs (1956). Lovestedt reported 16 cases, 8 of which had hypoplastic ridged or malformed teeth; 2 had premolars and molars with short stubby roots; 3 had several unerupted teeth and 1 was totally edentulous at 13 years. In spite of this Lovestedt made the surprising statement that 'clinical dental findings in cases of parathyroid insufficiency were rare'. Emerson, Walsh, and Howard (1941), Mortell (1946), and Miller (1957) each reported a case featuring hypoplastic teeth and unerupted teeth. Barr, McBryde, and Sanders (1938) recorded a case with gross hypoplasia. MacGregor and Whitehead (1954) and McLean (1954) each recorded one case having unerupted teeth and mention early loss of others. One of Drake *et al.*'s cases had premolars with short stubby roots. Hinrichs (1956) reviewed 5 cases, of which 4 had hypoplastic enamel and large pulps, 2 had premolars with short stubby roots, and 2 had unerupted teeth.

From this brief review, the similarity of dental abnormality in pseudohypoparathyroidism and idiopathic hypoparathyroidism is evident, and the cases reported here agree with this.

### Histological Findings in Cases of Idiopathic Hypoparathyroidism

The first to note microscopical histological changes in the dental tissues was Humphreys (1939), who drew attention to the similarity with those in parathyroprivic rats. A second case has been reported at some length by Sunde and Hals (1961).

Humphreys' case was a young woman of 23 years who had suffered tetany symptoms for 11 years. Parathormone had improved the clinical picture and had raised the serum calcium level to normal. Ground sections of the teeth showed hypoplasia of the enamel dating from the 6th year and disturbance of the dentine from the ninth year, which worsened after the twelfth year. There were alternating bands of normal dentine and dentine with a coarse granular matrix and interglobular spaces. The dentine nearest the pulp resembled osteodentine and contained vascular inclusions.

The case described by Sunde and Hals was a young woman aged 27 years who had suffered tetanic contractions since she was 15 months old. She had all the physical, mental, and radiographic features of idiopathic hypoparathyroidism including calcification of the basal ganglia. All the deciduous teeth were believed to have been present and erupted. At 11 years the following teeth were present. E D C | 1 2 E : these were mobile and there was

2 1 | 1 2

gingival hyperplasia. Eruption of the permanent teeth was delayed for about 2 to $2\frac{1}{2}$ years. Radiographs showed resorption of the roots of the retained deciduous teeth and that the lower second premolars were absent. Development was incomplete in both erupted and unerupted teeth with premature narrowing of the apical foramina. Ground and decalcified sections showed hypoplasia and hypomineralization of the enamel. The dentine matrix was irregular and granular with interglobular spaces. In the cervical parts of the teeth there were spaces containing vascular tissue. A lamella of bone-like tissue partially occluded the pulp chambers.

The histological findings in these cases are similar to those reported here from cases of pseudohypoparathyroidism, except for the site of the vascular inclusions.

### Discussion

Gottlieb (1920) reported that parathormone deficiency resulted in delayed eruption, though Schour *et al.* (1937) found it had no influence on the rate of eruption in rats. Albright and Strock (1933) maintained that eruption might be delayed or fail altogether and that the enamel was often deficient and ridged. Changes might also occur in the dentine. No decalcification of the teeth occurred in adulthood. Hinrichs (1956) stated there was no conclusive evidence that hypoparathyroidism prevented initiation of tooth germ formation, but that there was some evidence that deficiency was associated with delayed eruption and affected both matrix formation and calcification.

The effect of thyroparathyroidectomy in rats was studied by Ziskin, Salmon, and Applebaum (1940) and was found to cause severe retardation of growth and development generally and especially the length of the jaws rather than the width. Eruption time, dentine, and root development were retarded also. The size of the molar crowns, however, was not affected.

The effect of parathyroidectomy in rats has been extensively studied by Schour *et al.* (1937). Classically this results in a calcio-traumatic response in the dental tissues. However, deficiency of parathormone is not the only cause for this response which is characterized by bands of hyper- and hypocalcification in the dentine. In decalcified section the hypercalcified areas stain darkly with haematoxylin and the hypocalcified areas stain strongly with eosin. It has been suggested that the darker areas represent an increase in the amount of cement substance between the fibrils and that this cement substance takes up an increased quantity of calcium salts. If this is so, then presumably there is interference with the metabolism of both odontoblasts in calcification and in the pulp cells in laying down the matrix. Hypocalcification of the pre-dentine may result from changes in the metabolism of the odontoblasts or changes in the local composition of the tissue fluid. Hypercalcified areas on the other hand may result from temporary cessation of matrix production, so that the deposition of calcium salts is concentrated into a smaller area. Tooth studies in rats following parathyroidectomy have shown that no changes take place in the first three weeks following operation but thereafter the enamel is affected. The ameloblasts shorten and this is followed by a breakup of the enamel organ and the formation of epithelial cysts. The calcio-traumatic response was observed in the dentine with irregular areas of defective dentine formation, the layers or increments becoming progressively less well calcified. This was emphasized in animals on a calcium-deficient diet.

Disorganization of the odontoblast layer of the pulp results in folds in the dentine, which contain vascular and pulpal tissue. This tissue becomes trapped in the dentine, giving rise to the vascular inclusions. Except for the site of the vascular inclusions, the dental manifestations in pseudohypoparathyroidism are very similar to those in idiopathic hypoparathyroidism and in parathyroprivic rats.

Parathormone deficiency has an effect on the calcification of the dental tissues and to a lesser extent on matrix production also, but the mechanism is obscure.

In pseudohypoparathyroidism there is presumably a second hormone factor missing or a deficiency of some intermediate substance which is responsible for the manifestations common to the three conditions.

Vitamin D has two independent actions, first it increases calcium absorption from the gut, and secondly it increases phosphorus excretion in the urine. A.T.10 has the same action but gives a greater phosphorus excretion relative to the increase in calcium absorption. It is the hypocalcaemia that is responsible for such signs and symptoms as mental retardation, calcification of the basal ganglia, and tetany.

Albright (1938), quoting the work of J. S. L. Brown, stated that parathormone may produce somewhere in the body a lipoid substance similar to A.T.10 and differing in the same way that A.T.10 differs from vitamin D.

## Conclusions

Pseudohypoparathyroidism is a disease very similar to idiopathic hypoparathyroidism and having almost identical dental manifestations, clinical, radiographic, and histological.

Treatment with vitamin D or A.T.10 improves the medical condition by controlling the hypocalcaemia; dental tissues developed after the initiation of successful treatment are almost normal. No alteration, however, takes place in existing dental abnormalities. Careful correlation of the dental abnormalities in relation to the chronological development of the teeth can indicate the time of onset of the disease. It is possible that a deficiency of an unidentified principle in parathormone secretion, or an intermediate substance, is responsible for these characteristic manifestations.

## Summary

Four cases of pseudohypoparathyroidism are described. The dental findings are similar to those reported in cases of idiopathic hypoparathyroidism. The teeth have small crowns with thin hypoplastic enamel, the roots are often short with blunt apices, and the pulp chambers large but nearly occluded by calcified deposits. Some teeth may not be developed and others remain unerupted. Histologically, there are what appear to be vascular canals in the peripheral dentine and cementum of the root.

The published reports are reviewed, noting the references to dental manifestation in cases of idiopathic and pseudohypoparathyroidism, and correlating these with the reported findings in parathyroprivic rats.

The possible action of parathormone in these conditions is discussed briefly.

The author wishes to thank Professor A. S. Prophet of University College Hospital Dental School for advice in the preparation of this paper and Professor C. E. Dent of U.C.H. Medical School for help and encouragement during this work and for permission to investigate Cases 2 and 4; Dr. I. C. Wickes of the North Middlesex Hospital and Dr. W. A. Oliver and Mr. Alan Chapple of the Norwich and Norfolk Hospital, who made their records available and allowed investigation of Cases 1 and 3, respectively. Grateful thanks are also recorded to Dr. Sissons of the Royal National Orthopaedic Hospital for facilities to make the microradiographic study and to Mr. Dale for his guidance and assistance; finally to Dr. D. Quinsay of Jamaica for information concerning the changing conditions in Case 4 during part of the time this investigation was carried out, and to Mr. A. Lees for production of the illustrations.

BIBLIOGRAPHY


Albright, F. (1938). Metabolic effects of A.T.10 (dihydrotachysterol) compared with those of vitamin D and with those of parathyroid hormone. *Trans. Ass. Amer. Phycns*, **53**, 221.

——, Burnett, C. H., Smith, P. H., and Parson, W. (1942). Pseudohypoparathyroidism—an example of 'Seabright—Bantam syndrome'. *Endocrinology*, **30**, 922.

——, and Ellsworth, R. (1929). Studies on the physiology of the parathyroid glands. I. Calcium and phosphorus studies on a case of idiopathic hypoparathyroidism. *J. clin. Invest.*, **7**, 183.

——, and Reifenstein, E. C. (1948). *The Parathyroid Glands and Metabolic Bone Disease*. Williams and Wilkins, Baltimore.

——, and Strock, M. S. (1933). The association of acalcification of dentine with hypoparathyroidism in rats and the cure of same with parathormone, with some correlated observations in man. *J. clin. Invest.*, **12**, 974.

Alexander, S. B., and Tucker, H. St. G., Jr. (1949). Pseudohypoparathyroidism. Report of a case with late manifestations. *J. clin. Endocr.*, **9**, 862.

Bakwin, H., Gorman, W. F., and Ziegra, S. R. (1950). Pseudohypoparathyroid tetany. *J. Pediat.*, **36**, 567.

Barr, D. P., MacBryde, C. M., and Sanders, T. E. (1938). Tetany with increased intracranial pressure and papilledema—results from treatment with dihydrotachysterol. *Trans. Ass. Amer. Phycns*, **53**, 227.

Bishop, P. M. F., and de Mowbray, R. R. (1951). Pseudohypoparathyroidism. *Proc. roy. Soc. Med.*, **44**, 952.

Camp, J. D. (1947). Symmetrical calcification of cerebral basal ganglia: its roentgenologic significance in the diagnosis of parathyroid insufficiency. *Radiology*, **49**, 568.

Collip, J. B., Clark, E. P., and Scott, J. W. (1925). The effect of a parathyroid hormone on normal animals. *J. biol. Chem.*, **63**, 439.

Dent, C. E., Bishop, P. M. F., and de Mowbray, R. R. (1953). Discussion on the physiology and clinical disorders of the parathyroid glands. *Proc. roy. Soc. Med.*, **46**, 291.

Drake, T. G., Albright, F., Bauer, W., and Castleman, B. (1939). Chronic idiopathic hypoparathyroidism: report of six cases with autopsy findings in one. *Ann. intern. Med.*, **12**, 1751.

Ellsworth, R., and Howard, J. E. (1934). Studies on the physiology of the parathyroid glands. VII. Some responses of normal human kidneys and blood to intravenous parathyroid extract. *Bull. Johns Hopk. Hosp.*, **55**, 296.

Elrick, H., Albright, F., Bartter, F. C., Forbes, A. P., and Reeves, J. D. (1950). Further studies on pseudo-hypoparathyroidism: report of four new cases. *Acta endocr.* (*Kbh.*), **5**, 199.

——, Bartter, F. C., Sutphin, A., and Albright, F. (1949). Pseudohypoparathyroidism: a report of 2 new cases with special reference to the epiphyseal changes. *J. clin. Endocr.*, **9**, 665.

Emerson, K., Jr., Walsh, F. B., and Howard, J. E. (1941). Idiopathic hypoparathyroidism: a report of 2 cases. *Ann. intern. Med.*, **14**, 1256.

Erdheim, J. (1906). Tetania parathyreoprivea. *Mitt. Grenzgeb. Med. Chir.*, **16**, 632.

Gottlieb, B. (1920). Schmelzhypoplasie und Rhachitis. *Wien. Vjschr. Zahnheilk.*, **36**, 76.

Grette, K. (1955). A case of hypoparathyroidism in an 18 years old girl. *Acta. endocr.* (*Kbh.*), **18**, 506.

Hagberg, B., and Olsson, H. (1956). Tandutvecklingsrubbning vid underfunktion av parathyreoideakörtlarna. *Odont. Revy*, **7**, 197.

Hansted, C., and Holst, G. (1952). Changes in dental tissue in hypoparathyroidism. *Acta. odont. scand.*, **10**, 71.

Hinrichs, E. H., Jr. (1956). Dental changes in idiopathic juvenile hypoparathyroidism. *Oral. Surg.*, **9**, 1102.

Humphreys, H. F. (1939). The teeth from a case of hypoparathyroidism. *Proc. roy. Soc. Med.*, **32**, 633.

Keating F. R. Jr. (1947). Normal and pathologic physiology of the parathyroid glands. *Amer. J. Orthodont.*, **33**, 129P.

Lachmann, A. (1941). Hypoparathyroidism in Denmark. A clinical study. *Acta med. scand.*, suppl. 121.

Laing, J. K. (1960). Pseudo-hypoparathyroidism; report of a case. *N.Z. med. J.*, **59**, 156.

Learner, N., and Brown, C. L. (1943). Ectodermal disorders in chronic hypoparathyroidism. *J. clin. Endocr.*, **3**, 261.

Lovestedt, S. A. (1950). The dental picture of spontaneous parathyroid insufficiency. *Oral. Surg.*, **3**, 396.

Lowe, C. U., Ellinger, A. J., Wright, W. S., and Stauffen, H. M. (1950). Pseudohypoparathyroidism. (The Seabright Bantam syndrome). *J. Pediat.*, **36**, 1.

MacGregor, M. E., and Whitehead, T. P. (1954). Pseudo-hypoparathyroidism. A description of three cases and a critical appraisal of earlier accounts of the disease. *Arch. Dis. Childh.*, **29**, 398, 418.

Mackler, H., Fouts, J. R., and Birsner, J. W. (1952). Familial pseudohypoparathyroidism: a report of two cases. *Calif. Med.*, **77**, 332.

McLean, M. M. (1954). Chronic idiopathic hypoparathyroidism associated with moniliasis. *Arch. Dis. Childh.*, **29**, 419.

Miller, A. T. (1957). *Oral Diagnosis and Treatment*, 3rd ed., p. 649. The Blakiston Company, Philadelphia.

Moehlig, R. C., and Gerisch, R. A. (1950). Pseudohypoparathyroidism with decreased glucose tolerance: report of a case. *J. clin. Endocr.*, **10**, 1609.

Mortell, E. J. (1946). Idiopathic hypoparathyroidism with mental deterioration: effect of treatment on intellectual function. *ibid.*, **6**, 266.

de Mowbray, R. R., Smith, S. H. Llewellyn, and Symonds, W. J. C. (1954). Hypoparathyroidism and pseudo-hypoparathyroidism. *Brit. med. J.*, **1**, 903.

Nally, J. N., and Courvoisier, B. (1953). Étude des anomalies dentaires dans les syndromes d'insuffisance parathyroïdienne. *Schweiz. Mschr. Zahnheilk.*, **63**, 764.

Peterman, M. G., and Garvey, J. L. (1948). Pseudohypoparathyroidism; a case report. *J. Lab. clin. Med.*, **33**, 1620.

——, and —— (1949). Pseudohypoparathyroidism: case report. *Pediatrics*, **4**, 790.

Prentice, R. J. (1954). Pseudohypoparathyroidism: a case report. *J. clin. Endocr.*, **14**, 1069.

Schour, I., Chandler, S. B., and Tweedy, W. R. (1937). Changes in the teeth following parathyroidectomy. I. The effects of different periods of survival, fasting, and repeated pregnancies and lactations on the incisor of the rat. *Amer. J. Path.*, **13**, 945.

——, and Massler, M. (1943). Endocrines and dentistry. *J. Amer. dent. Ass.*, **30**, 595, 763, 943.

——, and —— (1945). The effects of dietary deficiencies upon the oral structures. II. *ibid.*, **32**, 871.

Selye, H. (1947). *Textbook of Endocrinology*, p. 570. Acta Endocrinologica, Univ. de Montreal, Montreal.

Sprague, R. G., Haines, S. F., and Power, M. H. (1945). Metabolic effects of parathyroid hormone, dihydrotachysterol and calciferol in a case of pseudohypoparathyroidism. *J. Lab. clin. Med.*, **30**, 363.

Steinberg, H., and Waldron, B. R. (1952). Idiopathic hypoparathyroidism: an analysis of 52 cases, including the report of a new case. *Medicine* (*Baltimore*), **31**, 133.

Sunde, O. E., and Hals, E. (1961). Dental changes in a patient with hypoparathyroidism. *Brit. dent. J.*, **111**, 112.

Sutphin, A., Albright, F., and McCune, D. J. (1943). Five cases (3 in siblings) of idiopathic hypoparathyroidism associated with moniliasis. *J. clin. Endocr.*, **3**, 625.

Talbot, N. B., Sobel, E. H., McArthur, J. W., and Crawford, J. D (1952). *Functional Endocrinology*, pp. 111-114. Harvard Univ. Press, Cambridge (Mass.).

Taubenhaus, M., and Engle, H. M. (1945). Clinical observations on a case of idiopathic tetany and epilepsy. *J. clin. Endocr.*, **5**, 147.

Toyofuku, T. (1911). Ueber die parathyreoprive Veränderung des Rattenzahnes. *Frankfurt. Z. Path.*, **7**, 249.

Trevathan, T. H. (1961). Delayed eruption of teeth in pseudohypoparathyroidism. *N.Z. dent J.*, **57**, 20.

Ziskin, D. E., Salmon, T. N., and Applebaum, E. (1940). The effect of thyroparathyroidectomy at birth and at 7 days on dental and skeletal development of rats. *J. dent. Res.*, **19**, 93.

# BOOK REVIEWS

**The Family and Individual Development.** By D. W. WINNICOTT. (Pp. viii + 181. 30s.) London: Tavistock Publications. 1965.

Even to the paediatrician who has acquired an adequate veneer of psychological understanding, the language of Freud is not always acceptable or at times even understandable. Yet most of these 18 lectures were delivered, over the course of the past decade, to various non-medical people concerned in some way with mothers and infants and families generally: and they read amazingly well. The writing is beautifully simple and easily understood and thereby gains immeasurably in its impact. Dr. Winnicott has profound respect for mothers and a deep instinctive understanding of the psychological and emotional situations that motivate and guide, and sometimes impede, the infant's development and growth, and it is this, rather than his avowed adherence to the psycho-analytical school, that makes what he says convincing. It is also important since, as he points out, doctors and nurses have so often to interfere with the mother-child relationship, and they ought to know what they are interfering with. But Freudian he is, and so 'emotional development starts at the beginning . . . and it is not possible to ignore the events of the first few days and hours . . . and even birth experience may be significant'.

Dr. Winnicott takes his reader through the story of human emotional development, from infancy to childhood and adolescence, into adult life, and delineates some of the pitfalls that may overtake the child on the way. The utterly dependent infant gradually acquires an awareness of his dependence and the capacity for letting the environment know when attention is needed. The environment is at first the mother, for whom Dr. Winnicott has such respect. During pregnancy, he says, she has gradually acquired a 'primary maternal preoccupation', almost like an illness, which gives her a special ability to do the right thing.

The environment extends to the father and the family circle and through them all to society. Gradually out of dependence emerges the beginnings of independence and by 5 years the child is 'emerging from an enclosure' into which it becomes increasingly difficult to return. Here the benefits of widening experience are discussed and the need for school, where more extensive facilities may exist than in the home, but where still 'someone is always present to supervise the child's first experiments in social life such as bashing the next child on the head with a spade'.

Several chapters are devoted to the integrative and disruptive factors at work in the family which, Dr. Winnicott points out, may work both ways. The child may himself 'contribute in' to the family situation or, if he is anti-social, may become a disrupting element even to the extent of having to be removed for the sake of the integrity of the family circle.

There is a delightful and, to worried parents, illuminating chapter on adolescence—'struggling through the doldrums'—for which Dr. Winnicott rightly says there exists no real cure other than the 'passage of time and the gradual maturation process', and here he makes some perhaps surprising remarks on what he considers to be the three main social developments that have altered the whole climate for adolescents; venereal disease, which is no longer a bogey and deterrent; the development of contraceptive techniques, which allows the adolescent to explore 'if she or he has a mind to the whole area of sensuous living without suffering the mental agony that accidental conception involves'; and the atom bomb which, he maintains, 'because we have to carry on now on the basis that *there is not going to be another war*' has profoundly altered the relationship between adult society and the everflowing adolescent tide. Dr. Winnicott does not develop this theme and leaves the reader frustrated and wanting to have it out with him.

The final chapter 'Some thoughts on the meaning of democracy' is perhaps less convincing than the rest, and Dr. Winnicott himself admits he is stepping outside his own speciality in attempting to equate what he has said about the family and individual development with the political state of the society within which families are situated and individuals develop. Nevertheless it is an interesting attempt to integrate political thought with developmental psychology.

These essays are packed with the author's very personal wisdom, humanity, and charm, and will illuminate the understanding of any adult who reads them. If one had half a dozen copies to whom would one give them? to a Sister in charge of a children's ward, a health visitor, a married couple embarking on a family, a children's officer, a midwife perhaps, and certainly to a paediatrician.

**The Advancement of Child Health.** (Heath Clark Lectures 1961). By A. V. NEALE. (Pp. 191; 49 tables. 25s.) London: University of London—The Athlone Press. 1964.

The Heath Clark Lectures for 1961, delivered by A. V. Neale in the University of London, are here published in book form. In reading these pages one can learn much of their writer, a man devoted to the welfare of children: patient, painstaking, erudite, and clear-thinking. The chapters contain a wealth of information on medical practice, public attitudes, and litigation regarding health and disease, especially of children, throughout the ages and over the world. The first chapter reviews in general terms the advances of thought on the education and medical care of children. The second chapter deals with human reproduction, and the importance of maternal health and care in relation to the welfare of the foetus and infant. In the following chapters Neale illustrates the ways in which advances have been made by reference to epidemiology, especially in relation to tuberculosis and juvenile rheumatism, and the final chapter surveys the interrelation of the many aspects of child health. Throughout the book there is evidence of much patient research, with valuable statistical tables and references to the many men whose teaching and writing have influenced the progress of humanity. There is an extensive bibliography. The writing is simple, direct, and non-technical, and the book can be read with profit and pleasure by all those, medical and lay, who are interested in the welfare of children, and of humanity as a whole.

**Assessment of Cerebral Palsy. I. Muscle Function, Locomotion and Hand Function.** By K. S. HOLT. (Pp. vi + 214; 103 figures + 4 tables. 40s.) London: Lloyd-Luke (Medical Books). 1965.

Here is a constructive contribution to the treatment of cerebral palsy. In a child with cerebral palsy there exists a dynamic situation in which the abnormalities of muscle function can lead to the development of deformities and disabilities, and great care is needed in interpreting the significance of what is taking place.

In this book, the result of work carried out at the Ryegate Cerebral Palsy Centre, Sheffield, Dr. Holt suggests ways of observing and assessing the many factors that contribute to the total disabilities of cerebral palsy.

It has a practical approach which should prove useful to specialists and therapists.

The assessments of muscle function are helpful to the understanding of the peculiar difficulties experienced in cerebral palsy in initiating and maintaining muscle contraction. While those on the range of joint movements contribute useful information as to how much any deformity may be responsible for disability, therefore what functional benefit can be expected from treatment, especially surgical.

The failure to appreciate the importance of this issue in the past has accounted for many disappointments in treatment which produced a good anatomical result without any improvement of function, and sometimes an actual deterioration, whereas probably the most rewarding result of physiotherapy comes from the anticipation and prevention of deformities which are likely to develop. The results in both instances depend upon adequate assessments to determine the right course of action at the optimum time. These sections are particularly well illustrated with clear informative pictures, as are also the assessments of arm and hand action.

Some of the assessments of posture and balance tend to be a little finicky and in carrying them out a few enthusiasts may lose sight of the child involved. Dr. Holt, however, never loses sight of the whole child, and stresses the importance of critical discussion at every opportunity between all the therapists and doctors concerned, for the most senior person present has only one pair of eyes, and judgement improves immensely as a result of frequent free comment and discussion. It is to be hoped that the publication of this book will likewise help all those concerned with the assessment of cerebral palsy.

**Infantile Spasms. A Review of the Literature and a Study of 112 Cases.** Clinics in Developmental Medicine No. 15. By PETER M. JEAVONS and BRIAN D. BOWER. (Pp. 82; 15 figures + 22 tables. 20s.; $3) London: The Spastics Society Medical Education and Information Unit in Association with William Heinemann Medical Books. 1964.

This admirable monograph is concerned with the syndrome—known by many names—of infantile spasms with mental subnormality and often a characteristic electroencephalographic abnormality. The book begins with a review of the literature, which is particularly valuable since many of the key papers are in foreign languages. The landmarks include Dr. W. J. West's account of his own son's 'salaam spasms' in 1841, the description of the EEG by Vazquez and Turner in 1951 and the results of corticotrophin treatment published by Sorel in 1958. The authors then review their own series of 112 cases followed for periods of up to 9 years. They distinguish clearly between symptomatic cases with a known underlying metabolic or cerebral abnormality, and cryptogenic cases where the prognosis is slightly better. In 16 infants the first spasm occurred within one week of pertussis immunization and though a causal relation is hard to establish with certainty it seems disturbingly likely that in some instances this tragic condition is iatrogenic.

The authors analyse in detail their extensive experience of steroid treatment. Though in most cases, particularly in the cryptogenic group, the spasms can quickly be stopped, there is little evidence of any improvement in subsequent mental development. The possible exceptions are some instances where steroid treatment was begun very soon after the onset of spasms. This emphasizes the need for early recognition of a condition where at present there is often delay in diagnosis. This monograph should help to spread knowledge and awareness of infantile spasms. It is exceptionally lucid and readable, sufficiently detailed to be of value to specialists in neurology or epilepsy, and at the same time readily comprehensible (even in the sections on electroencephalography) to any doctor concerned with infant care. It easily ranks with the best of the very good Little Club publications.

*Review Article*

*Arch. Dis. Childh.*, 1965, **40**, 575.

# THE LUNGS AT BIRTH

BY

L. B. STRANG

*From the Department of Paediatrics, University College Hospital Medical School, London*

(RECEIVED FOR PUBLICATION JUNE 20, 1965)

In order to obtain insight into disturbances of pulmonary function in newborn infants we have to consider the physiological changes that occur in the lungs at birth. By combining the information obtained from a variety of animal experiments with our clinical observations, we can construct a fairly coherent picture of some of these events and see the ways in which their normal course is disturbed by disease. The first breath of air also marks the beginning of individual life, an abrupt change in the mode of external respiration, and it stands in its own right as a subject of general interest.

The ultimate exchange of oxygen and carbon dioxide between cells and their environment occurs by molecular diffusion, but multicellular forms require a specialized organ of external respiration such as gills, placenta, or lungs, to and from which the gases are transported by a circulation. During foetal life the infant's gases exchange in the placenta between two liquids, the maternal and foetal bloods, but from the moment of birth this function is transferred to the lungs where the exchange is between liquid and gas. In this sense the evolutionary development from water to air is re-enacted each time an infant is born.

The foetal lungs are functionally inert. The alveoli are filled with liquid, and they are perfused by only 10% of the cardiac output. For the lungs to acquire their function as a gas exchanger a number of changes must take place. A gas-liquid interface has to be formed and the alveoli have to acquire a volume of gas which remains in the lungs even at the end of an expiration, and can be exchanged with the atmosphere by the movements of ventilation. It is also fundamental for normal gas exchange that the gas volume should be evenly distributed throughout the lungs. As the gas that enters the foetal lungs occupies a space formerly filled with liquid, we also have to consider how this liquid is removed.

On the other side of the interface a large increase in blood flow is required. Although the rates at which gases equilibrate in the lung depend on the area, thickness, and composition of the tissues lying between the gas and blood, the amounts exchanged depend on the flow of blood through the lungs. In the adult, pulmonary blood flow equals right ventricular output, but in the foetus most of the cardiac output bypasses the lungs. At the start of breathing an increase in pulmonary flow is achieved by a change in the distribution of cardiac output.

These various changes are all a consequence of the first breath of air, which depends on the activity of the respiratory muscles and the nervous system. The present account, however, is confined to events in the lungs. The formation of an alveolar gas volume, the removal of liquid from the foetal lungs, and the increase in pulmonary blood flow are functionally linked, but they can be separated for descriptive purposes.

### Formation of Alveolar Volume

FIG. 1A shows the relation between inflating pressure and lung volume when the lungs of a mature foetal lamb are inflated with air through the trachea. The same relationships apply when the inflating pressure is a negative pleural pressure and have been verified in a variety of other species. During inflation, an opening pressure of 18 cm. $H_2O$ is required before any air enters the lungs and then they inflate readily to their full volume with only a small further increase in pressure. The deflation curve is widely separated from the inflation curve, and at each pressure much more air remains in the lung during deflation than during inflation. Even at zero pressure about 25% of the lung volume remains. The second inflation of this lung is different because no opening pressure is now required and the lung inflates to 80% of its volume at a pressure that was



2

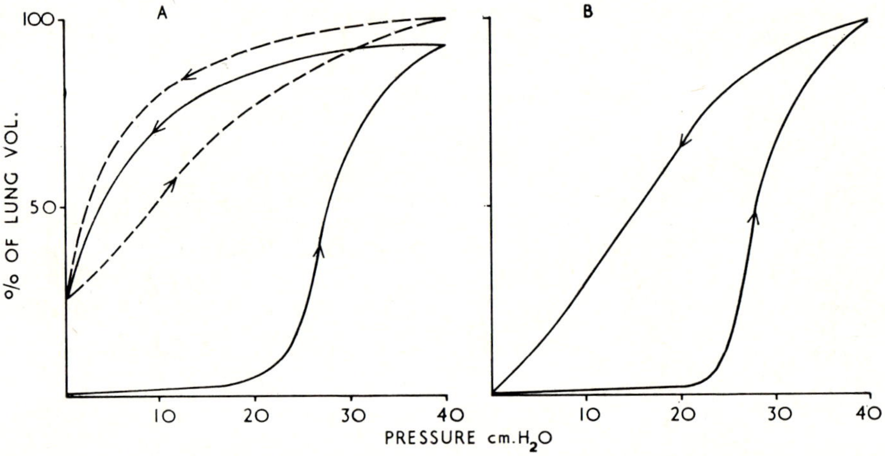


FIG. 1A.—Relationship between inflating pressure and the volume of gas in the lung during the first and second inflation of the lungs of a lamb of 140 days' gestation (term = 147 days). The first inflation and deflation are shown with a solid line, the second with an interrupted line. Direction (whether inflation or deflation) is indicated by arrows.

FIG. 1B.—Inflating pressure and gas volume of the lungs of a lamb of 122 days' gestation. In this case there is no difference between the first and second inflations.

insufficient to open it for the first time. Fig. 1B shows the relationship for an immature lamb. The inflation curve is similar to Fig. 1A, but the deflation limb is closer to the inflation curve, and at zero pressure the lung is empty of air. For this reason the lung has to be reopened with the second breath and with each succeeding breath. Figs. 2A and 2B represent these curves pictorially as steps in the inflation and deflation of an imaginary alveolus.

Thus in the mature lung a stable alveolar volume (Functional Residual Capacity—FRC) is formed after the first inflation, and normal ventilation can proceed with relatively small pleural pressure changes. Each succeeding tidal breath exchanges about 30% of this FRC for fresh air (Strang and McGrath, 1962), while oxygen and carbon dioxide exchange continuously between the gas and blood. In the immature lung, as almost no FRC is formed, ventilation requires abnormally large pressures to open the lungs with each new breath, and it seems likely that gas exchange can take place only during inspiration, while the alveoli are held open, instead of during the whole ventilatory cycle. A dynamic picture of ventilation in these two types of lung can be obtained by watching the surface of a lamb's lung during positive pressure ventilation. In the mature lung the first inflation converts the liver-like lung of the foetal lamb to the pale pink inflated appearance

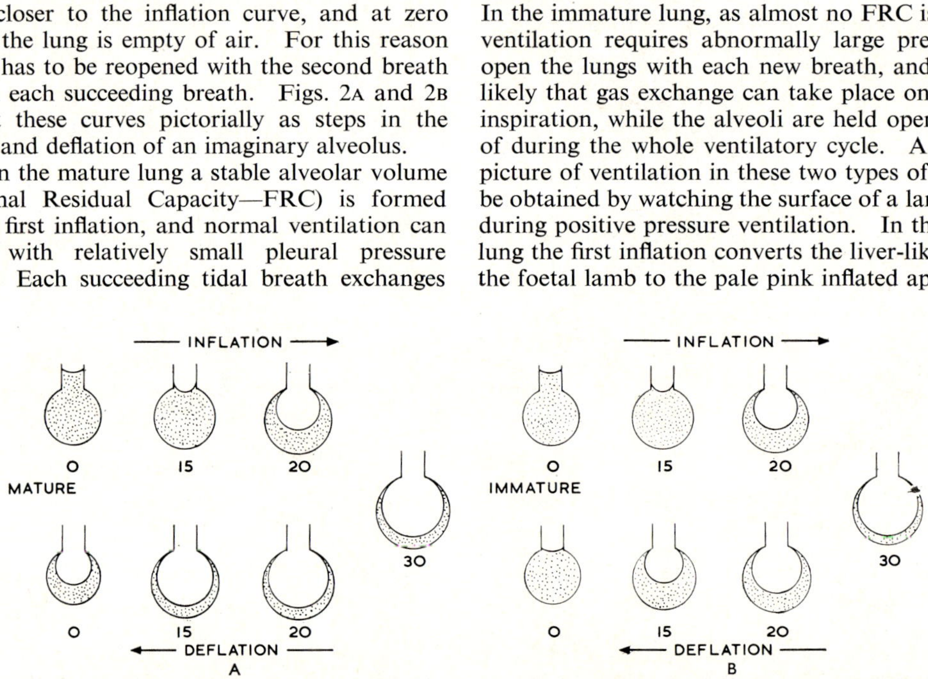


FIG. 2A.—Pictorial representation of stages during the initial inflation and deflation of an imaginary alveolus in a mature lung such as that represented in 1A. The alveolus is pictured as being filled with liquid (shaded) before air enters it, and the air is accommodated partly by displacement of the liquid. Numbers indicate inflating pressure in cm. $H_2O$.

FIG. 2B.—Inflation and deflation of imaginary alveolus from immature lung such as that represented in 1B.

characteristic of normal lungs, and during deflation this appearance is retained. By contrast the immature lung has the inflated appearance only at the peak of inspiration and returns to the foetal appearance during each expiratory phase.

The formation of a stable FRC in the mature lung can be explained by the properties of the surface film which forms in the alveoli. The alveoli of the normal lung are lined by a lipoprotein film which on compression has a very low surface tension, and prevents the alveoli from collapsing under the pressure generated by their surfaces (Pattle, 1955). To understand this statement we have to consider the effect of surface tension at a curved interface. The molecules of a liquid exert an attracting force on each other. At any depth in the liquid these forces balance, but at the surface there remains an unbalanced intermolecular attraction which creates the surface tension. The effect of this force is to pull the surface to as small an area as possible. When the surface is curved, surface tension will exert a force in the direction of the radius. In a sphere, for example a bubble in water, surface tension will produce a pressure difference across the wall. The relationship between the pressure generated in a sphere by the tension in its wall is given by an expression of La Place, $P = \frac{2\gamma}{r}$ (where P is pressure, $\gamma$ is tension, and r is radius). Consider an alveolus into which air has been forced by the first inspiration. If the air space which is formed is spherical with a radius of $5 \times 10^{-3}$ cm. and the surface tension is 55 dynes/cm. (the surface tension of most body fluids), the surface will exert a pressure of 22·5 cm. $H_2O$. In other words a negative pleural pressure of this amount would be required to hold the space open, and during expiration, when the inspiratory muscles are relaxed, the space would collapse. In the mature lung a surface film of lipoprotein is formed as soon as air enters the lung which, when compressed, yields a very low surface tension, probably of the order of 1-5 dynes/cm., whereas the same film when stretched gives a surface tension value of about 50 dynes/cm. (Clements, Brown, and Johnson, 1958). During inspiration, while the alveoli are enlarging, a considerable pressure is generated by the lung surface, but as soon as expiration starts and the alveolar surface is compressed a little, the surface tension falls and the retractive pressure generated by the surface becomes much less. For example in the alveolus considered above, a surface tension of 1 dyne per cm. would yield a pressure of about 0·5 cm. $H_2O$. The presence of lipoprotein (surfactant), which forms a film with these special characteristics, explains the pressure-volume characteristics of the lung illustrated in Fig. 1A, and in particular the small pressure generated during deflation. The surfactant material could not be demonstrated in the lung illustrated in Fig. 1B, which accounts for its different behaviour during deflation, including the failure to form an FRC.

Surfactant also tends to stabilize the distribution of air in the lungs. Because of the relationship between pressure and radius in the La Place equation, smaller alveoli would develop a higher pressure than larger alveoli and tend to empty into them, if the surface tension remained constant. However, as an alveolus decreases in size, its lining film becomes more compressed and its surface tension falls, thus tending to equalize the pressures in alveoli of differing size and consequently to equalize the alveolar sizes themselves.

Thus, the formation of a stable alveolar volume, and its equal distribution in the lungs, depends on the special properties of the surface film which is formed in alveoli when air first enters the lung. The lipoprotein from which the film is formed is probably present in functionally adequate amounts from about 30 weeks' gestation onwards in the human, but it appears relatively later in the gestations of lambs, rabbits, and mice. (For a review of this question see Strang and Reynolds, 1965.)

**Removal of Liquid from the Lungs**

The lungs of the foetus contain clear liquid which, in the foetal lamb, pours readily from the cut end of the trachea or bronchus. Its volume is about 50 ml. in a foetal lamb of 3·5 kg. (Howatt, Humphreys, Normand, and Strang, 1965), which is similar to the alveolar gas volume (FRC) in infants of similar weight (Strang and McGrath, 1962). Indeed the resting volume of the lungs, which depends on the position where the elastic recoil of the lungs is balanced by the elastic recoil of the chest wall, should be very similar before and after a breath of air if the surface force is small. With a large surface force the gas volume should be smaller than the liquid volume. Setnikar, Agostoni, and Taglietti (1959) and Adams and Fujiwara (1963) have shown that the lung liquid differs in composition from amniotic liquid and contains much less bicarbonate than a blood transudate, from which we may deduce that it is a lung secretion.

Where does the liquid go when breathing starts? Some can be squeezed out through the mouth during the second stage of labour, or drain by gravity when the newborn infant is held head down. The amount that remains in the lungs must vary with the circumstances of delivery and should be greatest after caesarean section. As the survival of mature infants after this mode of delivery is as good as after vaginal delivery (Strang, Anderson, and Platt, 1957) the volume drained from the lungs is probably unimportant for survival. The remaining fluid must be taken up when breathing starts, but there have been no direct studies of the rate at which this takes place. The mean weight of mature lambs' lungs falls by about 50 g. during the first six hours of life and then no further, suggesting that the liquid is cleared in this period (author's unpublished data). The liquid is usually assumed to be absorbed directly into the blood, but no change that would favour this transfer, such as a fall in pulmonary capillary pressure, is known to occur. Indeed the pulmonary vasodilatation at the onset of breathing should cause a rise in capillary pressure, if, as seems likely, the change in vasomotor tone is in precapillary arterioles.

Recent experiments have shown that a large increase in lymph flow from the lungs accompanies the onset of ventilation in mature lambs, and it seems likely that some of the lung liquid is cleared from the lungs by this route (Boston, Humphreys, Reynolds, and Strang, 1965). The mechanism envisaged is that air entering the alveoli displaces liquid (as in Fig. 2A) into the interalveolar spaces of the lung where lymphatic capillaries are abundant. A similar mechanism for the removal of lung liquid was suggested by Aherne and Dawkins (1964) from the histological appearance of rabbits' lungs. Boston *et al.* (1965) found a much smaller increase of lymph flow at the onset of ventilation in immature lambs. In the immature lung it may be that abnormally high surface tensions cause the alveoli to fill up with liquid during expiration (as pictured in Fig. 2B) and impede the transfer of liquid to the interalveolar spaces.

### Increase in Pulmonary Blood Flow

During foetal life most of the inflow from the great veins bypasses the lungs. About half the flow from the inferior vena cava passes directly through the foramen ovale to the left atrium, the left ventricle, and the aorta. The remaining inferior vena caval flow and the superior vena caval flow enters the right atrium, right ventricle, and pulmonary artery. From the pulmonary artery most of the flow goes to the aorta through the ductus arteriosus, and only a small fraction (say 10%) passes through the lungs. This distribution depends on the vascular resistance in the lungs being higher than the systemic vascular resistance. Dawes, Mott, Widdicombe, and Wyatt (1953) showed that a large decrease in pulmonary vascular resistance occurred when the lungs were first ventilated and that pulmonary blood flow increased by a factor of 5 or 10. Closure of the valve of the foramen ovale by a rise in left atrial pressure above inferior vena caval pressure is a consequence of the increased inflow to the left atrium from the lungs. Closure of the ductus arteriosus occurs by active constriction of the muscle in its wall, which contracts in response to a rise in the oxygen tension of the arterial blood leaving the newly ventilated lung. For a review of these changes see Dawes (1958). Thus all the changes in the circulation depend on the decrease in pulmonary vascular resistance at the onset of ventilation, and hence it is important to determine by what means the vascular resistance is lowered.

In experiments that aim to compare the vascular resistance of the lungs under various conditions, serious difficulties of interpretation may arise because the relationship between pulmonary artery pressure and flow is non-linear. Fig. 3 shows two pressure flow curves for the pulmonary vessels of a lamb. If the relationship were linear through zero, resistance, computed as pressure divided by flow, would be a constant, but this is not true of these grossly non-linear relations. As shown in Fig. 3, a change in perfusion pressure such as will occur during a change in vascular resistance, unless it is artificially controlled, can cause an apparent change in vascular resist-

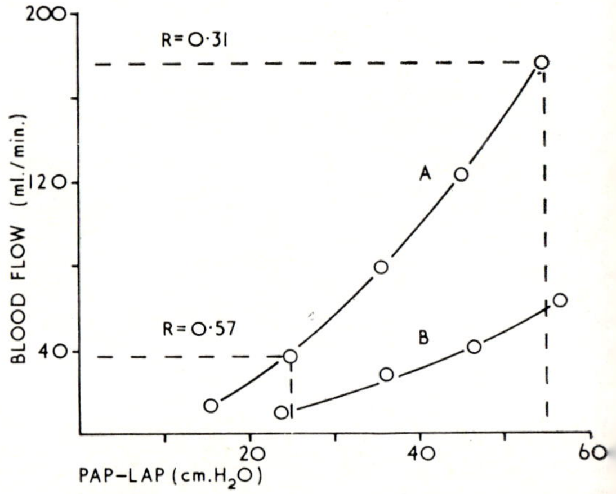


FIG. 3.—Pressure flow curves of the vasculature of the left lung of a lamb. Curve B was obtained during lung collapse and curve A during ventilation with air. The curves were obtained by perfusing the lung at a series of pulmonary artery pressures (PAP) while left atrial pressure (LAP) remained steady. As shown, calculated 'resistance' (R), obtained by dividing pressure by flow, gives lower values at a high PAP than at a low PAP. In one set of experiments differences such as that between curves A and B were investigated by comparing the flows at a constant PAP. In another set of experiments the comparison was made by drawing pressure flow curves using the device shown in Fig. 5. In Fig. 6 pressure flow curves have been simplified by showing straight lines fitted to the steepest part of the curves. (Reproduced from Cook *et al.* (1963) by permission of *J. Physiol.* (*Lond.*).)

ance when there is really no intrinsic change in the vessels themselves. For this reason, in the type of experiments to be considered now, some device has to be adopted that will allow comparisons between states of the vasculature, such as those depicted by the two curves in Fig. 3. There are three possible solutions: (i) to hold flow constant by some device and compare perfusion pressure, (ii) to hold pressure constant and compare flows, (iii) to draw some kind of pressure flow curve for each set of conditions. In the experiments to be described methods (ii) and (iii) have been used.

Experiments in which the left pulmonary artery of the lamb was perfused at a constant pressure showed that the pulmonary vessels could exhibit an extremely active vasomotor tone, and that lowering the oxygen tension or increasing the carbon dioxide tension of the ventilating gas had a strong vasoconstrictor effect (Fig. 4) (Cook, Drinker, Jacobson, Levison,

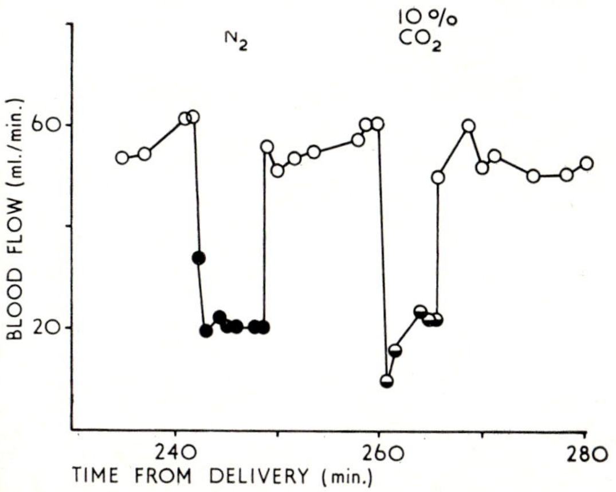


FIG. 4.—Measurement of left pulmonary artery flow in the lamb at a constant pulmonary artery pressure of 40 cm. $H_2O$. The open circles are blood flow during ventilation of the lung with air, the closed circles are flow during ventilation with nitrogen, and the half-closed circles are flow during ventilation with 10% carbon dioxide in air. The sharp decreases in flow at a constant perfusion pressure are due to powerful vasoconstriction. (Reproduced from Cook *et al.* (1963) by permission of *J. Physiol.* (*Lond.*).)

and Strang, 1963). The vasomotor tone of the foetal lung was also detected by the vasodilator effects of acetyl choline and histamine (Dawes and Mott, 1962). The vasoconstrictor effect of asphyxial gas tensions could also be produced in the unexpanded foetal lung by umbilical cord occlusion (Dawes and Mott, 1962) or by perfusing the lung with blood of high $P_{CO_2}$ and low $P_{O_2}$ (Cassin, Dawes, Mott, Ross, and Strang, 1964). There was some evidence that the changes in gas tension were effective mainly by a direct action on the pulmonary vascular muscle, rather than through chemoreceptors (Cook *et al.*, 1963).

The $P_{O_2}$ and $P_{CO_2}$ of the foetal lung are determined by the tensions of these gases in the pulmonary arterial blood. This implies that the areas with the highest $P_{O_2}$'s will have a tension between 20 and 30 mm. Hg, and the areas with the lowest $P_{CO_2}$'s, a tension between 40 and 50 mm. Hg. Ventilation with air will raise the highest $P_{O_2}$ areas to over 100 mm. Hg and decrease the $P_{CO_2}$ by an amount dependent on the extent to which blood flow increases in response to ventilation. Plainly the vasodilatation at the onset of breathing could be due to the effects of changes in gas tensions alone. Sensitivity of the vasomotor tone to $P_{CO_2}$ would, in particular, tend to match blood flow to ventilation, because alveolar $P_{CO_2}$ is an almost linear function of the ratio of ventilation to perfusion. For example, if a lung were well ventilated but poorly perfused (high ventilation-perfusion ratio), the $P_{CO_2}$ would fall and tend to increase perfusion by decreasing vasomotor tone.

The extent to which the changes in gas tension do in fact determine the effect of ventilation was investigated by Cassin *et al.* (1964). In these experiments the vascular 'resistance' of the lamb's lung was determined by drawing pressure-flow curves of the vasculature of the left lung under various conditions by the means described in the captions to Figs. 5 and 6. The lungs were first ventilated with a mixture of 7% carbon dioxide in nitrogen which has gas tensions very similar to those of the blood perfusing the foetal lung. In this way the effect of ventilation could be tested independently of the gas tension changes induced by ventilation with air. Subsequently, the ventilating gas was changed to air, or to nitrogen, or to 10% carbon dioxide in air, so that the effects of increasing $P_{O_2}$ and lowering $P_{CO_2}$ could be measured separately. Fig. 6 gives the maximum slopes of the pressure flow curves obtained, showing the relative effects of ventilation with 10% carbon dioxide in nitrogen and with the other gas mixtures. In general, 20% of the vasodilatation was associated with ventilation itself, and the remainder was due in approximately equal amounts to a decrease in $P_{CO_2}$ and an increase in $P_{O_2}$. The means by which ventilation, as distinct from gas tension change, causes vasodilatation is at present unknown, but the effects of $P_{O_2}$ and $P_{CO_2}$ are clearly identified as vasomotor. Naeye (1961) has shown that the muscular coat of pulmonary arterioles in the foetus is thicker than that of the systemic arterioles, and that this muscle atrophies during the first weeks of postnatal life. These arterioles are presumably the site of the observed vasomotor effects.

In summary, the increase in pulmonary blood flow and the redistribution of cardiac output at the start of ventilation are all due to a decrease in pulmonary

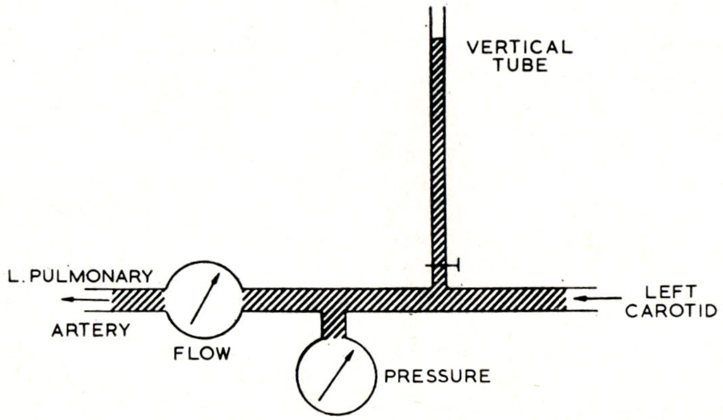


FIG. 5.—Arrangement for obtaining pressure flow curves of pulmonary vasculature in the lamb. The left lung is perfused from the left carotid artery and a vertical tube is placed in the circuit. At intervals this tube is filled with blood and the column of blood is then allowed to flow into the pulmonary artery while the carotid supply is occluded. By recording pressure and flow on the two axes of an oscilloscope or X-Y recorder, a graph of flow over a range of pressures is rapidly obtained. Curves of this kind can be drawn repeatedly. (Reproduced from Cassin *et al.* (1964) by permission of *J. Physiol.* (*Lond.*).)

vascular resistance, which is in large part due to the effects of changing $Po_2$ and $Pco_2$ on the tone of the pulmonary vessels.

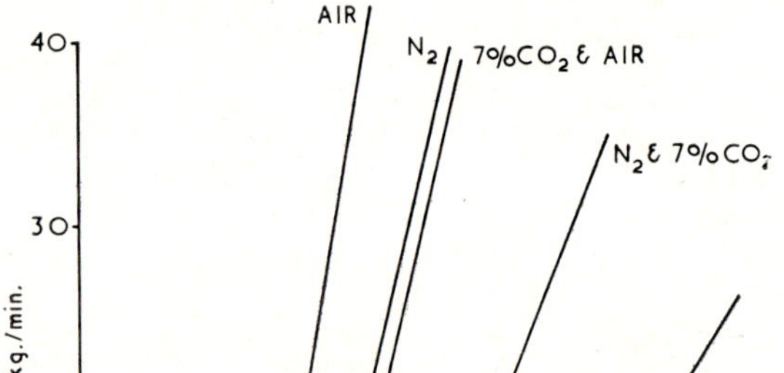


FIG. 6.—Mean pressure flow curves of the left lung of the foetal lamb. A straight line has been fitted to the maximum slope of each curve. The lower the vascular resistance, the more vertical the line and the more displaced to the left. The mean curve in the unventilated foetal lung is compared with the mean of the curves obtained after ventilation with a mixture of 7% $CO_2$ in $N_2$, with $N_2$, with 7% $CO_2$ in air, and with air as indicated on the diagram. The effect of ventilation unaccompanied by gas tension change is given by the difference between the 'foetal' line and the '7% $CO_2$ in $N_2$ line'. The effect of lowering $Pco_2$ is given by the difference between the '7% $CO_2$ in $N_2$' line and the '$N_2$' line, or by the difference between '7% $CO_2$ in air' and 'air'. Similarly the effect of raising $Po_2$ is the difference between the '$N_2$' and 'air' lines. (Reproduced from Cassin *et al.* (1964) by permission of *J. Physiol.* (*Lond.*).)

### Disturbances of the Physiological Changes in the Lungs at Birth

We have seen that important changes in the lungs at birth can be traced to two events: the formation of surface film with special properties and an active vasodilatation of pulmonary vessels. When we come to consider cardiopulmonary abnormalities in the newborn we find that the same two factors determine a large part of the abnormalities encountered.

**Respiratory Distress Syndrome.** Avery and Mead (1959) showed that pulmonary surfactant was absent or inactive in infants dying with hyaline membrane disease. The finding has been confirmed repeatedly (Pattle, Claireaux, Davies, and Cameron, 1962; Reynolds, Orzalesi, Motoyama, Craig, and Cook, 1965b), and hyaline membranes have been shown to develop in immature lambs delivered at 125-130 days' gestation (proportionally equivalent to about 34 weeks in humans), when the alveoli are fully formed, but when pulmonary surfactant cannot be detected by standard techniques (Reynolds, Jacobson, Motoyama, Kikkawa, Craig, Orzalesi, and Cook, 1965a). Indeed the absence of surfactant can account for all the findings in this condition. Extensive atelectasis due to the surfactant deficiency causes the low lung compliance (Gribetz, Frank, and Avery, 1959) which in turn leads to ventilatory insufficiency (Blystad, 1956; Strang and MacLeish, 1961) and to right-to-left shunting (Strang and MacLeish, 1961; Warley and Gairdner, 1962; Prod'hom, Levison, Cherry, Drorbaugh, Hubbell, and Smith, 1962). According to Pattle (1965) the presence of the hyaline membranes, which are mainly a blood transudate (Gitlin and Craig, 1956), can also be explained as an effect of a high alveolar surface tension which sets up a pressure gradient between the air space and the underlying capillary during any phase of ventilation in which the alveolus is held open. But variations in capillary permeability may also be an important factor in determining the amount of transudation that occurs. The development of respiratory acidosis is due to the underventilation, and the metabolic acidosis is caused by anaerobic glycolysis due to a deficient oxygen supply, itself the result of the right-to-left shunting. The oxygen deficiency may be aggravated by the excessive oxygen consumption of the overworked muscles of ventilation.

Since the whole chain of events can start with a deficiency of surfactant, the primary deficiency of this substance as a result of immaturity could be the whole cause of the disease. This theory is supported by the prevalence of the disease in prematures, perhaps the only really well-established aetiological factor as yet identified, and by the development of the disease in immature but otherwise undamaged lambs (Reynolds *et al.*, 1965a). On the other hand, the disease usually develops somewhat after the probable time of appearance of surfactant in humans (at about 30 weeks), and it seems likely that other factors can affect the surface, though this has not yet been proved.

**Right-to-left Shunting.** In general most pulmonary disturbances cause cyanosis by impairment of oxygen diffusion or by inequalities of ventilation with respect to blood flow. The breathing of pure oxygen eliminates these effects by massively increasing the gradient for diffusion and by eliminating the effects of uneven ventilation on alveolar oxygen tensions (for a more rigorous treatment of these statements see Berggren, 1942). Therefore, when cyanosis and arterial desaturation persist while the subject is breathing pure oxygen, it can only be because blood is passing through unventilated areas of the lungs or is bypassing them through extrapulmonary channels.

Newborn infants with ventilatory failure, whether caused by central depression or impaired lung mechanics, often remain deeply cyanosed even in high concentrations of oxygen. In hyaline membrane disease the finding of arterial desaturation in these circumstances is now well established and firmly attributed to right-to-left shunting. Plainly the shunting could be through unventilated atelectatic parts of the lungs, but, in the lamb at least, both lung collapse and underventilation cause an increase of pulmonary vascular resistance, presumably through their effect on alveolar gas tensions (Figs. 7 and 8) (Cook *et al.*, 1963), and this would shunt blood away from the lungs and particularly from any atelectatic areas. Thus it seems more likely to the present author that the large shunts take place through the ductus arteriosus and foramen ovale, i.e. that the circulation returns towards its foetal distribution. Just as a fall in vascular resistance determines the change from a foetal to a neonatal circulation, so will a rise in the resistance reverse the process. The finding of Chu, Clements, Cotton, Klaus, Sweet, Thomas, and Tooley (1965), that excised lungs of infants dying with hyaline membrane disease have a high vascular resistance, considerably strengthens this view of the situation. Indeed the reversibility of the circulatory changes at birth, and

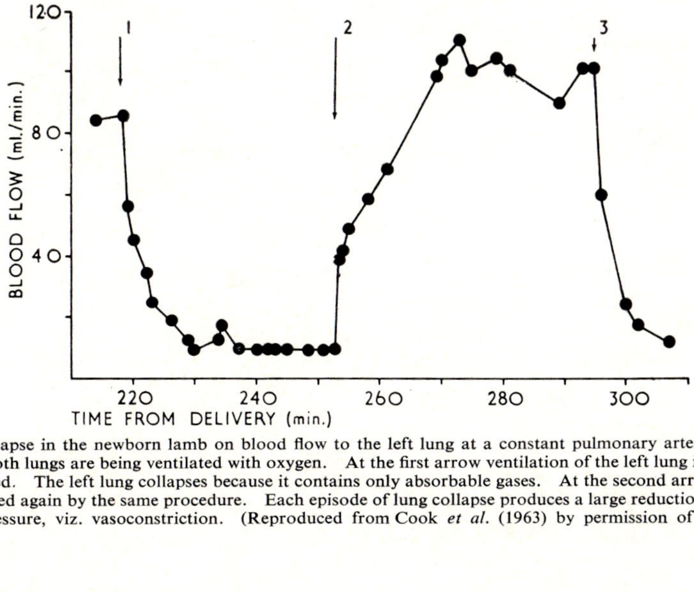


FIG. 7.—Effect of lung collapse in the newborn lamb on blood flow to the left lung at a constant pulmonary artery pressure of 40 cm. $H_2O$. At the start of the record both lungs are being ventilated with oxygen. At the first arrow ventilation of the left lung is stopped while ventilation of the right lung is continued. The left lung collapses because it contains only absorbable gases. At the second arrow the lung is reventilated, and at the third it is collapsed again by the same procedure. Each episode of lung collapse produces a large reduction of blood flow at constant pulmonary artery pressure, viz. vasoconstriction. (Reproduced from Cook *et al.* (1963) by permission of *J. Physiol.* (*Lond.*).)

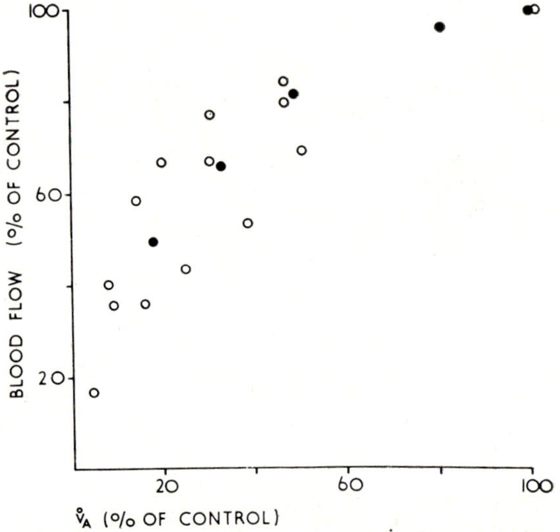


FIG. 8.—Effect of changing alveolar ventilation (V̇A) on blood flow to the left lung at constant pulmonary artery pressure. The open circles represent changes in tidal volume, the closed circles changes in frequency. Reducing pulmonary ventilation causes a more or less proportional reduction in blood flow in these circumstances. (Reproduced from Cook *et al.* (1963) by permission of *J. Physiol.* (*Lond.*).)

their dependence on ventilation of the lungs, means that severe hypoxia is a greater hazard of underventilation in the newborn infant than at other ages—a fact that may well be decisive in determining the high mortality of respiratory conditions in infants.

## Summary

When the normal infant starts to breathe there are at least three important changes in the lungs: they acquire a stable alveolar gas volume, lose the liquid with which they were filled in the foetal state, and increase their blood flow by five or ten times. The formation of the stable alveolar volume depends on the properties of the surface film (surfactant) which forms in the alveoli. The factors concerned in the uptake of liquid are still uncertain. The increase in blood flow is largely due to a decrease in pulmonary vasomotor tone brought about by an increase in $P_{O_2}$ and a decrease in $P_{CO_2}$.

Deficiency or inactivation of surfactant leads to atelectasis and all the abnormalities encountered in the respiratory distress syndrome. Maturity is one important factor in determining the amount of surfactant in the lungs at birth.

Underventilation for any reason causes a rise in pulmonary vascular resistance and a tendency to reverse the changes in the foetal circulation at birth, and hence right-to-left shunting is a common complication of respiratory failure in infants.

### REFERENCES

Adams, F. H., and Fujiwara, T. (1963). Surfactant in fetal lamb tracheal fluid. *J. Pediat.*, **63**, 537.

Aherne, W., and Dawkins, M. J. R. (1964). The removal of fluid from the pulmonary airways after birth in the rabbit, and the effect on this of prematurity and prenatal hypoxia. *Biol. Neonat.*, 7, 214.

Avery, M. E., and Mead, J. (1959). Surface properties in relation to atelectasis and hyaline membrane disease. *Amer. J. Dis. Child.*, **97**, 517.

Berggren, S. M. (1942). The oxygen deficit of arterial blood caused by non-ventilating parts of the lung. *Acta physiol. scand.*, **4**, suppl. 11.

Blystad, W. (1956). Blood gas determinations on premature infants. III. Investigations on premature infants with recurrent attacks of apnea. *Acta paediat.* (*Uppsala*), **45**, 211.

Boston, R. W., Humphreys, P. W., Reynolds, E. O. R., and Strang, L. B. (1965). Lymph flow and clearance of liquid from the lungs of the foetal lamb. *Lancet*, **2**, 473.

Cassin, S., Dawes, G. S., Mott, J. C., Ross, B. B., and Strang, L. B. (1964). The vascular resistance of the foetal and newly ventilated lung of the lamb. *J. Physiol.* (*Lond.*), **171**, 61.

Chu, J., Clements, J. A., Cotton, E., Klaus, M. H., Sweet, A. Y., Thomas, M. A., and Tooley, W. H. (1965). The pulmonary hypoperfusion syndrome. *Pediatrics*, **35**, 733.

Clements, J. A., Brown, E. S., and Johnson, R. P. (1958). Pulmonary surface tension and the mucus lining of the lungs: some theoretical considerations. *J. appl. Physiol.*, **12**, 262.

Cook, C. D., Drinker, P. A., Jacobson, H. N., Levison, H., and Strang, L. B. (1963). Control of pulmonary blood flow in the foetal and newly born lamb. *J. Physiol.* (*Lond.*), **169**, 10.

Dawes, G. (1958). Changes in the circulation at birth and the effects of asphyxia. In *Recent Advances in Paediatrics*, 2nd ed., ed D. Gairdner, pp. 1-49. Churchill, London.

——, and Mott, J. C. (1962). The vascular tone of the foetal lung. *J. Physiol.* (*Lond.*), **164**, 465.

——, ——, Widdicombe, J. G., and Wyatt, D. G. (1953). Changes in the lungs of the new-born lamb. *ibid.*, **121**, 141.

Gitlin, D., and Craig, J. M. (1956). Nature of the hyaline membrane in asphyxia of the newborn. *Pediatrics*, **17**, 64.

Gribetz, I., Frank, N. R., and Avery, M. E. (1959). Static volume-pressure relations of excised lungs of infants with hyaline membrane disease, newborn, and stillborn infants. *J. clin. Invest.*, **38**, 2168.

Howatt, W. F., Humphreys, P. W., Normand, I. C. S., and Strang, L. B. (1965). Ventilation of liquid by the fetal lamb during asphyxia. *J. appl. Physiol.*, **20**, 496.

Naeye, R. L. (1961). Arterial changes during the perinatal period. *Arch. Path.*, **71**, 121.

Pattle, R. E. (1955). Properties, function and origin of the alveolar lining layer. *Nature* (*Lond.*), **175**, 1125.

—— (1965). Surface lining of lung alveoli. *Physiol. Rev.*, **45**, 48.

——, Claireaux, A. E., Davies, P. A., and Cameron, A. H. (1962). Inability to form a lung-lining film: as a cause of the respiratory-distress syndrome in the newborn. *Lancet*, **2**, 469.

Prod'hom, L. S., Levison, H., Cherry, R. B., Drorbaugh, J. E., Hubbell, J. R., Jr., and Smith, C. A. (1962). Evolution of right-to-left shunt and acid-base balance in newborn infants with respiratory distress. *Amer. J. Dis. Child.*, **104**, 465.

Reynolds, E. O. R., Jacobson, H. N., Motoyama, E. K., Kikkawa, Y., Craig, J. M., Orzalesi, M. M., and Cook, C. D. (1965a). The effect of immaturity and prenatal asphyxia on the lungs and pulmonary function of newborn lambs: the experimental production of respiratory distress. *Pediatrics*, **35**, 382.

——, Orzalesi, M. M., Motoyama, E. K., Craig, J. M., and Cook, C. D. (1965b). Surface properties of saline extracts of the lungs of newborn infants. *Acta paediat. scand.* In the press.

Setnikar, I., Agostoni, E., and Taglietti, A. (1959). The fetal lung: a source of amniotic fluid. *Proc. Soc. exp. Biol.* (*N.Y.*), **101**, 842.

Strang, L. B., Anderson, G. S., and Platt, J. W. (1957). Neonatal death and elective Caesarian section. *Lancet*, **1**, 954.

——, and McGrath, M. W. (1962). Alveolar ventilation in normal newborn infants studied by air wash-in after oxygen breathing. *Clin. Sci.*, **23**, 129.

——, and MacLeish, M. H. (1961). Ventilatory failure and right-to-left shunt in newborn infants with respiratory distress. *Pediatrics*, **28**, 17.

——, and Reynolds, E. O. R. (1965). The alveolar surface properties of the newborn lung. *Brit. med. Bull.* In the press.

Warley, M. A., and Gairdner, D. (1962). Respiratory distress syndrome of the newborn—principles in treatment. *Arch. Dis. Childh.*, **37**, 455.

*Arch. Dis. Childh.*, 1965, **40**, 583.

# EXCRETION OF CORTICOSTEROIDS BY INFANTS OF DIABETIC AND PRE-DIABETIC MOTHERS*

BY

D. METHVEN CATHRO and CONSTANCE C. FORSYTH

*From The Department of Child Health, University of St. Andrews, Queen's College, Dundee*

(RECEIVED FOR PUBLICATION FEBRUARY 25, 1965)

Infants born to diabetic women are usually larger and heavier than average for their gestational age and often bear a superficial resemblance to cases of Cushing's syndrome (Åkerrén, 1954; Jackson, 1955; Farquhar, 1956a; Roszkowski and Janczewska, 1964).

On this account, various workers have investigated the excretion of adrenal steroids by these infants but the results have been inconclusive, possibly due to the fact that methods for the assay of groups of adrenocortical steroids have been used—methods primarily designed to measure the principal steroid metabolites excreted by adults and of limited application to studies of newborn infants with their unique steroid metabolism (Cathro, Birchall, Mitchell, and Forsyth, 1963). There is a further drawback to the use of these methods in analyses of urine obtained from newborn infants, in that accurate correction to exclude the contribution of the large quantities of non-specific chromogens that are characteristic of this age-group is somewhat difficult (Birchall and Mitchell, 1965).

Using such methods for the assay of groups of steroids, Rose (1960) found the corticosteroid excretion of infants of diabetic mothers to be normal, while Björklund (1954) and Farquhar (1956a) found it increased, and Field, Smith, and Reardon (1963) reported that the output of Porter-Silber chromogens in the urine of such infants when they developed respiratory distress was approximately twice as high as the output of these compounds in stressed premature infants born to women who did not suffer from diabetes.

Analysis of amniotic fluid has been no more rewarding. Hoet (1954) found appreciable quantities of corticoids in the amniotic fluid obtained from a pregnant diabetic woman, whereas the same techniques could not demonstrate the presence of corticosteroids in the amniotic fluid from normal controls. In contrast, Baird and Bush (1960) found no significant differences between the amniotic fluids obtained from normal pregnant women and from diabetics, when they estimated the levels of cortisol and cortisone.

Evidence from anatomical studies carried out on infants of diabetic women has also been inconclusive with regard to the degree of development of adrenal tissue. Miller and his colleagues (Miller, Johnson, and Durlacher, 1944; Miller, 1945) reported that occasionally the adrenal glands of such infants might be increased in size and weight, whereas this was not found in a large series of necropsies on infants of diabetic mothers reported by Driscoll, Benirschke, and Curtis (1960).

These inconsistent findings led us to investigate the individual neutral steroids excreted in the urine of infants born to diabetic mothers, since this approach, though technically more difficult, was considered preferable to the use of the group methods of steroid assay with their doubtful or, at best, limited, applicability at this period of life.

## Materials and Method

Urine was collected on days 1, 2, 3, and 6, from 8 infants born to women with diabetes mellitus and from 6 infants born to women with pre-diabetes. The average gestational age at the time of birth of the infants of diabetic mothers was 36·3 weeks (range 35-37·5 weeks) while the average gestational age of the infants born to pre-diabetic mothers was 37·3 weeks (range 36-38 weeks). Mothers were classified as *diabetic* if they required treatment with insulin or with drugs following the puerperium, and as *pre-diabetic* if drugs or insulin were unnecessary following the birth of the baby. In some cases, the diabetogenic tendency was so mild that only dietary measures were required during the pregnancy, but in all of these, the diagnosis of diminished tolerance to carbohydrate was confirmed by means of glucose tolerance tests.

* A preliminary communication on this subject was presented at the Tenth International Congress of Paediatrics at Lisbon in September 1962.

The control specimens of urine were obtained on days 1, 2, 3, and 6 from 14 healthy infants born uneventfully at term to mothers who had no endocrine abnormality. Specimens were also obtained from 10 full-term infants who were stressed at birth or in the neonatal period. Most of these suffered severe asphyxia at birth but 3 had haemolytic disease requiring exchange transfusion. A further 16 infants studied have been classified as premature on the basis of a birth weight of 2·5 kg. or less. Any 24-hour urine samples considered to be incomplete were discarded. In all but two instances the infants studied were male. Complete 24-hour specimens of urine were collected from the mothers during the period immediately following delivery.

Individual neutral steroids in the urine samples from infants were assayed by the method of Birchall, Cathro, Forsyth, and Mitchell (1963). In this method, an extract of the unconjugated steroids originally present in the urine and of steroids released by a two-stage enzyme hydrolysis, which will cleave steroid sulphates as well as steroid glucosiduronates, is subjected to preliminary purification and to chromatography, which allows subdivision of the steroids into three fractions on the basis of polarity. Fraction I contains 11-deoxy-17-oxosteroids and other relatively non-polar compounds, Fraction II contains the 11-oxy-17-oxosteroids, and Fraction III the corticosteroids. Final chromatography of the steroids in each fraction is followed by staining techniques which permit direct measurement on paper chromatograms. Corrections for losses of steroid during the estimations are applied on the basis of the recovery values for $4\text{–}^{14}C$ steroids added to the urine samples at the outset.

The specimens from the mothers were assayed for 17-hydroxycorticosteroids by the method of Appleby, Gibson, Norymberski, and Stubbs (1955). 17-oxosteroids were assayed by a modification of the method of Norymberski, Stubbs, and West (1953).

The number of infants of diabetic mothers studied was unavoidably small, since the region served by the obstetric units has a limited population, and since attempts at accurate collection of 24-hour urine specimens from female infants were found impracticable. For purposes of comparison it is fortunate that all the infants of diabetic mothers studied during days 1 to 6 were clinically satisfactory. None of them developed respiratory distress, which is the major danger to these infants in the neonatal period (Gellis and Hsia, 1959), but one of these infants was subjected to the stress of exchange transfusion on both day 1 and day 3 on account of haemolytic disease due to Rhesus incompatibility.

Most of the results presented were obtained by the estimation of Fraction III steroids, both that group of primary hormones retaining the 4-en-3-one group and giving sodium fluorescence, and the quantitatively more prominent group of adrenocortical steroid hormones reducing blue tetrazolium, including both these primary hormones and their metabolites. The estimation of the Fraction II blue tetrazolium-reducing steroid 3$\beta$ : 21-dihydroxypregn-5-ene-20-one in the urine of infants born to diabetic mothers has been described in detail elsewhere (Cathro, Birchall, Mitchell, and Forsyth, 1965).

## Results

Group analysis for 17-hydroxycorticosteroids in a few specimens of urine from diabetic and pre-diabetic women in the third trimester of pregnancy showed an excretion no different from that of normal pregnant women. Similarly, analysis of the urine obtained from mothers during the 24-hour period following delivery showed that the excretion levels of 17-hydroxycorticosteroids and of 17-oxosteroids in diabetic and pre-diabetic mothers were within the ranges found in normal women following childbirth. In both diabetic and pre-diabetic patients caesarean section was the mode of delivery for two-thirds of the mothers, and their corticosteroid excretion values during the ensuing 24 hours were not unduly high. The average value for 17-hydroxycorticosteroid excretion obtained from the diabetic women was 14·6 mg./24 hr. and that from the pre-diabetic women, 12·2 mg./24 hr. The respective values for the 17-oxosteroids were 8·2 mg./24 hr. and 9·3 mg./24 hr.

Measurement of the individual neutral steroids excreted by infants showed essentially the same patterns of steroid excretion in infants born to diabetic mothers as in full-term and premature infants born to women without endocrine disease. Although the unique excretion patterns during the first week of life are indicative of a different mode of steroid metabolism from that found in adults (Cathro *et al.*, 1963), the structure of many of the compounds which have been tentatively identified in infancy urine, and the probable structures of others, from theoretical considerations (Birchall, 1963; Cathro, 1964), are such that quantitative estimations of these individual compounds are considered likely to have provided a reasonably accurate indication of adrenocortical activity in early infancy.

Application of this technique revealed that there was much greater individual variation in the quantities of steroids excreted by healthy endocrinologically normal infants than is to be found with adults. In our view, satisfactory comparison of the steroid outputs of different infants may be made on a basis of the excretion per kg. birth weight per 24 hr. Since the steroid excretion patterns of premature infants and of those born at term were found to be similar, it was thought permissible to compare the steroid excretion values per kg. birth weight amongst infants of very different birth weights, irrespective of their estimated maturity at the time of birth. Although subsequent recordings of weight have been available, excretion values have been calculated per kg. birth weight per 24 hr. throughout the first week of life. The steroid excretion results individually determined for each 24-hour sample on days 1, 2,

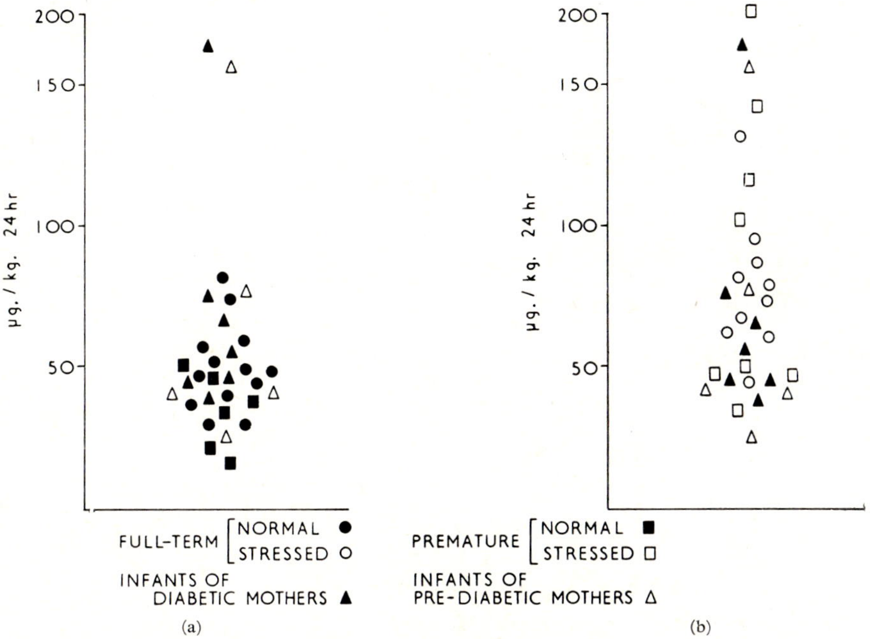


FIG. 1a.—Average excretion on days 1, 2, and 3, of total sodium-fluorescent steroids by *normal* full-term and premature infants and by infants of diabetic and pre-diabetic mothers.

FIG. 1b.—Average excretion on days 1, 2, and 3, of total sodium-fluorescent steroids by *stressed* full-term and premature infants and by infants of diabetic and pre-diabetic mothers.

and 3 have been used to present average 24-hour excretion values during the first three days for each infant. In some instances, results were obtained from the excretion values measured on only two of these days, and occasionally the output measured in an isolated 24-hour urine specimen was charted. This use of an average value for days 1 to 3 was thought justifiable in that the degree of development of renal function might differ in individual infants, and in some cases there might be a delay of at least 24 hours before evidence of increased corticosteroid production was shown in the urinary excretion of steroids.

For each infant, sodium-fluorescent steroids in Fraction III of the urinary extracts were measured individually and totalled. The principal constituents of this group of steroids, in descending order of polarity, are 6$\beta$-hydroxycortisol, a prominent unidentified compound with properties suggesting that it may be 6$\beta$-hydroxycorticosterone, cortisol, cortisone, and corticosterone. The total excretion of these compounds in 24 hours during days 1 to 3 is shown in Fig. 1a and b. The one infant born to an established diabetic mother to show a high output was the infant with concomitant haemolytic disease requiring an exchange transfusion on the day of birth and a second exchange at 68 hours. Fig. 1b shows that this high excretion value has been matched on occasion by that of acutely ill premature infants, and approached by the output of one stressed full-term infant whose mother had no endocrine abnormality. The one infant of a pre-diabetic mother to show a high output of sodium-fluorescent steroids was in excellent clinical condition from the moment of birth, and had an output of blue tetrazolium-reducing steroids which was within the normal range. This infant did, however, have a cushingoid appearance and a noticeably reddish colour.

During the first three days of life the sodium-fluorescent steroid excretion values for the other infants born to diabetic and pre-diabetic mothers were found unremarkable, and were lower than those of many of the stressed infants. Although not illustrated, a similar scatter of results for the sodium-fluorescent steroid excretion values from infants of diabetic mothers compared with those from healthy full-term control infants and from premature infants was found on the sixth day of life.

Increased corticosteroid output, or, certainly, a tendency towards increased adrenal activity in the infants born to diabetic mothers is suggested by the

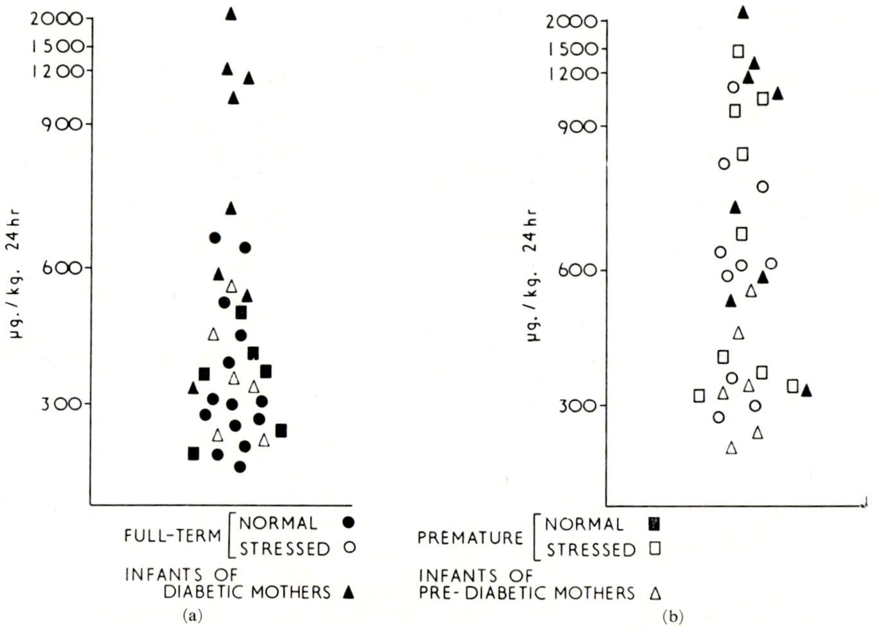


FIG. 2a.—Average excretion on days 1, 2, and 3, of blue tetrazolium-reducing steroids by *normal* full-term and premature infants and by infants of diabetic and pre-diabetic mothers.

FIG. 2b.—Average excretion on days 1, 2, and 3, of blue tetrazolium-reducing steroids by *stressed* full-term and premature infants and by infants of diabetic and pre-diabetic mothers.

excretion of blue tetrazolium-reducing steroids during the first three days of life, illustrated in Fig. 2a and b. The compounds measured are all the Fraction III steroids reducing blue tetrazolium. Evidence suggests that corticosteroids amongst the compounds measured are: 6β-hydroxylated and other highly polar metabolites of cortisol, tetrahydrocortisol, tetrahydrocortisone, cortisol, cortisone, dihydrocortisone, tetrahydrocorticosterone, allotetrahydrocorticosterone, and corticosterone, as well as other, yet unidentified, steroids. Again, the highest value was obtained from the infant subjected to exchange transfusion. However, none of the other infants of diabetic mothers could be classified as stressed on clinical grounds. Despite a scatter of results amongst those from healthy control infants, Figs. 3 and 4 illustrate that the corticosteroid output of infants born to diabetic women is generally raised, and in the same range as that from full-term and premature infants who have suffered birth asphyxia or other severe stress. In contrast, values obtained from infants born to pre-diabetic women are within the range of normal.

Fig. 3a and b show that, even on the sixth day of life, an undue proportion of the small series of infants born to diabetic mothers have shown an output of blue tetrazolium-reducing steroids in the upper part of the normal range, if not, in fact, above it. The isolated high value of 910 μg./kg. 24 hr. from an infant of a woman with pre-diabetes is not directly comparable with the others, but it is noteworthy in that it represents the day 7 excretion of an infant whose neonatal progress was poor following forceps delivery at 36 weeks, and who had all the manifestations of the respiratory distress syndrome despite a birth weight of 3·1 kg. Pre-eclamptic toxaemia had been diagnosed in the mother in a small outlying hospital and her pre-diabetes was only discovered following investigations during the puerperium—prompted by the poor condition of the infant. The highest value of all on day 6 was from an infant of a diabetic mother with no evidence at all of respiratory distress but in whom the characteristic red coloration was marked. One of the other three high values in infants born to diabetic mothers was given by the infant who had an exchange transfusion on the day of birth and again at 68 hours. As previously stated, none of the other infants born to diabetic or pre-diabetic mothers showed any signs of distress which could be detected clinically.

The excretion values for the relatively non-polar Zimmermann-reacting compounds occurring in

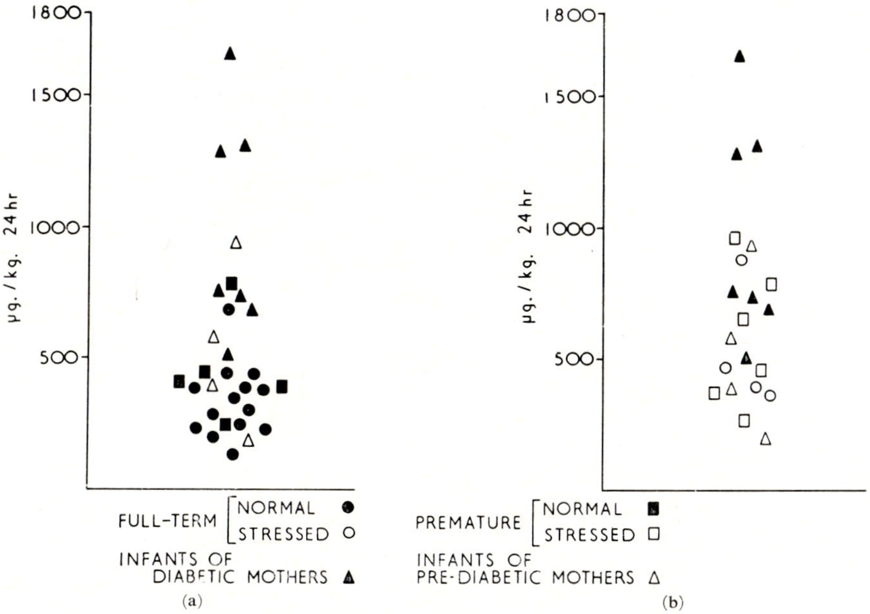


FIG. 3a.—Excretion on day 6 of blue tetrazolium-reducing steroids by *normal* full-term and premature infants and by infants of diabetic and pre-diabetic mothers.

FIG. 3b.—Excretion on day 6 of blue tetrazolium-reducing steroids by *stressed* full-term and premature infants and by infants of diabetic and pre-diabetic mothers.

Fraction I of the urinary extracts of the infants of different categories during the first three days of life are shown in Table 1. The characteristic compounds obtained in this fraction of urinary extracts from adults, namely, dehydroepiandrosterone, aetiocholanolone, and androsterone are almost inconspicuous in infancy urine, in which the typical Zimmermann chromogens are substances less polar than androsterone (Cathro *et al.*, 1963). An early impression from work on pooled urine that the excretion of Fraction I compounds seemed to be more marked in premature infants (Birchall, Cathro, Forsyth, and Mitchell, 1961) has been sustained.

The excretion of Fraction II Zimmermann chromogens of medium polarity is reported in Table 2. The highest results have been obtained in infants of diabetic mothers.

## Discussion

The results of this study indicate that infants born to women with diabetes mellitus show greater adrenocortical activity than control infants. This is

TABLE 1
EXCRETION OF FRACTION I ZIMMERMANN CHROMOGENS DURING DAYS 1-3 (μg./kg. 24 hr.)

| | Full-term Normal | Full-term Stressed | Premature | Mother Diabetic | Mother Pre-diabetic |
|---|---|---|---|---|---|
| Average .. .. | 26·1 (13) | 24·3 (10) | 46 (14) | 28·9 (8) | 60·4 (4) |
| Range .. .. .. | 11-76 | 9·1-55 | 14-95 | 22-48 | 22-96 |

The numbers of infants studied are given in parentheses.

TABLE 2
EXCRETION OF FRACTION II ZIMMERMANN CHROMOGENS DURING DAYS 1-3 (μg./kg. 24 hr.)

| | Full-term Normal | Full-term Stressed | Premature | Mother Diabetic | Mother Pre-diabetic |
|---|---|---|---|---|---|
| Average .. .. | 30·9 (14) | 35·0 (11) | 41·9 (12) | 54·2 (8) | 30·2 (5) |
| Range .. .. .. | 12-55 | 6-63 | 18-61 | 30-82 | 18-53 |

The numbers of infants studied are given in parentheses.

manifest in an increased excretion of reducing corticosteroids of all ranges of polarity and cannot be attributed merely to the prematurity of these infants. The increased output of corticosteroids found during the first three days of life in the admittedly small series of infants studied has not been associated with respiratory distress or with other illness during the neonatal period, since all the infants were in good condition at birth and maintained satisfactory progress thereafter. In Fig. 2a, if the symbol representing the corticosteroid excretion of the child requiring exchange transfusion is excluded, three of the four values from infants of diabetic mothers which are clearly above the normal range were from infants noted to have a cushingoid appearance. The one other infant of an established diabetic mother, who showed the classical physiognomy associated with maternal diabetes, had a blue tetrazolium-reducing steroid output of 557 μg./kg. 24 hr., in the upper part of the range obtained from control infants. Some degree of cushingoid appearance was observed in only one of the infants born to carefully controlled pre-diabetic mothers. This infant was the only one in his category who did not have a corticosteroid output during the first days of life which was in the normal range (Fig. 1a) and, even in his case, the high output of sodium-fluorescent steroids was countered by normal excretion of the blue tetrazolium-reducing compounds which are quantitatively more important. One other child born to an untreated pre-diabetic mother had a more obvious cushingoid appearance and developed respiratory distress. The excretion of corticosteroids by this child on day 7 (Fig. 3a) was very high. By far the highest excretion levels measured were in an infant with haemolytic disease born to a diabetic woman and subjected to two exchange transfusions. This is taken to indicate that the high corticosteroid secretion of infants of diabetic mothers, when they are in satisfactory clinical condition, is not maximum and that it increases when there is extraneous stress. This finding in one infant in the present series is therefore in support of the results of Field *et al.* (1963) who found a corticosteroid excretion in infants born to diabetic women and developing respiratory distress, which was approximately twice that of stressed premature control infants. Additional evidence suggesting increased adrenocortical activity in the infants of diabetic mothers has been provided in a previous study from this laboratory (Cathro *et al.*, 1965), in which it was noted that the urinary excretion of the steroid 21-hydroxypregnenolone, an intermediary compound in a pathway of corticosteroid biosynthesis of peculiar importance in the foetus and the newborn infant, tended to be higher in infants born to diabetic mothers than in most of the controls.

Our finding of an above average output of corticosteroids by the infants of diabetic mothers was not associated with a raised 17-hydroxycorticosteroid excretion in their mothers, nor was there an increase in individual compounds, including 21-hydroxypregnenolone, in the maternal urines in which they were measured.

This problem of the maternal contribution to the steroids measurable in the cord blood and in the urine of newborn infants has recently been examined by Aarskog (1965) who has not found the mean concentration of total cortisol in the cord plasma of infants born to diabetic mothers to be significantly different from that observed in the cord plasma of normal full-term and premature infants. Aarskog has verified earlier reports that the corticosteroid-binding globulin levels are much lower in cord plasma than in maternal plasma, and has demonstrated that binding of corticosteroids is less developed in the premature infant than in the infant born at term. He has further shown that though the mean ratio of maternal to cord total plasma cortisol is of the order 3 : 1, the mean ratio of maternal to cord unbound cortisol is about 1 : 1. The nine premature infants he studied showed a mean cord level of unbound (and, presumably, physiologically active) cortisol which was significantly higher than the mean cord level of unbound cortisol measured in the nine infants born at term. The mean concentration of unbound cortisol in the cord plasma of 11 infants born to diabetic mothers fell between the levels in the two categories of infants born to normal mothers. Aarskog has interpreted his findings to imply that during foetal life an equilibrium exists across the semi-permeable membrane of the placenta, whereby effective cortisol levels in the foetus are in homeostasis with those of the mother. He admits, however, that at delivery, maternal cortisol levels rise so substantially above the protein-binding capacity that there is likely to be considerable transfer to the foetus, and thus his finding of normal cord levels of unbound cortisol in infants born to diabetic mothers does not exclude the possibility of such infants having above-average levels of effective cortisol during intrauterine life.

In Aarskog's study, the possibility of the adrenal gland of the infant contributing significantly to the unbound cortisol levels on either side of the placenta is not discussed and, no doubt through caution, significance has not been attached to the fact that the mean value for unbound cortisol in the plasma of diabetic mothers was found to be slightly less than the mean value obtained from examination of the levels of unbound cortisol in the cord blood of their infants, though the ratio of unbound cortisol in maternal and cord plasma was approaching unity at 0·93 : 1. The equivalent ratios for mothers and full-term infants and mothers and premature infants were 1·15 : 1 and 1·05 : 1. In only 2 of the 11 cases of diabetic pregnancy examined were the maternal levels of unbound cortisol actually above the cord levels. Aarskog has suggested that the problem of whether the foetus of the diabetic woman produces, or is subjected to, above normal levels of effective cortisol *in utero* might best be revealed by a study of the unbound plasma cortisol of the mother throughout pregnancy. New significance is therefore given to an earlier study by Plotz, Davis, and Ricketts (1959) who found an increased output of urinary corticosteroids in 11 out of 13 diabetic women during the second trimester of pregnancy, though during the third trimester their average output was comparable with that of normal pregnant women.

Other recent work by Aarskog (1963, 1965) at first sight appears to be in disagreement with the results of the present study. His determination of the cortisol production rates by the isotope dilution method in 8 newborn infants of diabetic mothers and in 5 normal newborn infants, showed that when the results were corrected for body surface area the average cortisol production per square metre per 24 hours in the infants born to diabetic mothers was 26·89 mg. and that of the controls 21·96 mg. He found an overlap of values from both groups of infants and therefore did not think the difference between the mean values significant. It is of note that the tests were carried out on the controls on days 3 and 4 and on the infants of diabetic mothers on days 4 to 6, and even this relatively slight discrepancy in timing may have been enough to affect the results at a period of life when modes of steroid metabolism are undergoing rapid and progressive alteration (Bertrand, Loras, Gilly, and Cautenet, 1963; Cathro *et al.*, 1963). Moreover, the one infant in Aarskog's rather small series showing a low cortisol production rate would, in the present study, have been classed as the child of a pre-diabetic mother. Had our criteria been adopted, of the 7 infants of diabetic mothers he examined, one gave a value in the lower part of the normal range, 3 gave results in the upper part of the normal range, and the remaining 3 gave results well above the maximum control value. Two of the three high values were from infants who showed no clinical evidence of stress, and thus, though Aarskog has been more cautious in his interpretation of results from a small series, his findings are not completely at variance with those now reported. Aarskog carried out his studies later than the third day of life to exclude the steroid contribution from the mother, but there is nothing to suggest that this is any greater from a mother with diabetes than from a normal control. The present study has been carried out on infants newly released from a diabetic environment, and may thus have shown up differences between the two categories of infants, which become less evident day by day over the first week. Moreover, the present study has measured metabolites of corticosterone as well as of cortisol, and there is evidence that corticosterone is of relatively greater importance in early infancy than it is thereafter (Cathro *et al.*, 1963).

The method adopted in this study has revealed quantitative differences, which are quite definite, between the infants of diabetic mothers and control infants with regard to corticosteroid excretion. Qualitative differences have also been detected but these have been more subtle. The excretion patterns of neutral steroids have been found to be basically similar in all the newborn infants studied. Tetrahydrocortisol, a major cortisol metabolite in the adult, is not a prominent constituent of the urine of normal newborn infants during the first three days of life (Bertrand *et al.*, 1963) when a complex of steroids containing a major unknown compound as well as tetrahydrocortisone is characteristically dominant among reducing steroids of this order of polarity (Cathro *et al.*, 1963). However, in the urine of 4 of the infants of diabetic women included in this study, reducing steroid with the mobility of tetrahydrocortisol has been as prominent as, or more prominent than, the accumulation of steroid in the tetrahydrocortisone area of the chromatograms. The results of the present study cannot be compared directly with those of Grossman, Crigler, and Gold (1963), since these workers hydrolysed their urine specimens with purified $\beta$-glucuronidase, and probably measured tetrahydrocortisone uncontaminated either with hydroxylated $\Delta^5$-pregnene derivatives (Cathro *et al.*, 1965), or with other reducing steroids with a polarity similar to that of tetrahydrocortisone, which are likely to be released from conjugation by sulphatases present in the crude enzyme preparations used in the standard technique employed in this laboratory. Despite these technological differences, it is probably justifiable to state that the results of the present study support the belief of Grossman and his colleagues that either the tetrahydrocortisol to tetrahydrocortisone ratio is greatly increased in the urine of infants whose mothers have diabetes or, at least, that such infants show evidence of a steroid metabolism that is slightly different both qualitatively and quantitatively from that of normal newborn infants.

A further qualitative difference in the steroid

metabolism of infants born to diabetic mothers is suggested by the results in Table 2, in which the total output of Zimmermann chromogens of medium polarity from such infants is shown to be higher than can be attributable to their prematurity. So many of the prominent steroid compounds in this fraction of the urinary extracts from newborn infants are of an unknown nature (Cathro *et al.*, 1963) that there can be no rational speculation as to the specific significance of this finding. One of the dominant Zimmermann-reacting compounds in Fraction II of urinary extracts from newborn infants is the unidentified compound with the $R_F$ value of 0·19 in the Bush chromatography system LB 21/80 at 28°, described in previous papers (Cathro *et al.*, 1963; Cathro *et al.*, 1965), and this may be the same steroid as has been found in urine collected in later childhood (Gupta and Tanner, 1964). However, the output of this particular steroid in the urine of infants of diabetic mothers has been no higher than has been found in the urine of full-term or of premature infants, whether normal or stressed, and the difference in steroid output in infants of diabetic mothers is due to a general increase in other Zimmermann chromogens in this Fraction. This over-all increase in Zimmermann chromogen excretion in the infants of diabetic mothers lends support to the earlier study of Björklund and Jensen (1955) and is a further pointer to some degree of hyperadrenocorticism in these infants.

Osler and Pedersen (1960) have put forward convincing arguments against hyperadrenocorticism being a major cause of the foetal overgrowth in infants of diabetic mothers. They have assigned the changes in body composition in these infants with their increased proportion of fat as being essentially due to an increased supply of glucose being transmitted across the placenta from the mother during gestation (Osler, 1960; Roszkowski and Janczewska, 1964; Milner and Hales, 1965), with resultant hyperinsulinism as the primary endocrine response in the foetus (Pedersen, 1952; Farquhar, 1956b; Baird and Farquhar, 1962).

Although the cushingoid appearance of infants of diabetic mothers may, therefore, be in part due to a relative increase in their total fat, the results of the present study support Farquhar's (1962) belief that the adrenal gland is involved to some extent in producing the complicated endocrine state of these infants. In view of the high perinatal mortality in infants of diabetic mothers, it is tempting to speculate that their increased adrenal activity reflects an adaptation to stress in the form of some subtle biochemical abnormality, for example, as a response to the foetal hyperinsulinism. In addition, all 4 infants of diabetic mothers on whom electrolyte studies were performed as an ancillary part of the present study showed an above-average excretion of sodium, chloride, and potassium during the first three days and on the sixth day of life, suggesting an alteration in body composition.

Whatever the cause of the hyperadrenocorticism in these infants, evidence of its existence indicates that corticosteroid therapy has no useful place in their management. It is suggested that on the relatively rare occasions when such infants develop symptoms in association with hypoglycaemia, glucagon would be the rational adjuvant to therapy with glucose.

All the infants of diabetic mothers included in this study were in good condition at birth and progressed well thereafter. Only 4 of the 8 demonstrated some degree of the cushingoid appearance which typified such infants prior to the very careful management of diabetes during pregnancy, which is now standard practice (Gellis and Hsia, 1959; Brandstrup, Osler, and Pedersen, 1961; Deuil and Durand, 1961), and 3 of these had a high excretion of corticosteroids. One of the infants born to a pre-diabetic woman, whose underlying disorder had not been diagnosed during her pregnancy, showed a very high output of corticosteroids during recovery from respiratory distress. On the other hand, the corticosteroid excretion of infants of pre-diabetic women who were strictly controlled during pregnancy was consistently within the normal range, which provides further circumstantial evidence that strict control of diabetes and pre-diabetes during pregnancy is a major factor in reducing the endocrine abnormality in the foetus.

**Summary**

The urinary excretion of individually estimated neutral steroids on days 1, 2, 3, and 6, from 8 infants born to diabetic mothers, and from 6 infants born to pre-diabetic mothers, has been compared with the excretion of these compounds by full-term and by premature infants born to non-diabetic mothers.

The results suggest that infants born to women with diabetes show adrenocortical activity that is greater than that of control infants. This is manifest in an increased excretion of blue tetrazolium-reducing corticosteroids of all ranges of polarity. This increased excretion of corticosteroids shown by the infants of diabetic mothers is not attributable to their relative prematurity nor to clinically detectable stress.

While differences in the excretion of corticosteroids between infants of diabetic mothers and control infants have been essentially quantitative, more subtle qualitative differences have also been detected, but these defy interpretation in the present state of knowledge.

This research programme has been supported by a grant from the Scottish Hospital Endowments Research Trust.

We wish to thank Professor J. L. Henderson for his support and encouragement, also Professor J. Walker and Miss A. J. Herring of the Department of Midwifery of the University of St. Andrews for access to their patients. We also thank Dr. K. Birchall and Dr. F. L. Mitchell for biochemical advice.

We are indebted to the nursing staffs of the nurseries in the Maternity Units at Maryfield Hospital and at Dundee Royal Infirmary for their sustained co-operation.

Technical assistance is gratefully acknowledged from Mrs. J. Cameron, Mr. I. Roberts, and Miss F. Lumsden.

**Appendix**

The following terms have been used throughout the text.

| | |
|---|---|
| Aetiocholanolone | 3α-hydroxy-5β-androstan-17-one |
| Allotetrahydrocorticosterone | 3α : 11β : 21-trihydroxy-5α-pregnan-20-one |
| Androsterone | 3α-hydroxy-5α-androstan-17-one |
| Blue tetrazolium | 3 : 3′-dianisole-bis-4 : 4′ (3 : 5 diphenyl)-tetrazolium chloride |
| Corticosterone | 11β : 21-dihydroxypregn-4-ene-3 : 20-dione |
| Cortisol | 11β : 17α : 21-trihydroxy-pregn-4-ene-3 : 20-dione |
| Cortisone | 17α : 21-dihydroxypregn-4-ene-3 : 11 : 20-trione |
| Dehydroepiandrosterone | 3β-hydroxyandrost-5-ene-17-one |
| Dihydrocortisone | 17α : 21-dihydroxy-5β-pregnan-3 : 11 : 20-trione |
| 6β-Hydroxycortisol | 6β : 11β : 17α : 21-tetrahydroxypregn-4-ene-3 : 20-dione |
| 6β-Hydroxycorticosterone | 6β : 11β : 21-trihydroxy-pregn-4-ene-3 : 20-dione |
| 21-Hydroxypregnenolone | 3β : 21-dihydroxypregn-5-ene-20-one |
| Tetrahydrocorticosterone | 3α : 11β : 21-trihydroxy-5β-pregnan-20-one |
| Tetrahydrocortisol | 3α : 11β : 17α : 21-tetrahydroxy-5β-pregnan-20-one |
| Tetrahydrocortisone | 3α : 17α : 21-trihydroxy-5β-pregnan-11 : 20-dione |

References

arskog, D. (1963). Cortisol production rate in newborn infants of diabetic mothers. *J. Pediat.*, **62**, 807.

—(1965). Cortisol in the newborn infant. *Acta paediat.* (*Uppsala*), Suppl. 158.

Åkerrén, Y. (1954). A characteristic physiognomy, resembling that encountered in Cushing's syndrome, observed in newborn infants of diabetic mothers. *ibid.*, **43**, Suppl. 100, 185.

Appleby, J. I., Gibson, G., Norymberski, J. K., and Stubbs, R. D. (1955). Indirect analysis of corticosteroids. 1. The determination of 17-hydroxycorticosteroids. *Biochem. J.*, **60**, 453.

Baird, C. W., and Bush, I. E. (1960). Cortisol and cortisone content of amniotic fluid from diabetic and non-diabetic women. *Acta endocr.* (*Kbh.*), **34**, 97.

Baird, J. D., and Farquhar, J. W. (1962). Insulin-secreting capacity in newborn infants of normal and diabetic women. *Lancet*, **1**, 71.

Bertrand, J., Loras, B., Gilly, R., and Cautenet, B. (1963). Contribution à l'étude de la sécrétion et du métabolisme du cortisol chez le nouveauné et le nourrison de moins de trois mois. *Path. et Biol.*, **11**, 997.

Birchall, K. (1963). A Study of Adrenocortical Steroids in the Urine of Newborn Infants. Ph.D. Thesis, University of St. Andrews, Queen's College, Dundee.

——, Cathro, D. M., Forsyth, C. C., and Mitchell, F. L. (1961). Separation and estimation of adrenal steroids in the urine of newborn infants. *Lancet*, **1**, 26.

——, ——, ——, and —— (1963). A method for the separation and estimation of neutral steroids in the urine of newborn infants. *J. Endocr.*, **27**, 31.

——, and Mitchell, F. L. (1965). Investigation of the Zimmermann reaction when used for the assay of groups of steroids in infants. *Clin. Chim. Acta*, **12**, 125.

Björklund, S. -I. (1954). Infants of diabetic mothers with special reference to neonatal adrenocortical function as assessed by urinary excretion of corticoids and tests using adrenocorticotrophic hormones. *Acta endocr.* (*Kbh.*), **15**, 25.

——, and Jensen, C. C. (1955). Infants of diabetic mothers with special reference to neonatal adrenocortical function as assessed by urinary excretion of 17-ketosteroids. *ibid.*, **18**, 133.

Brandstrup, E., Osler, M., and Pedersen, J. (1961). Perinatal mortality in diabetic pregnancy. The relationship to management during pregnancy and to foetal age and weight. *ibid.*, **37**, 434.

Cathro, D. M. (1964). A Study of Adrenocortical Function in Newborn Infants. M.D. Thesis, University of Edinburgh.

——, Birchall, K., Mitchell, F. L., and Forsyth, C. C. (1963). The excretion of neutral steroids in the urine of newborn infants. *J. Endocr.*, **27**, 53.

——, ——, ——, and —— (1965). 3β: 21-dihydroxypregn-5-ene-20-one in the urine of normal newborn infants and in the third day urine of child with deficiency of 3β-hydroxysteroid-dehydrogenase. *Arch. Dis. Childh.*, **40**, 251.

Deuil, R., and Durand, A. (1961). Le traitment de la femme enceinte diabétique en function de ses conséquences pour l'enfant. *Thérapie*, **16**, 544.

Driscoll, S., Benirschke, K., and Curtis, G. W. (1960). Neonatal deaths among infants of diabetic mothers. *Amer. J. Dis. Child.*, **100**, 818.

Farquhar, J. W. (1956a). The possible influence of hyperadrenocorticism on the foetus of the diabetic woman. *Arch. Dis. Childh.*, **31**, 483.

—— (1956b). The significance of hypoglycaemia in the newborn infant of the diabetic woman. *ibid.*, **31**, 203.

—— (1962). Maternal hyperglycaemia and foetal hyperinsulinism in diabetic pregnancy. *Postgrad. med. J.*, **38**, 612.

Field, S. H., Smith, E. K., and Reardon, H. S. (1963). Dissimilarities in the respiratory distress syndrome of infants of diabetic and nondiabetic mothers. *J. Pediat.*, **63**, 863.

Gellis, S. S., and Hsia, D. Y. -Y. (1959). The infant of the diabetic mother. *Amer. J. Dis. Child.*, **97**, 1.

Grossman, M. S., Crigler, J. F., Jr., and Gold, N. I. (1963). Urinary cortisol metabolites excreted by newborn infants and infants born to diabetic mothers. *J. Pediat.*, **63**, 717.

Gupta, D., and Tanner, J. M. (1964). A new steroid found in the urine of children but not adults. *Nature* (*Lond.*), **203**, 187.

Hoet, J. P. (1954). Adrenocortical function in infants of diabetic mothers. *Cold Spr. Harb. Symp. quant. Biol.*, **19**, 182.

Jackson, W. P. U. (1955). A concept of diabetes. *Lancet*, **2**, 625.

Miller, H. C. (1945). Cardiac hypertrophy and extramedullary erythropoiesis in newborn infants of prediabetic mothers. *Amer. J. med. Sci.*, **209**, 447.

——, Johnson, R. D., and Durlacher, S. H. (1944). A comparison of newborn infants with erythroblastosis fetalis with those born to diabetic mothers. *J. Pediat.*, **24**, 603.

Milner, R. D. G., and Hales, C. N. (1965). Effect of intravenous glucose on concentration of insulin in maternal and umbilical-cord plasma. *Brit. med. J.*, **1**, 284.

Norymberski, J. K., Stubbs, R. D., and West, H. F. (1953). Assessment of adrenocortical activity by assay of 17-ketogenic steroids in urine. *Lancet*, **1**, 1276.

Osler, M. (1960). Body water of newborn infants of diabetic mothers. *Acta endocr.* (*Kbh.*), **34**, 261.

——, and Pedersen, J. (1960). The body composition of newborn infants of diabetic mothers. *Pediatrics*, **26**, 985.

Pedersen, J. (1952). *Diabetes and Pregnancy: Blood Sugar of Newborn Infants during Fasting and Glucose Administration.* Danish Science Press, Copenhagen.

Plotz, E. J., Davis, M. E., and Ricketts, H. T. (1959). Endocrine studies in pregnant diabetic women. *Diabetes*, **8**, 14.

Rose, V. (1960). Infants of diabetic mothers: clinical and pathological features in a series of 25 cases. *Canad. med. Ass. J.*, **82**, 306.

Roszkowski, I., and Janczewska, E. (1964). The daily glycemia profile in pregnancy. *Amer. J. Obstet. Gynec*, **88**, 204.

*Arch. Dis. Childh.*, 1965, **40**, 593.

# CORTICOSTEROIDS AND VARICELLA

## SIX-YEAR EXPERIENCE IN AN ASTHMATIC POPULATION

BY

CONSTANTINE J. FALLIERS and ELLIOT F. ELLIS

*Children's Asthma Research Institute and Hospital, Denver, Colorado, and Department of Pediatrics, University of Florida College of Medicine, Gainesville, Florida, U.S.A.*

(RECEIVED FOR PUBLICATION APRIL 5, 1965)

The ubiquitous nature of certain viral exanthematous diseases, particularly varicella and rubeola, results in the occasional occurrence of these illnesses in patients with disorders of a more chronic character (Gordon, 1962). This fortuitous association offers an opportunity to detect possible reciprocal influences and presents clinical problems, the solution of which may lead to a better understanding of both coexisting disorders. Moreover, it is frequent that a chronic illness requires the administration of a pharmacological agent which in itself can modify the patient's response to an infective disease. One such situation that has aroused considerable interest during the past decade has been the occurrence of varicella in patients receiving corticosteroids for a variety of diseases. This event has been looked upon ominously since the report of Haggerty and Eley (1956) of fatal outcome of varicella in steroid-treated patients. Since our experience with varicella in a large group of chronic asthmatic patients was at variance with this view, we undertook a review of the material published on this subject both here and abroad. The result of this review plus our own experience in this area over a six-year period forms the basis of this report.

### Material

Fifty-nine cases of varicella came under one or another of the authors' personal attention during the six-year period from July 1, 1957, to June 30, 1963. All patients were children in residence at the Children's Asthma Research Institute and Hospital (C.A.R.I.H.) (formerly the Jewish National Home for Asthmatic Children) in Denver, Colorado, for intractable asthma.

### Bibliographical Survey

In the decade from July 1953 to June 1963, 31 published reports appeared (Josserand, De L'Hermuzière, and Vacher, 1953; Shee and Fehrsen, 1953; Crisalli and Terragna, 1956; Cheatham, Weller, Dolan, and Dower, 1956; Bernheim, Larbre, Mouriquand, and Germain, 1956; Haggerty and Eley, 1956; Moulinier, Lartigaut, Cantonné, Martin, Geindre, and Traissac, 1956; Nichols, 1957; Le Tan Vinh, Canlorbe, Gentile, and Lelong, 1957; Gillot, Clausse, and de Peretti, 1958; Monnet, 1958; Kuipers and Van der Mei, 1958; Kaplan, 1958; Siegel, Lovin, Ely, and Kelley, 1959; Bernheim, Larbre, and Germain, 1959; Thoenes, 1959; Combe, Boineau, and Zannettacci, 1959; Kredba and Bradáčová, 1959; Hennemanne, 1960; Kirchhoff, 1960; Johnson and Nelson, 1960; Breton, Ponté, and Boniface, 1960; Falliers, Halberstein, and Bukantz, 1961; Pinkel, 1961; Finkel, 1961; Guazzelli and Calzolari, 1961; Celinska, Goledzinowska, Szpakowska, and Zychowicz, 1961; Viklický, Doutlík, and Kottová, 1961; Krajewska, 1961, 1962; Gerbeaux, Couvreur, Baculard-Beauchef, and Joly, 1963), describing cases of varicella in steroid-treated children (from 3 months to 16 years of age). There were several other reports where mention of this clinical problem was made, and others where some of the same cases were included for the second time. Such articles were noted but not included in the present bibliographical survey. The first reported fatal outcome of varicella 'during therapy with cortisone-ACTH' was in 1953, in France, by Josserand *et al.* (1953). This fatality occurred in a 6-year-old girl with rheumatic fever, in whom therapy with cortisone, 150 mg. daily, *was stopped* four days before varicella, because of 'marked obesity'. Following this, the patient received ACTH for three days. The disease terminated fatally in three days. In the same year, Shee and Fehrsen (1953) reported that cortisone, 100 mg. daily, given to an 11-year-old boy for urticaria, was associated with reactivation of varicella a month after the initial illness. Both courses of varicella were mild with the second one occurring immediately after discontinuation of cortisone.

TABLE 1

CORTICOSTEROIDS AND VARICELLA: REPORTED FATALITIES

| | Number of Publications* | Total Cases Reported | Deaths | Steroid Therapy in Cases Terminating Fatally | | | |
|---|---|---|---|---|---|---|---|
| | | | | Maintained | Increased | Decreased | Stopped |
| 1953-57 .. .. | 9 | 21 | 16 | 6 | 3 | 3 | 4 |
| 1958-63 .. .. | 22 | 253 | 22 | 13 | 3 | 4 | 2 |

* Editorials, reviews, or duplicate presentations excluded.

The incidence of relapses or second episodes of varicella attributable to corticosteroid therapy was further studied by Crisalli and Terragna (1956). These authors gave cortisone to 22 patients at varying time intervals (10-60 days) after varicella. Typical signs of varicella reappeared in 11 cases, but always after the sudden discontinuance of steroid therapy. These observations were considered as 'due to cortisone'. However, the significance of the steroid withdrawal was not discussed.

The literature of the decade following the reports of Josserand *et al.* and Shee and Fehrsen contained articles with diametrically contrasting data on the question of the effect of steroid therapy on varicella. While sound judgements are difficult to make under such circumstances, the bibliographical review does give an estimate of the magnitude of the problem and, in addition, provides data from which one may decide whether the severity of varicella in a steroid-treated patient is dependent upon (a) the nature of the initial disorder for which corticosteroids were administered, (b) the duration and dosage of steroid therapy, and (c) the therapeutic manipulations of the clinician in managing the situation (abrupt discontinuation, increase or decrease of steroid therapy) during both the incubation period and the acute phase of varicella.

A marked difference in the mortality figures in the reports appearing before and after 1958 was noted (Table 1). This may be attributed to several factors. (1) The intent of the early publications were seemingly to call attention to the life-threatening hazard of varicella in the steroid-treated patient. (2) Subsequent reports appeared to present a more comprehensive survey of the situation in which both mild and fatal cases were reported. (3) Management of the clinical situation and the therapeutic attitudes of the attending physicians may have been different during the two periods. Although cortisone was used more commonly before 1958, and prednisone more often thereafter, no significant differences in daily dosage were noted if dose equivalents were considered (Aceto, Blizzard, and Migeon, 1962). Of the 21 cases reported before 1958, 16 terminated fatally. The remaining 5 represent too small a number to permit meaningful comparisons with the 231 cases reported in articles published after 1958 that recovered uneventfully. It appeared, however, that there was no significant difference in the dose and duration of therapy in these two groups. To permit a $\chi^2$ analysis of the data (not possible otherwise with numbers of cases as small as these) the distribution was limited to two items: (1) therapy maintained or increased, and (2) therapy decreased or stopped. Considering only these two points, the difference in management before and after 1958 was not found to be statistically significant ($\chi^2 = 1 \cdot 12$, $p = 0 \cdot 1$).

Table 2 relates the outcome of varicella to the manner in which steroid therapy was managed before or during this illness. The majority of the reported cases were maintained on hormonal therapy. This fact was not always positively stated, but if no mention was made to the contrary it was assumed that the steroids were continued. It is of interest that in 49 of the 195 mild or average cases (25%) the dosage was increased, while in the 38 fatal cases an increase in steroid therapy was reported in 6 (16%). The daily dose of steroids was decreased in 21 cases, fairly evenly distributed among the various illness categories. In many more cases (excluding the instances of reactivation) therapy was abruptly discontinued.

The influence of the initial illness on the mortality rate is clearly shown in Table 3. Although in many instances the total number of cases is small, the data indicate that the deaths in cases of leukaemia, other haematological disorders, and in the rheumatic and connective tissue diseases significantly exceeded the mean of 14% for the total of the 274 cases reported. The dosage of steroid therapy varied considerably from case to case, and also within the groups of illnesses reviewed. In many cases the information available was only fragmentary. Calculations based on the available data indicated that the mean daily dose, expressed in milligrams of cortisone, was, in the cases of leukaemia and other haematological disorders, 160 mg. of cortisone or its equivalent.* The

* Equivalents were calculated by multiplying the given dose of the inflammatory steroid by an appropriate factor, as described elsewhere (Aceto *et al.*, 1962; Falliers, Tan, Szentivanyi, Jorgensen, and Bukantz, 1963).

TABLE 2

CORTICOSTEROIDS AND VARICELLA, 1953-1963: RELATIONSHIP OF OUTCOME OF VARICELLA TO STEROID MANAGEMENT

| | Corticosteroid Therapy | | | | | | | |
|---|---|---|---|---|---|---|---|---|
| | Maintained | Increased or Resumed | | Reduced | | Stopped | | Total |
| | | A | B | A | B | A | B | |
| Mild or average cases . . . . . . . . | 116 | 12 | 37* | 8† | 1 | 27† | 2 | 195 |
| Reactivation . . . . . . . . | — | — | — | — | — | 11 | 1 | 12 |
| Atypical or complicated cases . . . . | 26 | — | — | 2 | 3 | 8 | 2 | 41 |
| Fatalities . . . . . . . . . . | 19 | 1 | 5 | 4 | 3 | 3 | 3 | 38 |

A: Incubation period. B: Acute phase of varicella.

* Steroids stopped in incubation period and resumed during varicella in three cases.

† In the majority of these cases steroids were reduced or stopped as part of the therapeutic programme for the original illness and not because of the supervening varicella.

TABLE 3

CORTICOSTEROIDS AND VARICELLA, 1953-1963: IMPORTANCE OF THE PRIMARY DISEASE

| Disease | Total Cases Reported | Prolonged or Atypical Eruption | Compli-cations | Deaths | Mortality (%) | References |
|---|---|---|---|---|---|---|
| Asthma . . . . . . . . . . . . | 11 | 0 | 0 | 1 | 9 | Haggerty and Eley (1956) |
| Allergic disorders (other than asthma) . . | 8 | 1 | 0 | 1 | 12 | Haggerty and Eley (1956) |
| Leukaemia . . . . . . . . . . | 30 | 1 | 3 | 14 | 46 | Haggerty and Eley (1956); Nichols (1957); Le Tan Vinh *et al.* (1957); Kredba and Bradáčová (1959); Hennemanne (1960); Pinkel (1961); Finkel (1961); Krajewska (1962) |
| Other haematological disorders . . . . | 16 | 2 | 1 | 6 | 37 | Haggerty and Eley (1956); Kuipers and Van der Mei (1958); Celinska *et al.* (1961) |
| Rheumatic and connective tissue diseases | 30 | 1 | 3 | 9 | 30 | Josserand *et al.* (1953); Cheatham *et al.* (1956); Bernheim *et al.* (1956); Haggerty and Eley (1956); Kirchhoff (1960); Finkel (1961) |
| Nephrosis and nephritis . . . . . . | 13 | 0 | 0 | 0 | 0 | |
| Infectious hepatitis . . . . . . | 10 | 0 | 3 | 0 | 0 | |
| Metabolic and endocrine . . . . | 4 | 1 | 0 | 1 | 25 | Viklický *et al.* (1961) |
| Nutritional and gastro-intestinal disorders . . . . . . . . . . | 4 | 0 | 0 | 0 | 0 | |
| Tuberculosis . . . . . . . . . . | 115 | 8 | 11 | 3 | 2·6 | Gillot *et al.* (1958); Thoenes (1959); Johnson and Nelson (1960) |
| Misc. bacterial infections . . . . | 20 | 2 | 3 | 1 | 5 | Viklický *et al.* (1961) |
| Neurological disorders . . . . . . | 11 | 1 | 0 | 0 | 0 | |
| Diagnosis not stated . . . . . . | 2 | 0 | 0 | 2 | 100 | Haggerty and Eley (1956) |
| Totals . . . . . . . . . . | 274 | 17 | 24 | 38 | 14 | |

duration of therapy was not indicated in all cases. The figures reported ranged from two weeks to several years'. The period during which steroid therapy had been given continuously did not seem to have influenced the management of therapy during varicella nor was it found to bear a close relation to the outcome.

The ages of the patients varied considerably with a range from 3 months to 16 years, and median of 6 years. Age alone did not have any bearing on the mortality or morbidity figures.

**Experience at C.A.R.I.H. in Denver**

Table 4 shows the total number of admissions during the six-year period of this survey and indicates the frequency of pre-admission therapy with anti-inflammatory steroids, as reported in the protocols of the physicians and in the parents' application forms. It can be seen that almost half of these children came to the Institute receiving daily steroid therapy for periods ranging from 1 month to 8 years with a mean of 16 months. Steroid therapy given for less than one month was not considered as

TABLE 4

CORTICOSTEROID THERAPY IN INTRACTABLE ASTHMA PRE-ADMISSION RECORDS OF CHILDREN AT C.A.R.I.H. JULY 1, 1957-JUNE 30, 1963

| | No. of Patients | % |
|---|---|---|
| Total admissions . . . . . . . . . . | 515 | |
| One or more previous courses of steroids | 470 | 91·3 |
| No previous steroid therapy . . . . | 45 | 8·7 |
| Maintenance, daily therapy (months or years) . . . . . . . . . . | 242* | 47·0 |

* In 118 patients or 48·5% of the 242, steroid therapy was gradually reduced and stopped 3 to 12 weeks after admission to C.A.R.I.H

TABLE 5

VARICELLA AT C.A.R.I.H. FEVER IN RELATION TO STEROID THERAPY

| | Maximum Temperature Elevation (°C.) | | | Duration of Fever (days) | | |
|---|---|---|---|---|---|---|
| | Range | Median | Mean | Range | Median | Mean |
| (A) No steroid therapy (N = 34) . . . . . . | 37·8-40·2 | 39·0 | 38·7 | 2-6 | 3 | 3·23 |
| (B) Steroids* taken daily (N = 21) . . . . . . | 37·4-40·0 | 38·6 | 38·3 | 1-5 | 3 | 3·50 |
| (C) Steroids stopped 4-19 days before varicella (N = 4) | 38·8-39·2 | 38·8 | 38·9 | 3-5 | 3 | 3·75 |

* Prednisone, 2·5-15 mg. (mean 7·5 mg.) daily, or betamethasone, 0·3-1·8 (mean 1·0 mg.) daily, or dexamethasone phosphate inhalations, 2-9 daily.

TABLE 6

VARICELLA AT C.A.R.I.H. 1958-1963. MULTIPLE CORRELATIONS

| Steroids | Fever | | | Asthma | Fever | | | Exanthema | Fever | | | Age (yr.) |
|---|---|---|---|---|---|---|---|---|---|---|---|---|
| | A | B | C | | A | B | C | | A | B | C | |
| I | 0 | 3 | 0 | M | 0 | 1 | 0 | + | 0 | 8 | 4 | 6-9 |
| | 1 | 6 | 2 | S | 1 | 8 | 5 | ++ | 1 | 4 | 2 | 9½-12 |
| | 0 | 4 | 5 | L | 0 | 4 | 1 | +++ | 0 | 1 | 1 | 12½-16 |
| II | 0 | 3 | 1 | M | 0 | 4 | 1 | + | 1 | 10 | 1 | 6-9 |
| | 1 | 6 | 2 | S | 0 | 6 | 3 | ++ | 0 | 1 | 2 | 9½-12 |
| | 0 | 3 | 1 | L | 1 | 2 | 0 | +++ | 0 | 1 | 1 | 12½-16 |
| III | 0 | 5 | 2 | M | 0 | 2 | 2 | + | 3 | 6 | 2 | 6-9 |
| | 0 | 3 | 3 | S | 0 | 8 | 5 | ++ | 0 | 2 | 4 | 9½-12 |
| | 3 | 3 | 2 | L | 3 | 1 | 0 | +++ | 0 | 3 | 1 | 12½-16 |
| Total . . | 5 + | 36 + | 18 = 59 Pts. | | | | | | | | | |

Steroids: I, none; II, stopped within past 12 months; III, daily therapy.

Fever: A, 37·0-38·0; B, 38·1-39·0; C, 39·1-40·0 (°C.).

Asthma: M, more; S, same; L, less than before.

Exanthema: +, mild; ++, average; +++, severe.

Analysis of Variance

| | |
|---|---|
| Steroids vs. fever . . . . | F* = 0·20 (not significant) |
| Fever vs. asthma . . . . | F = 0·015 (not significant) |
| Steroids vs. exanthema . . | F = 0·81 (not significant) |
| Steroids vs. age . . . . . . | F = 0·58 (not significant) |

* F = 3·23 would be needed to achieve a 5% level of significance, with 2 and 56 degrees of freedom (F = 0·05 (2, 56) = 3·23).

maintenance therapy, and such cases were included under the category of 'one or more previous courses of steroids'. A cautious but persistent effort is made to withdraw therapy in as many cases as possible. It can be seen from the Table that this effort was successful in about half the children. In several more, therapy was discontinued several times, but only temporarily and had to be resumed as it provided the only means for acceptable control of the asthma. Of the 59 children at C.A.R.I.H., 21 were taking steroids daily at the time of varicella. There were two complications in the steroid group, a bacterial pneumonitis and a pyoderma. In the non-steroid group there was one case of pneumonitis and two of pyoderma. In all cases oral antimicrobial therapy was given, and recovery was uneventful. No fatalities, atypical eruptions, or any other reported complications were noted among the steroid-treated children during or after varicella.

There were 17 children in whom steroid therapy had been discontinued during the 12 months preceding varicella, and in 4 of them the therapy had been stopped during the incubation period. The course of these patients during the exanthematous disease was followed very closely with special attention to possible signs or symptoms of adrenal insufficiency. All of these children ran an uneventful course.

Despite the absence of obvious complications, the possibility was considered that the over-all severity of varicella might be different in the three groups of patients described, i.e. children who had not received steroid therapy for at least one year before varicella, children who were on maintenance therapy with steroids, and children in whom therapy was stopped within the 12 months preceding varicella. The magnitude of the febrile response and the duration of fever were thought worth investigating in view of the well-known antipyretic effect of the adrenocortical hormones. Table 5 relates the febrile responses noted to the steroid treatment state. The differences among the three treatment groups are not significant.

In order to carry out multiple statistical correlations between the severity of varicella (extent of eruption), febrile responses, steroid therapy, changes in asthma, and age of the patient, each one of the children observed was placed in an appropriate box, as shown in Table 6. The analysis of variance technique, used to evaluate the differences observed, was that of a single variable of classification, with unequal-sized subgroup samples (Dixon and Massey, 1957). The over-all severity of varicella and the extent and duration of the exanthema were not found to be affected by steroid therapy ($F = 0 \cdot 81$). Fever was also not affected by steroids in the dosage range employed ($F = 0 \cdot 20$). It was also noted that fever in these children was not accompanied by a consistent reduction in the severity of asthma, as had been noted and reported previously (Falliers *et al.*, 1961).

The initial inspection of the data gave the impression that older children, on steroid therapy, appeared more susceptible to varicella. In fact, the relation between age and steroid therapy was not found to be statistically significant ($F = 0 \cdot 58$). The three oldest children had a history of having had varicella in the past. This historical information could not be confirmed with absolute certainty, but the possibility exists that in these three the varicella observed by us represented a second attack in a steroid-treated child.

In all cases except one steroid therapy was maintained or slightly increased during varicella. The sole exception was the first case in this series seen by the authors. At this time we were influenced here by the grave prognosis indicated in the early published reports, and a discontinuance of therapy on the third day of the illness was considered advisable. A more 'physiological' thinking has prevailed since, and, summarizing an experience with 21 cases, we have found that varicella pursued its ordinary course in children in whom the daily dose of prednisone was maintained at the low levels usually sufficient for reasonable control of asthma.

## Discussion

Despite the great interest in the nature of viral agents and the diseases caused by them during the past few decades, the precise mechanisms of resistance to viral infection are unclear. One is still unable to assess the relative importance in viral immunity of humoral factors such as antibody, cellular factors, e.g. the interferons, and hypersensitivity of the delayed type (Friedman, Baron, Buckler, and Steinmuller, 1962; Wagner, 1963; Hale, 1961). Superimposing the effects of corticosteroids upon this already complex problem further beclouds the issue. There is a voluminous literature on the effects of corticosteroids on resistance to infection (Kass and Finland, 1958). In attempting to evaluate the experimental data that bear upon this question, it is well to consider the following points.

(1) The species of animal with which one deals is of great significance. The effects of cortisol on resistance to infection in the mouse, rat, and rabbit, whose major adrenal cortical hormones are not the 17-OH corticoids (Bush, 1951), may be quite different from the effects of these same steroids in the guinea-pig, monkey, and man. Experiments in the former group of animals, receiving 17-OH corticosteroids, which show heightened susceptibility to infection, must be interpreted in the light of the possibility that these 'foreign corticosteroids' have a more profound effect on their metabolism in general, and specifically on their resistance to infection. In species such as man, whose major corticosteroids are the 17-OH derivatives, the effect of addition of these hormones may be a quantitative one only (Long, 1960).

(2) The timing of the administration of the corticosteroids in relation to the giving of the antigenic stimulus (either natural or artificial) influences the effect of the steroid on antibody production. Given after antibody production is already underway, corticosteroids have little, if any, effect and are similar in this regard to the effect of *x*-irradiation and cytotoxic drugs (Berglund, 1956).

(3) As with other agents that affect antibody production, the factor of dosage is of great importance. The corticosteroid dosage used in many of the animal experiments was, when related to body weight, many times in excess of what ordinarily would be used in man.

Recent brief reports have indicated that the viral exanthematous diseases, rubeola and rubella, usually run an uneventful course when occurring in children treated with corticosteroids (Falliers *et al.*, 1961; Gerbeaux *et al.*, 1963). The opposite has been the case with varicella, where an increase in mortality has been alleged to occur and be a direct result of the steroid hormones. It seems clear that the corticosteroid-varicella combination may be lethal in those disorders in which an underlying defect in the immune mechanism is known to exist, e.g. malignancy (Miller, 1962). However, when the immune mechanism is not compromised by the primary disease, a corticosteroid-varicella hazard is unproven. In reviewing the deaths reported in this latter group, one is impressed by the lack of specific details, especially regarding the dose of corticosteroid at the time of death (Haggerty and Eley, 1956; Eley, 1961). It has been accurately noted that 'at the present time we are conditioned to associate the administration of corticosteroids or ACTH with an increased susceptibility of man to infectious agents' (Raffel, 1961). Since it has been recommended that corticosteroids be stopped in the face of varicella (Eley, 1961), it is quite possible that this course of action was followed in a number of the fatal cases. Death, then, may have resulted from adrenal insufficiency (Aceto *et al.*, 1962), precipitated by the stress of varicella, in a patient dependent upon exogenous corticosteroids. Mortality more likely occurred as a result of *not* using steroids rather than using them. Some of the catastrophic deaths occurring in steroid-treated asthmatics may likewise have resulted from a similar reluctance to reinstitute or increase steroid therapy in stressful situations, which, of course, would include severe asthma.

## Summary

Two hundred and seventy-four cases of varicella occurring in children who were receiving corticosteroids have been reported from all over the world between the years 1953 and 1963. Mortality was higher in the period before 1958 than thereafter. The reasons for this have been discussed. A significantly higher mortality was found in cases treated with steroids for leukaemia and other haematological disorders, as well as for rheumatic and connective-tissue diseases, than in illnesses in which the immune mechanism is not thought to be compromised.

Of the 59 cases of varicella seen at C.A.R.I.H. during a six-year period, 21 were on corticosteroid therapy. No fatalities and no serious complications attributable to the adrenal cortical hormones were noted; indeed, steroid therapy did not influence the degree of duration of pyrexia, nor the extent or severity of the exanthematous eruption, as compared to a group of controls. When a child receiving steroids for a chronic disorder is exposed to or becomes ill with varicella, therapy at physiological levels equivalent to 25-50 mg./day of cortisone should be continued. Abrupt withdrawal of corticosteroids in the face of any potentially stressful disease, such as varicella, is unphysiological and hazardous.

The contribution of the entire medical staff at C.A.R.I.H. in the care and study of the patients reported in this communication is gratefully acknowledged. K. Edward Dietiker, Clinical Psychologist of the Behavioral Science Division of C.A.R.I.H. offered valuable advice and assistance in the performance of the statistical studies. The tireless efforts of Mrs. Elizabeth Loomis, Interlibrary Loan Director of the Denison Library, Colorado University Medical Center, greatly facilitated the collection of references.

### References

Aceto, T., Jr., Blizzard, R. M., and Migeon, C. J. (1962). Varicella and steroid therapy. *Pediatrics*, **29**, 1029.

Berglund, K. (1956). Studies on factors which condition the effect of cortisone on antibody production. *Acta path. microbiol. scand.*, **38**, 311, 329.

Bernheim, M., Larbre, F., and Germain, D. (1959). Corticotherapie et varicelle. *Rev. Prat. (Paris)*, **9**, 2879.

——, ——, Mouriquand, C., and Germain, D. (1956). Deux cas de varicelle hémorragique a évolution mortelle chez deux enfants traités à la cortisone pour maladie de Bouillaud. *Pédiatrie*, **11**, 920.

Breton, A., Ponté, C., and Boniface, L. (1960). Que faut-il penser de l'influence aggravante des corticoïdes sur l'evolution des maladies virales contagieuses de l'enfance? *Lille méd.*, **5**, 358.

Bush, I. E. (1951). Paper-chromatographic study of the secretion of the adrenal cortex in various mammalian species. *J. Physiol. (Lond.)*, **115**, 12P.

Celinska, W., Goledzinowska, L., Szpakowska, W., and Zychowicz, C. (1961). Wpływ hormonów sterydowych na przebicg ospy Wietrzncj. [The effect of corticoids on the course of varicella.] *Pol. Tyg. lek.*, **16**, 1615.

Cheatham, W. J., Weller, T. H., Dolan, T. F., Jr., and Dower, J. C. (1956). Varicella: report of two fatal cases with necropsy, virus isolation, and serologic studies. *Amer. J. Path.*, **32**, 1015.

Combe, P., Boineau, N., and Mme. Zannettacci (1959). Manifestations pulmonaires de la varicelle au cours de la primo-infection tuberculeuse de nourrisson: considérations générales sur le poumon varicelleux. *Pédiatrie*, **14**, 503.

Crisalli, M., and Terragna, A. (1956). Modificazioni indotte dal cortisone sull' esantema varicelloso. *Gazz. sanit., milano*, **27**, 297.

Dixon, W. J., and Massey, F. J., Jr. (1957). *Introduction to Statistical Analysis*, 2nd ed., p. 145. McGraw-Hill, New York.

Eley, R. C. (1961). Varicella and steroid therapy. *Pediatrics*, **28**, 1027.

Falliers, C. J., Halberstein, S. G., and Bukantz, S. C. (1961). Effect of rubeola, rubella, varicella, and a viral upper respiratory infection upon the severity of childhood asthma: with a note on the role of corticosteroids. *J. Allergy*, **32**, 69.

——, Tan, L. S., Szentivanyi, J., Jorgensen, J. R., and Bukantz, S. C. (1963). Childhood asthma and steroid therapy as influences on growth. *Amer. J. Dis. Child.*, **105**, 127.

Finkel, K. C. (1961). Mortality from varicella in children receiving adrenocorticosteroids and adrenocorticotropin. *Pediatrics*, **28**, 436.

Friedman, R. M., Baron, S., Buckler, C. E., and Steinmuller, R. I. (1962). The role of antibody, delayed hypersensitivity, and interferon production in recovery of guinea pigs from primary infection with vaccinia virus. *J. exp. Med.*, **116**, 347.

Gerbeaux, J., Couvreur, J., Baculard-Beauchef, A., and Joly, J. B. (1963). Maladies infectieuses sous corticothérapie au long cours (194 observations dont 102 varicelles). *Sem. Hôp. Paris*, **39**, 61.

Gillot, F., Clausse, J., and de Peretti, E. (1958). Varicelle et cortisone (à propos de 7 observations). *Algérie méd.*, **62**, 273.

Gordon, J. E. (1962). Chickenpox: an epidemiological review. *Amer. J. med. Sci.*, **244**, 362.

Guazzelli, C., and Calzolari, C. (1961). Varicella e cotisonici. Russegna della letteratura con descrizione di un caso clinico. *Riv. Clin. pediat.*, **67**, 41.

Haggerty, R. J., and Eley, R. C. (1956). Varicella and cortisone. *Pediatrics*, **18**, 160.

Hale, J. H. (1961). Duration of immunity in virus disease. *Advanc. Immunol.*, **1**, 263.

Hennemanne, G. (1960). Varicelle et cortisone: quelle doit être, notre attitude thérapeutique. *Arch. franç. Pédiat.*, **17**, 38.

Johnson, R. W. P., and Nelson, A. M. (1960). Haemorrhagic chicken-pox: Two fatal cases. *Brit. med. J.*, **1**, 1183.

Josserand, P., De L'Hermuzière, and Mlle. Vacher (1953). Varicelle mortelle à forme hémorragique dans le décours d'un traitement par cortisone—ACTH. *Pédiatrie*, **8**, 947.

Kaplan, A. S. (1958). Faut-il interrompre ou intensifier le traitement lorsque survient une maladie infectieuse intercurrente chez un enfant traite par les hormones surrénaliennes? *Sem. Hôp. Paris*, **34**, 2078.

Kass, E. H., and Finland, M. (1958). Corticosteroids and infections. *Advanc. intern. Med.*, **9**, 45.

Kirchhoff, H. W. (1960). Kritische Bemerkungen zur Cortison-Therapie. *Mschr. Kinderheilk.*, **108**, 200.

Krajewska, B. (1961). Ospa wietrzna a leczenie hormonami nadnercza. [Chickenpox and the therapy by means of hormones of the suprarenals.] *Pediat. pol.*, **36**, 1067.

—— (1962). Corticotherapy in the course of varicella. *Helv. paediat. Acta*, **17**, 150.

Kredba, V., and Bradáčová, M. (1959). Atypischer Verlauf von Windpocken bei Kindern die mit steroiden Hormonen behandelt wurden. *Med. Klin.*, **54**, 2295.

Kuipers, F., and Van der Mei, J. (1958). Ernstige compicaties bij waterpokken. *Maandschr. Kindergeneesk.*, **26**, 294.

Le Tan Vinh, Canlorbe, P., Gentile, C., and Lelong, M. (1957). La varicelle maligne pluriviscérale; un cas avec mise en évidence des foyers de nécrose et des inclusions acidophiles intranucléaires. *Sem. Hôp. Paris*, **33**, 3989.

Long, D. A. (1960). Relationship between susceptibility to corticosteroids and resistance to infection and response to chemotherapy. *Antibiot. Chemother.* (*Basel*), **7**, 29.

Miller, D. G. (1962). Patterns of immunological deficiency in lymphomas and leukemias. *Ann. intern. Med.*, **57**, 703.

Monnet, M. P. (1958). Varicelle et cortisone. *Rev. lyon. Méd.*, **7**, 1127.

Moulinier, Lartigaut, Cantonné, Martin, Geindre, and Traissac (1956). Varicelle et leucose. *J. Méd. Bordeaux*, **133**, 180.

Nichols, W. W. (1957). Experiences with chickenpox in patients with hematologic disease receiving cortisone. *Amer. J. Dis. Child.*, **94**, 219.

Pinkel, D. (1961). Chickenpox and leukemia. *J. Pediat.*, **58**, 729.

Raffel, S. (1961). *Immunity*, 2nd ed., p. 270. Appleton-Century-Crofts, New York.

Shee, J. C., and Fehrsen, P. (1953). Reactivation of varicella virus by cortisone therapy. *Brit. med. J.*, **2**, 82.

Siegel, S. C., Lovin, B. J., Jr., Ely, R. S., and Kelley, V. C. (1959). Adrenal function in allergy. III. Effect of prolonged intermittent steroid therapy in allergic children. *Pediatrics*, **24**, 434,

Thoenes, F. (1959). Maligne Varicellen. *Mschr. Kinkerheilk.*, **107**, 422.

Viklický, J., Doutlík, S., and Kottová, A. (1961). Varicella a léčba kortikoidy (klinicko-morfologická studie). [Varicella and corticoid treatment (clinical and morphological investigation).] *Čas. Lék. čes.*, **100**, 1419.

Wagner, R. R. (1963). Cellular resistance to viral infection with particular reference to endogenous interferon. *Bact. Rev.*, **27**, 72.

*Arch. Dis. Childh.*, 1965, **40**, 600.

# E (16-18) TRISOMY SYNDROME: ANALYSIS OF 13 CASES

BY

L. J. BUTLER, G. J. A. I. SNODGRASS, N. E. FRANCE, L. SINCLAIR, and A. RUSSELL

*From the Queen Elizabeth Hospital for Children, London*

(RECEIVED FOR PUBLICATION MARCH 12, 1965)

The syndrome of multiple congenital abnormalities associated with an additional autosome in the Denver Group 16-18 (E) was first described by Edwards, Harnden, Cameron, Crosse, and Wolff (1960). Its documentation has gradually been accumulated since, notably by Smith, Patau, Therman, and Inhorn (1960), Smith, Patau, Therman, and Inhorn (1962), Smith (1963), and Hecht, Bryant, Motulsky, and Giblett (1963). Morphological evidence is cited to show that the additional autosome is unequivocally No. 18 in all cases of our series, with one exception, where a possible small duplication in the long arms of the additional chromosome is postulated.

The data on all 13 cases are presented in tabular form, and the individual anomalies discussed in order that their over-all pattern may be appreciated. Case 13 has been reported by Sinclair (1963).

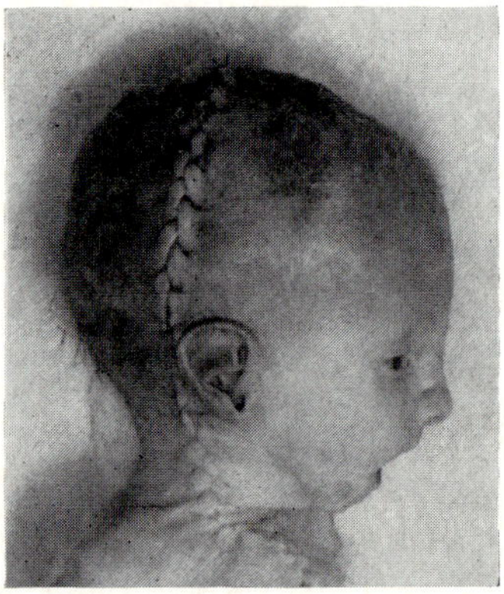

FIG. 1a.—Case 5. Face in profile to demonstrate the 'Grecian nose', micrognathia, and flattened 'stretched-out' upper segment of pinna.

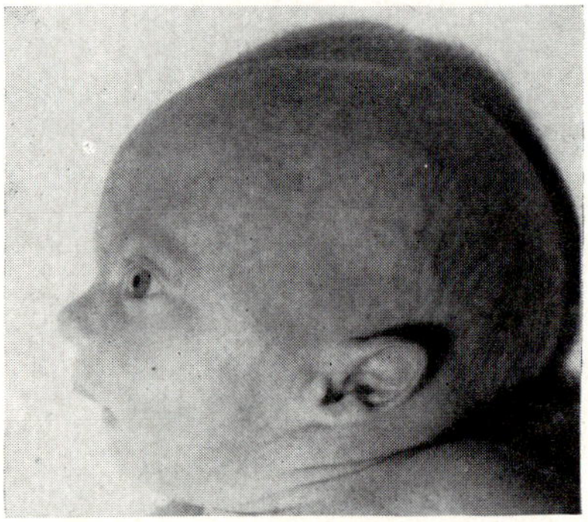

FIG. 1b.—Case 7. Elfin appearance of the second of two facial categories.

## Analysis of Anomalies in 13 Cases

### (i) Anomalies Evident on Clinical Examination (Table 1).

*Cranio-facial.*—In 6 cases the skull circumference was less than the normal range. The bifrontal diameter was reduced in all cases, and in the most marked examples this gave a false impression of widening of the parietal region. Although some degree of microcephaly was present in 6 cases, this was not immediately obvious on inspection because of the considerable relative retardation of facial growth and variable degree of hypoplasia of both maxillae and mandible. The supra-orbital ridges were poorly developed in most cases, and the orbits were shallow. Abnormal occipital prominence is reported as being common (Finley, Finley, and Carte, 1963; Voorhess, Vaharu, and Gardner, 1962; Smith *et al.*, 1962; Smith, 1963). None of the present series showed this finding. It is probable that the marked retardation of facial growth is responsible for this impression. The occipito-frontal circumference was below the lowest limits of normality in relation to birth weight in 6 of the 11 cases in which it was ascertained and in no case was it greater than the mean. In the extreme instances (Fig. 1a) there appeared to be complete continuity of frontal and nasal bones, a so-called Grecian nose, while in others nasal bridge development was normal (Fig. 1b). Where no true bridge exists, the association of this with the other cranio-facial features constitutes an unmistakable face. Radiography of

TABLE 1

CLINICAL FINDINGS

| | Case No. | | | | | | | | | | | | | Total |
|---|---|---|---|---|---|---|---|---|---|---|---|---|---|---|
| | 1 | 2 | 3 | 4 | 5 | 6 | 7 | 8 | 9 | 10 | 11 | 12 | 13 | |
| Sex | M | F | F | F | F | F | F | M | F | F | F | F | M | 10 F<br>3 M |
| Race | C | C | C | N | C | C | C | N | C | C | C | C | C | 2 N<br>11 C |
| Gestation (wk.) | 36 | 42 | 40 | 36 | 37 | 42 | 42 | 42 | 40 | 43 | 40 | 38 | 42 | — |
| Birth weight (g.) | 1332 | 2097 | 1998 | 1445 | 1700 | 2607 | <2267 | 3402 | 2097 | 2295 | 1756 | 2239 | 2182 | — |
| Resuscitation difficulty | + | + | + | – | + | + | – | – | + | + | + | + | – | 9/13 |
| Age at death (days) | 4 | 66 | 31 | SB | 18 | 9 | 60 | 31 | 49 | 22 | 21 | 29 | 8 | — |
| *Craniofacial* | | | | | | | | | | | | | | |
| Narrow bifrontal diameter | + | + | + | + | + | + | + | + | + | + | + | + | + | 13/13 |
| Small face | + | + | + | + | + | + | + | + | + | + | + | + | + | 13/13 |
| Micrognathia | + | + | + | + | + | + | + | + | + | + | + | + | + | 13/13 |
| Hypoplasia of orbital ridges | + | + | + | – | – | – | + | + | – | + | – | + | + | 8/13 |
| Mild microcephaly | – | + | + | ? | + | – | – | – | + | – | + | + | ? | 6/11 |
| Epicanthic folds | + | + | ? | ? | + | – | – | + | ? | – | + | + | + | 7/10 |
| Narrow palpebral fissures | + | + | + | + | + | + | + | + | ? | + | + | + | + | 12/12 |
| Ocular defect | – | – | ? | – | + | + | – | – | – | – | – | + | – | 3/12 |
| Low-set ears | + | – | + | + | – | + | + | – | – | + | + | + | + | 9/13 |
| Cartilaginous deficiency ears | + | + | + | – | + | + | + | – | – | + | + | + | + | 10/13 |
| Atretic auditory meatus | – | – | + | – | – | – | – | – | – | + | – | – | – | 2/13 |
| Abnormally situated auditory meatus | + | – | + | – | + | – | – | – | – | + | + | + | – | 6/13 |
| Small mouth | + | + | + | + | + | + | + | + | + | + | + | + | + | 13/13 |
| High arched palate | – | – | – | + | – | – | – | – | – | + | – | – | – | 2/13 |
| Neck webbing | – | + | + | – | – | – | + | – | – | + | + | + | + | 7/13 |
| Facial palsy | – | – | + | ? | + | – | – | – | ? | + | – | – | – | 3/11 |
| *Thorax and Abdomen* | | | | | | | | | | | | | | |
| Hypermobile shoulders | + | + | + | ? | + | + | + | ? | ? | + | + | + | + | 10/10 |
| Partial agenesis of clavicles | – | + | – | – | – | – | – | – | – | – | – | – | + | 2/13 |
| Short sternum | – | + | – | – | + | + | + | + | ? | – | – | – | + | 6/12 |
| Wide-set nipples | + | + | ? | ? | – | – | + | ? | ? | + | + | – | + | 6/9 |
| Para-umbilical hernia | – | – | – | – | – | – | – | – | – | – | + | + | – | 2/13 |
| Imperforate anus | + | – | – | – | – | – | – | – | – | – | – | – | – | 1/13 |
| Abnormal genitalia | – | – | – | – | – | – | – | – | – | – | + | + | – | 2/13 |
| *Limbs* | | | | | | | | | | | | | | |
| Flexion deformity of fingers | + | + | + | + | – | – | + | + | + | – | + | + | + | 10/13 |
| Flexion deformity of wrists | + | – | – | – | + | – | – | + | + | – | – | – | + | 5/13 |
| Flexion deformity of elbows | – | – | – | – | – | – | – | – | – | + | + | + | – | 3/13 |
| Flexion deformity of hips | – | – | – | – | – | – | – | – | – | – | + | + | – | 2/13 |
| Aplasia radius | – | – | – | – | – | – | – | – | + | – | – | – | – | 1/13 |
| Aplastic or hypoplastic thumb | – | + | – | + | + | – | – | + | + | + | + | + | + | 9/13 |
| Short hallux | + | + | + | + | + | + | + | + | + | + | + | + | + | 13/13 |
| Syndactyly 2nd and 3rd toes | + | + | ? | – | – | – | + | + | ? | + | + | + | + | 8/11 |
| Lobster claw deformity | – | – | – | – | – | – | – | + | – | – | – | – | – | 1/13 |
| Protuberant heels | + | – | + | – | – | + | + | + | – | + | + | + | + | 9/13 |
| Hypoplasia of nails | + | – | – | ? | – | – | – | ? | ? | + | + | + | ? | 4/9 |
| Hypertonia | + | + | + | ? | + | + | + | + | + | + | – | + | + | 11/12 |

+ = Presence ascertained. – = Absent. ? = Not known. Race C = Caucasian. N = Negro. SB = Stillborn.
M = Male. F = Female.

the skull (Fig. 2) showed no typical defect, apart from poor facial growth; the occiput seems prominent, but this was not apparent clinically. All but one case had narrow palpebral fissures. The impression of 'ptosis' derived from an inability to separate completely the eyelids. In some cases, the impression of proptosis, contributed to by shallowness of the orbits, was exaggerated by the hypoplasia of the supra-orbital ridges. Case 5 had microphthalmus on the left, and Case 6 had bilateral hazy corneal opacities. Case 12 showed a coloboma of the choroid involving the optic disc on the right, while the coloboma was confined to the disc on the left. Optic abnormalities do not appear to be common in Group E trisomy, though optic atrophy and glaucoma (Townes, Manning, and DeHart, 1962), corneal opacity (Smith, 1963), and lens opacity (Smith *et al.*, 1960) have been described. The ears were considered to be low set in 9 cases where the uppermost point of the pinna lay below the outer canthus of the eye. Deficiencies in cartilaginous formation of the external ear varied from a rudimentary skin ridge (Fig. 3), to being paper thin and rather elephantine (Fig. 1a), to flattening of the pinna superiorly with primitive helical development. In Case 1 the skin of the scalp was directly reflected over the pinna which could not be pulled forward. Abnormalities of the external auditory meatus were found in 7 cases, ranging from complete atresia (Fig. 3), or an extremely low location, to small size and excessive anterior direction. Unilateral meatal atresia was present in 2 cases, and

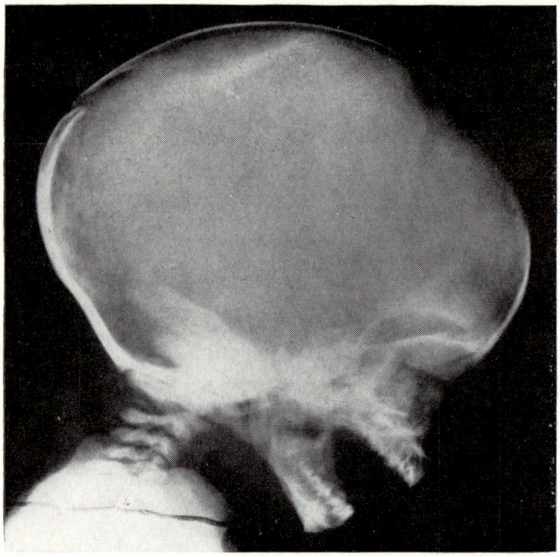

FIG. 2.—Case 10. Skull radiograph showing non-canalization of petrous temporal bone.

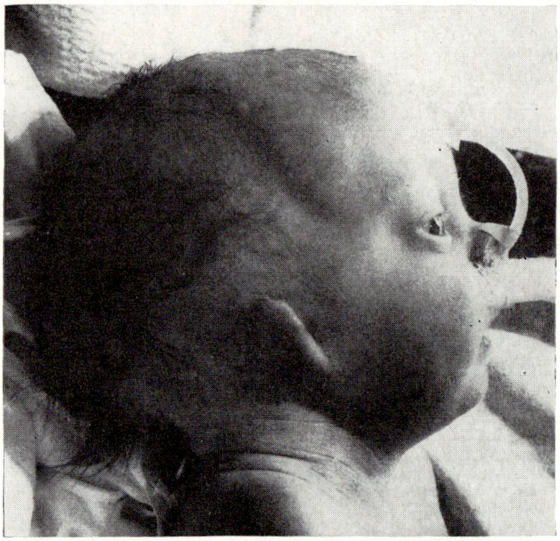

FIG. 3.—Case 10. Cartilaginous deficiency of ear with atretic external auditory meatus.

was associated with a rudimentary external ear. Fig. 2 illustrates absence of canalization of the petrous temporal bone on radiography. In only two cases were the ears normal. The mouth was small in all our cases and tended to be triangular in some. In Cases 4 and 10 the palate was high and arched, but there were no cases of cleft lip or palate. Peripheral right-sided facial palsy was seen in 3 cases. Seventh nerve palsy has been noted previously (Smith *et al.*, 1962; Holman, Erkman, Zacharias, and Kock, 1963), and has invariably been right-sided. In 2 cases there was associated atresia of the right external auditory meatus, and it is possible that this could affect the course of the 7th nerve, as sometimes seen in the first visceral arch syndrome. Neck webbing was bilateral in 6 cases and unilateral in 1; a recent review (Finley *et al.*, 1963) revealed this in 6 of 8 cases where sought.

*Thorax.* The most common clinical anomaly in this series was hypermobility of the shoulders which could be unduly approximated. The sternum was short, with a 'shield like' thorax and wide subcostal angle in half the cases; Finley *et al.* (1963) noted these features in the records of 13 of 15 cases where sought, while Smith (1963) found them in 14 out of 16. In 2 (Cases 2 and 13) the medial third of both clavicles was absent and the lateral portions were extremely thin. Unusually thin clavicles have been noted previously (German, Rankin, Harrison, Donovan, Hogan, and Bearn, 1962). One or both nipples were displaced well outside the mid-clavicular line in half of our cases, and showed varying degrees of hypoplasia.

*Cardiovascular System.* A systolic murmur was noted in the 12 born alive, in all but one appearing within the first three days of life.

*Abdomen.* Inguinal herniae were noted in 11 of 16 cases in Smith's review (1963). No inguinal hernia was found in this series, but two examples of para-umbilical hernia occurred and were associated with marked diastasis recti and gross bulging of the epigastric area on crying. Clinical evidence of pyloric stenosis emerged in 2, Cases 3 and 12, with post-mortem confirmation in Case 3.

*Limbs.* Hypertonia was extremely marked in some infants, and was present in 11 of 12 cases. It is a constant feature in the reviews, but in one case (Finley *et al.*, 1963) there was striking hypotonia. Anomalies of the limbs, particularly of distal segments, are consistent in this syndrome and emphasized in all the published reviews. A curiously frequent posture adopted by 6 cases was created by abduction of the arms at the shoulder and flexion at the elbow, the so-called 'surrender position'. Flexion deformities of the fingers with abduction of the thumb across the palm and the index finger over-riding one or more of the other fingers are extremely common (Smith *et al.*, 1962; Finley *et al.*, 1963; Gottlieb, Hirschhorn, Cooper, Lusskin, Moloshok, and Hodes, 1962) and were found in most of our

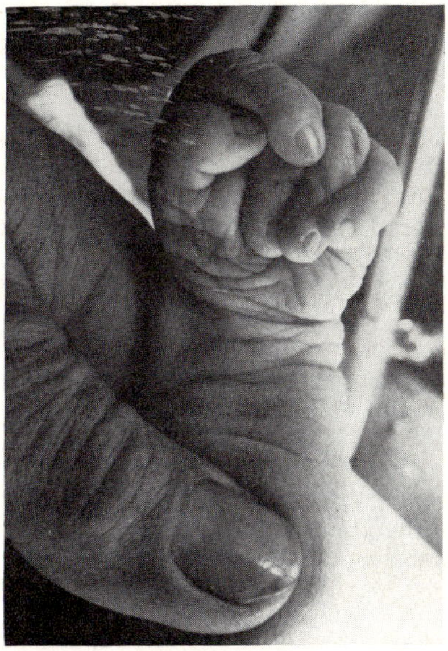

FIG. 4.—Case 10. Characteristic flexion deformity of fingers.

cases. The fifth finger often overrides the fourth (Fig. 4). The fingers of these cases could only be straightened with great difficulty, and in one case barely at all. Characteristically this forcible extension of the fingers was attended by their gross ulnar deviation (Fig. 5) and instability of the interphalangeal and metacarpophalangeal joints. The flexion deformities were associated with varying degrees of apparent hypoplasia of the long flexor muscles and tendons to the fingers, as seen in arthrogryposis, and often with hypoplasia of thenar and hypothenar muscles. Aplasia and hypoplasia of thenar musculature has been the subject of comment by Smith *et al.* (1962), who also noted a decrease of muscle mass generally in these patients. The thumb was hypoplastic in 8 cases and completely absent in one (Case 9): this was associated with shortening of the first metacarpal, and in 2 infants with aplasia (Cases 9 and 13). Hypoplasia or aplasia of the first metacarpal was invariably associated with hypoplasia of thenar musculature. There was considerable splaying of the metacarpal heads on forcible extension in most cases.

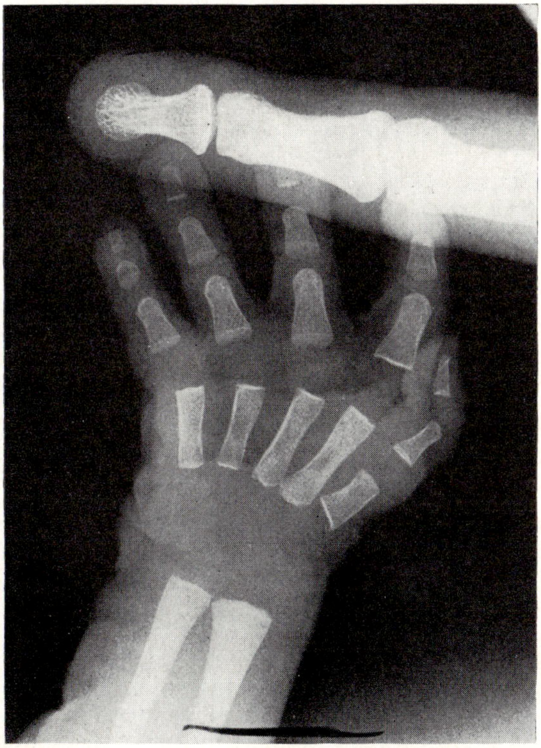

FIG. 5.—Case 1. Radiograph of hand after forcible extension of fingers, especially illustrating the 1st metacarpal hypoplasia.

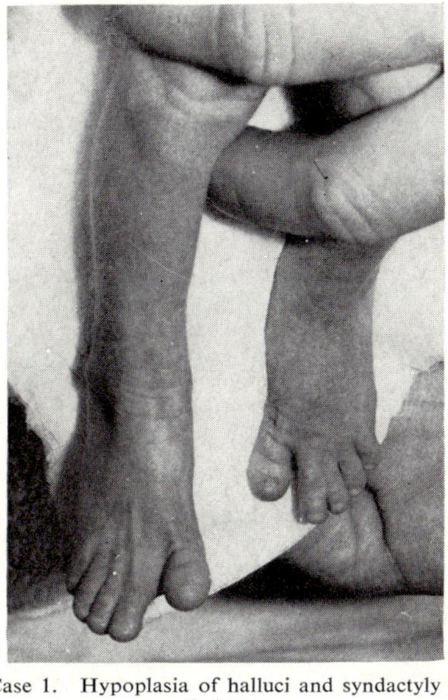

FIG. 6.—Case 1. Hypoplasia of halluci and syndactyly of 2nd and 3rd toes.

Hypoplasia of the hallux (Fig. 6) was invariable, and intermittent dorsiflexion found in 10 instances was not associated with hypoplasia of the long extensor muscles. In some shortening of the first metatarsal was noted (Fig. 7). Varying degrees of syndactyly of the second and third toes were seen (Fig. 6), a common enough anomaly in otherwise

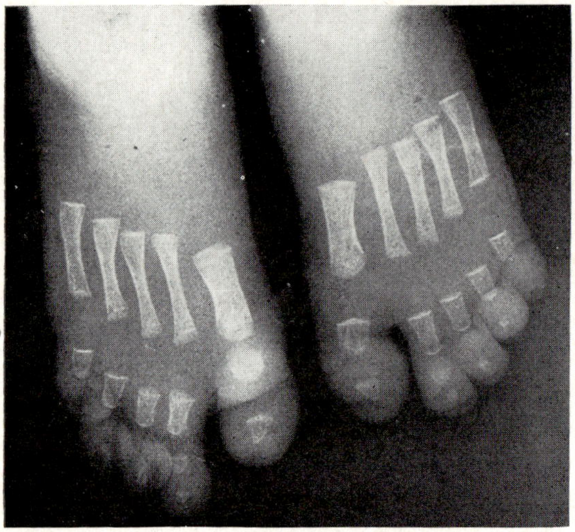

FIG. 7.—Case 1. Radiograph of feet illustrating hypoplasia of 1st metatarsals.

normal people, presumably because these toes derive from a single developmental bud. Protuberance of the heels was present in 9 infants, but not in association with a vertical talus in the 5 where radiographs were available. In Case 8 (Fig. 8) there was a bizarre cleft between the right hallux and toes 4 and 5 with absence of the second and third toes. A similar smaller cleft was present on the left foot. In Case 12 this defect was present to a mild degree also, but was not associated with aplasia of any toes. A vertical skin crease between the first and second toes was found in 4 other infants but no skin cleft was present. Hypoplasia of the nails was found in 4 but aplasia was not observed.

The dermal ridges characteristically show a predominance of the simple arch pattern. Uchida and Soltan (1963) found that in 20 patients, 18 had 6 or more simple arches, and in 8 arches were present on all 10 digits. In the present series prints were obtained only from Cases 10, 11, and 12, and examined by Professor L. S. Penrose. These conformed to the criteria of Uchida and Soltan (1963), and in Cases 11 and 12 this pattern was found on all 20 digits. Hallucal and palmar patterns are so far non-contributory. A single flexion crease on the fifth finger is also a frequent finding (11 out of 18 in Uchida's series), 2 of our series showing this feature. Obtaining prints during life is technically extremely difficult in these cases owing to the flexion deformities.

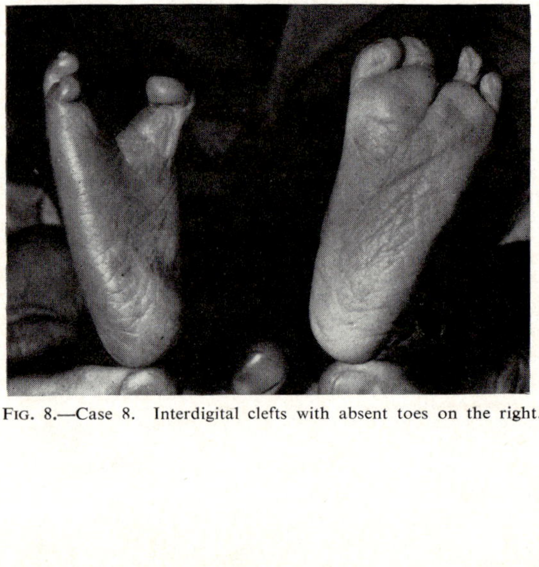

FIG. 8.—Case 8. Interdigital clefts with absent toes on the right.

Flexion deformities of the large joints of the upper limbs were progressively less frequent the more proximal the joint and did not appear to be secondary to hypertonia since complete extension could not be obtained passively. In Cases 11 and 12 the hips could not be fully abducted. This did not seem to be associated with skeletal muscle hypoplasia but was related to curiously tight skin folds and hypertonia. In both cases there was some clitoridal hypertrophy similar to that illustrated by Hecht *et al.* (1963). No other abnormalities of the external genitalia were found.

Defective ossification of the skull was noted in 3 of 5 cases where radiography was performed; the knee epiphyses were present in all 5. In one (Fig. 7) there was lack of ossification of the middle phalanges of the 3rd and 4th toes bilaterally and of the distal phalanges of the 5th toes. In the longest-lived cases of the series, osseous development remained at birth level.

(ii) **Anomalies Found at Necropsy (Table 2).**

*Cardiovascular System.* The most consistent anomaly was wide patency of the ductus arteriosus usually associated with a high ventricular septal defect. In Case 2 a second ventricular septal defect was present below and posterior to the higher defect, while in 3 the aortic valve was partially transposed. Only minor defects of valves were found: in 2 instances both aortic and pulmonary valves were bicuspid and in 3 others there was one bicuspid semilunar valve. A single umbilical artery was associated with low rectal atresia in Case 1, and Case 8 showed a left superior vena cava draining into a dilated coronary sinus.

Changes in the pulmonary vessels were noted histologically in Cases 2 and 7 (Fig. 9). In arteries of 3-400 μ external diameter, there were scattered eccentric patches of intimal thickening due to relatively acellular fibroelastic tissue. In arteries of

TABLE 2
NECROPSY FINDINGS

| | Case No. | | | | | | | | | | | | Total |
|---|---|---|---|---|---|---|---|---|---|---|---|---|---|
| | 1 | 2 | 3 | 4 | 5 | 6 | 7 | 8 | 9 | 10 | 11 | 13 | |
| *Cardiovascular* | | | | | | | | | | | | | |
| Ventricular septal defect | + | + | – | + | + | + | + | + | – | + | + | + | 10/12 |
| Dextroposition of aortic valve | + | – | – | – | – | + | – | + | – | – | – | – | 3/12 |
| Bicuspid aortic valve | – | + | – | – | – | + | – | + | – | – | + | – | 4/12 |
| Bicuspid pulmonary valve | – | + | – | – | + | – | – | – | – | – | + | – | 3/12 |
| Patent ductus arteriosus | + | + | – | + | + | + | + | + | + | + | + | + | 11/12 |
| Single umbilical artery | + | – | ? | – | – | – | – | ? | ? | – | – | – | 1/9 |
| Left superior vena cava | – | – | – | – | – | – | – | + | – | – | – | – | 1/12 |
| Pulmonary hypertensive changes | – | + | – | – | – | – | + | – | – | – | – | – | 2/12 |
| *Urogenital* | | | | | | | | | | | | | |
| Cysts of kidneys | – | – | – | – | – | – | – | – | – | + | – | – | 1/12 |
| Horseshoe kidney | – | – | – | – | – | – | – | + | – | + | – | – | 2/12 |
| Anomalous shape of kidney | – | – | – | – | – | – | – | – | – | – | + | – | 1/12 |
| Hypoplasia of ovaries | M | – | ? | + | – | + | – | M | ? | – | – | M | 2/7 |
| *Alimentary* | | | | | | | | | | | | | |
| Pyloric stenosis | – | + | – | – | – | – | – | – | – | – | – | – | 1/12 |
| Meckel's diverticulum | – | – | + | – | – | – | – | – | – | – | + | – | 2/12 |
| Fibrocystic liver | – | + | – | – | – | – | – | – | – | – | – | – | 1/12 |
| *Other anomalies* | | | | | | | | | | | | | |
| Prosencephaly | – | – | – | + | – | – | – | – | – | – | – | – | 1/12 |
| Diaphragmatic hernia | – | – | – | + | – | – | – | – | – | – | – | – | 1/12 |
| Eventration of diaphragm | – | + | – | – | – | – | – | – | + | – | – | – | 2/12 |

+ = Presence ascertained. – = Absent. ? = Not known. M = Male.

80-200 μ diameter marked cellular intimal proliferation of both concentric and nodular type severely reduced the size of the lumen and sometimes totally occluded the vessel. These changes were often prominent where a small artery was given off from a medium-sized vessel. The cellular lesions consisted of fairly large cells with vesicular nuclei and clear cytoplasm. The media was of normal thickness for the age and well defined in vessels as small as 40 μ external diameter. Only in some vessels was the internal elastic lamina lacking or interrupted.

Rubin and Strauss (1961) described similar obliterative changes of small pulmonary arteries in 5 infants who died during the perinatal period with multiple anomalies. Though no chromosomal studies were made, the anomalies present in their Cases 1, 3, and 4 are suggestive of trisomy 13-15 and include many features found in trisomy 18.

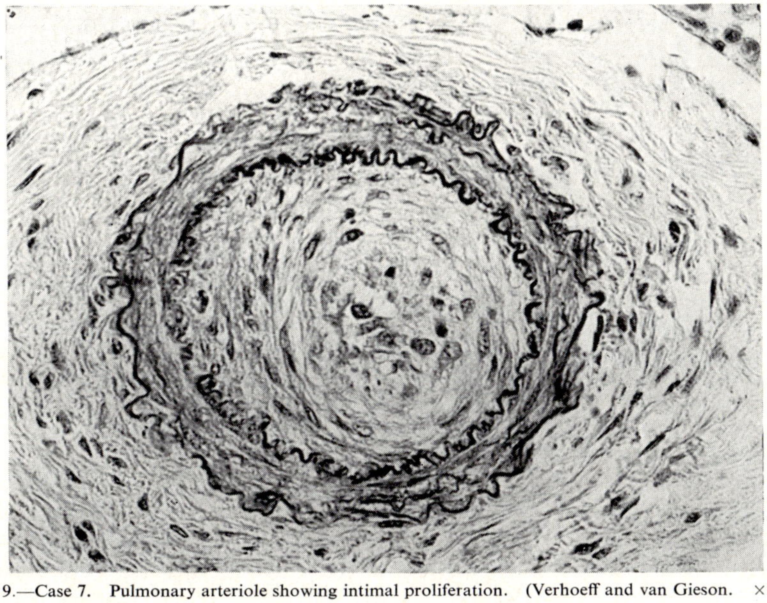

FIG. 9.—Case 7. Pulmonary arteriole showing intimal proliferation. (Verhoeff and van Gieson. × 390.)

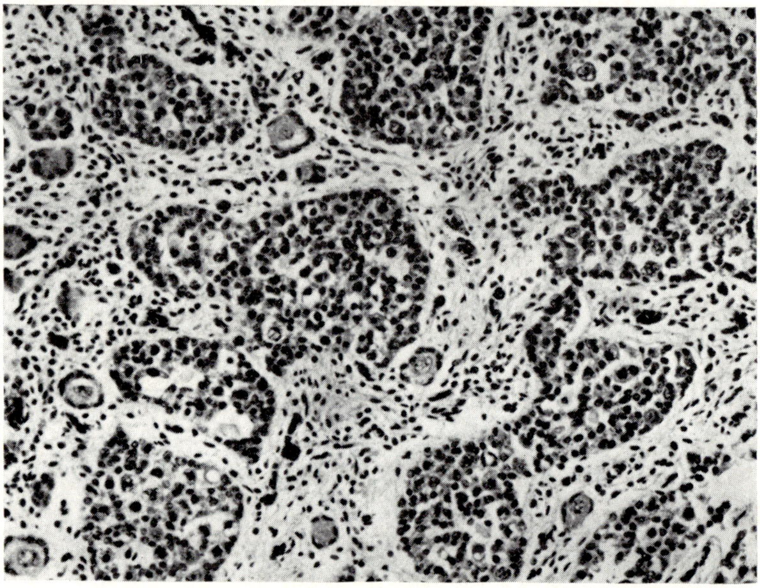

FIG. 10.—Case 11. Ovary showing 'granulosaballen' and scattered normal primordial follicles. (H. and E. × 160.

*Urogenital.* Two infants had horseshoe kidneys, both being associated with a number of microscopical cysts in the renal cortex. The lower pole of the left kidney in Case 11 extended to the midline but was not fused with the right kidney. In 7 cases the ovaries were examined microscopically, and 2 showed considerable reduction in the number of primordial follicles associated with marked proliferation of granulosa cells to form irregular small masses of deeply staining cells (Fig. 10). Similar 'granulosaballen' were seen in Cases 5 and 11, but in these infants primordial follicles were present in normal numbers.

*Neurological.* Only the stillborn infant (Case 4) showed gross abnormalities of the central nervous system. The whole brain weighed only 136 g. and showed incomplete separation into two cerebral hemispheres; the frontal lobes were separate for a distance of about 3 cm., but, more posteriorly, there was an area of fusion 4·5 cm. long with divergence of the hemispheres posteriorly; the frontal and occipital lobes were underdeveloped with relatively large temporal and parietal lobes, and the gyral pattern was abnormal with rather stout convolutions. The olfactory nerves and grooves were lacking but all other cranial nerves appeared to be present. The tuber cinereum was unusually prominent and the cerebellum appeared normal.

*Diaphragmatic.* There was partial fibrosis of the left dome of the diaphragm in 2 infants. It was almost completely absent in Case 4 where the left pleural sac contained the greater part of small and large intestines together with the stomach, spleen, and left lobe of liver; the left lung was hypoplastic.

## Obstetric Factors

**Family History.** The mean maternal age in this series (32·2 years) was higher than in the general population (Table 3). It was less than in the review of 37 cases (34·4 years) by Hecht *et al.* (1963), but was greater than that reported by Weiss, Di George, and Baird (1962) in their 4 cases (22·4 years). The mean maternal age is considerably less than that for trisomy 21 (Penrose, 1961). The mean paternal age of this series (37 years) is comparable with the figure of 36 years quoted by Hecht *et al.* (1963). As they noted, there are two peaks of maternal age incidence, one in the mid-twenties, and one in the mid-thirties. More significantly, the mean of the sum of the ages of the parents is increased. In our series this mean value was greater than 30 years in 8 of 11 cases, a figure that agrees with the findings of Hecht *et al.* (1963).

In only 3 instances was any kind of congenital anomaly traceable in the family history. A maternal aunt of Case 2 died at the age of 3 days from renal agenesis, and a female sib of Case 7 had a haeman-

TABLE 3

OBSTETRIC FEATURES

| | Case No. | | | | | | | | | | | | |
|---|---|---|---|---|---|---|---|---|---|---|---|---|---|
| | 1 | 2 | 3 | 4 | 5 | 6 | 7 | 8 | 9 | 10 | 11 | 12 | 13 |
| Maternal age (yr.) | 43 | 31 | 35 | 25 | 23 | 35 | 32 | 25 | 37 | 42 | 19 | 44 | 28 |
| Paternal age (yr.) | 50 | 31 | 41 | ? | 27 | ? | 39 | 38 | 41 | 54 | 22 | 45 | 28 |
| Years married | 25 | 7 | 2·5 | 1 | 2·5 | 14 | 10 | ? | 13 | 10 | 0·8 | 5 | ? |
| Parity | 4 | 1 | – | 5 | – | 3 | 2 | 1 | 3 | 2 | – | 2 | 1 |
| Previous abortions | 1 | – | – | – | – | – | – | – | 1 | – | – | 1 | – |
| Years of previous pregnancies or subsequent pregnancies | 1942<br>1944<br>1949<br>1959* | 1956 | 1963 | 1953<br>1955<br>1958<br>1960<br>1961 | 1963 | 1946<br>1949<br>1958 | 1954<br>1957 | 1961 | 1951<br>1954*<br>1955 | 1957<br>1960 | – | 1960<br>1961* | 1961 |
| Year of birth of affected infant | 1962 | 1961 | 1961 | 1963 | 1962 | 1963 | 1961 | 1962 | 1962 | 1963 | 1963 | 1963 | 1962 |
| Pre-eclampsia | + | – | + | + | + | – | – | – | + | + | + | ? | ? |
| Polyhydramnios | + | – | + | + | + | – | – | – | – | – | – | – | – |
| Placenta praevia | + | – | – | + | – | – | – | – | – | – | – | – | – |
| Persistent breech lie | – | + | – | – | – | – | + | – | – | + | – | – | – |
| Blood-stained liquor | + | – | + | + | – | + | – | – | – | + | – | – | ? |
| Small for dates | + | + | + | + | + | + | + | – | + | – | + | + | – |
| Placental size (g.) | 340 | 368 | S | 368 | ? | S | ? | 396 | 368 | 488 | S | S | ? |

+ = Presence ascertained. – = Absent. ? = Not known. * = Abortion. S = Small.

gioma of the lower lip. The father of Case 10 had been married previously, and the second child by his first wife, who died in the neonatal period, had a cleft palate and hare-lip. In previously reported series the incidence of familial congenital abnormality was also not above the normal.

**Previous Obstetric History.** Maternal parity did not appear to be significant in this series. There were 3 primigravidae, 2 under 25 years of age: 2 (Cases 3 and 5) have since given birth to normal children. There was no evidence of relative subfertility. Where the interval between any two pregnancies was high, the maternal and paternal ages were also high. This can be taken as the normal decline in fertility related to age. Abnormalities of previous pregnancies were few. In contrast to Smith's series (1963) the incidence of abortion in our cases was low, and was confined to the eldest mothers. Placenta praevia occurred in previous pregnancies of Cases 1 and 9.

**Present Pregnancy and Delivery.** There was a high incidence of severe pre-eclamptic toxaemia, and three instances of persistent breech presentation requiring external version. Drainage of blood-stained liquor was relatively common, but only two cases of foetal distress occurred. Placenta praevia was present in two cases. Polyhydramnios occurred in 4, and was acute in onset in 2 of them. The association of this condition, coupled with an extremely small placenta, was noted by Smith *et al.* (1960) and Smith (1963). Apart from iron, no drugs were taken except in Case 11 in which antihistamines and phenobarbitone were presented because of hyperemesis. In no case was either parent exposed to ionizing radiation or X rays. Intrauterine growth retardation was marked, and even before delivery 10 out of 13 infants were said to be small for the period of gestation. The birth weights were low, and in only 3 were they greater than 5 lb. (2,267 g.). Gestation was prolonged in 6 instances, and labour was induced at term in 3.

Delivery was normal in 10 cases, by caesarean section in one (Case 1), and by the breech in one (Case 10).

This report agrees with the predominance of females noted by most authors (Ferguson-Smith, 1962). 2 of the 3 males were the shortest lived of the series, but the proportion of males is not sufficient to draw comparisons as to survival in the sexes; Ferguson-Smith (1962) states that there is no difference. Studies on spontaneous abortions and stillbirths may provide the ultimate answer to this question.

## Clinical Progress

Resuscitation difficulties were experienced in 9 infants, in all of whom endotracheal intubation was required following failure of spontaneous respirations at 5 minutes.

All except Case 4 required continuous tube feeding from the first few days of life, and all but one of the live-born infants (Case 8) developed respiratory distress or cardiac failure in the first 3 days of life. None gained more than 1 lb. (453 g.) in weight throughout life. All but Case 11 underwent progressive cardiopulmonary failure before death. It is of interest that 3 infants were very sensitive to digoxin (Cases 2, 6, and 7) in a digitalizing dose of 0·02 mg./lb. body weight, all developing varying degrees of atrioventricular heart block. This seems a high incidence (20%), and considering the relative tolerance of newborn infants to the drug, might suggest a specific defect in these cases. In a number of instances the cardiac condition did not seem to be severe enough to account for early death. Death was sudden and unexplained, even after necropsy data were available. Compared with trisomy 13-15 and trisomy 21, this condition appears to carry a poor prognosis. Of the series reported by Smith *et al.* (1962), only one survived the age of 6 months, ultimately succumbing at 16 months; this is the longest lived case so far recorded, excluding mosaic forms. Smith (1963) comments that the failure to thrive and death seem to be due to a summation of anomalies, rather than to any specific one.

In 5 cases chromatography of the urine was performed, and no abnormality was found. Electrolyte, calcium, and phosphorus estimations were normal in 9 cases on which they were performed. No specific biochemical abnormality has yet been found in this condition. Case 2 had a transient glucose tolerance of diabetic type, but was the only case tested.

### Cytogenetic Findings

Preparations of chromosomes were obtained by using cultures of leucocytes from peripheral blood and tissue cultures of skin fibroblasts. The methods were based on those of Moorhead, Nowell, Mellman, Battips, and Hungerford (1960), of Tjio and Puck (1958), Rothfels and Siminovitch (1958), and Harnden (1960), but with some important modifications which are the subject of a separate publication.

The results of chromosome studies are summarized in Table 4. The chromosome count in all cases was consistently 47 in the tissues sampled, all cells with a count less than the modal number being broken during preparation. Most of the cells with 46 chromosomes contained 7 in Group E. Those cells from skin cultures with a count greater than 48 were tetraploid with 94 chromosomes. Other excess counts were due to chromosome breakage.

At least 6 complete karyotypes were prepared for each tissue, the Group E chromosomes identified in photographs of the remainder, and arranged in order. Despite the variation in the degrees of contraction between homologous chromosomes, which is sometimes encountered and which can be quite marked in Group E, especially in the case of No. 16, the majority could be matched satisfactorily so that a trisomic condition for No. 18 resulted. Measurements on photographs magnified to $\times$ 8,000 were made as a standard procedure to check the visual arrangement. Because of the variations referred to above, they could not be arranged in order by reference to over-all length. There is considerable overlap in the range of relative lengths in normal karyotypes as shown in Table 5. These figures have been derived from a study of a series of 50 normal karyotypes, mostly from clinically normal subjects, and the results compare with the lower limits of those published in Table 2 of the Denver Report (1960), being closely similar to those of Fraccaro and Lindsten (1960) and Buckton, Jacobs, and Harnden (1960).

It has been found much more reliable to consider both the relative length of the short arms (i.e. the centromeric index), and the arm ratio. Chromosome 16, having the longest short arms, has a greater centromeric index and smaller arm ratio than chromosome 18 which has the shortest short arms of the Group. Using these criteria, a consistent pattern has emerged and all patients with one exception showed a regular trisomy for 18. Occasional cells in some patients could be interpreted, both visually and by measurement, as trisomy 17, while other cells contained an extra chromosome which could not be matched accurately. In assessing their probable identity, the average of several cells is taken into consideration.

Case 9, however, could not be interpreted as a straightforward trisomy 18. The measurements of

TABLE 4
CASES WITH A DIAGNOSIS OF TRISOMY 18

| Case No. | Culture | Chromosome Count | | | | | No. of Karyotypes Analysed |
|---|---|---|---|---|---|---|---|
| | | $\leqslant 45$ | 46 | 47 | 48 | $> 48$ | |
| 1 | Blood | 5 | 2 | 44 | — | — | 23 |
| | Skin | 1 | 5 | 53 | — | 1 | 32 |
| 2 | Blood | 1 | 1 | 46 | — | — | 15 |
| 3 | Blood | 2 | 1 | 33 | 1 | — | 14 |
| 4 | Skin | 2 | 1 | 35 | — | 1 | 15 |
| 5 | Blood | 1 | 3 | 21 | — | 1 | 8 |
| 6 | Skin | 1 | 2 | 44 | — | 1 | 22 |
| 7 | Skin | — | 3 | 21 | — | — | 6 |
| 8 | Blood | 5 | 3 | 51 | — | — | 34 |
| | Skin | 1 | 2 | 30 | — | — | 15 |
| 9* | Blood | 6 | 3 | 52 | — | — | 26 |
| 10 | Blood | 3 | 2 | 56 | — | — | 26 |
| | Skin | 1 | 2 | 47 | — | 1 | 21 |
| 11 | Blood | 1 | 2 | 51 | — | — | 18 |
| 12 | Blood | 1 | 2 | 45 | 2 | — | 20 |
| | Skin | 3 | 1 | 54 | — | — | 34 |
| 13 | Blood | 1 | 1 | 54 | — | — | 23 |
| | Skin | 1 | 1 | 50 | — | — | 26 |

* In this case there was partial duplication of long arms of the additional chromosome.

TABLE 5
MEASUREMENT OF GROUP E CHROMOSOMES

| | Normal Karyotype Measurements (50 cells) | | | Karyotype Measurements of Case 9 (26 cells) | | | |
|---|---|---|---|---|---|---|---|
| Chromosome number | 16 | 17 | 18 | 16 | 17 | 18 | Extra Chromosome |
| Relative length .. .. | 33 (± 4) | 30 (± 4·5) | 29 (± 5·5) | 31 (± 4) | 29·0 (± 4) | 26 (± 5) | 30 (± 5·5) |
| Arm ratio .. .. .. | 1·3 (± 0·3) | 1·7 (± 0·4) | 2·2 (± 0·4) | 1·4 (± 0·2) | 1·9 (± 0·4) | 2·3 (± 0·5) | 2·8 (± 0·7) |
| Centromeric index .. | 43 (± 6) | 37 (± 5) | 31 (± 8) | 41·0 (± 3) | 34 (± 6) | 30 (± 5) | 26 (± 5) |

*Note:* Most values were, in fact, close to the mean, and when a value for one particular chromosome was at the extreme end of the range, then other chromosomes in the group had a value at the same extreme, depending on the relative degree of contraction. The mean figures, therefore, represent a true guide as to the relationship of one chromosome to another, and thus statistically the extra chromosome in Case 9 is significantly different from both '17' and '18'.

Group E chromosomes from 26 cells from Case 9 are shown in Table 5, and their appearance in Fig. 11. The relative length of the extra chromosome was similar to that of No. 16 but with significantly different arm ratio and centromeric index values, the long arm length exceeding that of both 17 and 18. It is possible that in this case the long arm of the extra chromosome contains extra chromatin which could be of homologous or non-homologous origin. The anomaly might exist in one of the parents or could have arisen during gametogenesis and could be a factor in non-disjunction. Muldal (1961) has suggested an explanation for the origins of apparent trisomy 17 and of deletion of 18, by considering a duplication of the short arms of a No. 18. He further suggests that this would explain how, at that time, trisomy for 17 and 18 had been reported with equal frequency. From this series, however, there has been no indication that half of the patients could be interpreted as trisomy 17. In fact, since 1961, most reported cases have been interpreted as either trisomy 18 or, less dogmatically, trisomy 17-18 pointing to the fact that duplications are of rare occurrence. Recent autoradiographic studies (Yunis, Hook, and Mayer, 1964) have pinpointed 18 as a late DNA-replicating chromosome compared with 17 which replicates early. This behaviour pattern is a valuable one, but the distinction between the two still hinges on morphological differences.

## Comment

Clinical recognition of the syndrome is not difficult. There appears to be a gradation of facial

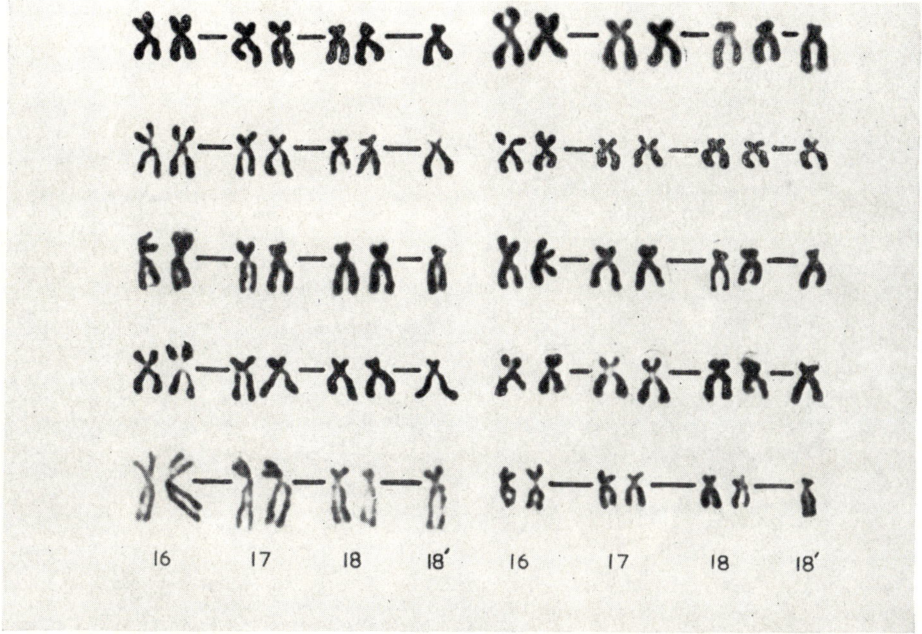


FIG. 11.—Case 9. Group E from 10 cells showing the abnormal additional chromosome 18. (Approximately × 2,500.)

types with those at each end of the range being quite distinct. At one extreme the facies is unmistakable with the 'Grecian' nose, round face, and extreme narrowing of the palpebral fissures (Fig. 1a). At the other end there is a well-developed nasal bridge, with an upturned nose and only slight narrowing of the palpebral fissures, giving rise to a rather elfin appearance (Fig. 1b). None of the cases of this type (Cases 6, 7, and 10) had microcephaly, and 2 of them were the largest infants in the series. Good examples of this type are seen in the series of Smith *et al.* (1962, Fig. 3) and the paper of German *et al.* (1962, Fig. 1). There was no specific combination of anomalies that correlated with either facial type.

The aural and facial abnormalities have many features of the first arch syndrome (McKenzie, 1958), and it is possible that insufficiency of the blood supply between the third and fifth weeks of intrauterine life may be responsible. McKenzie (1958) states that during this phase, following the disappearance of the first aortic arch, the first visceral arch depends on only the stapedial artery, and the developing external carotid artery. If this delicate balance is disturbed then the typical spectrum of cranio-facial anomalies of the syndrome will occur.

As can be seen from Table 1, the clinically obvious anomalies occur in the limbs and cranio-facial areas. Limb anomalies are progressively more frequent from the proximal to distal direction. A combination of the above anomalies should raise the suspicion of trisomy E as a clinical diagnosis.

The chromosome studies produced a consistent pattern despite variation in the clinical appearance.

## Summary

The clinical features of 13 cases of 'E' trisomy are presented, and the pattern of anomalies is discussed. Consideration of the facies together with the other anomalies permits a reasonably accurate clinical diagnosis.

The major necropsy findings are presented and analysed. The most consistent anomaly on internal examination was wide patency of the ductus arteriosus, usually associated with a high ventricular septal defect. In two cases there was intimal proliferation of small pulmonary arteries.

No specific antenatal factor could be held responsible in any case. Dysmaturity was common, and associated with small placental size.

Apparent hypersensitivity to the standard dose of digoxin was encountered in two cases, with resulting atrioventricular heart block.

The only biochemical abnormality discovered was that of a transient glucose intolerance, with glycosuria, in one case.

Morphologically the extra chromosome is considered to be No. 18 in all cases but one. The exception shows an extra chromosome with increased length of the long arms.

This investigation required the co-operation and encouragement of many individuals. We wish to thank the following physicians for permission to publish clinical details of cases under their care:
Dr. I. M. Anderson (Cases 10 and 13), Dr. R. J. K. Brown (Cases 1, 4, and 11), Dr. R. H. Dobbs (Cases 7 and 12), Dr. C. G. Fagg (Case 6), Dr. N. F. O'Reilly (Case 8), and Dr. M. J. Wilmers (Cases 3 and 9).

We are grateful to the following pathologists for allowing us to examine specimens from their cases and to quote their necropsy findings:
Dr. B. S. Cardell (Case 3), Dr. I. M. P. Dawson (Case 13), Dr. A. Gibson (Case 9), and Dr. T. E. W. Goodier (Case 8).

We are further indebted to Dr. L. Crome for his report of the brain of Case 4, Dr. J. D. A. Delhanty for chromosome studies of Case 7, Dr. W. J. Harrison for his opinion of the arterial changes in Cases 2 and 7, Dr. C. J. Hodson for the radiological studies, Dr. B. Levin for various biochemical investigations, and Professor L. S. Penrose for the dermatoglyphic studies of Cases 10 and 12.

## References

Buckton, K. E., Jacobs, P. A., and Harnden, D. G. (1960). In Denver Report.

Denver Report (1960). A proposed standard system of nomenclature of human mitotic chromosomes. *Cerebr. Palsy Bull.*, **2**, Suppl., and *Lancet*, **1**, 1063.

Edwards, J. H., Harnden, D. G., Cameron, A. H., Crosse, V. M., and Wolff, O. H. (1960). A new trisomic syndrome. *Lancet*, **1**, 787.

Ferguson-Smith, M. A. (1962). Abnormal sex ratio in the autosomal trisomy syndromes. *ibid.*, **2**, 357.

Finley, W. H., Finley, S. C., and Carte, E. T. (1963). 17-18 trisomy syndrome. Review and report of a case. *Amer. J. Dis. Child.*, **106**, 591.

Fraccaro, M., and Lindsten, J. (1960). In Denver Report.

German, J. L., III, Rankin, J. K., Harrison, P. A., Donovan, D. J., Hogan, W. J., and Bearn, A. G. (1962). Autosomal trisomy of a group 16-18 chromosome. *J. Pediat.*, **60**, 503.

Gottlieb, M. I., Hirschhorn, K., Cooper, H. L., Lusskin, N., Moloshok, R. E., and Hodes, H. L. (1962). Trisomy-17 syndrome: report of three cases and review of the literature. *Amer. J. Med.*, **33**, 763.

Harnden, D. G. (1960). A human skin culture technique used for cytological examinations. *Brit. J. exp. Path.*, **41**, 31.

Hecht, F., Bryant, J. S., Motulsky, A. G., and Giblett, E. R. (1963). The No. 17-18 (E) trisomy syndrome. *J. Pediat.*, **63**, 605.

Holman, G. H., Erkman, B., Zacharias, D. L., and Kock, H. F. (1963). The 18 trisomy syndrome—two new clinical variants. *New Engl. J. Med.*, **268**, 982.

McKenzie, J. (1958). The first arch syndrome. *Arch. Dis. Childh.*, **33**, 477.

Moorhead, P. S., Nowell, P. C., Mellman, W. J., Battips, D. M., and Hungerford, D. A. (1960). Chromosome preparations of leukocytes cultured from human peripheral blood. *Exp. Cell Res.*, **20**, 613.

Muldal, S. (1961). Trisomy and group V. *Lancet*, **2**, 879.

Penrose, L. S. (1961). Mongolism. *Brit. med. Bull.*, **17**, 184.

Rothfels, K. H., and Siminovitch, L. (1958). An air-drying technique for flattening chromosomes in mammalian cells grown *in vitro*. *Stain Technol.*, **33**, 73.

Rubin, E., and Strauss, L. (1961). Occlusive intrapulmonary vascular anomaly in the newborn. A cause of congenital pulmonary hypertension. *Amer. J. Path.*, **39**, 145.

Sinclair, L. (1963). Some recent congenital anomalies. *Broadway*, **R.19**, Clin. Suppl., **6**, 39.

Smith, D. W. (1963). The No. 18 trisomy and $D_1$ trisomy syndromes. *Pediat. Clin. N. Amer.*, **10**, 389.

——, Patau, K., Therman, E., and Inhorn, S. L. (1960). A new autosomal trisomy syndrome: multiple congenital anomalies caused by an extra chromosome. *J. Pediat.*, **57**, 338.

——, ——, ——, and —— (1962). The No. 18 trisomy syndrome. *ibid.*, **60**, 513.

Tjio, J. H., and Puck, T. T. (1958). The somatic chromosomes of man. *Proc. nat. Acad. Sci. (Wash.)*, **44**, 1229.

Townes, P. L., Manning, J. A., and DeHart, G. K., Jr. (1962). Trisomy 18 (16-18) associated with congenital glaucoma and optic atrophy. *J. Pediat.*, **61**, 755.

Uchida, I. A., and Soltan, H. C. (1963). Evaluation of dermatoglyphics in medical genetics. *Pediat. Clin. N. Amer.*, **10**, 409.

Voorhess, M. L., Vaharu, T., and Gardner, L. I. (1962). Trisomy 16-18 syndrome. *Lancet*, **2**, 992.

Weiss, L., Di George, A. M., and Baird, H. W., III (1962). Four infants with the trisomy 18 syndrome and one with trisomy 18 mosaicism. *Amer. J. Dis. Child.*, **104**, 533.

Yunis, J. J., Hook, E. B., and Mayer, M. (1964). Deoxyribosenucleic-acid replication pattern of trisomy 18. *Lancet*, **2**, 286.

*Arch. Dis. Childh.*, 1965, **40**, 612.

# ELECTROENCEPHALOGRAPHIC STUDIES IN INFANTS AND CHILDREN WITH HYPOTHYROIDISM

BY

R. HARRIS, M. DELLA ROVERE,* and P. F. PRIOR†

*From the Department of Electroencephalography and Clinical Neurophysiology, The Hospital for Sick Children, London*

(RECEIVED FOR PUBLICATION MARCH 8, 1965)

Congenital hypothyroidism, or cretinism, is a condition believed to be present at birth or possibly prenatally, and due to absence, or a defect in the development, of the thyroid gland, or to a defect in hormone synthesis. Acquired hypothyroidism arises some time after birth and may be due to primary atrophy of the gland, operative removal, infection, auto-immune processes, or infiltrating conditions affecting the gland, or to deficiency of thyrotropic hormone as in diseases of the hypophysis cerebri. In infancy and childhood the manifestations of hypothyroidism consist of a general retardation of both growth and mental development in association with the physical stigmata affecting the face, tongue, larynx, skin, and umbilicus that have been described amongst others by Wilkins (1957). Confirmation may be given by the findings of a low basal metabolic rate and protein-bound iodine (PBI) and by the radiographic appearances of abnormalities of epiphysial development.

While it is well known that abnormalities in the electroencephalogram (EEG) may be seen in endocrine disorders (Rohmer, Wackenheim, and Kurtz, 1959; Faure, 1959), few studies of the EEG in hypothyroid children have been made (Avignon and Melin, 1949; Chaptal, Passouant, Jean, Cadilhac, and Carli, 1956; Passouant, Cadilhac, and Jean, 1956; Tangheroni and Pardelli, 1957; Nieman, 1961). These authors have reported, amongst other EEG features, sporadic slow activity and rather little or no alpha rhythm. A proportional relation has been described between the severity of the clinical signs of mental defect and the degree of EEG abnormality (Topper, 1951; Mai and Schaper, 1953). The EEG abnormality has been said to improve in relation to appropriate hormone replacement therapy, but not usually in those cases where there were focal EEG abnormalities (Passouant *et al.*, 1956). In these children the clinical signs of hypothyroidism would regress, but not the coexisting neurological signs.

The present study is based on a group of 34 children suffering from hypothyroidism, who were referred by their physicians for EEG examination either as part of the routine investigation of mental defect or because of a neurological disorder unrelated to the endocrine condition. In some cases EEG examinations were made particularly for the study of the relation between thyroid function and changes in cerebral electrical activity. In all patients the clinical diagnosis was confirmed by metabolic investigations and all the patients required maintenance therapy with thyroid hormone.

## Material and Methods

A total of 63 EEGs was obtained from the 34 children, 15 having had two or more records at variable time intervals. Of the patients, 15 were very young children under 18 months of age (Table 1). Almost one-third of the children had, in addition to the hypothyroidism, some associated clinical condition which might have altered the EEG in some way (Table 2). It was not possible to make systematic EEG studies in relation to the effects of administration of thyroid hormone, as some children were only seen as part of the preliminary investigations, while others were only referred after receiving some treatment. The patients were under the care of various physicians and were treated according to individual plans.

TABLE 1
AGES AT TIME OF THE FIRST EEG

| Age range | 2-5 mth. | 9-18 mth. | 2-3 yr. | 3-4 yr. | 6-14 yr. |
|---|---|---|---|---|---|
| No. of cases . . | 8 | 7 | 5 | 2 | 12 |

* Present address: Ospedale Psichiatrico Provinciale Santa Maria della Pieta, Rome.

† Present address: The E.E.G. Department, The London Hospital, E.1.

TABLE 2

HYPOTHYROIDISM AND ASSOCIATED CONDITIONS (10 CASES)

| Case No. | Condition |
|---|---|
| 8 | Epilepsy, pyridoxine deficiency, and cerebral atrophy |
| 12 | Webbing of the neck (but no other stigmata of Turner's syndrome) |
| 19 | Renal insufficiency |
| 16 | Fractured skull |
| 9 | Congenital syphilis, encephalitis, progressive cerebral degeneration |
| 3 | Severe headaches described as 'migraine' |
| 32 | Epilepsy |
| 29 | Cerebral atrophy involving the left more than right hemisphere |
| 18 | Epilepsy |
| 2 | Tuberculous meningitis and epilepsy |

15 children had their first EEG before any drugs were given and 6 of these were followed up in relation to the effects of thyroid treatment. 3 other cases were studied only in relation to test doses of tri-iodothyronine and will be considered separately. 16 were seen only at various time intervals after treatment had begun.

A standardized technique of electrode placement was used (Pampiglione, 1956) with silver, silver-chlorided cup electrodes held in position on the scalp with collodion. The majority of the records were taken on Type D or Type T Offner Electroencephalographs, the remaining few being taken on Ediswan apparatus.

The appearances of the EEGs were then evaluated in relation to the child's age, therapy, and the presence of any condition coexisting with the hypothyroidism; variations in frequency and amplitude of the cerebral activity were examined in relation to what we would have considered appropriate to the child's years and the state of wakefulness or sleep at the time of recording.

**Definition of Terms.** The activity was defined as being of small amplitude when no waves of more than $50\mu V$ occurred and when the greater part of the activity was of less than $25\mu V$ in amplitude. The relative amounts of various frequencies present were assessed visually and in particular the presence of an excess of slow wave activity was noted. In view of the maturational changes that occur in the EEG in the first decade of life, it is not possible to define concisely what we have considered to be an excess of slow wave activity, but in general terms it should be noted that both the slow ($< 3\frac{1}{2}$ c/s) and the intermediate slow (4-7 c/s) frequency bands were separately evaluated in most cases.

## Results

**EEGs Before Treatment.** The main features of the EEGs taken from 15 children before treatment are summarized in Tables 3 and 4. An excess of slow activity was found in 12 and the traces were also of small amplitude in 5 children. Small amplitude activity was mainly seen in the younger children.

Sharp waves or discharges were seen in 3 children. In one, a child of 7 years (Case 4, Table 3), sharp waves were present over both temporo-occipital regions, and there was an asymmetry in the distribution of the excessive slow wave activity posteriorly. Only 1 (Case 8, Table 4) of the 3 children whose preliminary EEGs showed abnormal discharges had other complicating factors in addition to the hypothyroidism. He had epilepsy, and on investigation a cerebral atrophy was found; in addition the child was said to have pyridoxine deficiency.

Thus in untreated cases an excess of slow wave activity was often present, especially in those children who were over 2 years of age, while the younger children tended to show small amplitude records. Abnormal discharges were seen infrequently and were associated with a history of epilepsy in one.

**EEGs Before and After a Test Dose of Tri-iodothyronine.** The hormone tri-iodothyronine has a very rapid action when compared with thyroxine and can produce clinical improvement in a hypothyroid subject soon after administration. This property of tri-iodothyronine has led to its use in a clinical test designed to judge the potential efficiency of thyroid treatment in particular cases. EEGs were recorded during these tests to see if changes appeared parallel with the clinical improvement. A test dose (5 $\mu$g.) of

TABLE 3

EEG FEATURES OF CASES WITH RECORDS TAKEN ONLY BEFORE THYROID TREATMENT (9 CASES)

| Case No. | Age (yr.) | Slow Activity | Small Amplitude | Fast Activity | Discharges | Comment |
|---|---|---|---|---|---|---|
| 34 | 2/12 | + | + | – | – | |
| 24 | 3/12 | – | + | – | – | |
| 15 | 1 2/12 | + | – | – | – | Drowsy during test |
| 5 | 1 | + | + | – | – | |
| 14 | 2 | – | – | – | – | Slight asymmetry posteriorly |
| 7 | 2 3/12 | + | – | + | – | Sleep record after quinalbarbitone |
| 7 | 2 6/12 | + | + | + | – | Sleep record after quinalbarbitone |
| 4 | 7 | + | – | – | Sharp waves | |
| 13 | 8 | – | – | – | Sharp waves | |
| 13 | 8 | + | – | – | – | |
| 2 | 11 | + | – | – | – | Previous tuberculous meningitis and epilepsy |

TABLE 4

EEG FEATURES IN CASES WITH RECORDS TAKEN BEFORE AND AFTER TREATMENT (6 CASES)

| Case No. | Before Treatment | | | | | After Treatment | | | | | Comment |
|---|---|---|---|---|---|---|---|---|---|---|---|
| | Age (yr.) | Slow Activity | Small Amplitude | Fast Activity | Discharges | Age (yr.) | Slow Activity | Small Amplitude | Fast Activity | Discharges | |
| 17 | 2/12 | – | + | – | – | 2 11/12 | – | – | – | – | Thyroid gr. 1 daily for 2 years |
| 25 | 3/12 | + | + | – | – | 4/12 | – | – | – | – | Rhythmic activity present at 4 months; thyroid gr. 1 daily for 3 wk. EEG improved |
| 26 | 3 10/12 | + | + | – | – | 3 11/12 | + | – | – | Sharp waves | Thryroid gr. ¼ daily for 1 mth. |
| | | | | | | 4 | + | – | + | – | Thyroid gr. 1 daily for 1 mth.; EEG improved less slow activity present |
| 8 | 8 10/12 | + | – | + | + | 9 | + | – | + | + | 3 similar records before treatment and 2 after thyroxine; 6 mg. daily without change 2 mth. later; epilepsy, cerebral atrophy, and pyridoxine deficiency |
| 11 | 10 | + | – | – | – | 10 | + | – | – | + | Thyroid gr. 1 daily for 2 days |
| 9 | 13 | – | Anterior | – | – | 13 4/12 | + | – | – | + | Tri-iodothyronine trial, then maintained on thyroid gr. 3 daily; congenital syphilis, previous encephalitis, progressive cerebral degeneration |
| | | | | | | 14 | + | – | – | – | |

tri-iodothyronine was given to 3 of the patients in this series. The first two were sisters aged 18 months and 2 months whose preliminary EEGs had shown rather small amplitude activity. Five further records were taken from each child during the 24 hours after the test dose of tri-iodothyronine and, apart from some fluctuations in relation to drowsiness and sleep, these did not show any significant change, though clinically both children were obviously brighter and the older child appeared more playful. The third child aged 2 years and 2 months, whose preliminary record had shown an excess of slow activity, showed no change in the EEG appearances 5 hours after the test dose of tri-iodothyronine, though there was a similarly good clinical response.

**EEGs Taken Before and After Treatment with Thyroid Hormone.** Replacement therapy with thyroid hormone or in some cases thyroxine was given in all the children studied and in 6 instances serial recordings were taken before and after treatment. The findings are summarized in Table 4. In 2 of them (Cases 25 and 26 in Table 4, see also Fig.) there was an improvement in the EEG appearances. In one (Case 17, Table 4) there was probably improvement: however, only two records were obtained, and these were separated by a time interval that made comparison difficult in a young child. Another (Case 11, Table 4) had an EEG taken only two days after beginning therapy. It showed no change when compared with the preliminary tracing, both showing an excess of slow wave activity. The remaining 2 children (Case 8 and 9, Table 4) showed no improvement in serial EEGs in relation to thyroid administration: both presented a complex clinical picture and treatment began comparatively late. Case 8, who has been mentioned previously with regard to the many abnormal electroencephalographic features, was known to have pyridoxine deficiency, cerebral atrophy, and epilepsy; 5 records over a period of 4 months all showed a similar pattern and degree of abnormality. Case 9 showed deterioration in the EEG over a period of 8 months after beginning thyroid treatment, but this was most probably due to the progressive cerebral degeneration which was present. Thus, it is apparent that in children with uncomplicated hypothyroidism who are treated with thyroid or thyroxine it may be some time before any improvement in the EEG features occurs.

**EEGs Taken Only After Treatment.** 16 children had an EEG taken after thyroid replacement therapy had begun, there being no previous records available for comparison. The main features of these records and details of therapy are given in Table 5. Four cases (Cases 28, 33, 10, and 20, Table 5) had only been treated for one week or less when the EEG was recorded, and an excess of slow wave activity was present in the records of three of them. Abnormal features were not usually present in children who had been treated for more than a few weeks, unless there was evidence of some associated cerebral lesion. One child of 13 (Case 32, Table 5) in this group who suffered from epilepsy showed both an excess of slow wave activity and abnormal discharges in the EEG.

TABLE 5

EEG FEATURES OF CASES WITH RECORDS TAKEN ONLY AFTER THYROID TREATMENT (16 CASES)

| Case No. | Age (yr.) | Slow Activity | Small Amplitude | Fast Activity | Discharges | Comment |
|---|---|---|---|---|---|---|
| 30 | 3/12 | – | – | – | – | On ½ gr. thyroid daily for 2 wk. |
| 28 | 3/12 | – | – | – | – | On ¼ gr. thyroid daily for 1 wk. |
| 33 | 4/12 | + | – | – | – | On thyroid for 2 days |
| | 5/12 | – | – | – | – | Thyroid for 1 mth. |
| 18 | 9/12 | – | – | – | – | Thyroid 1 gr. daily for 3½ mth. |
| 19 | 1 | – | – | | – | Thyroid 2½ gr. daily for 5 mth.; renal insufficiency |
| 6 | 1 1/12 | – | – | – | – | Thyroxine for 9 mth. |
| 29 | 1 5/12 | – | – | – | – | Thyroid gr. 2 daily for 6 mth.; cerebral atrophy |
| 21 | 2 | – | – | – | – | Thyroid 1½ gr. daily for 1 7/12 yr. |
| 27 | 2 2/12 and 2 9/12 | – | – | – | – | Thyroid 1½ gr. daily from 2 mth. |
| 10 | 4 6/12 | + | + | – | – | Thyroid ¾ gr. for 3 days; more rhythmic |
| | 4 6/12 | + | – | – | – | activity after 15 days of treatment |
| 3 | 6 | + | – | – | – | Treated for 3 yr.: thyroid 1½ gr. and |
| | 8 | + | – | – | – | 25 µg. tri-iodothyronine alternate days; no change 2 yr. later; severe headaches |
| 20 | 8 | + | – | – | – | Thyroid gr. ½ daily for 2 days |
| 12 | 9 | – | + | – | – | Thyroid gr. 1 daily for 6 yr.; webbed neck |
| 16 | 12 | – | – | – | – | Thyroid gr. 1 daily from 4 mth.; previous skull fracture; some asymmetry in EEG |
| 22 | 12 | – | – | – | – | Thyroid gr. ¼ daily since 6 yr. |
| 32 | 13 | + | – | – | + | On thyroid; no details of duration; epilepsy |

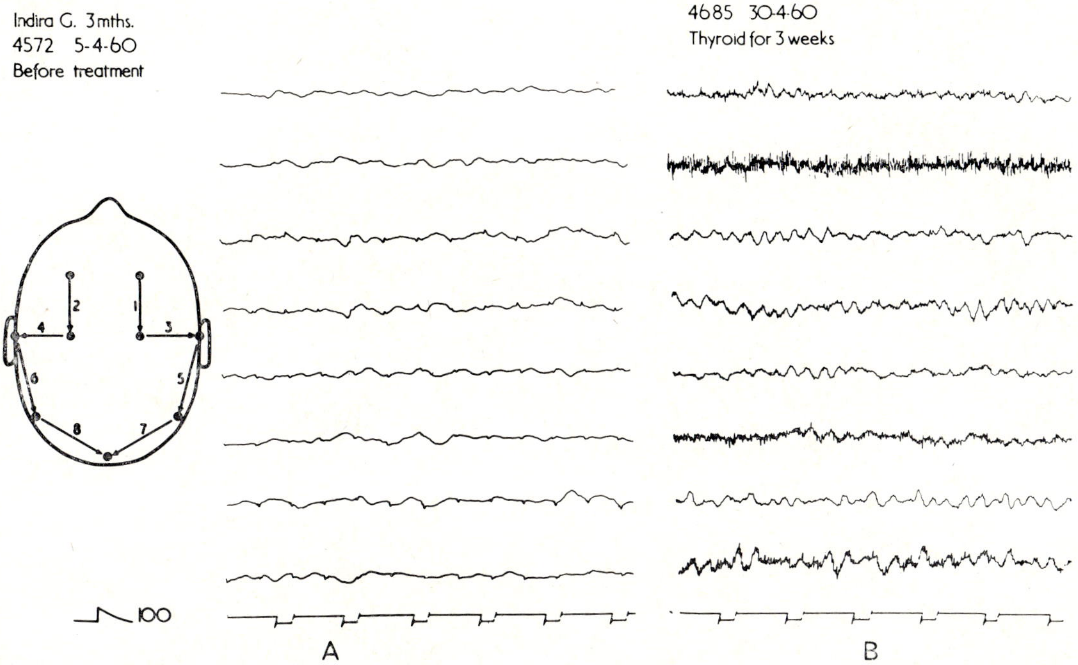


FIG.—Electroencephalogram of Case 25, a cretin. A. At 3 months, taken immediately before treatment began, showing irregular slow activity of small amplitude over all regions. The electrode placement and calibration signal are shown in the diagram. B. The same baby after 3 weeks' treatment with thyroid hormone, showing an increase in the frequency amplitude and rhythmicity of the activity. The baby lay quietly and was awake on both occasions.

## Discussion

Although the group of children studied is not large nor particularly uniform as regards age or stage of treatment, we had the opportunity to examine a relatively high proportion of untreated infants and to carry out serial recordings on many occasions. Some general trends are apparent from the results presented, which are of interest clinically, particularly in view of the recent experimental work on the abnormalities of development of cerebral activity in thyroid deficiency (Bradley, Eayrs, and Schmalbach, 1960).

The older children suffering from hypothyroidism in this series have tended to show an excess of slow components in their EEG. We have less often seen this feature in the EEG of babies of a few months of age before treatment; in this age-group the activity is more likely to be of small amplitude. This feature is difficult to evaluate as there may sometimes be little activity present in the EEG of a restless wakeful baby, and it was not always possible to obtain records during sleep. However, the activity found in these babies was of smaller amplitude than is usual in our experience of other babies of comparable age. No change was seen in the EEG features immediately after a test dose of tri-iodothyronine or where treatment had only been given for a few days. Improvement was seen after a few weeks or months of thyroid hormone therapy and some of the abnormal EEG features still present in older children treated for a long time were often probably due to some associated cerebral lesion.

These findings should be considered in the light of the experimental work done by Faure (1959) and by Eayrs and Taylor (1951), Eayrs (1955, 1960), and Bradley *et al.* (1960). Faure showed the changes of cerebral activity in relation to various hormones. Eayrs and Bradley and their co-workers showed that ablation of the thyroid gland in newborn rats caused histological cerebral changes only after a period of time. The neurones appear to be immature for the chronological age, and at the same stage small amplitude activity was seen in the EEG. If the ablation was done at a later stage of development, however, the neuronal and EEG changes were less marked. If the results of this animal work can be applied to man, it should follow that the EEG changes would be more marked in cases of congenital or early acquired hypothyroidism than in cases arising in older age-groups where the nervous system is mature. It has been shown by Lansing and Trunnell (1963) that in adults with acquired hypothyroidism the EEG changes are not very great and that they are reversible. The alpha rhythm, which tended to be relatively slow before treatment, increased in frequency when thyroid hormone was given; however, the EEG would return to the original state if the hormone was withdrawn. It is likely, therefore, that these changes seen in adult patients were due to metabolic rather than structural changes in the central nervous system. In the present study, the patients were children in whom, as shown by Bradley *et al.* (1960) in the rat, the effect of thyroid hormone deprivation is greater on the immature brain than on the mature brain from both the EEG and the histological aspects. Improvement in the EEG occurred when thyroid had been given for more than a few days in the younger patients. No EEG change, however, was seen in response to a test dose of tri-iodothyronine or in older children who had been successfully treated with thyroid. This might indicate that the time taken for the EEG to improve in response to thyroid replacement therapy in the immature human brain may also depend on structural as well as metabolic changes in the central nervous system. It is unlikely that sufficient histopathological studies combined with EEG documentation could be obtained in children with hypothyroidism to elucidate the problem of subsequent cerebral maturation in relation to the duration of the hypothyroid state in the immature human brain. However, in the light of present knowledge, the experimental findings quoted might be considered to offer a reasonable explanation for the EEG changes in relation to age and treatment found in the children in this study.

## Summary

Studies were carried out on 63 EEGs taken from 34 hypothyroid children, aged 2 months to 14 years, in relation to age, therapy, and associated disorders. Most of the EEGs on the untreated cases showed an excessive amount of slow activity, though this feature was less prominent in young babies than in older children. Babies tended to have records of unusually low amplitude. No EEG changes occurred in relation to a test dose of tri-iodothyronine in 3 children, in spite of clinical response. With thyroid replacement therapy for more than a few days, uncomplicated cases usually showed a return to normal in the EEG. The implications of these findings are discussed in relation to the experimental findings in young rats deprived of thyroid hormone.

We should like to thank Dr. E. M. Creak, Dr. R. H. Dobbs, Dr. P. R. Evans, Dr. A. White Franklin, Dr. R. Lightwood, Professor Sir Alan A. Moncrieff, Dr. G. H. Newns, Dr. A. P. Norman, and Sir Wilfrid Sheldon who referred the children for EEG studies. We are grateful to Dr. G. Pampiglione for his help and advice in the preparation of this paper. One of us (M.D.R.) was holding a Fellowship of the World Health Organization.

REFERENCES

Avignon, M. d', and Melin, K. A. (1949). The electroencephalogram in congenital hypothyreosis. *Acta paediat. (Uppsala)*, **38**, 37.

Bradley, P. B., Eayrs, J. T., and Schmalbach, K. (1960). The electroencephalogram of normal and hypothyroid rats. *Electroenceph. clin. Neurophysiol.*, **12**, 467.

Chaptal, J., Passouant, P., Jean, R., Cadilhac, J., and Carli, N. (1956). La souffrance cérébrale dans le myxoedème de l'enfant; étude electro-encephalographique. *Presse méd.*, **64**, 2257.

Eayrs, J. T. (1955). The cerebral cortex of normal and hypothyroid rats. *Acta anat. (Basel)*, **25**, 160.

—— (1960). Influence of the thyroid on the central nervous system. *Brit. med. Bull.*, **16**, 122.

——, and Taylor, S. H. (1951). The effect of thyroid deficiency induced by methyl thiouracil on the maturation of the central nervous system. *J. Anat. (Lond.)*, **85**, 350.

Faure, J. (1959). Études expérimentales de l'influence des facteurs hormonaux et métaboliques sur l'activité électrique de cerveau. *Rev. neurol.*, **100**, 255.

Lansing, R. W., and Trunnell, J. B. (1963). Electroencephalographic changes accompanying thyroid deficiency in man. *J. clin. Endocr.*, **23**, 470.

Mai von H., and Schaper, G. (1953). Beitrag zur Klinik der Hypothyreose. Studie über die nach langdauernder Thyreodinbehandlung erreichte Intelligenz und über das Verhalten des Hirnstrombildes. *Ann. paediat. (Basel)*, **180**, 65.

Nieman, E. A. (1961). The electroencephalogram in congenital hypothyroidism: a study of 10 cases. *J. Neurol. Neurosurg. Psychiat.*, **24**, 50.

Pampiglione, G. (1956). Some anatomical considerations upon electrode placement in routine EEG. *Proc. Electrophysiological Technologists Ass.*, **7**, 80.

Passouant, P., Cadilhac, J., and Jean, R. (1956). Les anomalies EEG selon l'origine thyroïdienne ou cérébrale du myxoedème de l'enfant. *Rev. neurol.*, **95**, 569.

Rohmer, F., Wackenheim, A., and Kurtz, D. (1959). L'EEG dans les syndromes endocriniens, hypophysaires, thyroïdiens, surrénaux et dans la tétanie de l'adulte. *ibid.*, **100**, 297.

Tangheroni, W., and Pardelli, L. (1957). Rilievi comparativi fra sviluppo psichico e attività bioelettrica cerebrale nell'ipotiroidismo. *Minerva pediat.*, **9**, 1631.

Topper, A. (1951). Mental achievement of congenitally hypothyroid children; a follow-up study of 20 cases. *A.M.A. Amer. J. Dis. Child.*, **81**, 233.

Wilkins, L. (1957). *The Diagnosis and Treatment of Endocrine Disorders in Childhood and Adolescence*, 2nd ed., pp. 88-109. Blackwell, Oxford.

*Arch. Dis. Childh.*, 1965, **40**, 618.

# HYALINE MEMBRANE DISEASE: A PATHOLOGICAL STUDY OF 55 INFANTS

BY

J. M. LAUWERYNS

*From the Department of Pathology B, 12, Minderbroedersstraat, Leuven, Belgium*

(RECEIVED FOR PUBLICATION MARCH 9, 1965)

This study concerns the pathological changes found in the lungs of 55 newborn infants with hyaline membrane disease (HMD). The accepted appearances are a widespread resorption of air with collapse of many alveolar ducts and most alveoli, producing a severe atelectasis. The alveolar ducts and alveoli that remain open are distended and lined by a variable amount of homogeneous acidophilic material. There is intense vascular engorgement (Morison, 1952; Potter, 1953; Nesbitt, 1957).

Numerous hypotheses have been proposed to explain the formation of the hyaline membranes: these include the aspiration of amniotic fluid (Farber and Sweet, 1931; Farber and Wilson, 1933; Blystad, Landing, and Smith, 1951; MacGregor, 1953), defect in pulmonary circulation with plasma transudate (Rudolph, Auld, Drorbaugh, Rudolph, Nadas, and Smith, 1959; Neligan, 1959), and a disturbance of alveolar surface tension (Avery and Mead, 1959; Klaus, Reiss, Tooley, Piel, and Clements, 1962).

In this study an attempt has been made to determine the relation between the possible aetiological factors and the morphological findings. Particular attention has been paid to the degree of pulmonary maturation, the degree of pulmonary expansion or atelectasis, the extent of the hyaline membranes, the pulmonary lymphatics, the amount of aspirated amniotic fluid, the presence of alveolar oedema, the occurrence of pulmonary haemorrhages, and the relation of the hyaline membranes to the alveolar septa.

## Material and Methods

Studies were carried out on 55 babies with HMD, born in the University Maternity Unit of Louvain (Belgium) during the past 6 years, during which period there were 15,000 deliveries. The distribution of the cases related to foetal age is shown in Table 1.

The frequency of HMD was maximal (22·9%) in the group of foetal age 29-30 weeks.

Necropsy included systematic histology of the lungs, heart, liver, spleen, kidney, pancreas, adrenal, and thymus. Afterwards, each case was discussed at the weekly seminar on perinatal mortality, when the obstetric, paediatric, and pathological data were correlated.

The lungs were fixed in Bouin's fluid. To allow extensive study, blocks were taken covering the complete cut surface of a lobe. In 22 cases blocks were taken from each of the five lobes.

Lung sections were stained with haematoxylin and eosin, haematoxylin and eosin and saffranin, Masson's trichromic, Mayer's mucicarmine, PAS, Mallory's phosphotungstic acid-haematoxylin, Verhoeff-van Gieson elastica stain, and Bielschowsky's method as modified by Foot for the staining of the reticular fibres. These methods are described in the *Manual of Histologic and Special Staining Technics* (1957).

## Results

**Naked-eye Appearance.** The lungs had a dark-red, purplish colour. Their consistency was usually firm. On gentle manual palpation no crepitation could be felt. A 'hydrostatic lung test' was carried out on each lung and lobe in 25 cases. All the lobes sank in water in 17 cases; all the lobes floated in 2 cases; and in 7 cases parts only of the lungs floated.

**Histology.** *Pulmonary Maturation.* One can easily distinguish lung parenchyma that is either

TABLE 1

DISTRIBUTION OF 55 CASES OF HYALINE MEMBRANE DISEASE (HMD) RELATED TO FOETAL AGE

| Foetal Age (wk.) | Number of Live Births | Deaths from HMD* |
|---|---|---|
| 26 | 33 | 5 (15) |
| 26-28 | 42 | 5 (12) |
| 29-30 | 61 | 14 (23) |
| 31-32 | 91 | 13 (14) |
| 33-34 | 156 | 7 (4) |
| 35-36 | 250 | 5 (2) |
| 37-38 | 1,200 | 1 (0·8) |
| 39 + | 13,167 | 5 (0·4) |
| | 15,000 | 55 |

* Percentages are given in parentheses.

*bronchiolar* or immature, *canalicular* and *canaliculo-alveolar* or premature, and *aveolar* or mature. The pulmonary parenchyma of the 11 babies born before the 29th week of gestation showed a canalicular structure. Alveolar differentiation occurred in our series about the 29th to 30th week of gestation (Potter, 1953).

*Pulmonary Expansion.* The pulmonary parenchyma always showed the classical picture of secondary or resorption atelectasis, distended emphysematous alveolar ducts and alveoli alternating with extensive atelectatic areas. In large sections covering a whole lobe, areas with other varieties of disturbed pulmonary expansion were present. For example, localized areas of interstitial emphysema were seen in 7 cases: in each instance the baby's foetal age was more than 30 weeks.

*Hyaline Membranes.* The membranes stained red with haematoxylin and eosin, purple-brown with phosphotungstic acid haematoxylin, and varying shades of purple with a predominance of either red or blue, with Masson's aniline blue trichromic stain. The PAS stain yielded either a positive reaction (21 cases), a slightly positive reaction (22 cases), or a negative reaction (12 cases). The membranes are usually not stained positively with Mayer's mucicarmine, but a positive reaction was noted in 7 cases.

The hyaline membranes varied in extent, as described by Latham, Nesbitt, and Anderson (1955), who placed them in four grades according to their individual thickness and extent and their distribution in large lung sections. The membranes of the 55 cases have been classified according to the same criteria. It was found that the hyaline membranes were nearly always less extensive and less developed (grades 1 and 2) in the very premature group of less than 28 weeks, while the more developed and more extensive membranes (grades 3 and 4) were observed in more mature infants.

*Pulmonary Oedema.* A conspicuous, homogeneous or slightly granular fibrinous exudate was present in the alveoli and alveolar ducts. It was seen in nearly all cases (45), but with varying intensity: slight in 24 cases, moderate in 12 cases, severe and diffuse in 9 cases.

*Pulmonary Haemorrhage.* Pulmonary haemorrhages were common. They were usually localized, either in the alveoli (10 cases), in the alveoli and septa (7 cases), or in the alveoli, septa, and bronchi (10 cases).

*Aspirated Amniotic Material.* Numerous cells and debris of amniotic fluid origin were seen in the alveoli or alveolar ducts in only 7 cases. No correlation between the extent of this aspiration on the one hand and the degree of the hyaline membranes on the other could be established. Nor was there any relation between the degree of aspiration and the foetal age.

*Relationship of Hyaline Membranes to the Inter-alveolar Septum.* We have investigated the relation of the hyaline membranes to the walls of the alveoli and alveolar ducts, and in particular their relation to the reticular fibres. After silver impregnation, it was clearly seen that the hyaline membranes were directly apposed to the reticular fibres of the alveolar walls and alveolar ducts (Figs. 1, 2, 3, and 4). The membranes frequently contained necrotic cellular material (Figs. 1 and 5) which likewise appeared to rest directly upon the reticular fibres. To our knowledge this phenomenon has not been described previously; its possible significance is discussed below.

*Pulmonary Lymphatics.* Impregnation of the reticular fibres is also an established method for outlining the lymphatic vessels (Lauweryns, 1962, 1964). In most of the cases the lymphatic vessels were strikingly distended with fluid, sometimes appearing angiectatic and congested (Figs. 6, 7, 8, and 9). Their lumina contained eosinophilic material, which was sometimes granular and sometimes homogeneous fibrinous. These ectatic lymphatic vessels were observed at all sites, including the peribronchial, periarterial (Fig. 6), and perivenous (Fig. 7) and pleural (Figs. 8 and 9) lymphatics. Lymphatic angiectasis was most conspicuous in cases where the hyaline membranes were extensive (Table 2). This observation has, to our knowledge, not been recorded in the literature.

TABLE 2

LYMPHANGIECTASIS RELATED TO HYALINE MEMBRANES

| No. of Cases | Degree of Lymphangiectasis | Case Distribution According to Grade of HMD | |
|---|---|---|---|
| | | Grades 1-2 | Grades 3-4 |
| 28 | Severe | 12 | 16 |
| 15 | Moderate | 6 | 9 |
| 9 | Slight | 8 | 1 |

## Discussion

**Importance of Histological Examination.** This has to be emphasized once again, since the so-called hydrostatic lung test is still used in forensic medicine to determine whether a baby found dead has breathed or not, and as evidence in possible cases of

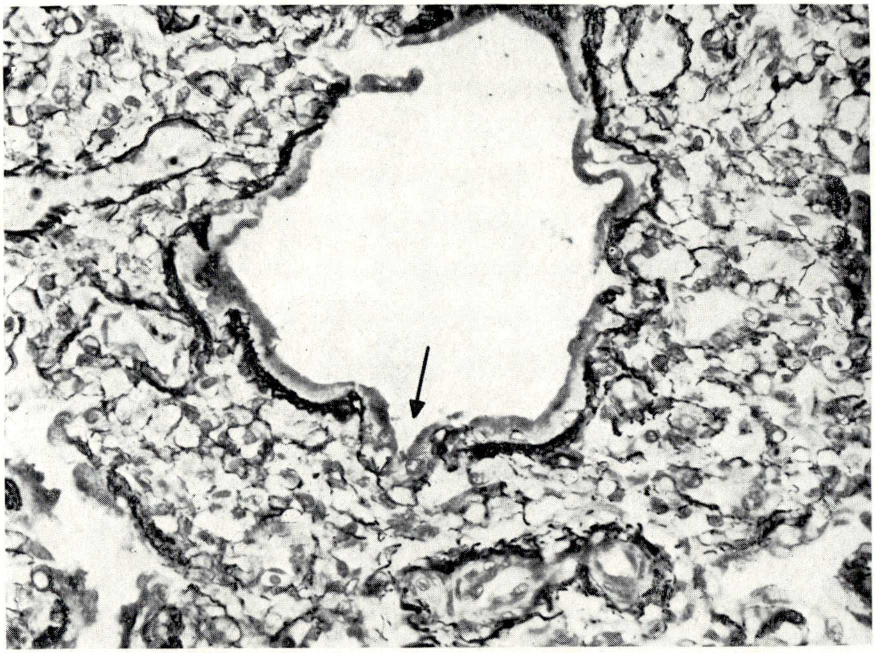

FIG. 1.—Hyaline membranes directly apposed to the reticular fibres; cellular material containing prominent nuclei enmeshed within the hyaline membranes themselves (marked with arrow). (Reticular fibres impregnated according to the method of Bielschowsky as modified by Foot; eosin counterstain. × 250.)

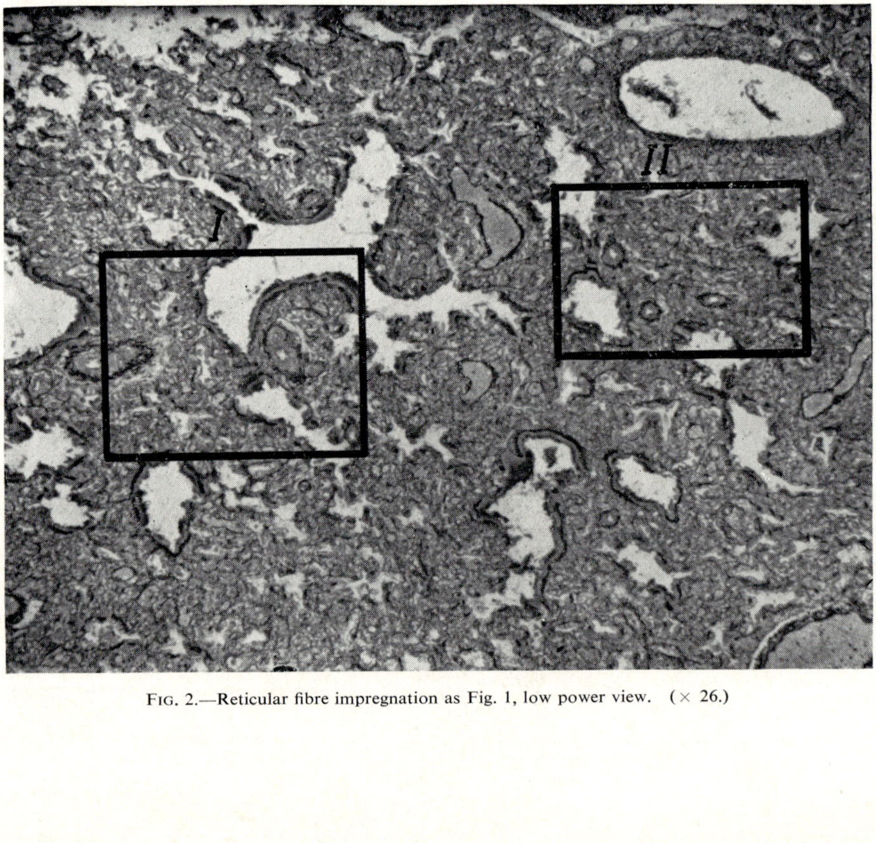


FIG. 2.—Reticular fibre impregnation as Fig. 1, low power view. (× 26.)

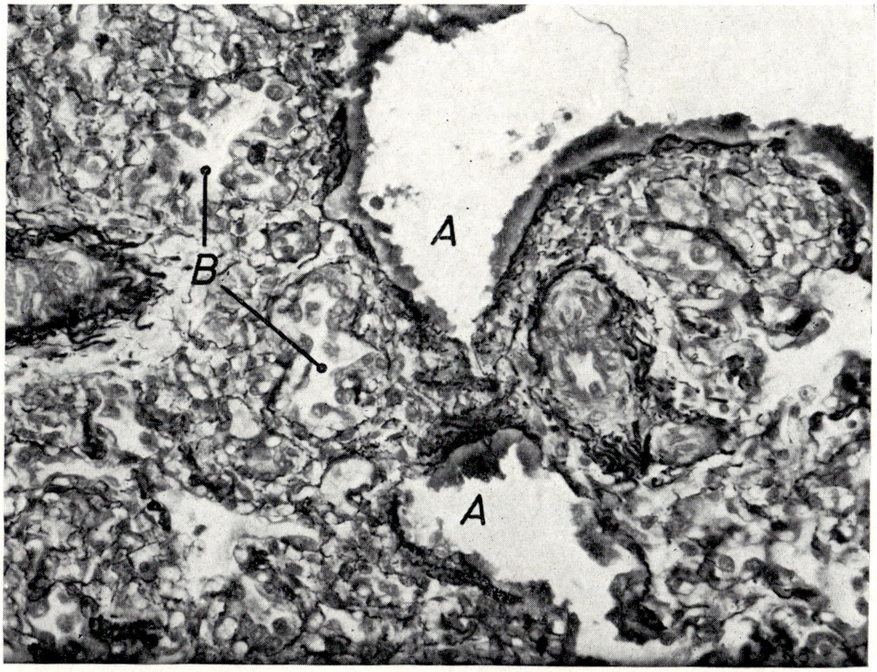


FIG. 3.—Magnified area I of Fig. 2; direct apposition (A) of hyaline membranes to the reticular fibres. Compare on the same field with the reticular fibre structure of normal alveoli (B) where the alveolar epithelial cells rest upon the reticular fibres. (Staining as Fig. 1. × 200.)

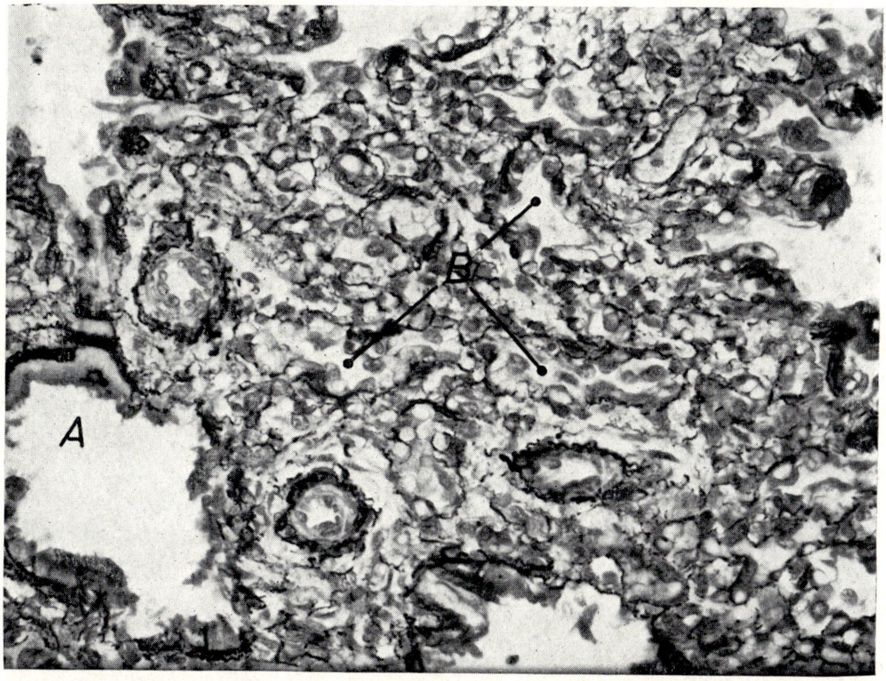


FIG. 4.—Magnified area II of Fig. 2. Compare the reticular fibre structure of an alveolar duct (A) lined by a hyaline membrane, with that of the normal (but collapsed) alveoli (B). (Staining as Fig. 1. × 200.)

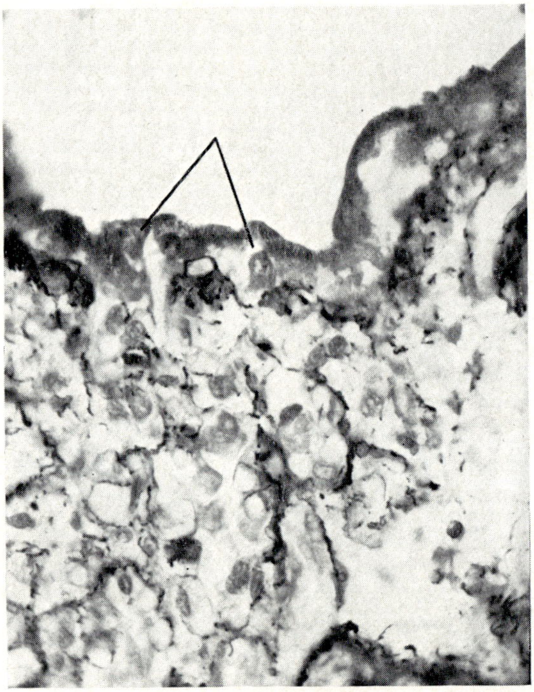

FIG. 5.—Nuclear material (marked with pointers) enmeshed within a hyaline membrane, apposed to the reticular fibres. (Staining as Fig. 1. × 314.)

infanticide. The complete fallibility of the test has been pointed out by others (Gonzales, Vance, Helpern, and Umberger, 1954; Fournier, 1957; Parmentier, 1962) and has been confirmed here.

**Pulmonary Expansion.** In addition to the so-called secondary or resorption atelectasis, localized areas of interstitial emphysema were observed in 7 cases. As this phenomenon was observed only in the more mature group (with a foetal age of more than 30 weeks), interstitial emphysema is perhaps partially due to the greater strength of respiratory movements in these babies as compared to the younger age-group (E. Eggermont, personal communication, 1964). (In 3 of the 7 cases showing interstitial emphysema it was known that positive-pressure resuscitation had been used, and in 3 it was known that it had not.)

**Pulmonary Oedema.** Though the intensity and distribution of pulmonary oedema varied in individual cases, its constant presence strongly favours some failure of the 'alveolocapillary barrier' in hyaline membrane disease. (This same phenomenon is also discussed in relation to the pulmonary lymphatics—see below.)

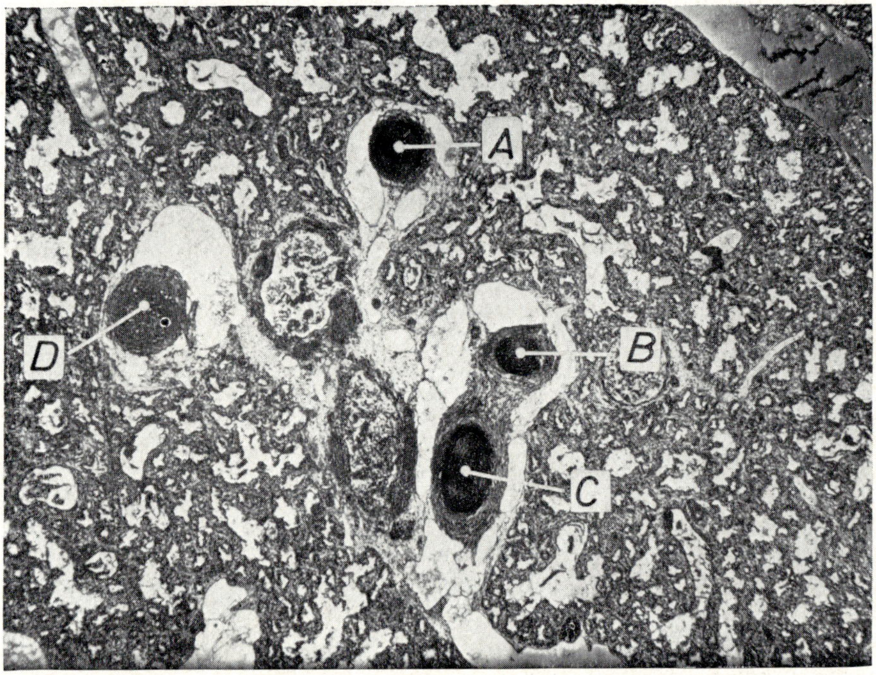


FIG. 6.—Marked distension and ectasia of many peri-arterial lymphatic vessels; some lymphatic vessels contain a granular precipitate. A, B, C, D are pulmonary arteries. (Staining as Fig. 1. × 26.)

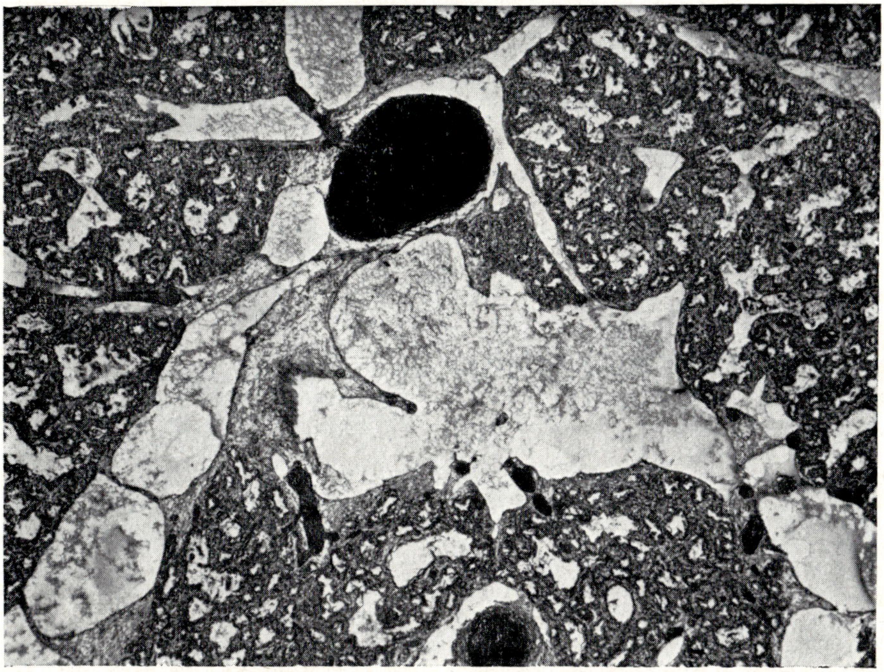

FIG. 7.—Unusual case of extreme peri-venous and septal lymphangiectasia and lymphatic congestion, mimicking congenital pulmonary lymphangiectasis. (Staining as Fig. 1. × 26.)

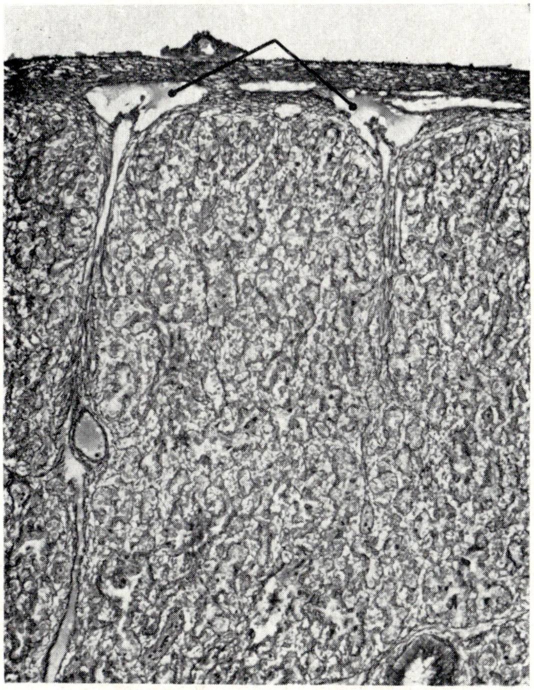

FIG. 8.—Collapsed area of lung with neonatal hyaline membrane disease; pleural lymphatic congestion; lymphatic vessels contain a fibrinous fluid, and valves pointed to the pleura (marked with pointers). (Staining as Fig. 1. × 31.)

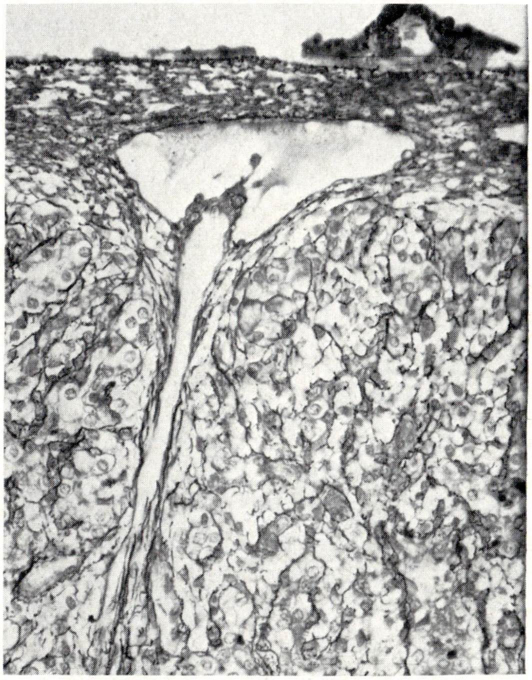

FIG. 9.—Magnified area from Fig. 8. Pleural lymphatic vessel, congested and containing a fibrinous exudate. Valves pointed to the pleura. (Staining as Fig. 1. × 190.)

**Pulmonary Haemorrhages.** These were observed in about half the cases. In a recent review of 30 cases of primary neonatal pulmonary haemorrhage, pulmonary haemorrhage was found in a broad variety of fatal neonatal conditions (Lauweryns, Eggermont, and Romelart, 1963). Here also, these haemorrhages probably represent merely a terminal complication of severe neonatal distress.

**Aspiration of Amniotic Fluid.** Intra-alveolar aspiration of amniotic fluid was in the past considered an important factor in the formation of hyaline membranes (Farber and Wilson, 1933; Farber and Sweet, 1931; Blystad *et al.*, 1951; MacGregor, 1953). The hypothesis is not supported by these observations. Aspirated amniotic material in considerable amounts was observed in only 7 cases, and there was no close correlation between the extent of this aspiration and the degree of hyaline membrane formation.

**Relation of Hyaline Membranes to Alveolar Wall.** The observed relation of the hyaline membranes to the reticular fibres of the walls of the alveoli and alveolar ducts (Figs. 1, 3, and 4) seemed important in connexion with the pathogenesis of the disease. The relation is clear and well defined. A comparison in the same microscopic field of alveoli lined by hyaline membranes with normal alveoli shows how in a normal alveolus it is the alveolar epithelial cells that are resting upon the reticular fibres, while the hyaline membranes are directly apposed to these fibres (Figs. 3 and 4).

The precise histological structure of the alveolar wall, as revealed by the electron microscope (Low, 1953; Karrer, 1956; Bargmann and Knoop, 1956; Schulz, 1957; Policard, Collet, and Pregermain, 1957; Divertie and Brown, 1964) shows that the 'alveolo-capillary membrane' is made up of three continuous and distinct layers: (1) external, the alveolar cells (both small and large), (2) the interstitium, (3) the capillary endothelium (Weibel, 1963). The interstitium, limited on one side by the endothelial and on the other by the epithelial basement membrane, contains the reticular fibres.

The hyaline membranes as seen by conventional microscopy lie directly upon the reticular fibres of the alveoli and alveolar ducts, so it follows that there must be necrosis of the epithelial part of the wall. This hypothesis is strengthened by the finding in the same sections of areas with hyaline membranes and absent epithelium, along with normal alveoli with an epithelial lining but no membranes.

This view is also supported by the well-known fact, confirmed by this study, that the hyaline membranes often include necrotic nuclear and cellular material, DNA-positive (Buckingham and Sommers, 1960). Moreover, some of these nuclei and cell remnants have the cytological characteristics of alveolar cells and macrophages (Figs. 1 and 5). This interpretation is supported by the electron microscope studies of Van Breemen, Neustein, and Bruns (1957) and Campiche, Jaccottet, and Julliard (1962), which demonstrated necrotic changes in the alveolar epithelial cells in cases of HMD.

It is of course impossible by light microscopy to specify if this superficial necrosis of the alveolar wall also involves the alveolar basement membrane. Indeed the hyaline membrane cannot be certainly differentiated from the alveolar basement membrane, which covers superficially the alveolar interstitium as such. The intimate relationship of the hyaline membranes to the reticular fibres does suggest also that there is necrosis (at least partial) of the basement membrane, and this receives some support from the work of Van Breeman *et al.* (1957), who observed a partial disintegration and necrosis of the basement membranes in electron micrographs.

**Pulmonary Lymphatics.** The ectasia and congestion of the pulmonary lymphatic vessels (Figs. 6, 7, 8, and 9) observed in most of our cases, particularly in those with extensive hyaline membranes, are perhaps a consequence of transudation through the alveolo-capillary wall. The demonstration of fibrin as a constituent part of the hyaline membranes (Gitlin and Craig, 1956) provided the first evidence of such alveolo-capillary transudate. The pulmonary congestion and oedema, demonstrated by Shanklin (1963) and also observed in the present cases, are in keeping with such a process.

## Summary

A detailed analysis has been made of the pathological lesions in the lungs of 55 human newborn infants with hyaline membrane disease.

The highest incidence in this series was in the groups of foetal age, 29-30 weeks.

At necropsy, a hydrostatic lung test was often negative. The inconsistency of this test as evidence of live-birth is re-emphasized.

Histology included total sections of the different lung lobes. In addition to the accepted lesions of hyaline membrane disease, this study stresses the following features.

(1) Localized areas of interstitial emphysema in 7 babies who were relatively mature. This may be the result of the greater force of their inspiratory movements.

(2) Hyaline membranes were less extensive and less developed in the very young premature age-group (less than 28 weeks).
(3) Pulmonary oedema was almost constant.
(4) Localized or extensive pulmonary haemorrhages were present in approximately half the cases, and were thought to be a terminal complication.
(5) Aspiration of amniotic fluid was usually not impressive; when present, it did not correlate with the extent of the hyaline membranes.

In addition, two previously undescribed features have been observed. The hyaline membranes are directly apposed to the reticular fibres of the alveolar walls and alveolar ducts which they line, suggesting a superficial necrosis of the walls of alveoli and alveolar ducts in hyaline membrane disease. The lymphatic vessels of the lungs were in most cases distended with fluid and often appeared angiectatic and congested. This, and the pulmonary oedema, are in keeping with the concept of an abnormal alveolo-capillary transudation in hyaline membrane disease.

This work was supported by a research grant from the Nationaal Fonds voor Wetenschappelijk Onderzoek (Belgium).

We are much indebted to Dr. A. H. Cameron (Birmingham) for his advice and help with the manuscript. We wish also to acknowledge the stimulating clinical help of Dr. E. Eggermont and Dr. A. Van den Driessche, the valuable technical help of Mrs. M. R. Van Hamme, and the analysis of the different morphological data by Mrs. Cl. De Coninck.

## References

Avery, M. E., and Mead, J. (1959). Surface properties in relation to atelectasis and hyaline membrane disease. *Amer. J. Dis. Child.*, **97**, 517.

Bargmann, W., and Knoop, A. (1956). Vergleichende elektronenmikroskopische Untersuchungen der Lungenkapillaren. *Z. Zellforsch.*, **44**, 263.

Blystad, W., Landing, B. H., and Smith, C. A. (1951). Pulmonary hyaline membranes in newborn infants. Statistical, morphologic and experimental study of their nature, occurrence and significance. *Pediatrics*, **8**, 5.

Buckingham, S., and Sommers, S. C. (1960). Pulmonary hyaline membranes: a study of the infant disease and experimental hyaline membranes induced pharmacologically. *Amer. J. Dis. Child.*, **99**, 216.

Campiche, M., Jaccottet, M., and Julliard, E. (1962). La pneumonose à membranes hyalines; observations au microscope électronique. *Ann. paediat.* (*Basel*), **199**, 74.

Divertie, M. B., and Brown, A. L., Jr. (1964). The fine structure of the normal alveolo-capillary membrane. *J. Amer. med. Ass.*, **187**, 938.

Farber, S., and Sweet, L. K. (1931). Amniotic sac contents in the lungs of infants. *Amer. J. Dis. Child.*, **42**, 1372.

——, and Wilson, J. L. (1933). Atelectasis of the new-born: a study and critical review. *ibid.*, **46**, 572.

Fournier, É. (1957). *Eléments de Médecine Légale et Législation Médicale.* Flammarion, Paris.

Gitlin, D., and Craig, J. M. (1956). The nature of hyaline membrane in asphyxia of the newborn. *Pediatrics*, **17**, 64.

Gonzales, T. A., Vance, M., Helpern, M., and Umberger, C. J. (1954). *Legal Medicine, Pathology and Toxicology*, 2nd ed. Appleton, New York.

Karrer, H. E. (1956). An electronmicroscopic study of the fine structure of pulmonary capillaries and alveoli of the mouse. *Bull. Johns Hopk. Hosp.*, **98**, 65.

Klaus, M., Reiss, O. K., Tooley, W. H., Piel, C., and Clements, J. A. (1962). Alveolar epithelial cell mitochondria as a source of the surface-active lung lining. *Science*, **137**, 750.

Latham, E. F., Nesbitt, R. E. L., Jr., and Anderson, G. W. (1955). A clinical pathological study of the newborn lung with hyaline-like membranes. *Bull. Johns Hopk. Hosp.*, **96**, 173.

Lauweryns, J. (1962). *De Longvaten: Hun Architectoniek en Hun Rol bij de Longontplooiing.* Arscia, Brussels.

—— (1964). Les vaisseaux lymphatiques du poumon néonatal normal et pathologique (atélectasie secondaire avec membranes hyalines)—description d'une nouvelle technique et résultats. *C. R. Ass. Anat., Madrid.* In the press.

——, Eggermont, E., and Romelart, G. (1963). Les hémorragies pulmonaires au cours de la période périnatale. *Bull. Soc. roy. belge Gynéc. Obstét.*, **33**, 35.

Low, F. N. (1953). The pulmonary alveolar epithelium of laboratory mammals and man. *Anat. Rec.*, **117**, 241.

MacGregor, A. R. (1953). Some observations on aspiration on liquor amnii and the so-called "vernix membrane". In *Anoxia of the Newborn Infant: a Symposium Organized by the C.I.O.M.S.*, p. 97. Blackwell, Oxford.

*Manual of Histologic and Special Staining Technics* (1957). Armed Forces Institute of Pathology, Washington, D.C.

Morison, J. E. (1952). *Foetal and Neonatal Pathology.* Butterworth, London.

Neligan, G. (1959). The systolic blood pressure in neonatal asphyxia and the respiratory distress syndrome. *Amer. J. Dis. Child.*, **98**, 460.

Nesbitt, R. E. L. (1957). *Perinatal Loss in Modern Obstetrics.* Davis, Philadelphia.

Parmentier, R. (1962). L'aération néonatale du poumon; contribution expérimentale et anatomo-clinique. *Rev. belge. Path.*, **29**, 121.

Policard, A., Collet, A., and Pregermain, S. (1957). Étude au microscope éléctronique des capillaires pulmonaires. *Acta anat.* (*Basel*), **30**, 624.

Potter, E. L. (1953). *Pathology of the Fetus and the Newborn.* Year Book Publishers, Chicago.

Rudolph, A. M., Auld, P. A. M., Drorbaugh, J. E., Rudolph, A. J., Nadas, A. S., and Smith, C. A. (1959). Studies on the circulation of infants with hyaline membrane disease. *Amer. J. Dis. Child.*, **98**, 630.

Schulz, H. (1957). Elektronenmikroskopische Untersuchungen des experimentellen Lungenödems. Electron. Micros. Proc. Stockholm, Congr. Syst., p. 240. Almquist and Wiksell, Uppsala.

Shanklin, D. R. (1963). Abstr. Amer. ped. Soc., Atlantic City, p. 100.

Van Breemen, V. L., Neustein, H. B., and Bruns, P. D. (1957). Pulmonary hyaline membranes studied with the electron microscope. *Amer. J. Path.*, **33**, 769.

Weibel, E. (1963). *Morphometry of the Human Lung.* Springer, Berlin.

*Arch. Dis. Childh.*, 1965, **40**, 626.

# ACID-BASE CHANGES FOLLOWING EXCHANGE TRANSFUSION WITH CITRATED BLOOD

BY

MARY CALLADINE, DOUGLAS GAIRDNER, B. T. NAIDOO, and D. H. ORRELL

*From the Cambridge Maternity Hospital and the John Bonnett Laboratories, United Cambridge Hospitals*

(RECEIVED FOR PUBLICATION MARCH 26, 1965)

The acid-citrate-dextrose (ACD) solution used to preserve blood consists in effect of 2 parts trisodium citrate to 1 part citric acid. It forms a buffer solution such that the *p*H of bank blood less than 5 days old is, in our experience, $6 \cdot 6 \pm 0 \cdot 2$. It can be predicted, therefore, that infusion of ACD blood must lead to an initial *acidosis*, and that this will in due course be replaced by a metabolic *alkalosis* as citrate is metabolized to form 3 moles of sodium bicarbonate for each mole of trisodium citrate retained. In the individual subject, the rates at which these two effects operate will determine the severity of the initial acidosis, and the stage at which the later alkalosis develops.

## Material and Methods

The babies studied received exchange transfusion for Rh or ABO haemolytic disease, or, in one case, for unexplained hyperbilirubinaemia. Their ages varied between 3 hours and 7 days. Two blood volumes (i.e. 180 ml./kg.) were exchanged in the course of 2 hours. In about half the cases both umbilical artery and vein were utilized for the transfusion, the baby's blood being allowed to drip from a catheter placed in an umbilical artery, while being replaced by donor blood dripped into a catheter placed in the umbilical vein. In the remaining cases the conventional intermittent method was used, with 20 ml. aliquots taken and given via the umbilical vein. Calcium gluconate 0·1 g. was given with every 100 ml. transfused.

Donor blood was less than 5 days old. The ACD routinely used in this area has the composition shown in Table 1. This provides rather more citrate than the formula commonly used which has 2 g. disodium citrate.

The donor blood was usually concentrated by the removal of about 150 ml. supernatant plasma. The final analysis varied somewhat on account of the variable haematocrit of the donor's blood, but from analyses of 24 bottles (8 analyses for citrate) the average composition of bank blood after concentration was as given in Table 2 (values for a normal baby are quoted for comparison).

Blood samples were obtained during the course of transfusion either from the aorta via umbilical artery catheter, or from the umbilical vein when the artery had not been catheterized. In practice there was little difference between the analyses of samples from the two sources, as blood from the region of the portal vein is almost arterial in character. Furthermore, plasma bicarbonate, with which we were chiefly concerned, is substantially the same in venous and arterial blood (Gandy, Grann, Cunningham, Adamsons, and James, 1964). After the end of transfusion, samples of 'arterialized' blood were obtained by skin-prick of the well-warmed foot. Samples were analysed without delay by the Astrup technique for *p*H, $Pco_2$, and bicarbonate; the latter has been expressed throughout this paper in terms of *standard bicarbonate* (Astrup, Jørgensen, Siggaard Andersen, and Engel, 1960), as this provides a convenient measure of metabolic acidosis and alkalosis. Chloride was measured by electrometric titration. Citrate was measured by the method of McArdle (1955).

TABLE 1

COMPOSITION OF ACID-CITRATE-DEXTROSE

| | |
|---|---|
| Disodium citrate ($Na_2H.C_6H_5O_7,1\frac{1}{2}H_2O$) | 2·85 g. (12 mm.) |
| Glucose | 3·27 g. |
| Water | 120 ml. |
| Blood | 420 ml. |

TABLE 2

AVERAGE COMPOSITION OF BANK BLOOD AFTER CONCENTRATION

| | Donor Blood | Blood of Normal Baby (1st week) |
|---|---|---|
| Plasma Na (mEq/l.) | 160 | 134 |
| Plasma K (mEq/l.) | 6·8 | 4·0 |
| Plasma Cl (mEq/l.) | 63 | 104 |
| Plasma bicarbonate (mEq/l.) | 6 | 23 |
| Plasma citrate (mg./100 ml.) | 620 | <4 |
| (mM/l.) | 32·3 | <0·2 |
| Plasma protein (g./100 ml.) | 6·7 | 6·2 |
| Blood Hb (g./100 ml.) | 13 | 19 |
| Blood haematocrit (%) | 42 | 57 |
| Blood *p*H | 6·6 | 7·4 |

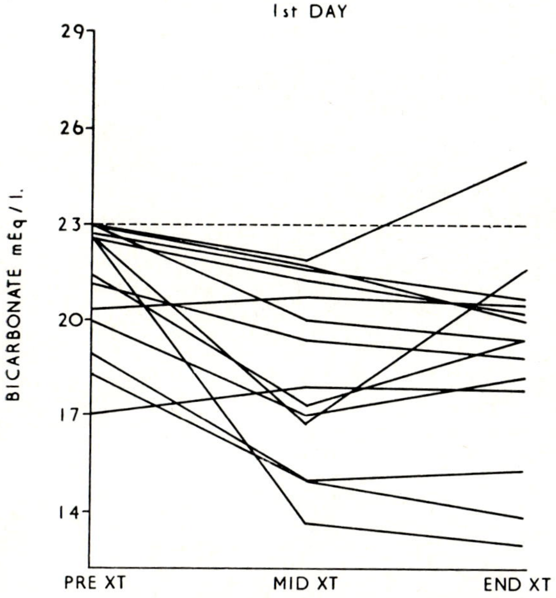


FIG. 1.—Plasma bicarbonate during exchange transfusion on 1st day of life in 14 babies (normal level 23 mEq/l. indicated).

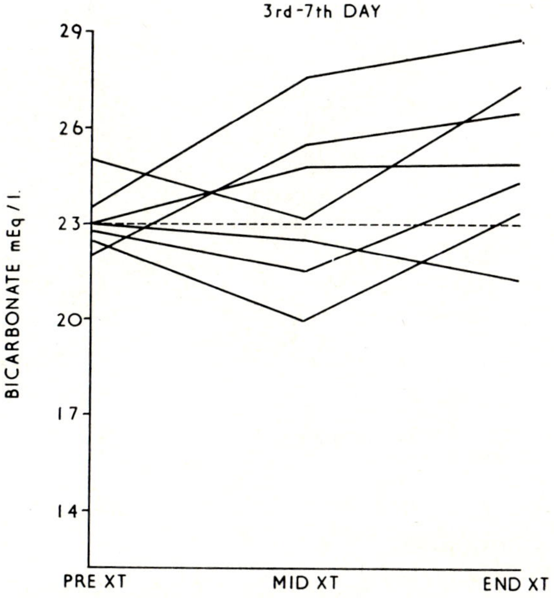


FIG. 2.—Plasma bicarbonate during exchange transfusion in 7 babies 3-7 days old.

## Results

**Plasma Bicarbonate During Exchange Transfusion.** 21 babies were studied, of between 37 and 40 weeks' gestation. They fell into two groups: (a) 14 babies transfused on the first day of life; many of these babies were anaemic, the Hb varying from 5·4 to 13·8, mean 10·5 g./100 ml.; (b) 7 babies transfused at 3-7 days old; the Hb level was higher in this group, ranging from 12·5 to 16·5, mean 14·6 g./100 ml.

Fig. 1 shows the change in plasma bicarbonate in the 14 babies transfused on day 1. The pre-exchange value ranged from 17 to 23 mEq/l. During the first half of the 2-hour exchange transfusion the bicarbonate fell in 12 of the 14 cases. During the second half it continued to fall in some and rose in others, but with one exception the final value was less than 21·5 mEq/l.

Fig. 2 shows comparable results for the 7 babies transfused when 3-7 days old. In 3 babies there was an initial fall in bicarbonate, but in 6 of the 7 the bicarbonate rose during the second half of the transfusion so that the final value was, with a single exception, higher than the pre-exchange value, and more than 23 mEq/l.

**Plasma Citrate During Exchange Transfusion.** This was followed in 8 cases (Table 3). Despite the fact that the plasma citrate in the donor blood was about 620 mg./100 ml., the highest level recorded during transfusion was 96 mg./100 ml.

TABLE 3

PLASMA CITRATE LEVELS IN 8 BABIES RECEIVING EXCHANGE TRANSFUSION

| Case | Age (days) | Plasma Citrate Level: mg./100 ml. (and mM/l.) | |
|---|---|---|---|
| | | Mid-exchange (1 hour) | End-exchange (2 hours) |
| 1 | 1 | — | 59·5 (3·1) |
| 2 | 1 | 44 (2·3) | 96 (5·0) |
| 3 | 1 | 36 (1·9) | 51 (2·7) |
| 4 | 1 | 96 (5·0) | 39 (2·0) |
| 5 | 3 | 13 (0·65) | 27 (1·4) |
| 6 | 4 | 58 (3·0) | 77 (4·0) |
| 7 | 4 | 48 (2·5) | 78 (4·1) |
| 8 | 6 | — | 57 (3·0) |

**Plasma Chloride During Exchange Transfusion.** Plasma chloride levels before and after transfusion were measured in 10 cases. Before transfusion the mean value was 104 mEq/l. (range 97-107), after transfusion it was 95 mEq/l. (range 81-101). In every case there was a fall in chloride, which averaged 9 mEq/l.

It is useful to calculate the approximate amount of chloride removed from the body as a result of exchange transfusion. The mean concentration of

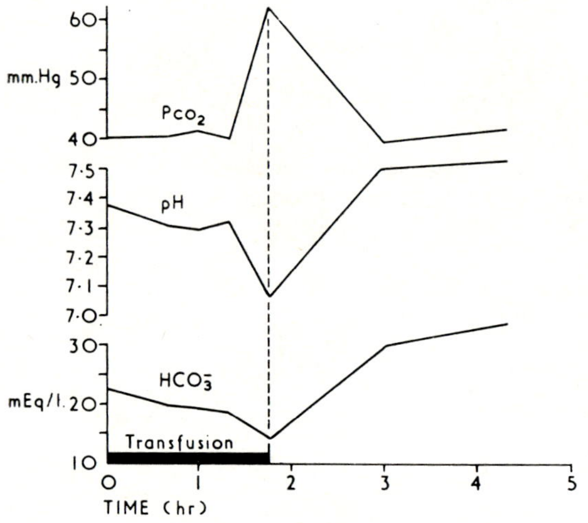


FIG. 3.—$Pco_2$, *p*H, and bicarbonate of plasma in a premature baby who became ill towards the end of exchange transfusion. Note development of severe acidosis during transfusion, rapid correction after transfusion terminated, followed by development of alkalosis.

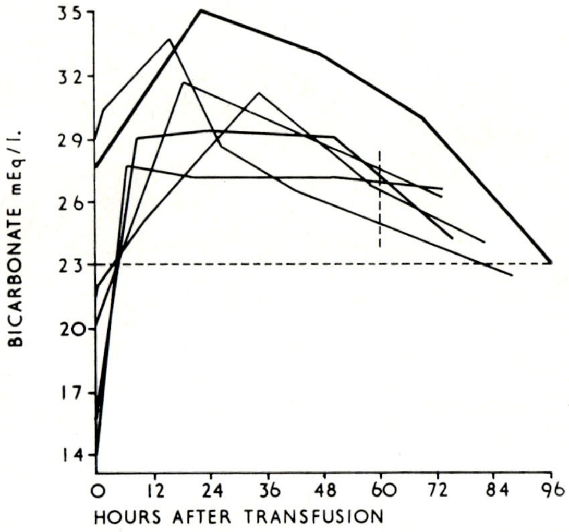


FIG. 4.—Plasma bicarbonate following exchange transfusion in 5 babies receiving one transfusion (——), and in one baby (——) receiving a second transfusion 36 hours after a transfusion on day 1. At 60 hours bicarbonate is still raised.

chloride in the effluent (10 cases) was 98 mEq/l., and in the donor blood 63 mEq/l. Since 180 ml./kg. of blood was exchanged, and assuming a haematocrit of 42% for both donor and recipient blood, the net loss of chloride was (98-63) × 180/1000 × (100-42) /100 = 3·7 mEq. per kg. body weight.

**Blood *p*H and $Pco_2$ During Exchange Transfusion.** Values for *p*H and $Pco_2$ were obtained at the same time as those for bicarbonate in the 21 cases shown in Figs. 1 and 2, but have not been detailed here as they would have added little of importance. With few exceptions $Pco_2$ remained near normal and within the range 37-46 mm.Hg, so that changes in *p*H ran parallel with changes in bicarbonate. The *p*H seldom fell below 7·2 and never below 7·1.

A different pattern was recorded, however, in a baby not included in the above series because it was premature, 36 weeks' gestation, 2·4 kg. (Fig. 3). Haemolytic disease was of moderate severity, the Hb being 10 g./100 ml.; exchange transfusion was carried out at 3 hours. During the first $1\frac{1}{4}$ hours of the transfusion a mild metabolic acidosis developed, $HCO_3^-$ falling from 22·5 to 18·5 mEq/l., but the clinical state occasioned no anxiety until $1\frac{3}{4}$ hours, when the baby's breathing became laboured and his colour pale. This abrupt clinical deterioration coincided with the development of a severe respiratory acidosis superimposed on a sharply increased metabolic acidosis, the $Pco_2$ rising to 65 mm.Hg, and $HCO_3^-$ falling to 13 mEq/l. and *p*H to 7·03. The transfusion was stopped and the baby's condition thereafter improved rapidly, as did both the respiratory and metabolic acidosis (Fig. 3).

**Plasma Sodium and Potassium During Exchange Transfusion.** These remained within the normal range in 13 cases investigated. In no case did potassium reach 5 mEq/l.

**Plasma Bicarbonate Following Exchange Transfusion.** This was determined in 5 cases after a single exchange transfusion, and in 1 case after a second exchange transfusion carried out 36 hours after an initial exchange at 4 hours old (Fig. 4).

The plasma bicarbonate rose rapidly after transfusion in all cases, so that the acidosis that was often present at the end of transfusion was replaced by an alkalosis within an hour or so (see also Fig. 3). During the first 24 hours after transfusion the bicarbonate in the 5 single-transfusion cases rose to between 27 and 33 mEq/l., and to 35 mEq/l. in the case receiving a second transfusion. The maximum *p*H in the same period was between 7·48 and 7·53 in 5 of these 6 cases, and was 7·43 in the remaining case.

Thereafter the bicarbonate level slowly fell, a period of more than 72 hours elapsing before a normal level of 23 mEq/l. was reached.

It was pointed out to us by Dr. John Davies that the rate at which post-transfusion alkalosis was corrected might be limited by the amount of chloride

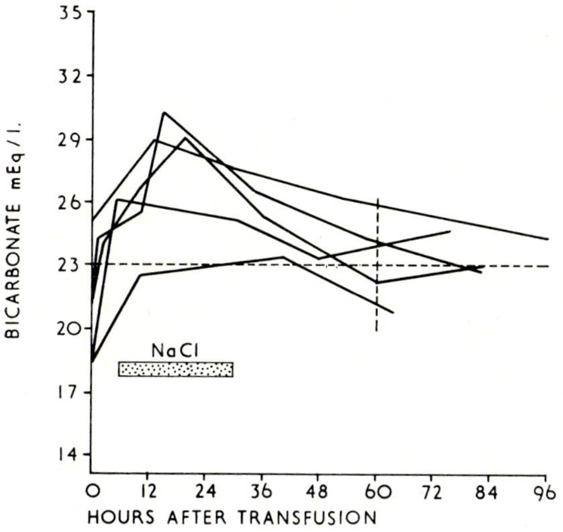


FIG. 5.—Plasma bicarbonate following exchange transfusion in 5 babies, to whom a supplement of NaCl (6-10 mEq/kg.) was given. At 60 hours the mean plasma bicarbonate is almost normal.

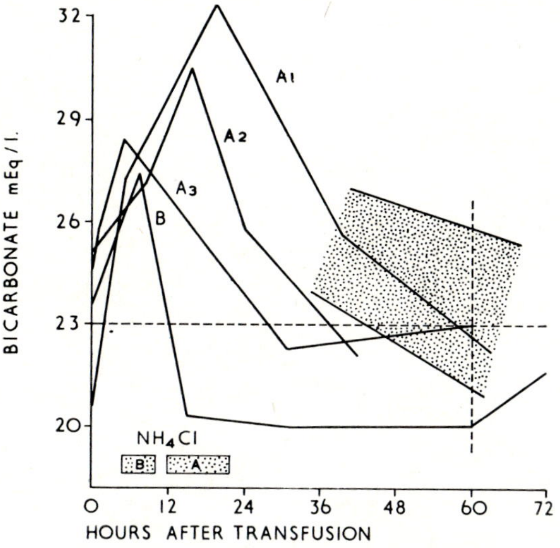


FIG. 6.—Plasma bicarbonate following exchange transfusion in 3 babies ($A_1$, $A_2$, $A_3$) given $NH_4Cl$ 5-8 mEq/kg., and in 1 baby (B) given $NH_4Cl$ 15 mEq/kg. within the periods of time indicated. The shaded area includes the values for the 5 babies receiving NaCl as shown in Fig. 5.

available to the baby, since the chloride content of milk, both human (12 mEq/l.) and cows' (29 mEq/l.), is low. To test this idea we gave a supplement of NaCl, 6-10 mEq/kg., to a series of 5 babies. The salt was given during the period 6-30 hours after transfusion, along with the ordinary feed. The 5 babies who received NaCl were comparable with the 5 who did not, 4 babies in each group having been transfused on the first day and 1 in each group on the fourth day of life.

Results are shown in Fig. 5. The babies receiving NaCl corrected the post-transfusion alkalosis somewhat more quickly. Comparing the two groups of babies at 60 hours after transfusion (Figs. 4, 5), in 4 out of the 5 babies receiving NaCl the bicarbonate level had by this time fallen below 24, while in 4 of the 5 controls the level was still above 27 mEq/l. At 60 hours the mean bicarbonate level was 23·3 mEq/l. (SD 1·62) for the babies receiving NaCl, and 26·6 mEq/l. (SD 0·85) for the controls. The difference between the two means is highly significant ($p < 0{\cdot}001$).

An alternative and more logical way of correcting a hypochloraemic alkalosis is to give $NH_4Cl$ rather than NaCl, and the former was, therefore, given to a further 4 babies after transfusion. In 3 babies the dosage and timing of the $NH_4Cl$ administration was essentially similar to that of the group receiving NaCl, 5-8 mEq/kg. being given along with the baby's milk feeds between 12 and 21 hours after transfusion (Fig. 6, Cases $A_1$, $A_2$, $A_3$). Comparing the rate at which the bicarbonate level of these babies fell to normal with the results for the NaCl-treated group (shaded area in Fig. 6), it is seen that in one case ($A_1$) the rate of fall was similar and in two cases ($A_2$, $A_3$) it was faster. A fourth case received a dose of $NH_4Cl$ which was both much larger (15 mEq/l.) and was given early, within 10 hours of the transfusion. This resulted (Case B, Fig. 6) in the post-transfusion alkalosis being rapidly overcorrected, the bicarbonate falling to 20 mEq/l.

## Discussion

**Acid-base Changes During Exchange Transfusion.** The acidosis occurring during exchange transfusion with citrated blood has been recorded by Povey (1964), who measured the *p*H of blood withdrawn from the umbilical vein. In 3 of his 6 cases the *p*H fell below 7·1, which contrasts with the fact that in none of our 21 cases of more than 37 weeks' gestation did the *p*H fall below 7·1; indeed values below 7·2 were exceptional. His paper contains no description of the age, gestational age, or degree of anaemia of the cases, but one factor probably explaining the lower *p*H values occurring during transfusion in his series is that transfusions were usually completed in 50 to 90 minutes, as against the 120 minutes of our series.

Plasma citrate levels during exchange transfusion have been recorded by several authors, with divergent results. In our cases the highest citrate level recorded was 96 mg./100 ml., and comparable values were found by Wexler, Pincus, Natelson, and Lugovoy (1949) and by Anderson, Marks, Tomlinson, and Walker (1963). The latter authors in an earlier study (Anderson, Smith, and Walker, 1961) had found much higher levels up to 350 mg./100 ml., with the highest levels tending to occur in premature babies; the different results in the two studies were attributed to the fact that in the earlier study the rate of transfusion was faster (J. Anderson, personal communication). In Farquhar and Smith's (1958) series, levels of 100-200 mg./100 ml. were common, and in one case with a severe haemolytic disease the level rose to 346 mg./100 ml.

Since for every 3 moles of citrate in ACD transfused (and retained) 2 moles when metabolized reappear as bicarbonate, the rate at which citrate is metabolized can conveniently be measured in terms of plasma bicarbonate. So measured, our results show that this rate is a function of a baby's age and/or its clinical status, since first-day babies, who in this series tended also to be moderately anaemic, metabolized citrate a good deal less rapidly than 3-7-day-old babies who were not anaemic (Figs. 1, 2). Thus at the end of transfusion, first-day babies showed a metabolic acidosis, while a metabolic alkalosis had usually already developed by the end of transfusion in the babies of 3-7 days old.

These facts can best be explained in terms of the functional efficiency of the liver, infused citrate being mainly metabolized in the liver. In our series, the younger group of babies was also the more severely affected by haemolytic disease (in terms of anaemia), so that we have been unable to separate two factors that may influence hepatic function—the age of the baby, and liver damage resulting from haemolytic disease. As regards the age factor, there is evidence that certain aspects of hepatic function (activity of glucuronyl transferase, bromsulphalein excretion) improve during the first few days after birth (see Smith, 1959), and it seems not unlikely that the capacity to metabolize citrate may behave similarly. That liver damage impairs the ability to metabolize citrate has been concluded both from observations on adult patients and from experiments on animals (Bunker, Stetson, Coe, Grillo, and Murphy, 1955; Sjöström, 1937).

In summary of this section: our own data, taken in conjunction with those of other workers quoted, are consistent with a conclusion that the severity of the acidosis developing during exchange transfusion is inversely related to the rate at which citrate is metabolized, and that this rate is probably slower in the premature than in the mature baby, in the anaemic or otherwise sick baby than in the well baby, and in the baby a few hours old than in the baby of a few days.

**Acid-base Changes After Exchange Transfusion.** Two components of the alkalosis developing after transfusion can be distinguished. One is the depletion of body chloride resulting from the use of donor blood with a chloride concentration only two-thirds that of plasma: this was reflected in a lowering of plasma chloride by an average of 8 mEq/l. by the end of transfusion. The other is the build-up of plasma bicarbonate as citrate is metabolized. The combined effect is to produce a hypochloraemic alkalosis, *p*H in our series rising to 7·5 or more, with plasma bicarbonate levels of up to 35 mEq/l. In due course the alkalosis is corrected by the kidneys excreting $HCO_3^-$ and retaining $Cl^-$ in its place, and the rate at which this takes place is limited by the supply of chloride.

The amount of chloride removed as a result of exchange transfusion has been assessed at about 3·7 mEq/kg. body weight, representing about 7% of the total body chloride, which is 50 mEq/kg. at birth (Forbes, Reid, Bondurant, and Etheridge, 1956). The depletion of chloride for a 3·5 kg. baby must thus amount to 13 mEq, requiring for its replacement the ingestion by the baby of about 1 litre of human milk, or $\frac{1}{2}$ litre of cows' milk. These figures make it clear that the relatively small amount of chloride ingested by a baby in the first few days of life, particularly when taking breast milk, necessarily limits the rate at which the post-transfusion alkalosis can be corrected. Supplying additional chloride as NaCl, or better as $NH_4Cl$, is shown to hasten correction of the alkalosis (Figs. 5, 6).

**Practical Implications.** The wisdom of employing a slow rate of transfusion is underlined, particularly in first-day babies and those with anaemia. Slow transfusion gives time for the initial acidosis to be offset by the alkalinizing effect of metabolized citrate. A slower rate of transfusion would probably have prevented the severe acidosis and clinical deterioration which developed in the case shown in Fig. 3.

There is some evidence to suggest that acidosis favours the passage of bilirubin from plasma, where it is largely bound to albumin, into cells, alkalosis favouring the reverse trend. Martin (1949), for instance, provides data showing that albumin binds 30% more bilirubin at *p*H 7·6 than at 7·4. Odell (1964) studied the partition of bilirubin *in vitro* between mitochondria and a solution of albumin, and concluded that 'any reduction in extracellular *p*H or addition of organic anions would favour intracellular diffusion of bilirubin displaced from albumin'. These facts imply that in any hyperbilirubinaemic situation it is particularly important to avoid acidosis developing during exchange transfusion. For the same reason, the post-transfusion alkalosis may be a positive advantage in hyperbilirubinaemia.

In the light of these facts, the pros and cons of concentrating citrated blood by removal of some plasma are worth considering.

The effects of concentrating donor blood are four:

(1) The baby will be left with a higher haematocrit and Hb level at the end of transfusion, which may obviate the need for a later top-up transfusion for anaemia.

(2) To the extent that the haematocrit at the end of transfusion is higher, the total circulating plasma protein is lower, and hence its binding capacity for bilirubin is lower.

(3) The amount of citrate administered will be less, hence the acidosis developing during transfusion will be lessened.

(4) The post-transfusion alkalosis will be diminished, which may perhaps be disadvantageous if there is hyperbilirubinaemia.

The first and third of these effects are advantageous and will usually be considered to outweigh the more marginal disadvantages of the second and fourth effects.

With the idea of offsetting the metabolic acidosis developing during exchange transfusion (Fig. 1). Boda, Tóth, Eck, and Murányi (1965) have advised giving an intravenous dose of sodium lactate to babies before transfusion, especially if an acidosis is already present. Povey (1964) suggested adding $NaHCO_3$ or tris-buffer (THAM) to the donor blood. These approaches seem logical, particularly so if the baby is premature or affected by a severe degree of haemolytic disease. However, such procedures might well cause an exaggeration of the post-transfusion alkalosis, similar to that observed in the baby receiving a second exchange transfusion (Fig. 4). Although we have not discerned any clinical disorder resulting from the alkalosis (*p*H up to 7·53) after transfusion with ACD blood, it would be unwise to assume that more severe degrees of alkalosis would be harmless.

## Summary

Acid-base changes have been followed in 21 babies during exchange transfusion with citrated blood.

During exchange transfusion a metabolic acidosis developed initially. In the babies transfused on the first day of life, many of whom were also anaemic, the acidosis persisted throughout the course of a 2-hour transfusion. In older babies, 3-7 days of age, the initial acidosis was corrected by the end of transfusion.

Following exchange transfusion a hypochloraemic alkalosis developed and was not corrected until about the fourth day after transfusion.

Correction of post-transfusion alkalosis was accelerated by providing supplementary chloride, either as NaCl or $NH_4Cl$, because the amount of chloride available to the milk-fed baby is small relative to the depletion of chloride caused by exchange transfusion.

Certain practical implications of these findings are discussed.

Dr. John Davies's contribution, referred to in the text, is gratefully acknowledged. B.T.N. held a British Council Scholarship, and M.C. was supported by a Medical Research Council grant.

### References

Anderson, J., Marks, V., Tomlinson, R. W. S., and Walker, W. (1963). Changes in the blood concentration of glucose, α-oxoglutarate, pyruvate and citrate during exchange transfusion in haemolytic disease of the newborn. *Arch. Dis. Childh.*, **38**, 481.

——, Smith, B. M., and Walker, W. (1961). Certain biochemical changes during exchange transfusion. *Vox Sang. (Basel)*, **6**, 525.

Astrup, P., Jørgensen, K., Siggaard Andersen, O., and Engel, K. (1960). The acid-base metabolism: a new approach. *Lancet*, **1**, 1035.

Boda, D., Tóth, G., Eck, E., and Murányi, L. (1965). pH changes in exchange transfusion. *ibid.*, **1**, 164.

Bunker, J. P., Stetson, J. B., Coe, R. C., Grillo, H. C., and Murphy, A. J. (1955). Citric acid intoxication. *J. Amer. med. Ass.*, **157**, 1361.

Farquhar, J. W., and Smith, H. (1958). Clinical and biochemical changes during exchange transfusion. *Arch. Dis. Childh.*, **33**, 142.

Forbes, G. B., Reid, A. F., Bondurant, J., and Etheridge, J. (1956). Changes in total body chloride during growth. *Pediatrics*, **17**, 334.

Gandy, G., Grann, L., Cunningham, N., Adamsons, K., and James, L. S. (1964). The validity of pH and $P_{CO_2}$ measurements in capillary samples in sick and healthy newborn infants. *ibid.*, **34**, 192.

McArdle, B. (1955). A modified method for the microdetermination of citric acid. *Biochem. J.*, **60**, 647.

Martin, N. H. (1949). Preparation and properties of serum and plasma proteins. XXI. Interactions with bilirubin. *J. Amer. chem. Soc.*, **71**, 1230.

Odell, G. B. (1964). The influence of pH on the distribution of bilirubin between albumin and mitochondria. *J. Pediat.*, **65**, 1108.

Povey, M. J. C. (1964). pH changes during exchange transfusion. *Lancet*, **2**, 339.

Sjöström, P. (1937). Der Citratgehalt im Blutserum als Diagnosticum bei Krankheiten der Leber und der Gallenwege: eine methodologische, tierexperimentelle und klinische studie. *Acta chir. scand.*, Suppl. 49.

Smith, C. A. (1959). *The Physiology of the Newborn Infant*, 3rd ed., pp. 183-202. Blackwell, Oxford.

Wexler, I. B., Pincus, J. B., Natelson, S., and Lugovoy, J. K. (1949). The fate of citrate in erythroblastotic infants treated with exchange transfusion. *J. clin. Invest.*, **28**, 474.

*Arch. Dis. Childh,.* 1965, **40**, 632.

# METABOLIC AND CHROMOSOMAL STUDIES IN LEPRECHAUNISM

BY

ANATOLE DEKABAN

*From Section on Child Neurology, National Institutes of Health, Bethesda, Maryland, U.S.A.*

(RECEIVED FOR PUBLICATION MARCH 8, 1965)

Donohue and Uchida (1954) described two sisters with grotesque facial appearance, extreme emaciation, and death occurring under 3 months of age. Based on the assumed resemblance of these children to dwarf cobblers from Irish folklore, the authors called the condition leprechaunism. It is hoped that this term will be changed to a more appropriate name when the underlying lesion is better understood. Until the present time four additional cases of leprechaunism have been described (Evans, 1955; Patterson and Watkins, 1962; Salmon and Webb, 1963). Findings on physical examination suggested to all these investigators an endocrine or metabolic disorder as the possible cause. However, laboratory studies as well as post-mortem examinations in three patients have failed to reveal the basic abnormality. The seventh patient here reported has characteristics typical of leprechaunism. To further the investigation of this condition we have performed most of the metabolic and endocrinological tests currently available, as well as the chromosome studies in the patient and in his parents.

## Case Report

E.H. is a 14-month-old boy. The mother was 32 years of age at his birth and she was well except for recurrent episodes of eczematous dermatitis; the father was 35 years of age and healthy. There were no hereditary disorders or the birth of abnormal children in the parents' families. The mother's first pregnancy ended in miscarriage in the third month of gestation; the second, third, and fourth resulted in three normal children, two boys and one girl. The fifth pregnancy, from which the patient was born, was complicated by mild polyhydramnios. The delivery was spontaneous at an estimated 37 weeks of gestation with a birth weight of 3·6 kg. The male infant was noted to be grossly abnormal: his face was grotesque, he had large nares, low-set ears, somewhat sunken and widely-spread eyes, and a short neck. The abdomen was relatively large but the extremities appeared short with ulnar deviation of both hands and equinovarus position of feet. He developed neonatal jaundice but Coombs test was negative and his peripheral blood was essentially normal. Deficient food intake was noted early and he failed to gain weight. At 4 months of age he weighed only 3·5 kg. His nipples appeared enlarged and his body was wasted. Because of difficulty in feeding and generally frail condition he has spent most of his life in hospitals.

Examination at the age of 7 months showed an undersized and emaciated infant of unusual appearance (Fig.). His weight was 4·5 kg., body length 57 cm., and head circumference 43 cm. The skin on the extremities and buttocks was redundant and was thrown into deep folds on his palms. The subcutaneous adipose tissue was almost completely absent. His hair was sparse, the anterior fontanelle was widely open, and the eyes were sunken. The respirations were frequent with intercostal retraction but the chest was clear to auscultation. The heart rate was 116 a minute with a faint systolic murmur which was considered to be functional. The abdomen was protuberant but liver and spleen were not enlarged. He had small umbilical and pronounced bilateral inguinal hernias as well as a diastasis of the rectus muscles. Both testicles were present in the lower part of the inguinal canals and their consistency was normal. He looked at faces and followed objects with his eyes from side to side and funduscopic examination was normal. His best performance consisted of briefly lifting his head up about 3 inches from the mattress while in prone position. Muscle strength was greatly deficient throughout but muscle tone was normal. Tendon reflexes were present and equal, and plantar responses were predominantly flexor. He was weaned from tube feeding, and vigorous but largely unsuccessful attempts were made to increase his weight. There has been some progress, however, in his motor and mental development.

At 14 months of age he was readily turning over and was able to keep his head and chest up while supporting himself on his forearms in prone position. He keenly observed the activity around him showing jealousy if attention was given to the other child in his room and smiled occasionally in response to appropriate stimulation. However, he gave no evidence of understanding spoken words or gestures. In spite of all efforts to increase his food intake and in spite of a well-balanced

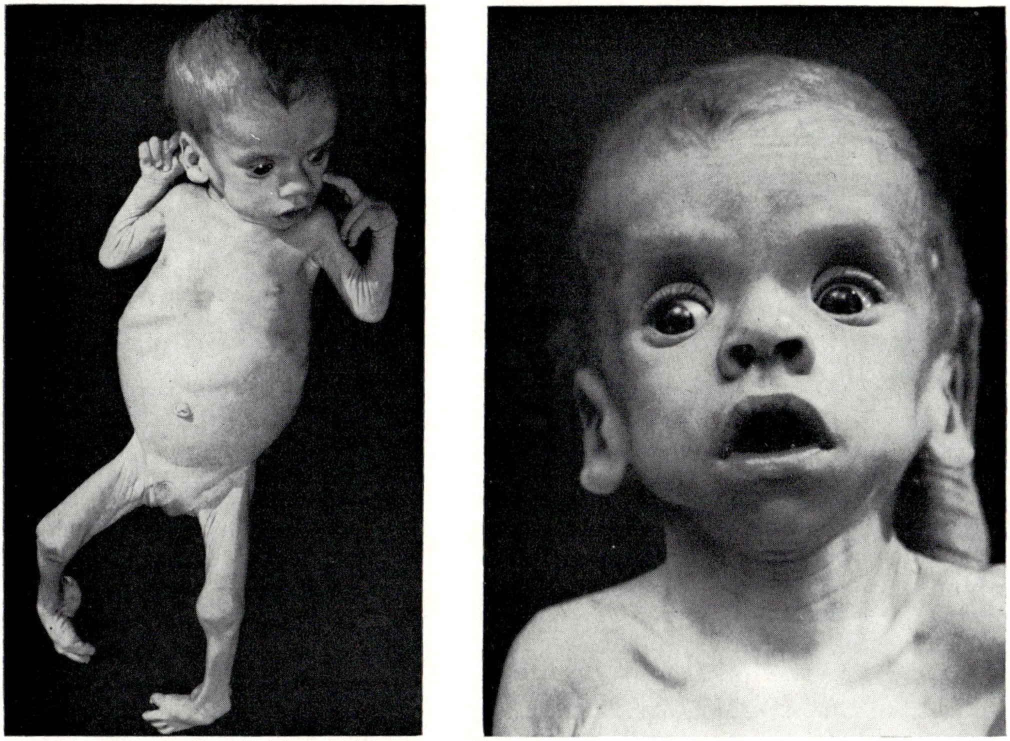

A B

FIG. A and B.—Photograph of the patient at the age of 7 months. Note low-set ears, sunken eyes, deformity of feet, and extreme emaciation.

diet, his weight was only 5 kg. and his height 64 cm. Persisting failure to gain weight was puzzling, especially as there was no evidence that he was losing protein and sugar in urine or fat and protein in the stools. He was subject to frequent staphylococcal infections of the skin and eyelids.

**Laboratory Investigations.** Routine urinalysis and haemogram were normal on repeated examination. BUN was 17 mg., urinary total α-amino nitrogen was 9 and 7 mg./24 hours on two occasions; quantitative estimation of amino acids in urine (Spinco amino acid analyser) gave normal values. Liver function tests were largely negative. Plasma electrolytes as well as the results of serum protein and γ-globulin electrophoresis were normal. Serology was negative. Electrocardiogram and electroencephalogram were both within normal limits. Radiographs of skull, chest, and skeleton were normal except for a retardation of bone-age and equinovarus deformity of feet. Intravenous pyelogram was normal.

*Carbohydrate Metabolism.* Blood glucose levels varied from normal to low depending on the duration of fasting. This is well demonstrated in Tables 1 and 2. Similarly, the adrenaline and glucagon tests were normal if he

TABLE 1

ORAL GLUCOSE TOLERANCE TEST (2·2 g./kg. body weight) AT 8 MONTHS OF AGE FOLLOWING A FAST LASTING 10 HOURS

| | Blood Sugar Levels |
|---|---|
| Fasting | 33 |
| At 30 min. | 92 |
| At 1 hour | 120 |
| At 2 hours | 141 |
| At 3 hours | 46 |
| At 4 hours | 42 |

Blood sugar levels are in mg./100 ml.

TABLE 2

GLUCAGON TEST (1 mg. intramuscularly), AND L-LEUCINE TEST (0·15 mg./kg. body weight orally) AT 8 MONTHS

| Glucagon Test (7 hours fast) | | L-Leucine Test (10 hours fast) | |
|---|---|---|---|
| Fasting blood sugar | 61 | Fasting blood sugar | 43 |
| 15 min. | 110 | 20 min. | 38 |
| 30 min. | 129 | 40 min. | 39 |
| 60 min. | 129 | 60 min. | 38 |
| | | 80 min. | 42 |

Blood sugar levels are in mg./100 ml.

fasted for 6 hours and deficient if he fasted for 10 hours (Table 3). Combined insulin-adrenaline test showed excessive and prolonged fall of glucose after insulin and a slow response to adrenaline as compared with values in a normal child (Table 5). The L-leucine tolerance test was not associated with a fall of plasma glucose (Table 2).

TABLE 3

RESULTS OF ADRENALINE TOLERANCE TEST (0·15 mg. subcutaneously) AT 8 MONTHS; FIRST, WHEN THE PATIENT WAS FASTING FOR 10 HOURS, AND TWO DAYS LATER AFTER FASTING FOR 6 HOURS

| | Fasting 10 hours | Fasting 6 hours |
|---|---|---|
| Fasting blood sugar | 32·5 | 41·3 |
| 15 min. | — | 56·1 |
| 30 min. | 35·2 | 54·4 |
| 45 min. | — | 53·0 |
| 60 min. | 35·3 | 55·2 |
| 90 min. | 36·0 | 51·0 |
| 120 min. | 35·2 | — |

Blood sugar levels are in mg./100 ml.

TABLE 4

VALUES OF PLASMA LIPIDS ESTIMATED ON THREE DIFFERENT OCCASIONS FOLLOWING VARIABLE LENGTH OF FAST

| | Age 8 months: 11 hours' fast | Age 9 months: 8 hours' fast | Age 14 months: 7 hours' fast |
|---|---|---|---|
| Total lipids (mg./100 ml.) | 338 | 396 | 573 |
| Cholesterol (mg./100 ml.) | 105 | 146 | 192 |
| Phospholipids (mg./100 ml.) | 139 | 166 | 196 |
| Triglycerides (mg./100 ml.) | 113 | 107 | 212 |
| TFA (μg./100 ml.,) .. | 702 | 745 | 1,020 |
| FFA (μg./100 ml.) .. | 199 | 88 | 86 |

TABLE 5

INSULIN (0·25 u./kg. body weight subcutaneously) AND ADRENALINE (0·15 mg. subcutaneously) TOLERANCE TESTS AFTER 5 HOURS OF FASTING IN THE PATIENT, AND AFTER 10 HOURS OF FASTING IN A NORMAL CONTROL INFANT (Plasma glucose is in mg./100 ml.)

| | Patient | Normal Control Infant |
|---|---|---|
| Fasting blood sugar .. .. | 70 | 85 |
| *Insulin* | | |
| 30 min. later .. .. .. | 49 | 58 |
| 60 min. later .. .. .. | 42 | 59 |
| 90 min. later .. .. .. | 47 | 62 |
| 2 hours later .. .. .. | 37 | 69 |
| *Adrenaline* | | |
| 30 min. later .. .. . | 41 | 76 |
| 60 min. later .. .. .. | 56 | 88 |

*Lipid Studies.* Serum lipids after 11 hours of fasting were low, especially cholesterol, but the values were normal after 7 hours of fasting (Table 4). Quantitative estimations of fat in stools collected on 9 consecutive days and divided into 3-day samples gave consistently normal values of 2·1 to 2·5 g./day. The fat intake during this period varied from 20-30 g. daily. Blood vitamin A was 33 units and carotene was 35 units/100 ml.

*Endocrinological and Other Studies.* Protein-bound iodine (PBI) was 8·5 μg./100 ml.; urinary 17-ketosteroids 0·5 mg./24 hours; urinary oestrogen 8 μg./24 hours, and urinary gonadotrophins less than 3 mouse units per 24 hours. Human growth hormone in plasma was 7 mμ/ml. (normal or slightly raised). Sex chromatin was typical of a male. Alkaline phosphatase was 12 and 14 K-A units on two occasions. Urine was negative for mucopolysaccharides.

*Chromosome Studies in Short-term Blood Cultures.* The patient and his father had a modal number of 46 chromosomes and normal karyotypes. The mother had likewise 46 chromosomes; however, they exhibited a high rate of chromatid- and chromosome-type of breaks. Thus, among 80 mitoses scored in three separate blood cultures there were 19 (24%) breaks encountered (normal 0-1·5%).

## Discussion

There was relatively little laboratory work done on the two patients with leprechaunism described by Donohue and Uchida (1954), but the authors provided detailed records of necropsy examination. Two patients of Evans (1955) were alive at the time of his report. However, his second patient (Case 2) did not have features common to other patients with leprechaunism and probably should not be included in this group. The patient of Patterson and Watkins (1962) is still alive and the authors performed a considerable number of laboratory studies. The patient of Salmon and Webb (1963) died at age of 7 months and a detailed necropsy report is available.

The main unifying features of these patients including the present child consist of a grotesque and old facial appearance, dwarfism, extreme emaciation, almost complete failure to gain weight, and mental and motor retardation. The facial characteristics include low-set and generally large ears, beaked nose with flaring nostrils, widely-spaced eyes, thick lips, mostly open mouth, and short neck. Among less consistent physical findings are enlargement of breasts and external genitalia and a variable degree of hirsutism.

The following is the synopsis of the laboratory findings pertinent to studies of endocrine and metabolic disorders in these patients. Low and prolonged response to insulin was noted in all 3 children in whom this test was performed; low fasting blood sugar levels were recorded in most but not all patients. Alkaline phosphatase was low in patients of Patterson and Watkins (1962), Salmon and Webb (1963), and ours, but the values were not known in other cases. Retarded bone-age was noted in all, but this may be a secondary finding which depends on grossly deficient nutritional state and poor motor activity. Urinary amino acids were estimated in 4 patients; in 2 of these they were normal and in 2 raised. 17-ketosteroids were determined in 5 patients and they were normal in all. Urinary oestrogens in Case 1 of Evans (1955) and in the present patient were normal. Urinary gonadotrophins and plasma growth hormone in our patient were within normal limits.

Results of post-mortem examination in 3 patients and organ biopsies in another 3 can be stated as follows. The brains in the 2 children of Donohue and Uchida (1954) were normal, whereas the patient of Salmon and Webb (1963) had severe malformation of the brain in a form of agyria of cerebral hemispheres and rudimentary cerebellum; no histological details are given. Examinations of the pancreas in 4 cases (one of which was biopsy) showed hypertrophy of islets of Langerhans in 3 and normal histological structure in one (Evans, Case 1). The liver was examined histologically in 5 patients: no abnormality was found in 2 biopsy specimens, and in 3 patients who died the lesions were largely unspecific and consisted of focal degeneration or necrosis. In Donohue and Uchida's (1954) patients there was in addition focal increase of glycogen and iron deposits. Ovaries were examined in 3 patients and in all cyst formation was present; in 2 male patients histological studies of the testicles were considered to be normal. Kidneys showed dilatation of tubules in 3 patients who came to necropsy. The pituitary gland was reported as normal in 2 patients and as showing absence of D basophil cells in the patient described by Salmon and Webb (1963). Thyroid, thymus, and other tissues did not disclose any specific abnormality of note. Thus, even with the aid of the necropsy and biopsy examination no uniform abnormality could be demonstrated. Moreover, it appears that we might be dealing rather with a syndrome than with a disease entity. For instance, the patient of Salmon and Webb (1963) had severe cerebral malformation which could account for retardation of development and deficient growth, whereas the brains in the patients of Donohue and Uchida (1954) were normal.

Having repeated carbohydrate and lipid studies in our patient at various occasions, we came to the conclusion that the values were within normal limits or close to normal limits when the fasting period was in the range of 6-7 hours; when the fasting was extended to 11 hours most of the glucose and lipid reserves appeared depleted, as indicated by their low blood levels (Tables 1 and 4). It is evident that the biochemical and endocrinological studies performed in this patient, as well as the results of tests reported by other investigators, did not disclose any consistent metabolic abnormality. However, a possibility of a generalized 'dyscrasia' of a kind seen in mongolism cannot be denied. At the present time we can distinguish only the very gross chromosomal abnormality. Most inversions and small deficiencies of chromosomes in man generally escape detection.

The abnormalities found in the chromosomes of the mother were of two types: the first consisted of random chromosome breaks in about 6% of the mitoses; the second consisted of a 'weak' region involving long arms of the same chromosome, which led to high frequency breaks (about 18%) in this segment. The first type of abnormality is commonly seen in the peripheral blood of individuals exposed to radiation (Tough, Buckton, Baikie, and Court-Brown, 1960; Bender and Gooch, 1962; Buckton, Jacobs, Court Brown, and Doll, 1962); the second type of chromosome abnormality is complex and it will be the subject of a separate communication. On questioning the mother, it was disclosed that she had received x-radiation treatments for eczematous dermatitis. Thus, in 1947 at the age of 16 years she was given 5 irradiations to both ankles, in 1951 3 irradiations to the neck and back of her head, between 1956 and 1957 15 irradiations to various parts of her body, and in 1964 4 irradiations to both hands and wrists. Using *Depth Dose Tables for Use in Radiotherapy* (Scientific Sub-Committee of the Hospital Physicists' Association, 1961), the radiation factors supplied by the respective physicians were individually converted into skin dose and then summed up to arrive at a total skin dose of 1,550r. All radiations were estimated as being for soft tissue and therefore the dose to the bone-marrow and the lymphoid tissue must be reduced by a factor of about 0·6. Although the history of radiation may tempt speculations, the evidence of the present data does not permit us to ascribe the clinical syndrome of the offspring to the chromosomal aberration encountered in the maternal blood.

## Summary

An infant with persisting failure to gain weight is described under the title of leprechaunism. Scanty literature pertaining to this condition is reviewed. Exhaustive biochemical and endocrinological studies conducted in this patient added new data but failed to reveal the cause of the underlying abnormality.

The blood levels of certain constituents were subnormal when fasting extended over 10-11 hours, but these values were within normal limits when the blood was drawn after 6 to 8 hours of fasting. The child has 46 chromosomes of normal appearance, but his mother has a high incidence (24%) of chromosome- and chromatid-type breaks. She has received repeated x-ray treatments to various parts of her body for eczematous dermatitis during the past 14 years.

### Addendum

When this article was ready for publication, two sisters with leprechaunism were reported from Hungary (Kálló, Lakatos, and Szijártó, 1965); they both died under 6 weeks of age. As in other females with leprechaunism, their ovaries showed follicular maturation with cystic formation. In general, the clinical and pathological findings corresponded closely to those described previously.

Sincere thanks are due to my associates and colleagues at the National Institutes of Health for stimulating discussions during the study of this patient. I am especially grateful to Dr. L. Laster for quantitative estimation of fat in stools and to Dr. J. Roth for the analysis of plasma growth hormone. Dr. S. Suddarth referred this child to us and supplied valuable clinical and laboratory data on the initial six months of life.

### References

Bender, M. A., and Gooch, P. C. (1962). Persistent chromosome aberrations in irradiated human subjects. *Radiat. Res.*, **16**, 44.

Buckton, K. E., Jacobs, P. A., Court Brown, W. M., and Doll, R. (1962). A study of the chromosome damage persisting after x-ray therapy for ankylosing spondylitis. *Lancet*, **2**, 676.

Donohue, W. L., and Uchida, L. (1954). Leprechaunism, a euphuism for a rare familial disorder. *J. Pediat.*, **45**, 505.

Evans, P. R. (1955). Leprechaunism. *Arch. Dis. Childh.*, **30**, 479.

Kálló, A., Lakatos, I., and Szijártó, L. (1965). Leprechaunism (Donohue's syndrome). *J. Pediat.*, **66**, 372.

Patterson, J. H., and Watkins, W. L. (1962). Leprechaunism in a male infant. *ibid.*, **60**, 730.

Salmon, M. A., and Webb, J. N. (1963). Dystrophic changes associated with leprechaunism in a male infant. *Arch. Dis. Childh.*, **38**, 530.

Scientific Sub-Committee of the Hospital Physicists' Association (1961). Depth Dose Tables for Use in Radiotherapy. *Brit. J. Radiol.*, Suppl. **10**.

Tough, I. M., Buckton, K. E., Baikie, A. G., and Court-Brown, W. M. (1960). X-ray-induced chromosome damage in man. *Lancet*, **2**, 849.

*Arch. Dis. Childh.*, 1965, **40**, 637.

# OBSERVATIONS ON BLOOD PRESSURE IN NEWBORN INFANTS

BY

J. M. GUPTA and J. W. SCOPES

*From the Nuffield Neonatal Research Unit, Institute of Child Health, Hammersmith Hospital, London W.12*

(RECEIVED FOR PUBLICATION MARCH 29, 1965)

The measurement and recording of blood pressure in newborn babies is fraught with technical difficulties. Direct measurement from an artery is certainly the most accurate method (de Bono, 1963) but has obvious limitations, particularly if repeated observations over a period of hours or days are required. It involves entering an artery, strict asepsis, and expensive equipment for recording. Repeated measurements by indirect means are at best time consuming and tiring for both baby and observer (Ashworth, Neligan, and Rogers, 1959), and at worst upsetting to the baby and, therefore, inaccurate and valueless. Many ingenious methods of measuring blood pressure indirectly have been devised, but all of them have their limitations. The subject was reviewed by Young (1961) who discussed the various means employed and reviewed the findings.

In this unit we have recently had special opportunities to measure blood pressure. First, an apparatus has been devised that automatically records a baby's blood pressure at 2-minute intervals. This has made possible an assessment of blood pressure changes over the course of hours and days, and the patterns of blood pressure variations, including any circadian or shorter rhythms. Secondly, babies who require frequent sampling of blood for clinical reasons (for example, premature babies with the respiratory distress syndrome) have an umbilical arterial catheter inserted soon after birth, and we have taken advantage of the opportunity to make direct measurements of blood pressure in a variety of babies with different clinical conditions, and of varying size and gestation.

### Automatic Recorder

With this instrument, which is an adaptation of that described by Ball, Pallett, and Shillingford (1961) for recording digital blood pressure in adults, blood pressure is recorded indirectly from an arm or leg, and all the technical hazards of such indirect recording apply. The apparatus consists of two cuffs placed on the baby's arm (or leg), a sensing device for detecting pulsations, a pump which operates automatically at 2-minute intervals, and a mechanical recorder (a diagram of the mechanical connexions is shown in Fig. 1). At 2-minute intervals the proximal occluding cuff is blown up to 150 mm.Hg over the course of 10 seconds and at the same time the distal sensing cuff is blown up to a pressure 10 mm.Hg below that of the occluding cuff to render it turgid. The pressures fall in parallel over the next 45 seconds by a controlled leak to air. As soon as pulsation is detected in the distal cuff, the mechanical recorder whose needle is moving on the surface of a drum begins to write. There is then an interval of about 1 minute when the pressure of both cuffs is nil to rest the arm before the cycle is repeated.

The cuffs used are standard 2·5 cm. × 15 cm. size ('Neligan' cuffs, supplied by Charles Thackray Ltd.). Pulsation is detected by the method of Pallett (1962), which depends on the small movement of air caused by pulsation being led through a capillary tube and playing on a heated thermistor bead. The bead is cooled sufficiently by this tiny puff of wind to alter its electrical resistance and give a signal. To reduce artefacts caused by the child moving his arm, it is arranged that the signal must be synchronous with pulsation taken in the same way from the occluding cuff before the recorder will write. The needle on the recorder moves vertically over the drum with each cycle and the drum rotates slowly over a 12-hour period. One is thus presented with a series of dotted lines, the vertical length of which is proportionate to the pressure being recorded. Calibration is achieved simply by having a mercury manometer attached on the side arm of the occluding cuff pressure lead.

The pressures recorded by this apparatus read somewhat lower than simultaneous measurement by auscultation or the xylol bead technique, and somewhat higher than those recorded by the 'flush'

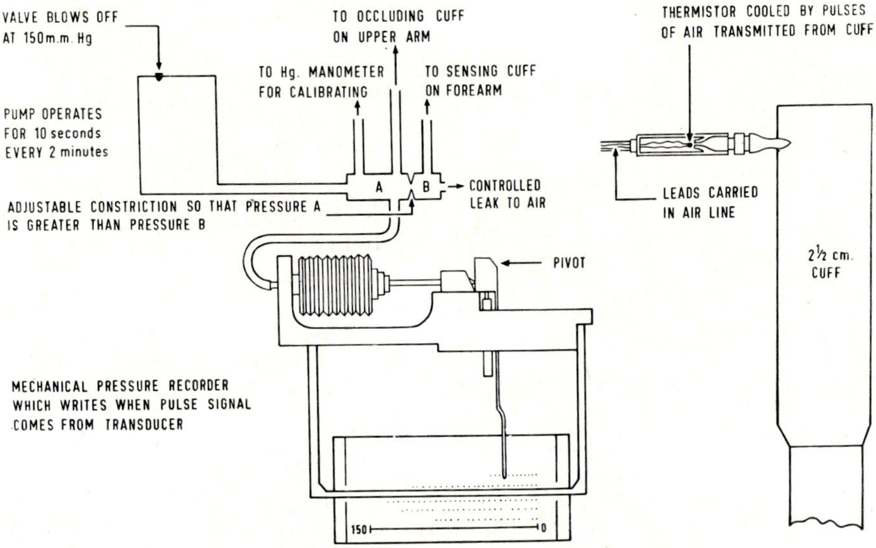


FIG. 1.—The automatic recorder—diagram of mechanical parts.

technique. On six occasions the readings have been compared with direct arterial pressure from an umbilical artery, when the pressure recorded was within 5 mm. of the *mean* blood pressure. Although measurement of absolute levels of blood pressure are not entirely satisfactory by this method, variations are well shown and represent the main concern of this part of the paper.

In full-term infants, the child's arm is unaffected by up to 12 hours of recording. In premature infants the hand sometimes begins to become oedematous after about 6 hours' recording, but this may be obviated by changing from one arm to another at intervals of 4 to 6 hours.

The results of the use of this instrument on just over 50 babies in the Neonatal Ward are presented here. These babies varied in weight from 1,200 to 3,600 g. and from 29 to 41 weeks' gestation. The interest in using this instrument lies not in the absolute levels of blood pressure obtained (which were in general agreement with levels obtained by other indirect techniques (Young, 1961)) but in the variations occurring during the day.

Fig. 2 shows a typical example of a tracing from a 3-day-old baby. The blood pressure of a baby fluctuates widely with the innumerable stimuli to which he is subject. Many minor procedures are accompanied by a large rise in blood pressure, and apart from periods when the baby is very quiet, a single blood pressure recording can be

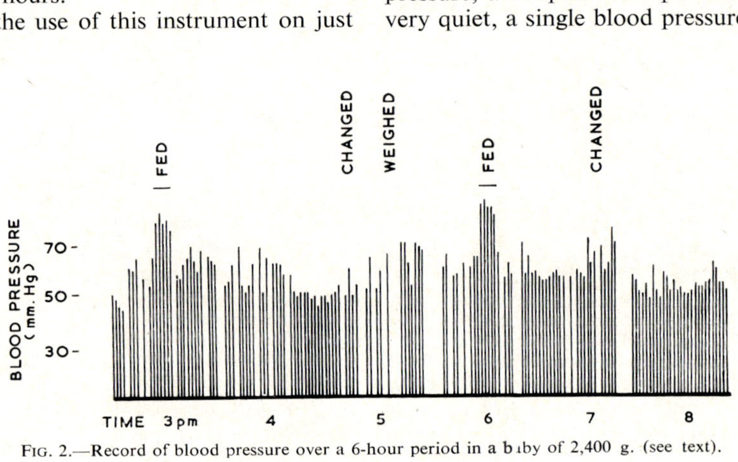


FIG. 2.—Record of blood pressure over a 6-hour period in a baby of 2,400 g. (see text).

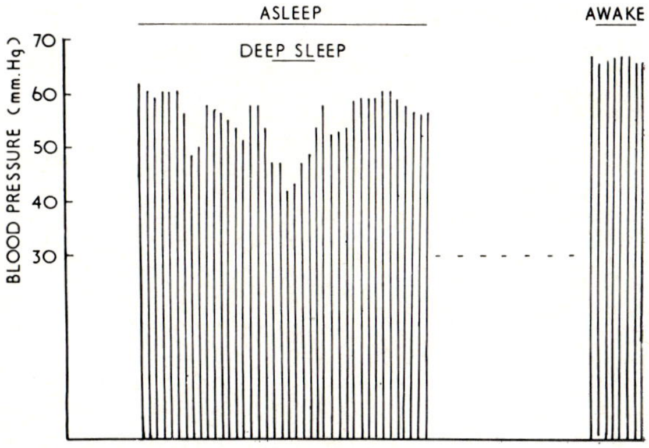


FIG. 3.—Record of blood pressure illustrating the fall that occurs in deep sleep. Each vertical line denotes an interval of two minutes. The dotted line indicates a broken time scale.

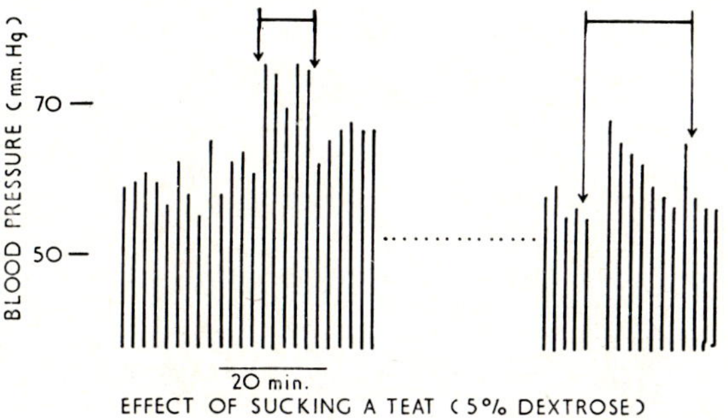


FIG. 4.—Effect on blood pressure of sucking a teat flavoured with 5% dextrose (see text).

far from representative of his 'basal' level. Normal babies do not stay in the Neonatal Ward for longer than a week or ten days, and in this time no circadian rhythm appeared. Premature babies were tested up to the age of 6 weeks, and under the somewhat artificial conditions of such a baby in hospital no circadian rhythm was seen. A series of changes related to feeding and sleeping were seen in almost all babies and a typical example is represented by Fig. 2. The blood pressure rises impressively by up to 20 mm. Hg during the feed, and settles after the feed to a 'resting' level. It tends to remain at this level for $\frac{1}{2}$ to 1 hour and then, as the child becomes deeply asleep, the level falls profoundly (Figs. 3 and 6). This fall appears to be related to the deep sleep phase described by Goldie (1964), for in it eye movements are absent, respiration is quite regular, and there is no movement apart from an occasional jerk. As the child emerges from this deep phase of sleep the blood pressure again rises to approximately the resting level. With the next feed, there is again a large rise in blood pressure. Almost any interference tends to cause a temporary rise in blood pressure.

The rise in blood pressure during a feed is the most striking feature of these variations. It was quite consistent and frequently as large as 20 mm. Hg. Some of the factors that might be responsible for this were investigated individually. Fig. 4 shows that when a child is allowed to suck a teat flavoured with 5% dextrose there is a substantial rise in blood pressure. This rise did not occur on insertion of the teat into the mouth unless the child sucked. The changes in blood pressure in Fig. 4 were noticed to be directly related to the vigour of the baby's sucking. In Fig. 4 (right hand section), there was no sucking for two minutes after insertion of the teat when vigorous sucking was observed. This sucking became progressively less until just before the teat was removed. A feed through a gastrostomy tube caused no rise in blood pressure in one infant. When a child is being fed by gavage, the tube being inserted through the mouth, there is a rise in blood pressure, not as well sustained as in an ordinary feed (see Fig. 5), and, in general, the rise occurs when the child is sucking on the tube through his mouth.

Other factors that may add to the rise in blood pressure during a feed include sitting the baby up and general arousal. Tilting to a head-up position causes a rise in blood pressure, and feeding a baby lying in his incubator causes a smaller rise in blood pressure than when he sits up for the feed. 'Arousal' is difficult to define, but a baby with his eyes open and a small amount of physical activity has a higher blood pressure than when he is completely quiet (see Figs. 2, 3, and 6).

The effect of mild cooling was examined, but it was difficult to separate the effect of the cooling from the slight arousal which is almost always produced.

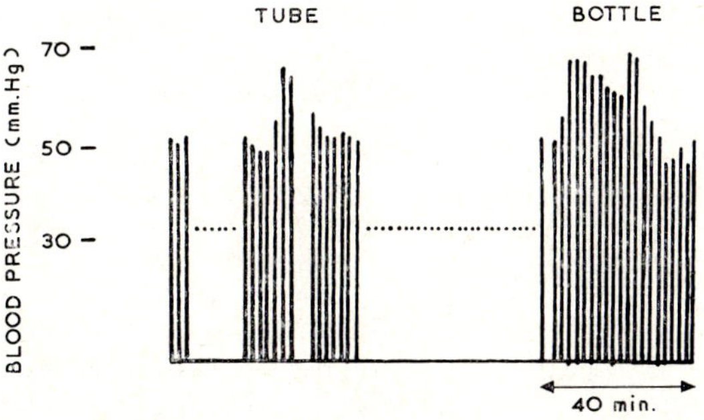


FIG. 5.—Effect on blood pressure of feeding by gavage and by bottle. The dotted line indicates a broken time-scale.

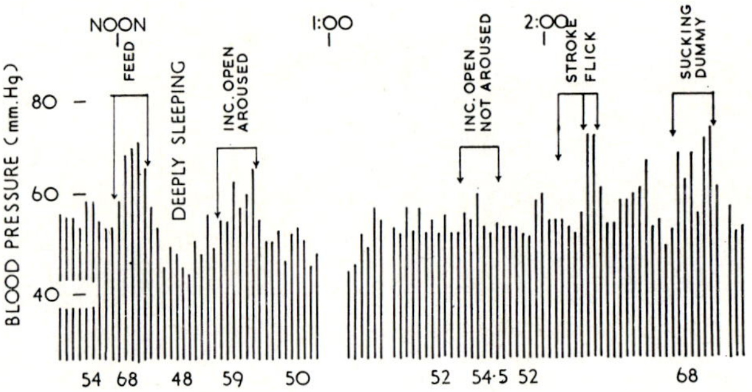


FIG. 6.—The blood pressure of a 1-week-old baby weighing 1,650 g. and its variation with various stimuli. The figures under the tracing refer to the average blood pressure over the ten-minute period concerned.

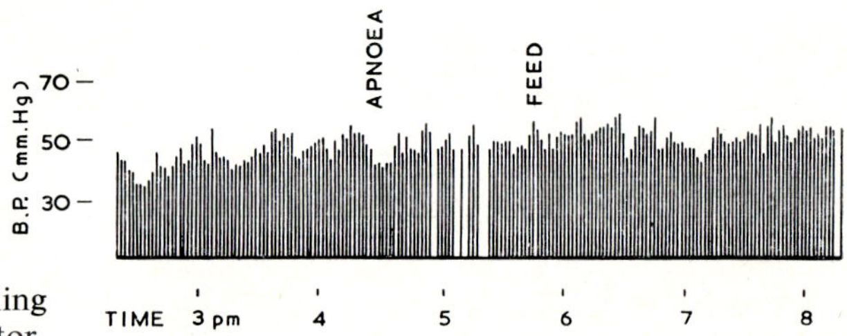


FIG. 7.—Blood pressure record of a baby of 1,880 g. with respiratory distress syndrome, aged 12 hours at the beginning of the record. Note gradual rise in blood pressure during the period of 5 hours when recovery from the respiratory distress was taking place.

Fig. 6 shows an example of such a test where cooling was achieved crudely by opening the incubator. (This obviously involves stimuli other than that of cooling.) During the period of cooling when there was no clinical arousal the blood pressure was slightly, but not statistically significantly, higher.

Neligan and Smith (1960) have reported a small steady rise in blood pressure in babies with respiratory distress after the first few hours of life. This was seen on a number of occasions and is illustrated by the tracing in Fig. 7 in a 1,880 g. baby, aged 12 hours and in Fig. 10. The fall in blood pressure at 4.30 p.m. in Fig. 7 was associated with a period of apnoea. A tube feed was given at 5.45 p.m. without any obvious change in blood pressure. This baby also showed a curious cycling of blood pressure approximately every $\frac{1}{4}$ to $\frac{1}{2}$ hour for which no obvious explanation was apparent.

### Direct Blood Pressure from the Umbilical Artery

The umbilical arterial catheter was connected to an Electro-Scholander transducer which was calibrated against a mercury manometer. The blood pressure was recorded on paper at a speed of 5 mm. per second in the form of a pulse wave, and thus it was possible to measure both systolic and diastolic pressures with each heart beat. Damping was reduced by making sure that there were no air bubbles in the transducer or in the arterial catheter. Mean pressures (i.e. average pressure in the artery with respect to time) were recorded directly, by abolishing the pulse wave with damping. Whenever possible an electrocardiogram was taken simultaneously. At first the recording was done with the baby flat in the incubator. This was followed by the baby in the sitting position for two minutes. The baby was then laid flat for two minutes. The blood pressure was then recorded for two minutes with the baby's head down at an inclination of 30°. If the baby cried during any of these observations the whole procedure was repeated. In a number of cases where it was not possible to keep the infant quiet with the head up or down the procedure was abandoned. Recordings were also done while the infant was being fed either by the bottle or the tube. In all these measurements the transducer was kept at the level of the infant's heart. All the recordings were done before the age of 24 hours and in most of the cases it was between 6 to 18 hours after birth.

A total of 43 infants was studied (Table 1). 15 of them weighed more than 2,500 g. Of these 15 infants, 6 were of diabetic mothers, 3 had respiratory distress syndrome, 2 had severe perinatal anoxia with convulsions, and the other 4 had haemolytic disease of the newborn. The blood pressure in the latter 4 was recorded during an exchange transfusion (done via the umbilical vein). The babies of diabetic mothers were not hypoglycaemic at the time of recording the blood pressure. The remaining 28 infants weighed less than 2,500 g. These are divided into those that weighed 1,501-2,500 g. and those that weighed less than 1,500 g. These two groups were further subdivided into infants small for their gestation (i.e. arbitrarily defined as those weighing 750 g. or more below the mean for their gestation) and infants within the normal weight range. Some of the infants referred to as normal in both Tables had blood glucose concentrations of less than 20 mg./100 ml. at some time during the neonatal period though not at the time when the blood pressure was recorded.

Results are shown in Table 2.

**Infants of Birth Weight More than 2,500 g.** Infants of diabetic mothers had an average blood pressure of 71/48 mm. Hg when lying flat, which rose to 80/57 mm. Hg when sitting up and fell to 65/44 mm. Hg with head down. The mean pressure when flat was 58 mm. Hg. During feeding the blood pressure rose to 78/56 mm. Hg and during crying it rose to 92/53 mm. Hg.

The average blood pressure (63/45 mm. Hg) in the infants with respiratory distress syndrome was less than the above-mentioned infants. Again there was a rise in blood pressure with raising the head (68/46 mm. Hg), feeding (72/52 mm. Hg), and crying (80/50 mm. Hg). There was a fall in blood pressure with lowering the head (55/40 mm. Hg). The mean blood pressure when flat was 49 mm. Hg. The two infants with convulsions due to perinatal anoxia behaved similarly.

Blood pressure recordings during exchange transfusion (Fig. 8) showed that the blood pressure dropped when the blood was withdrawn and it rose when blood was injected. The average rise or fall in systolic blood pressure on injecting or withdrawing 20 ml. of blood was 8 mm. Hg, but on many occasions much higher rises or falls (up to 15 mm. Hg) were noted. Changes in diastolic blood pressure were of a lesser magnitude, the average being 6 mm. Hg, though at times there was a rise or fall of 10 mm. Hg. It was noted also that this change in blood pressure was less often seen towards the end of an exchange transfusion suggesting that the circulation was becoming adjusted to the rapid changes in blood volume (Fig. 8).

**Infants of Birth Weight 1,501-2,500 g.** The 'normal' babies in this group had similar blood pressure readings to the infants of diabetic mothers weighing more than 2,500 g. Thus their blood pressure when flat was 70/46 with a mean blood pressure of 60 mm. Hg. This rose to 75/57 mm. Hg when sitting up, 86/46 mm. Hg when feeding, and 93/51 mm. Hg when crying. It fell to 65/44 mm. Hg when the head was lowered. There was no significant change in the blood pressure of one infant during a tube feed. Babies with respiratory distress syndrome also showed no significant change from those babies with the respiratory distress syndrome

TABLE 1

CLINICAL CONDITION OF BABIES WHOSE UMBILICAL ARTERIAL BLOOD PRESSURE WAS RECORDED

| Patient | | Number |
|---|---|---|
| *Birth weight more than* 2,500 *g.* | | |
| Infants of diabetic mothers | | 6 |
| Infants with respiratory distress syndrome (RDS) | | 3 |
| Infants with fits due to perinatal anoxia | | 2 |
| Infants with haemolytic disease of the newborn | | 4 |
| *Birth weight* 1,501-2,500 *g.* | | |
| Small for gestation: | 'Normal'* | 5 |
| | RDS | 5 |
| Normal weight for gestation: | RDS | 6 |
| *Birth weight less than* 1,500 *g.* | | |
| Small for gestation: | 'Normal'* | 2 |
| | RDS | 2 |
| Normal weight for gestation: | RDS | 6 |
| | Cardiac arrest | 1 |
| | IVH | 1 |
| | Total | 43 |

* See text.
RDS = respiratory distress syndrome.
IVH = intraventricular haemorrhage.

weighing more than 2,500 g. (see Table 2). There was no difference in blood pressure between infants of normal weight for their gestation and those that were small for their gestation.

**Infants of Birth Weight Less than 1,500 g.** In contrast to infants weighing more than 1,500 g., these infants had a low blood pressure with an average of 66/43 mm. Hg when flat and a mean of 54 mm. Hg. They also showed a rise in blood pressure with crying and on sitting up. The blood pressure fell when the head was held low. Babies with the respiratory distress syndrome in this group similarly had low blood pressures compared with those weighing more than 1,500 g. with the respiratory distress syndrome. On tube feeding there was no change in the blood pressure except during the process of passing the tube if the baby struggled.

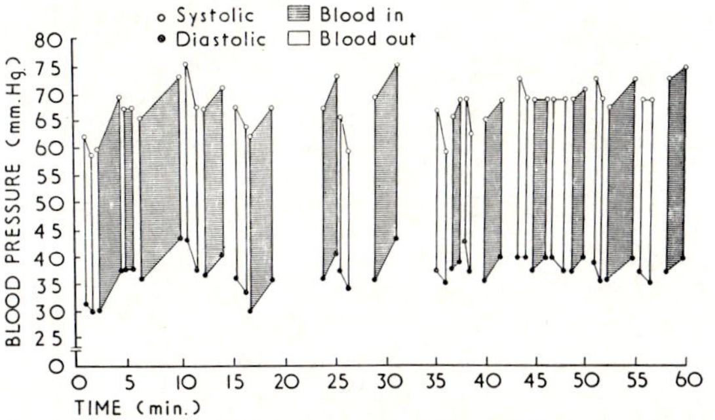


FIG. 8.—Direct blood pressure recording from umbilical artery during an exchange transfusion in a baby of 2,780 g. Open circles—systolic pressure. Closed circles—diastolic pressure. Shaded areas—during injection of 20 ml. blood. Unshaded areas—during withdrawal of 20 ml. blood.

TABLE 2

AVERAGES OF DIRECT ARTERIAL BLOOD PRESSURE MEASUREMENTS FROM UMBILICAL ARTERY

| Type of Patient | Blood Pressures (mm. Hg) | | | | | | |
|---|---|---|---|---|---|---|---|
| | Flat | Head up | Head down | Mean | Feed | Tube-feed | Crying |
| *Birth weight more than* 2,500 *g.* | | | | | | | |
| Infants of diabetic mothers .. | 71/48 | 80/57 | 65/44 | 58 | 78/56 | — | 92/53 |
| RDS .. .. .. .. | 63/45 | 68/46 | 55/40 | 49 | 72/52 | — | 80/50 |
| Fits due to perinatal anoxia .. | 62/39 | 63/43 | 58/35 | 51 | — | — | — |
| *Birth weight* 1,501-2,500 *g.* | | | | | | | |
| Small for gestation: 'Normal'* | 70/46 | 75/57 | 65/44 | 60 | 86/46 | — | 93/51 |
| RDS .. | 61/36 | 64/38 | 54/30 | 46 | 75/55 | — | 67/32 |
| Normal for gestation: RDS .. | 62/39 | 67/47 | 60/35 | 46 | — | — | 64/46 |
| *Birth weight less than* 1,500 *g.* | | | | | | | |
| Small for gestation: 'Normal'* | 66/43 | 73/49 | 66/43 | 54 | — | — | 75/50 |
| RDS .. | 51/33 | 58/46 | — | 41 | — | 48/34 | 66/39 |
| Normal for gestation: RDS .. | 50/30 | 58/38 | 40/20 | 39 | — | — | — |

* See text.

There was no change in blood pressure with the different periods of respiration in one infant with periodic breathing.

Fig. 9 shows the effect of external cardiac massage in an infant who had cardiac arrest following an apnoeic attack. The external cardiac massage always produced a large pulse wave. Following the cardiac massage the heart began to beat spontaneously and the blood pressure, which was unrecordable previously, rose to 44/32 mm. Hg.

## Discussion

A striking feature of the blood pressure of newborn babies is its variability (Figs. 2, 6, and 7), a fact that impinges on its use as a clinical measurement of any value. For instance, like Moss, Duffie, and Emmanouilides (1963) but unlike Young and Holland (1958), we found that crying, even in the first day of life, produced a large rise in both systolic and diastolic pressures (Table 2). Apart from the inaccuracies inherent in inadequate attention to technical details such as cuff size and pulse detection, a single estimation of blood pressure is clearly inadequate unless proper attention is given to ensuring that the child is quiet and comfortable during the examination. A continuous recorder has the advantage that a basal level is clearly seen after an hour or two of recording, a procedure that would be too time consuming for ordinary clinical use.

The rise in blood pressure during feeding is

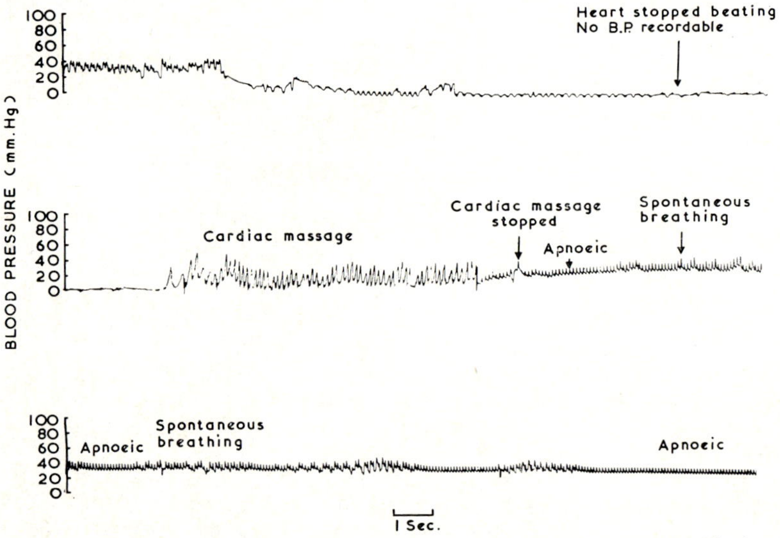


FIG. 9.—Direct blood pressure recording from umbilical artery in a baby during an episode of cardiac arrest. The three lines of tracing are in chronological order but the time scale is not continuous.

particularly obvious. It is a fairly common practice to measure a baby's blood pressure during a feed, because then the child is comparatively quiet. It is clear from our data that such a practice will not give a 'basal' blood pressure. It certainly appears that sucking, tilting, and 'arousal' contribute to this rise in blood pressure.

Tilting up a baby increases noradrenaline output (Greenberg, Lind, and von Euler, 1960) and sucking may also do so. Hakulinen, Hirvonen, and Peltonen (1962) found a rise in blood pressure during sucking and attributed it to the physical work involved, but it might equally well be a consequence of emotional excitement engendered by feeding. The rise in blood pressure provides one very good reason for feeding babies in cardiac difficulty by gavage.

The absence of a circadian rhythm is an interesting finding. Most normal babies are showing a circadian rhythm in wakefulness, pulse rate, and body temperature by about 3-6 weeks (Hellbrugge, 1960). We did not examine normal babies of 1 month, and the absence of circadian rhythm in premature babies of 6 weeks could be due to their prematurity (Hellbrugge, 1960) or to the abnormal environment of a premature unit where attendants, artificial light, and feeds are available throughout the night.

The rhythmic changes observed were related to the artificial rhythm of feeds and the natural rhythm of sleep (Goldie, 1964). The rhythm can be disturbed by external stimuli, and in our experience babies in hospital, especially premature babies, seldom have many consecutive hours without interference such as physical examination, blood tests, weighing, nappy change, and other nursing procedures.

The absolute levels recorded by direct measurements are in general agreement with the findings of other workers (Rudolph, Drorbaugh, Auld, Rudolph, Nadas, Smith, and Hubbell, 1961; Moss *et al.*, 1963). There are, however, one or two interesting features. The blood pressures of babies between 1,500 and 2,500 g. are not materially different from those of bigger babies. In babies below 1,500 g. the blood pressure is, however, lower (Table 2), as it is in babies suffering from respiratory distress syndrome. The blood pressure of babies who are 'small for dates' is more clearly related to the weight of the baby rather than to its gestational age. In animals, the blood pressure at birth is related to length of gestation (Dawes, 1961) but there is no information about the 'small for dates' animal (runts) in his figures.

There are conflicting reports regarding the effect of posture on blood pressure. Young and Holland (1958), measuring blood pressure indirectly by palpation, reported that there was no change on tilting the baby in the first three days of life, but a rise in systolic pressure which was maintained for at least two minutes on tilting to the head-up position occurred after the third day. Moss *et al.* (1963), measuring blood pressure directly via the umbilical artery, showed a small immediate increase on tilting to a head-up position followed by a short drop in both systolic and diastolic pressures with a subsequent rapid (within 20 seconds) return to the pre-tilt level, and this occurred even in the first day of life. Our own observations showed that there was a rise in both systolic and diastolic pressures on tilting to the head-up position, which was maintained for at least two minutes. This occurred even during the first day of life and also in premature, sometimes ill, babies. Unlike Young, we also found a fall in blood pressure on tilting to the head down position.

External cardiac massage is of undoubted value in resuscitating asphyxiated newborn animals (Adamsons, Behrman, Dawes, James, and Koford, 1964) and babies (personal observation and Fig. 9). In one patient in whom blood pressure was being recorded, there was cardiac standstill. External cardiac massage produced a good pulse pressure and the heart began to beat spontaneously again (Fig. 9). This was followed by spontaneous respiration which can be seen on the tracing by the respiratory fluctuations in blood pressure. The magnitude of the pulse wave and the efficiency of the treatment are demonstrated by this tracing.

Babies with the respiratory distress syndrome were consistently found to have low blood pressures (systolic and diastolic) compared with 'normal' term and premature babies of similar birth weight. The

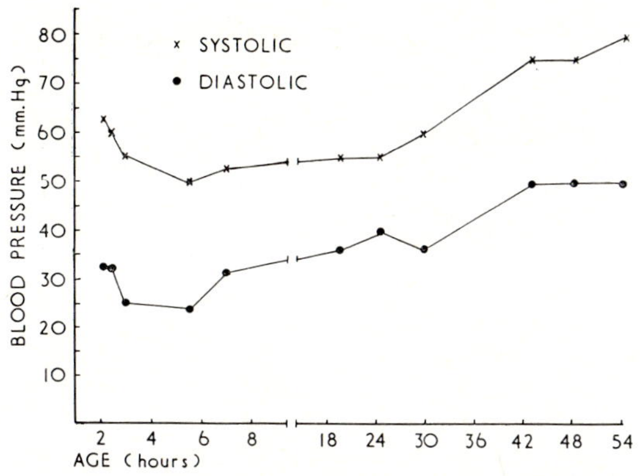


FIG. 10.—Direct blood pressure recording from the umbilical artery in a baby of 2,100 g. who developed and recovered from respiratory distress syndrome. All points plotted refer to records taken when the child was quiet. Note the discontinuous time scale.

fall in blood pressure coincided with the deterioration in the child's condition in the first hours of life. Subsequently, a steady rise occurred as the condition ameliorated (Fig. 10). A low systemic pressure in the presence of an open ductus arteriosus may well account for part of the right-to-left shunt known to occur in infants with severe respiratory distress (Strang and MacLeish, 1961; Warley and Gairdner, 1962). The low blood pressure in babies with respiratory distress has been reported by other authors (Neligan and Smith, 1960; Rudolph *et al.*, 1961).

Exchange transfusion produces large rapid fluctuations in blood pressure, though it is our practice to perform each individual manoeuvre slowly (e.g. two minutes to inject 20 ml. blood). The blood pressure, however, rapidly returned to 'basal' level if one stopped for a minute or two, and it was a common finding that towards the end of the procedure the fluctuations were less wide. This again suggests that vasomotor control at this age is far from inadequate.

**Summary**

An apparatus which automatically records blood pressure at 2-minute intervals in babies is described. The fluctuations and rhythms in a baby's blood pressure are demonstrated. Although there is no circadian rhythm in babies, there is a rhythm related to feeds. Feeding itself causes a large rise in blood pressure and the reasons for this rise are analysed. Direct arterial blood pressure readings from a number of babies are reported and analysed according to weight, gestation, and clinical condition. In 'small for dates' babies, the blood pressure is more closely related to the size of the baby than to his gestational age. The efficiency of external cardiac massage in producing a pulse pressure is demonstrated. The general contention that vasomotor regulatory mechanisms are functioning in babies is supported.

We are grateful to the trustees of the Sir William Coxen fund for equipment and laboratory facilities, and to the Nuffield Foundation and the Clothworkers Company for grants, which made this work possible. We also wish to thank Mr. J. E. Pallett, Dr. Gordon Ball, and Mr. K. T. Lanning for their invaluable help in the design and construction of the automatic recorder.

REFERENCES

Adamsons, K., Jr., Behrman, R., Dawes, G. S., James, L. S., and Koford, C. (1964). Resuscitation by positive pressure ventilation and trishydroxymethylaminomethane of rhesus monkeys asphyxiated at birth. *J. Pediat.*, **65**, 807.

Ashworth, A. M., Neligan, G. A., and Rogers, J. E. (1959). Sphygmomanometer for the newborn. *Lancet*, **1**, 801.

Ball, G. R., Pallett, J., and Shillingford, J. P. (1961). An automatic finger blood-pressure recorder. *ibid.*, **2**, 1178.

Dawes, G. S. (1961). Changes in the circulation at birth. *Brit. med. Bull.*, **17**, 148.

de Bono, E. F. (1963). A simple method of intra-arterial pressure measurement. *Lancet*, **1**, 1142.

Goldie, L. (1964). Innate sleep rhythms in newborn infants. Paper read at The Paediatric Research Society Meeting 20.3.64.

Greenberg, R. E., Lind, J., and von Euler, U. S. (1960). Effect of posture and insulin hypoglycemia on catecholamine excretion in the newborn. *Acta paediat. (Uppsala)*, **49**, 780.

Hakulinen, A., Hirvonen, L., and Peltonen, T. (1962). Response of blood presure to sucking and tilting in the newborn infant. *Ann. Paediat. Fenn.*, **8**, 56.

Hellbrugge, T. (1960). The developmert of circadian rhythms in infants. *Cold Spr. Harb. Symp. quant. Biol.*, **25**, 311.

Moss, A. J., Duffie, E. R., Jr., and Emmanouilides, G. (1963). Blood pressure and vasomotor reflexes in the newborn infant. *Pediatrics*, **32**, 175.

Neligan, G. A., and Smith, C. A. (1960). The blood pressure of newborn infants in asphyxial states and in hyaline membrane disease. *ibid.*, **26**, 735.

Pallett, J. E. (1962). A new transducer for recording finger pulsation. *J. sci. Instrum.*, **39**, 489.

Rudolph, A. M., Drorbaugh, J. E., Auld, P. A. M., Rudolph, A. J., Nadas, A. S., Smith, C. A., and Hubbell, J. P. (1961). Studies on the circulation in the neonatal period—the circulation in the respiratory distress syndrome. *Pediatrics*, **27**, 551.

Strang, L. B., and MacLeish, M. H. (1961). Ventilatory failure and right-to-left shunt in newborn infants with respiratory distress. *ibid.*, **28**, 17.

Warley, M. A., and Gairdner, D. (1962). Respiratory distress syndrome of the newborn—principles in treatment. *Arch. Dis. Childh.*, **37**, 455.

Young, I. M., and Holland, W. W. (1958). Some physiological responses of neonatal arterial blood pressure and pulse rate. *Brit. med. J.*, **2**, 276.

Young, M. (1961). Blood pressure in the newborn baby. *Brit. med. Bull.*, **17**, 154.

*Arch. Dis. Childh.*, 1965, **40**, 645.

# SERIAL ACID-BASE DETERMINATIONS IN NORMAL PREMATURE AND FULL-TERM INFANTS DURING THE FIRST 72 HOURS OF LIFE

BY

A. F. MALAN,* A. EVANS, and H. DE V. HEESE

*From the Neonatal Respiratory Unit, Department of Child Health, University of Cape Town*

(RECEIVED FOR PUBLICATION APRIL 5, 1965)

Considerable interest and research is centred on the acid-base homeostasis and on its disturbances in newborn infants. Most reports have concerned the acid-base status at birth and the changes during the first few hours of life (Oliver, Demis, and Bates, 1961; Weisbrot, James, Prince, Holaday, and Apgar, 1958; Fischer and Toussaint, 1963). Several authors have published values for normal infants at different ages (Reardon, Graham, Wilson, Baumann, Tsao, and Murayama, 1950; Graham and Wilson, 1954; Reardon, Baumann, and Haddad, 1960; Prod'hom, Levison, Cherry, Drorbaugh, Hubbell, and Smith, 1964; Kildeberg, 1964a, b), but only Reardon *et al.* (1960) have made a serial survey beyond the first 24 hours. It therefore seemed worth while to study the acid-base status on the same infants serially at predetermined times over a period of 72 hours. No such published data are available for premature infants. The opportunity also presented itself to re-evaluate the role of *p*H and $P_{CO_2}$ in infants with a respiratory frequency over 60/min. but without respiratory distress (Branning, 1942; Prod'hom *et al.*, 1964.

## Material and Methods

An unselected group of premature and full-term infants was studied in the Peninsula Maternity Hospital. The total number of infants was 36, of whom 20 were premature and 16 were full term. The series of estimations was largely completed on 17 of the premature and all the full-term infants. However, as only normal and healthy infants were to be considered, 3 premature babies who developed respiratory distress were excluded. Seven children were discharged between 48-72 hours and their final readings were, therefore, not obtained. The majority of the group studied were normal vertex deliveries, with 6 caesarean sections and 2 breech extractions, of which equal numbers were premature and full term. The decision as to maturity was made on birth weight alone. The average premature birth weight was 2·25 kg. and for full-term infants it was 3·09 kg. The premature group was not further subdivided because of the small number of cases below 2·0 kg. Premature babies were starved for the first 24 hours. They were then given two 5% dextrose water feeds followed by half-strength expressed breast milk (EBM). The strength of EBM was increased to 75% on the 3rd day. Full-term infants were given one or two 5% dextrose feeds at about 12 hours and then taken to the mothers for breast feeding. If the mother was not able to breast feed, e.g. after caesarean section, the infant then also received half-strength EBM which was increased to 75% on the 3rd day. In 15 premature and 6 full-term infants the respiratory rate was recorded every half-hour for the first 18 hours.

Arterialized capillary blood was collected from each infant at 2, 4, 6, 12, 24, 48, and 72 hours of age. Blood samples were taken from heel stabs after warming the foot for 15 minutes (Gambino, 1961). 224 acid-base values were immediately determined by means of the Astrup method (Siggaard Andersen, Engel, Jørgensen and Astrup, 1960). The *p*H and $P_{CO_2}$ were corrected for the temperature of the patient (Rosenthal, 1948; Siggaard Andersen, 1963): this was of importance, as some premature infants had subnormal temperatures. Care was taken to avoid crying before and during the procedure and we were successful on all but 12 of the 224 occasions. The collection of the blood and the determinations were carried out by two of the authors. Throughout the study there was good correlation between the findings of the two operators. Very good blood flow was obtained from these infants compared with experience in ill infants suffering from respiratory distress. Gandy, Grann, Cunningham, Adamsons, and James (1964) have drawn attention to this finding and to the necessity for warming the foot.

In all our calculations we used the standard chart and nomogram for adults according to Siggaard Andersen (1963) whose terminology has been adopted here.

* C.S.I.R. Senior Bursar, Department of Child Health, University of Cape Town.

TABLE 1

SUMMARY OF BLOOD VALUES AT VARIOUS AGES IN PREMATURE AND FULL-TERM INFANTS

| | Age (hr.) | Premature | | | Full-term | | |
|---|---|---|---|---|---|---|---|
| | | Mean | Standard Deviation | Range | Mean | Standard Deviation | Range |
| *p*H | 2 | 7·33 | 0·06 | 7·27-7·42 | 7·34 | 0·06 | 7·26-7·43 |
| | 4 | 7·35 | 0·04 | 7·28-7·42 | 7·38 | 0·04 | 7·33-7·46 |
| | 6 | 7·36 | 0·04 | 7·30-7·42 | 7·38 | 0·04 | 7·31-7·47 |
| | 12 | 7·38 | 0·03 | 7·33-7·44 | 7·40 | 0·03 | 7·33-7·46 |
| | 24 | 7·39 | 0·04 | 7·33-7·48 | 7·41 | 0·04 | 7·32-7·48 |
| | 48 | 7·37 | 0·05 | 7·29-7·46 | 7·42 | 0·05 | 7·31-7·50 |
| | 72 | 7·37 | 0·05 | 7·28-7·45 | 7·42 | 0·04 | 7·32-7·48 |
| $Pco_2$ (mm.Hg) | 2 | 42·8 | 6·8 | 31·7-52·0 | 41·4 | 8·8 | 24·5-60·0 |
| | 4 | 43·4 | 8·2 | 31·7-58·5 | 36·7 | 5·3 | 24·3-45·7 |
| | 6 | 40·9 | 9·6 | 29·5-60·5 | 36·5 | 3·6 | 27·5-42·0 |
| | 12 | 38·4 | 6·4 | 27·0-50·2 | 36·6 | 3·3 | 31·7-43·0 |
| | 24 | 35·8 | 4·0 | 27·6-43·0 | 34·9 | 4·0 | 28·5-43·0 |
| | 48 | 39·5 | 6·1 | 33·0-57·0 | 34·0 | 4·5 | 27·0-41·5 |
| | 72 | 36·8 | 5·2 | 29·0-45·0 | 35·5 | 5·4 | 25·0-46·0 |
| Base excess (mEq/l.) | 2 | − 3·7 | 2·9 | − 8·5 + 2·1 | − 3·8 | 2·4 | − 8·7 + 0·9 |
| | 4 | − 2·3 | 2·6 | − 6·6 + 2·9 | − 2·5 | 1·6 | − 5·9 + 0·9 |
| | 6 | − 2·1 | 3·0 | − 8·6 + 4·2 | − 2·5 | 1·8 | − 5·8 + 2·2 |
| | 12 | − 2·3 | 1·8 | − 6·1 + 0·3 | − 1·4 | 1·8 | − 4·5 + 4·0 |
| | 24 | − 2·6 | 1·8 | − 7·4 0 | − 1·4 | 1·8 | − 4·3 + 3·7 |
| | 48 | − 2·7 | 1·2 | − 7·5 + 0·6 | − 1·2 | 1·7 | − 5·3 + 2·0 |
| | 72 | − 3·3 | 2·9 | − 9·6 − 0·5 | − 0·8 | 2·4 | − 4·8 + 3·1 |
| Buffer base (mEq/l.) | 2 | 46·1 | 2·7 | 43·2-51·8 | 46·6 | 3·0 | 42·5-51·9 |
| | 4 | 47·8 | 3·0 | 44·0-53·2 | 47·5 | 1·8 | 45·0-51·2 |
| | 6 | 48·3 | 3·5 | 40·5-53·2 | 47·1 | 2·9 | 43·2-51·0 |
| | 12 | 46·7 | 2·7 | 41·1-50·3 | 47·6 | 2·6 | 44·4-53·0 |
| | 24 | 46·6 | 2·7 | 40·8-50·3 | 47·6 | 2·7 | 43·8-55·3 |
| | 48 | 46·2 | 2·8 | 41·8-51·0 | 47·8 | 3·2 | 39·6-51·5 |
| | 72 | 46·5 | 3·3 | 40·6-50·2 | 49·0 | 3·3 | 42·5-54·0 |
| Standard $HCO_3^-$ (mEq/l.) | 2 | 21·2 | 1·8 | 17·6-25·6 | 21·1 | 1·8 | 17·7-24·6 |
| | 4 | 22·2 | 2·2 | 19·2-26·2 | 22·0 | 1·3 | 19·7-24·6 |
| | 6 | 22·5 | 1·4 | 17·6-26·0 | 21·9 | 1·6 | 19·7-25·7 |
| | 12 | 22·1 | 1·6 | 19·4-24·2 | 22·9 | 1·7 | 21·3-27·2 |
| | 24 | 21·9 | 1·6 | 18·4-24·0 | 22·8 | 1·6 | 20·5-26·8 |
| | 48 | 21·9 | 1·7 | 18·4-24·4 | 23·0 | 1·6 | 19·9-25·5 |
| | 72 | 21·4 | 2·0 | 17·1-23·5 | 23·3 | 2·1 | 20·0-26·0 |
| Actual $HCO_3^-$ (mEq/l.) | 2 | 21·8 | 2·9 | 17·0-26·1 | 21·3 | 4·3 | 18·5-27·5 |
| | 4 | 22·9 | 3·7 | 17·0-30·5 | 21·4 | 1·4 | 18·0-23·4 |
| | 6 | 23·3 | 4·3 | 15·4-30·5 | 21·4 | 1·9 | 17·5-24·7 |
| | 12 | 21·7 | 2·6 | 17·2-26·0 | 22·1 | 2·0 | 19·5-27·4 |
| | 24 | 20·8 | 1·9 | 16·2-24·6 | 21·7 | 1·9 | 18·1-26·4 |
| | 48 | 21·6 | 1·6 | 17·6-24·6 | 21·3 | 2·0 | 19·4-26·0 |
| | 72 | 20·6 | 2·7 | 14·4-23·6 | 22·2 | 3·1 | 17·0-28·0 |

## Results

The values for *p*H, $Pco_2$, base excess, buffer base, standard bicarbonate, and actual bicarbonate at the times given above are summarized in Table 1.

The results of other authors are set out in Table 2. To enable a more direct comparison between the various studies, the relevant base excess has been calculated where not given. Fischer and Toussaint (1963) did not warm the foot before sampling, so that their figures are not strictly comparable. When allowances are made for different ages, methods of sampling, technique of determination, and calculations, the measurements of the present study approximate to those of other authors.

In Table 3 the comparative figures in premature infants with sustained respiratory rates (RR) over 60/min. (neonatal tachypnoea) and RR $< 60$ are set out. Neonatal tachypnoea is defined as a sustained RR $> 60$ for more than 3 hours in the absence of other signs of respiratory distress. 7 premature and 3 full-term infants fulfilled these criteria. Of the 7 prematures, 6 still had a RR $> 60$ at 12 hours. There was no significant difference between the two groups ($p > 0{\cdot}05$). This confirms the findings of Branning (1942) and Prod'hom *et al.* (1964). Nor could any correlation be found in the full-term infants between the RR and the acid-base values. Both groups had a similar distribution of acid-base status.

**Acid-base Distribution.** One of the objects was to study the acid-base changes in the same infant with relation to time. The changing patterns are demonstrated in Tables 4 and 5. We have again used the normal adult values and acid-base distribution as the basis of grouping (Siggaard Andersen,

TABLE 2
ACID-BASE VALUES REPORTED BY VARIOUS INVESTIGATORS

| Author | Infants | Age | Blood | *p*H | $P_{CO_2}$ (mm.Hg) | 'BE'* (mEq/l.) | Total $CO_2$ (mEq/l.) | BB† (mEq/l.) |
|---|---|---|---|---|---|---|---|---|
| Reardon *et al.* (1950) .. .. | 1·1-2·3 kg. | 1-65 day | Arterial | 7·31 | 39·0 | – 6·0 | 20·2 | |
| Graham and Wilson (1954) .. | > 2·4 kg. | 4-24 hr. | Capillary | 7·43 | 30·0 | – 2·8 | 19·9 | |
| Weisbrot *et al.* (1958) .. .. | > 2·5 kg. | 3 hr. | Arterial | 7·34 | 38·3 | – 4·6 | 21·87 | 43·94 |
| | | 24 hr. | Arterial | 7·408 | 33·6 | – 2·5 | 21·38 | 44·74 |
| Reardon *et al.* (1960) .. .. | Full-term | 1 hr. | Arterial | 7·30 | 39·1 | – 7·0 | 20·0 | 42·3 |
| | | 4 hr. | Arterial | 7·33 | 37·7 | – 5·7 | 20·7 | 44·3 |
| | | 24 hr. | Arterial | 7·38 | 33·4 | – 4·2 | 20·5 | 44·7 |
| | | 48 hr. | Arterial | 7·39 | 34·1 | – 3·4 | 21·1 | 45·0 |
| | | 72 hr. | Arterial | 7·38 | 34·8 | – 3·6 | 21·5 | 44·8 |
| | | 96 hr. | Arterial | 7·39 | 36·4 | – 2·3 | 22·5 | 46·0 |
| | Premature | 48 hr. | Arterial | 7·31 | 38·9 | – 6·3 | 20·3 | |
| Fischer and Toussaint (1963) .. | > 2·1 kg. | 24 hr. | Capillary | 7·28 | 35·5 | – 8·8 | | |
| Prod'hom *et al.* (1964) .. | IDM‡ | 4 hr. | Arterial | 7·37 | 40·0 | – 1·9 | 24·7 | |
| | | 24 hr. | Arterial | 7·43 | 36·0 | 0 | 23·8 | |
| Kildeberg (1964a) .. .. | <2·5 kg. | 0-7 day | Capillary | 7·37 | 37·7 | – 2·6 | 22·4 | 46·8 |
| | Full-term | 0-7 day | Capillary | 7·40 | 35·4 | – 1·94 | 22·3 | 49·0 |

* Base excess. † Buffer base. ‡ Infants of diabetic mothers.

TABLE 3
COMPARISON OF 15 PREMATURE INFANTS WITH AND WITHOUT NEONATAL TACHYPNOEA

| Age (hr.) | 7 Cases With Tachypnoea | | | | 8 Cases Without Tachypnoea | | |
|---|---|---|---|---|---|---|---|
| | No. with RR > 60 | *p*H | $P_{CO_2}$ (mm.Hg) | BE* (mEq/l.) | *p*H | $P_{CO_2}$ (mm.Hg) | BE* (mEq/l.) |
| 2 | 7 | 7·34 | 43·2 | – 3·2 | 7·30 | 42·8 | – 4·1 |
| 4 | 7 | 7·34 | 40·4 | – 2·2 | 7·35 | 43·2 | – 2·2 |
| 6 | 6 | 7·35 | 45·8 | – 1·1 | 7·36 | 42·1 | – 2·2 |
| 12 | 6 | 7·37 | 38·7 | – 2·9 | 7·37 | 39·5 | – 2·1 |

* Base excess.

TABLE 4
COURSE OF ACID-BASE STATUS IN 16 FULL-TERM INFANTS DURING FIRST 3 DAYS OF LIFE

| | Combined Acidosis | Respiratory Acidosis | Non-respiratory Acidosis | Normal | Respiratory Basosis |
|---|---|---|---|---|---|
| 2 hours .. .. .. | N | A G | C D E F I M | B K L O | H* |
| 4 hours .. .. .. | | | C D E F H L M N O | A B G I J K | |
| 6 hours .. .. .. | | | A H K M N O | B D E F G I J L P | C* |
| 12 hours .. .. .. | | | B C D M N P | A E F G I † K L | H O |
| 24 hours .. .. .. | | | F M N | B D E H I † L P | A C* G K* O |
| 48 hours .. .. .. | | | J M | A B D E G L P | C F H I K* |
| 72 hours .. .. .. | | | P | A B C † † H | I L* |

* Crying. † Non-respiratory basosis.

TABLE 5

COURSE OF ACID-BASE STATUS IN 16 PREMATURE INFANTS DURING FIRST 3 DAYS OF LIFE

| | Combined Acidosis | Respiratory Acidosis | Non-respiratory Acidosis | Normal | Respiratory Basosis |
|---|---|---|---|---|---|
| 2 hours .. .. .. | F<br>I<br>O P | A B<br>M | C D<br>E<br>J K L<br>N | G H | |
| 4 hours .. .. .. | F | A B<br>H<br>M O P | E<br>I J K L<br>N | C D<br>G | |
| 6 hours .. .. .. | | B<br>F H<br>O P | D<br>I J K<br>M N | A C<br>E G<br>L | |
| 12 hours .. .. .. | | B<br>F<br>M | A<br>G<br>J K<br>N O | C D<br>E<br>I<br>P | H*<br>L |
| 24 hours .. .. .. | | | A<br>E F G<br>I J K<br>O | B C D<br>H<br>L<br>P | M* N |
| 48 hours .. .. .. | I K | | A B C<br>E F<br>J<br>M | D<br>G H<br>L<br>N P | |
| 72 hours .. .. .. | | | A C<br>F<br>I K<br>M | B D<br>E<br>J<br>N P | L* |

* Crying.

1963). Each infant was designated by a letter of the alphabet and charted in the same position at each successive reading according to the acid-base status at that moment. It is, therefore, possible to follow individual infants as well as the over-all pattern. It is of interest to note that 9 of the 12 infants who were crying at the time of blood sampling were in respiratory basosis. These readings were not excluded from the study because it is not always possible to prevent crying in newborn infants, which can be regarded as part of the normal pattern.

(a) *Full-term Infants.* In this group, the striking finding is the normality of their acid-base status. Infants are born with a combined respiratory and non-respiratory acidosis. The full-term infants corrected this acidosis very rapidly and no respiratory acidosis persisted beyond 2 hours of life. Even the residual non-respiratory acidosis is of a minor degree and is virtually absent at 72 hours. These results are in accordance with Graham and Wilson (1954), Prod'hom *et al.* (1964), and Kildeberg (1964a). Weisbrot *et al.* (1958) and Reardon *et al.* (1960) found a greater degree of non-respiratory acidosis. The normal range forms the largest over-all group in Table 4. Seven infants had a respiratory basosis at some stage, usually after 24 hours. Reardon *et al.* (1960) found this in 18% of their infants. 3 infants were in mild non-respiratory basosis. Throughout the 72 hours the same infant tended to follow the same pattern, either of normality or of mild non-respiratory acidosis. This stability was very different from the premature group.

(b) *Premature Infants.* Some of the essential differences between premature and full-term infants are seen in Table 5. The wider scatter and greater degree of individual variation is in agreement with the findings of Reardon *et al.* (1950). Respiratory acidosis is much more persistent, and apparently healthy prematures often have quite high levels of $P_{CO_2}$. Kildeberg (1964a) has remarked on the same finding. Non-respiratory acidosis forms the largest single group, which is in accordance with all other published figures. At 72 hours there were still as many in the non-respiratory acidosis group as in the normal range. Only 2 premature infants showed a spontaneous respiratory basosis. Reardon *et al.* (1950) found no prematures with respiratory basosis. The two infants at 48 hours with combined acidosis underline the acid-base instability of the premature infant (Reardon *et al.*, 1950).

## Discussion

**Prematurity.** Because of the greater scatter of acid-base disturbances among premature infants, it would be of value in future to assess such variation according to gestational age. It is widely accepted that birth weight alone is not a reliable index of premature birth (Gruenwald, 1964). Some of our infants may well have been of low birth weight for age. Reardon *et al.* (1950), in their group of prematures between 1 and 65 days, found no statistical correlation of acid-base values to birth weight or age of sampling. It may well be that the greater degree of non-respiratory acidosis reported by them was due to the lower birth weights. On the other hand, their group would include infants with late non-respiratory acidosis developing after the first few weeks of life (Kildeberg, 1964b). In the present study the differences between the two groups are striking enough to indicate different populations.

The lowest mean base deficit was found at 6 hours corresponding to the highest standard bicarbonate levels. Whereas the standard bicarbonate levels in the full-term infants rose steadily with increasing age, those of the prematures appeared to fall again. This would be in keeping with their greater tendency to non-respiratory acidosis.

**Neonatal Tachypnoea.** Branning (1942) studied a group of acidotic (hyperpnoea) infants and found no difference between their acid-base status and that of 'normal' infants. Prod'hom *et al.* (1964) in their elegant study on infants of diabetic mothers (IDM), came to the conclusion that there was no difference in the *p*H, $PaCO_2$, and total ventilation between infants with RR of over 60/min. and those with a lower rate. These infants represent an extreme of the normal range with altered dead space/tidal volume ratios. The phenomenon of neonatal tachypnoea is more common in premature infants and may represent a form of structural immaturity. We agree entirely with other workers that a high RR alone is not indicative of respiratory distress. Our clinical experience with neonatal tachypnoea is to be the subject of a future publication.

**Carbon Dioxide Tension.** Contrary to the experience of others (Reardon *et al.*, 1960), little difference was found in this series in either the $Pco_2$ or *p*H of the premature and full-term groups at 2 hours. At 4 hours the premature infants showed a greater degree of hypoventilation. Our figures for $Pco_2$ correspond more closely to those of Prod'hom *et al.* (1964) than they do to other series, but this is probably the reflection of determination at different ages. Reardon *et al.* (1960) recorded their lowest $Pco_2$ values at 24 hours, and this corresponds to our premature group. The lowest value for full-term infants in the present series was found at 48 hours.

In all studies, the lowered $Pco_2$ of the full-term newborn and, to a lesser extent, premature infants is confirmed. The possible causes for this are discussed by Weisbrot *et al.* (1958). It is apparent from all the published data that the acid-base nomograms for adults are not entirely acceptable for the newborn and that allowance should be made for this (Oliver *et al.*, 1961; Prod'hom *et al.*, 1964). Sufficient data are, however, not available to define and delineate clearly the normal range of *p*H, $Pco_2$, base excess, and standard bicarbonate in the newborn premature and full-term infant.

**Caesarean Section.** There were not sufficient numbers in the present series to compare the acid-base status of infants delivered by different routes.

## Summary

Serial acid-base values for 17 premature and 16 full-term infants during the first 72 hours of life are presented. There is good agreement between the present study and comparable published data.

Premature infants have a more prolonged respiratory acidosis and a greater tendency towards non-respiratory acidosis. They exhibit a more variable and unstable acid-base pattern. No published reports of serial acid-base studies in premature infants are available for comparison.

Full-term infants are found to be in relatively normal and stable acid-base status; 37% have respiratory basosis at some time.

No correlation is found between neonatal tachypnoea (sustained respiratory rate $> 60$) and the acid-base status.

We wish to thank the Matron and staff of the Peninsula Maternity Hospital for their assistance and interest; Dr. A. W. Falconer, Medical Superintendent of the Peninsula Maternity Hospital for permission to publish; the Council for Scientific and Industrial Research for financial assistance; the Teaching Hospitals Staff Research Fund and the C. L. Herman Bequest Award for equipment used; Professor F. J. Ford for helpful criticism; and Mrs. O. M. Cartwright for her help in the preparation of this paper.

REFERENCES

Branning, W. S. (1942). The acid-base balance of premature infants. *J. clin. Invest.*, **21**, 101.

Fischer, W. M., and Toussaint, W. (1963). Über den Säure—Base-Haushalt beim Neugeborenen: Untersuchungen in den ersten Lebensminuten. *Arch. Gynäk.*, **199**, 182.

Gambino, S. R. (1961). Collection of capillary blood for simultaneous determinations of arterial pH, $CO_2$ content, $pCO_2$, and oxygen saturation. *Amer. J. clin. Path.*, **35**, 175.

Gandy, G., Grann, L., Cunningham, N., Adamsons, K., Jr., and James, L. S. (1964). The validity of pH and $Pco_2$ measurements in capillary samples in sick and healthy newborn infants. *Pediatrics*, **34**, 192.

Graham, B. D., and Wilson, J. L. (1954). Chemical control of respiration in newborn infants. *Amer. J. Dis. Child.*, **87**, 287.

Gruenwald, P. (1964). Infants of low birth weight among 5,000 deliveries. *Pediatrics*, **34**, 157.

Kildeberg, P. (1964a). Disturbances of hydrogen ion balance occurring in premature infants. I. Early types of acidosis. *Acta paediat.* (*Uppsala*), **53**, 505.

—— (1964b). Disturbance of hydrogen ion balance occurring in premature infants. II. Late metabolic acidosis. *ibid.*, **53**, 517.

Oliver, T. K., Jr., Demis, J. A., and Bates, G. D. (1961). Serial blood-gas tensions and acid-base balance during the first hour of life in human infants. *ibid.*, **50**, 346.

Prod'hom, L. S., Levison, H., Cherry, R. B., Drorbaugh, J. E., Hubbell, J. P., Jr., and Smith, C. A. (1964). Adjustment of ventilation, intrapulmonary gas exchange, and acid-base balance during the first day of life. *Pediatrics*, **33**, 682.

Reardon, H. S., Baumann, M. L., and Haddad, E. J. (1960). Chemical stimuli of respiration in the early neonatal period. *J. Pediat.*, **57**, 151.

——, Graham, B. D., Wilson, J. L., Baumann, M. L., Tsao, M. U., and Murayama, M. (1950). Studies of acid base equilibrium in premature infants. *Pediatrics*, **6**, 753.

Rosenthal, T. B. (1948). The effect of temperature on the *p*H of blood and plasma *in vitro*. *J. biol. Chem.*, **173**, 25.

Siggaard Andersen, O. (1963). The acid-base status of the blood. *Scand. J. clin. Lab. Invest.*. **15**, Suppl. 70.

——, Engel, K., Jørgensen, K., and Astrup, P. (1960). A micro method for determination of pH, carbon dioxide tension, base excess and standard bicarbonate in capillary blood. *ibid.*, **12**, 172.

Weisbrot, I. M., James, L. S., Prince, C. E., Holaday, D. A., and Apgar, V. (1958). Acid-base homeostasis of the newborn infant during the first 24 hours of life. *J. Pediat.*, **52**, 395.

*Arch. Dis. Childh.*, 1965, **40**, 651.

# EFFECT OF PENICILLAMINE ON SERUM IRON

BY

J. M. WALSHE and VALERIE PATSTON

*From the Department of Experimental Medicine, University of Cambridge, and the Biochemical Section, John Bonnett Clinical Laboratories, Addenbrooke's Hospital, Cambridge*

(RECEIVED FOR PUBLICATION MARCH 9, 1965)

In recent years there has been an increasing interest in toxic reactions to drugs, and a number of these have been reported following the treatment of Wilson's disease with penicillamine, particularly the D-L racemic mixture. Purified L-penicillamine has been shown to be a pyridoxine antimetabolite in rats (Kuchinskas and du Vigneaud, 1957; Kuchinskas, Hovarth, and du Vigneaud, 1957) and more recently evidence for this activity has been reported in man (Tu, Blackwell and Lee, 1963). The nephrotic syndrome and renal failure have also been reported following the use of D-L penicillamine (Adams, Goldman, Maxwell and Latta, 1964; Yonis and Karp, 1963) and also bone-marrow depression (Sternlieb and Scheinberg, 1964). Originally D-penicillamine was thought to be completely non-toxic but recently there have been suggestions that even this isomer, in large doses, can also act as a pyridoxine antagonist not only in rats* (Asatoor, 1964; Gibbs and Walshe, 1965) but also in man (Jaffe, Altman, and Merryman, 1964), though work in this laboratory (Gibbs and Walshe, 1965) does not support the latter observations. Surprisingly there has been little mention of the possible action of penicillamine depleting the body of other divalent cations besides copper, though zinc has received some attention (Schouwink, 1961). It has been shown that a significant fall in the serum copper occurs in patients with Wilson's disease after less than a year's treatment (J. M. Walshe, 1964, unpublished observations). Boulding mentioned the possibility of metal depletion (Boulding, 1961) and suggested that a 'trace metal cocktail' should be given weekly to all patients on maintenance doses of penicillamine. However, there are no published reports to suggest that this precept has been followed, and none of the reports on the use of penicillamine in the treatment of Wilson's disease have included any data on serum iron levels (Sternlieb and Scheinberg, 1964; Richmond, Rosenoer, Tompsett, Draper, and Simpson, 1964; Goldstein, Randall, Gross, Rosevear, and McGuckin, 1962; Walshe, 1960). We have therefore investigated the effect of maintenance doses of penicillamine, given to patients with Wilson's disease, on the concentration of serum iron, iron-binding capacity, and haemoglobin formation, and compared these with the changes in the serum copper and clinical status of the patients.

* Dose in rats was 300 mg./kg., equivalent to approximately 20 g./day for an adult patient.

## Material and Methods

Ten patients with Wilson's disease (3 male and 7 female) were selected because samples of their serum before the start of treatment were available in the deep freeze; all were clinically and biochemically typical of Wilson's disease and all had Kayser-Fleischer rings at the start of treatment. The mean duration of time between tests was 19·2 months.

Serum iron and iron-binding capacity were estimated by the methods of Ramsay (1957a, b) and serum copper by a modification of the dithiocarbamate method already described (Walshe, 1963). All patients received D-penicillamine in doses varying from 900 to 1,800 mg. daily.

## Results

The details are given in the accompanying Table. Briefly it can be seen that there was no significant change in the mean concentration of iron in the serum, or in the mean haemoglobin values. There was, however, a fall in the percentage saturation of the transferrin, which was due to a rise in the total iron-binding capacity of the sera from 377 μg./100 ml. to 479 μg./100 ml. Two patients call for special mention, J.Ba. and A.W. When J.Ba. was seen at one of her routine visits 29 months after she had started penicillamine treatment she was found to have severe hypervitaminosis D, with vomiting, weight loss, a raised blood urea, and polyuria, and this probably accounted for her low haemoglobin which rapidly returned to normal when the hypercalcaemia was controlled by vitamin D withdrawal

TABLE

SERUM IRON AND COPPER LEVELS AFTER PENICILLAMINE

| Subject | Age at First Test (yr.) | Sex | Months Between Tests | Penicil-lamine Dose (mg./day) | Serum Fe (µg./100 ml.) | | % Saturation of Transferrin | | Haemoglobin (g./100 ml.) | | Serum Cu (µg./100 ml.) | | Response to Treatment |
|---|---|---|---|---|---|---|---|---|---|---|---|---|---|
| L.H. | 10 | F | 4 | 1,000 | 136 | 109 | 83 | 30 | 11·1 | 12·5 | 42 | 28 | Symptom free |
| W.McC. | 42 | M | 7 | 1,350 | 138 | 114 | 42 | 25 | 14·8 | — | 50 | 20 | Symptom free |
| C.B. | 17 | F | 8 | 1,350 | 93 | 111 | 20 | 17 | 14·3 | 13·2 | 97 | 4 | Much improved |
| J.H. | 13 | F | 18 | 1,350 | 122 | 148 | 28 | 33 | 13·2 | 13·0 | 33 | 19 | Symptom free |
| N.Y. | 15 | F | 24 | 1,800 | 112 | 154 | 32 | 30 | — | 15·0 | 17 | 6 | Much improved |
| F.Ty. | 15 | F | 26 | 1,200 | 175 | 89 | 42 | 11 | 14·5 | 13·4 | 45 | 13 | Symptom free |
| A.K. | 14 | M | 27 | 900 | 147 | 100 | 40 | 23 | 13·2 | 14·0 | 32 | 17 | Much improved |
| H.L. | 15 | F | 28 | 1,350 | 111 | 102 | — | 26 | 12·7 | 14·0 | 38 | 17 | Symptom free |
| A.W. | 22 | M | 34 | 1,200 | 37 | 93 | 8 | 20 | — | 14·4 | 56 | 24 | Much improved |
| J.Ba. | 26 | F | 29 | 900 | 94 | 116 | 23 | 46 | 13·4 | 8·0 | 44 | 33 | Much improved |
| | | | 6 | 1,350 | — | 61 | — | 29 | — | 11·7 | — | 21 | |
| Means | | | 19·2 | 1,250 | 116·5 ± 11·8 | 108·8 ± 7·8 | 35·2 | 26·4 | 13·4 | 12·9 | 45·3 ± 6·67 | 18·4 ± 3·0 | |
| Normal range | | | | | 80-180 male<br>60-160 female | | 30-45 adult | | | | 90-150 | | |

and steroid therapy. The relatively rapid synthesis of haemoglobin in a patient with a history of prolonged vomiting, weight loss, and renal impairment may well have taxed the body stores of iron leading to the subsequent fall in the concentration of this metal in the serum to 61 µg./100 ml. 6 months later. During this time no iron preparation was given and penicillamine was continued at an increased dosage. The very low serum iron found in A.W. before the start of penicillamine could have been due to previous treatment with BAL but was more probably due to a chronic staphylococcal osteomyelitis of the spine which led to his admission to hospital. Again the serum iron levels returned to normal without additional iron treatment. Contrary to the apparent stability of the serum iron in the face of chelation therapy, there was a sharp and significant fall in the serum copper from 45·3 ± 6·7 µg./100 ml. to 18·4 ± 3·0 µg./100 ml. Corresponding with the fall in the serum copper there was a marked clinical improvement in all patients whether the symptoms were neurological (J.Ba., C.B., J.H., W.McC., H.L., A.K., A.W., and N.Y.) or hepatic (L.H. and F.T.).

## Discussion

These results leave little doubt that the serum iron and haemoglobin formation are not significantly affected by prolonged treatment with D-penicillamine, either in children, adolescents, or adults. In only one patient was there a fall in the concentration of serum iron to the lowest level of the normal range as determined by the method employed (60 to 160 µg./100 ml. for females), and in this case the clinical picture was obscured by moderately severe vitamin D intoxication. Similarly, except for this one patient, haemoglobin levels were also well maintained. There was, however, a fall in the percentage saturation of the transferrin due to a rise in the serum concentration of this protein. While this could have been an indication of slow progression of the liver lesion of Wilson's disease, it seems unlikely in view of the general clinical improvement of all the patients, even those presenting with liver damage. Corresponding with the clinical improvement there was a return to normal of the serum flocculation tests and transaminases. On the other hand all patients showed a progressive and highly significant fall in the serum copper levels, and these observations, taken in conjunction with findings of a fall in the serum caeruloplasmin reported elsewhere (Walshe, 1964), leave little doubt that this treatment is effective in depleting the abnormal body stores of copper which are found in this disease. Failure to achieve and maintain such a fall in the serum copper and caeruloplasmin (cf., Richmond *et al.*, 1964) probably means inadequate maintenance dosage of D-penicillamine and re-accumulation of excess copper stores. It is interesting that, as with iron, penicillamine does not appear to be able to deplete the body of copper for normal requirements of caeruloplasmin formation (Walshe, 1964) or in the formation of hair (Gibbs and Walshe, 1965). Thus the stability of iron stores for normal haemoglobin formation does not necessarily mean that the pathological accumulations which are found in haemochromatosis or haemosiderosis would necessarily be resistant to treatment with penicillamine. However, the therapeutic possibilities of penicillamine in these conditions seem to have attracted remarkably little attention, which is perhaps surprising as there is still no effective chelating agent for iron which is active when given by mouth (Gross, 1964).

## Summary

We have studied the effect of maintenance doses of D-penicillamine (mean 1,250 mg./day for 19·2 months) on the concentrations of serum iron and copper and on the haemoglobin values of 10 patients with Wilson's disease.

The mean serum iron before the start of treatment was 116·5 μg./100 ml. and after treatment it was 108 μg./100 ml. There was also a small fall in the level of haemoglobin from 13·4 to 12·9 g./100 ml.

There was a fall in the percentage saturation of the transferrin from 35·2 to 26·4% due to a rise in the total iron-binding capacity from 377 to 479 μg./100 ml.

There was a highly significant fall in the concentration of mean serum copper from 45·3 μg./100 ml. to 18·4 μg./100 ml., which corresponded with a marked clinical improvement in all cases.

It is concluded that D-penicillamine does not deplete essential body stores of iron.

We wish to thank all those physicians who have most generously allowed us to study patients under their care.

### References

Adams, D. A., Goldman, R., Maxwell, M. H., and Latta, H. (1964). Nephrotic syndrome associated with penicillamine therapy of Wilson's disease. *Amer. J. Med.*, **36**, 330.

Asatoor, A. M. (1964). Pyridoxine deficiency in the rat produced by D-penicillamine. *Nature (Lond.)*, **203**, 1382.

Boulding, J. E. (1961). Treatment of Wilson's disease with D-penicillamine. In *Wilson's Disease: Some Current Concepts*, ed. J. M. Walshe and J. N. Cumings, pp. 224-226. Blackwell, Oxford.

Gibbs, K., and Walshe, J. M. (1965). Copper content of hair in normal families and those with Wilson's disease. *J. med. Genet.*, **2**, 181.

Goldstein, N. P., Randall, R. V., Gross, J. B., Rosevear, J. W., and McGuckin, W. F. (1962). Treatment of Wilson's disease (hepatolenticular degeneration) with DL-penicillamine. *Neurology (Minneap.)*, **12**, 231.

Gross, F. (1964). *Iron Metabolism: an International Symposium.* Springer, Berlin.

Jaffe, I. A., Altman, K., and Merryman, P. (1964). The antipyridoxine effect of penicillamine in man. *J. clin. Invest.*, **43**, 1869.

Kuchinskas, E. J., and du Vigneaud, V. (1957). An increased vitamin $B_6$ requirement in the rat on a diet containing L-penicillamine. *Arch. Biochem.*, **66**, 1.

——, Hovarth, A., and du Vigneaud, V. (1957). An anti-vitamin $B_6$ action of L-penicillamine. *ibid.*, **68**, 69.

Ramsay, W. N. M. (1957a). The determination of iron in blood plasma or serum. *Clin. chim. Acta*, **2**, 214.

—— (1957b). The determination of total iron-binding capacity of serum. *ibid.*, **2**, 221.

Richmond, J., Rosenoer, V. M., Tompsett, S. L., Draper, I., and Simpson, J. A. (1964). Hepato-lenticular degeneration (Wilson's disease) treated by penicillamine. *Brain*, **87**, 619.

Schouwink, G. (1961). *De Hepato-cerebrale Degeneratie.* G. W. Van der Wiel, Arnhem.

Sternlieb, I., and Scheinberg, I. H. (1964). Penicillamine therapy for hepatolenticular degeneration. *J. Amer. med. Ass.*, **189**, 748.

Tu, J., Blackwell, R. Q., and Lee, P.-F. (1963). DL-penicillamine as a cause of optic axial neuritis. *ibid.*, **185**, 83.

Walshe, J. M. (1960). Treatment of Wilson's disease with penicillamine. *Lancet*, **1**, 188.

—— (1963). Filterable and non-filterable serum copper. 1. The action of penicillamine. *Clin. Sci.*, **25**, 405.

—— (1964). Endogenous copper clearance in Wilson's disease: a study of the mode of action of penicillamine. *ibid.*, **26**, 461.

Yonis, I. Z., and Karp, M. (1963). Chelating agents in Wilson's disease. *Lancet*, **2**, 689.

*Arch. Dis. Childh.*, 1965, **40**, 654.

# FATAL HAEMOLYTIC URAEMIC SYNDROME AND IDIOPATHIC HYPERLIPAEMIA IN MONOZYGOTIC TWINS

BY

S. CAMPBELL and I. J. CARRÉ

*From the Department of Child Health, the Queen's University of Belfast, and the Royal Belfast Hospital for Sick Children*

(RECEIVED FOR PUBLICATION APRIL 20, 1965)

In 1932 Bürger and Grütz described a previously unrecognized disorder characterized by triglyceride hyperlipaemia with variable clinical features, including attacks of abdominal pain, xanthomatous skin lesions, and hepatosplenomegaly. This condition is now usually called 'idiopathic hyperlipaemia' (Hsia, 1959).

More recently, Gasser, Gautier, Steck, Siebenmann, and Oechslin (1955) have defined the haemolytic-uraemic syndrome in young children. The features of this condition are renal damage with uraemia, a haemolytic anaemia with fragmentation of red blood cells, and thrombocytopenia.

In this report we record the association of these two relatively rare conditions in monozygotic twins.

## Case Reports

Twin girls, the first children of young unrelated parents, were born in hospital on March 3, 1961. The mother was told the twins were identical; each weighed 4 lb. (1·8 kg.). The neonatal period was uneventful and they were discharged from the maternity hospital when 5½ lb. (2·5 kg.).

**Twin I.** On August 30, 1961, she was admitted to the Royal Belfast Hospital for Sick Children. She had been ill for 12 hours with a cough, vomiting, and rapid breathing. On examination her temperature was 102° F. (38·9° C.) due to a chest infection; this was treated with a 5-day course of sulphadimidine. The haemoglobin on admission was 8 g./100 ml.; 6 days later this had fallen to 6·2 g./100 ml. (Fig. 1).

By September 7, 8 days after admission, she had become extremely pale and was passing blood-stained urine. There was no evidence of oedema.

*Investigations.* Urinalysis showed albumin +++, red cells ++. There was no evidence of a urinary infection. Blood urea 120 mg./100 ml. Plasma proteins, total 4 g./100 ml.: albumin 2·06 g./100 ml., globulin 1·94 g./100 ml. ($\alpha_1$, 0·33; $\alpha_2$, 0·51; $\beta$, 0·51, $\gamma$, 0·59). Haemoglobin 3 g./100 ml. Red cells 1·2 × $10^6$/c.mm., PCV 12%, MCV 100 $\mu^3$, MCHC 25%, reticulocytes 27%, white cells 18,000/c.mm., mostly lymphocytes; platelet count 136,000/c.mm. Serum bilirubin 0·2 mg./100 ml. A blood film showed bizarre poikilocytosis with fragmentation of red cells and the presence of 'burr' forms (Fig. 2).

A blood transfusion of 100 ml. raised the haemoglobin to 6·4 g./100 ml. Within 5 days of the transfusion the haemoglobin had fallen to 4·8 g./100 ml., and the blood urea had risen to 156 mg./100 ml.; a second transfusion (130 ml.) was given, which raised the haemoglobin to 6·7 g./100 ml.

By September 21, the haemoglobin had fallen to 4·9 g./100 ml. and a third transfusion of 100 ml. was given. At this time the blood urea was 162 mg./100 ml. and a platelet count 88,000/c.mm.; her blood pressure was recorded as 150/95 mm.Hg. Following transfusion the haemoglobin rose to 8 g./100 ml. During the next week the child became very ill; she developed oedema and oliguria, a further rise in blood urea to 250 mg./100 ml., a severe acidosis ($CO_2$CP 7·5 mEq/l.), and a drop in haemoglobin to 4·9 g./100 ml. Resonium A was given rectally because of a rise in serum potassium to 7·5 mEq/l. She died suddenly on October 1.

**Twin II.** The other twin was admitted to hospital on September 11, 1961, 12 days after her sister (Fig. 1). She had been ill for two days with an upper respiratory tract infection and vomiting. Apart from pallor there were no abnormal clinical findings.

*Investigations.* Urinalysis showed albumin ++ with microscopic haematuria; there was no evidence of a urinary infection. Blood urea 87 mg./100 ml. Plasma proteins, total 4 g./100 ml.: albumin 2 g./100 ml., globulin 2 g./100 ml. ($\alpha_1$, 0·35, $\alpha_2$, 0·53, $\beta$, 0·59, $\gamma$, 0·53). Haemoglobin 4·2 g./100 ml. Red cells 1·5 × $10^6$/c.mm., PCV 16%, MCV 106 $\mu^3$, MCHC 26%, reticulocytes 12%, white cells 19,400/c.mm., platelets 88,000/c.mm. Serum bilirubin 0·2 mg./100 ml. A blood film showed the same bizarre poikilocytosis of the red cells as in Twin I.

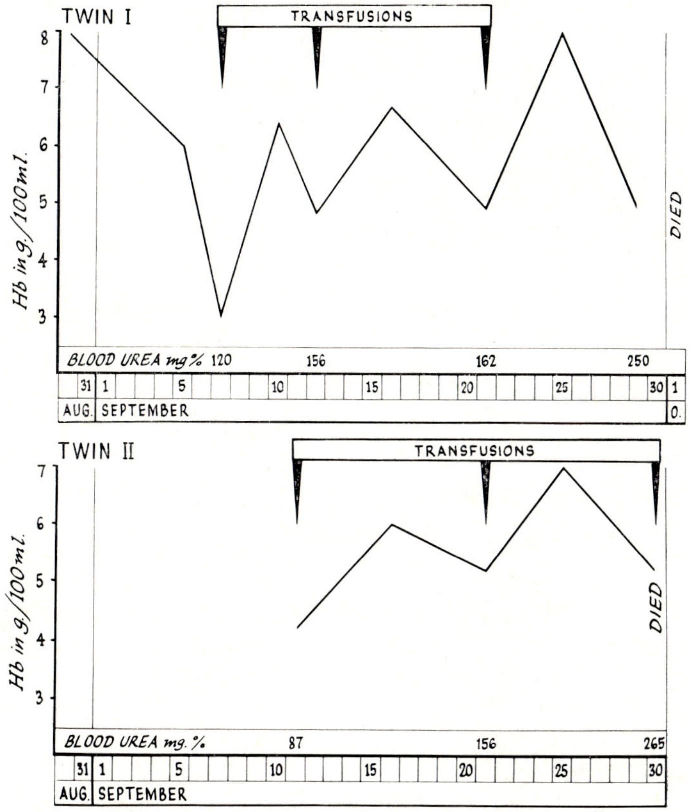


FIG. 1.—Summary of the terminal illness in twins I and II.

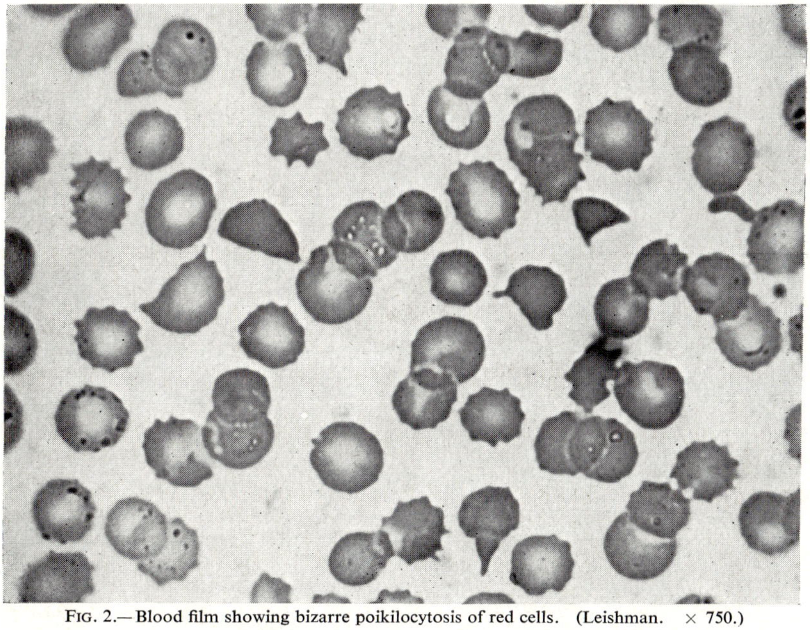

FIG. 2.—Blood film showing bizarre poikilocytosis of red cells. (Leishman. × 750.)

A blood transfusion (160 ml.) raised the haemoglobin to 6 g./100 ml.

By September 21, the haemoglobin had fallen to 5·2 g./100 ml. and the reticulocyte count had risen to 34%; her blood pressure was recorded as 200/150 mm.Hg and the blood urea as 156 mg./100 ml. A further transfusion (160 ml.) was given and the haemoglobin rose to 7 g./100 ml. Nine days after transfusion the haemoglobin had fallen to 5·2 g./100 ml. and the blood urea had risen to 265 mg./100 ml. She was given a third transfusion (100 ml.). She died the same evening.

**Comment**

No purpura, jaundice, xanthomata, hepatosplenomegaly, or retinal changes were noted in either twin during their illness. There was no history of drug therapy before admission to hospital. No evidence was obtained of a streptococcal infection. Except for a slight increase in red cell fragility, investigations aimed at defining a cause for the haemolytic anaemia in both babies were unrewarding: direct Coombs test was negative; no atypical red cell antibodies or abnormal haemoglobin were detected; no deficiency of glucose-6-phosphate dehydrogenase was demonstrated; the blood Wassermann reaction was negative.

Shortly after the admission to hospital of twin II it was noted that the serum of both infants was milky white. Biochemical estimation of serum lipids on pooled serum confirmed a marked increase in triglycerides associated with an increase in cholesterol and phospholipids (serum from each infant was inadvertently pooled before analysis). The fasting serum lipids of the father and of a sister born subsequent to the death of the twins were normal. Serum from the mother, who was symptom free, showed an increase in triglyceride, cholesterol, and phospholipid values (Table).

TABLE

SERUM LIPIDS OF FAMILY

| | Triglycerides (mEq/l.) | Cholesterol (mg./100 ml.) | Phospholipids (mg./100 ml.) |
|---|---|---|---|
| Normal range* | 2·78 ± 0·9 | 206 ± 26 | 241 ± 35 |
| Father .. .. .. | 2·21 | 172 | 183 |
| Mother .. .. .. | 8·38 | 280 | 324 |
| Twins' pooled serum .. | 52·09 | 354 | 552 |
| Sister .. .. .. | 0·68 | 94 | 132 |

* Normal range for methods used (Hayes and Neill, 1964).

No information was available regarding the placenta or foetal membranes. However, the results of blood group typing on the twins supported the statement made to the mother while in the maternity hospital that the babies were identical twins; no differences were found in the ABO, Rhesus, MN, S, P, Kell, Cellano, Lewis and Duffy blood groups.

**Pathology.** Permission was obtained for a limited examination only. Necropsy findings were the same in the two children. The pancreas, heart, and coronary vessels showed no abnormality. Fatty globules were present in the alveolar wall capillaries of the lungs, and in some liver and Kupffer cells, though no great intracellular increase in fat was evident. In the spleen fine droplets of fat were seen in cells lining veins and sinuses. There was no evidence of abnormal fat storage in the bone-marrow.

The kidneys showed marked pathological changes. In both children they were swollen to about twice the normal size. The capsule stripped easily revealing a smooth surface with fine purple mottling.

Histologically, primitive glomeruli where present were normal. All the definitive glomeruli, however, were damaged. Some were enlarged with swollen individual capillary loops; many showed necrotic changes while others were atrophic. Many glomerular tufts were occluded by fibrin plugs. Tubular changes appeared to be mostly secondary to the glomerular damage. Some were atrophied and others dilated; many contained casts of protein and red cells. There was no histological evidence of infection or glomerulonephritis.

Staining with Scharlach R showed the glomerular tufts to be full of lipid contained within the glomerular capillaries (Fig. 3). Further staining with Smith-Dietrich stain suggested that some of this fatty material was phospholipid. Schultz stain for cholesterol was indefinite. In contrast with the glomerular findings there was very little lipid in the tubular epithelium.

The lipid in the kidneys was shown by biochemical analysis to be mainly cholesterol, the cholesterol content of the kidneys being four times greater than that of the kidneys of another child of the same age. On the other hand, there was no biochemical evidence of an increase in renal phospholipid or triglyceride content. These observations differ noticeably from the blood findings of a very high triglyceride level with only moderate increases in phospholipid and cholesterol values. We have no satisfactory explanation for these findings.

**Discussion**

The diagnosis of idiopathic hyperlipaemia in these 6-month-old monozygotic twins was made on the basis of a milky serum with the typical biochemical findings of a marked increase in serum triglycerides associated with a moderate increase in phospholipid and cholesterol levels. The disorder is thought to be transmitted by an autosomal recessive gene. The observations noted in our family agree with this explanation. The occurrence of the disease in both members of monozygotic twins would be expected. The finding of raised serum lipids in the mother points to her being a heterozygote carrier of the gene (Boggs, Hsia, Mais, and Bigler, 1957). On the other hand, the normal serum lipid levels recorded in the father do not rule out the heterozygote state, since fat loading tests may be necessary to unmask a carrier of the abnormal gene. These tests may show an abnormally high serum lipid or slow rate of clearance of chylomicrons from the plasma (Bialkin,

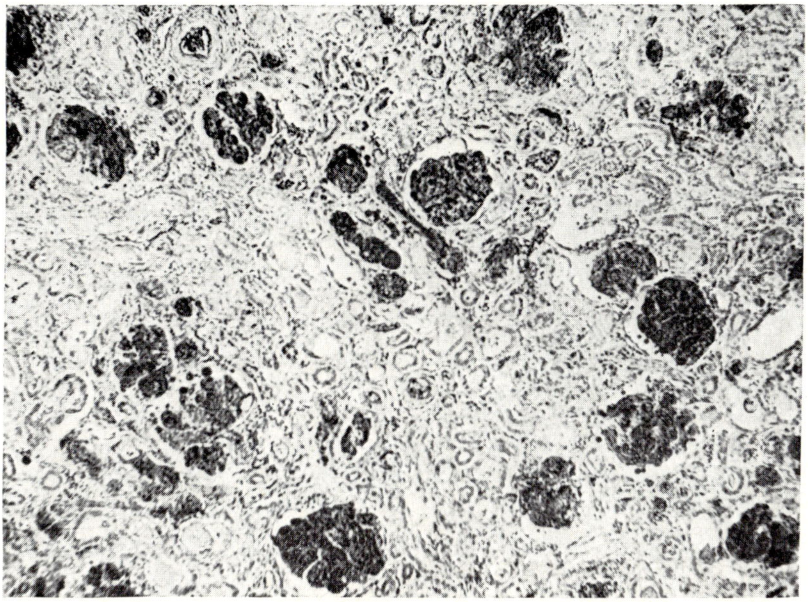

FIG. 3.—Lipid (stained black) in capillaries of renal glomeruli. (Scharlach R. × 60.)

Zucker, Sklarin, Hirschhorn, and Davidson, 1962). Unfortunately it proved impossible to carry out such studies on this family as permission for further investigation was refused by the parents and other relatives.

There have been few reports of idiopathic hyperlipaemia in childhood (Rausen and Adlersberg, 1961) and death in infancy seems to be exceedingly rare. Only two necropsy reports on young children have been traced. Chapman and Kinney (1941) described the post-mortem findings in a boy aged 21 months who was known to have had idiopathic hyperlipaemia: no adequate cause for his death was found. Baba and Volk (1964) reported the findings in a female infant aged 7 months who was dead on arrival at hospital. The diagnosis of idiopathic hyperlipaemia was made at necropsy. This infant died of an 'overwhelming pneumococcal septicaemia secondary to myelophthisic anaemia and leukopenia caused by replacement of the bone-marrow by severe deposition of lipids'.

The fatal malignant hyperlipaemia described by Hagberg, Hultquist, Svennerholm, and Voss (1964) in sibs of 9 and 15 weeks and by Lusher and Farber (1964) in a $4\frac{1}{2}$-month-old boy probably constitutes a different entity. The characteristic features of the disorder as described by Hagberg *et al.* were a familial occurrence, triglyceride hyperlipaemia, a clinical picture of acute reticuloendotheliosis with progressive pancytopenia and hepatosplenomegaly, and neutral fat-containing granuloma-like cell infiltrations in different organs. Hepatosplenomegaly, pancytopenia, and granulomatous infiltrations did not occur in our patients.

Although it is plain that the twins described in this report died from the haemolytic-uraemia syndrome, the relation of this disorder to their idiopathic hyperlipaemia is uncertain. Khachadurian and Obeid (1964) have recently reported a male patient of 35 years with idiopathic hyperlipaemia who, during crises of abdominal pain, had albuminuria. Clinical evidence of renal involvement does not seem to have been previously described and we have been unable to trace a single necropsy report of renal damage in this disease. In the two children with idiopathic hyperlipaemia reported by Chapman and Kinney (1941) and Baba and Volk (1964) the kidneys were recorded as normal.

The cause of the haemolytic-uraemic syndrome is unknown, though a viral aetiology has been suggested (Gianantonio, Vitacco, Mendilaharzu, Rutty, and Mendilaharzu, 1964). Reported necropsy findings in the kidneys of children dying from this condition have varied widely. However, a striking feature in many has been widespread patchy glomerular damage characterized by intracapillary thrombi and necrosis (Alison, 1957; Gianantonio *et al.*, 1964; Shinton, Galpine, Kendall, and Williams, 1964).

With so little known regarding the pathogenesis of the haemolytic-uraemic syndrome we can only speculate on the course of events in our patients. The terminal illness in each twin started with an upper respiratory infection, of probable viral aetiology. It is tempting to postulate glomerular damage occurring in association with this infection with lipid being subsequently deposited in damaged glomerular capillaries due to the coincidental existence of idiopathic hyperlipaemia. This deposition of lipid may well have converted a potentially reversible renal disorder into an irreversible one. An alternative explanation, though in our opinion a less likely one, is that glomerular capillaries were primarily occluded by lipid which secondarily resulted in the development of the haemolytic-uraemic syndrome. Either explanation would imply that idiopathic hyperlipaemia may not be as benign a disorder in children as is generally believed.

## Summary

Monozygotic twin girls with idiopathic hyperlipaemia who died with the haemolytic-uraemic syndrome at 6 months of age are reported. Serum lipid levels in the parents and a younger sister are recorded.

Histologically, glomerular tufts were shown to be full of lipid. It is postulated that this deposition of lipid occurred within damaged glomerular capillaries.

Attention is drawn to the fact that idiopathic hyperlipaemia may not be as benign a disease in childhood as is usually believed.

We wish to thank Dr. D. Carson for the pathology report and Dr. D. Hayes and Mr. D. W. Neill for the serum lipid estimations.

### References

Alison, A. C. (1957). Acute haemolytic anaemia with distortion and fragmentation of erythrocytes in children. *Brit. J. Haemat.*, **3**, 1.

Baba, N., and Volk, T. L. (1964). Idiopathic hyperlipemia. *Amer. J. Dis. Child.*, **108**, 633.

Bialkin, G., Zucker, S., Sklarin, B. S., Hirschhorn, K., and Davidson, M. (1962). A genetic and metabolic study of a family with hyperlipemia. *Pediatrics*, **29**, 566.

Boggs, J. D., Hsia, D. Y.-Y., Mais, R. F., and Bigler, J. A. (1957). The genetic mechanism of idiopathic hyperlipemia. *New Engl. J. Med.*, **257**, 1101.

Bürger, M., and Grütz, O. (1932). Über hepatosplenomegale Lipoidose mit xanthomatösen Veränderungen in Haut und Schleimhaut. *Arch. Derm. Syph. (Berl.)*, **166**, 542.

Chapman, F. D., and Kinney, T. D. (1941). Hyperlipemia: "idiopathic lipemia". *Amer. J. Dis. Child.*, **62**, 1014.

Gasser, C., Gautier, E., Steck, A., Siebenmann, R. E., and Oechslin, R. (1955). Hämolytisch-urämische Syndrome. Bilaterale Nierenrindennekrosen bei akuten erworbenen hämolytischen Anämien. *Schweiz. med. Wschr.*, **85**, 905.

Gianantonio, C., Vitacco, M., Mendilaharzu, F., Rutty, A., and Mendilaharzu, J. (1964). The hemolytic-uremic syndrome. *J. Pediat.*, **64**, 478.

Hagberg, B., Hultquist, G., Svennerholm, L., and Voss, H. (1964). Malignant hyperlipemia in infancy. *Amer. J. Dis. Child.*, **107**, 267.

Hayes, D., and Neill, D. W. (1964). Serum cholesterol and triglycerides in ischaemic heart disease. *Clin. Sci.*, **26**, 185.

Hsia, D. Y.-Y. (1959). *Inborn Errors of Metabolism.* Year Book Publishers, Chicago.

Khachadurian, A. K., and Obeid, A. I. (1964). Neuropathy in essential familial hyperlipaemia. *Lancet*, **2**, 911.

Lusher, J., and Farber, S. D. (1964). Another case of malignant hyperlipemia in infancy? *Amer. J. Dis. Child.*, **108**, 211.

Rausen, A. R., and Adlersberg, D. (1961). Idiopathic (hereditary) hyperlipemia and hypercholesteremia in children. *Pediatrics*, **28**, 276.

Shinton, N. K., Galpine, J. F., Kendall, A. C., and Williams, H. Parry (1964). Haemolytic anaemia with acute renal disease. *Arch. Dis. Childh.*, **39**, 455.

*Arch. Dis. Childh.*, 1965, **40**, 659.

# NEPHROSIS: A CLINICAL AND HISTOLOGICAL STUDY OF 38 CHILDREN

BY

R. McLAREN TODD and M. J. BOUTON
*From the Department of Child Health, Liverpool University, and Alder Hey Children's Hospital, Liverpool*

(RECEIVED FOR PUBLICATION MARCH 29, 1965)

Many attempts have been made to classify renal diseases in general and glomerulonephritis in particular since Richard Bright (1836) reported his classical researches into the clinical and pathological changes in his patients suffering from kidney disease. The word *nephrosis* was coined by Müller (1905) to define a clinical condition characterized by oedema, albuminuria, and hypoproteinaemia. Volhard and Fahr (1914) classified Bright's disease into three groups, (A) nephrosis, (B) nephritis, and (C) arteriosclerosis. The best known classification in this country is that of Ellis (1942) who divided nephritis into types 1 and 2: its great merit was that it attempted to correlate clinical features with histological changes. In our experience, however, it is often impossible to divide renal lesions into these two types, for there are often transitions from one type to another, and even the correlation between histological features and clinical findings is poor. The attempts by Dodge, Daeschner, Rosenberg, Brennan, Travis, and Hopps (1962) to introduce modifications of the Ellis system only lead to further confusion, especially when comparing their results with those of other workers. We have, therefore, come to the conclusion that the only helpful classification of nephritis is one based on descriptive morphology; in our experience this classification is of considerable help in prognosis, though it might not be of as much assistance in unravelling the aetiology of this group of diseases. It is likely that the kidney responds in much the same way to a variety of insults, but some of the changes may be permanent, some may develop slowly over a period of years, some may be progressive, and yet others may resolve completely. We believe that renal biopsy may be of considerable help in prognosis by providing evidence of the types of changes occurring in the kidney.

The patients we have studied have all shown clinical evidence of nephrosis. We apply this term to patients presenting a characteristic group of symptoms, signs, and biochemical features, i.e. oedema, albuminuria, hypoproteinaemia, and hypercholesterolaemia; all are often of insidious onset and vary in degree over a period of years. This clinical view of nephrosis is well described by Kramer, Goldman, and Cason (1952), who add that nephrosis occupies a position shared by few diseases in medicine: its aetiology is unknown, its course unpredictable, its prognosis uncertain, and its treatment unsatisfactory.

Over the past decade knowledge of the natural history of nephrosis has increased, due in no small measure to the improved biochemical and histological techniques which have been employed, and treatment has been more satisfactory since corticosteroids became available. It is our purpose in presenting the clinical, biochemical, and histological features of 38 children suffering from nephrosis to suggest that a more accurate diagnosis is possible, a more valid prognosis can be made, and the response to corticosteroids can be predicted.

## Clinical Features

The patients were all seen at Alder Hey Children's Hospital, Liverpool; 25 were boys and 13 were girls. The age at onset of the illness varied from 14 months to 13½ years, but as is shown in Fig. 1, 25 of the children were below the age of 6 years when first admitted to hospital; they have been followed up in the out-patient department for periods up to 10 years. The illness did not have a seasonal incidence and was not more common in the winter months when respiratory infections were prevalent, the onset of symptoms in half the patients being in the months of October to March and in the other half from April to September. There was, however, a history of pyrexial illness within 1 month of the onset of nephrosis in 27 of the 38 patients; 24 of them gave a history of a cold, tonsillitis, or otitis, 2 of them had

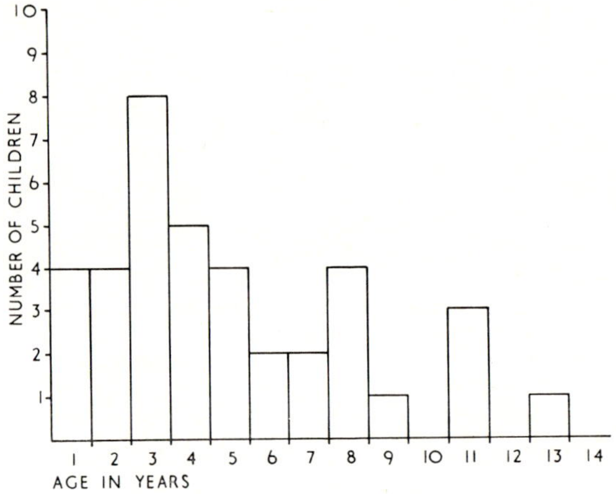


FIG. 1.—Age distribution of 38 children suffering from nephrosis.

recently recovered from gastro-enteritis, and 1 had suffered from boils.

The *presenting symptoms* were oedema in 36 patients, pallor in 17, abdominal pain in 11, vomiting in 7, and a rash in 3.

At the initial *clinical examination* all patients except 2 had oedema of variable degree: in 3 patients it was minimal, i.e. slight puffiness of the eyelids; in 13 it was moderate, i.e. pitting oedema of shins or feet; and in 20 it was severe, i.e. there were localized collections of fluid either in the peritoneal cavity, pleural cavity, or scrotum. Blood pressure was normal in 21 and raised in 17 patients. Albuminuria was present in all 38 patients: it was recorded as + in 5, ++ in 4, and +++ in 29 patients; red blood cells in excess of 10 per 1/6 field were present in 6 patients (Table 1).

### Investigations

*Throat swabs* were taken from 32 patients: in 27 no pathogenic organisms were grown, in 4 haemolytic streptococci were isolated, and in 1 *Haemophilus parainfluenzae* was isolated.

*Blood urea* was below 40 mg./100 ml. in all patients except 7, in whom it was between 40 and 50 mg./100 ml.

*Total serum protein* estimations and electrophoretic fractionations were carried out in all 38 patients and serum cholesterol values were measured in 34 patients. The total serum protein levels were subnormal in all except 2 patients; there was marked reduction in the levels of albumin, some reduction in $\gamma$-globulins, and an increase in $\alpha_2$-globulins. These changes are recorded in Fig. 2 and are related to the histological features obtained at renal biopsy. It will be seen that in the membranous type of nephrosis the total serum protein levels were not as low as in the other types, and the $\gamma$-globulin levels were normal or above normal in 4 of the 6 patients with membranous nephrosis.

*Renal biopsy* was performed in all 38 patients. Jungmann in 1924 was the first person to report his results of renal biopsies which were obtained during the course of abdominal operations. Percutaneous needle biopsy was first used by Nils Alwall of the University of Lund in 1944, but publication of his results was delayed until 1952. A relatively small amount of renal tissue is obtained by percutaneous biopsy, and the specimen may be torn or fragmented.

TABLE 1

DETAILS OF 38 CASES OF NEPHROSIS GROUPED ACCORDING TO RENAL HISTOLOGY

| | Proliferative | Membranous | Minimal | Mixed | Total |
|---|---|---|---|---|---|
| Number of patients | 20 | 6 | 8 | 4 | 38 |
| History of recent infection | 11 | 4 | 6 | 3 | 24 |
| *Haem. strep.* in throat | 2 | 1 | 1 | — | 4 |
| Oedema—minimal | 1 | 2 | — | — | 3 |
| moderate | 4 | 2 | 5 | 2 | 13 |
| severe | 14 | 1 | 3 | 2 | 20 |
| Albuminuria + | 2 | 1 | 2 | — | 5 |
| ++ | 2 | 1 | — | 1 | 4 |
| +++ | 16 | 4 | 6 | 3 | 29 |
| Urine—RBC over 10 per 1/6 field | — | 2 | — | 4 | 6 |
| Blood pressure—normal | 8 | 4 | 6 | 3 | 21 |
| raised | 12 | 2 | 2 | 1 | 17 |
| Blood urea < 40 mg./100 ml. | 15 | 6 | 6 | 4 | 31 |
| 40-50 mg./100 ml. | 5 | — | 2 | — | 7 |
| Blood cholesterol—normal | 5 | 2 | — | — | 7 |
| 240-350 mg./100 ml. | 7 | 2 | 2 | 2 | 13 |
| over 350 mg./100 ml. | 7 | 2 | 4 | 1 | 14 |
| not done | 1 | — | 2 | 1 | 4 |
| Deaths | 1 | 2 | — | 1 | 4 |
| Still active clinically | 2 | 2 | — | — | 4 |
| In remission—clinical | 1 | — | 1 | 2 | 4 |
| clinical and urine | 2 | — | 1 | — | 3 |
| clinical, urine, and biochemistry | 14* | 2† | 6 | 1 | 23 |

* Four off treatment. † One off treatment.

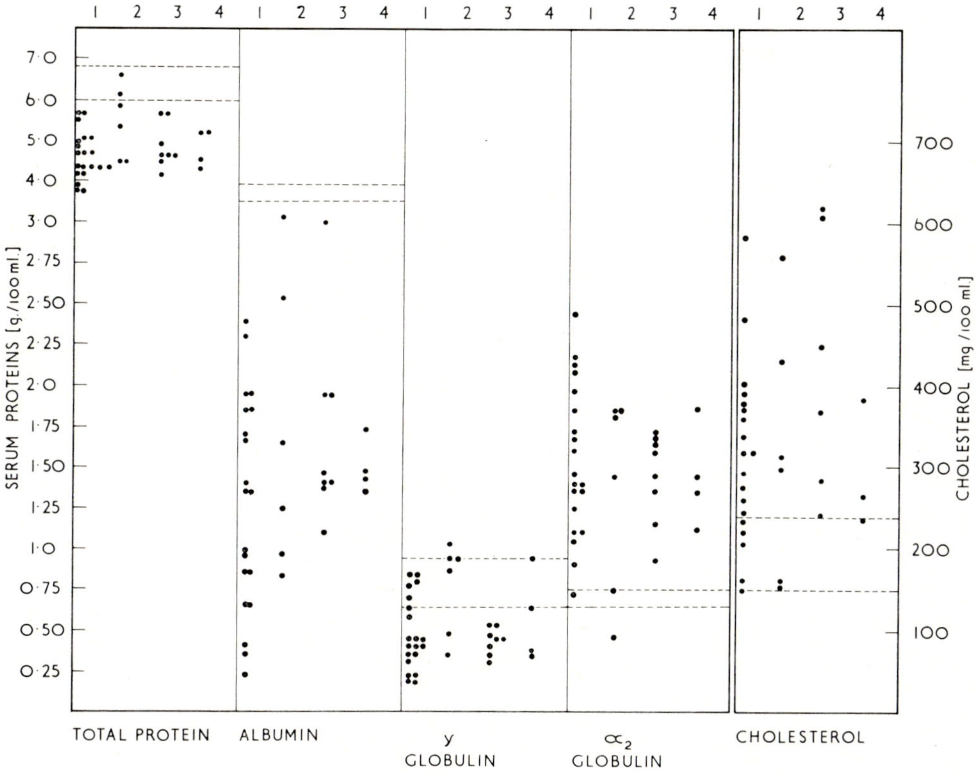


FIG. 2.—Serum proteins—total and fractional, and cholesterol levels in 38 cases of nephrosis grouped according to renal histology. (1) Proliferative. (2) Membranous. (3) Minimal. (4) Mixed. Broken lines indicate normal ranges.

It has been our practice to enlist the help of our surgical colleague, Mr. Herbert Johnston, to obtain a specimen of renal tissue by open biopsy. This entails a small incision in the loin not more than 1 in. (2·5 cm.) long, exposure of the kidney, and removal of 0·25 in. (0·6 cm.) cube of renal cortex under direct vision. The renal tissue contains 25 to 30 glomeruli per section, the specimen is not fragmented, and no serious complications have been observed. There was some delay in wound healing in a few patients who at the time of biopsy had massive oedema and who were already on treatment with corticosteroids. The histological features enabled us to divide the material into 4 types.

*Minimal proliferative.* This is probably identical with 'lipoid nephrosis'. The glomeruli show very little histological abnormality, but careful analysis will often show that there may be proliferation of nuclei in some of the glomeruli, or some reduction in the number of open capillary loops. They are filled by an eosinophilic material which probably represents a swelling of the mesangium.

*Proliferative.* All the changes described above are present but are more marked. The number of nuclei in the glomerular tuft is increased, but we have not found it possible to differentiate those of endothelial from those of epithelial origin. There is increased staining of the mesangium and the capillary lumen no longer appears patent. There is some rigidity of the basement membrane, which may be slightly thickened focally. There is diminution of the capsular space and synechiae are quite frequent. In a minority of cases there is proliferation of the cells lining Bowman's capsule, and crescents can be seen. We do not consider their presence to have any sinister significance, as implied by Ellis, but only that they indicate a more severe reaction. Nor could their frequency be correlated with the length of the disease process.

Periodic acid-Schiff staining reveals an increase in PAS-positive material in the tuft, which is mainly deposited like fibrils throughout the mesangium. They are probably the early stages of fibrillary scars. This group is very heterogeneous and probably contains aetiologically different diseases. It is not surprising, therefore, that it is this group that has given rise to most controversy, and has a less clear prognosis. But if it is remembered that the disease is in a state of 'flux' and can resolve or progress, much of the controversy is easily explained. In our experience with children the prognosis, as will be seen later, is good; but in adults the prognosis may be different (Kark, Pirani, Pollak, Muehrcke, and Blainey, 1958; Blainey, Brewer, Hardwicke, and Soothill, 1960).

Proliferative changes are sometimes focal, that is to say they are confined to one or two lobules of the glomerulus and often to only a few glomeruli. Although we have found these changes more often in patients who present with haematuria (Bouton and Todd—to be published), they also occur in some patients with the clinical and biochemical features of nephrosis.

This focal lesion is basically the same as that which occurs in Schönlein-Henoch purpura (Heptinstall, 1960), but when nephrotic features arise the glomerular lesion may become more generalized and epithelial crescents may be seen; it is still possible, however, to recognize focal scars in areas of focal lobular accentuation of proliferation, and differences between the glomeruli in the degree of involvement.

*Membranous.* This group is the easiest to recognize. Our criteria have been diffuse thickening of the basement membrane without any accompanying proliferation of nuclei. The thickening is usually marked and must not be confused with the rigidity which is often present in mainly proliferative cases. This thickening stains positively with PAS, but not infrequently the original basement membrane stains distinctly and the 'thickening' appears to consist of a material that has been deposited against the basement membrane, rather than a thickening of the original membrane. This type of lesion is permanent and can be progressive.

*Mixed.* It is not surprising that a number of cases show changes that are mainly proliferative in some glomeruli but mainly membranous in others. Two patients with clinical features of nephrosis also had evidence of Schönlein-Henoch purpura, and histological examination showed that mixed changes were present. They showed clinical improvement after prolonged steroid therapy, the serum proteins became normal, but a small amount of albumin persisted in the urine. It is pertinent here to point out that the proliferative changes in these patients and in other patients who did not have nephrosis were very marked, and included proliferation of extracapillary Bowman's membrane epithelium and numerous crescents. These changes were indistinguishable from those described in the so-called progressive form of Ellis type I subacute nephritis, and are further evidence that this classification is unworkable, as most of them have recovered clinically and have not yet developed chronic nephritis.

## Treatment

The main objectives in the treatment of our patients have been (i) to increase the level of serum proteins; (ii) to eliminate oedema; (iii) to prevent infections, especially those caused by pneumococci and streptococci; and (iv) to sustain the morale of patients and their parents in what is a long-term illness, often punctuated by exacerbations and remissions. We have attempted to achieve these objectives by the following four methods: (a) the provision of a high-protein, low-salt diet, supplemented in 3 patients by intravenous infusions of salt-free plasma; (b) the prophylactic use of penicillin given orally, in a dosage of 200,000 units twice daily, for a period of years; (c) the use of diuretics: hydrochlorothiazide was given to 9 patients, chlorothiazide to 6, spironolactone to 8, and frusemide to 1; and (d) the use of corticosteroids.

Prednisolone was the only corticosteroid given to 23 patients; in a further 9 patients it was given initially but changed to a water-soluble corticosteroid, e.g. prednisol, triamcinolone, because of lack of clinical response; in a further 3 patients prednisolone was given after a short course of ACTH, and in 3 patients corticosteroids other than prednisolone were given. The corticosteroid used reflected the preference of the paediatrician in charge of the patient, but prednisolone was usually preferred.

The initial dosage of prednisolone was 50 to 75 mg. daily and it was continued as a rule for 2 weeks until clinical response was obtained, and then gradually reduced over a period of 4 to 6 weeks to a maintenance dose of 7½ to 10 mg.; the maintenance dose was continued usually for years until the results of urine and blood analysis showed normality; in one patient prednisolone was discontinued after 10 weeks and during the subsequent 4 years he has not had a relapse either clinical or biochemical.

## Response to Treatment

Initial clinical response to steroid therapy occurred within a month in all patients except two, one with membranous changes and one with proliferative changes and necrotizing glomerulitis, and both these patients died. Relapse, indicated by recurrence of oedema and increase of albuminuria, was a common feature in all 4 groups. Relapse occurred on 58 occasions in 20 survivors in the *proliferative* group over an aggregate period of 91 patient years, i.e. an average of 1 relapse per patient every 18 months; in the *membranous* group of 6 patients, there were 2 deaths, 2 patients remained active clinically, 2 responded initially but 1 of them relapsed; in the *minimal* group there were 17 relapses in 8 patients in 31 years, i.e. 1 relapse per patient every 23 months; in the 4 patients showing *mixed* changes there was 1 death and relapse occurred in 2 of the survivors within 1 year of initial diagnosis.

*Complications* were observed in 3 patients; one patient developed osteoporosis of the spine after he had been on prednisolone for 4 years, and 2 patients developed pneumococcal peritonitis in spite of prophylactic penicillin therapy.

*Recovery* was judged by three criteria, namely clinical disappearance of oedema, cessation of albuminuria, and return to biochemical normality. Complete clinical, urinary, and biochemical recovery occurred in 14 patients in the *proliferative* group and 4 of these patients have stopped steroids; in a further 2 patients, clinical and urinary examination was negative but serum protein levels were not completely normal, and in 2 patients there was no oedema but albuminuria persisted and serum proteins were abnormal; 2 patients continued to have active clinical disease.

Complete recovery occurred in 2 of the 6 patients with *membranous* changes, 6 of 8 patients with *minimal* changes, and 1 of 3 patients with *mixed* changes. Death occurred in 4 of the 38 patients. One patient, a girl of 2 years, had proliferative changes with necrotizing glomerulitis: she was unresponsive to steroids and died in cardiac failure 5½ months after the onset of symptoms. The second death was in a girl aged 13½ years with membranous changes which failed to respond to steroids: she became hypertensive and died 18 months after the onset of the illness. The third death occurred in a boy aged 5 years with mixed changes, who was treated with steroids but who died 3 months after onset of symptoms. The fourth death occurred in a boy with membranous changes with a clinical history of 6 months' duration, who was unresponsive to steroids.

## Discussion

The main problems encountered in patients suffering from nephrosis are those concerned with (a) diagnosis, (b) treatment, and (c) prognosis.

(a) **Diagnosis**. Oedema, albuminuria, hypoproteinaemia, and hypercholesterolaemia are the clinical features of nephrosis, but these four abnormalities do not give any indication of the underlying cause. Kark *et al.* (1958) state that in adults there are 40 disease states which can produce nephrosis: in 46 of their 98 patients nephrosis was due to intrinsic renal disease, i.e. glomerulo-nephritis, but in others it was due to systemic diseases such as lupus erythematosus, amyloidosis, diabetes mellitus, Schönlein-Henoch purpura, drugs, e.g. mercury, gold, tridione, in which the renal involvement was but one element. Thus renal biopsy enables a more accurate diagnosis to be made.

Estimation of the levels of $\gamma$- and $\alpha_2$-globulins together with level of blood cholesterol may indicate whether membranous changes are present; in the membranous type $\gamma$-globulin may be above normal, $\alpha_2$-level may not be raised excessively, and cholesterol may be normal. In contrast, in patients showing proliferative changes at biopsy, the $\alpha_2$-level is raised often in excess of 1 g./100 ml., $\gamma$-globulin level is reduced and serum cholesterol level is often raised to 300 mg./100 ml. or more.

(b) **Treatment**. Many forms of therapy have been advocated for nephrosis; in their review of treatment used at the Children's Medical Center, Boston, Mass. during the years 1926 to 1948, Barness, Moll, and Janeway (1950) list 64 forms of treatment. There is general agreement that steroids have proved of considerable value in the treatment of nephrosis in childhood, and in most patients oedema disappears, and other clinical and biochemical changes indicate a favourable response to steroids. In adults, however, the outlook is not so favourable. Ross and Smith (1963) followed for a period of 5 years the progress of 26 adults treated with steroids; 4 responded by complete loss of proteinuria, in 7 proteinuria was reduced to less than 1 g. per litre, but in 15 patients failure to respond to steroids was reported. There are certain disadvantages in the prolonged use of steroids, such as stunting of growth, moon face, striae, osteoporosis, hypocalcaemia, and eye changes. Renal biopsy may be of help in deciding whether response to steroids is likely to occur; when proliferative changes are present, response to steroids usually occurs, but when membranous changes are already present it is unlikely that they will be influenced by steroids.

Relapses are frequently encountered in patients suffering with nephrosis and they are often provoked by certain infections. Respiratory tract infections will often be followed by reappearance of oedema and other signs of activity; when these infections are bacterial in origin, e.g. streptococcal, penicillin may be helpful in prophylaxis, but when epidemic viral infections are prevalent no form of chemoprophylaxis is of avail.

(c) **Prognosis.** It is extremely difficult in children suffering from nephrosis to give a direct answer to

TABLE 2

OUTCOME OF 590 CASES OF NEPHROSIS ACCORDING TO VARIOUS TYPES OF TREATMENT

| Author | Area | Date | No. of Patients | Well | | Active | | Deaths | |
|---|---|---|---|---|---|---|---|---|---|
| | | | | No. | % | No. | % | No. | % |
| Barness *et al.* (1950) .. | Boston, Mass. | 1926 to 1938 (pre-chemotherapy) | 40 | 17 | 42·5 | 6 | 15 | 17 | 42·5 |
| | | 1939 to 1942 (sulphonamides) | 32 | 9 | 28 | 2 | 7 | 21 | 65 |
| | | 1943 to 1948 (penicillin) | 64 | 18 | 28 | 17 | 27 | 29 | 45 |
| Schwarz, Kohn, and Weiner (1943) .. | New York | 1922 to 1942 | 40 | 12 | 30 | 6 | 15 | 22 | 55 |
| Lawson *et al.* (1960) .. | London | 1917 to 1938 (pre chemotherapy) | 78 | ?41 | 53 | — | — | ?37 | 47 |
| | | 1945 to 1957: no steroids | 62 | 33 | 53 | 9 | 15 | 20 | 32 |
| | | steroids | 40 | 16 | 40 | 6 | 15 | 18 | 45 |
| Arneil (1961) .. .. | Glasgow | 1929 to 1936 (low sodium diet, pre-sulphonamide) | 11 | 3 | 28 | 4 | 36 | 4 | 36 |
| | | 1937 to 1945 (sulphonamides) | 41 | 13 | 32 | 14 | 34 | 14 | 34 |
| | | 1946 to 1950 (penicillin, etc.) | 37 | 18 | 48 | 5 | 14 | 14 | 38 |
| | | 1951 to 1955 (cortisone, ACTH) | 53 | 26 | 42 | 18 | 39 | 9 | 19 |
| | | 1955 to 1957 (prednisolone) | 22 | 14 | 64 | 6 | 27 | 2 | 9 |
| Todd (1957) .. .. | Liverpool | 1948 to 1955 (50% given steroids) | 32 | 14 | 44 | 7 | 22 | 11 | 34 |
| Todd and Bouton (this investigation) .. | Liverpool | 1956 to 1964 (steroids) | 38 | 30 | 78 | 4 | 11 | 4 | 11 |
| | | | 590 | 264 | 44 | 104 | 18 | 222 | 38 |

the parents' request to indicate the probable course of the illness or its length, but certain factors are of considerable help in forming a prognostic judgement. A severe degree of oedema by no means indicates a bad prognosis, neither is prognosis worse if albuminuria is marked. In 6 patients red blood cells were present in the urine in excess of 10 per 1/6 field, and in many of these red cells exceeded 100 per 1/6 field, in 4 of these 6 patients there was either no response or a poor response to steroids; thus in our experience haematuria is a poor prognostic sign. Serum cholesterol levels were usually raised, but in 8 patients levels were normal; the response of all but 1 of these 8 patients to treatment was poor and suggests that estimation of the cholesterol level is of prognostic value. Blainey *et al.* (1960) in their study of nephrotic syndrome in adults found that the highest values for serum cholesterol were obtained in those patients who responded best to treatment.

Long-term follow up of patients suffering from nephrosis indicates the improved prognosis, as judged by mortality, resulting from the introduction first of sulphonamides and later of antibiotics; further improvement in prognosis has resulted from the introduction of steroids. Table 2 lists the results of treatment of 590 children suffering from nephrosis, and relates the results to the form of therapy used. The over-all mortality rate is 38% and the 'cure' rate 44%, using the term 'cure' for absence of clinical evidence of disease when assessed at least 3 years after the onset of the illness. Following the introduction of chemotherapeutic agents there was a slight improvement in prognosis, while with the introduction of steroids the mortality rate has been reduced by half and the 'cure' rate has increased. The percentage of deaths in the series of patients recorded in Table 2 was 45% before chemotherapy, 43% with chemotherapy but without steroids, and 21% with chemotherapy and steroids. The 'cure' rates in the three corresponding groups were 38%, 40%, and 54%. The only anomalous report is that from Great Ormond Street Children's Hospital (Lawson, Moncrieff, and Payne, 1960) in which the 'cure' rate without steroids was 53% and with steroids 40%, and the death rate 32% without steroids and 45% with steroids. In Alder Hey Children's Hospital, comparison of experience for 1948 to 1955 (Todd, 1957) with the present series (1956 to 1964) shows a reduction in mortality from 34% to 11% and an increase of 'cure' from 44% to 78%. There may well be an increase in the mortality rate and a decrease in the 'cure' rate as the follow-up period lengthens, but judging from our further observation of patients reported in 1957 (Todd) the cure rate should approach 70% after a minimum observation period of 3 years.

## Conclusions and Summary

The clinical and biochemical features and the histological appearances of the biopsied kidney have been studied in 38 children, varying in age from 14 months to 13½ years, who were suffering from nephrosis.

Renal biopsy has contributed to our knowledge of this illness in three main ways. First, it has led to a more accurate *diagnosis*, not only by excluding such diseases as lupus erythematosus, Schönlein-Henoch purpura, amyloidosis etc., but also by demonstrating the nature of the renal changes, whether proliferative or membranous, and their extent. Secondly, it has influenced *treatment*, steroid therapy being likely to be successful in patients showing proliferative changes, whereas the value of steroids is doubtful when membranous changes are already present. Thirdly, *prognosis* can be more accurate; in general, patients showing proliferative changes have a better prognosis, largely because of the value of steroids in a lesion which is potentially reversible, whereas the prognosis is poor in patients already showing membranous changes.

Alterations in the levels of serum proteins can be related to some extent to the histological picture. In the proliferative group, the total serum protein levels are often very reduced, and $\gamma$-globulin is low, whereas in the membranous group, the total serum proteins are not reduced so much, and $\gamma$-globulin level is often normal or even raised.

The long-term prognosis for nephrosis is discussed in the light of the published reports; it has improved considerably over the past 4 decades and the three-year 'cure' rate in children treated with antibiotics and steroids now approaches 70%.

We wish to thank all our colleagues for their help in this study, especially the Consultant Paediatricians for allowing us access to their patients, Mr. Herbert Johnston who performed the renal biopsies, and Mr. J. T. Ireland for the biochemical investigations.

## References

Alwall, N. (1952). Aspiration biopsy of the kidney. *Acta med. scand.*, **143**, 430.

Arneil, G. C. (1961). 164 children with nephrosis. *Lancet*, **2**, 1103.

Barness, L. A., Moll, G. H., and Janeway, C. A. (1950). Nephrotic syndrome. I. Natural history of the disease. *Pediatrics*, **5**, 486.

Blainey, J. D., Brewer, D. B., Hardwicke, J., and Soothill, J. F. (1960). The nephrotic syndrome. *Quart. J. Med.*, **29**, 235.

Bright, R. (1836). Cases and observations, illustrative of renal disease accompanied with the secretion of albuminous urine. *Guy's Hosp. Rep.*, **1**, 3838.

Dodge, W. F., Daeschner, C. W., Jr., Rosenberg, H. S., Brennan, J. C., Travis, L. B., and Hopps, H. C. (1962). Percutaneous renal biopsy in children. III. The nephrotic syndrome. *Pediatrics*, **30**, 459.

Ellis, A. (1942). Natural history of Bright's disease. *Lancet*, **1**, 1.

Heptinstall, R. H. (1960). Chapter 4. In *Recent Advances in Pathology*, 7th ed., ed. C. V. Harrison, p. 89. Churchill, London.

Jungmann, P. (1924). Über chronische Streptokokkeninfektionen. *Dtsch. med. Wschr.*, **50**, 71.

Kark, R. M., Pirani, C. L., Pollak, V. E., Muehrcke, R. C., and Blainey, J. D. (1958). The nephrotic syndrome in adults: a common disorder with many causes. *Ann. intern. Med.*, **49**, 751.

Kramer, B., Goldman, H., and Cason, L. (1952). The treatment of the nonedematous nephrotic child with ACTH. *J. Pediat.*, **41**, 792.

Lawson, D., Moncrieff, A., and Payne, W. W. (1960). Forty years of nephrosis in childhood. *Arch. Dis. Childh.*, **35**, 115.

Müller, F. (1905). Morbus Brightii. *Verh. dtsch. path. Ges.*, **9**, 64.

Ross, E. J., and Smith, J. F. (1963). The use of steroids in the treatment of the nephrotic syndrome in adults. *Quart. J. Med.*, **32**, 65.

Schwarz, H., Kohn, J. L., and Weiner, S. B. (1943). Lipid nephrosis. *Amer. J. Dis. Child.*, **65**, 355.

Todd, R. McL. (1957). The natural history of nephrosis. *Arch. Dis. Childh.*, **32**, 99.

Volhard, F., and Fahr, T. (1914). *Die Brightsche Nierenkrankheit*. Springer, Berlin.

*Arch. Dis. Childh.*, 1965, **40**, 666.

# EFFECT OF BLUE LIGHT ON HYPERBILIRUBINAEMIA

BY

P. M. G. BROUGHTON, E. J. R. ROSSITER, C. B. M. WARREN, G. GOULIS, and P. S. LORD

*From St. John's Hospital, Chelmsford; the Department of Medicine, Royal Free Hospital, London; and the Department of Chemical Pathology, University of Leeds*

(RECEIVED FOR PUBLICATION MARCH 25, 1965)

Neonatal hyperbilirubinaemia, of any cause, is potentially dangerous and may produce kernikterus. The standard method of treatment is by exchange transfusion, carried out as often as necessary to keep the serum bilirubin below an arbitrary danger level of between 20 and 30 mg./100 ml. There is, however, no clear evidence that any absolute value in serum bilirubin concentration *per se* constitutes a danger (Trolle, 1964). On the other hand it seems that certain additional factors, such as prematurity, asphyxia, and the respiratory distress syndrome, may potentiate the toxic action of bilirubin on brain cells (Wood, Culley, Waterhouse, and Powell, 1962). Exchange transfusion is not without risk and, as was suggested by Trolle (1964), the mortality rate from this method of treatment may exceed the incidence of kernikterus. A simpler and safer alternative is, therefore, desirable for cases that are not anaemic.

Cremer, Perryman, and Richards (1958) showed that in some cases of neonatal jaundice the serum bilirubin level could be reduced by exposure of the infant to sunlight or to an artificial blue light. Several groups of South American workers have described their experiences with this method of treatment (Ferreira, Cardim, and Mellone, 1960; Ferreira, Berezin, Barbieri and Larrubia, 1960a, b, c; Mellone, 1960; Peluffo, Beltran, Malinger, Giguens, Vila Vidal, and Lorenzo de Ibarreta, 1962), but it has not found general acceptance, mainly because of doubts as to its effectiveness and ignorance of the nature and possible toxicity of the products of the photochemical decomposition of bilirubin (Franklin, 1958; Blondheim, Zabriskie, and Lathrop, 1962b).

This paper records the results of *in vivo* and *in vitro* experiments which were designed to obtain more information about this method of treatment. Its effectiveness in lowering the serum bilirubin was investigated in a clinical trial on a group of infants with neonatal jaundice. Gunn rats have a similar unconjugated hyperbilirubinaemia, due to a deficiency of the enzyme glucuronyl transferase (Lathe and Walker, 1958), and the effect of blue light on their serum bilirubin levels was also studied. Signs of toxicity were looked for in both infants and rats. Ernster, Herlin, and Zetterström (1957) demonstrated that bilirubin uncoupled the oxidative phosphorylation of brain and liver mitochondria, and suggested that this was the basis of its toxicity. We have examined the possible toxicity of the photochemical decomposition products of bilirubin by studying their effect on oxidative phosphorylation. Biesold, Liebold, and Theile (1962) showed that, in the absence of soluble protein, uncoupling takes place at very low bilirubin concentrations. In order to match the conditions in the newborn infant, our experiments have been conducted in the presence of serum.

## Experimental

**Clinical Material and Methods.** The results of Cremer *et al.* (1958) and Perryman (personal communication) suggested that sunlight was more effective than artificial light in reducing serum bilirubin levels, but in Britain the former source is too unpredictable for a clinical trial. We have, therefore, used a light cradle, similar to that described by Cremer *et al.* (1958), containing 8 light blue fluorescent tubes (G.E.C. Ltd.,) which emit blue light with a peak emission at 480 m$\mu$, close to the absorption maximum of bilirubin.

The naked infant was placed in a Sorrento cot under this cradle, and the eyes were covered with a simple shield. The infant was turned every hour and the rectal temperature was recorded. This did not exceed 100·2° F. (37·9° C.) in any of the treated cases. The baby was removed for feeding, and treatment was not restarted until 30 minutes after the completion of the feed. The light exposure was continued for a maximum of 6 hours at a time, with an interval of 2 hours before further treatment.

The work of Cremer *et al.* (1958) suggested that light treatment was likely to be ineffective when the serum bilirubin was rising rapidly, as in haemolytic disease. It was, therefore, necessary to exclude such cases, and to restrict the trial to infants in whom there was no evidence of haemolytic disease. When light treatment is used in an individual case it is difficult to prove that a fall in serum bilirubin level is due to the effect of light, and not to experimental error or physiological variations. A scheme was therefore devised to test whether there were significant differences between a group of infants treated with light, and a similar untreated group. The following criteria were adopted for the selection of cases for this clinical trial.

(1) There was no clinical contraindication to the use of light treatment, e.g.—the use of continuous oxygen or an incubator.

(2) Cases of Rh haemolytic disease were excluded by choosing only those infants with a negative Coombs' test and a capillary blood haemoglobin level, at the age of more than 24 hours, of not less than 100% (13·8 g./100 ml.).

(3) All infants who were selected had a total serum bilirubin level of not less than 12 mg./100 ml., with not more than 2·5 mg./100 ml. in the conjugated form, at a time which is denoted by the point A in Fig. 1. Infants with a rapidly rising serum bilirubin level (e.g. 10 mg./100 ml. at the age of 24 hours) were excluded, since these were likely to need an exchange transfusion.

In those infants who fulfilled these criteria a second serum bilirubin estimation was made 12 hours later (point B). If this result was greater than that at A, and not less than 13·0 mg./100 ml., the infant was allocated by random selection to either the treated or the control group. Two further serum bilirubin estimations (points C and D) were made at 12-hourly intervals in all cases. Serum bilirubin was measured by the method of Lathe and Ruthven (1958) on blood collected from the heel of the infant.

Treated cases were irradiated with light for about 8 hours during the 12-hour period between points B and C. Cases in the control group were nursed in exactly the same way in the same ward, but received no light treatment.

**Gunn Rats.** Six shaved male Gunn rats, weighing 250-350 g., were kept in a cage placed directly under a lamp holder similar to that used for the infants. They were continuously exposed to blue light and received a mean value of 530 foot-candles for 10 days. The air temperature remained between 26 and 28° C. Blood was taken from the tail vein before light exposure, and on the 2nd, 4th, 6th, and 10th days, and the plasma bilirubin concentration was determined using the Malloy and Evelyn method (1937). The changes in plasma level were compared with those observed in 8 male Gunn rats kept under normal laboratory conditions.

**Rat Mitochondria.** A concentrated bilirubin solution was prepared by the method of Ruthven and Lathe (Rozdilsky and Olszewski, 1961) and contained a molar ratio of bilirubin to bovine albumin of 36 : 1. The solution was diluted with 9·0 volumes of 0·154 M potassium chloride containing 13·3% (V/V) fresh human serum, and centrifuged at 15,000 *g* for 20 minutes. The clear supernatant was drawn into glass tubes (600 mm. × 4 mm.), stoppered at both ends and suspended vertically in front of the blue light source for 32 hours. The diazo test, which is specific for bilirubin, was applied using the Lathe and Ruthven (1958) and the King and Coxon (1950) methods, allowing 1 hour for colour development in the latter. Inorganic phosphate was determined by the method of Fiske and Subbarrow (1925).

Oxidative phosphorylation was determined according to Lardy and Wellman (1952), using brain and liver mitochondria prepared from male Wistar rats by the method of Aldridge (1957). Each Warburg flask contained mitochondria equivalent to 1 mg. nitrogen (liver) or 0·5 mg. nitrogen (brain), in 0·2 ml. 0·25 M sucrose solution, together with 0·8 ml. incubation medium (*p*H 7·6) and 3·0 ml. light-treated or untreated bilirubin solution. In the control flasks, the bilirubin solution was replaced by 3·0 ml. 13·3% (V/V) serum in isotonic potassium chloride solution. The incubation medium was similar to that used by Aldridge (1957), supplemented with co-factors for brain mitochondria (Christie, Judah, and Rees, 1953).

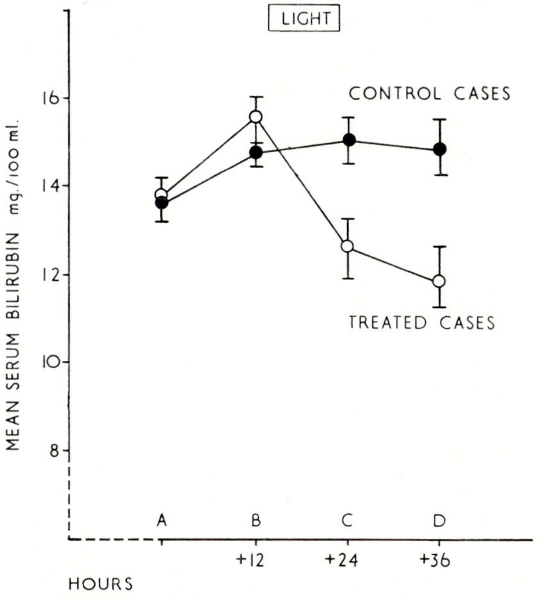


FIG. 1.—Mean serum bilirubin levels in treated and control groups of infants. The standard errors of the means are indicated by vertical bars.

## Results

**Clinical Trial.** The serum bilirubin concentrations of both the treated and the control groups of infants, together with their birth weights, are given in Table 1. If the light treatment is effective the serum bilirubin of the treated infants at Point C (Fig. 1) should be lower than that at B. Individual values of C—B for all cases are illustrated in Fig. 2. It can be seen that there is some overlap between these two groups, which is undoubtedly due to the

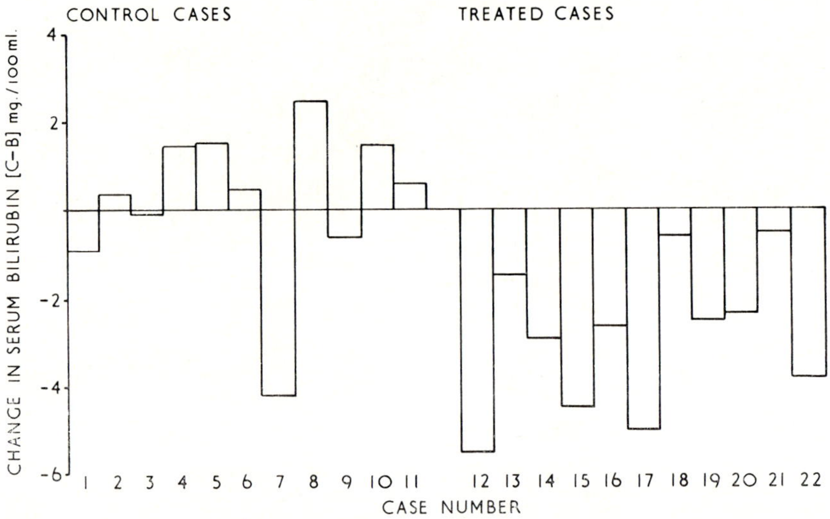


FIG. 2.—Changes in serum bilirubin levels of infants during the 12-hour period between B and C.

fact that the bilirubin level of some cases in the control group fell during this period. The mean fall in bilirubin level (C—B) in the treated group was 2·9 mg./100 ml., whereas the control group showed a mean rise of 0·2 mg./100 ml. in the same period. Student's 't' test showed that the difference between these two means was highly significant ($p < 0{\cdot}001$).

After the end of light treatment the serum bilirubin level of some cases showed a rebound. This is indicated in Table 1 by D—C, but there was no significant difference between the mean values of the two groups.

TABLE 1

RESULTS OF BILIRUBIN ESTIMATIONS, AT 12-HOURLY INTERVALS, ON TREATED AND CONTROL INFANTS

| Case No. | Wt. (lb.) | Hours Light | Age (hr.) | Serum Bilirubin (mg./100 ml.)* | | | | | |
|---|---|---|---|---|---|---|---|---|---|
| | | | | Point A | Point B | Point C | Point D | C-B | D-C |
| | *Control Cases* | | | | | | | | |
| 1 | 3·8 | Nil | 78 | 14·4 | 15·8 | 15·0 | 11·2 | − 0·8 | − 3·8 |
| 2 | 2·10 | | 77 | 13·4 | 14·7 | 15·0 | 15·0 | 0·3 | 0 |
| 3 | 7·2 | | 46 | 12·4 | 14·9 | 14·8 | 14·9 | − 0·1 | 0·1 |
| 4 | 5·0 | | 61 | 13·7 | 16·6 | 18·1 | 18·1 | 1·5 | 0 |
| 5 | 4·15 | | 83 | 14·0 | 15·0 | 16·6 | 16·9 | 1·6 | 0·3 |
| 6 | 5·10 | | 66 | 12·5 | 13·5 | 14·0 | — | 0·5 | — |
| 7 | 6·9 | | 142 | 15·1 | 16·2 | 12·0 | 14·5 | − 4·2 | 2·5 |
| 8 | 7·3 | | 62 | 13·7 | 14·6 | 17·0 | 15·4 | 2·4 | − 1·6 |
| 9 | 3·11 | | 121 | 13·0 | 15·1 | 14·4 | 14·4 | − 0·7 | 0 |
| 10 | 4·11 | | 76 | 12·1 | 13·1 | 14·6 | — | 1·5 | — |
| 11 | 5·5 | | 92 | 12·6 | 13·3 | 13·9 | 13·1 | 0·6 | − 0·8 |
| Mean | 5·2 | | 82 | 13·4 | 14·8 | 15·0 | 14·8 | 0·2 | − 0·4 |
| | *Treated Cases* | | | | | | | | |
| 12 | 5·2 | 9 | 103 | 14·1 | 15·4 | 9·9 | 10·1 | − 5·5 | 0·2 |
| 13 | 6·14 | 9 | 67 | 12·7 | 13·7 | 12·2 | 9·5 | − 1·5 | − 2·7 |
| 14 | 3·3 | 7½ | 79 | 13·8 | 17·2 | 14·3 | 14·9 | − 2·9 | 0·6 |
| 15 | 3·9 | 9 | 57 | 12·6 | 16·4 | 11·9 | 11·8 | − 4·5 | − 0·1 |
| 16 | 3·2 | 9 | 109 | 16·1 | 18·8 | 16·1 | 14·2 | − 2·7 | − 1·9 |
| 17 | 4·10 | 9½ | 83 | 13·1 | 14·0 | 9·0 | 10·8 | − 5·0 | 1·8 |
| 18 | 4·5 | 7 | 80 | 12·2 | 16·1 | 15·4 | 15·0 | − 0·7 | − 0·4 |
| 19 | 7·3 | 9 | 70 | 16·4 | 18·7 | 16·1 | — | − 2·6 | — |
| 20 | 5·0 | 8 | 89 | 12·1 | 13·6 | 11·2 | 11·1 | − 2·4 | − 0·1 |
| 21 | 6·10 | 9 | 70 | 13·1 | 13·8 | 13·2 | 13·5 | − 0·6 | 0·3 |
| 22 | 8·7 | 9 | 70 | 12·5 | 13·3 | 9·5 | 7·4 | − 3·8 | − 2·1 |
| Mean | 5·4 | 8 | 80 | 13·5 | 15·5 | 12·4 | 11·8 | − 2·9 | − 0·4 |

* The timing of points A, B, C, D, is given in the text, and illustrated in Fig. 1.

At the age of 1 year the treated infants were developing normally and showed no signs of neurological or other disorder.

**Gunn Rats.** The initial plasma bilirubin concentrations of the Gunn rats ranged from 6·7 to 12·6 mg./100 ml., all the pigment being in the unconjugated form. Exposure to blue light caused an immediate and significant fall in the bilirubin levels of all animals, as shown in Fig. 3. Further slight decreases were observed on subsequent days, but in no animal was it possible to reduce the plasma concentration to less than 36% of the initial value, even when exposure was continued for as long as 20 days. Similar changes were observed in female rats. No detectable ill effects due to the light were observed: the animals ate well, maintained their body weight, and suffered no apparent deterioration of vision.

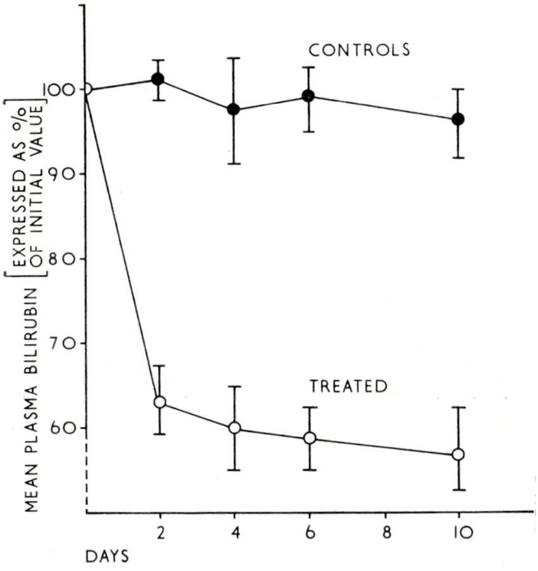


FIG. 3.—Effect of blue light on the mean plasma bilirubin levels of Gunn rats. The standard errors of the means are indicated by vertical bars.

**Mitochondria.** Results of typical experiments with liver and brain mitochondria are given in Table 2. These show that untreated bilirubin uncoupled oxidative phosphorylation, as demonstrated by a reduction in the P/O ratio. Light treatment of bilirubin, sufficient to reduce the concentration to about half its original value, restored the P/O ratio to that of the control flask. After 32 hours irradiation the bilirubin concentration had fallen to less than 20 mg./100 ml., and other experiments (P. S. Lord, 1965, unpublished results), which did not involve irradiation, showed that this concentration, in a solution containing fresh human serum, did not uncouple oxidative phosphorylation. The products of bilirubin irradiation have failed to show any effect on oxidative phosphorylation in the experiments described here.

TABLE 2

EFFECT OF BILIRUBIN AND LIGHT TREATED BILIRUBIN ON THE PHOSPHORUS/OXYGEN (P/O) RATIO OF RAT LIVER AND BRAIN MITOCHONDRIA, IN A MEDIUM CONTAINING 10% SERUM

| Addition to Flask | Liver Mitochondria: Bilirubin Concentration in Medium (mg./100 ml.) | Liver Mitochondria: P/O Ratio | Brain Mitochondria: Bilirubin Concentration in Medium (mg./100 ml.) | Brain Mitochondria: P/O Ratio |
|---|---|---|---|---|
| Nil .. .. .. | Nil | 1·54 | Nil | 1·47 |
| Bilirubin stored in dark at 22° C. for 32 hours | 34·6 | 0·54 | 35·4 | 0·85 |
| Bilirubin, light treated at 26° C. for 32 hours | 18·0 | 1·59 | 17·4 | 1·60 |

Each value represents the mean of duplicate estimations. P/O refers to the ratio of μ moles of inorganic phosphate esterified per μatom of oxygen consumed.

## Discussion

These experiments show clearly that the serum bilirubin levels of both jaundiced infants and Gunn rats can be reduced by irradiation with blue light.

All the 11 irradiated infants described in this paper showed a decrease in serum bilirubin level, averaging 2·9 mg./100 ml., after approximately 8 hours of treatment, and this fall was significantly different from that of the control group. Cremer *et al.* (1958) found that serum bilirubin concentrations fell in all 9 premature infants with jaundice who were treated with artificial blue light, and Franklin (1958) obtained similar results in 8 out of 10 treated cases. Blondheim *et al.* (1962b), however, considered the method disappointing, and noted that serum levels rose slightly in 3 out of 8 cases treated with light of an unspecified type.

Light treatment of jaundiced infants can only be recommended if the products of irradiation are less toxic than bilirubin. The toxic effect of bilirubin on tissue respiration has previously been demonstrated by its inhibition of oxygen uptake by brain (Day, 1954) and by the uncoupling of oxidative phosphorylation in both liver and brain mitochondria (Zetterström and Ernster, 1956; Biesold *et al.*, 1962). The experiments reported here, in which mitochondria were incubated with irradiated solutions of bilirubin, indicate that the products of this photodecomposition have no effect on oxidative phosphorylation, whereas untreated bilirubin was highly active.

The nature of these products is unknown, though Cremer *et al.* (1958) and Brodersen and Vind (1963) obtained evidence that biliverdin was formed when jaundiced serum was irradiated with blue light. Most reports have indicated that this substance has no effect on tissue respiration (Day, 1956; Ebnöter and Vest, 1959) or oxidative phosphorylation (Zetterström and Ernster, 1956), though Biesold *et al.* (1962) found an inhibition of respiration due to biliverdin. Larson, Evans, and Watson (1947) described the presence of biliverdin in the serum of jaundiced adults, and did not associate this with any toxic effects. Blondheim, Lathrop, and Zabriskie (1960, 1962a) studied the spectral changes that occur when jaundiced serum is exposed to light, and found that the products were more diffusible than bilirubin. Other workers have shown that they are more polar and therefore more water-soluble than bilirubin (Ostrow, Hammaker, and Schmid, 1961; Brodersen and Vind, 1963). Blondheim *et al.* (1962b) inferred from this that they might cross the blood brain barrier and be potentially toxic. But the toxicity of bilirubin has been attributed to its fat solubility, and it seems probable that the water-soluble products would, therefore, be less toxic, and also more easily excreted. From our results, there was no evidence that the products of light treatment were toxic to infants or rats, and the loss of toxicity to mitochondria after irradiation of bilirubin was striking.

The usefulness of exposure to light as a treatment for hyperbilirubinaemia in an individual case will depend on the rate at which the serum bilirubin is rising, upon the duration of treatment, and probably on other factors. This method provides a possible alternative to exchange transfusion in selected cases of 'physiological' jaundice in both premature and full-term infants, who require treatment. In such cases the rate of rise of serum bilirubin is usually slow, allowing time for lengthy exposure to light. It might also have a limited application in the treatment of some mildly affected cases of haemolytic disease, where the serum bilirubin is only rising slowly. In more severe cases, which have been given an initial exchange transfusion, light treatment could occasionally be considered as an alternative to a difficult second or third transfusion. It should, however, be emphasized that light treatment is ineffective when the serum bilirubin level is rising rapidly, and it follows that the method should not be considered unless serum bilirubin determinations are readily available.

**Summary**

A group of 11 infants with 'physiological' jaundice, chosen by random selection, have been treated by irradiation with an artificial blue light. The serum bilirubin concentration of the treated infants fell by an average of 2·9 mg./100 ml. during treatment, and this was significantly greater than the change in bilirubin level in a similar untreated group of infants.

Jaundiced Gunn rats were exposed to a similar light source for 10 days, and their plasma bilirubin concentrations fell significantly when compared with an untreated control group of rats.

Bilirubin in the presence of serum uncouples oxidative phosphorylation of rat liver and brain mitochondria. Photodecomposition of the bilirubin destroys this uncoupling effect, and the products of the reaction showed no effect on oxidative phosphorylation.

These results show that treatment of a jaundiced subject with blue light can reduce the serum bilirubin level, and that there is no evidence that the products of light treatment are toxic.

We are grateful to Mr. P. W. Perryman for advice in the construction of the light cradle and for valuable information about its use; to the General Electric Co., Ltd., for information about the light source used; and to Dr. B. H. Billing, Professor G. H. Lathe, and Dr. C. Toothill for their helpful advice and criticism of this work.

REFERENCES

Aldridge, W. N. (1957). Liver and brain mitochondria. *Biochem. J.*, **67**, 423.

Biesold, D., Liebold, F., and Theile, H. (1962). Die Wirkung von Bilirubin auf den Hirnstoffwechsel in vitro. *Acta biol. med. germ.*, **9**, 652.

Blondheim, S. H., Lathrop, D., and Zabriskie, J. (1960). A diffusible bilirubin(oid) produced by exposure of jaundiced serum to light. *Gastroenterology*, **38**, 798.

——, ——, and Zabriskie, J. (1962a). Effect of light on the absorption spectrum of jaundiced serum. *J. Lab. clin. Med.*, **60**, 31.

——, Zabriskie, J., and Lathrop, D. (1962b). Kernicterus and prematurity. *Brit. med. J.*, **1**, 52.

Brodersen, R., and Vind, I. (1963). Chloroform extraction of serum bilirubin in relation to its binding to proteins. *Scand. J. clin. Lab. Invest.*, **15**, 107.

Christie, G. S., Judah, J. D., and Rees, K. R. (1953). Cofactor and metal requirements of brain mitochondria. *Proc. roy. Soc. B* **141**, 523.

Cremer, R. J., Perryman, P. W., and Richards, D. H. (1958). Influence of light on the hyperbilirubinaemia of infants. *Lancet*, **1**, 1094.

Day, R. L. (1954). Inhibition of brain respiration *in vitro* by bilirubin. Reversal of inhibition by various means. *Proc. Soc. exp. Biol. (N.Y.)*, **85**, 261.

—— (1956). Kernicterus: further observations on the toxicity of heme pigments. *Pediatrics*, **17**, 925.

Ebnöter, P., and Vest, M. (1959). Zum Problem der Hyperbilirubinämie und des Kernikterus. *Ann. paediat. (Basel)*, **193**, 279.

Ernster, L., Herlin, L., and Zetterström, R. (1957). Experimental studies on the pathogenesis of kernicterus. *Pediatrics*, **20**, 647.

Ferreira, H. C., Berezin, A., Barbieri, D., and Larrubia, N. M. (1960a). A super iluminação no tratamento das hiperbilirrubinemias do recém-nascido. *Rev. Ass. méd. bras.* **6** **201**

——, ——, ——, and —— (1960b). A super-iluminação na hiperbilirrubinemia do recém-nascido. *J. Pediát. (Rio de J.)*, **25**, 12.
——, ——, ——, and —— (1960c). A super-iluminação na hiperbilirrubinemia do recém-nascido. *An. bras. Ginec.*, **49**, 147.
——, Cardim, W. H., and Mellone, O. (1960). Fototerapia: novo recurso terapêutico na hiperbilirrubinemia do recém-nascido. *J. Pediát. (Rio de J.)*, **25**, 347.
Fiske, C. H., and Subbarrow, Y. (1925). The colorimetric determination of phosphorus. *J. biol. Chem.*, **66**, 375.
Franklin, A. W. (1958). Influence of light on the hyperbilirubinaemia of infants. *Lancet*, **1**, 1227.
King, E. J., and Coxon, R. V. (1950). Determination of bilirubin with precipitation of the plasma proteins. *J. clin. Path.*, **3**, 248.
Lardy, H. A., and Wellman, H. (1952). Oxidation phosphorylations: role of inorganic phosphate and acceptor systems in control of metabolic rates. *J. biol. Chem.*, **195**, 215.
Larson, E. A., Evans, G. T., and Watson, C. J. (1947). A study of the serum biliverdin concentration in various types of jaundice. *J. Lab. clin. Med.*, **32**, 481.
Lathe, G. H., and Ruthven, C. R. J. (1958). Factors affecting the rate of coupling of bilirubin and conjugated bilirubin in the van den Bergh reaction. *J. clin. Path.*, **11**, 155.
——, and Walker, M. (1958). The synthesis of bilirubin glucuronide in animal and human liver. *Biochem. J.*, **70**, 705.
Malloy, H. T., and Evelyn, K. A. (1937). The determination of bilirubin with the photoelectric colorimeter. *J. biol. Chem.*, **119**, 481.
Mellone, O. (1960). Tratamento da hiperbilirrubinemia do recém-nascido por foco de luz intensa. *Rev. paul. Med.*, **57**, 47.
Ostrow, J. D., Hammaker, L., and Schmid, R. (1961). The preparation of crystalline bilirubin-$C^{14}$. *J. clin. Invest.*, **40**, 1442.
Peluffo, E., Beltran, J. C., Malinger, A., Giguens, W., Vila Vidal, P. and Lorenzo de Ibarreta, J. (1962). Luminoterapia en las ictericias del recien nacido. *Arch. Pediat. Urug.*, **33**, 98.
Rozdilsky, B., and Olszewski, J. (1961). Experimental studies of the toxicity of bilirubin in newborn animals. *J. Neuropath. exp. Neurol.*, **20**, 193.
Trolle, D. (1964). Incidence and possible relation to athetosis of neonatal jaundice of unknown aetiology. *Arch. Dis. Childh.*, **39**, 85.
Wood, B. S. B., Culley, P. E., Waterhouse, J. A. H., and Powell, D. J. (1962). Factors influencing neonatal jaundice. *ibid.*, **37**, 371.
Zetterström, R., and Ernster, L. (1956). Bilirubin, an uncoupler of oxidative phosphorylation in isolated mitochondria. *Nature (Lond.)*, **178**, 1335.

## Addendum

G.E.C. Ltd., have recently informed us that a similar intensity of illumination, but with less heating effect, could be obtained by the use of ten 2 foot 20 watt lamps instead of the eight 40 watt lamps used here. We have not tried this.

*Arch. Dis. Childh.*, 1965, **40**, 672.

# HEAD CIRCUMFERENCE OF INFANTS RELATED TO BODY WEIGHT

BY

R. S. ILLINGWORTH and W. LUTZ

*From the Department of Child Health, and the Department of Statistics, the University of Sheffield*

(RECEIVED FOR PUBLICATION FEBRUARY 24, 1965)

The measurement of the maximum circumference of the head is a part of the routine physical examination of any baby, just as much as examination of the heart, chest, and abdomen, as examination of the hips for subluxation, of the urine for phenylpyruvic acid, and of the hearing after the age of 3 or 4 months, The importance of measuring the head circumference lies partly in the early detection of hydrocephalus, which is now amenable to surgical procedures, and partly in the early diagnosis of mental subnormality. When there are indications for a careful developmental assessment, measurement of the maximum head circumference is a vital part of the examination.

Though the maximum head circumference is of great importance in developmental and neurological assessment, there are several difficulties in its interpretation. A large head may be merely a familial feature. It is rarely due to megalencephaly, and still more rarely to hydranencephaly. The diagnosis of the obvious cause, hydrocephalus, is normally supported by other clinical signs, such as a bulging fontanelle or undue separation of the sutures. In the very young baby with a spina bifida, air studies may demonstrate a fairly considerable degree of hydrocephalus before its presence is revealed by an excessive head size or excessive increase in its size (Lorber, 1961).

A small head is not strictly synonymous with microcephaly. It may, for instance, be a familial feature. A true microcephalic head is characterized not only by the small head circumference, but by its shape, and in particular by the excessive tapering off toward the vertex.

Microcephaly is usual in children suffering from mental subnormality (unless there be hydrocephalus, megalencephaly, or hydranencephaly), and if a mentally subnormal child has developed normally during the early months, the head will by then have attained much of its eventual size. By the age of 9 months the brain has reached half its adult size, and by the age of 2 years, three-quarters its adult size. To put it another way, if mental subnormality dates from birth or before birth, the head is usually small. The later in the first year at which the mental subnormality develops, the less will be the evidence of microcephaly. If it develops after the first year there will be no significant evidence of microcephaly.

A broad head (brachycephaly), with a flat occiput, may have an average head circumference, but it is nevertheless commonly associated with mental subnormality. The head in generalized craniostenosis may be unduly small, but craniostenosis is distinguished from microcephaly by palpation of the sutures and by radiological examination.

Serial measurements are more important than isolated measurements. A changing relationship between the head circumference and its placing on the percentile head chart may well indicate the development of hydrocephalus or microcephaly (Fig. 1). On the other hand, a placing above or below the upper or lower percentile respectively will be seen to be normal when serial measurements indicate that the position in relation to the percentile is not changing (Fig. 2).

A minor difficulty in interpretation of the head circumference lies in the fact that the younger the baby (or foetus) the larger the head size in relation to the size of the rest of the baby.

A major difficulty is the obvious fact that at any given age a large baby is likely to have a larger head than a small baby, and vice versa. It is necessary, therefore, to relate the size of the head to the size of the baby—and a convenient index of the size of the baby is his weight. Up to the present, we have plotted the head circumference on a chart which gives the 10th, 50th, and 90th percentiles, and his weight against a weight chart which gives the same percentiles for the relevant sex at the age in question. One can then determine whether his head size corresponds with (i.e. occupies the same relative percentile position as) his weight. This method

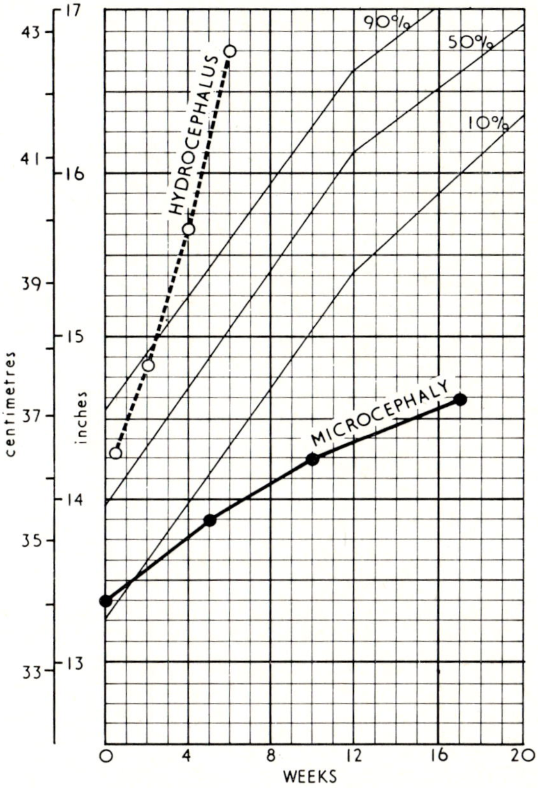


FIG. 1.—Head circumference: serial measurements in a case of hydrocephalus and a case of microcephaly.

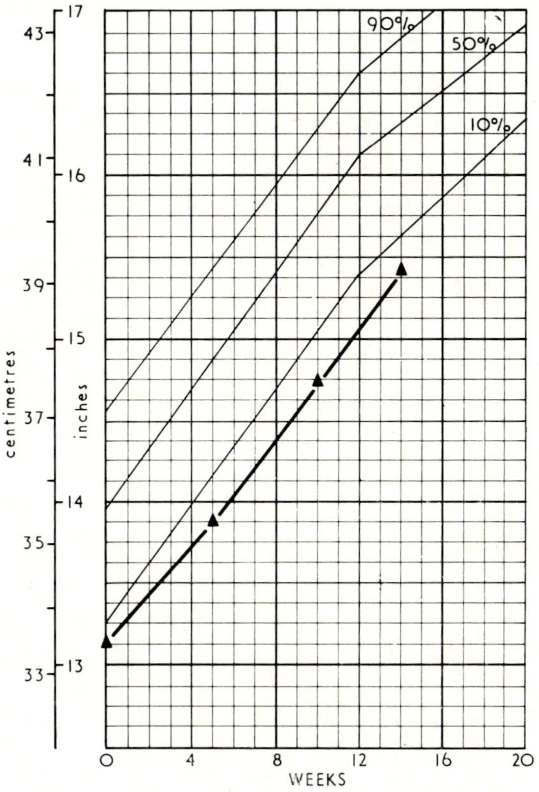


FIG. 2.—Head circumference in a normal small child; serial measurements indicate normal rate of head growth.

involves the use of two charts for each child. Our present study was intended to provide a more accurate method of relating the head size to the weight, using a single graph for each child.

## Material and Methods

During a joint obstetrical and paediatric study made with a different object, we kept a record of certain physical measurements including the child's weight and maximum head circumference. The children were seen at birth, and followed up as nearly as possible at the ages of 6 weeks, 6 months, and 10 months. Those ages were chosen because it was felt that they were the best for developmental assessment. The total number of children for whom we have the necessary measurements is shown in the statistical addendum (Table A).

The nude weight was recorded. The maximum head circumference was measured by a non-elastic soft tape which was checked for accuracy at frequent intervals. Infants who were suspected on developmental testing of being mentally subnormal, or of having hydrocephalus, were excluded from this investigation. Table 1 gives the average head circumference and weight of the boys and girls studied in this investigation. The figures indicate that there is a direct relationship between body weight and head circumference.

## Results

We had hoped to obtain one graph for each sex, covering the four age periods, but it was found that the data available would not permit this. Consequently we have prepared eight graphs, four for each sex, covering the periods of birth, 6 weeks, 6 months, and 10 months (Figs. 3 and 4). From these graphs it is immediately possible to determine the expected head circumference for a child of given sex, age, and weight.

It can be seen from the graphs that the expected head circumference can be calculated with reasonable accuracy by subtracting (or adding) the following measurements from (or to) the head circumference for each pound above (or below) the average weight (Table 2).

We emphasize that the head circumference of most children will not coincide with these average values.

TABLE 1

HEAD CIRCUMFERENCE RELATED TO WEIGHT AT DIFFERENT AGES

| | Boys | | | Girls | | | Weight | | | |
|---|---|---|---|---|---|---|---|---|---|---|
| | Average Head Circumference | | Regression Coefficient Head Circumference on Weight | Average Head Circumference | | Regression Coefficient Head Circumference on Weight | Boys | | Girls | |
| | Inch | Cm. | | Inch | Cm. | | lb. oz. | g. | lb. oz. | g. |
| Birth | 13·7 | 34·8 | 0·343 | 13·8 | 35·0 | 0·231 | 7 5½ | 3,180 | 7 5¼ | 3,180 |
| 6 weeks | 15·3 | 38·9 | 0·235 | 14·9 | 37·8 | 0·262 | 10 13 | 4,860 | 10 0 | 4,500 |
| 6 months | 17·5 | 44·4 | 0·122 | 17·0 | 43·2 | 0·124 | 18 12¼ | 8,520 | 17 7¼ | 7,840 |
| 10 months | 18·4 | 46·7 | 0·114 | 17·9 | 45·5 | 0·099 | 22 2½ | 10,460 | 20 10½ | 9,380 |

There are considerable normal variations, and it is essential to take into account the 95% confidence limits, and all the relevant clinical features mentioned.

TABLE 2

CALCULATION OF EXPECTED HEAD CIRCUMFERENCE FROM AGE AND WEIGHT*

| | Boys | | Girls | |
|---|---|---|---|---|
| | Inch | Cm. | Inch | Cm. |
| Birth | 0·3 | 0·8 | 0·25 | 0·6 |
| 6 weeks | 0·25 | 0·6 | 0·25 | 0·6 |
| 6 months | 0·125 | 0·3 | 0·125 | 0·3 |
| 10 months | 0·1 | 0·3 | 0·1 | 0·3 |

* The figures show the amount to be added to or subtracted from the head circumference for each lb. above or below the average weight.

There is bound to be some degree of error in head and weight measurements. In practice, allowance for the influence of body weight will be made in older infants of over 6 months, only in extreme cases of overweight or underweight. It is important to note that a sudden loss of weight, such as may occur with acute dehydration, will disturb the relation between head circumference and weight. A sudden increase of weight will normally be accompanied by a corresponding increase in head size. At first sight this might lead the unwary, relying on a head chart alone, to make the erroneous diagnosis of hydrocephalus.

The relationship of head size to weight in grossly underweight children with the 'failure to thrive' picture, is still uncertain. Dean (1965) found that

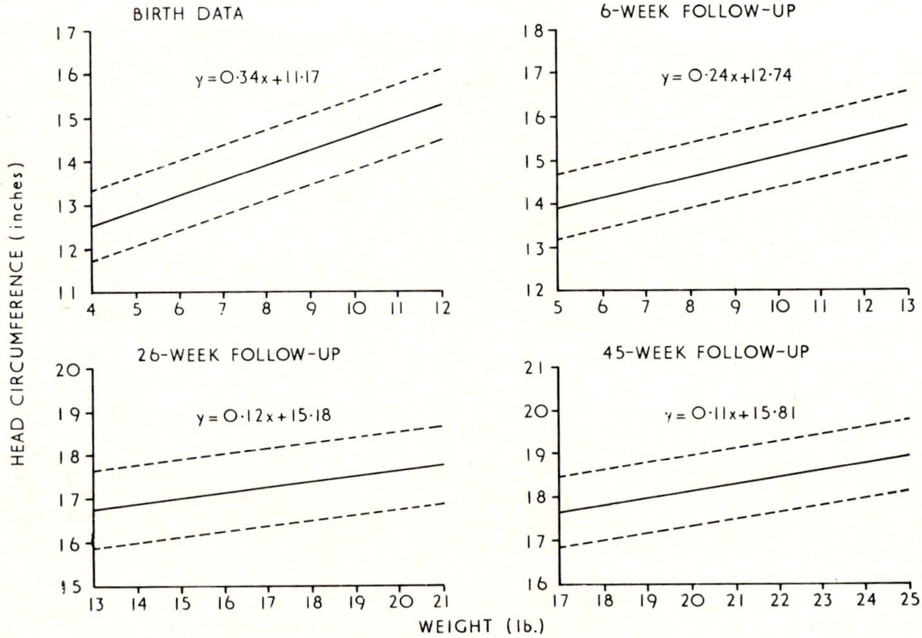


FIG. 3.—Relationship of head circumference to weight (boys).

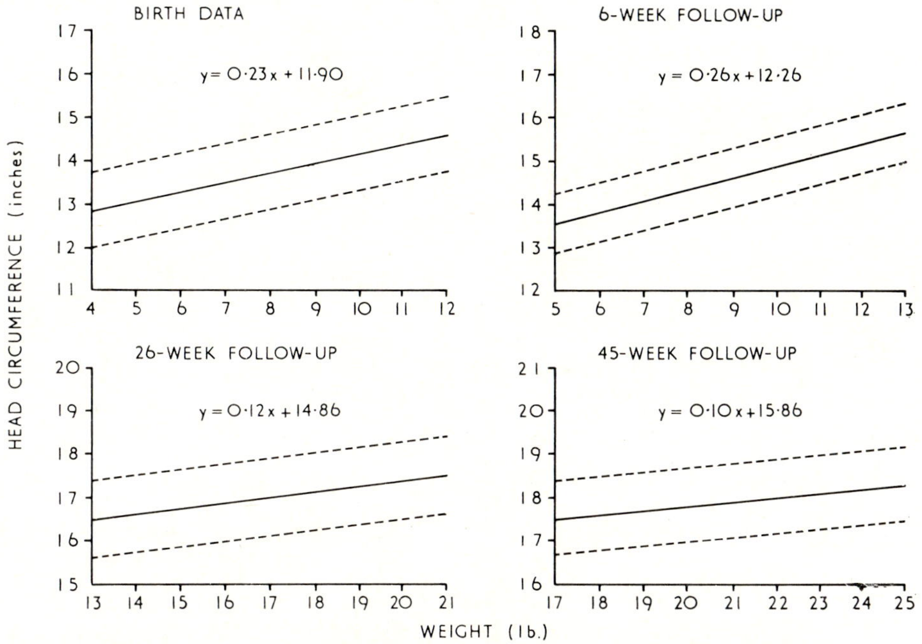


FIG. 4.—Relationship of head circumference to weight (girls).

the relationship between the circumference of the head and that of the chest was useful in assessing children with severe malnutrition, such as kwashiorkor. Whereas the circumference of the head is normally greater than that of the chest until the age of 6 months, that of the chest is normally greater after that age. Dean found that in malnutrition the measurement affected least was the head circumference, and that the head was nearly always larger than it should be in relation to the size of the body. In malnourished children the extent of the difference between the circumference of the head and the thorax was related in a statistically significant way.

## Discussion

Too much must not be read into an unusual head size, but in conjunction with other clinical features, it is of the utmost importance in developmental assessment. Thus, if a child is developmentally retarded, and the head circumference is found to be low in relation to his weight, one will be very suspicious that he may prove to be mentally subnormal. If, on the other hand, the child is developmentally retarded and yet the head circumference corresponds well with the weight, the child may be an example of delayed maturation, and later prove to be normal. In doubtful cases serial measurements can throw a great deal of light on the problem.

## Summary

The measurement of the maximum head circumference must be part of the routine examination of any baby.

It must be related to the size of the baby, and the weight is a good index of this.

Graphs have been constructed in which the head circumference is related to the size of the baby. A table, which enables a rough correction to be made in order to relate the head size to the weight, is given.

Difficulties in interpreting the results are discussed.

We wish to thank the Spastics Society for support in the joint obstetrical and paediatric study, from which the figures were obtained for this investigation.

### References

Dean, R. F. A. (1965). Effects of malnutrition, especially of slight degree, on the growth of young children. *Courrier*, **15**, 73.

Lorber, J. (1961). Systematic ventriculographic studies in infants born with meningomyelocele and encephalocele: the incidence and development of hydrocephalus. *Arch. Dis. Childh.*, **36**, 381.

## Statistical Addendum

The data for boys and girls were analysed separately and the subsequent results showed that the boys had a slightly larger head circumference at all ages after birth. We realized that a linear regression over the whole period of 45 weeks was unlikely to be realistic. On the other

TABLE A

| | No. of Cases | | Mean Age (wk.) | | Standard Deviation of Age | | Range of Ages (wk.) (sexes combined) | Regression Coefficient Head Circumference on Weight | |
|---|---|---|---|---|---|---|---|---|---|
| | Boys | Girls | Boys | Girls | Boys | Girls | | Boys | Girls |
| Birth .. .. .. | 397 | 311 | — | — | — | — | — | 0·343 | 0·231 |
| 1st follow-up .. | 362 | 307 | 6·7 | 6·7 | 1·27 | 1·28 | 4-15 | 0·235 | 0·262 |
| 2nd follow-up .. | 353 | 295 | 26·7 | 26·8 | 1·50 | 2·06 | 21-36 | 0·122 | 0·124 |
| 3rd follow-up .. | 356 | 312 | 44·6 | 44·8 | 2·02 | 2·52 | 35-57 | 0·114 | 0·099 |

hand, fitting a curve to data concentrated at 4 points only (0, 6, 26, and 45 weeks) was not advisable.

Hence each of the four stages, birth, and the follow-up studies at 6, 26, and 45 weeks, was treated separately.

A comparison of the linear regression lines of head circumference on gestation and birth weight, with the regression line on birth weight only (both sexes treated separately), clearly showed that gestation did not reduce the sum of squares about the regression curve to any worth-while degree. Thus gestation, as a predictor of head circumference, was unsatisfactory for the birth data and would obviously be of even less value at older ages.

Mothers were requested to bring their children in for examination at the three stated ages. Not all were able to comply, resulting in a varying number of cases at the different follow-ups. Moreover, mothers were not always able to adhere precisely to the times requested, resulting in a variation of age at each of the follow-up periods.

Table A shows the extent of these variations in numbers and age.

Analysis showed that the variable 'age' at each follow-up study did not reduce the sum of squares about the regression line by more than a minute fraction. Since gestation as a predictor had already been eliminated, we finally used the regression line of head circumference on weight only at each of the four age stages, and for each sex.

It is not claimed that there is no relationship between age and head circumference. In fact, there must exist, at least in the first year, a fairly strong relationship between head circumference on the one hand with age and weight on the other. However, the limited age variation at each single follow-up study added little to the ability to predict head circumference. The regression studies, therefore, seem applicable to children whose ages vary a few weeks either side of the mean ages 6½, 26, and 45 weeks.

Cases of hydrocephalus and microcephalus (not included in the series) showed their head circumferences to lie well outside the 95% confidence belts as shown on the graphs, in nearly all instances.

Table A also shows the regression coefficients of head circumference on weight at the four periods studied. The regression coefficient 0·343 for boys and 0·231 for girls at birth was significantly different at the 95% level. At later ages the regression coefficients for boys and girls were not significantly different. The decline in the regression coefficients with age clearly indicates that weight alone becomes an increasingly poor predictor of head circumference with age, at least on its own. For older children a combination of several variables will have to be considered if a good predictor of head circumference is desired.

*Arch. Dis. Childh.*, 1965, **40**, 677.

# MASTOCYTOSIS

## REPORT OF A CASE IN A 15½-WEEK-OLD INFANT WITH CUTANEOUS AND GENERALIZED SKELETAL CHANGES

BY

ARTHUR R. C. COLE

*From The Princess Margaret Hospital, and Hospital for Sick Children, Toronto, Canada*

(RECEIVED FOR PUBLICATION APRIL 13, 1965)

The evolution of medicine has seen the concept of urticaria pigmentosa, as first described nearly 100 years ago by Nettleship (1869), expand to a wide spectrum of disease extending from the simple benign mastocytoma (Marshall, Walker, Lurie, Hansen, and Mackenzie, 1957) to the malignant generalized fatal mastocytosis (Ellis, 1949). Sagher and Even-Paz (1960) cite 15 synonyms which may be included under this heading.

At first the disease was considered to be entirely in the field of dermatology, and many references come from that speciality. However, since Ellis (1949) described a necropsy on a fatal case in a male infant, showing the invasion of many organs by mast cells, and Sagher, Cohen, and Schorr (1952), Sagher, Liban, Ungar, and Schorr (1956), and Sagher and Schorr (1956) noted the radiographic changes associated with this condition, the interest has spread to radiologists, hospital doctors, and paediatricians (Marshall *et al.*, 1957; Rider, Stein, and Abbuhl, 1957; Waters and Lacson, 1957; Lees and Stroud, 1959; Poppel, Gruber, Silber, Holder, and Christman, 1959; Stutzman, Zsoldos, Ambrus, and Asboe-Hansen, 1960; Stutzman and Urbach, 1961; Bigelow, 1961; Szweda, Abraham, Fine, Nixon, and Rupe, 1962; Pastras and Beerman, 1962).

The first descriptions of the basic mast cell were made by Thin (1877) and Ehrlich (1877). Sangster (1878) coined the term urticaria pigmentosa. Unna (1887) described the mast cell infiltrate in the then only known cutaneous lesion. More recently attempts have been made to understand the functions of the basic cell and its evolution from basic cell types (Remy and Herzberg, 1961; Nickel, 1957; Beare, 1958; West, 1958; Head, 1958; Degos, 1960; Padawer, 1963). Bigelow (1961) compares the histiocytoses and mastocytoses, their similarities and differences.

Many unusual findings are noted in patients with mastocytosis, which are not common to all patients and may not be present at all times in any particular patient. Among them are hyperhistaminaemia, hyperhistaminuria, hyperheparinaemia, capillary changes, gastro-enteric symptoms, spontaneous histamine shock, aspirin sensitivity, coagulation changes, and abnormalities of lipoprotein metabolism. Mastocytosis may also occur without cutaneous lesions and constitutes a diagnostic challenge (Friedman, Will, Freiman, and Braunstein, 1958; Ende and Cherniss, 1958).

The surgical removal of an isolated mastocytoma in a patient with generalized symptoms due to excess histamine release may lead to a dramatic cure of their complaints. There is no specific treatment for other forms of the disease at the present time. Paediatricians should be acquainted with the condition and its vagaries, as 75% of reported cases (which includes benign urticaria pigmentosa) are seen in this age-group: of the paediatric cases, 50% begin in the first six months of life. The majority of these patients have multiple cutaneous lesions which clear completely at puberty.

Eight classifications were offered recently (Ellis, 1949; Sagher, 1956; Nickel, 1957; Marshall *et al.*, 1957; Beare, 1958; Poppel *et al.*, 1959; Sagher and Even-Paz, 1960; Szweda *et al.*, 1962), of which Sagher and Even-Paz (1960) provides the most comprehensive one. He divides the patients into 3 groups: (a) cutaneous, (b) cutaneo-systemic, and (c) systemic.

*The radiological changes* that may occur are divided into a *generalized* or a *localized type*. The *generalized* type shows generalized cystic osteoporosis of the ribs with thickening of the bony trabeculae, stippling of the bony structures of the skull, and thickening of the skull tables and osteosclerosis of the pelvic bones and vertebrae. The *localized* type shows calcified and decalcified areas which may

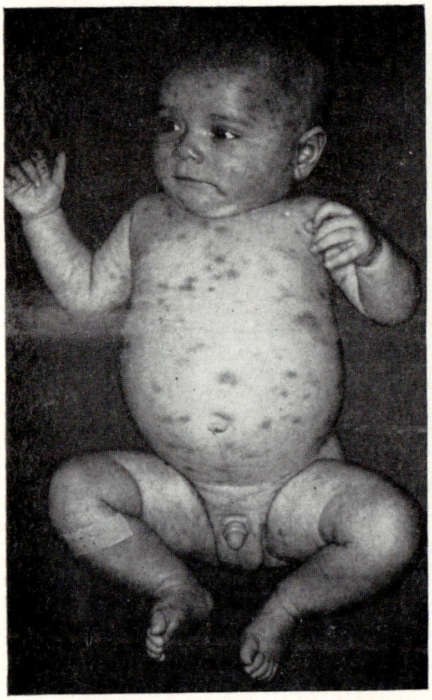

FIG. 1.—Anterior view of the patient.

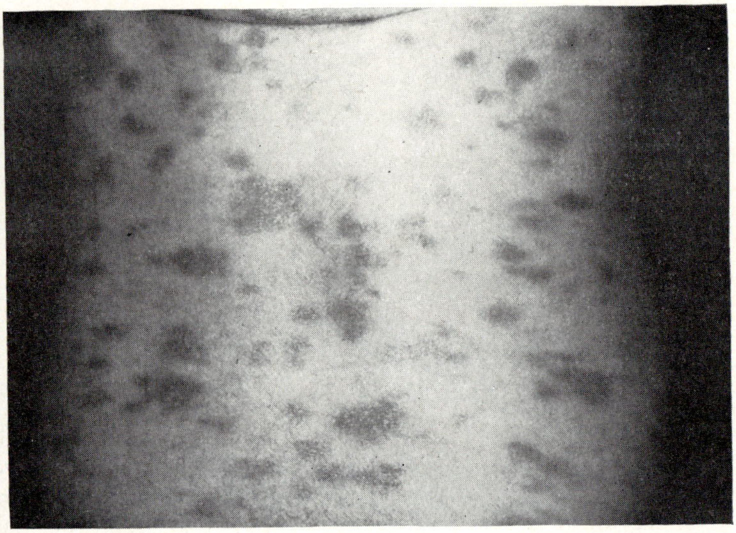

FIG. 2.—Close-up view of lesions on the back of the patient.

occur in humerus, radius, femur, skull, clavicle, and scapula.

The following report is of an infant with disseminated cutaneous and generalized skeletal changes.

### Case Report

B.P. (548, 648 H.S.C.), a male infant, born February 3, 1963, after a normal pregnancy lasting 37-38 weeks, birth weight 3·29 kg., was admitted on May 21, 1963, to the Hospital for Sick Children, Toronto, at 15½ weeks of age, because a rash had appeared at 1 month of age. The rash had erupted following the introduction of cereal and orange juice into the diet. The stools became loose and the buttocks reddened at this time. The rash continued to spread; the early pink lesions did not disappear, and as they aged, they became pale brown in colour (Figs. 1 and 2). With the exception of two colds with associated diarrhoea, the infant had had no illness.

Family history indicated that the mother had hay fever and both maternal and paternal grandmothers had asthma.

Examination revealed a body length of 59·7 cm.; head and chest each measured 39·4 cm. The liver was palpable 2·5 cm. below the right costal margin. The cutaneous lesions varied from 4 mm. to 2·5 cm. in diameter. The surface of the lesions was slightly rough. Urtication occurred on stroking the lesions (Darier's sign) which were mauvish brown to pale brown and were distributed over the whole body, but more densely over the head and trunk. No red or pink lesions were apparent, and there were no haemorrhages or bullae.

Laboratory findings are reported in Tables 1 to 4. A skeletal survey in May 1963 revealed a diffuse disturbance of bone growth with dense zones of provisional calcification at the metaphyses of the long bones and dense perimeters around the vertebral bodies, iliac crests, and small bones of the extremities (Fig. 3a-c). Biopsy of one of the cutaneous lesions showed diffuse infiltration of the subepidermis with mast cells. The enlargement of the liver was not apparent at follow-up examination in July 1963, but a small firm raised area, 0·25 cm. in diameter, appeared at the vertex of the skull In January 1964 the body weight was 10 kg. The liver was again palpable 1 cm. below the right costal margin. The lesion at the vertex had disappeared. Radiographs taken in March 1964 (Fig. 4a-c) showed complete clearing of the bony changes described above. In July 1964, the cutaneous lesions were unchanged, the liver and spleen were not palpable, and the baby was well.

### Discussion

As the diverse nature of mastocytosis has become known and since there was a fatality in infancy, there has been reason to admit these patients for investigation.

A review of the patients seen at the Hospital for Sick Children, Toronto, revealed 14 (Tables 1-4). The first was admitted in 1938 and the remainder in the past 10 years. Before 1949 it was felt that most cases occurring in early childhood had a good prognosis and a spontaneous recovery occurred from 6 to 10 years of age. No record of out patients seen

TABLE 1
MASTOCYTOSIS: HISTORY AND PHYSICAL FINDINGS

| History No. (H.S.C.) | Year of Diagnosis | Age (yr.) on Admission | Age at Onset of Rash | Family History of Allergy | Allergic Disease in Patient | Other Disease in Patient | Urticaria Pigmentosa | Description of Rash |
|---|---|---|---|---|---|---|---|---|
| 94759 | 1938 | 1 10/12 | 2 wk. | – | – | Localized convulsive disorder | + | Profuse general maculopapular lesions 1-2 to 5-10 mm. in diameter, light melanotic tint, small raised areas of erythema |
| 189576 | 1953 | 3 4/12 | 8 mth. | – | – | Rt. ptosis, rt. meiosis | + | Rash in diaper area extending to face, trunk, and extremities |
| 251593 | 1953 | 2 3/12 | 4 mth. | – | Eczema | Secondary infection of eczema | + | Generalized rash of irregularly rounded papular brownish lesions |
| 298486 | 1954 | 1 | Birth | – | – | – | + | Reddish-brown discrete, slightly raised spots on back, chest, neck, and trunk; diaper area and limbs clear |
| 318131 | 1955 | 1 4/12 | 1 mth. | Hay fever, asthma | – | – | + | Generalized rash except palms of hands |
| 339173 | 1956 | 4/12 | 2 mth. | – | Urticaria | – | + | Rash on chest, trunk, neck, upper arms, and legs |
| 389993 | 1958 | 6 | | – | – | Convulsive disorder | + | Pigmented papules, pink to brown over scalp, trunk, neck, forearms, and thighs |
| 412417 | 1959 | 1 6/12 | | – | – | – | Solitary lesion | Rough slightly raised reddish area on left foot (mastocytosis) |
| 430824 | 1959 | 6 3/12 | 3 yr. | – | Urticaria | ? Addison's disease | + | Spotty brown rash |
| 433742 | 1959 | 6 7/12 | 18 mth. | – | – | Nephrosis | + | Rash over trunk, upper parts of arm, around neck, a few papules over trunk |
| 449701 | 1960 | 1 2/12 | 3 mth. | – | – | Pyloric stenosis | + | Small macular reddish to yellowish-brown rash on trunk, limbs, lower face, and neck |
| 502944 | 1961 | 3/12 | 6 mth. | – | – | – | + | Red macular rash in diaper area, spreading over body, more numerous in creases |
| 481643 | 1961 | 7/12 | 4 mth. | – | – | – | + | Rash in diaper area and chest, nodular in nature, lesions 2 to 8 mm. diameter; also fine macular rash on chest and abdomen |
| 548648 | 1963 | 4/12 | 1 mth. | Hay fever, asthma | – | – | + | Macular, profuse, discrete, pink to mauvish brown rash; lesions 6 mm. to 2·5 cm. diameter, on trunk, scalp, and face; few lesions on extremities |

TABLE 2
PHYSICAL AND LABORATORY FINDINGS

| History No. (H.S.C.) | Urtication (Darier's sign) | Pruritis | Dermographism | Spleen | Liver | Biopsy | Radiographs | Wassermann | TB Test | Urine | EEG |
|---|---|---|---|---|---|---|---|---|---|---|---|
| 94759 | Yes | – | + | – | | 0 | 0 | – ve | – ve | – ve | |
| 189576 | Yes | – | – | – | | + ve | Chest – ve; long bones – ve | 0 | – ve | – ve | |
| 251593 | – | – | – | 2 cm. | 2 cm. | + ve | 0 | 0 | – ve | – ve | |
| 298486 | – | – | – | – | | – ve | 0 | 0 | – ve | | |
| 318131 | – | – | – | – | | 0 | 0 | 0 | – ve | – ve | |
| 339173 | – | – | – | – | – | 0 | 0 | 0 | 0 | Albumin trace; occas. WBC | |
| 389993 | Yes | – | – | – | | 0 | Skull – ve; ankle – ve | 0 | – ve | – ve | 'Non-specific changes' |
| 412417 | No | – | – | – | – | + ve | 0 | 0 | 0 | – ve | |
| 436824 | No | – | – | – | | 0 | Chest – ve; IVP – ve; skull – ve | 0 | – ve | – ve | |
| 433742 | Yes | – | – | – | | ± | Hands – ve; skull – ve; chest – ve; IVP – ve | 0 | 0 | Albumin + +; occas. epith. cells | |
| 449701 | – | – | – | – | | 0 | 0 | 0 | 0 | – ve | |
| 502944 | Yes | – | – | – | 3 cm. | + ve | Chest – ve; long bones – ve | 0 | – ve | – ve | |
| 481643 | – | – | – | – | 2 cm. | + ve | Chest – ve; skull – ve | 0 | – ve | – ve | |
| 548648 | Yes | – | – | – | 2·5 cm. | + ve | Skeletal survey + ve | 0 | – ve | – ve | |

HAEMATOLC

| History No. (H.S.C.) | Hb (g./100 ml.) | RBC $10^6$ | WBC $10^3$ | Platelets $10^3$ | Neutrophils | Bands (%) | Eosin (%) | Lymphocytes (%) | M |
|---|---|---|---|---|---|---|---|---|---|
| 94756 | | 4·5 | 8·5 | | 35 | | | 65 | |
| 189576 | 12·4 | 4·3 | 8·4 | N | 41 | 2 | 2 | 42 | |
| 257893 | 9·5 | | 19·6 | | | | | | |
| 298486 | 13·6 | | 20·3 | N | 53 | 1 | 2 | 38 | |
| 318131 | 12·9 | | 17·2 | N | 60 | 5 | 2 | 32 | |
| 339173 | 12·7 | | 9·8 | 214 | 28 | 0 | 1 | 68 | |
| 389993 | 12·8 | | 10·5 | N | 54 | | | 45 | |
| 412417 | | | | | | | | | |
| 430824 | 12·0 | | 5·3 | | 48 | | 2 | 49 | |
| 433742 | 13·9 | | 9·2 | 370 | | | | | |
| 449701 | 11·8 | | 9·5 | | 41 | 3 | | 51 | |
| 502944 | 8·6 | | 12·8 | | | | | | |
| 481643 | 12·3 | | 14·9 | | 33 | | 1 | 61 | |
| 548648 | 10·6 | | 19·0 | 603 | 25 | 7 | 5 | 55 (11% atypical) | |

but not admitted has been kept, and more cases have been seen at this hospital than this report indicates.

One child had a solitary mastocytoma, the remainder had urticaria pigmentosa. The age range at the time of admission was 4 months to 6 years and 7 months. There were 9 boys and 5 girls. The onset of the rash was recorded in 12 cases: 8 were 6 months or under, 2 were 6 to 12 months, one was 18 months, and one was 3 years. A family history of hay fever with asthma was recorded in 2 patients. One patient showed dermographism, none had pruritis, 2 had simple urticaria, and one had eczema in addition to urticaria pigmentosa. Other organic disease was present in 6 patients, 2 with

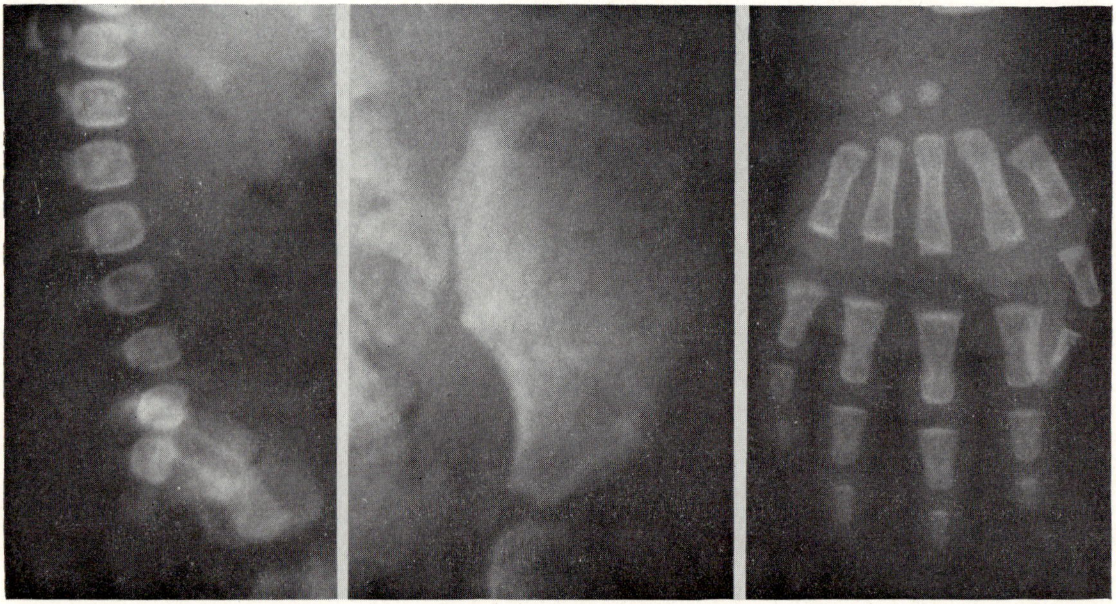

(a) (b) (c)

FIG. 3.—Radiographs taken May 1963, showing dense perimeters of calcification around the vertebral bodies (a); the iliac crests (b); and around the small bones of the hands (c).

TIGATIONS

| a<br>%) | Basophils (%) | Metamyelo-cytes (%) | Smear | Reticulocyte Count | ESR (mm./hr.) | Bleeding Time | Clotting Time | PTT (sec.) |
|---|---|---|---|---|---|---|---|---|
| | | | RBC, slight anisocytosis; WBC, atypical; lymphocytes present | | | | | |
| | | | RBC, slight hypochromasia; WBC occas. atypical lymphocyte | | | 2 min. 45 sec. | 6 min. 25 sec. | |
| | | | RBC normal WBC neutrophilia | | | | | |
| | | | Smear normal | | | | | |
| | | | Slight lymphocytosis | | 8<br>30 | 1 min. 15 sec. | 5 min. 30 sec. | |
| | | | Differential normal | 2·6 | | | | |
| | 2 | 1 | RBC, slight hypochromia; occas. poikilocytosis and polychromasia | | | | | 53 |

TABLE 4

BONE-MARROW DIFFERENTIAL COUNTS PER 100 CELLS IN 2 CASES*

| History No. (H.S.C.) | Bone-marrow | Myelo-cytes | Meta-myelo-cytes | Bands | Eosino-phils | Poly-morphs | Lympho-cytes | Mast Cells | Erythroid Elements | Blasts |
|---|---|---|---|---|---|---|---|---|---|---|
| 433742 | Positive | 10 | 13 | 22 | 4 | 16 | 12 | 3 | 20 | 0 |
| 548648 | Negative | 9 | 16 | 21 | 0 | 13 | 23 | 0 | 17 | 1 |

* In one other case (251593) bone-marrow cell count showed normal proportions of white cells, megakaryocytes, platelets, and red blood cells.

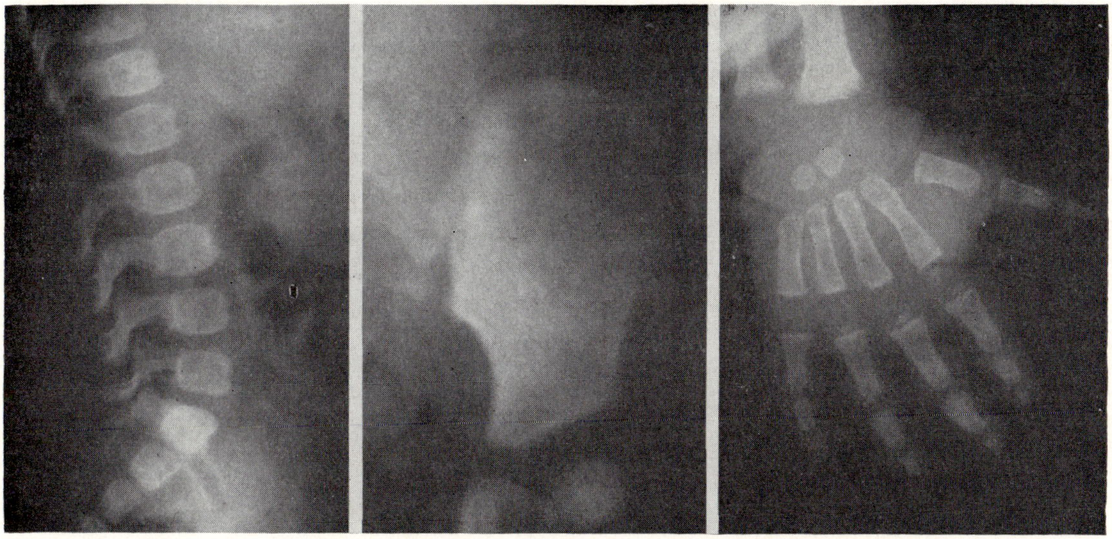

(a) (b) (c)

FIG. 4a-c.—Radiographs taken in March 1964, showing complete clearing of the bony changes.

convulsive disorder, one with nephrosis, one with possible Addison's disease, one with secondarily infected eczema, and one with pyloric stenosis. In 8 patients, the central portions of the body (head and trunk) were more affected. In 3 patients the rash was more prominent in the diaper area. In one, none was present in this area. The nodular or papular nature of the rash was mentioned in 7 patients. Red, reddish, pink, mauve, brown, and melanotic colorations were described. Enlargement of the spleen was noted in one and an enlarged liver in 4 patients. Albuminuria was noted in 2 (one with nephrosis). Biopsy was performed in 8 patients and was positive in 6, negative in one, and questionable in one. Bone-marrow study of 3 patients gave positive findings (excessive mast cells) in one, and negative findings in 2. Radiographs in 7 patients revealed one with bony change. Anaemia was present in 2 and a leucocytosis of more than 10,000 cells/c.mm. in 7. An excess of platelets was observed in one patient. Eosinophils were raised in one; another showed plasma cells in the peripheral blood smear; and atypical lymphocytes were described in 3 patients.

A search of the published reports revealed 12 paediatric patients with cutaneous and bone lesions. Of these, 9 showed solitary or localized skeletal lesions (Asboe-Hansen, 1953; Grupper, 1954; Shair and Casper, 1955; Gulden and Niebauer, 1956; Edelstein, 1956; Remy, 1957; Hasselmann and Scholder-Oehmichen, 1957; Lees and Stroud, 1959; Niordson, 1962); and 3 showed the generalized type of skeletal lesion, the youngest of whom was 2 years old (Rider *et al.*, 1957; Lees and Stroud, 1959). The case reported here appears to be the youngest to show generalized skeletal lesions, and is unusual in that the radiographic changes completely disappeared by 17 months of age.

On reviewing the description of patients with mastocytosis but without cutaneous lesions, one wonders if some of the infants or small children with general or local pruritis, but no cutaneous lesions other than self-inflicted scratch marks, may not have systemic mastocytosis without skin lesions. Complaints such as flushing, sweating, and fainting, frequently may suggest this diagnosis and warrant more investigation than these symptoms are commonly accorded.

## Summary

A brief discussion of mastocytosis is presented.

An infant less than 4 months old with cutaneous and skeletal asymptomatic mastocytosis is described.

The skeletal lesions in this patient apparently cleared entirely with growth.

The records of 14 patients with this condition admitted to the Hospital for Sick Children (1938-1963) are reviewed.

I wish to thank Dr. J. H. Ebbs for reviewing this report.

### References

Asboe-Hansen, G. (1953). Urticaria pigmentosa with bone lesions. *Acta derm-venereol.* (*Stockh.*), **33**, 471.
Beare, M. (1958). Urticaria pigmentosa and allied disorders. *Brit. J. Derm.*, **70**, 418.
Bigelow, E. L. (1961). Changing concepts concerning mastocytosis. *J. Pediat.*, **58**, 499.
Degos, R. (1960). Mastocitos—mastocitosis-mastocitoma. *Rev. argent. Dermatosif.*, **44**, 25.
Edelstein, A. J. (1956). Urticaria pigmentosa with bone changes. *Arch. Derm.*, **74**, 676.
Ehrlich, P. (1877). Beiträge zur Kenntnis der Anilinfärbungen and ihrer Verwendung in der mikroskopischen Technik. *Arch. mikr. Anat.*, **13**, 263.
Ellis, J. M. (1949). Urticaria pigmentosa: a report of a case with autopsy. *Arch. Path.*, **48**, 426.
Ende, N., and Cherniss, E. I. (1958). Splenic mastocytosis. *Blood*, **13**, 631.
Friedman, B. I., Will, J. J., Freiman, D. G., and Braunstein, H. (1958). Tissue mast cell leukemia. *ibid.*, **13**, 70.
Grupper, C. (1954). In discussion on Sobel, N. Urticaria pigmentosa. *Arch. Derm. Syph.* (*Chic.*), **69**, 109.
Gulden, K., and Niebauer, G. (1956). Vorläufige Mitteilung zum Urticaria pigmentosa-Problem. *Wien. klin. Wschr.*, **68**, 52.
Hasselmann, C. M., and Scholder-Oehmichen, C. (1957). Zum Problem der Urticaria pigmentosa. *Arch. klin. exp. Derm.*, **205**, 261.
Head, K. W. (1958). Cutaneous mast-cell tumours in the dog, cat and ox. *Brit. J. Derm.*, **70**, 389.
Lees, M. H., and Stroud, C. E. (1959). Bone lesions in urticaria pigmentosa in childhood. *Arch. Dis. Childh.*, **34**, 205.
Marshall, J., Walker, J., Lurie, H. I., Hansen, J. D. L., and Mackenzie, D. (1957). Solitary mastocytoma and the mastocytoses: a discussion of the mastocytoses and a report of two cases of solitary mastocytoma showing an unusual phenomenon of generalized flushing. *S. Afr. med. J.*, **31**, 867.
Nettleship, E. (1869). Rare forms of urticaria. *Brit. med. J.*, **2**, 323.
Nickel, W. R. (1957). Urticaria pigmentosa; mastocytosis: a consideration of various manifestations. *Arch. Derm.*, **76**, 476.
Niordson, A. M. (1962). Urticaria pigmentosa: age of onset and prognosis. *Acta derm.-venereol.* (*Stockh.*), **42**, 433.
Padawer, J. (1963). Mast cells and basophils. *Ann. N.Y. Acad. Sci.*, **103**, 1.
Pastras, T., and Beerman, H. (1962). Mastocytosis: some contributions to the recent literature. *Amer. J. med. Sci.*, **244**, 510.
Poppel, M. H., Gruber, W. F., Silber, R., Holder, A. K., and Christman, R. O. (1959). The roentgen manifestations of urticaria pigmentosa (mastocytosis). *Amer. J. Roentgenol.*, **82**, 239.
Remy, D. (1957). Die Mastocytose. *Dtsch. med. Wschr.*, **82**, 719.
——, and Herzberg, J. J. (1961). Symposion 2 (a) Die Physiologie der Mastzelle. (b) Klinik und Therapie der Mastocytosen. *Arch. klin. exp. Derm.*, **213**, 544.
Rider, T. L., Stein, A. A., and Abbuhl, J. W. (1957). Generalized mast cell disease and urticaria pigmentosa: report of a case. *Pediatrics*, **19**, 1023.
Sagher, F. (1956). Mast cell disorders: the changing aspect of urticaria pigmentosa from a pure cutaneous to a systemic disease. *Excerpta med.* (*Amst.*), *Sect. XIII*, **10**, 311.
——, Cohen, C., and Schorr, S. (1952). Concomitant bone changes in urticaria pigmentosa. *J. invest. Derm.*, **18**, 425.
——, and Even-Paz, Z. (1960). Mastocytosis (urticaria pigmentosa). In *Cutaneous Manifestations of the Reticuloendothelial Granulomas*, ed. S. M. Bluefarb, p. 268. Charles C. Thomas, Springfield, Illinois.
——, Liban, E., Ungar, H., and Schorr, S. (1956). Urticaria pigmentosa with bone involvement: mast cell aggregates in bones and myelosclerosis found at autopsy in a case dying of monocytic leukemia. *J. invest. Derm.*, **27**, 355.

——, and Schorr, S. (1956). Bone lesions in urticaria pigmentosa. *ibid.*, **26**, 431.
Sangster, A. (1878). An anomalous mottled rash, accompanied by pruritus, factitious urticaria, and pigmentation, "urticaria pigmentosa (?)". *Trans. clin. Soc. Lond.*, **11**, 161.
Shair, H. M., and Casper, S. L. (1955). Personal communication to Sagher and Schorr (1956).
Stutzman, L., and Urbach, F. (1961). Mast cell disease. *Pediat. Clin. N. Amer.*, **8**, 857.
——, Zsoldos, S., Ambrus, J. L., and Asboe-Hansen, G. (1960). Systemic mast cell disease: physiological considerations and report of a patient treated with nitrogen mustard. *Amer. J. Med.*, **29**, 894.
Szweda, J. A., Abraham, J. P., Fine, G., Nixon, R. K., and Rupe, C. E. (1962). Systemic mast cell disease: a review and report of three cases. *ibid.*, **32**, 227.
Thin, G. (1877). On the microscopic appearances of the skin of a patient whose case is described by Mr. Morrant Baker in the 8th volume of this Society's Transactions. *Trans. clin. Soc. Lond.*, **10**, 198.
Unna, P. G. (1887). Beiträge zur Anatomie und Pathogenese der Urticaria simplex und pigmentosa. *Derm. Stud. Hamburg*, 3.
Waters, W. J., and Lacson, P. S. (1957). Mast cell leukemia presenting as urticaria pigmentosa: report of a case. *Pediatrics*, **19**, 1033.
West, G. B. (1958). Pharmacology of the tissue mast cell. *Brit. J. Derm.*, **70**, 409.

*Arch. Dis. Childh.*, 1965, **40**, 684.

# ACCURACY OF THE SWEAT TEST: ADVANTAGE OF A MICROMETHOD

BY

R. DE HALLER*, J. DE HALLER, and P. SIEGENTHALER†

*From the Institute of Diseases of the Chest, Brompton Hospital, London, and the Policlinique Universitaire de Médecine, Geneva (Switzerland)*

(RECEIVED FOR PUBLICATION APRIL 26, 1965)

The high sweat electrolyte concentration in cystic fibrosis is most important in the diagnosis of this disease. The method used for its determination should be simple to perform, harmless to the patient, and accurate. The widely-used method of collecting sweat on a filter paper (Shwachman, Leubner, and Catzel, 1955) after pilocarpine iontophoresis (Gibson and Cooke, 1959) fulfils the first two conditions but not the latter. Both weighing and elution may introduce serious errors, and the method is known to be unreliable for samples weighing under 20 mg. Moreover, the sweat sample is not transportable and has to be analysed rapidly in order to avoid evaporation.

A simple, harmless, and accurate method of collecting and estimating sweat electrolyte concentration is described, which has given satisfactory results for over three years (de Haller, Siegenthaler, Hampaï, Spahr, Vulliet, and Favre, 1962; Siegenthaler, de Haller, de Haller, Hampaï, and Muller, 1964).

## Material and Methods

The skin area (palmar aspect of the forearm in adults, or epigastrium in small children) is cleaned with distilled water and alcohol ether. Sweat secretion is stimulated by the iontophoresis of 5 drops of a 0·2% pilocarpine nitrate solution placed on a filter paper 4 cm. in diameter, which is covered with the positive electrode 3·5 cm. in diameter (Gibson and Cooke, 1959). The negative electrode trapped in gauze soaked in electrolyte, is held in the patient's hand. A current of 2 mAmp. is maintained for 5 minutes. If large sweat samples are needed, they can easily be obtained by increasing the area of the electrode, the amount of pilocarpine, and the electrical intensity. After stimulation, the skin is washed with distilled water and thoroughly dried. It is then covered with a glass or plastic cup 4·5 cm. in diameter and, in order to avoid contact with the sweat, at least 0·5 cm. high (the cap of a standard screw-topped bottle was used). The cup, washed with distilled water and dried, is fixed to the skin with tape, and to prevent condensation is kept at body temperature by an electric pad or a warm hand. After 20 minutes the cup is removed. If condensation has occurred in the cup, the sample should be discarded. The sweat drops are collected by drawing a capillary tube gently over the skin surface. There will be no significant evaporation if this collection takes place within 30 seconds, which is easy to achieve. By inclining the tube at an appropriate angle the sweat ascends spontaneously, and air bubbles, which would complicate sampling, are avoided. The tube is then sealed in a low flame (the pilot light of a Bunsen burner is ideal) 2 cm. beyond the extremities of the sweat column. The tightness of the first sealing can be tested by holding the tube vertically, open end down. The capillary tube, 1-2 mm. in diameter, is made of ordinary laboratory glass, washed with chromic acid and tap water, rinsed with distilled water, and dried. For estimation, no weighing is required, as the sweat sample is then aspirated directly into a plastic micropipette (Sanz, 1957). The same pipette is used for both sweat and standard solution. This is not possible with a glass ultramicropipette (Kirk type), with which an additional error of 1-4% must be taken into account (Sanz, 1957). 5 $\mu$l. are required for one estimation of Na or Cl, and 20 $\mu$l. for K. Na and K are estimated by a flame photometer (Beckman), providing a direct reading after dilution with 1 ml. distilled water delivered by an automatic syringe;* chloride is estimated by a Beckman and Spinko microburette (Sanz, 1957) as titrated by Schales and Schales (1941). Only values for sodium will be reported here.

The accuracy of the method was checked with a series of NaCl solutions of 7 different strengths obtained by diluting a solution of approximately 120 mEq/l. Na. Their exact concentration is given in the Table. The majority contained over 50 mEq/l. Na, as it was more

* Research fellow 1963-1964, Institute of Diseases of the Chest, Brompton Hospital, London. Present address: Basle Sanatorium, 7260 Davos (Switzerland).

† Policlinique universitaire de médecine, Geneva (Switzerland).

* An identical experiment, as described below, was performed on standard solutions of NaCl with an Evans Electrode Photometer (Eel), as this type is more widely used. 5 $\mu$l. samples were adequately diluted with an ordinary pipette so that the values could be read on the 100 U scale. Accuracy of the results was of a similar order to that of the original experiment.

TABLE

ACCURACY OF CAPILLARY TUBE METHOD TESTED AGAINST 7 SOLUTIONS OF NaCl, WITH 2 TUBES (a AND b) FOR EACH SOLUTION

| Standard Solution (mEq/l. Na) | Capillary Tube | Na Concentration (mEq/l.) | | | | | Maximum Difference in Percentage of Mean |
|---|---|---|---|---|---|---|---|
| | | Dry End | | Wet End | | Mean | |
| | | a | b | a | b | | |
| I: 118·0 | a | 116·0 | 117·0 | 117·0 | 120·0 | 118·0 | 3 |
| | b | 117·0 | 119·0 | 116·0 | 120·0 | | |
| II: 96·5 | a | 97·5 | 96·5 | 96·0 | 100·0 | 97·0 | 5 |
| | b | 95·0 | 96·0 | 97·0 | 97·5 | | |
| III: 81·0 | a | 79·0 | 81·0 | 80·0 | 82·0 | 80·5 | 4 |
| | b | 81·0 | 80·0 | 79·5 | 82·0 | | |
| IV: 57·5 | a | 58·0 | 58·0 | 57·0 | 57·0 | 58·5 | 7 |
| | b | 58·0 | 60·0 | 59·5 | 61·0 | | |
| V: 48·5 | a | 52·0 | 49·0 | 48·0 | 48·0 | 49·0 | 8 |
| | b | 48·0 | 49·0 | (42·0) | 49·0 | | |
| VI: 16·0 | a | 16·0 | 16·0 | 16·0 | 16·5 | 16·5 | 9 |
| | b | 16·5 | 17·5 | 16·0 | 16·0 | | |
| VII: 8·0 | a | 8·0 | 8·0 | 7·5 | 7·5 | 8·0 | 6 |
| | b | 8·0 | 8·0 | 7·5 | 8·0 | | |
| Mean (solutions I-V) | | 80·43 ± 1·23 | | 80·38 ± 2·50 | | | |

*Note:* The values have been rounded up to the nearest half unit. Statistical calculations were applied only to solutions I-V.

important to assess the accuracy of the method in borderline and pathological values (upper limit of the normal = 70-80 mEq/l. Na). Two capillary tubes (a and b) were filled with each solution and sealed, and 4 estimations were performed for each tube: the first two from the end which was wetted when drawing up the solution, the second two from the dry end. This was done to ensure that higher concentrations of sodium did not occur in the wetted end as a result of evaporation during sealing (Table).

## Results and Discussion

In columns 3 and 4 of the Table the results of the double estimations made at the dry end of each capillary tube are listed, and in columns 5 and 6 those made at the wet end. The respective mean values are not significantly different (difference of the means = 0·05 ± 2·40), even though the standard deviation of the mean value at the wet end is larger than that found at the dry one. This means that by sealing the capillary tube 2 cm. beyond the sweat column, the minute evaporation that may occur at the wet end has no significant effect on the final result. Closing the tube with plasticine failed to give satisfactory results, as this substance loses its plastic properties with drying or cooling. Once sealed, the tube can be transported and stored for weeks, the electrolyte concentration of the sweat remaining unaltered. This is valuable for paediatricians living far away from laboratory centres.

Column 8 shows that below 50 mEq/l. Na the maximum experimental error of this method is 9% (the single incidental extreme value of 42 mEq/l. in solution V not being taken into account), and that above 50 mEq/l. it does not exceed 7%.

In contrast, paediatricians find the error of occasional sweat tests with the filter paper method to be ± 15%; in trained hands the maximum error remains as much as ± 10%, reaching ± 25% when samples are minute or poorly concentrated (Lobeck and Huebner, 1962). With the capillary tube method, the electrolyte concentration of small amounts of sweat can be estimated accurately. This is valuable for the study of sweat physiology (Siegenthaler *et al.*, 1964), and is very useful in small children whose sweat production may be limited.

In addition to its accuracy, the capillary tube method has the advantage that it uses techniques and apparatus available in most routine laboratories. This is not the case with other methods suggested recently, which have been based on electrical conductivity of sweat, using conductivity cells (Shwachman, Dunham, and Phillips, 1963) and sodium electrodes (Goldbloom and Sekelj, 1963), the accuracy of which, moreover, is not better than that of the filter paper.

In conclusion the capillary tube method is simple to perform and provides accurate results, even for minute amounts of sweat. As the capillary tube is sealed after collection, it may be transported and stored. For estimation of sodium and other sweat electrolytes ordinary laboratory equipment is suitable.

## Summary

A new capillary tube method is described for the analysis of sodium and other electrolytes in sweat. This is shown to be reliable and more accurate than other methods. Furthermore, standard laboratory equipment can be used, and the capillary tube containing the sweat sample can be sealed, transported, and stored.

We wish to thank Mr. P. M. Payne, director of the South Metropolitan Cancer Registry, Sutton (Surrey), for the statistical investigation, and Dr. D. G. Jones and Dr. J. C. Batten of the Brompton Hospital for their help.

REFERENCES

Gibson, L. E., and Cooke, R. E. (1959). A test for concentration of electrolytes in sweat in cystic fibrosis of the pancreas utilizing pilocarpine by iontophoresis. *Pediatrics*, **23**, 545.

Goldbloom, R. B., and Sekelj, P. (1963). Cystic fibrosis of the pancreas: diagnosis by application of a sodium electrode to the skin. *New Engl. J. Med.*, **269**, 1349.

de Haller, R., Siegenthaler, P., Hampaï, A., Spahr, A., Vulliet, V., and Favre, R. (1962). Étude critique du test de la transpiration pour le dépistage des hétérozygotes de la mucoviscidose. *Schweiz. med. Wschr.*, **92**, 1493.

Lobeck, C. C., and Huebner, D. (1962). Effect of age, sex, and cystic fibrosis on the sodium and potassium content of human sweat. *Pediatrics*, **30**, 172.

Sanz, M. C. (1957). Ultramicro methods and standardization of equipment. *Clin. Chem.*, **3**, 406.

Schales, O., and Schales, S. S. (1941). A simple and accurate method for the determination of chloride in biological fluids. *J. biol. Chem.*, **140**, 879.

Shwachman, H., Dunham, R., and Phillips, W. R. (1963). Electrical conductivity of sweat. A simple diagnostic test in children. *Pediatrics*, **32**, 85.

——, Leubner, H., and Catzel, P. (1955). Mucoviscidosis. *Advanc. Pediat.*, **7**, 297.

Siegenthaler, P., de Haller, J., de Haller, R., Hampaï, A., and Muller, A. F. (1964). Effect of experimental salt depletion and aldosterone load on sodium and chloride concentration in the sweat of patients with cystic fibrosis of the pancreas and of normal children. *Arch. Dis. Childh.*, **39**, 61.

*Arch. Dis. Childh.*, 1965, **40**, 687.

# LARYNGEAL STRIDOR AND RESPIRATORY OBSTRUCTION ASSOCIATED WITH MENINGOMYELOCELE

BY

J. S. FITZSIMMONS*

*From the Royal Aberdeen Hospital for Sick Children*

(RECEIVED FOR PUBLICATION MARCH 11, 1965)

Laryngeal stridor in infancy may be associated with a variety of disorders including abnormalities of the nervous system. The association of stridor with meningomyelocele, however, has received only scant attention in published reports, and in view of this the following cases may be of interest.

## Case Reports

**Case 1.** A male infant, birth weight 6 lb. 6 oz. (2,891 g.), had a lumbar meningomyelocele which was repaired on the second day of life. At the age of 10 days, the infant's anterior fontanelle was tense and an air ventriculogram showed some dilatation of the lateral ventricles. However, subsequent head growth was not excessive, and by 5 months the skull circumference was 17⅜ in. (44 cm.). At the age of 2 months the child developed laryngeal stridor which worsened over a period of one week. Laryngoscopy revealed no local cause for this symptom, but two weeks later tracheostomy was necessary for severe respiratory obstruction. Following operation, there were repeated episodes of vomiting and respiratory infection. It was six months before the infant could manage without the tracheostomy tube. Stridor has not recurred and the infant remains well without evidence of hydrocephalus. The only abnormality is paralytic talipes of the left foot.

**Case 2.** A male infant, birth weight 6 lb. 7 oz. (2,919 g.), had a lumbar meningomyelocele which was repaired on the first day of life. Hydrocephalus subsequently developed and a Spitz-Holter valve was inserted when the patient was 6 weeks old. From birth he showed a flaccid paraplegia of both lower limbs and double sphincter paralysis.

Laryngeal stridor and difficulty in swallowing were noticed when he was 4 months old, and he was admitted to hospital at the age of 5 months with increasing respiratory obstruction. Laryngoscopy revealed bilateral adductor spasm of the vocal cords and urgent tracheostomy was necessary. The tracheostomy tube had to be maintained in position for six months, though frequent attempts to remove it were made. The severe difficulty in swallowing persisted during this period and the patient had to be tube-fed for several weeks. Now, at the age of 2 years, he has only slight stridor after crying but he still has difficulty in swallowing solids. There have been no further episodes of respiratory obstruction.

**Case 3.** A male infant, birth weight 5 lb. 8 oz. (2,494 g.), had a lumbar meningomyelocele which was repaired within 24 hours of birth. Following operation, transient cyanotic attacks occurred without obvious cause, and at the age of 5 weeks he developed laryngeal stridor. This was never very severe, but at this time he had an attack of pneumonia which responded to antibiotics. Hydrocephalus developed and a Spitz-Holter valve was inserted at 7 weeks of age. At operation, inspection of the larynx revealed no local lesion. Now, at the age of 6 months, the infant is well and the head circumference is 16¾ in. (42·5 cm.). There is still obvious, but variable, stridor. Except for the period when he had pneumonia, this child did not have significant respiratory distress.

## Discussion

The cause of laryngeal stridor in these patients is uncertain. Examination of the larynx revealed no local lesion, but the presence of congenital abnormalities of the nervous system suggested the possibility of faulty nervous control of the vocal cords. Graham (1963) reported two cases of bilateral vocal cord paralysis associated with meningomyelocele and suggested that the stridor resulted from traction on the vagus nerve. Both his cases required tracheostomy for respiratory obstruction and both died: at necropsy they were found to have the Arnold-Chiari malformation with caudal displacement of the brainstem. Smith (1959) reported two cases of stridor with meningomyelocele, and at necropsy one of these infants had hydrocephalus without the Arnold-Chiari malformation. He suggested that 'coning' of the medulla might cause disordered vagal action and, hence, stridor. In our Case 3, the possibility of 'coning' was considered. This infant's stridor was thought to be most marked when the anterior fontanelle was very tense. However, removal of

* Present address: Mansfield and District General Hospital, West Hill Drive, Mansfield, Notts.

cerebrospinal fluid from the lateral ventricles produced no dramatic change and the stridor persisted after the insertion of a Spitz-Holter valve.

Kiger, Kohlmoos, and May (1964) described an infant with bilateral vocal cord paralysis and an occipital meningomyelocele. Stridor developed at the age of 9 days and the infant required tracheostomy for respiratory obstruction at 6 months. The child still had the tracheostomy tube in position at the age of 2½ years; there was no evidence of hydrocephalus. The authors mentioned Graham's cases and also discussed the Arnold-Chiari malformation as a cause of the vocal cord paralysis.

In a survey of 80 infants with stridor, Apley (1953) reported 2 with associated meningomyelocele. They had persistent stridulous breathing and opisthotonus. Necropsy revealed no obvious cause for the respiratory symptoms and there was no mention of the Arnold-Chiari malformation. It was suggested that the stridor resulted from central nervous system dysfunction. Approximately half of these 80 infants had frequent choking attacks and difficulty with swallowing. This is of interest in view of the marked feeding difficulty encountered in Case 1. There was no obvious cause for this additional complication, but it suggested the possibility of brain-stem involvement. Bigler, Holinger, Johnston, and Schiller (1954), reporting respiratory obstruction with meningomyelocele, mentioned that their two patients had associated cranial nerve abnormalities. They did not, however, elaborate on these other lesions.

In Apley's series, 16 infants had mental retardation, and the association of stridor with low intelligence has been confirmed by Benians, Benson, Sherwood, and Spector (1964).

Graham (1963) commented on how seldom stridor has been reported in association with meningomyelocele and hydrocephalus, despite the frequency of these congenital malformations. However, the association may be commoner than the literature suggests, but unless the respiratory symptoms were severe they would be overshadowed by the other lesions. In Case 3 the stridor caused some concern, but in the other two patients the respiratory symptoms were of major importance and required urgent surgical treatment.

## Summary

Three cases of laryngeal stridor associated with meningomyelocele are reported. Two required tracheostomy for respiratory obstruction and both recovered. The mechanism of production of the stridor is discussed.

I am grateful to Professor R. G. Mitchell and Dr. N. S. Clark for their help and advice in the preparation of this paper.

### References

Apley, J. (1953). The infant with stridor: a follow-up survey of 80 cases. *Arch. Dis. Childh.*, **28**, 423.

Benians, R. C., Benson, P. F., Sherwood, T., and Spector, R. G. (1964). Intellectual impairment in congenital laryngeal stridor. *Guy's Hosp. Rep.*, **113**, 360.

Bigler, J. A., Holinger, P. H., Johnston, K. C., and Schiller, F. (1954). Tracheostomy in infancy. *Pediatrics*, **13**, 476.

Graham, M. D. (1963). Bilateral vocal cord paralysis associated with meningomyelocele and the Arnold-Chiari malformation. *Laryngoscope (St. Louis)*, **73**, 85.

Kiger, J. R., Kohlmoos, H. W., and May, I. A. (1964). Bilateral vocal cord paralysis in infancy. *Amer. J. Dis. Child.*, **108**, 648.

Smith, M. E. N. (1959). The association of laryngeal stridor with meningo-myelocele. *J. Laryng.*, **73**, 188.

*Arch. Dis. Childh.*, 1965, **40**, 689.

# FOETUS IN FOETU

BY

EDMUND Y. C. LEE

*From the University of Hong Kong, Department of Surgery, Queen Mary Hospital*

(RECEIVED FOR PUBLICATION APRIL 26, 1965)

Foetus in foetu, a term coined by Meckel (quoted by Lewis, 1961), is applied to those cases where a parasitic twin is found included within its bearer. It is rightly regarded as a rarity. Since Young reported a detailed study of a case in 1809, only sporadic case reports appeared from time to time, only 13 having been traced since 1900. Lord (1956) reported 2 personally studied cases and reviewed 7 others from published reports. In most of these, only one foetus was found, and nearly all were intra-abdominal in situation (Lord, 1956; Lewis, 1961; Janovski, 1962). In this communication, an example of inclusion quadruplets is reported with unusual and perhaps unique features.

## Case Report

A 2-month-old Chinese male infant was admitted to the Professorial Surgical Unit, Queen Mary Hospital, Hong Kong, on May 10, 1964. The complaint was that of gradual abdominal distension for 10 days with no symptoms of obstruction either in the gastro-intestinal tract or in the genito-urinary tract. He had been taking feeds well and weight gain had been normal. The child was the last sib in a family of 11. There was no history of twin pregnancy.

*On examination* the infant appeared well nourished and healthy. His weight was 12 lb. (5,443 g.). There was no sign of dehydration or anaemia. The abdomen was grossly distended across the midline with dilated superficial veins coursing vertically and upwards. An irregular but circumscribed firm mass was palpable in the abdomen extending into the pelvis. On rectal examination, the same mass was felt to the right of the rectum and was ballotable bimanually. It was slightly mobile but could not be pushed out of the pelvis. Emptying the bladder failed to alter the physical characteristics of the mass.

**Investigations.** Haemoglobin was 11·5 g./100 ml. WBC count 8,900/c.mm. Blood group A. Urinalysis was normal. A plain radiograph of the abdomen was taken; complete spinal columns and other skeletal parts were seen in a large soft tissue mass (Fig. 1).

**Operation.** Three foetuses were found bathing in clear fluid inside a single thin wall sac to which they were attached by umbilical cords (Fig. 2). The sac itself was situated in the pelvis behind the bladder. The rectum was pushed to the right. On cutting the umbilical cords, arterial blood was found spurting from the distal ends and on tracing them further, they were found to lead to the mid-sacral artery, to which the sac was adherent. The three foetuses with the sac were easily removed. The abdomen was closed in layers without drainage. Post-operative course was uneventful and normal feeding was rapidly re-established. The infant was discharged on the 8th post-operative day. The patient has shown normal progress when seen in the follow-up clinic.

**Pathology.** A detailed study of the specimens was made by dissection and microscopy. The sac was found to be lined by one layer of endothelial cells. No placenta was found. The largest specimen, measuring 15 cm. × 6·2 cm. and weighing 1,262 g. was the most developed of the 3. It was covered by skin with hair-bearing areas in front and at the shoulders, 4 well-formed limbs were present, bearing 5 and 6 digits on the upper limbs and 7 and 6 on the lower limbs. There was no face or skull discernible, but a well-formed central nervous system with differentiation into cerebrum and cerebellum covered with meninges and in continuity with an exposed spinal cord was found. The skeletal system appeared to be of the highest development. The radiograph of the specimens (Fig. 3) and dissection showed a well-developed spine composed of a series of vertebrae with characteristic cranio-caudal differentiation, namely, well-formed thoracic, lumbar, and sacral parts. The thoracic part showed related ribs on either side and the sacrum was found attached to a well-formed pelvic girdle. Scapulae were well developed, so were the limb bones as distal as the digits. Thus, excepting the skull and facial bones, all other parts of the skeleton were as well developed as those of a full-term infant.

The nervous system also showed a high degree of differentiation (Fig. 4), two cerebral hemispheres with enclosed ventricles were found. The cerebellum was identified. The spinal cord, enclosed in a spinal canal lined by meninges, was exposed at its upper half. Spinal nerves with ganglia were found to be given off segmentally.

Loops of intestine were found suspended in mesentery within an endothelium-lined cavity (Fig. 5). The caecum and appendix were identified, and, therefore, small and large bowels were easily differentiated. No

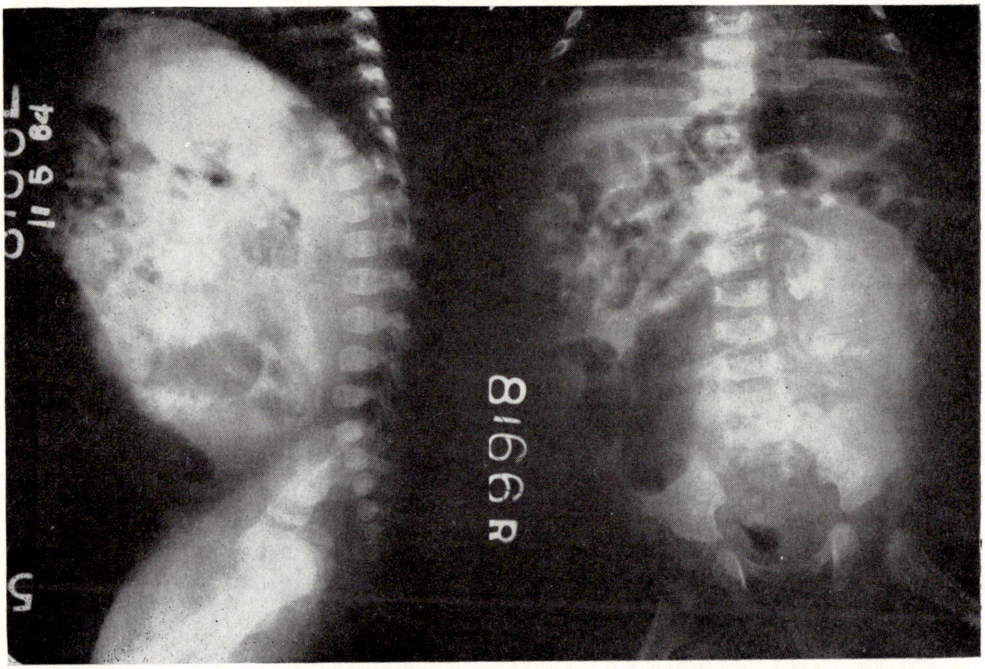

FIG. 1.—Radiograph of abdomen showing well-formed spinal columns and other skeletal parts.

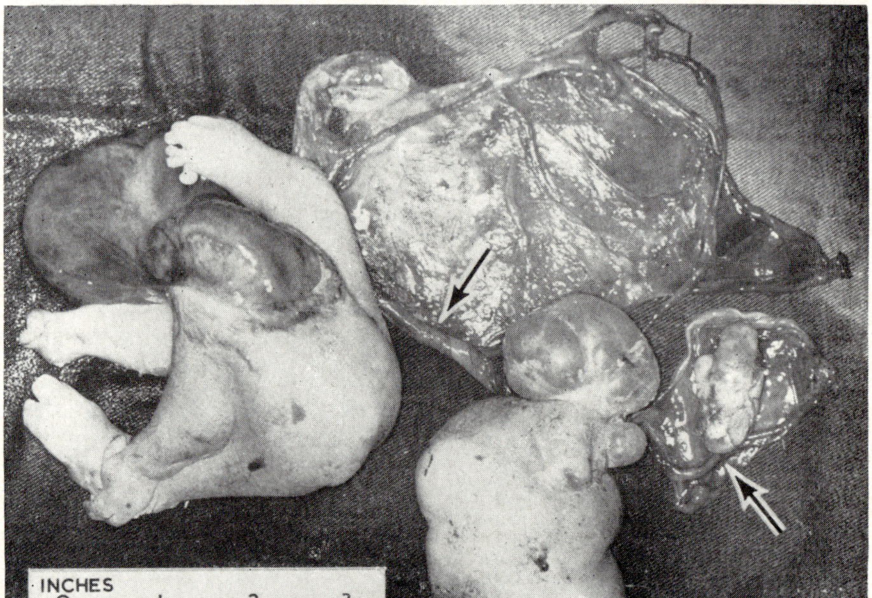


FIG. 2.—The three foetuses with their ruptured sac. Arrows show the umbilical cords attached to the foetuses.

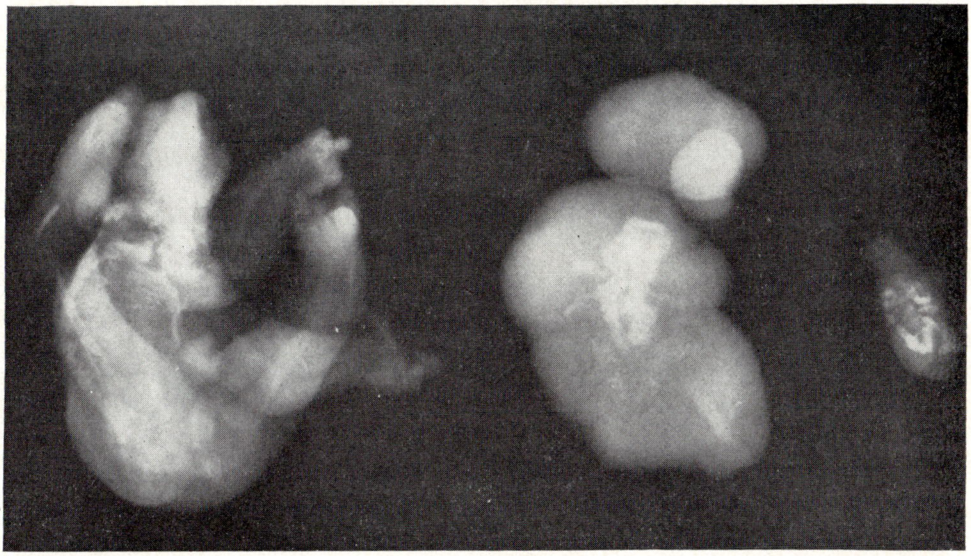

FIG. 3.—Radiograph of the specimens showing spinal columns and other skeletal parts, including thoracic cages.

derivatives of the genito-urinary tract were discovered, though what appeared to be a genital tubercle was found in the perineum. The organs described were all well supplied with blood vessels, but no heart or aorta was found, though a particularly large artery was found in the umbilical cord.

The other two foetuses were much less developed, weighing 52 g. and 13 g., respectively; nevertheless, they showed well-formed skeletal parts, coelomic cavities with intestinal loops, umbilical cords, and nervous tissues. There was little doubt that they were foetuses of a more primitive development than their companion. All three were included in a single sac and all three had the same blood group as their bearer.

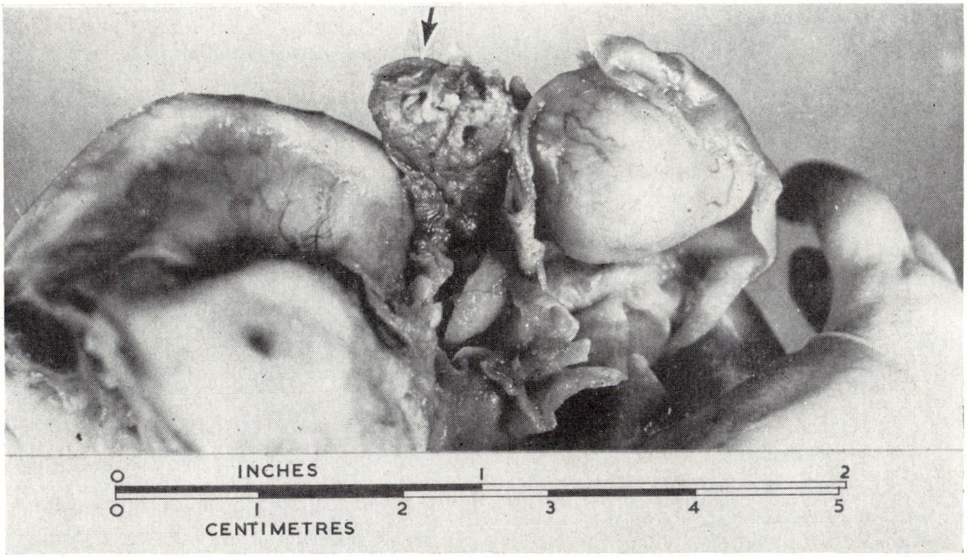


FIG. 4.—Dissected specimen showing well-formed central nervous system, including cerebrum, cerebellum, spinal cord, and their meninges. Arrow points to a part of the cerebellum.

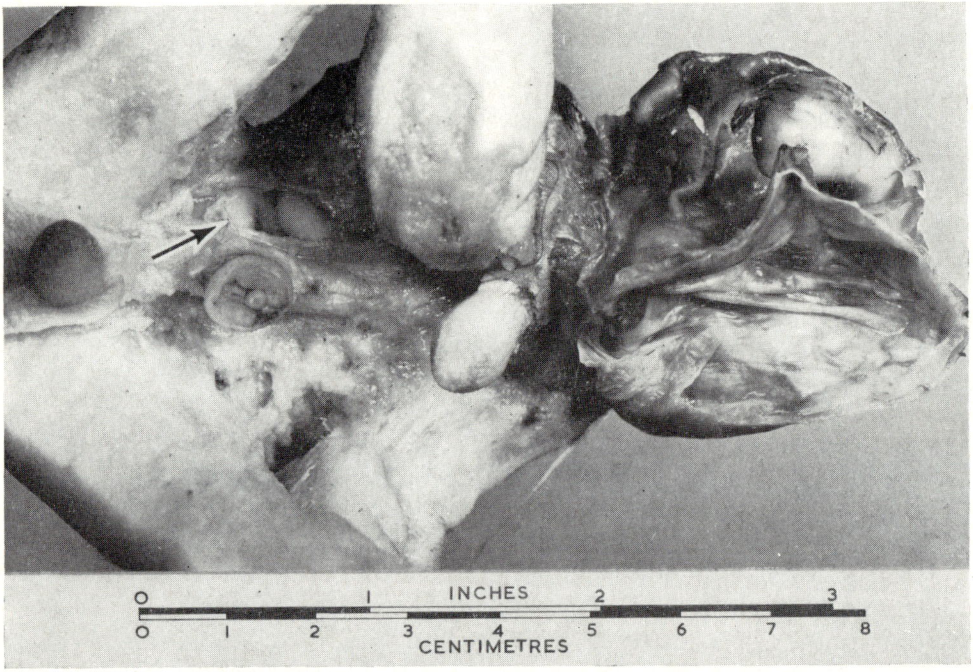


FIG. 5.—Dissected specimen showing loops of intestine in an abdominal cavity as shown by the arrow. The umbilical cord shows two large vessels and several intestinal loops. A scrotum-like nodule seen at the perineum.

## Discussion

Willis (1935) adopted the criterion of diagnosing foetus in foetu, in distinguishing it from teratoma by the presence of a vertebral axis and by an appropriate arrangement of other organs or limbs with respect to the axis. When this criterion was adopted, probably many of the recorded cases were not true examples of foetus in foetu. Lord (1956) found 31 reports of alleged cases before 1900 and 11 reports since that year. Of the 11 more recent cases, only 4 had unequivocal evidence of the condition. Most of these were intra-abdominal foetus in foetu. Examples of foetus in foetu at other sites were less common. Kimmel, Moyer, Peale, Winborne, and Gotwals (1950) described a cerebral tumour in which 5 foetuses were found. Older writers customarily subdivided cases of abdominal foetus in foetu into two groups, extra- and intra-abdominal. But those reports of allegedly extra-abdominal origin (Taruffi, 1885; Curtis, 1826) are far from clear in their descriptions.

In all cases of intra-abdominal foetus in foetu in which the sites of origin were specified, the retroperitoneal tissues in the upper abdomen were found to be the sites. In many of the surgically treated cases, the site was not ascertained. In the present case the sac was found to be attached to the midsacral artery by a pedicle in the retroperitoneal space in front of the sacrum. It appears to be the only case of pelvic origin.

Another unique feature in this case was the number of foetuses found within a sac. Gross and Clatworthy (1951) reported a case of twin foetuses. All other examples of intra-abdominal foetus in foetu consisted of only one foetus. All three foetuses in this case showed separate umbilical cords, all showed well-formed spinal columns and skeletal parts, and all had well-developed intestinal elements.

**Pathogenesis.** Many theories have been advanced to elucidate the pathogenesis of foetus in foetu. It has been repeatedly emphasized not to confuse them with highly differentiated teratomata. Teratoma, though it may contain highly organized structures, is a true neoplasm (Willis, 1953) which arises from embryonic pleuripotential cells with benign or malignant propensities. Whereas a foetus in foetu, as its name implies, is a parasitic twin within its fellow. The most plausible explanation is that it is a monozygotic twin of its bearer. White (1956), as quoted by Lord (1956), suggests that it is included as a consequence of the anastomosis of the vitelline circulations. In the present case, though the sex of the malformed foetuses is not externally discernible, they are all confined in one sac and have the same blood group. The two smaller masses are examples of amorphous twins which had been overshadowed in development by their larger co-twins.

## Summary

A unique example of foetus in foetu is described. Three foetuses of various stages of development in a single sac were found at operation in the pelvis of a 2-month-old Chinese male infant. The child survived.

Careful dissection of the foetuses revealed well-formed skeletal, intestinal, and nervous parts in all three members, all of which had umbilical cords attached to the host.

The published material is briefly reviewed and the diagnosis and pathogenesis of the condition are discussed.

I wish to record my gratitude to Professor G. B. Ong for permission to publish this case, and to Mr. James Ho for the photographs.

### References

Curtis, E. (1826). Physiological anomaly. [A study of fetus in fetu.] *New Engl. J. Med. Surg.*, **15**, 31.

Gross, R. E., and Clatworthy, H. W., Jr. (1951). Twin fetuses in fetu. *J. Pediat.*, **38**, 502.

Janovski, N. A. (1962). Fetus in fetu. *ibid.*, **61**, 100.

Kimmel, D. L., Moyer, E. K., Peale, A. R., Winborne, L. W., and Gotwals, J. E. (1950). A cerebral tumor containing five human fetuses: a case of fetus in fetu. *Anat. Rec.*, **106**, 141.

Lewis, R. H. (1961). Foetus in foetu and the retroperitoneal teratoma. *Arch. Dis. Childh.*, **36**, 220.

Lord, J. M. (1956). Intra-abdominal foetus in foetu. *J. Path. Bact.*, **72**, 627.

Taruffi, C. (1885). *Storia della Teratologia*, Vol. 3, Chap. 55. Regia Tipografia, Bologna.

White, L. L. R. (1956). Quoted by Lord (1956).

Willis, R. A. (1935). The structure of teratomata. *J. Path. Bact.*, **40**, 1.

—— (1953). *Pathology of Tumours*, 2nd ed. Butterworth, London.

Young, G. W. (1809). Case of a foetus found in the abdomen of a boy. *Med.-chir. Trans.*, **1**, 234.

*Arch. Dis. Childh.*, 1965, **40**, 694.

# SYNDROME OF INCOMPLETE REGIONAL ACHONDROPLASIA (ILIUM AND RIBS) WITH ABDOMINAL MUSCLE DYSPLASIA

BY

EMMANUEL SHAPIRA, EFRAIM FISCHEL, SHIMON MOSES, and STANLEY LEVIN

*From the Department of Pediatrics B and Radiological Department, Kaplan Hospital, Rehovoth, Israel*

(RECEIVED FOR PUBLICATION APRIL 6, 1965)

The classical picture of achondroplasia with abnormal formation of bone from cartilage involves mainly the long bones, and is well described in medical literature. In its incomplete form, the disease has been reported as affecting one side of the body, one extremity, or even a single bone (Caffey, 1948). We have recently come across a case of an infant with regional achondroplasia of only the pelvis and ribs, together with pronounced weakness of the abdominal muscles. In this child's family the syndrome is fully encountered in the proband, and appears partially in several others.

## Case Report

K.M. was born following an uncomplicated pregnancy and delivery, weighing 3·2 kg. She was first admitted to our department on the day after birth because of marked deformity of the chest and suspected congenital lack of abdominal muscles. The outline of the stomach and intestines were very apparent, and peristalsis could easily be seen through the skin of the abdomen. On subsequent admissions, usually due to recurrent respiratory tract infections, gradual development of the abdominal muscles was observed, though, when last examined at the age of 4 years, a considerable degree of hypoplasia was still evident together with a muscle defect in the area between the rectus abdominis and obliquus externus muscles on the left side. There were umbilical and bilateral inguinal herniae. The child had always been small for her age, of asthenic build with narrow chest, wide at the base and tapering towards the apex. The abdomen was protuberant (Fig. 1a and b). Mental development appeared to be entirely normal.

**Laboratory Findings.** Haemoglobin and differential blood counts were found to be normal on successive examinations. Blood proteins, glucose, and urea were within normal limits as were calcium, phosphorus, and phosphatase.

**X-ray Examinations.** Repeated radiological examinations of the skull, limbs, and vertebrae showed no abnormalities. The pelvis and ribs, however, showed the typical deformities of achondroplasia (Caffey, 1958). In the radiological examination carried out at the age of 3 days, the lower part of the ilium was missing. The acetabular angle of inclination was found to be zero (normal 28°), and the greater sciatic notch was deep and narrow. At the ages of $2\frac{1}{2}$ and 4 years, progressive development of the pelvic bones was plainly discernible (Fig. 2a, b), though the above-mentioned deformity was still present. In addition, an almost complete closure of

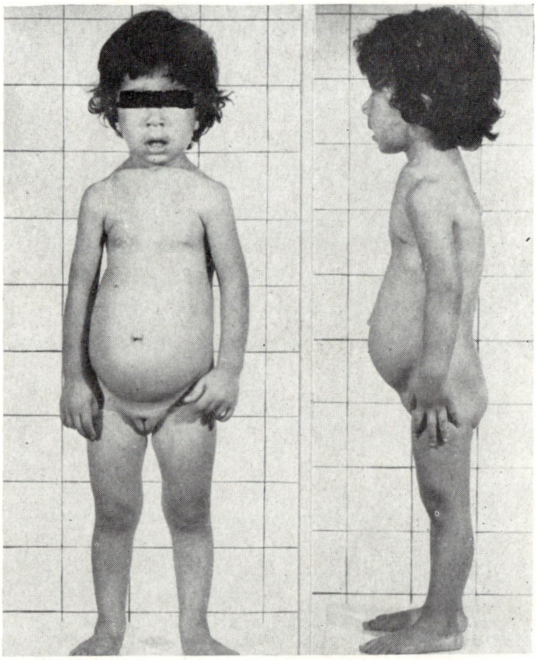

FIG. 1a, b.—A child with achondroplasia of pelvis and ribs and hypoplastic abdominal musculature at the age of $2\frac{1}{2}$ years. Note protuberant abdomen, short pelvis, deformed chest, and normal body limb proportions.

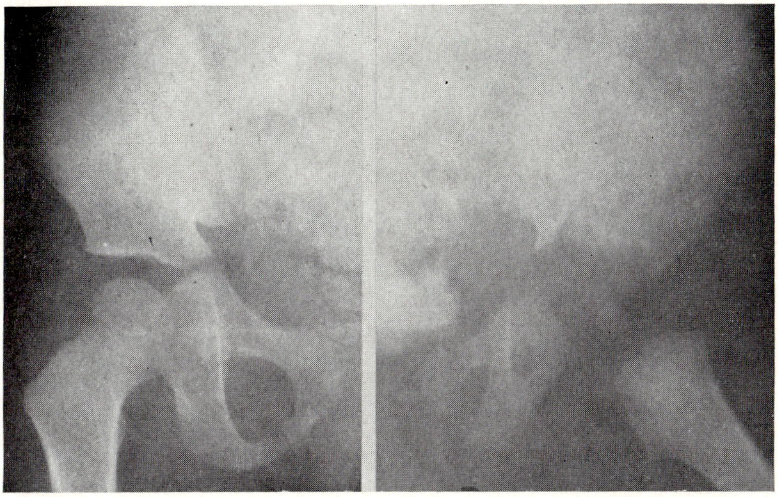

(a) (b)

FIG. 2.—Radiographs showing typical achondroplastic changes in the pelvis: (a) at birth; (b) at $2\frac{1}{2}$ years.

the ischio-pubic synchondrosis was present at the age of $2\frac{1}{2}$ years (normal at about 6 years). The chest radiographs showed deformity of all ribs with flattening of the tips, which accounted for the chest deformation as a whole (Fig. 3a, b). Intravenous pyelography on two occasions was normal.

**Family History.** The parents were first cousins (Fig. 4). On the father's side (III. 4-16), 3 brothers and 2 sisters died in childhood of unknown causes. Another brother (III. 6) died of congenital heart disease at the age of 22 years. There were also two spontaneous miscarriages. In the patient's generation (IV. 1-8), one sister and one brother (IV. 4, 6) died on delivery and another child died on the 6th day of life. In these last three cases a good many skeletal deformities were noticed, one infant having 'hydrocephalus'. Two pregnancies of the patient's mother ended in spontaneous abortions.

Of 16 members of this family (II, III + IV) surviving infancy, 8 had either umbilical, femoral, or inguinal herniae. 3 had chest deformities similar to those of the patient (IV. 3 and III. 6, 12), though in 2 of them, an aunt and an elder sister of the patient, chest and pelvic radiographs showed no abnormalities.

Details of generation I and the offspring of II.1 are unknown.

## Discussion

Whereas achondroplasia in its classical form has been found in a skeleton of the Neolithic period some 7,000 years old, as well as in pictures of ancient Egyptian gods, it was Parrot in 1878 who described it clearly as an entity for the first time.

Among the known cartilaginous dysplasias, achondroplasia is the most frequent, being in fact a hypoplasia and not an aplasia. The pathological

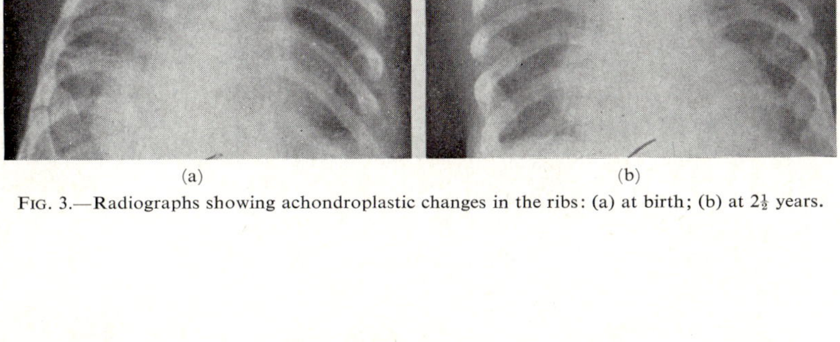

(a) (b)

FIG. 3.—Radiographs showing achondroplastic changes in the ribs: (a) at birth; (b) at $2\frac{1}{2}$ years.

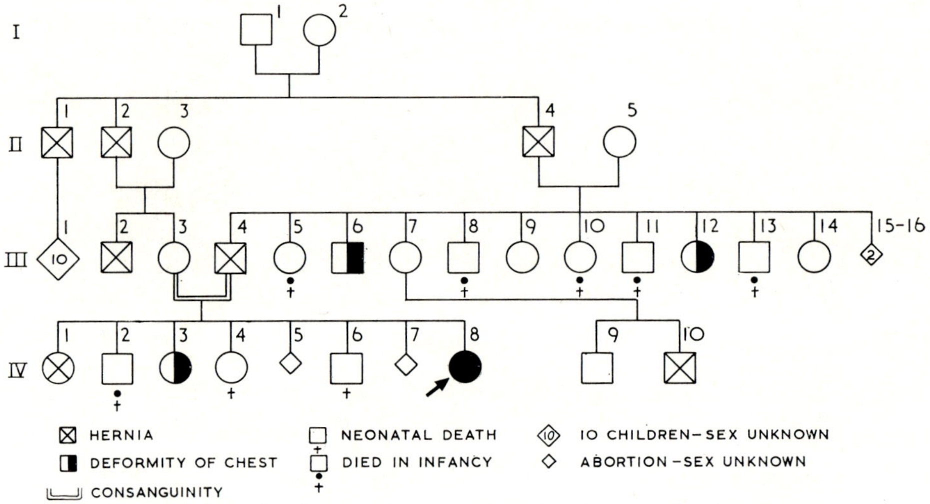


FIG. 4.—Pedigree of family with regional achondroplasia and abdominal muscular defects.

picture indicates a defect in cartilaginous growth and in bone formation from cartilage (Lane, 1960).

In its complete form the disease affects mainly the long bones. Other bones involved are the ribs, vertebrae, scapulae, skull—particularly at its base, and pelvis—particularly the ilium. For patients surviving the first year of life, prognosis is favourable.

In our case, the disease affected only the pelvis and ribs and was accompanied by congenital hypoplasia of the abdominal muscles. The radiological picture of the pelvis was identical to that described by Caffey in 1958 (Fig. 5): on studying the radiographs, he expressed the opinion that this was a unique case of regional achondroplasia of the pelvis and ribs.

Among animals the disease appears both in its complete and its regional form. As an example of the complete form, Irish cattle may be cited, and of the regional form, the bulldog, where the effect appears in the spinal column and the skull (Lane, 1960). Transmission of the disease among some animals such as cattle appears as a dominant trait.

A similar disease has been described in rabbits where transmission is recessive. The homozygote being non-vital dies *in utero* or shortly after delivery, whereas the heterozygote develops entirely normally (Brown and Pearce, 1945).

In the human, genetic transmission is accepted as being dominant (Mörch, 1940). Evidence of genetic transmission can be ascertained in only 20% of patients, the remainder being sporadic cases apparently due to spontaneous mutation. The spontaneous mutation rate in this disease has been

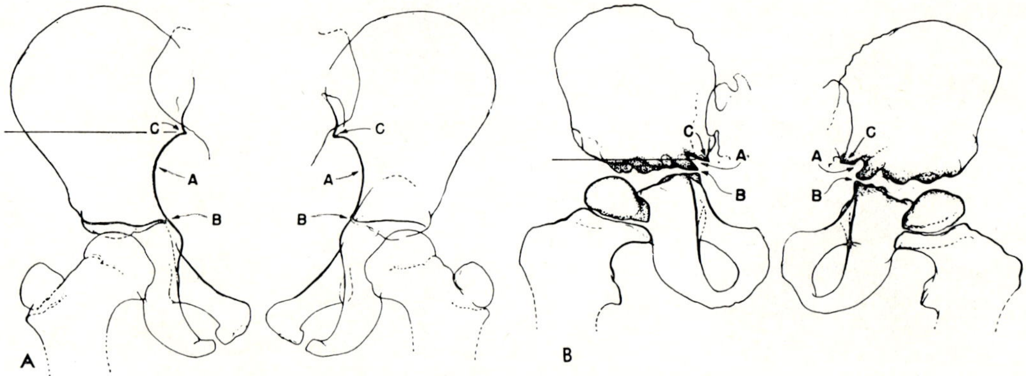


FIG. 5.—Comparison of normal (A) and achondroplastic pelves (B) at 5 years of age. Letters A mark the greater sciatic notches; B the Y cartilages; and C the postero-inferior iliac spines. In the achondroplast practically all the ilium below these spines is missing and the greater sciatic notches are reduced to narrow deep clefts. Iliums are square with elongated flat lower edges.
(Reprinted from Caffey, J. (1958). Achondroplasia of pelvis and lumbosacral spine; some roentgenographic features. *Amer. J. Roentgenol.*, 80, 449.)

estimated to be $4 \times 10^{-5}$ or one mutant birth in 12,000 (Mörch, 1941). Catherine de Medici is known to have made unsuccessful attempts to breed achondroplastic dwarfs by intermarriage (Rischbieth, 1912).

In both the complete and the regional forms of achondroplasia, the typical pot-belly is explained by the effect on posture of the changes in the vertebrae and pelvis. A normal development of skeletal muscles is usually emphasized in achondroplastic dwarfs. In our case, the hypoplastic abdominal musculature was the cause of the protuberant abdomen, a feature not previously described.

Another striking feature in this family was the high incidence of herniae. It seems possible, therefore, that the muscular and skeletal defects are related. According to the data available from this pedigree no conclusion about linkage can be drawn, though the mode of inheritance, both of the hernia and the chest deformity, seems compatible with autosomal dominant transmission with incomplete penetrance.

Since chondrodystrophy occurs in phenotypically different forms, different genes may be involved and recessive inheritance could occasionally occur. This could be the case in this family, where consanguinity may have been a factor in producing affected homozygotes in generation IV. The high mortality rate seen in the generation of the patient's father, may have been due to severely affected patients, though the combination of chest deformity with a tendency to recurrent pulmonary infections, which were successfully treated in our patient, may well have been the cause of death in others. However, the high mortality rate could have been the result of poor health conditions in their homeland, the family having migrated later to Israel from a middle-eastern country with a high infant mortality rate.

The gradual improvement over the years in the radiological findings and of the abdominal musculature in our case provides us with a possible explanation for the lack of abnormal radiological findings in both the older sister and the aunt of the patient, in spite of the marked resemblance from the clinical point of view.

## Summary

An infant with extreme hypoplasia of the abdominal muscles and skeletal deformities was found to have achondroplasia of the ribs and ilium. The rest of the skeleton was normal. Follow-up examination at the age of 4 years showed fair development of the abdominal muscles and good growth of the affected bones. Bilateral direct inguinal hernias were repaired at this time.

A study of the family indicated several persons with chest deformity, and 50% of grown-up survivors with herniae.

Regional achondroplasia of the ribs and ilium is rare, and its occurrence with abdominal muscle weakness as a specific syndrome is reported here for the first time. The pedigree is compatible with autosomal dominant transmission with incomplete penetrance.

We should like to thank Professor John Caffey for reviewing the radiographs.

### References

Brown, W. H., and Pearce, L. (1945). Hereditary achondroplasia in the rabbit. *J. exp. Med.*, **82**, 241.

Caffey, J. (1948). Achondroplasia. In *Practice of Pediatrics*, Vol. IV, chap. 28, ed. J. Brennemann. W. F. Prior Co., Hagerstown, Maryland.

—— (1958). Achondroplasia of pelvis and lumbo-sacral spine. *Amer. J. Roentgenol.*, **80**, 449.

Lane, J. W. (1960). Roentgenographic manifestations of the cartilaginous dysplasias. *Amer. J. med. Sci.*, **240**, 636.

Mörch, E. T. (1940). Achondroplasia is always hereditary and is inherited dominantly. *J. Hered.*, **31**, 439.

—— (1941). Chondrodystrophic dwarfs in Denmark. *Op. Domo Biol. hered. hum., Kbh.*, **3**.

Parrot, M. J. (1878). Sur la malformation achondroplasique et le dieu Ptah. *Bull. Soc. Anthrop. Paris*, **1** (3rd series), 296.

Rischbieth, H. (1912). Dwarfism. *Treas. hum. Inher.*, **1**, 355.

# BOOK REVIEWS

**Concepts of Development in Early Childhood Education.** An Institute Conducted by The Child Development Center New York City. Edited by PETER B. NEUBAUER. (Pp. ix + 149. $6.50) Springfield, Illinois: Charles C. Thomas. 1965.

This book consists of papers and discussions at a two-day conference in 1962 in a Child Development Centre in New York. The speakers were psychologists, psychiatrists, and educationalists, and the topic was 'Development and Education'. The papers were those of Ausubel on 'Stages of Intellectual Development and their Implications for early Childhood Education'; Lili Peller on 'Language and Development'; Irving Sigel on 'Development Considerations of the Nursery School Experience'; and Jules Henry on 'Death Fear and Climax in Nursery School Play'.

The book is definitely more suitable for psychologists than it is for simple-minded paediatricians, who will find much of it difficult to understand. For instance, Ausubel, in a section entitled 'The concrete abstract dimension of cognitive development' wrote: 'The concrete abstract dimension of intellectual development may be divided into three qualitatively distinct developmental stages—the preoperational stage, the stage of concrete operations, and the stage of abstract operations.' 'This dependence upon concrete—empirical props obviously limits his (the elementary school pupil's) ability meaningfully to group and manipulate relationships between abstractions, since he can only acquire these understandings and perform those logical operations which do not go beyond the concrete and particularized representation of reality in his use of props.'

Mrs. Lili Peller's contribution is a psychoanalytical account of language development. Some ignorant paediatricians, like the writer, will find her explanations difficult to follow. She wrote 'Through the highly libidinized, incessant, and tremendously repetitive motor and sensory activity of the sadistic—anal phase, the child develops the image of his self and of his body functions. He creates the world of things anchored in space'. She goes on to say, 'A psychoanalytic symbol carries an intense affect, which originally belonged to a body part, a body function, a basic family relationship, or to facts of life and death. The shift of affect from the symbolized, e.g. urination to the symbol, e.g. water—is due to repression.' She declares that 'It is narcissism and the drive for mastery which accounts for all early play.'

Elsewhere in the book there is an interesting discussion on the age at which children can learn, and the question of whether they can learn anything that adults can. Ausubel contends that children cannot learn as much as adults, though they are at certain advantages over adults: the latter may have to unlearn things if they have been taught badly, they are more apt to have emotional blocks with respect to subjects, and 'there is a marked falling off of intellectual enthusiasm as one moves up the academic ladder'.

Psychologists and educationalists will find much of interest in this book.

**The Syndrome of Stuttering.** Clinics in Developmental Medicine No. 17. By GAVIN ANDREWS and MARY HARRIS with ROGER GARSIDE and DAVID KAY. (Pp. 191; 16 figures + 92 tables + Appendices. 40s.; $6) London: The Spastics Society Medical Education and Information Unit in association with William Heinemann Medical Books. 1964.

The main core of this book consists of a report of an epidemiological survey of stuttering in schoolchildren. For the purposes of the survey a representative sample of stutterers and their mothers was matched with a group of controls. A comprehensive battery of questions and tests was put to each and the results both compared simply, and analysed statistically. In this way several factors which differentiated the stutterers from the control group emerged. These should prove of considerable practical value.

The scoring of stutterers was then examined separately to highlight intergroup differences. From this emerged four factors which the authors pinpointed as appearing singly or jointly in all but a small minority of cases studied.

The book is concluded with an account of an interesting but unfinished experiment conducted with 35 stutterers of all ages, into the inhibition of stuttering by the use of syllable-timed speech.

In addition to the main studies in the book, there are two smaller, but no less interesting sections, one reviewing concisely the existing literature on the subject and the other dealing with the genetics of stuttering.

This important book should be of value to all those who are interested in a methodical approach to the syndrome of stuttering. The authors themselves admit the value of a detailed observation of a limited number of cases, as a first stage in research. The next is essentially a formal attempt to validate the hypotheses so formed, and it is as a part of this stage that the work was carried out. The authors have succeeded in producing a clear, concise, and readable report on their contribution to the present knowledge of the syndrome of stuttering.

**Biochemical Approaches to Mental Handicap in Children.** A Symposium of the Society for the Study of Inborn Errors of Metabolism, held at Liverpool University on September 16, 1964. Edited by J. D. ALLAN and K. S. HOLT. (Pp. vii + 84; illustrated. 15s.) London: E. & S. Livingstone. 1965.

This is the report of a third symposium held in the North of England on 'Neurometabolic disorders of childhood', containing the communications given at that meeting. Although the general standard was not as high as that achieved in Sheffield the previous year, several interesting papers were offered. A full description of the biochemical survey of mental handicap which is being carried out in Northern Ireland was given by Dr. Carson, and Dr. Brian Bower described the study undertaken in Birmingham of tryptophan metabolism in infantile spasms. The treatment of maple syrup urine disease in two patients was described by Mr. Ireland of Liverpool using a relatively inexpensive diet.

Then followed three papers reviewing in detail the published material on heterozygotes in neurometabolic disorders, the biochemical aspects of Down's disease, and the problems of infantile autism. Finally there was an interesting review of special diets in the treatment of biochemical disorders, followed by some personal observations by Dr. Margaret Wilson on the effect of varying vitamin intakes on growth in young rats, which emphasized the need for full well-balanced vitamin intake when special milks are prescribed for infants and growing children.

This book does not contain any new information concerning mental handicap in children, but it will be of assistance to students and paediatric residents who are anxious to acquaint themselves with recent work in this aspect of mental handicap.

**Nutricia Symposium on the Adaptation of the Newborn Infant to Extra-Uterine Life.** Editors: J. H. P. JONXIS, H. K. A. VISSER, and J. A. TROELSTRA. (Pp. xiii + 331; illustrated. fl.38.) Leiden: H. E. Stenfert Kroese N.V. 1964.

This book contains the proceedings of a symposium held at the University of Groningen in February 1964. The four subjects considered are nutrition, water and electrolyte metabolism, respiratory problems, and temperature control.

Inevitably one must compare this volume with the previously published Ciba Foundation Symposium on Somatic Stability of the Newborn, and indeed there is considerable overlap particularly in the realms of renal function and temperature regulation. However, most of the material presented is from data on human infants and there is a fair balance between pure physiology and its application to clinical situations. The discussions following each section are helpful, and as a source of information the references should prove useful.

The nutrition section covers body composition before and after birth, nutritional problems in low birth weight infants, the effects of prolonged starvation in surgical patients, and neonatal hypoglycaemia. R. A. McCance reviews water and electrolyte metabolism, and there is an excellent account of some aspects of adrenocortical function in normal infants as well as those with congenital adrenal hyperplasia in the early months of life. A rational approach to the practical management of neonatal dehydration is also presented. In the respiratory section the changes taking place in the lung at birth are summarized and some of the factors influencing pulmonary blood flow are described from an experimental point of view. The ever baffling problem of respiratory distress syndrome is presented from the standpoints of diagnosis, disordered respiratory function, and treatment with bicarbonate and THAM. The section on temperature control, which is perhaps the best, contains much information on chemical thermogenesis and the possible role of brown fat in its mediation; the importance of providing a suitable thermal environment for the premature is stressed once more.

**Year Book of Pediatrics** (1964-1965 Year Book Series). Edited by SYDNEY S. GELLIS. (Pp. 537; 114 figures. 64s.) London: Lloyd Luke. 1965.

The editor of this attractive volume has made an interesting and well-balanced selection of some of the paediatric publications that have appeared during the year ending September 1964. The coverage is wide and includes most subjects of general paediatric interest, though with some bias towards clinical problems rather than basic research. The extracts are, in the main, well written but in a few instances condensation of the original has led to some loss of clarity; something which is probably inevitable in this type of publication.

Although the abstractors remain anonymous many of the more important and controversial topics have attracted comments from the editor or from named contributors. Some of these critical evaluations are invaluable for they impart a sense of caution and balance which is occasionally lacking in the original articles. This practice, which over the years has given the Year Book series a character of its own, should be commended, since nowadays many medical journals are without correspondence columns and their contents are immune from criticism. An interesting and helpful improvement, perhaps, would be to allow the original authors to add their own remarks.

This book has a high standard of production with good clear print, acceptable illustrations, and diagrams and a useful author and subject index. It can be recommended for all those who wish to gain a broad view of recent paediatric literature, especially the busy doctor whose reading time is severely restricted.

**Tay-Sachs' Disease.** Edited by BRUNO W. VOLK. (Pp. viii + 158; illustrated. \$5·75.) London and New York: Grune and Stratton. 1964.

When the National Tay-Sachs' Association in New York encouraged the establishment of a small clinical unit to study this disease in detail they created an opportunity for an enthusiastic team of workers to make a major contribution to medical knowledge. This excellent comprehensive monograph is evidence that the initial hopes have been fulfilled, as it demonstrates the value of collecting together cases of a rare disease and investigating them in great detail.

The material, which is well presented, is in five sections; historical, clinical, pathological, biochemical, and epidemiological. In each section the bibliography is full and up to date (end of 1963). In the clinical section 15 cases are described in great detail and the pathological section contains detailed histopathological and histochemical information. The biochemical section starts with very clear formulae and then continues with a full description of enzymatic activity and the structure and biosynthesis of gangliosides. One minor criticism concerns Fig. 12 (page 94) on the distribution of serum sialic acid levels associated with various protein functions, where the key is incorrect. The epidemiological section is fascinating as it details the value of fructose-1-phosphate aldolase as a method of detecting heterozygotes and gives information about the frequency and carrier rates for the disease amongst the Jewish and non-Jewish populations.

This monograph is recommended to University or Research departments in paediatrics and pathology, as it is an excellent reference book containing information essential to anyone working in this field. Dr. Volk and his colleagues are to be congratulated on their presentation.

**Current Research in Leukaemia.** A Symposium edited by F. G. J. Hayhoe. (Pp. xii + 306; illustrated. 120s.) London: Cambridge University Press. 1965.

This book contains most of the papers given at a postgraduate Symposium in Cambridge in August 1964. The editor and publishers are to be congratulated on producing the written record of the meeting so quickly and elegantly. Of the 22 papers, over half are on aspects of cytology, electron microscopy, and cell growth and division, while only one is concerned with the therapy of leukaemia, this being a paper by Mathé and Amiel on the treatment of acute leukaemia by bone-marrow grafting. Unfortunately the speed of publication necessitated the exclusion of a paper on the clinical use of Vinca alkaloids, and contributions on the drug treatment of leukaemia are conspicuously absent—a reflection, perhaps, of the slow rate of advance in this subject in recent years.

Those concerned with the clinical care of leukaemia will find much else to interest them, however, notably an excellent short critical review by E. G. Knox on the space-time distribution of leukaemia, stressing the limitations of the statistical methods employed, and a review of other epidemiological aspects by Richard Doll. There are three papers on cytogenetic aspects of leukaemias and related conditions, a short critical survey by R. J. C. Harris of work on the pathology and aetiology of Burkitt's lymphoma, and two papers on virus and mycoplasma studies in human and animal leukaemias by Dmochowski and Harris—the former beautifully illustrated by 75 electron micrographs which have unfortunately been arranged in the wrong order, so that they are difficult to relate to the test.

This volume serves a most useful purpose in bringing together the results of recent leukaemia research by workers in many different disciplines. It will be welcomed by all those who are actively concerned in this broad subject, and can be recommended as stimulating reading to anyone with a general interest in the problems of leukaemia.

**Differentialdiagnose seltener Lungenerkrankungen im Röntgenbild. Ein Atlas.** 2nd enlarged edition. Edited by Karl Musshoff and Jürgen Weinreich. (Pp. vii + 272; 137 figures + 2 tables. Dm. 108,) Berlin, Göttingen, Heidelberg, New York: Springer-Verlag. 1964.

This beautifully illustrated atlas depicts the radiological differential diagnosis of rare pulmonary and mediastinal diseases. Only two years have elapsed since the first edition appeared, clearly indicating the popularity of this work in Germany.

A logical approach to the analysis of the radiographs has been attempted by arranging the material according to the radiographic appearances, which has lost something of its effectiveness by the indefinite terms employed. An excellent feature is the summary of the clinical presentation and results of other special investigations which accompany each radiograph.

Selection of material for a book of this nature presents obvious difficulties and not everyone will agree with the authors' choice and emphasis. It would perhaps have been an improvement to have listed at the beginning of each chapter both common and rare causes of the various radiographic appearances under which the diseases are segregated. As it is, a number of rare pulmonary lesions such as histoplasmosis and other mycoses have been omitted. The method of classification of the index is also an unusual one, and not easy to use.

On the whole this book contains a valuable store of illustrative material which should be useful to radiologists, physicians, and surgeons interested in chest diseases. It is obviously of limited value to a paediatrician.

**Lung Function: Assessment and Application in Medicine.** By J. E. Coles. (Pp. x + 154; 39 figures. 63s.) Oxford: Blackwell Scientific Publications. 1965.

With the disappearance in many countries of destructive diseases of the lung, such as tubercle, chest physicians have been able to devote their attention to those disorders of the lung where more subtle disturbances of function were responsible for the patients' symptoms, conditions such as emphysema or the effect on the lung of heart disorders. This has brought about a revolution in chest medicine over the past 10 or 15 years; and the surprisingly long neglected subject of pulmonary physiology has made rapid strides.

Many paediatricians, brought up in an era before this renaissance took place, will be largely ignorant of what means now exist, beyond the use of their five senses aided by the stethoscope and x-ray, for the appraisal of lung disorders.

This book provides a useful guide to the subject so that the paediatrician wishing to discover which tests might help him with a particular clinical problem would readily find the answer. The author has incorporated a good deal of information about lung function in children, though hardly any about that in infants, and the special instrumentation required. However, it is with basic principles that the author is mainly concerned, and here he writes with admirable clarity. (Does bubbling oxygen through water really humidify it?)

This book is strongly recommended as a reference text, which it would be sensible to have easily available in every children's hospital.

The printing is a delight to the eye, and the method of arranging references both novel and good, but the binding is less sound.

# AUTHOR INDEX

## 1965, Volume XL


ABERDEEN, E. and WATERSTON, D.: Preductal coarctation of the aorta, 228, *P.*
ABRAHAMOV, A., *see* FREIER, S. *et al.*
ACHARYA, P. T. and PAYNE, W. W.: Blood chemistry of normal full-term infants in the first 48 hours of life, 430
—— *see also* PAYNE, W. W. and ACHARYA, P. T.
ADAMS, J. H. and CAMERON, H. M.: Obstetrical paralysis due to ischaemia of the spinal cord, 93
ADLER, T., *see* DANIEL, F. and KÖTELES, G.
AHERNE, W.: Fat infiltration in the tissues of the newborn infant, 406
—— *see also* CORNEY, G. and AHERNE, W.
ALBERMAN, E. D.: The causes of congenital club foot, 548
ANDERSON, C. M., KERRY, K. R., and TOWNLEY, R. R. W.: An inborn defect of intestinal absorption of certain monosaccharides, 1
ANTHONY, P. P., COLES, H. M. T., PRYSE-DAVIES, J., and SINCLAIR, L.: Biochemical, pharmacological, and histochemical studies in neuroblastoma, 411

BÄCKLUND, L., GROTTE, G., and REUTERSKIÖLD, A.: Functional stenosis as cause of pelvi-ureteric obstruction and hydronephrosis, 203
BAIN, A. D., INSLEY, J., DOUGLAS, D. M., GAULD, I. K., and SCOTT, H. A.: Normal/trisomy 13-15 mosaicism in two infants, 442
BARNETT, H.: Paediatric nephrology (George Frederic Still Memorial Lecture), 451, *P.* (*title only*)
BARRIE, D.: Incubator-borne *Pseudomonas pyocyanea* infection in a newborn nursery, 555
BAUCHE, P., *see* DUHAMEL, J. and BAUCHE, P.
BAXTER, T. J.: Cysts arising in the renal corpuscle, a microdissection study, 455
—— Cysts arising in the renal tubules, a microdissection study, 464
BECROFT, D. M. O., COSTELLO, J. M., and SCOTT, P. J.: A-β-Lipoproteinaemia (Bassen-Kornzweig syndrome), 40
BELLMANN, G.: Congenital diaphragmatic hernia, 229, *P.*
BENIRSCHKE, K., *see* HOEFNAGEL, D. and BENIRSCHKE, K.
BENSON, P. F., GOUGH, M. H., and POLANI, P. E.: Lymphangiography and chromosome studies in females with lymphoedema and possible ovarian dysgenesis, 27
BENSON, S., *see* HAZRA, M., *et al.*
BIRCHALL, K., *see* CATHRO, D. M., *et al.*
BLUHM, M. M., *see* INALL, J. A., *et al.*
BOBINSKI, H., *see* MACIEJEWSKI, A. and BOBINSKI, H.
BOIX-OCHOA, J. and REHBEIN, F.: Oesophageal stenosis due to reflux oesophagitis, 197
BOOGAARD, H. M. P. van den, *see* NOORDIJK, J. A., *et al.*
BOROWICZ, K. and BOROWICZ, J.: The mouse placenta in experimental toxoplasmosis, 336, *P.*
BOUTON, M. J., *see* TODD, R. MCL. and BOUTON, M. J.
BRANDESKY, G.: On treatment and prognosis of severe head injuries in children, 230, *P.*
BROCK, SIR RUSSELL: The development of heart surgery in children, 123
BROM, A. G., SCHAAR, H. V. D., and NAUTA, J.: The surgery of transposition of the great vessels, 128
BROOKFIELD, R. W., *see* WORSLEY, H. E., *et al.*
BROUGHTON, P. M. G., ROSSITER, E. J. R., WARREN, C. B. M., GOULIS, G., and LORD, P. S.: Effect of blue light on hyperbilirubinaemia, 666
BROWNE, D.: Orthopaedics of the foetus, 230, *P.*
BURMAN, D.: The jejunal mucosa in kwashiorkor, 526
BURNELL, R. H. and MARKEY, G. B.: Choledochal cyst: a case report and discussion of aetiology, 329
BUTLER, E. B., *see* GRAY, O. P. and BUTLER, E. B.
BUTLER, L. J., SNODGRASS, G. J. A. I., FRANCE, N. E., SINCLAIR, L., and RUSSELL, A.: E (16-18) trisomy syndrome: analysis of 13 cases, 600

CABAK, V. and NAJDANVIC, R.: Effect of undernutrition in early life on physical and mental development, 532
CAHALANE, S. F.: Pinealoma with aldosterone-like activity, 336, *P.*
CALLADINE, M., GAIRDNER, D., NAIDOO, B. T., and ORRELL, D. H.: Acid-base changes following exchange transfusion with citrated blood, 626
CAMERON, A. H.: Malformations of the thymus and cardiovascular system, 334, *P.*
CAMERON, H. M., *see* ADAMS, J. H. and CAMERON, H. M.
CAMPBELL, S. and CARRÉ, I. J.: Fatal haemolytic uraemic syndrome and idiopathic hyperlipaemia in monozygotic twins, 654
CARRÉ, I. J., *see* CAMPBELL, S. and CARRÉ, I. J.
CATHRO, D. M., BIRCHALL, K., MITCHELL, F. L., and FORSYTH, C. C.: 3β:21-dihydroxypregn-5-ene-20-one in urine of normal newborn infants and in third day urine of child with deficiency of 3β-hydroxysteroid-dehydrogenase, 251
—— and FORSYTH, C. C.: Excretion of corticosteroids by infants of diabetic and pre-diabetic mothers, 583
CLAIREAUX, A. E.: Congenital renal anomalies in the newborn, 335, *P.*
CLAYTON, B. E., *see* FITSCHEN, W. and CLAYTON, B. E.
CLAYTON, J. E., *see* HOCKADAY, T. D. R., *et al.*, *also* MANN, T. P., *et al.*
COHEN, S. J.: Diagnostic aids for the unusual types of oesophageal atresia and tracheo-oesophageal fistulae, 229, *P.*
COLE, A. R. C.: Mastocytosis. Report of a case in a 15½-week-old infant with cutaneous and generalized skeletal changes, 677
COLEMAN, E. N.: Infantile hypercalcaemia and cardiovascular lesions, evidence, hypothesis, and speculation, 535
COLES, H. M. T., *see* ANTHONY, P. P., COLES, H. M. T., PRYSE-DAVIES, J., and SINCLAIR, L.
CONEN, P. E. and ERKMAN, B.: Chromosome studies in paediatric intersex problems, 335, *P.*
CORNEY, G. and AHERNE, W.: The placental transfusion syndrome in monozygous twins, 264
COSTEFF, H.: Methods of routine haemoglobinometry in childhood: evaluation of copper sulphate densitometry, 309
COSTELLO, J. M., *see* BECROFT, D. M. O., *et al.*
COTTOM, D. and YOUNG, M.: Venous pressure measurement in exchange transfusion, 323
CRAIG, W. S.: An unusual case of subcutaneous fat necrosis in a newly born infant, 326
CREAK, E. M.: Some aspects of mental handicap studied in the 'Thousand Families Survey', 451, *P.*
CROME, L. and WELLER, S. D. V.: Infantile neuroaxonal dystrophy, 502

DANIEL, F., ADLER, T., and KÖTELES, G.: Surgical complications of staphylococcal pneumonia in infants, 229, *P.*

DAVIS, J. A., HARVEY, D. R., and YU, J. S.: Neonatal fits associated with hypomagnesaemia, 286
DEKABAN, A.: Metabolic and chromosomal studies in leprechaunism, 632
DELIVORIA-PAPADOPOULOS, M., LEVISON, H., and SWYER, P. R.: Intermittent positive pressure respiration as a treatment in severe respiratory distress syndrome, 474
DENT, C. E., SMELLIE, J. M., and WATSON, L.: Studies in osteopetrosis, 7
DEVENS, K.: Atresia of the deferent duct (vas deferens), 227, *P.*
DEVI, B., *see* MORE, J. R. S. and DEVI, B.
DILLING, L., *see* HAWORTH, J. C., *et al.*
DODSON, M. E. and STEAD, A. L.: Correction of acidosis in the resuscitation of the collapsed child, 385
DOUGLAS, D. M., *see* BAIN, A. D., *et al.*
DOUGLAS, T. A., *see* INALL, J. A., *et al.*
DRESCHER, E.: Some remarks on congenital atresia of the oesophagus, 229, *P.*
DRUKKER, A., *see* LONDON, R., *et al.*
DUBOWITZ, V.: Intellectual impairment in muscular dystrophy, 296
——, LORBER, J., and ZACHARY, R. B.: Lipoma of the cauda equina, 207
DUHAMEL, J. and BAUCHE, P.: Polyps of the colon beyond the reach of the sigmoidoscope, 173
DUNN, P. M.: The respiratory distress syndrome of the newborn: immaturity versus prematurity, 62
DYGGVE, H. V. and MIKKELSEN, M.: Partial deletion of the short arms of a chromosome of the 4-5 group (Denver), 82

ECKSTEIN, H. B.: Urethral valves: A review of 104 cases, 227, *P.*
EDWARDS, J. H.: Classification of malformations, 335, *P.*
EDWARDS, R. W. H., *see* MCKENDRICK, T. and EDWARDS, R. W. H.
EHRENPREIS, T.: Acquired megacolon as a complication of recto-sigmoidectomy for Hirschsprung's disease, 180
—— Pseudo-Hirschsprung's disease, 177
EKESPARRE, W. VON: The operative treatment of diaphragmatic hernia and relaxation, 229, *P.*
EL-AKKARI, EL-SAYED, EL-DIN, M., KAMAL BADR, and KASSEM, A. S.: Diverticulum of the left ventricle, report of a case, 545
EL-DIN, M., KAMAL BADR, *see* EL-AKKARI, EL-SAYED, *et al.*
ELLIS, E. F., *see* FALLIERS, C. J., and ELLIS, E. F.
ELVES, M.: Recent studies on the thymus, 333, *P.*
ELWOOD, J. S., *see* WORSLEY, H. E., *et al.*
EMERY, J. L.: Nuclear abnormality and cytomegaly in the islets of Langerhans of newborns, 332, *P.*
ERKMAN, B., *see* CONEN, P. E. and ERKMAN, B.
EVANS, A., *see* MALAN, A. F., *et al.*

FALLIERS, C. J. and ELLIS, E. F.: Corticosteroids and varicella, six-year experience in an asthmatic population, 593
FISHEL, E., *see* SHAPIRA, E., *et al.*
FITSCHEN, W. and CLAYTON, B. E.: Urinary excretion of gonadotrophins with particular reference to children, 16
FITZSIMMONS, J. S.: Laryngeal stridor and respiratory obstruction associated with meningomyelocele, 687
FORSYTH, C. C., LLOYD, J. K., and FOSBROOKE, A. S.: A-β-Lipoproteinaemia, 47
—— *see also* CATHRO, D. M. and FORSYTH, C. C.
CATHRO, D. M., *et al.*
FOSBROOKE, A. S., *see* FORSYTH, C. C., *et al.*
FOSS, G. L.: The influence of androgen treatment on ultimate height in males, 66
FOX, H.: The villous cytotrophoblast as an index of placental ischaemia, 334, *P.*
FRANCE, N. E., *see* BUTLER, L. J., *et al.*
SWAIN, V. A. J., *et al.*
FREEMAN, R.: Reversible myocarditis due to chronic lead poisoning in childhood, 389
FREIER, S., MAYER, K., LEVENE, C., and ABRAHAMOV, A.: Neonatal jaundice associated with familial G6PD deficiency in Israel, 280

GADEKAR, N. G., *see* GHAI, O. P., *et al.*
GAIRDNER, D. M. T.: Acid-base changes following exchange transfusion with citrated blood, 450, *P.*
—— *see also* CALLADINE, M., *et al.*
GAULD, I. K., *see* BAIN, A. D., INSLEY, J., DOUGLAS, D. M., GAULD, I. K., and SCOTT, H. A.
GENEL, M., *see* VERHAGEN, A. D., *et al.*
GHAI, O. P., SINGH, M., WALIA, B. N. S., and GADEKAR, N. G.: An assessment of gastric acid secretory response with 'maximal' augmented histamine stimulation in children with peptic ulcer, 77
GODBER, SIR GEORGE: The development of paediatric services, 451, *P.* (*title only*)
GOUGH, M. H., *see* BENSON, P. F., *et al.*
GOULIS, G., *see* BROUGHTON, P. M. G., *et al.*
GRAY, O. P. and BUTLER, E. B.: Megaloblastic anaemia in premature infants, 53
GREEP, J. M., *see* HENDREN, W. H., *et al.*
GROTTE, G., *see* BÄCKLUND, L., *et al.*
GULYAS, J., *see* SZÖTS, I. and GULYAS, J.
GUPTA, J. M. and SCOPES, J. W.: Observations on blood pressure in newborn infants, 637

HALLER, R. DE, HALLER, J. DE, and SIEGENTHALER, P.: Accuracy of the sweat test: advantage of a micromethod, 684
HAMILTON, J., *see* VERHAGEN, A. D., *et al.*
HAMILTON, W.: Aldosterone and 17-hydroxycorticosteroid excretion following Ramstedt's operation, 261
HARRIS, R., ROVERE, M. DELLA, and PRIOR, P. F.: Electroencephalographic studies in infants and children with hypothyroidism, 612
HARTL, H.: Intrathoracic duplications of the gastro-intestinal tract and their complications, 229, *P.*
HARVEY, D. R., *see* DAVIS, J. A., *et al.*
HASSE, W.: Intrahepatic vascular and bile-duct systems as related to operative treatment of bile-duct atresia, 162
HAWORTH, J. C., NORRIS, M., and DILLING, L.: A study of the immunoglobulins in premature infants, 243
HAZRA, M., BENSON, S., and SANDLER, M.: Blood 5-hydroxytryptamine levels in the newborn, 513
HEESE, H. DE V., *see* MALAN, A. F., *et al.*
SUTIN, G. J., *et al.*
HENDREN, W. H., GREEP, J. M., and PATTON, A. S.: Pancreatitis in childhood: experience with 15 cases, 132
HINDEN, E.: External injury causing foetal deformity, 80
HOCKADAY, T. D. R., CLAYTON, J. E., and SMITH, L. H.: The metabolic error in primary hyperoxaluria, 485
HOEFNAGEL, D. and BENIRSCHKE, K.: Dyscephalia mandibulo-oculo-facialis (Hallerman-Streiff syndrome), 57
HOLT, J. M. and SLADDEN, R. A.: Favism in England —two more cases, 271
HOPE, C. S., *see* INALL, J. A., *et al.*
HORNER, R., *see* SUTIN, G. J., *et al.*
HOUSTON, I. B.: Urinary white cell excretion in childhood, 313
HOWARD, R.: Actinomycin D in Wilms' tumour: treatment of lung metastases, 200
HUBER, J.: Hereditary 18-oxidation defect in the biosynthesis of aldosterone, 332, *P.*

Hugh-Jones, K., Wallace, S. J., Thornber, J. M., and Atkin, N. B.: Gonadal dysgenesis with unusual abnormalities, 274
Hutchison, J. H., *see* Inall, J. A., *et al.*

Ifekwunigwe, A., *see* Yu, J., *et al.*
Illingworth, R. S. and Lutz, W.: Head circumference of infants related to body weight, 672
Inall, J. A., Bluhm, M. M., Kerr, M. M., Douglas, T. A., Hope, C. S., and Hutchison, J. H.: Blood volume and haematocrit studies in respiratory distress syndrome of the newborn, 480
Insley, J., *see* Bain, A. D., *et al.*
Ivemark, B. and Robertson, B.: Pulmonary microangiography in congenital malformations of the heart, 333, *P.*
Iwai, S., *see* Suruga, K., *et al.*

Jackson, R. H.: Tuberous sclerosis in childhood, 450, *P.*
Johnston, J. H.: The undescended testis, review article, 113
Johnstone, G.: Accessory lobe of liver presenting through a congenital deficiency of anterior abdominal wall, 541

Kafka, V., Krolupper, M., and Paleček, L.: Rhabdomyosarcoma of the bladder in childhood, 227, *P.*
Kalpaktsoglou, P. K.: Crown-rump length in vital statistics of the newborn, 334, *P.*
Kamel, I., *see* Loutfi, A. H. and Mehrez, I.
Kassem, A. S., *see* AL-Akkari, El-Sayed, *et al.*
Kay, J. M., *see* Norman, R. M. and Kay, J. M.
Kerr, M. M., *see* Inall, J. A., *et al.*
Kerry, K. R., *see* Anderson, C. M., *et al.*
Kincannon, W. N., *see* Meeker, I. A. and Kincannon, W. N.
Kirkland, I.: Chylothorax in infancy and childhood, 186
Koteles, G., *see* Adler, T., *et al.*
Krolupper, M., *see* Kafka, V., *et al.*
Kubicz, S., *see* Reszke, S., *et al.*

Laird, A. P.: Operative treatment for failed cases of talipes equinovarus, 230, *P.*
Lake, B. D.: A reliable rapid screening test for sulphatide lipidosis, 284
Langley, F. A.: Thymic hyperplasia and the choice of a suitable biometric framework, 333, *P.*
Laurence, K. M.: Progressive familial infantile cerebral cortical degeneration, 335, *P.*
Laurence, M.: Survey of major central nervous system abnormalities in South Wales, 451, *P.*
Lauweryns, J. M.: Hyaline membrane disease: a pathological study of 55 infants, 618
Lee, E. Y. C.: Foetus in foetu, 689
Leonard, B. J.: White cell alkaline phosphatase in the developing foetus, 450, *P.*
Levene, C., *see* Freier, S., *et al.*
Levin, B., *see* Peonides, A., *et al.*
Levin, S., *see* Shapira, E., *et al.*
Levison, H., *see* Delivoria-Papadopoulos, M., *et al.*
Lincoln, J. C. R.: Cervico-auricular fistulae, 218
Lloyd, J. K., *see* Forsyth, C. C., *et al.*
London, R., Drukker, A., and Sandbank, U.: Fanconi's anaemia with hydrocephalus and thyroid abnormality, 89
Lorber, J., *see* Dubowitz, V., *et al.*
Lord, P. S., *see* Broughton, P. M. G., *et al.*
Loutfi, A. H., Mehrez, I., and Kamel, I.: Masses in the spermatic cord in children, 228, *P.*
Lutz, W., *see* Illingworth, R. S., and Lutz, W.

MacDonald, A. M.: A case of apparent adrenal hypoplasia in the neonate, 336, *P.*
Maciejewski, A. and Bobinski, H.: Serum lactic dehydrogenase and ribonuclease in the diagnosis of malignant tumours in children, 183
MacKellar, A.: Mycobacterial lymphadenitis in childhood, 450, *P.*
McKendrick, T. and Edwards, R. W. H.: The excretion of 4-hydroxy-3-methoxy-mandelic acid by children, 418
—— and Newns, G. H.: Thyrotoxicosis in children: a follow-up, 71
Maier, W. A.: Thalidomide embryopathy and limb defects, experiences in habilitation of children with ectromelias, 154
Malan, A. F., Evans, A., and Heese, H. de V.: Serial determinations in normal premature and full-term infants during the first 72 hours of life, 645
—— *see also* Sutin, G. J., *et al.*
Mann, T. P., Wilson, K. M., and Clayton, B. E.: A deficiency state arising in infants on synthetic foods, 364
Markey, G. B., *see* Burnell, R. H. and Markey, G. B.
Marsden, H. B.: Addison's disease and cerebral sclerosis, 332, *P.*
Martin, A. G.: The challenge of xeroderma pigmentosum, 228, *P.*
Mayer, K., *see* Freier, S., *et al.*
Meadow, S. R.: Hand, foot, and mouth diseases, 560
Meeker, I. A. and Kincannon, W. N.: The role of ventral hernia in the correction of diaphragmatic defects in the newborn, 146
Mehrez, I., *see* Loutfi, A. H., *et al.*
Mellick, S. A. and Phelan, P. D.: Internal carotid artery occlusion in a child, 224
Meulen, J. C. H. M. van der and Raadsveld, J. C.: Hypospadias, 228, *P.*
Mikkelsen, M., *see* Dyggve, H. V. and Mikkelsen, M.
Mitchell, F. L., *see* Cathro, D. M., *et al.*
More, J. R. S. and Devi, B.: A case of bilateral pulmonary agenesis, 334. *P,*
Mori, W., *see* Suruga, K., *et al.*
Moses, S., *see* Shajira, E., *et al.*
Moutsouris, C., *see* Tsakayannis, E., *et al.*

Nagashima, K., *see* Suruga, K., *et al.*
Naidoo, B. T., *see* Calladine, M., *et al.*
Najdanvic, R., *see* Cabak, V. and Najdanvic, R.
Nauta, J., *see* Brom, A. G., *et al.*
Neugebauerová, L., *see* Poláček, E., *et al.*
Newman, R. L. and Stewart, G. T.: The use of fibrinolytic activators in meningitis and similar conditions, 235
Newns, G. H., *see* McKendrick, T. and Newns, G. H.
Nixon, H. H.: Hepatic tumours in childhood and their treatment by major hepatic resection, 169
Noble, R. L., *see* Worsley, H. E., *et al.*
Noordijk, J. A., Oey, F. T. I., and Boogaard, H. M. P. van den: Late results of the operation for coarctation in the growing child, 192
Norman, R. M. and Kay, J. M.: Cerebello-thalamo-spinal degeneration in infancy: an unusual variant of Werdnig-Hoffman disease, 302
Norris, M., *see* Haworth, J. C., *et al.*

Oberniedermayr, A.: Adrenal surgery, 228, *P.*
Ockenden, B.: Absent abdominal muscles and associated genito-urinary abnormalities, 335, *P.*
Oey, F. T. I., *see* Noordijk, J. A., *et al.*
Orrell, D. H., *see* Calladine, M., *et al.*
Osborne, G. R.: Congenital diabetes, 332, *P.*

Paleček, L., *see* Kafka, V., *et al.*
Pampiglione, G.: Some neurophysiological and neuropathological observations in infantile spasms, 451, *P.*

PATSTON, V., *see* WALSHE, J. M. and PATSTON, V.
PATTON, A. S., *see* HENDREN, W. H., *et al.*
PAYNE, W. W. and ACHARYA, P. T.: The effect of abnormal birth on blood chemistry during the first 48 hours of life, 436
—— *see also* ACHARYA, P. T. and PAYNE, W. W.
YU, J., *et al.*
PEONIDES, A., LEVIN, B., and YOUNG, W. F.: The renal excretion of hydrogen ions in infants and children, 33
PHELAN, P. D., *see* MELLICK, S. A. and PHELAN, P. D.
PLUM, P.: Aetiology of athetosis with special reference to neonatal asphyxia, idiopathic icterus, and ABO-incompatibility, 376
POLÁČEK, E., VOCEL, J., NEUGEBAUEROVÁ, L., ŠEBKOVÁ, M., and VĚCHETOVÁ, E.: The osmotic concentrating ability in healthy infants and children, 291
POLANI, P. E., *see* BENSON, P. F., *et al.*
PRIOR, P. F., *see* HARRIS, R., *et al.*
PRYSE-DAVIES, J., *see* ANTHONY, P. P., *et al.*

RAADSVELD, J. C.: Hypospadias
—— *see also* MEULEN, J. C. H. M. and RAADSVELD, J. C.
RAISCH, O. E.: Treatment of fractures of head of radius in childhood, 230, *P.*
RAPANT, V., SERY, Z., and VOJTEK, V.: Indications and results of pulmonary resections in children, 229, *P.*
REHBEIN, F., *see* BOIX-OCHOA, J. and REHBEIN, F.
RESZKE, S., RONDIO, Z., and KUBICZ, S.: Suppurative lesions of the pulmonary tissue in children due to presence of foreign body in the bronchus, 229, *P.*
REUTERSKIÖLD, A., *see* BÄCKLUND, L., *et al.*
RITCHIE, G. MACL.: Dental manifestations of pseudohypoparathyroidism, 565
ROBERTSON, B., *see* IVEMARK, B. and ROBERTSON, B.
RONDIO, Z., *see* RESZKE, S., *et al.*
ROSSITER, E. J. E., *see* BROUGHTON, P. M. G., *et al.*
ROVERE, M. DELLA, *see* HARRIS, R., *et al.*
RUSSELL, A., *see* BUTLER, L. J., *et al.*
RUTHVEN, C. R. J., *see* SANDLER, M. and RUTHVEN, C. R. J.

SALZBERG, R., *see* VEST, M. F. and SALZBERG, R.
SANDBANK, U., *see* LONDON, R., *et al.*
SANDLER, M. and RUTHVEN, C. R. J.: Catecholamine-metabolites in neuroblastoma, 333, *P.*
—— *see also* HAZRA, M., *et al.*
SCHAAR, H. V. D., *see* BROM, A. G., *et al.*
SCOPES, J. W., *see* GUPTA, J. M. and SCOPES, J. W.
SCOTT, H. A., *see* BAIN, A. D., *et al.*
SCOTT, J. E. S.: Upper ureteric obstruction in childhood, 228, *P.*
SCOTT, J. M.: Histological observations on glycogen reserves of the foetus and newborn infant, 317
—— Iatrogenic lesions in babies following umbilical vein catheterization, 426
SCOTT, P. J., *see* BECROFT, D. M. O., *et al.*
SEBKOVÁ, M., *see* POLÁČEK, E., *et al.*
SEPHTON SMITH, R., *see* SMITH, R. SEPHTON
SERY, Z., *see* RAPANT, V., *et al.*
SHAPIRA, E., FISHEL, E., and LEVIN, S.: Intrathoracic kidney in a premature infant, 86
—— —— —— and MOSES, S.: Syndrome of incomplete regional achondroplasia (ilium and ribs) with abdominal muscle dysplasia, 694
SHAW, N.: The primary treatment of congenital talipes equinovarus, 230, *P.*
SIEGENTHALER, P., *see* HALLER, R. DE, *et al.*
SINCLAIR, L., *see* ANTHONY, P. P., *et al.*
BUTLER, L. J., *et al.*
SINGH, M., *see* GHAI, O. P., *et al.*
SLADDEN, R. A., *see* HOLT, J. M. and SLADDEN, R. A.
SMELLIE, J. M., *see* DENT, C. E., *et al.*
SMITH, J. L. S. and STEWART, J. K.: Spontaneous regression of retinoblastoma, 336, *P.*
SMITH, L. H., *see* HOCKADAY, T. D. R., *et al.*
SMITH, R. SEPHTON: Iron deficiency and iron overload, 343
SNODGRASS, G. J. A. I., *see* BUTLER, L. J., *et al.*
STEAD, A. L., *see* DODSON, M. E. and STEAD, A. L.
STEVENS, J., *see* YU, J., *et al.*
STEWART, G. T., *see* NEWMAN, R. L. and STEWART, G. T.
STEWART, J. K., *see* SMITH, J. L. S. and STEWART, J. K.
STIMMLER, L., *see* SWAIN, V. A. J., *et al.*
STRANG, L. B.: The lungs at birth, 575
SURUGA, K., YAMAZAKI, Z., IWAI, S., NAGASHIMA, K., and MORI, W.: The surgery of infantile obstructive jaundice, 158
SUTIN, G. J., HORNER, R., HEESE, H. DE V., and MALAN, A. F.: The electrocardiogram in respiratory distress syndrome; the praecordial P wave as an aid to assessment, 402
SWAIN, V. A. J., STIMMLER, L., FRANCE, N. E., and TUCKER, S.: Perinatal ascites with extravasation of urine from the kidneys, 228, *P.*
SWYER, P. R., *see* DELIVORIA-PAPADOPOULOS, M., *et al.*
SZÖTS, I. and GULYAS, J.: Bronchial adenoma in children, 230, *P.*

TAYLOR, W. H., *see* WORSLEY, H. E., *et al.*
TEMPANY, E.: Peptic ulceration in childhood, 451, *P.*
THORNBER, J. M., *see* HUGH-JONES, K., *et al.*
TOBIN, J. O'H. and WHITE, L. L. R.: Virus isolation from Manchester children with acute respiratory disease, 334, *P.*
TODD, R. MCL. and BOUTON, M. J.: Nephrosis: a clinical and histological study of 38 children, 659
TOWNLEY, R. R. W., *see* ANDERSON, C. M., *et al.*
TRYGSTAD, O.: The insulin-glucose tolerance test in pituitary growth retardation, 508
TSAKAYANNIS, E., MOUTSOURIS, C., and VALAES, T.: Divided liver: twisted pediculated left half, 228, *P.*
TUCKER, S., *see* SWAIN, V. A. J., *et al.*

VALAES, T., *see* TSAKAYANNIS, E., *et al.*
VĚCHETOVÁ, E., *see* POLÁČEK, E., *et al.*
VERHAGEN, A. D., HAMILTON, J. P., and GENEL, M.: Renal vein thrombosis in infants, 214
VEST, M. F. and SALZBERG, R.: Conjugation reactions in the newborn infant: the metabolism of para-aminobenzoic acid, 97
VESTERMARK, S.: Osteochondrodystrophia deformans with mucopolysaccharidosis, 106
VOCEL, J., *see* POLÁČEK, E., *et al.*
VOJTEK, V., *see* RAPANT, V., *et al.*

WALIA, B. N. S., *see* GHAI, O. P., *et al.*
WALKER, C. H. M.: Partial perfusion for neonatal respiratory distress, 450, *P.*
WALLACE, S. J., *see* HUGH-JONES, K., *et al.*
WALSHE, J. M. and PATSTON, V.: Effect of penicillamine on serum iron, 651
WARREN, C. B. M., *see* BROUGHTON, P. M. G., *et al.*
WATERSTON, D., *see* ABERDEEN, E. and WATERSTON, D.
WATSON, L., *see* DENT, C. E., *et al.*
WELLER, S. D. V., *see* CROME, L. and WELLER, S. D. V.
WHITE, L. L. R., *see* TOBIN, J. O'H. and WHITE, L. L. R.
WHITE, R. H. R.: The pathology of the nephrotic syndrome, 451, *P.*
WILKINSON, A. W.: Biochemical aspects of neonatal surgery, 228, *P.*
—— Giant haemangiolymphangioma, 450, *P.*
WILLIAMS, C. D.: Populations and paediatrics, 450, *P.*
WILSON, K. M., *see* MANN, T. P., *et al.*
WOODS, G. E.: Some clinical notes and electroencephalographic findings in cerebral palsy, 394

WORSLEY, H. E., BROOKFIELD, R. W., ELWOOD, J. S., NOBLE, R. L., and TAYLOR, W. H.: Lactic acidosis with necrotizing encephalopathy in two sibs, 492
WYSOCKA, K.: Some remarks concerning the surgical palliative treatment of tetralogy of Fallot in children, 230, *P.*

YAMAZAKI, Z., *see* SURUGA, K., *et al.*
YOUNG, M., *see* COTTOM, D. and YOUNG, M.
YOUNG, W. F., *see* PEONIDES, A., *et al.*
YU, J., PAYNE, W. W., IFEKWUNIGWE, A., and STEVENS, J.: Biochemical status of healthy premature infants in the first 48 hours of life, 516
—— *see also* DAVIS, J. A., *et al.*

ZACHARY, R. B., *see* DUBOWITZ, V., *et al.*
ZEBEN, W. VAN: Cervical lymph node tuberculosis caused by atypical mycobacteria, 228, *P.*

# SUBJECT INDEX

## 1965, Volume XL

Absorption, intestinal, of certain monosaccharides, inborn defect, 1
Achondroplasia, regional incomplete (ilium and ribs) with abdominal muscle dysplasia, 694
Acid-base balance, of healthy premature infants in first 48 hours of life, 516
—— changes following exchange transfusion with citrated blood, 626, 450, *P.*
—— determination in normal premature and full-term infants during the first 72 hours of life, 645
Acidosis, correction, in resuscitation of collapsed child, 385
—— lactic, with necrotizing encephalopathy in two sibs, 492
Actinomycin D in Wilms' tumour, treatment of lung metastases, 200
Addison's disease and cerebral sclerosis, 332, *P.*
Adenoma, bronchial, childhood, 230, *P.*
Adrenal hypoplasia, in newborn, 336, *P.*
Adreno-genital syndrome, surgery, 228, *P.*
Agenesis, pulmonary, bilateral, and total tracheopulmonary agenesis, 334, *P.*
Albers-Schönberg disease, *see* Osteopetrosis
Aldosterone, excretion following Ramstedt's operation, 261
—— hereditary 18-oxidation defect in biosynthesis, 332, *P.*
Anaemia, Fanconi's, with hydrocephalus and thyroid abnormality, 89
—— megaloblastic, in premature infants, 53
Androgens, influence on height in males, 66
Artery, carotid, occlusion, internal, child, 224
Ascites, perinatal, and extravasation of urine from kidneys, 228, *P.*
Asphyxia, neonatal, in aetiology of athetosis, 376
Asthma, occurrence of varicella with, and corticosteroids, 593
Athetosis, aetiology, with special reference to neonatal asphyxia, idiopathic icterus, and ABO- incompatibility, 376

Bassen-Kornzweig syndrome, *see* Lipoproteinaemia
Bile-duct atresia, surgery, and intrahepatic vascular and bile-duct systems, 162
Biochemistry, of healthy premature infants in first 48 hours of life, 516
—— *see also* Acid-base; Blood chemistry
Birth, lungs at, review article, 575
Bladder, rhabdomyosarcoma, childhood, 227, *P.*
Blood chemistry, during first 48 hours of life, effect of abnormal birth, 436
—— ——, normal full-term infants, 430
—— groups, ABO-incompatibility in aetiology of athetosis, 376
—— pressure in newborn infants, 637
—— volume, in respiratory distress syndrome, 480
Body, foreign, causing suppurative lesions in bronchus, children, 229, *P.*

BOOK REVIEWS: ALLAN, J. D. and HOLT, K. S., *eds.:* Biochemical approaches to mental handicap in children, 1965, 699; ANDREWS, G., HARRIS, M., GARSIDE, R., and KAY, D.: The syndrome of stuttering, 1964, 698; BECKER, P., *ed.:* Humangenetik. Ein kurzes Handbuch in fünf Bänden, Band II, 1964, 341; BIRMINGHAM, THE CHILDREN'S HOSPITAL: The Children's Hospital medical vade-mecum, 5th ed., 1964, 452; BOSE, S. K. and DEY, A. K., *eds.:* Asian paediatrics, The Scientific Proceedings of the First All-Asian Congress of Paediatrics New Delhi, January, 1961, 1965, 453; CATZEL, P.: The paediatric prescriber, 2nd ed., 1963, 231; CATEL, W.: Die Pflege des gesunden und des kranken Kindes. Zugleich ein Lehrbuch der Ausbildung zur Sauglings- und Kinderkrankenschwester, 1964, 112; CIBA: Iron metabolism, Symposium, July 1963, 1964, 339; CIBA FOUNDATION GENERAL SYMPOSIUM: Control of glycogen metabolism, 1964, 233; CIBA FOUNDATION STUDY GROUP No. 17. Diet and bodily constitution, edited by Wolstenholme and O'Connor, 1964, 232; COLES, J. E.: Lung function: assessment and application in medicine, 1965, 700; FARMER, T. W., *ed.:* Pediatric neurology, 1964, 337; FARROW, R. and FORREST, D.: The surgery of childhood for nurses, 2nd ed. 1964, 112; FISCH, L., *ed.:* Research in deafness in children, 1964, 340; GAIRDNER, D., *ed.:* Recent advances in paediatrics, 3rd ed., 1965, 452; HAYHOE, F. G. J., *ed.:* Current research in leukaemia, 1965, 700; HILSON, D.: Practical paediatrics, 1964, 453; HOLMES, D. J.: The adolescent in psychotherapy, 1964, 453; HOLT, K. S.: Assessment of cerebral palsy. I. Muscle function, locomotion and hand function, 1965, 574; HUTCHISON, J. A.: Practical paediatric problems, 1964, 338; ILLINGWORTH. R. and ILLINGWORTH, C.: Babies and young children, Feeding, management and care, 3rd ed., 1964, 342; JEAVONS, P. M. and BOWER, B. D.: Infantile spasms. A review of the literature and a study of 112 cases, 1964, 574; JONXIS, J. H. P., VISSER, H. K. A., and TROELSTRA, J. A., *eds.:* Nutricia symposium on the adaptation of the newborn infant to extra-uterine life, 1964, 699; KAPLAN, S. A.: Growth disorders in childhood and adolescents, 1964, 232; KELLAWAY, P. and PETERSEN, I., *eds.:* Neurological and encephalographic correlative studies in infancy, 1964, 337; KOECHER, P. H.: Klinische Diagnostik für den Kinderarzt, Heute gebräuchliche Funktionsprüfungen und Laboruntersuchungen, 1964, 232; LEVIN, A. K.: Cerebral palsy. The pioneer years of occupational therapy in Scotland, 1964, 341; LOWENFELD, B.: Our blind children, growing and learning with them, 2nd ed., 1964, 340; MARGET, W. and KIENITZ, M., *eds.:* Praxis der Antibiotikatherapie im Kindesalter ihre Anwendung, 1964, 338; MARTI, H. R.: Pathologie und Klinik in Einzeldarstellungen. Band XIII: Normale und Anomale Menschliche Hämoglobine, 1963, 233; MILLER, M. H. and POLISNAR, I. A.: Audiological evaluation of the pediatric patient, 1964, 231; MOESCHLIN, S.: Klinik und Therapy der Vergiftungen, 4th ed., 1964, 339; MUSSHOFF, K. and WEINREICH, J., *eds.*: Differentialdiagnose seltener Lungenerkrankungen im Rontgenbild. Ein Atlas, 2nd enlarged edition, 1964, 700; NEALE, A. V.: The advancement of child health, 1964, 574; Nelson textbook of pediatrics, 8th ed., 1963, 338; NEUBAUER, P. B., *ed.*: Concepts of development in early childhood education, 1965, 698; RENFREW, C. and MURPHY, K., *eds.*: The child who does not talk (Clinics in Developmental Medicine, No. 13), 1963, 341; ROSSI, E., *ed.*: Postgraduate courses in pediatrics. Blutkrankheiten im Kindesalter. Vol. 11-12, 1964, 454; ROSSI, E., *ed.*: Tumoren im Kindesalter, Postgraduate courses in Pediatrics, Vol. 13, 1964, 234; ROSSI, E., *ed.*: Postgraduate courses in pediatrics. Vol. 15. Leberkrankheiten beim Lind, 1965, 453; SACHARIN, R. M. and HUNTER, M. H. S.: Paediatric nursing procedures, 1964, 112; SIMONDS, B.: Tuberculosis in twins, 1964, 341; VOLK, B. W., *ed.*: Tay-Sachs' disease, 1964, 699; WALTON, J. N., *ed.*: Disorders of voluntary muscle, 1964, 234; WENGER, R.: Endokardfibrosen. Klinik-Therapie-Pathologie, 1964, 454; WILLIAMSON, B. and MAYON-WHITE, R. M.: A handbook on diseases of children including dietetics and the common fevers, 9th ed., 1964, 111; WINNICOTT, D. W.: The family and individual development, 1965, 573; Year Book of Pediatrics, 1964-1965, 1965, 699.

British Association of Paediatric Surgeons, 11th Annual Meeting, 227
British Paediatric Association, Proceedings of the 36th annual meeting, 446
Bronchus, foreign bodies causing suppurative lesions in children, 229, *P.*

Cardiovascular system, malformations, and of the thymus, 334, *P.*
Cauda equina, lipoma, 207
Cells, white, urinary, excretion, childhood, 313
Cerebral palsy, clinical notes and electroencephalographic findings, 394
Child care, and over-population, 450, *P.*
Chromosome(s), 4-5 group (Denver), partial deletion of short arms, 82
—— E (16-18) trisomy syndrome, analysis of 13 cases, 600
—— in leprechaunism, 632
—— in lymphoedema and possible ovarian dysgenesis, 27
—— normal/trisomy 13-15 mosaicism, two infants, 442
—— in paediatric intersex problems, 335, *P.*
Chylothorax in infancy and childhood, 186
Citrate, acid-base changes following exchange transfusion with citrated blood, 626, 450, *P.*
Club foot, congenital, causes, 548
Coarctation, late results of operation, growing child, 192
—— preductal, aorta, 228, *P.*
Collapse, correction of acidosis in resuscitation of children, 385
Copper sulphate densitometry, evaluation, routine haemoglobinometry methods, 309
Cord, spermatic, masses, in children, 228, *P.*
—— spinal, obstetrical paralysis due to ischaemia of, 93
Corpuscle, renal, *see* Renal
Corticosteroids, excretion by infants of diabetic and pre-diabetic mothers, 583
—— and varicella, in asthmatic children, 593
Curriculum, undergraduate, paediatrics in discussion, 451, *P.* (*title only*)
Cushing's syndrome, surgery, 228, *P.*
Cyst(s) arising in the renal corpuscle, microdissection, 455
—— arising in the renal tubules, microdissection, 464
—— choledochal, case report and aetiology, 329
Cytomegaly, in islets of Langerhans, newborn, 332, *P.*
Cytotrophoblast, villous, index of placental ischaemia, 334, *P.*

Deficiency state arising in infants on synthetic foods, 364
—— *see also* Iron
Degeneration, cerebello-thalamo-spinal, infancy, unusual variant of Werdnig-Hoffmann disease, 302
—— progressive familial infantile cerebral cortical, 2 sisters, 335
Desferrioxamine, in iron overload, 343
Development, physical and mental, effect of undernutrition in early life on, 532
Diabetes, congenital, 14-day-old infant, 332, *P.*
—— and pre-diabetes, excretion of corticosteroids by infants of mothers with, 583
Diaphragm, defects, role of ventral hernia, newborn, 146
Diverticulum of the left ventricle, case report, 545
Donald Paterson Prize Essay, 1965, 234
DTPA, in iron overload, 343
Duct, deferent, atresia, 227, *P.*
Dwarfism, pituitary, insulin-glucose tolerance test in, 508
Dyscephalia mandibulo-oculo-facialis (Hallermann-Streiff syndrome), 57
Dysgenesis, ovarian, possible, and lymphoedema, lymphangiography and chromosome studies, 27
Dystrophy, infantile neuroaxonal, 502

Ectromelia, habilitation, thalidomide embryopathy, 154
Electrocardiography in respiratory distress syndrome, praecordial P wave in assessment, 402
Electroencephalography in cerebral palsy, 394
—— studies in infants and children with hypothyroidism, 612
Encephalopathy, necrotizing, lactic acidosis, in two sibs, 492

Fat infiltration in the tissues of the newborn infant, 406
—— necrosis in a newly-born infant, 326
Favism, in England, two more cases, 271
Fibrin, use of activators in meningitis and similar conditions, 235
Fistulae, cervico-auricular, review and report, 218
—— tracheo-oesophageal, some remarks, 229, *P.*
—— —— and oesophageal atresia, unusual types, 229, *P.*
Fits, neonatal, associated with hypomagnesaemia, 286
Fluid, cerebrospinal, use of fibrinolytic activators in meningitis and similar conditions, 235
Foetus, developing, white cell alkaline phosphatase in, 450, *P.*
—— external injury to, causing deformity, 80
—— in foetu, 689
—— glycogen reserves, histology, 317
—— orthopaedics, 230, *P.*
Foods, synthetic, infant, deficiency state arising during feeding, 364

Gastric acid secretory capacity in peptic ulcer, 77
Genito-urinary abnormalities, and absent abdominal muscles, 335, *P.*
George Frederic Still Memorial Lecture: Paediatric nephrology: the scientific study of the kidneys and their diseases in infants and young children (Barnett), 451, *P.* (*title only*)
Glucose-6-phosphate dehydrogenase deficiency, neonatal jaundice associated with, Israel, 280
Glycogen reserves of foetus and newborn infant, histology, 317

Gonadal dysgenesis with unusual abnormalities, 274
Gonadotrophins, urinary excretion, especially children, 16

Haemangiolymphangioma, giant, 450, *P.*
Haematocrit studies in respiratory distress syndrome, 480
Haemoglobinometry, routine in childhood, evaluation of copper sulphate densitometry, 309
Haemolytic uraemia syndrome, fatal, and idiopathic hyperlipaemia in monozygotic twins, 654
Hallermann-Streiff syndrome (dyscephalia mandibulo-oculo-facialis), 57
Hand, foot, and mouth diseases, 560
Head circumference of infants related to body weight, 672
—— injuries, severe, treatment and prognosis, children, 230, *P.*
Heart, congenital malformations, pulmonary microangiography in, 333, *P.*
—— surgery in children, development, 123
Height, influence of androgen treatment, males, 66
Hernia, diaphragmatic, congenital, 229, *P.*
—— —— operative treatment, and relaxation, 229, *P.*
—— ventral, role in diaphragmatic defects, newborn, 146
Hirschsprung's disease, acquired megacolon as a complication of recto-sigmoidectomy, 180
—— —— pseudo, 177
Hormone, human growth, insulin-glucose tolerance test in pituitary dwarfism, 508
Hyaline membrane disease, pathological study of 55 infants, 618
Hydrocephalus, in a case of Fanconi's anaemia, with thyroid abnormality, 89
Hydrogen ions, renal excretion in infants and children, 33
Hydronephrosis, and pelvi-ureteric obstruction, functional stenosis causing, 203
17-Hydroxycorticosteroid, and aldosterone excretion following Ramstedt's operation, 261
4-Hydroxy-3-methoxy-mandelic acid (HMMA), excretion by children, 418
21-Hydroxypregnenolone excretion, in normal, and child with deficiency of 3β-hydroxysteroid-dehydrogenase, 251
3β-Hydroxysteroid-dehydrogenase, deficiency, 21-hydroxypregnenolone excretion in, 251
5-Hydroxytryptamine levels, blood, in the newborn, 513
Hyperbilirubinaemia, effect of blue light on, 666
Hypercalcaemia, idiopathic, and cardiovascular lesions, evidence, hypothesis, and speculation, 535
Hyperlipaemia, idiopathic, and fatal haemolytic uraemia syndrome in monozygotic twins, 654
Hyperoxaluria, primary, metabolic error in, 485
Hypomagnesaemia, and neonatal fits, 290
Hypospadias, 228, *P.*
Hypothyroidism, electroencephalographic studies in infants and children, 612

Iatrogenic lesion following umbilical vein catheterization, babies, 426
Icterus, idiopathic, in aetiology of athetosis, 376
Immaturity, respiratory distress syndrome in, 62
Immunoglobulins, in premature infants, 243
Infants, premature, megaloblastic anaemia in, 53
Infection, *Pseudomonas pyocynea*, incubator-borne, in a newborn nursery, 555
Insulin-glucose tolerance test in pituitary growth retardation, 508
Intersex problems, chromosomes in, 335, *P.*
Iron deficiency and iron overload, 343
—— serum, effect on penicillamine, 651
Ischaemia, of spinal cord, causing obstetrical paralysis, 93
Islets of Langerhans, nuclear abnormality and cytomegaly in, newborn, 332, *P.*

Jaundice, neonatal, associated with familial G6PD deficiency, in Israel, 280

Ketovite tablets and syrup, use in deficiency states arising from synthetic foods in infancy, 364
Kidney(s), congenital anomalies, newborn, 335, *P.*
—— excretion of hydrogen ions in infants and children, 33
—— intrathoracic, premature infant, 86
—— osmotic concentrating ability in healthy infants and children, 291
Kwashiorkor, jejunal mucosa in, 526

Lactic dehydrogenase, serum, and ribonuclease in diagnosis of malignant tumours, childhood, 183
Lead poisoning, chronic, causing reversible myocarditis, 389
Length, crown-rump, of newborn, 334, *P.*
Leprechaunism, metabolic and chromosomal studies, 632
Lesions, cardiovascular, and infantile hypercalcaemia, evidence, hypothesis, and speculation, 535
Light, blue, effect on hyperbilirubinaemia, 666
Limb defects, and thalidomide embryopathy, 154
Lipidosis, sulphatide, reliable rapid screening test, 284
Lipoma, of the cauda equina, 207
Lipoproteinaemia, A-β-, 40, 47
Liver, divided, twisted pediculated left half, 228, *P.*
—— intrahepatic vascular and bile-duct systems in surgery of bile-duct atresias, 162
—— lobe, accessory, presenting through a congenital deficiency of anterior abdominal wall, 541
—— tumours, treatment by major hepatic resection, 169
Lungs at birth, review article, 575
—— metastases, treatment, Actinomycin D in Wilms' tumour, 200
—— pulmonary microangiography in congenital malformations of the heart, 333, *P.*
—— resections, results, children, 229, *P.*
Lymph nodes, cervical, tuberculosis, caused by atypical mycobacteria, 228, *P.*
Lymphadenitis, mycobacterial, in childhood, 450, *P.*
Lymphoedema, and possible ovarian dysgenesis, lymphangiography and chromosome studies, 27

Malformations, classifications, 335, *P.*
—— *see also* individual organs affected
Mastocytosis, cutaneous and generalized skeletal changes, 15½-week-old infant, 677
Megacolon, acquired, complication of recto-sigmoidectomy for Hirschsprung's disease, 180
Meningitis, use of fibrinolytic activators in, 235
Meningomyelocele, laryngeal stridor and respiratory obstruction associated with, 687
Mental handicap, aspects studied in the 'Thousand Families Survey', 451, *P.*
—— retardation in muscular dystrophy, 296
Metabolism in leprechaunism, 632, *P.*
Metabolites, catecholamine, in neuroblastoma, 333, *P.*
Microangiography, pulmonary, in congenital malformation of the heart, 333, *P.*
Monosaccharides, inborn defect of intestinal absorption, 1
Mosaicism, 13-15, normal/trisomy, two infants, 442
—— *see also* Trisomy
Mucosa, jejunal, in kwashiorkor, 526
Muscle(s), abdominal, absent, and associated genito-urinary abnormalities, 335, *P.*
—— —— dysplasia, with incomplete regional achondroplasia (ilium and ribs), 694
Muscular dystrophy, intellectual impairment in, 296
Mycobacteria, atypical, cervical lymph node tuberculosis caused by, 228, *P.*

Myocarditis, reversible, due to chronic lead poisoning in childhood, 389

Nephrosis, a clinical and histological study, 38 children, 659
Nephrotic syndrome, pathology, 451, *P.*
Nervous system, central, abnormalities, South Wales, 451, *P.*
Neuroblastoma, biochemical, pharmacological, and histochemical studies, 411
—— catecholamine metabolites in, 333, *P.*
Newborn, surgery, biochemistry, 228, *P.*
Nuclei, abnormality in islets of Langerhans, newborn, 332, *P.*

Obstruction, pelvi-ureteric, and hydronephrosis, functional stenosis causing, 203
—— respiratory, and laryngeal stridor, associated with meningomyelocele, 687
—— ureteric, childhood, 228, *P.*
Occlusion, carotid artery, internal, child, 224
Oesophagitis, reflex, due to oesophageal stenosis, 197
Oesophagus, atresia, some remarks, 229, *P.*
—— —— and tracheo-oesophageal fistulae, unusual types, 229, *P.*
Orthopaedics of the foetus, 230, *P.*
Osmotic concentrating ability in healthy infants and children, 291
Osteochondrodystrophia deformans with mucopolysaccharidosis, 106
Osteopetrosis, 7

Paediatric Pathology Club, Proceedings of 10th Annual Meeting, 332
—— Research Society, 6th meeting, October, 1964, 342
—— services, development, 451, *P.* (*title only*)
—— in the undergraduate curriculum, discussion, 451, *P.* (*title only*)
Palsy, cerebral, *see* Cerebral palsy
Pancreatitis in childhood, 15 cases, 132
Para-aminobenzoic acid, metabolism, conjugation reactions in newborn infant, 97
Paralysis, obstetrical, due to ischaemia of the spinal cord, 93
Penicillamine, effect on serum iron, 651
Perfusion, partial, for neonatal respiratory distress, 450, *P.*
Phaeochromocytoma, surgery, 228, *P.*
Phosphatase, alkaline, white cell, in developing foetus, 450, *P.*
Pinealoma, with aldosterone-like activity, 336, *P.*
Placenta in experimental toxoplasmosis, mouse, 336, *P.*
—— ischaemia, villous cytotrophoblast as an index of, 334, *P.*
Placental transfusion syndrome in monozygous twins, 264
Plasminogen, in meningitis and similar conditions, 235
Pneumonia, staphylococcal, surgical complications, in infants, 229, *P.*
Poisoning, lead, *see* Lead
Polyps, of colon, beyond reach of sigmoidoscope, 173
Populations and paediatrics, 450, *P.*
Pressure, venous, measurement in exchange transfusion, 323
Pseudo-Hirschsprung's disease, 177
Pseudohypoparathyroidism, dental manifestations in, 565
*Pseudomonas pyocyanea* infection, incubator-borne, in a newborn nursery, 555

Radius, head of, fractures, treatment, 230, *P.*
Ramstedt's operation, aldosterone and 17-hydroxycorticosterone excretion following, 261
Recto-sigmoidectomy, acquired megacolon complicating, in Hirschsprung's disease, 180
Renal corpuscle, cysts arising in, microdissection, 455
—— tubules, cysts arising in, microdissection, 464
Respiration, intermittent positive pressure, as a treatment in severe respiratory distress syndrome, 474
Respiratory disease, acute, virus isolation from Manchester children, 334
Respiratory distress syndrome, blood volume and haematocrit studies, 480
—— —— —— electrocardiogram in, praecordial P wave, 402
—— —— —— in immature and premature newborns, 62
—— —— —— intermittent positive pressure treatment, 474
—— —— —— neonatal, partial perfusion, 450, *P.*
Resuscitation, of collapsed child, correction of acidosis in, 385
Retinoblastoma, spontaneous regression, 336. *P.*
Rhabdomyosarcoma, bladder, childhood, 227, *P.*
Ribonuclease, serum, and lactic dehydrogenase, in diagnosis of malignant tumours, childhood, 183

Sclerosis, cerebral, and Addison's disease, 332
—— tuberous, in childhood, 450, *P.*
Spasms, infantile, neurophysiological and neuropathological observations, 451, *P.*
Stenosis, functional, as a cause of pelvi-ureteric obstruction and hydronephrosis, 203
—— oesophageal, due to reflux oesophagitis, 197
Stridor, laryngeal, and respiratory obstruction associated with meningomyelocele, 687
Surgery, adrenal, 228, *P.*
—— heart, in children, development, 123
—— neonatal, biochemistry, 228, *P.*
—— transposition of great vessels, 128
Sweat test, accuracy, advantage of a micromethod, 684

Talipes equinovarus, congenital, primary treatment, 230, *P.*
—— —— operative treatment for failed cases, 230, *P.*
Teeth, in pseudohypoparathyroidism, 565
Testis, undescended, review article, 113
Tetralogy of Fallot, palliative surgical treatment, children, 230, *P.*
Thalidomide embryopathy, and limb defects, especially ectromelias, 154
Thousand Families Survey, study of mental handicap in, 451, *P.*
Thrombosis, renal vein, in infants, 214
Thymus, hyperplasia, and the choice of suitable biometric framework, 333, *P.*
—— malformations, and of cardiovascular system, 334, *P.*
—— recent studies, 333, *P.*
Thyroid abnormality, in a case of Fanconi's anaemia with hydrocephalus, 89
Thyrotoxicosis in children: follow-up study, 71
Toxoplasmosis, experimental, mouse placenta in, 336
Tract, gastro-intestinal, intrathoracic duplications, complications, 229, *P.*
Transfusion, exchange, with citrated blood, acid-base changes following, 626, 450, *P.*
—— —— venous pressure measurement, 323
Transposition, great arteries, pulmonary microangiography in, 333, *P.*
—— great vessels, surgery, 128
Trisomy syndrome, E (16-18): analysis of 13 cases, 600
——, *see also* Mosaicism
Tuberculosis, cervical lymph node, caused by atypical mycobacteria, 228, *P.*
Tubules, renal, *see* Renal
Tumours, hepatic, treatment by resection, 169
—— Wilms', Actinomycin D in, treatment of lung metastases, 200

Twins, monozygotic, fatal haemolytic uraemic syndrome and idiopathic hyperlipaemia in, 654
—— —— placental transfusion syndrome in, 264

Ulcer, peptic, assessment of gastric acid secretory response with 'Maximal' augmented histamine stimulation, 77
—— —— in childhood, 451, *P.*
Undernutrition, in early life, effect on physical and mental development, 532
Ureters, obstruction, childhood, 228, *P.*
Urine, extravasation from kidneys, and perinatal ascites, 228, *P.*

Valves, urethral, review of 104 cases, 227, *P.*
Varicella, occurrence in asthma, and corticosteroid treatment, 593
Vas deferens, atresia, 227, *P.*
Vein, renal, thrombosis, in infants, 214
—— umbilical, catheterization, iatrogenic lesions in babies following, 426
Ventricle, left, diverticulum, case report, 545
Vessels, great, transposition, surgery, 128
Virus isolation from Manchester children with acute respiratory disease, 334, *P.*
Vitamin supplements, use in conjunction with synthetic infant foods, 364

Wall, abdominal, anterior, accessory lobe of liver presenting through a congenital deficiency of, 541
Wave, praecordial P, in respiratory distress syndrome, 402
Weight, body, relationship to head circumference, 672
Werdnig-Hoffmann disease, unusual variant, cerebello-thalamo-spinal degeneration, 302

Xeroderma pigmentosa, treatment, 228, *P.*

PRINTED IN GREAT BRITAIN BY HEADLEY BROTHERS LTD
109 KINGSWAY LONDON WC2 AND ASHFORD KENT